DAVI-ELLEN CHABNER, BA, MAT

The Language of Medicine

ELSEVIER
SAUNDERS

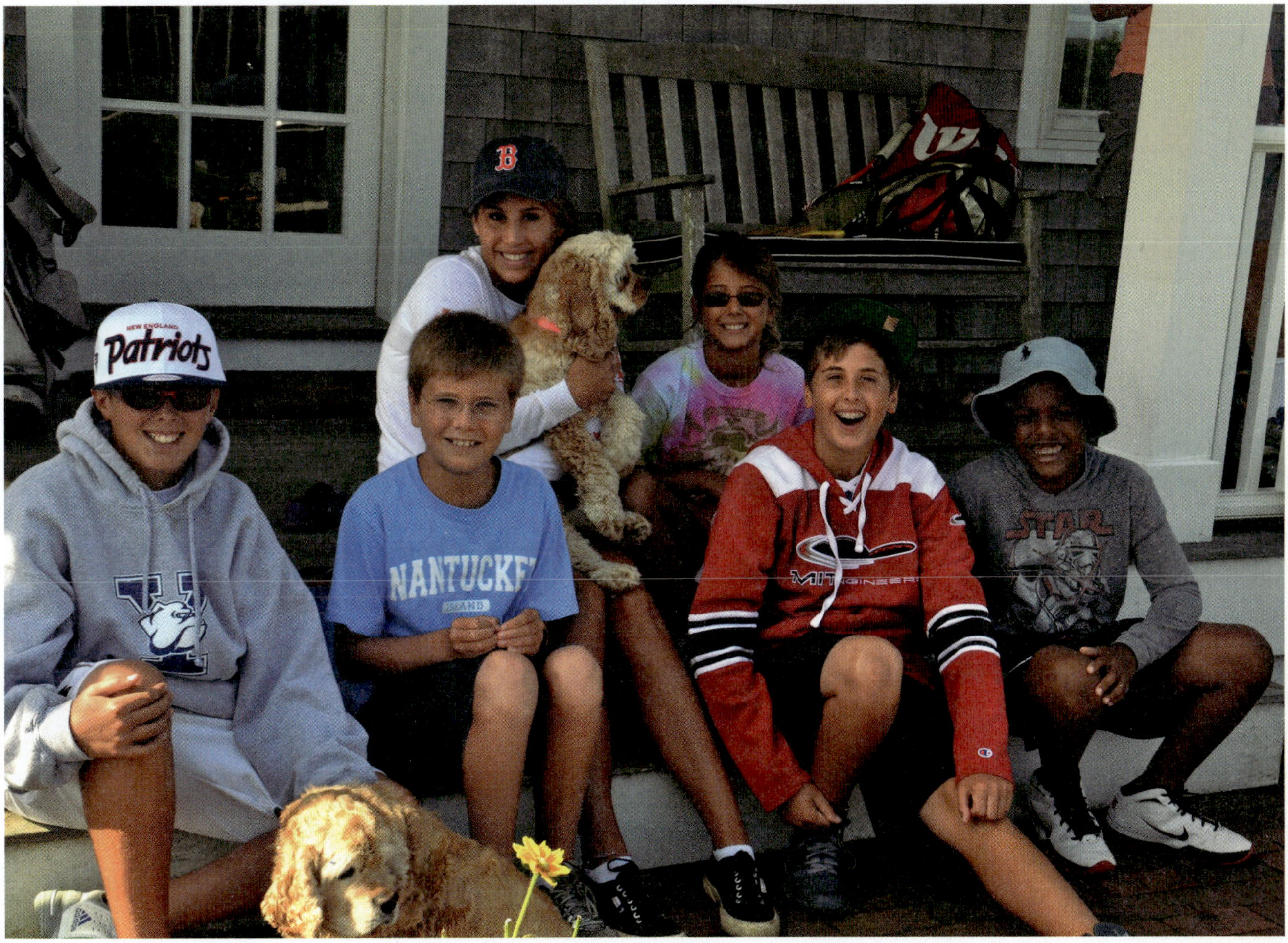

For Gus, Ben, Bebe, Louisa, Solomon, and Amari…

and of course, Owen & Greta.

Here are the kids and canines whose affection and love relax and inspire me every day.

ELSEVIER
SAUNDERS

3251 Riverport Lane
St. Louis, Missouri 63043

THE LANGUAGE OF MEDICINE, TENTH EDITION ISBN: 978-1-4557-2846-6

ISBN: 978-1-4557-2846-6

Vice President and Publisher: Andrew Allen
Content Strategy Director: Jeanne Olson
Content Strategist: Linda Woodard
Senior Content Development Specialist: Luke Held
Publishing Services Manager: Julie Eddy
Senior Project Manager: Celeste Clingan
Design Direction: Ellen Zanolle

Printed in Canada

Last digit is the print number: 9 8 7 6 5 4 3 2 1

PREFACE

WELCOME TO THE 10TH EDITION OF THE LANGUAGE OF MEDICINE

The enhanced focus of this new edition is its relevance to real-life medical situations. Drawing on current technology, state-of-the-art medical practice, and the latest procedures and treatments, *The Language of Medicine* brings medical terminology to life. The dynamic images and compelling patient stories further illustrate medical terminology in action.

I am honored that this text continues to be the book instructors return to, year after year, because their students tell them that it works! As a student, you will find that *The Language of Medicine* speaks to you no matter what your background or level of education. It is written in simple, non-technical language that creates an exceptionally accessible pathway to learning. Since it is a workbook-text combination, you engage and interact on practically every page through writing and reviewing terms, labeling diagrams, and answering questions. Terminology is explained so that you understand medical terms in their proper context, which is the structure and function of the human body in health and disease.

Throughout the process of writing this text over its 10 editions, I have listened to hundreds of students and instructors and incorporated their insightful suggestions. Expert medical reviewers have once again helped me to ensure that the terminology included reflects cutting edge clinical practice. New information and illustrations throughout are the result of recommendations from all those who have so generously provided feedback. My continuing goal in writing *The Language of Medicine* is to help you not only learn medical terminology but also to enjoy learning! You will find that medical terminology comes alive and stays with you when you use my interactive, logical, and easy-to-follow method. Undeniably, the study of this language requires commitment and hard work, but the benefits are great. Knowledge of medical terminology will give you a strong start in your career.

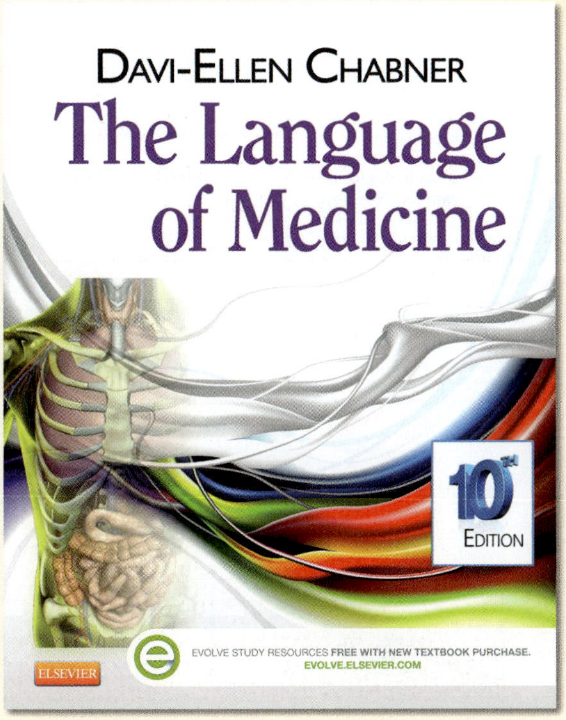

NEW TO THE 10TH EDITION

While the essential elements of *The Language of Medicine* remain in place, the new 10th edition is even more relevant to real-life medical situations.

The 10th edition includes 20 new, first-hand stories of medical conditions and procedures. These personal accounts make medical terminology more understandable.

IN PERSON

This first-person narrative was written by a woman living with Crohn disease ("Crohn's").

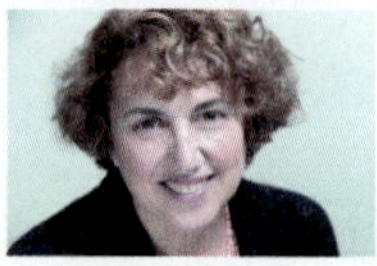

he flu yesterday, I was jealous. To
ving something acute always seems
, take over-the-counter meds, sleep
. I have Crohn disease, a chronic
s characterized by flare-ups and remission. During flare-ups, I've
and intestinal obstruction. Even in remission I am never "okay."
years after a third surgery to remove yet another portion of my
rather rare symptom of Crohn's, necessitated the surgery. I was
urned into bimonthly blood transfusions, as my hemoglobin
y to live. After the surgery, the bleeding stopped, but I had bouts
was no way to live either, and unfortunately, as wonderful as my
ddress after-effects of small bowel surgery. After visiting several
ot these symptoms under control with codeine, Lomotil, and
vitamin B_{12}, so I must inject it monthly for the rest of my life. In
aving less and less small bowel, I take medicine in the hopes of
ic medicine, Humira, but I must
e effects, the scariest of which is
d to think of valuing my present
e.
loctor hadn't told my parents that
e caused by "nerves?" By the time
n pain after every meal. My dad
at showed I had Crohn's and that
oo late for even prednisone (then
to open up the inflamed passage,
se times—as well as all the other
remember what it felt like. In my
tender gut.
y mark on the world, but I spent
oothing strains of "Make Believe
ompanied the pain, I lay with my
with two young children, I would
ot take part.
on of those around me: husband,
things get unbearable. It's not the
approximate those times of being
a night's sleep to get "better." You
hat you will likely end up in the

in is a writer, editor, and food columnist.

IN PERSON

This first-person narrative was written by a kidney donor.

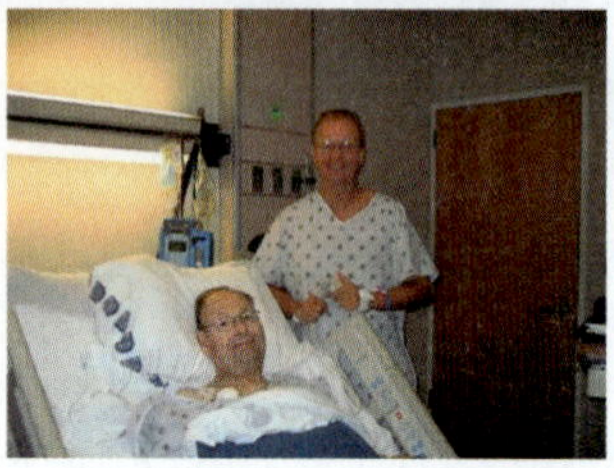

When my 64 year-old father-in-law announced to my wife and me that his kidney function was failing, it didn't really enter our minds that one of us might ultimately have a part to play in his survival. Five years later, dialysis was taking its toll on his organ systems, and there had been no success in obtaining a cadaveric kidney. Things had reached the point where he needed a kidney in short order, before his health deteriorated to the point where he would no longer be a candidate for transplantation.

My wife's blood type ruled out the possibility of her being a
direct donor, so I voluntee
were a match on 5 of the 7 k
function—was able to be do
provide a full liter of urine i
The results of those tests
center at the University of \
recipient—the entire proce
RN) was assigned specificall
to me, the donor. Similarly,
My visit involved some m
enough for major surgery. M
being a donor—the inhere
recovery time, and the possib
The discussions that aftern
positively impact someone e
The events around the
Wednesday evening, with th
night—I watched my favori
in the morning. As you migh
for all of us. We shed a lot
beginning for my father-in-l
so I was taken back first. A r
is of one last hug for my wif
When I woke up in recove
through which the surgeon
which the kidney was remo
the kidney had immediately
return home the next Frida
All told, I was out of work
following a major surgery, i
weekly blood tests to chart t
at the 6 week mark. I was re
capacity. Blood tests contin
center's care six months aft

IN PERSON

This first-person narrative describes the symptoms and treatment of a 42-year-old woman with gallbladder stones.

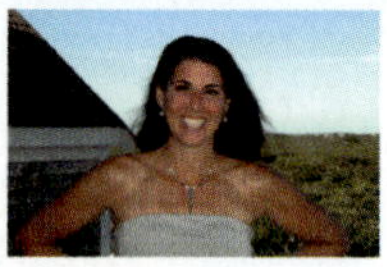

Everyone enjoys a little dessert after dinner, but when the ice cream or a creamy tart leads to pain, most would avoid it. I loved sweets, and despite the revenge they took on my waistline, I still would not pass up an ice cream cone—until my gallbladder decided it had had enough. After several late nights spent doubled over in pain, I tried to steer clear of fatty foods but could not resist the temptation of frozen yogurt.

With one hand I pushed my cart through the supermarket; with the other hand I fed myself some delicious low-fat (not non-fat) frozen yogurt. I never dreamed that the attendant at the quick service window actually gave me soft-serve ice cream. Within 10 minutes of eating the questionable yogurt, I broke out into a sweat; a wave of nausea took me, over and a knifelike pain stabbed me in my right upper quadrant. It hurt even more when I pressed my hand on the area in an attempt to brace the pain.

Several months earlier, after a similar painful episode, I had undergone an ultrasound of my gallbladder, and the surgeon then recommended cholecystectomy. The U/S showed multiple stones in my gallbladder. Most of the stones were just the right size to lodge in the common bile duct and cause blockage of the outflow of bile that occurs after a fatty meal. When I heard the ultrasound results, I swore off all fatty foods.

I just did not imagine that ice cream masquarading as "low-fat yogurt"would be the straw that broke the camel's back! Soon enough, I abandoned my shopping cart and apologized to the manager of the store for vomiting all over aisle 4. The unrelenting pain did not cease when I vomited—it only intensified. I have no idea how I made it home and into bed, but my husband found me several hours later in a deep sweat. I managed to call my surgeon and arrange for "semiemergent" surgery the next morning.

Dr. Fernandez and his team performed a laparoscopic cholecystectomy and relayed to me as I came out of anesthesia that I no longer had a "bag of marbles" for a gallbladder. I had a gassy, distended feeling in my abdomen over the two weeks after surgery (carbon dioxide gas is injected into the abdomen before surgery to allow space between abdominal organs). I felt "tight as a drum" for the first few days and the day by day it went away. My four tiny incisions healed just fine, and in about 2 weeks I was feeling back to "normal". Now I can eat ice cream to my heart's content, only suffering the padding on my waistline, not the stabbing pain just above. Without missing a beat, my liver now delivers the bile into my small intestine right after I eat a fatty meal. The bile emulsifies (breaks down) the fat. I just don't have a storage bag to hold bile in reserve.

I've had an appendectomy, my wisdom teeth removed, and now I gave up my gallbladder! How many more "useless" body parts are there to go?

Elizabeth Chabner Thompson is the CEO/Founder of BFFL Co a company devoted to improving the patient experience. She is also a physician, ultra-marathoner, wife, and the proud mother of four children ages 9-15.

Molecularly Targeted Drugs

Examples are:

Gleevec (imatinib mesylat)—blocks bcr-abl tyrosine kinase in chronic myelogenous leukemia cells.
Tarceva (erlotinib)—blocks epidermal growth factor (EGFR) in lung cancer cells.
Zelboraf (ven

Types of melanin: Eumelanin and Pheomelanin

Eumelanin (eu- = true) is more common and is a brown-black pigment. **Pheomelanin** (pheo- = dusky) is a red-yellow pigment. People with darker skin have more eumelanin, whereas people with lighter skin have more pheomelanin. Pheomelanin is a photo-sensitizer (doesn't protect the skin from damaging ultraviolet rays) and makes lighter-skin individuals more susceptible to skin cancer.

New content on cutting-edge procedures enhances the relevance of medical terms.

New clinical photographs and drawings dynamically illustrate medical terminology, conditions, and treatments.

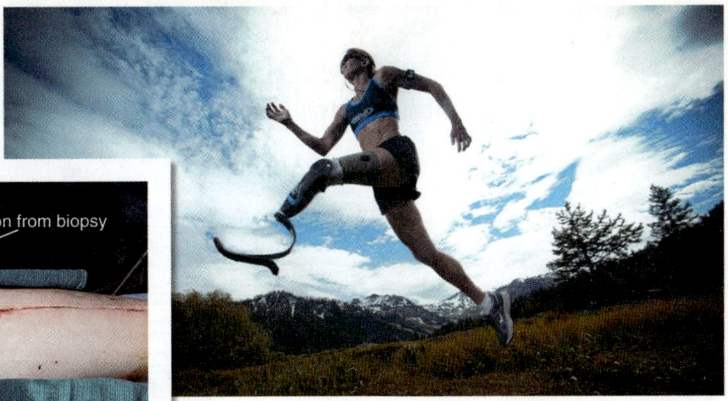

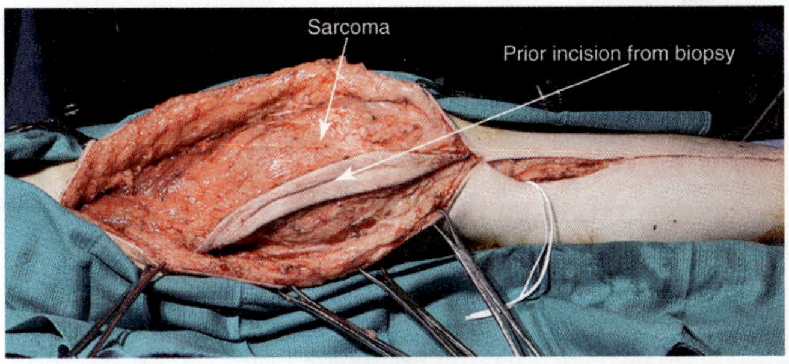

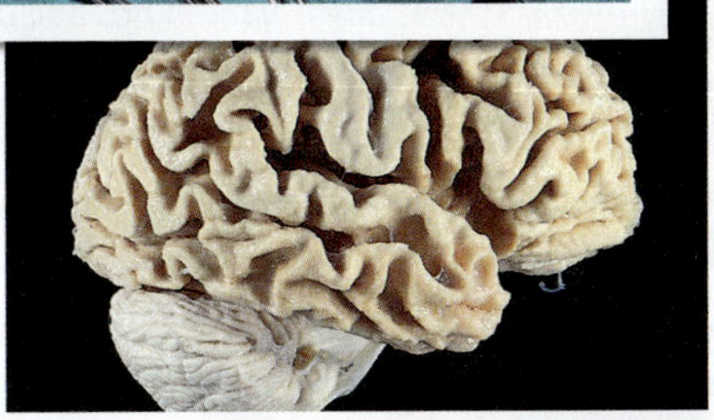

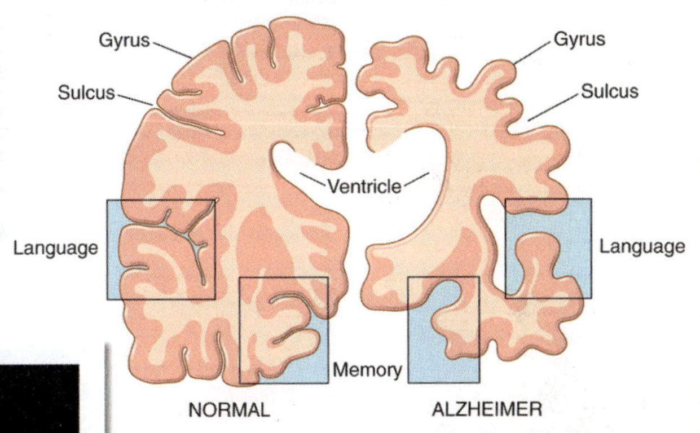

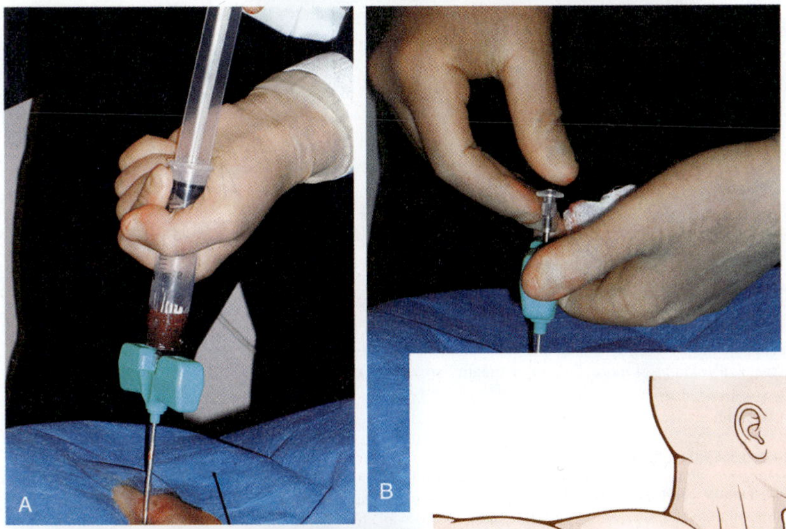

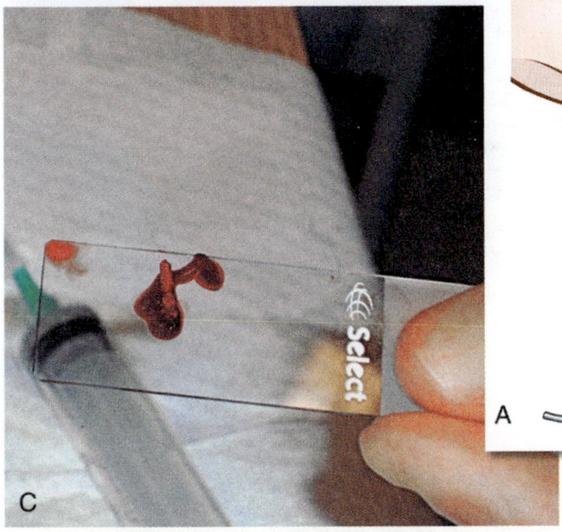

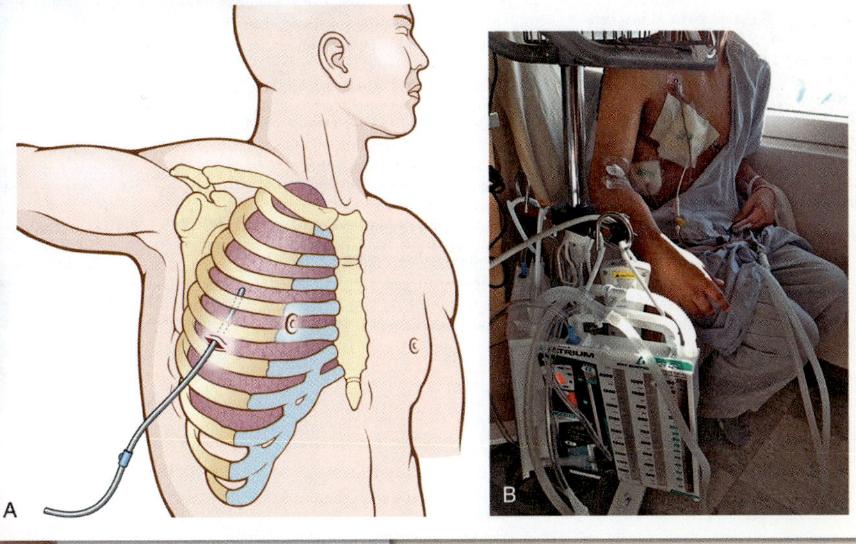

HOW TO USE THE BOOK

The Language of Medicine makes learning easy. The book guides and coaches you step by step through the learning experience. Don't get overwhelmed! Approach learning systematically, step by step. I've helped you study each chapter by organizing the information in small pieces. Icons are provided to help you navigate the sections of the text.

VOCABULARY

This list reviews new terms introduced in the text. Short definitions reinforce your understanding of the terms. See page 449 of this chapter for pronunciation of terms.

aorta	Largest artery in the body.
apex of the heart	The lower tip of the heart.
arteriole	Small artery.
artery	Largest type of blood vessel; carries blood away from the heart to all parts of the body. Notice that artery and away begin with an "a."
atrioventricular bundle (bundle of His)	Specialized muscle fibers connecting the atria with the ventricles and transmitting electrical impulses between them. His is pronounced "hiss."
atrioventricular node (AV node)	Specialized tissue in the wall pass from the pacemaker (SA atrioventricular bundle or bu

After basic material in the chapter is introduced, the key terms you need to learn are presented in Vocabulary lists. These lists help you study and stay focused.

TERMINOLOGY

Write the meanings of the medical terms in the spaces provided.

COMBINING FORMS

COMBINING FORM	MEANING	TERMINOLOGY	MEANING
adenoid/o	adenoids	adenoidectomy	______
		adenoid hypertrophy	______
alveol/o	alveolus, air sac	alveolar	______
bronch/o bronchi/o	bronchial tube, bronchus	bronchospasm *This tightening of the bronchus is a chief characteristic of asthma and bronchitis.*	______
		bronchiectasis *Caused by weakening of the bronchial wall from infection.*	______
		tion, or enlargement, of the opening of a ventilation to the lungs. An example is ia an inhaler.	______
		tula is an abnormal connection between the he pleural cavity (space). Occurring as a or surgical complication, this can cause an ral space.	______

You cannot get lost using *The Language of Medicine*. You learn and engage in small incremental steps. The book imparts the most important concepts, allowing you to concentrate on what is essential.

PRACTICAL APPLICATIONS

This section contains an x-ray report, an orthopedic operating room schedule, a case report with findings presented in SOAP format, and a short clinical case. Explanations of more difficult or unfamiliar terms are given in brackets.

Answers to the matching questions are found on page 640.

MEDICAL REPORT: RESULTS OF CHEST X-RAY EXAMINATION

PA [posteroanterior] and lateral chest: The heart is enlarged in its transverse diameter. The lungs are fully expanded and free of active disease.

Thoracic spine shows a scoliosis of the upper thoracic spine convex to the left. There is 50% wedge compression fracture of T6 and slight wedge compression fracture of T5. There is also anterior wedge compression fracture of T12.

Lumbar spine shows 90% compression fractures of L1 and L3 with 30% compression fractures of L2 and L5. All bones are markedly osteoporotic. There is calcification within the aortic arch. There are gallstones in the right upper quadrant. The findings in the spine are most compatible with osteoporotic compression fractures. During the procedure, the patient had a sickable [syncopal—this word was incorrectly transcribed!] episode and fell, striking her head. A skull series, done at no cost to the patient, shows no evidence of bony fracture. The pineal gland is calcified and has a midline location. The sella turcica is normal.

OPERATING ROOM SCHEDULE I

Match the operation in Column I with an accompanying diagnosis or indication for surgery from Column II.

COLUMN I		COLUMN II
1. Excision, osteochondroma, R calcaneus	____	A. Fracture of the ankle
2. TMJ arthroscopy with probable arthrotomy	____	B. ACL rupture
3. L4–5 laminectomy and diskectomy	____	C. Neoplastic lesion in brain
4. Arthroscopy, left knee	____	D. Exostosis on heel bone
		E. Pelvic fracture
		F. Pain and malocclusion of jawbones

Medical terminology is connected to real life with case reports and case studies throughout the text and on the companion Evolve website.

As you study with *The Language of Medicine,* you are engaged in each step of the learning process. On nearly every page, you are actively involved in labeling diagrams, dividing words into component parts, writing meanings to terms, testing, reviewing, and evaluating your learning.

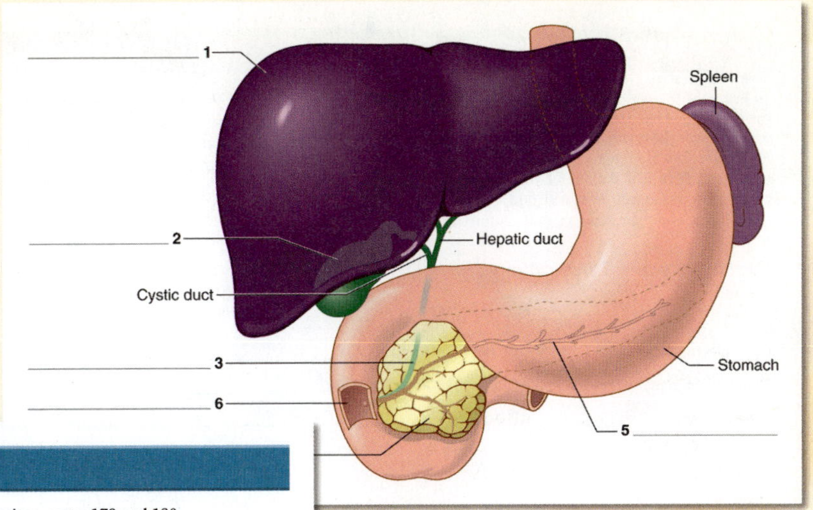

EXERCISES

Remember to check your answers carefully with the Answers to Exercises, pages 179 and 180.

A Match the following digestive system structures with their meanings below.

anus	esophagus	liver
cecum	gallbladder	pancreas
colon	ileum	pharynx
duodenum	jejunum	sigmoid colon

1. consists of ascending, transverse, descending, and sigmoid sections ____________
2. small sac under the liver; stores bile ____________
3. first part of the large intestine ____________
4. end of the digestive tract opening to the outside of the b
5. second part of the small intestine ____________
6. tube connecting the throat to the stomach ____________
7. third part of the small intestine ____________
8. large organ in the RUQ; secretes bile, stores sugar, produ
9. throat ____________
10. lowest part of the colon ____________
11. first part of the small intestine ____________
12. organ under the stomach; produce

Abbreviations are listed and explained in each body system chapter.

ABBREVIATIONS

alk phos	alkaline phosphatase	**HBV**	hepatitis B virus
ALT, AST	alanine transaminase, aspartate transaminase—enzymes measured to evaluate liver function	**IBD**	inflammatory bowel disease (Crohn disease and ulcerative colitis)
		LAC	laparoscopic-assisted colectomy
BE	barium enema	**LFTs**	liver function tests—alk phos, bilirubin, AST, ALT
BM	bowel movement		
BRBPR	bright red blood per rectum—hematochezia (Latin per means through)	**MRI**	magnetic resonance imaging
		NG tube	nasogastric tube
CD	celiac disease	**NPO**	nothing by mouth (Latin nil per os)
			ic gastrostomy
			ic jejunostomy
			atic
			on
			ions typically se), proteins olytes (sodium, , and vitamins.
			duct for drainage bile bag) on the

A Review Sheet at the end of each chapter helps you organize and test yourself on what you have learned!

REVIEW SHEET

Write the meanings of each word part in the space provided. Check your answers with the information in the chapter or in the Glossary (Medical Word Parts—English) at the end of the book.

Combining Forms

COMBINING FORM	MEANING	COMBINING FORM	MEANING
aneurysm/o	____________	ox/o	____________
angi/o	____________	pericardi/o	____________
aort/o	____________	phleb/o	____________
arter/o, arteri/o	____________	pulmon/o	____________
ather/o	____________	rrhythm/o	____________
atri/o	____________	sphygm/o	____________
axill/o	____________	steth/o	____________
brachi/o	____________	thromb/o	____________
cardi/o	____________	valv/o	____________
cholesterol/o	____________	valvul/o	____________
coron/o	____________	vas/o	____________
cyan/o	____________	vascul/o	____________
isch/o	____________	ven/o, ven/i	____________
my/o	____________	ventricul/o	____________
myx/o	____________		

PRONUNCIATION OF TERMS

To test your understanding of the terminology in this chapter, write the meaning of each term in the space provided. In addition, you may wish to cover the terms and write them by looking at your definitions. Make sure your spelling is correct. The page number after each term indicates where it is defined or used in the book, so you can easily check your responses. You will find complete definitions for all of these terms and their audio pronunciations on the Evolve website.

Pronunciation Guide

ā as in āpe	ă as in ăpple
ē as in ēven	ĕ as in ĕvery
ī as in īce	ĭ as in ĭnterest
ō as in ōpen	ŏ as in pŏt
ū as in ūnit	ŭ as in ŭnder

Vocabulary and Terminology

TERM	PRONUNCIATION	MEANING
adenoidectomy (••)	ăd-ĕ-noyd-ĔK-tō-mē	______
adenoid hypertrophy (••)	ĂD-ĕ-noyd hī-PĔR-trō-fē	______
adenoids (••)	ĂD-ĕ-noydz	______
alveolar (••)	ăl-VĒ-ō-lăr	______
alveolus; alveoli (••)	ăl-VĒ-ō-lŭs; ăl-VĒ-ō-lī	______
anosmia (••)	ăn-ŎS-mē-ă	______
apex of the lung (••)	Ā-pĕkz of the lŭng	______
apical (••)	Ā-pĭ-kăl	______
apnea (••)	ĂP-nē-ă	______
asphyxia (••)	ăs-FĬK-sē-ă	______
atelectasis (••)	ă-tĕ-LĔK-tă-sĭs	______
base of the lung (••)	bās of the lŭng	______
bronchiectasis (••)	brŏng-kē-ĔK-tă-sĭs	______
bronchioles (••)	BRŎNG-kē-ōlz	______
bronchiolitis (••)	brŏng-kē-ō-LĪ-tĭs	______

The Pronunciation of Terms section shows you how to pronounce each new term in the chapter and gives you the chance to practice writing its meaning. You can also hear these terms pronounced on the companion Evolve website. The answers to the Pronunciation of Terms section are found on the Evolve website as well.

ALSO AVAILABLE

STUDENT EVOLVE RESOURCES
(complimentary access included with purchase of this text)

All student resources are now available online on the Evolve website. The student website accompanying this new edition is packed with activities, games, additional information, and video clips to expand your understanding and test your knowledge. Chapter by chapter you will find quizzes, case studies, examples of medical records, and a wealth of images to illustrate terminology. Additionally, on the website, you can hear the terms corresponding to the Pronunciation of Terms section in each chapter (more than 3,000 terms in all). Access your resources at: http://evolve.elsevier.com/Chabner/language.

New to the Student Evolve Website for the 10th Edition

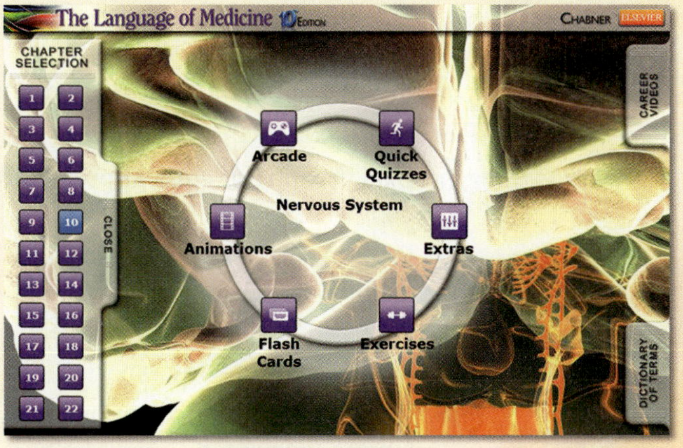

- Updated interface enabling convenient online access to your resources.
- A Mobile Dictionary has been added for this edition. Access this complimentary resource from the Evolve site on your desktop or mobile device and have easy access to definitions of all terms found in the text. This resource helps you study each chapter and also will be a reference for you in the workplace. Each definition has been crafted carefully to explain terms using plain, nontechnical language.
- A Quick Quiz feature has also been added, enabling students to get a snapshot assessment of their knowledge of a chapter's content.
- The new Mobile Dictionary, Quick Quizzes, and updated Flash Cards have been optimized for use on mobile devices, providing convenient access for on-the-go studying.

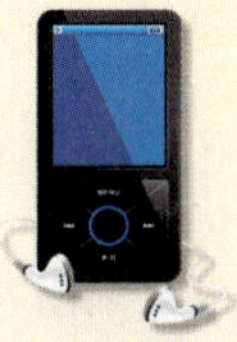

iTerms Study Companion (for sale separately)

The iTerms audio study guide provides pronunciation and enables you to hear each term pronounced with its definition, in a portable format. This audio companion is available for download. Also included are short review quizzes and coaching tips to help you make the most of your study.

MEDICAL LANGUAGE INSTANT TRANSLATOR (for sale separately)

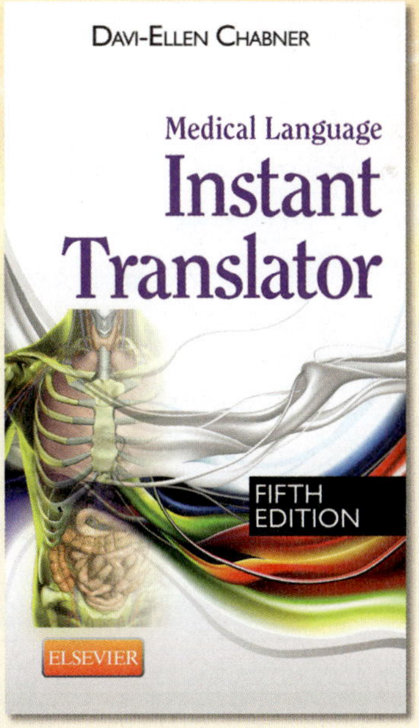

The *Medical Language Instant Translator* is a uniquely useful resource for all allied health professionals and students of medical terminology. It is a pocket-sized medical terminology reference with convenient information at your fingertips!

- NEW updates to correlate with the revision of *The Language of Medicine*

INSTRUCTOR'S RESOURCE MANUAL

The Language of Medicine Instructor's Resource Manual (includes instructor's manual, PowerPoints, and an image collection) is available with even more new quizzes, teaching suggestions, crossword puzzles, medical reports, and reference material. The image collection contains all figures and photos from the 10th edition. The instructor materials plus a test bank can be accessed online at http://evolve.elsevier.com/Chabner/language.

The fundamental features you have come to trust in learning and teaching medical terminology remain strong in this new edition. These are:

- Simple, nontechnical explanations of medical terms.
- Workbook format with ample space to write answers.
- Explanations of clinical procedures, laboratory tests, and abbreviations related to each body system.
- Pronunciation of Terms sections with phonetic spellings and spaces to write meanings of terms.
- Practical Applications sections with case reports, operative and diagnostic tests, and laboratory and x-ray reports.
- Exercises that test your understanding of terminology as you work through the text step by step (answers are included).
- Review Sheets that pull together terminology to help you study.
- Comprehensive glossaries and appendices for reference in class and on the job.

Each student and teacher who selects *The Language of Medicine* becomes my partner in the exciting adventure of learning medical terms. Continuity is crucial. Continue to communicate with me through email (daviellenchabner@gmail.com) with your suggestions and comments so that future printings and editions may benefit. A website connected to *The Language of Medicine* and dedicated to helping students and teachers is located at http://evolve.elsevier.com/Chabner/language. I hope you will tell me about additional resources you would like to see on that website so that we can make it an even more useful part of the learning process. You should know that I still experience the thrill and joy of teaching new students. I love being in a classroom and feel privileged to continue to write this text. I hope that my enthusiasm and passion for the medical language are transmitted to you through these pages.

Work hard, but have fun with
The Language of Medicine!

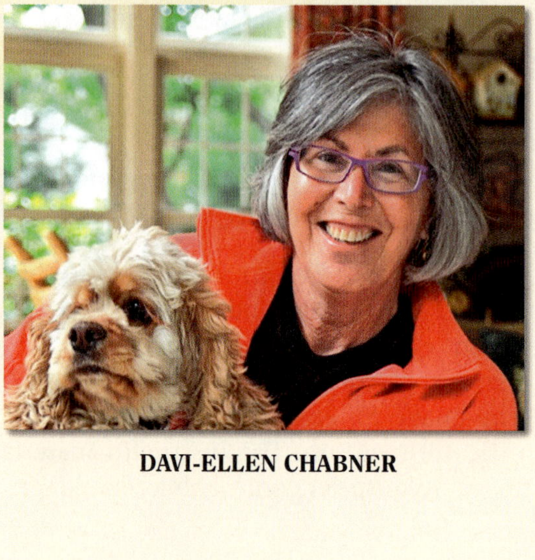

DAVI-ELLEN CHABNER

ACKNOWLEDGMENTS

Maureen Pfeifer has been my extraordinary editorial partner for the last 15 years. Her phenomenal expertise in all facets of communication, coordination, production, editing, updating, and management is amazing. She has the unique ability to "make things happen" and "make things right." Both personally and professionally, I am grateful for her unique insight and capabilities. She is intelligent, calm, and upbeat in the face of any issue affecting *The Language of Medicine* and its ancillaries. Most of all, I rely on her loyalty and her confidence that we are creating an eminently useful and valuable textbook and resource for both students and instructors. Thank you, Maureen, for everything you do for me.

Ellen Zanolle, Senior Book Designer, Art and Design, continues to astound me with her fresh and vibrant presentation for the cover and interior of this new edition. Her creative genius is evident on every page. She is always responsive and innovative in presenting a complex layout and coordinating multiple elements of the text. Ellen, I am so grateful for your fierce dedication to all of my books! Bill Donnelly, page layout designer, once again did an excellent job arranging and crafting each page to make learning easier for students. Bill, thanks for all your hard work.

Jim Perkins, Assistant Professor of Medical Illustration, Rochester Institute of Technology, has been associated with *The Language of Medicine* since its 6th edition. He has worked with me to create drawings that are not only attractive but also essential in making the terminology more understandable. I have come to rely on his unique talent for clarity, accuracy, and detail.

Elizabeth Galbraith copyedited and proofread the manuscript with her characteristic attention to grammatical detail and medical accuracy. Thanks to her, students will read and study the text with greater ease.

Bruce A. Chabner, MD, and Elizabeth Chabner Thompson, MD, MPH, continue to be an amazing resource to me for expert and up-to-date medical advice. Their contributions were essential in reviewing and editing all chapters and glossaries. In addition, Elizabeth, once again recorded the iTerms for the book, an invaluable accessory to the text for help in pronunciation and understanding terminology. Dan Longo, MD, never turned me down for valuable medical advice and editing of chapters. He was also a wonderful resource for helping me identify expert reviewers.

I am indebted to the many medical reviewers listed on pages xv-xvi who offered essential advice and comments on specific chapters. Their insights and expertise make this 10th edition reflect what is current, accurate, and cutting edge in medicine today.

The classroom instructors listed on pages xvi-xvii extensively and carefully reviewed the text, and I have listened to their comments, which are integrated into this new edition. Many other instructors contacted me personally through email with helpful suggestions. Special thank you to Madellaine Bart, Joyce Y. Nakano, Rosemary Van Vranken, PhD, Martha J. Payne, Christine Urata, RN, Kabir Chuttani, Dr. Chabed Kutani, Dorothy Flood-Granat, Chanthon Hang, Lydia Chari, Susanne Smith, and Heather LaJoie.

I am always pleased to hear from students who comment on the book and ask important questions. I try to answer each as quickly and accurately as possible. Thanks to Michael Moschella, Peter Nguyen, Tracey Elsberry-Gladney, Nicole Zarber, Ginny Henderson, Beth Gutridge, Mike Westva, Sheila Cross, Charlene Kelley, Brenda Gardiner, Michael Mazano, Elizabeth Ramirez, Sara Kleinfelder, Samie Lim, Robert Boyd, and Christopher Halldorson.

Kathleen Carbone, CPC, Massachusetts General Hospital medical coder, and one of my former medical terminology students, has been a valuable resource for coding information, not only for *The Language of Medicine* but the *Medical Language Instant Translator*. She is always willing to help, and I count on her advice and expertise.

I am particularly excited about the addition of In Person stories beginning in Chapter 5. These are first-person accounts of experiences with illness and medical procedures. The writers of these stories were extraordinarily generous to share their insights and reactions so that we all might benefit. A very special thank you to: Stan Ber, Nancy J. Brandwein, Mary Braun, Bruce A. Chabner, Sidra DeKoven Ezrahi, Elizabeth F. Fideler, Tanzie Johnson, Kevin Mahoney, Frank McGinnis, Brenda Melson, John Melson, Laura Claridge Oppenheimer, Bob Rowe, Ruthellen Sheldon, Elizabeth Chabner Thompson, and Cathy Ward.

The superb staff at Elsevier Health Sciences continues to be vital to the success of *The Language of Medicine*. Luke Held, Senior Content Development Specialist, was always responsive, available, and effective in managing the many details of the project. Rachel Allen, Content Coordinator, coordinated countless facets of this edition. I appreciate Linda Woodard, Content Strategist, and Jeanne Olson, Content Strategy Director, for their expert management and their steadfast support of my books.

I am grateful to Sally Schrefer, Executive Vice President, Nursing and Health Sciences, and to Andrew Allen, Vice President and Publisher, Health Professions II, for their continuing confidence and support for *The Language of Medicine*. Thanks to Peggy Fagen, Director of Publishing Services, Gayle May, Book Production Manager, and Julie Eddy, Publishing Services Manager, for their superb production efforts. Celeste Clingan, Senior Project Manager, tirelessly and effectively handled the day-to-day aspects of the production process. Thank you, Celeste! I continue to be impressed by the talents of the entire marketing team, especially Janet Blanner, Vice President Nursing and Health Professions Marketing, Julie Burchett, Director of Content Marketing, Pat Crowe, Group Segment Manager, and Danielle LeCompte, Project Manager, Health Sciences Marketing. They do a phenomenal job keeping *The Language of Medicine* in-step with the needs of instructors and students.

Thanks to Tyson Sturgeon, Manager of Multimedia Production, Jeanne Crook, Team Lead, Multimedia Production, and Jennifer Presley, Producer, for their work on the electronic products associated with this new edition.

A very special note of gratitude to the extraordinary and devoted sales team at Elsevier Health Sciences, which is beyond compare! Led by Terri Allen, Vice President of US Academic Sales, and Linda Morris, Director of Sales Operations, Nursing and Health Professions, they work tirelessly to bring my books and learning system to the marketplace. You are the best!

My family and friends continue to be my greatest comfort and support. The kids, Brandon, Marla, Noonie, and Dave, are always “in my corner.” The grandkids, Bebe, Solomon, Ben, Gus, Louisa, and Amari make me feel “on top of the world.” Juliana Do Carmo, by managing so many day-to-day responsibilities, allows me the luxury of being able to work and concentrate. Bruce, my husband of nearly 50 years, has always encouraged my passion for teaching and writing, and given me the space and time to enjoy it. His calm and reassurance trumps any doubt or angst. Lastly, our canine kids, Owen and Greta, remain the love of our lives, providing countless hours of relaxation.

REVIEWERS

The following persons reviewed the text and/or the ancillaries:

MEDICAL REVIEWERS

Elizabeth Chabner Thompson, MD, MPH
CEO/Founder of BFFL Co
Scarsdale, New York

Bruce A. Chabner, MD
Director of Clinical Research
Massachusetts General Hospital Cancer Center
Professor of Medicine
Harvard Medical School
Boston, Massachusetts

Michael F. Greene, MD
Professor of Obstetrics, Gynecology, and Reproductive Biology
Harvard Medical School
Vincent Department of Obstetrics and Gynecology
Massachusetts General Hospital
Boston, Massachusetts

Thomas K.Fehring, MD
Co-Director Orthocarolina Hip and Knee Center
Charlotte, North Carolina

Morris A. Fisher, M.D.
Attending Neurologist
Edward Hines Jr. Veterans Hospital
Hines, Illinois
Professor of Neurology Loyola University
Chicago Stritch School of Medicine
Maywood, Illinois

Lisa Grodsky Delmonico, MSPT
Boston, Massachusetts

Lipika Goyal, MD
Boston, Massachusetts

Carlos A. Jamis-Dow, M.D.
Associate Professor of Radiology
Penn State
Milton S. Hershey Medical Center
Hershey, Pennsylvania

Jay Loeffler, MD
Chief of Radiation Oncology
Massachusetts General Hospital Cancer Center
Herman and Joan Professor
Harvard Medical School
Boston, Massachusetts

Dan L. Longo, MD
Deputy Editor
New England Journal of Medicine
Professor of Medicine
Harvard Medical School
Boston, Massachusetts

W. Scott McDougal, MD
Chief Emeritus, Urology Service
Massachusetts General Hospital
Boston, Massachusetts

Ann Sacher, MD
Scarsdale, New York

Henry E. Schniewind, MD
Boston, Massachusetts

Noëlle S. Sherber, MD, FAAD
Consultant Dermatologist
Johns Hopkins Scleroderma Center
Baltimore, Maryland

Leigh H. Simmons, MD
General Medicine Division
Massachusetts General Hospital
Boston, Massachusetts

Daniel I. Simon, MD
Chief, Division of Cardiovascular Medicine
Director, Harrington Heart & Vascular Institute
University Hospitals Case Medical Center
Herman K. Hellerstein Professor of Cardiovascular Research
Case Western Reserve University School of Medicine
Cleveland, Ohio

Norman M. Simon, MD
Evanston Northwestern Healthcare
Professor of Medicine
Northwestern University
Feinberg School of Medicine
Chicago, Illinois

Jill Smith, MD
Chief of Ophthalmology
Newton-Wellesley Hospital
Newton, Massachusetts

Sheila Thomas, OD
20/20 Vision
McDonough, Georgia

INSTRUCTOR REVIEWERS

Francine Armenth-Brothers, EdD, MS, ATC/L
Associate Professor of Health
Heartland Community College
Normal, Illinois

Janet S. Barnard, RN, BSN, CCMA-AC
Medical Careers Instructor
Central Sierra ROP
Placerville, California

Bradley S. Bowden
Professor of Biology
Alfred University
Alfred, New York

Shawnmarie Carpenter, MEd, AKMFT
University of Alaska SE
Ketchikan, Alaska

Ericha Clare, ND
Naturopathic Physician
Clark College
Vancouver, Washington

Sherie Courchaine RN, BSN
Crystal Falls, Michigan

Beth A. Crow, BSEd
Financial Aid Officer and A&P Instructor
American Commercial College
Abilene, Texas

Amy M. DeVore, MSTD, CEHRS, CPC, CMA (AAMA)
Butler County Community College
Butler, Pennsylvania

Rick Durling, BS, CMA (AAMA, CPC, CPC-I)
Faculty
Linn Benton Community College
Albany, Oregon

Shandra Esparza, MEd, ATC, LAT
Clinical Coordinator and Instructor in Athletic Training Education
The Universaity of the Incarnate Word
San Antonio, Texas

Suzanne B. Garrett, MSA, RHIA
HIT Program Director
College of Central Florida
Ocala, Florida

Janice Hess, MA, RMT
HIMS Coordinator
Metropolitan Community College
Omaha, Nebraska

Joseph A. Mamatz, Jr., MAEd, RT(R)(T)(ARRT)
Academic Chairman and Radiography Program Director
Radiography Education Program
Bergen Community College
Paramus, New Jersey

Susan Newton, MT (ASCP)
Franklin County High School
Rocky Mount, Virginia

Alice M. Noblin, PhD, RHIA, CCS
Health Informatics and Information Management Program Director and Instructor
University of Central Florida
Orlando, Florida

Yvette E. Pawlowski, BA, CMT, RHIT
Faculty Instructor
Central Texas College
Killeen, Texas

David Rice, RMA, BA
Medical Instructor
Milan Institute
Sparks, Nevada

Jenny E. Torchia
Instructor
Spanish Medical Interpreter Program MIP
Southwest Skill Center at Estrella Mountain Community College
Avondale, Arizona

Kasey Waychoff, AOS, CMA, CPT
Allied Health Curriculum Specialist
Centura College
Virginia Beach, Virginia

Mandie Wilkerson-McMahon, MD, MBA
Clinical Externship Coordinator, Clinical Instructor
American Commercial College
Lubbock, Texas

Barbara Wortman, RN, MSN, CPhT
Bossier Parish Technical School
Bossier City, Louisiana

CONTENTS

CHAPTER 1

Basic Word Structure

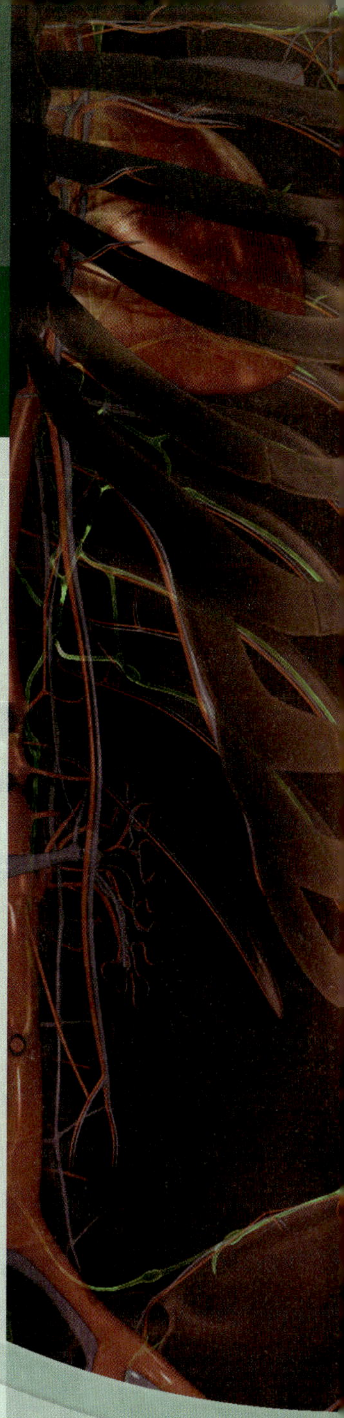

This chapter is divided
into the following sections:

CHAPTER GOALS

- Identify basic objectives to guide your study of the medical language.
- Divide medical words into their component parts.
- Learn the meanings of basic combining forms, suffixes, and prefixes of the medical language.
- Use these combining forms, suffixes, and prefixes to build medical words.

OBJECTIVES IN STUDYING THE MEDICAL LANGUAGE

There are three objectives to keep in mind as you study medical terminology:

- **Analyze words by dividing them into component parts.**
  Your goal is to learn the *tools* of word analysis that will make understanding complex terminology easier. Do not simply memorize terms; think about dividing terms into component parts. This book will show you how to separate both complicated and simple terms into understandable word elements. Medical terms are much like jigsaw puzzles in that they are constructed of small pieces that make each word unique, with one major difference: The pieces can be shuffled up and used in lots of combinations to make other words as well. As you become familiar with word parts and learn what each means, you will be able to recognize those word parts in totally new combinations in other terms.
- **Relate the medical terms to the structure and function of the human body.**
  Memorization of terms, although essential to retention of the language, should not become the primary objective of your study. A major focus of this book is to *explain* terms in the context of how the body works in health and disease. Medical terms explained in their proper context also will be easier to remember. Thus, the term **hepatitis,** meaning inflammation **(-itis)** of the liver **(hepat),** is better understood when you know where the liver is and how it functions. No previous knowledge of biology, anatomy, or physiology is needed for this study. Explanations in this book are straightforward and basic.
- **Be aware of spelling and pronunciation problems.**
  Some medical terms are pronounced alike but are spelled differently, which accounts for their different meanings. For example, **ilium** and **ileum** have identical pronunciations, but the first term, **ilium**, means a part of the hip bone, whereas the second term, **ileum**, refers to a part of the small intestine (Figure 1-1). Even

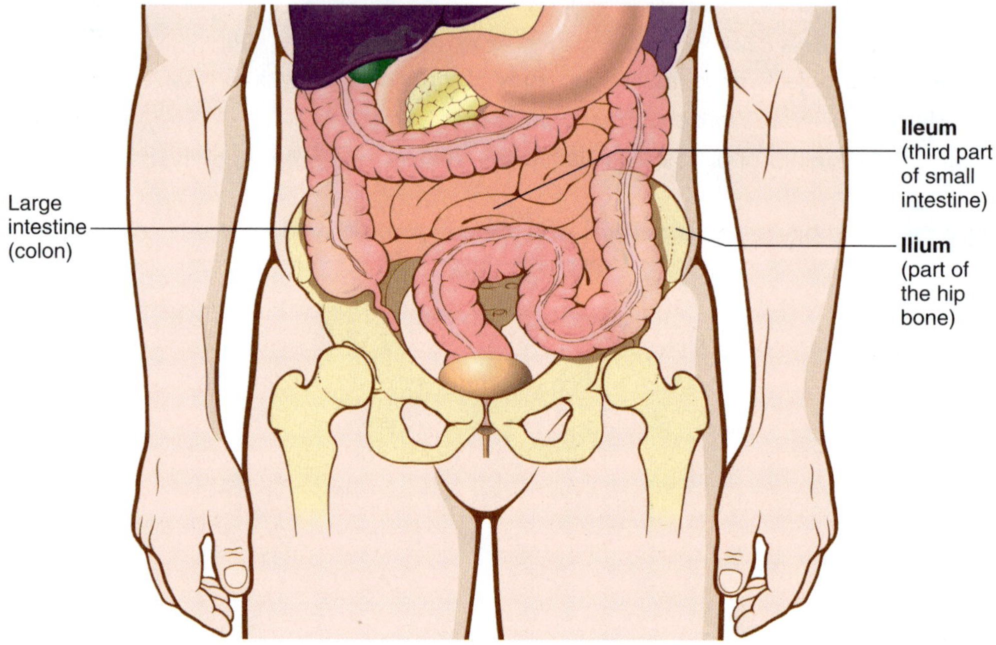

FIGURE 1-1 The terms **ileum** and **ilium** can be confusing because they are pronounced alike and located in the same region of the body.

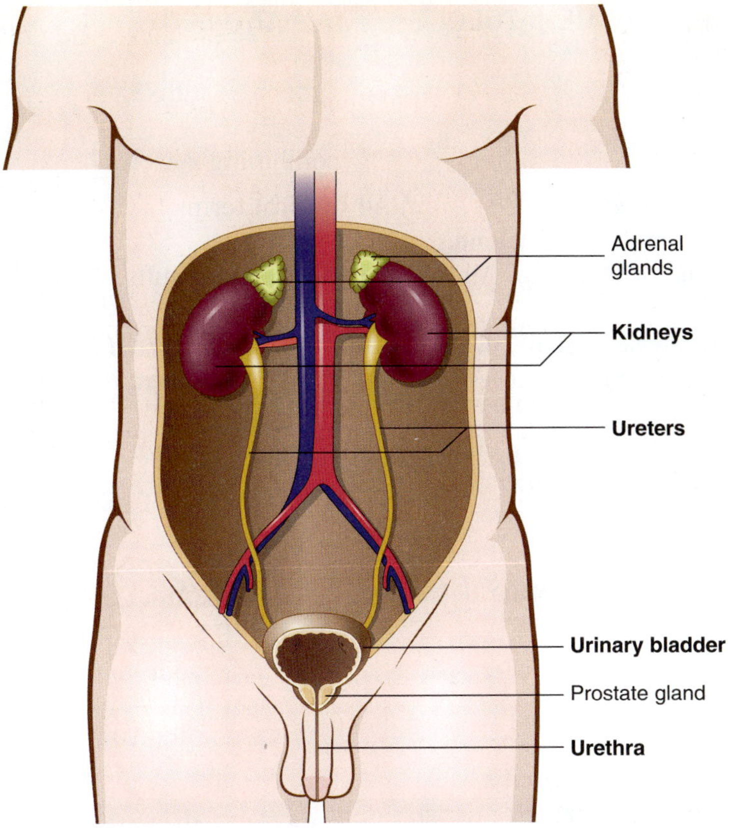

FIGURE 1-2 **Male urinary tract.** The terms **urethra** and **ureter** can be confusing because they are both tubes of the urinary system, but the spellings and pronunciations are different. Notice the locations: **two** ureters between the kidneys and urinary bladder and **one** urethra between the urinary bladder and the outside of the body.

when terms are spelled correctly, they can be misunderstood because of incorrect pronunciation. For example, the **urethra** (ū-RĒ-thrăh) is the tube leading from the urinary bladder to the outside of the body, whereas a **ureter** (ŪR-ĕ-tĕr) is one of two tubes each leading from a single kidney and inserting into the urinary bladder. Figure 1-2 illustrates the difference between the urethra and the ureters.

WORD ANALYSIS

Studying medical terminology is very similar to learning a new language. At first, the words sound strange and complicated, although they may stand for commonly known disorders and terms. For example, **cephalgia** means "headache," and an **ophthalmologist** is an "eye doctor."

Your first job in learning the language of medicine is to understand how to divide words into their component parts. Logically, most terms, whether complex or simple, can be broken down into basic parts and then understood. For example, consider the following term:

HEMATOLOGY HEMAT/O/LOGY

root: HEMAT; combining vowel: O; suffix: LOGY

The **root** is the *foundation of the word.* All medical terms have one or more roots. For example, the root **hemat** means **blood.**

The **suffix** is the *word ending*. All medical terms have a suffix. The suffix **-logy** means **process of study.**

The **combining vowel**—usually **o,** as in this term—*links the root to the suffix or the root to another root*. A combining vowel has no meaning of its own; it joins one word part to another.

It is useful to read the meaning of medical terms *starting from the suffix and then going back to the beginning of the term*. Thus, the term **hematology** means **process of study of blood.**

Here is another familiar medical term:

ELECTROCARDIOGRAM ELECTR/O/CARDI/O/GRAM

root: ELECTR; combining vowel: O; root: CARDI; combining vowel: O; suffix: GRAM

The root **electr** means **electricity.**

The root **cardi** means **heart.**

The suffix **-gram** means **record.**

The entire word, reading from the suffix back to the beginning of the term, means **record of the electricity in the heart.**

Notice that there are two combining vowels—both **o**—in this term. The first o links the two roots **electr** and **cardi**; the second o links the root **cardi** and the suffix **-gram.**

Try another term:

GASTRITIS GASTR/ITIS

root: GASTR; suffix: ITIS

The root **gastr** means **stomach.**

The suffix **-itis** means **inflammation.**

The entire word, reading from the end of the term (suffix) to the beginning, means **inflammation of the stomach.**

Notice that the combining vowel, o, is missing in this term. This is because the suffix, **-itis,** begins with a vowel. The combining vowel is dropped before a suffix that begins with a vowel. It is retained, however, between two roots, even if the second root begins with a vowel.

Consider the following term:

GASTROENTEROLOGY GASTR/O/ENTER/O/LOGY

root: GASTR; combining vowel: O; root: ENTER; combining vowel: O; suffix: LOGY

The root **gastr** means **stomach.**

The root **enter** means **intestines.**

The suffix **-logy** means **process of study.**

The entire term means **process of study of the stomach and intestines.**

Notice that the combining vowel is used between **gastr** and **enter,** even though the second root, **enter,** begins with a vowel. When a term contains two or more roots related to parts of the body, anatomic position often determines which root goes before the other. For example, the stomach receives food first, before the small intestine—so the word is formed as **gastroenterology,** not "enterogastrology."

In summary, remember **three general rules:**

1. Read the meaning of medical terms from the suffix back to the beginning of the term and across.
2. Drop the combining vowel (usually o) before a suffix beginning with a vowel: **gastritis,** *not* "gastroitis."
3. Keep the combining vowel between two roots: **gastroenterology,** *not* "gastrenterology."

In addition to the root, suffix, and combining vowel, two other word parts are commonly found in medical terms. These are the **combining form** and the **prefix.** The combining form is simply the root plus the combining vowel. For example, you already are familiar with the following combining forms and their meanings:

HEMAT/O means **blood**

root + combining vowel = COMBINING FORM

GASTR/O means **stomach**

root + combining vowel = COMBINING FORM

CARDI/O means **heart**

root + combining vowel = COMBINING FORM

Combining forms are used with many different suffixes. Remembering the meaning of a combining form will help you understand different medical terms.

The **prefix** is a small part that is attached to the *beginning of a term*. Not all medical terms contain prefixes, but the prefix can have an important influence on the meaning. Consider the following examples:

HYPO/GASTR/IC means **pertaining to below the stomach**

prefix (**below**) root (**stomach**) suffix (**pertaining to**)

EPI/GASTR/IC means **pertaining to above the stomach**

prefix (**above**) root (**stomach**) suffix (**pertaining to**)

In summary, the **important elements of medical terms** are the following:

1. **Root:** foundation of the term
2. **Suffix:** word ending
3. **Prefix:** word beginning
4. **Combining vowel:** vowel (usually o) that links the root to the suffix or the root to another root
5. **Combining form:** combination of the root and the combining vowel

TERMINOLOGY

In previous examples you have been introduced to the combining forms **gastr/o** (stomach), **hemat/o** (blood), and **cardi/o** (heart). This section of the chapter presents a list of additional combining forms, suffixes, and prefixes, with examples of medical words using those word parts. (Similar lists are included for each chapter in the book.) Write the *meaning* of the medical term in the space provided. Then check the correct pronunciation for each term with the Pronunciation of Terms list on pages 27 to 30. The Evolve website for *The Language of Medicine* contains definitions and audio pronunciations for each term. Use it!

Most medical terms are derived from Greek and Latin roots. Greek, Roman, and Arabic physicians had developed medically useful concepts and associated vocabularies long before the 21st century. Greek and Latin derivations for medical terms are presented for your interest on the Evolve website.

CHAPTER STUDY GUIDE

1. **Use slashes to divide each term** into component parts *(aden/oma)*, and **write its meaning** *(tumor of a gland)* in the space provided. Although most medical terms are divided easily into component parts and understood, others defy simple explanation. Information in *italics* under a medical term helps you define and understand the term. You can check meanings on the Evolve site.
2. **Complete the Exercises,** pages 17 to 23, and **check your answers against those provided** on pages 24 to 26.
3. **Write meanings for terms on the Pronunciation of Terms list,** pages 27 to 30. Definitions are on the Evolve site.
4. **Complete the Review Sheet,** pages 31 and 32. Check your answers with the Glossary, page 961. Then, **test yourself** by writing Review Sheet terms and meanings on a separate sheet of paper.
5. **Make your own flash cards.** Using the Review Sheet as a guide, create flash cards that can be transported wherever you study!
6. **Create your own book tabs** to have easy access to key concepts and frequently used sections; for example the **Glossary of Word Parts,** beginning on page 961.
7. **Review terms** using the audio pronunciations found on the Evolve website.

Notice that you are actively engaging in the learning process by writing terms and their meanings and testing yourself repeatedly. Here is your study mantra: **R**ead, **WR**ite, **R**ecite, and **R**eview. I guarantee success if you follow these simple steps. This is a proven method—it really works!

COMBINING FORMS

Remember: You will find every term phonetically pronounced starting on page 27, and you can hear the pronunciations on the Evolve website.

COMBINING FORM	MEANING	TERMINOLOGY	MEANING
aden/o	gland	adenoma	*tumor of a gland*
		The suffix -oma means tumor or mass.	
		adenitis	
		The suffix -itis means inflammation.	
arthr/o	joint	arthritis	
bi/o	life	biology	
		The suffix -logy is composed of the root log (study) and the final suffix -y (process or condition).	
		biopsy	
		The suffix -opsy means process of viewing. Living tissue is removed from the body and viewed under a microscope.	
carcin/o	cancerous, cancer	carcinoma	
		A carcinoma is a cancerous tumor. Carcinomas grow from the epithelial (surface or skin) cells that cover the outside of the body and line organs, cavities, and tubes within the body (Figure 1-3).	
cardi/o	heart	cardiology	
cephal/o	head	cephalic	
		(sĕ-FĂL-ĭk) The suffix -ic means pertaining to. A cephalic presentation describes a "head first" position for the delivery of an infant.	

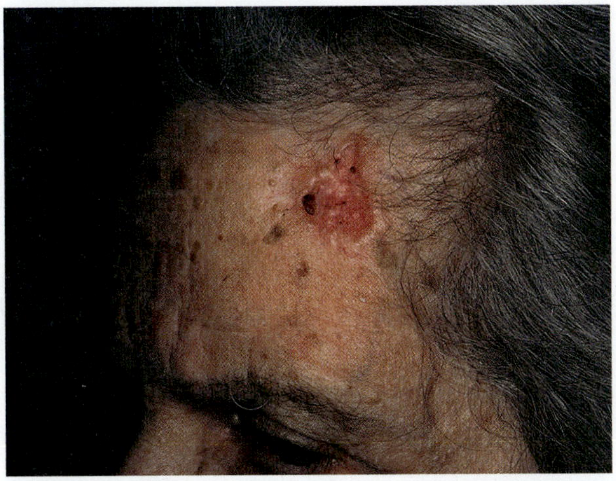

FIGURE 1-3 **Carcinoma** of the skin. This is a **basal cell carcinoma,** the most common form of skin cancer. It usually occurs on sun-damaged skin.

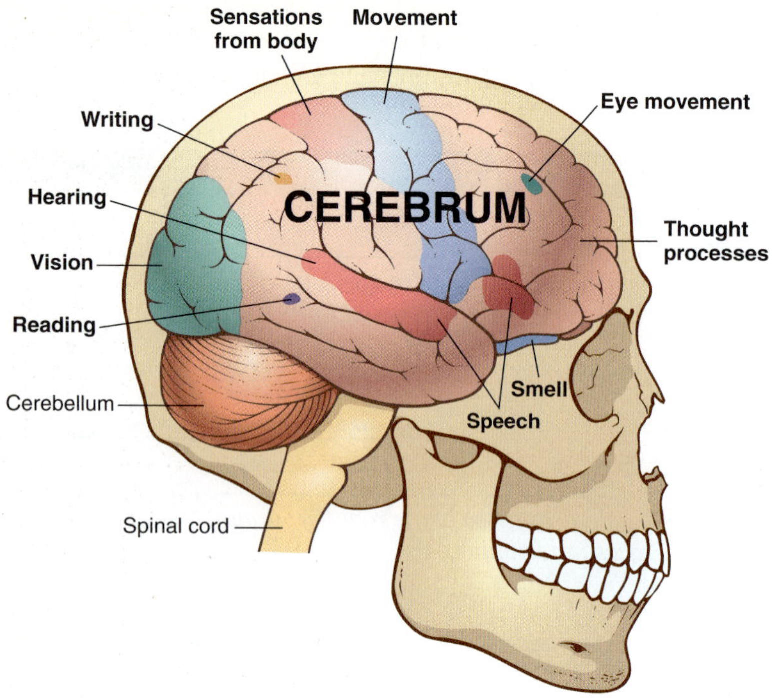

FIGURE 1-4 **Cerebrum** and the functions it controls. A **cerebrovascular accident (CVA)**, or **stroke,** occurs when blood vessels (vascul/o means blood vessel) are damaged in the cerebrum and blood is prevented from reaching functional areas of the brain. Cells, deprived of oxygen and nutrients, are damaged, causing loss of movement, speech, and other signs and symptoms of a CVA.

COMBINING FORM	MEANING	TERMINOLOGY	MEANING
cerebr/o	cerebrum (largest part of the brain)	cerebral *The suffix -al means pertaining to. Figure 1-4 shows the cerebrum and its many functional areas.*	
cis/o	to cut	incision *The prefix in- means into, and the suffix -ion means process.* excision *The prefix ex- means out.*	
crin/o	to secrete (to form and give off)	endocrine glands *The prefix endo- means within; endocrine glands (e.g., thyroid, pituitary, and adrenal glands) secrete hormones directly within (into) the bloodstream. Other glands, called exocrine glands, release their secretions (e.g., saliva, sweat, tears) through tubes (ducts) to the outside of the body.*	
cyst/o	urinary bladder; a sac or a cyst (sac containing fluid)	cystoscopy *(sĭs-TŎS-kō-pē) The suffix -scopy is a* ***complex suffix*** *that includes the root scop, meaning visual examination, and the final suffix -y, meaning process.*	

Complex suffixes

Many suffixes, like **-scopy,** contain an embedded root word. Other examples are **-opsy** (ops is a root) and **-logy** (log is a root).

COMBINING FORM	MEANING	TERMINOLOGY	MEANING
cyt/o	cell	cytology *See Figure 1-5 for examples of blood cells.*	____________
derm/o	skin	dermatitis	____________
dermat/o		hypodermic *The prefix hypo- means under or below.*	____________
electr/o	electricity	electrocardiogram *The suffix -gram means record. Abbreviated ECG (or sometimes EKG).*	____________
encephal/o	brain	electroencephalogram *Abbreviated EEG.*	____________
enter/o	intestines (usually the small intestine)	enteritis *The small intestine is narrower but much longer than the large intestine (colon). See Figure 1-1 on p. 2, which shows the small and large intestines.*	____________
erythr/o	red	erythrocyte *The suffix -cyte means cell. Erythrocytes carry oxygen in the blood.*	____________
gastr/o	stomach	gastrectomy *The suffix -ectomy means excision or removal. All or, more commonly, part of the stomach is removed.*	____________
		gastrotomy *The suffix -tomy is another complex suffix, which contains the root tom, meaning to cut, and the final suffix -y, meaning process of.*	____________

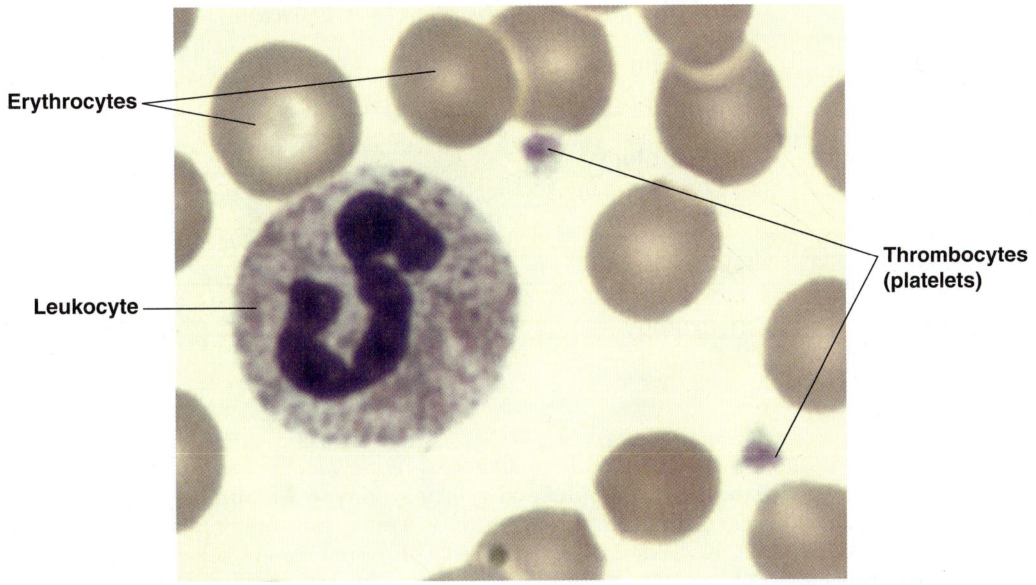

FIGURE 1-5 Blood cells. Notice red blood cells (erythrocytes), a white blood cell (leukocyte), and clotting cells (thrombocytes or platelets).

COMBINING FORM	MEANING	TERMINOLOGY	MEANING
glyc/o	sugar	hyperglycemia *The prefix hyper- means excessive, above, or more than normal. The suffix -emia means blood condition.*	________
gnos/o	knowledge	diagnosis *The prefix dia- means complete. The suffix -sis means state or condition of. A diagnosis is made after sufficient information has been obtained about the patient's condition. Literally, it is a "state of complete knowledge."*	________
		prognosis *The prefix pro- means before. Literally "knowledge before," a prognosis is a prediction about the outcome of an illness, but it is always given after the diagnosis has been determined.*	________
gynec/o	woman, female	gynecology	________
hemat/o	blood	hematology	________
hem/o		hematoma *In this term, -oma means a mass or collection of blood, rather than a growth of cells (tumor). A hematoma forms when blood escapes from blood vessels and collects as a clot in a cavity or organ or under the skin. See Figure 1-6.*	________
		hemoglobin *The suffix -globin means protein. Hemoglobin carries oxygen in red blood cells.*	________
hepat/o	liver	hepatitis	________
iatr/o	treatment, physician	iatrogenic *The suffix -genic means pertaining to producing, produced by, or produced in. Iatrogenic conditions are adverse effects that result from treatment or intervention by a physician.*	________
leuk/o	white	leukocyte *This blood cell helps the body fight disease.*	________
log/o	study of	dermatology	________
nephr/o	kidney	nephritis	________
		nephrology	________
neur/o	nerve	neurology	________

Hyperglycemia and Diabetes

Hyperglycemia (high blood sugar) most frequently is associated with **diabetes.** People with diabetes have high blood sugar levels because they **lack insulin** (in **type 1 diabetes**) or have **ineffective insulin** (in **type 2 diabetes**). Insulin is the hormone normally released by the pancreas (an endocrine gland near the stomach) to "escort" sugar from the bloodstream into cells. Sugar (glucose) is then broken down in cells to release energy. When insulin is not present, sugar cannot enter cells and builds up in the bloodstream (hyperglycemia).

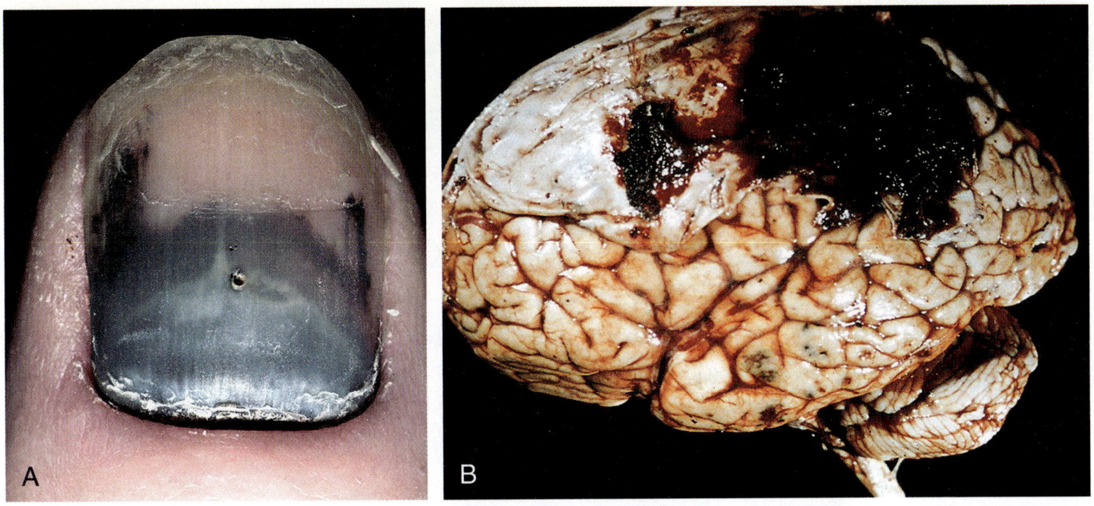

FIGURE 1-6 **A,** Notice the **hematoma** under the nail. **B, Hematoma** caused by external trauma to the brain (cerebrum). Blood collects above the brain's outermost (epi-) covering (dura). It is an **epidural hematoma.** (**B,** *Courtesy of Dr. Raymond D. Adams, Massachusetts General Hospital, Boston.*).

COMBINING FORM	MEANING	TERMINOLOGY	MEANING
onc/o	tumor	oncology	________________
		oncologist *The suffix -ist means one who specializes in a field of medicine (or other profession).*	________________
ophthalm/o	eye	ophthalmoscope *(ŏf-THĂL-mō-skōp) The suffix -scope means an instrument for visual examination. (To help with spelling, notice that just as there are two eyes, there are two "h"s in this term.)*	________________
oste/o	bone	osteitis	________________
		osteoarthritis *This condition of aging is actually a degeneration of bones and joints often accompanied by inflammation.*	________________
path/o	disease	pathology	________________
		pathologist *A pathologist examines biopsy samples microscopically and examines dead bodies to determine the cause of death.*	________________
ped/o	child	pediatric *Notice that ped/o is also in the term orthopedist. Orthopedists once were doctors who straightened (orth/o means straight) children's bones and corrected deformities. Nowadays, orthopedists specialize in disorders of bones and muscles in people of all ages.*	________________

COMBINING FORM	MEANING	TERMINOLOGY	MEANING
psych/o	mind	psychology	______________
		psychiatrist	______________
radi/o	x-rays	radiology	______________
		Low-energy x-rays are used for diagnostic imaging.	
ren/o	kidney	renal	______________
		Ren/o (Latin) and nephr/o (Greek) both mean kidney. Ren/o is used with -al (Latin) to describe the kidney, whereas nephr/o is used with other suffixes such as -osis, -itis, and -ectomy (Greek) to describe abnormal conditions and operative procedures.	
rhin/o	nose	rhinitis	______________
sarc/o	flesh	sarcoma	______________
		This is a cancerous (malignant) tumor. A ***sarcoma*** *(Figure 1-7) grows from cells of "fleshy" connective tissue such as muscle, bone, and fat, whereas a* ***carcinoma*** *(another type of cancerous tumor) grows from epithelial cells that line the outside of the body or the inside of organs in the body.*	
sect/o	to cut	resection	______________
		The prefix re- means back. A resection is a cutting back in the sense of cutting out or removal (excision). A gastric resection is a gastrectomy, or excision of the stomach.	
thromb/o	clot, clotting	thrombocyte	______________
		Also known as platelets, these cells help clot blood. A ***thrombus*** *is the actual clot that forms, and* ***thrombosis*** *(-osis means condition) is the condition of clot formation.*	
ur/o	urinary tract, urine	urology	______________
		A urologist is a surgeon who operates on the organs of the urinary tract and the organs of the male reproductive system.	

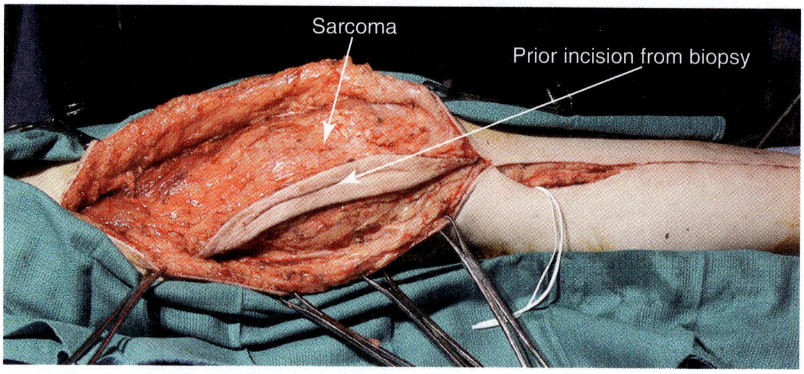

FIGURE 1-7 **Sarcoma of muscle** in the thigh. *(Courtesy Dr. Sam Yoon, Massachusetts General Hospital, Boston.)*

SUFFIXES

SUFFIX	MEANING	TERMINOLOGY	MEANING
-ac	pertaining to	cardiac	
-al	pertaining to	neural	
-algia	pain	arthralgia	
		neuralgia	
-cyte	cell	erythrocyte	
-ectomy	excision, removal	nephrectomy	
-emia	blood condition	leukemia *Literally, this term means "a blood condition of white (blood cells)." Actually, it is a condition of blood in which cancerous white blood cells proliferate (increase in number).*	
-genic	pertaining to producing, produced by, or produced in	carcinogenic *Cigarette smoke is carcinogenic.*	
		pathogenic *A virus or a bacterium is a pathogenic organism.*	
		iatrogenic *In this term, -genic means produced by.*	
-globin	protein	hemoglobin	
-gram	record	electroencephalogram	
-ic, -ical	pertaining to	gastric	
		neurologic *Log/o means study of.*	
-ion	process	excision	
-ist	specialist	ophthalmologist	
-itis	inflammation	cystitis	
-logy	process of study	endocrinology	
-oma	tumor, mass, swelling	hepatoma *A hepatoma (hepatocellular carcinoma) is a malignant tumor of the liver.*	
-opsy	process of viewing	biopsy *Biopsy specimens are obtained and viewed under a microscope.*	

Ophthalmologist, Optometrist, Optician

An **ophthalmologist** is a **physician** who specializes in diagnosing and treating (surgically and medically) disorders of the eye. An **optometrist** is a **healthcare professional** who examines (metr/o = to measure) eyes and prescribes corrective lenses, and may treat eye diseases. An **optician** grinds lenses and fits glasses but does not examine eyes, prescribe corrective lenses, or treat eye diseases.

SUFFIX	MEANING	TERMINOLOGY	MEANING
-osis	condition, usually abnormal (slight increase in numbers when used with blood cells)	nephrosis	____________
		leukocytosis *This condition, a slight increase in normal white blood cells, occurs as white blood cells multiply to fight an infection. Don't confuse **leukocytosis** with **leukemia,** which is a cancerous (malignant) condition marked by high levels of abnormal, immature white blood cells.*	____________
-pathy	disease condition	enteropathy *(ĕn-tĕ-RŎP-ă-thē)*	____________
		adenopathy *(ă-dĕ-NŎP-ă-thē)*	____________
-scope	instrument to visually examine	endoscope *Endo- means within. A cystoscope is a type of endoscope.*	____________
-scopy	process of visually examining	endoscopy *(ĕn-DŎS-kō-pē)* *Endoscopy is performed with an endoscope.*	____________
-sis	state of; condition	prognosis	____________
-tomy	process of cutting, incision	osteotomy *(ŏs-tē-ŎT-tō-mē)*	____________
-y	process, condition	gastroenterology	____________

PREFIXES

PREFIX	MEANING	TERMINOLOGY	MEANING
a-, an-	no, not, without	anemia *Anemia is a decreased number of erythrocytes or an abnormality of the hemoglobin (a chemical) within the red blood cells. This results in decreased delivery of oxygen to cells of the body. Anemic patients look so pale that early physicians thought they were literally "without blood."*	____________
aut-, auto-	self, own	autopsy *This term literally means "process of viewing by oneself." Hence, an autopsy is the examination of a dead body with one's own eyes to determine the cause of death and nature of disease.*	____________
dia-	complete, through	diagnosis *The plural of diagnosis is diagnoses.*	____________

Plurals

Terms ending in -is (diagnos**is**, prognos**is**) form their plural by dropping the **-is** and adding **-es.** See **Appendix I,** page 981, for other rules on formation of plurals.

PREFIX	MEANING	TERMINOLOGY	MEANING
endo-	within	endocrinologist	______
epi-	above, upon	epigastric	______
		epidermis *This outermost layer of skin lies above the middle layer of skin, known as the dermis.*	______
ex-, exo-	out, outside of, outward	excision	______
		exocrine glands	______
hyper-	excessive, above, more than normal	hyperthyroidism *The suffix -ism means process or condition.*	______
hypo-	deficient, below, under, less than normal	hypogastric *When hypo- is used with a part of the body, it means below.*	______
		hypoglycemia *In this term, hypo- means deficient.*	______
in-	into, in	incision	______
peri-	surrounding, around	pericardium *The suffix -um means a structure. The pericardium is the membrane that surrounds the heart.*	______
pro-	before, forward	prostate gland *This exocrine gland "stands" (-state) before or in front of the urinary bladder (see Figure 1-2). It produces semen, which contains fluid and sperm cells.*	______
re-	back, backward, again	resection *This is an operation in which tissue is "cut back" or removed. The Latin resectio means a trimming or pruning.*	______
retro-	behind	retrocardiac	______
sub-	below, under	subhepatic	______
trans-	across, through	transhepatic	______

Understanding Hyperthyroidism

In **hyperthyroidism,** a **hyperactive thyroid gland** (an endocrine gland in the neck) secretes a greater than normal amount of **thyroxine** (thyroid hormone, or T_4). Because thyroxine causes cells to burn fuel and release energy, signs and symptoms of hyperthyroidism are **increased energy level** and **nervousness, tachycardia** (increased heart rate), **weight loss,** and **exophthalmos** (bulging eyeballs).

PRACTICAL APPLICATIONS

This section provides an opportunity for you to use your skill in understanding medical terms and to increase your knowledge of new terms. Be sure to check your answers with the Answers to Practical Applications on page 26. You should find helpful explanations there.

SPECIALISTS

Match the **abnormal condition** in Column I with the **physician (specialist)** who treats it in Column II. Write the letter of the correct specialist in the space provided.

COLUMN I		COLUMN II
1. heart attack	D	A. gastroenterologist
2. ovarian cysts	F	B. hematologist
3. bipolar (manic-depressive) disorder	J	C. nephrologist
4. breast adenocarcinoma	E	D. cardiologist
5. iron deficiency anemia	B	E. oncologist
6. retinopathy	H	F. gynecologist
7. cerebrovascular accident; stroke	I	G. urologist
8. renal failure	C	H. ophthalmologist
9. inflammatory bowel disease	A	I. neurologist
10. cystitis	G	J. psychiatrist

EXERCISES

The exercises that follow are designed to help you learn the terms presented in the chapter. **Writing terms** over and over again is a good way to study this new language. You will find the answers to these exercises starting on page 24. This makes it easy to **check your work.** As you check each answer, you not only will reinforce your understanding of a term but often will gain additional information from the answer.

Each exercise is designed not as a test, but rather as an opportunity for you to learn the material.

A Complete the following sentences.

1. Word beginnings are called prefixes.
2. Word endings are called suffixes.
3. The foundation of a word is known as the root word.
4. A letter linking a suffix and a root, or linking two roots, in a term is the combining form.
5. The combination of a root and a combining vowel is known as the __________.

B Give the meanings of the following combining forms.

1. cardi/o __________
2. aden/o __________
3. bi/o __________
4. cerebr/o __________
5. cephal/o __________
6. arthr/o __________
7. carcin/o __________
8. cyst/o __________
9. cyt/o __________
10. derm/o or dermat/o __________
11. encephal/o __________
12. electr/o __________

C Give the meanings of the following suffixes.

1. -oma __________
2. -al __________
3. -itis __________
4. -logy __________
5. -scopy __________
6. -ic __________
7. -gram __________
8. -opsy __________

D Using slashes, divide the following terms into parts, and give the meaning of the entire term.

1. cerebral ______
2. biopsy ______
3. adenitis ______
4. cephalic ______
5. carcinoma ______
6. cystoscopy ______
7. electrocardiogram ______
8. cardiology ______
9. electroencephalogram ______
10. dermatitis ______
11. arthroscopy ______
12. cytology ______

E Give the meanings of the following combining forms.

1. erythr/o ______
2. enter/o ______
3. gastr/o ______
4. gnos/o ______
5. hemat/o ______
6. cis/o ______
7. nephr/o ______
8. leuk/o ______
9. iatr/o ______
10. hepat/o ______
11. neur/o ______
12. gynec/o ______

F Complete the medical term, based on its meaning as provided.

1. white blood cell: ______cyte
2. inflammation of the stomach: gastr______
3. pertaining to being produced by treatment: ______genic
4. study of kidneys: ______logy
5. red blood cell: ______cyte
6. mass of blood: ______oma
7. process of viewing living tissue (using a microscope): bi______
8. pain of nerves: neur______
9. process of visual examination of the eye: ______scopy
10. inflammation of the small intestine: ______itis

G **Select from the combining forms below to match each English term. Write the correct combining form in the space provided.**

onc/o	path/o	ren/o	sect/o
ophthalm/o	psych/o	rhin/o	thromb/o
oste/o	radi/o	sarc/o	ur/o

English Terms

1. kidney ______________________
2. disease ______________________
3. eye ______________________
4. to cut ______________________
5. nose ______________________
6. flesh ______________________
7. mind ______________________
8. urinary tract ______________________
9. bone ______________________
10. x-rays ______________________
11. clotting ______________________
12. tumor ______________________

H **Underline the suffix in each term, and then give the meaning of the term.**

1. ophthalmoscopy ______________________
2. ophthalmoscope ______________________
3. oncology ______________________
4. osteitis ______________________
5. psychosis ______________________
6. thrombocyte ______________________
7. renal ______________________
8. nephrectomy ______________________
9. osteotomy ______________________
10. resection ______________________
11. carcinogenic ______________________
12. sarcoma ______________________

I **Match the suffix in Column I with its meaning in Column II. Write the correct meaning in the space provided.**

COLUMN I *Suffix*	**COLUMN II** *Meaning*
1. -algia ______	condition, usually abnormal
2. -ion ______	blood condition
3. -emia ______	cell
4. -gram ______	disease condition
5. -scope ______	process of cutting, incision
6. -osis ______	inflammation
7. -ectomy ______	instrument to visually examine
8. -genic ______	pain
9. -pathy ______	pertaining to producing, produced by, or produced in
10. -tomy ______	process
11. -itis ______	record
12. -cyte ______	excision, removal (resection)

J **Select from the listed terms to complete the following sentences.**

arthralgia	hematoma	iatrogenic
carcinogenic	hepatoma (hepatocellular carcinoma)	leukemia
cystitis	enteropathy	leukocytosis
endocrine		neuralgia
exocrine		

1. When Paul smoked cigarettes, he inhaled a ______ substance with each puff.
2. Sally's sore throat, fever, and chills made her doctor order a white blood cell count. The results, indicating infection, showed a slight increase in normal cells, a condition called ______.
3. Mr. Smith's liver enlarged, giving him abdominal pain. His radiologic tests and biopsy revealed a malignant tumor, or ______.
4. Mrs. Rose complained of pain in her hip joints, knees, and shoulders each morning. She was told that she had painful joints, or ______.
5. Dr. Black was trained to treat disorders of the pancreas, thyroid gland, adrenal glands, and pituitary gland. Thus, he was an expert in the ______ glands.
6. Ms. Walsh told her doctor she had pain when urinating. After tests, the doctor's diagnosis was inflammation of the urinary bladder, or ______.

7. Elizabeth's overhead tennis shot hit David in the thigh, producing a large ________________. His skin looked bruised and was tender.

8. Mr. Bell's white blood cell count is 10 times higher than normal. Examination of his blood shows cancerous white blood cells. His diagnosis is ________________.

9. Mr. Kay was resuscitated (revived from potential or apparent death) in the emergency department after experiencing a heart attack. Unfortunately, he suffered a broken rib as a result of the physician's chest compressions. This is an example of a/an ________________ fracture.

10. After coming back from a trip during which he had eaten unfamiliar foods, Mr. Cameron had a disease of his intestines called ________________.

K Give the meanings of the following prefixes.

1. dia- ________________
2. pro- ________________
3. aut-, auto- ________________
4. a-, an- ________________
5. hyper- ________________
6. hypo- ________________
7. epi- ________________
8. endo- ________________
9. retro- ________________
10. trans- ________________
11. peri- ________________
12. ex-, exo- ________________
13. sub- ________________
14. re- ________________

L Underline the prefix in the following terms and give the meaning of the entire term.

1. diagnosis ________________
2. prognosis ________________
3. subhepatic ________________
4. pericardium ________________
5. hyperglycemia ________________
6. hypodermic ________________
7. epigastric ________________
8. resection ________________
9. hypoglycemia ________________
10. anemia ________________

M Complete the following terms (describing areas of medicine), based on their meanings as given.

1. study of the urinary tract: ____________________logy
2. study of women and women's diseases: ____________________logy
3. study of blood: ____________________logy
4. study of tumors: ____________________logy
5. study of the kidneys: ____________________logy
6. study of nerves: ____________________logy
7. treatment of children: ____________________iatrics
8. study of x-rays in diagnostic imaging: ____________________logy
9. study of the eyes: ____________________logy
10. study of the stomach and intestines: ____________________logy
11. study of glands that secrete hormones: ____________________logy
12. treatment of the mind: ____________________iatry
13. study of disease: ____________________logy
14. study of the heart: ____________________logy

N Give the meaning of the underlined word part and then define the term.

1. cerebrovascular accident ____
2. encephalitis ____
3. cystoscope ____
4. transhepatic ____
5. iatrogenic ____
6. hypogastric ____
7. endocrine glands ____
8. nephrectomy ____
9. exocrine glands ____
10. neuralgia ____

O Select from the terms listed below to complete the sentences on the following page.

anemia
biopsy
diagnosis
leukemia
nephrologist
neuropathy

oncogenic
oncologist
osteoarthritis
pathogenic
prognosis

psychiatrist
psychologist
thrombocyte
thrombosis
urologist

1. Pamela Crick is 72 years old and suffers from a degenerative joint disease that is caused by the wearing away of tissue around her joints. This disease, which literally means "inflammation of bones and joints," is ____________________.
2. The ____________________ sample was removed during surgery and sent to a pathologist to be examined under a microscope for a proper diagnosis.
3. A/An ____________________ performed surgery to remove Mr. Simon's cancerous kidney.
4. Ms. Rose has suffered from diabetes with hyperglycemia for many years. This condition can lead to long-term complications, such as the disease of nerves called diabetic ____________________.
5. A virus or a bacterium produces disease and is therefore a/an ____________________ organism.
6. Jordan has a disease caused by abnormal hemoglobin in his erythrocytes. The erythrocytes change shape, collapsing to form sickle-shaped cells that can become clots and stop the flow of blood. His condition is called sickle cell ____________________.
7. Dr. Max Shelby is a physician who treats carcinomas and sarcomas. He is a/an ____________________.
8. Bill had difficulty stopping the bleeding from a cut on his face while shaving. He knew his medication caused him to have decreased platelets, or a low ____________________ count, and that probably was the reason his blood was not clotting very well.
9. Dr. Susan Parker told Paul that his condition would improve with treatment in a few weeks. She said his ____________________ is excellent and he can expect total recovery.
10. After fleeing the World Trade Center on September 11, 2001, Mrs. Jones had many problems with her job, her husband, and her family relationships. She went to see a ____________________, who prescribed drugs to treat her depression.

P **Circle the correct term to complete each sentence.**

1. Ms. Brody had a cough and fever. Her doctor instructed her to go to the **(pathology, radiology, hematology)** department for a chest x-ray examination.
2. After she gave birth to her fourth child, Ms. Thompson had problems holding her urine (a condition known as urinary incontinence). She made an appointment with a **(gastroenterologist, pathologist, urologist)** to evaluate her condition.
3. Dr. Monroe told a new mother she had lost much blood during delivery of her child. She had **(anemia, leukocytosis, adenitis)** and needed a blood transfusion immediately.
4. Mr. Preston was having chest pain during his morning walks. He made an appointment to discuss his new symptom with a **(nephrologist, neurologist, cardiologist).**
5. After my skiing accident, Dr. Curtin suggested **(cystoscopy, biopsy, arthroscopy)** to visually examine my swollen, painful knee.

ANSWERS TO EXERCISES

A

1. prefixes
2. suffixes
3. root
4. combining vowel
5. combining form

B

1. heart
2. gland
3. life
4. cerebrum, largest part of the brain
5. head
6. joint
7. cancer, cancerous
8. urinary bladder
9. cell
10. skin
11. brain
12. electricity

C

1. tumor, mass, swelling
2. pertaining to
3. inflammation
4. process of study
5. process of visual examination
6. pertaining to
7. record (image)
8. process of viewing

D

1. cerebr/al—pertaining to the cerebrum, or largest part of the brain
2. bi/opsy—process of viewing life (removal of living tissue and viewing it under a microscope)
3. aden/itis—inflammation of a gland
4. cephal/ic—pertaining to the head
5. carcin/oma—tumor that is cancerous (cancerous tumor)
6. cyst/o/scopy—process of visually examining the urinary bladder
7. electr/o/cardi/o/gram—record of the electricity in the heart
8. cardi/o/logy—process of study of the heart
9. electr/o/encephal/o/gram—record of the electricity in the brain
10. dermat/itis—inflammation of the skin
11. arthr/o/scopy—process of visual examination of a joint
12. cyt/o/logy—process of study of cells

E

1. red
2. intestines (usually small intestine)
3. stomach
4. knowledge
5. blood
6. to cut
7. kidney
8. white
9. treatment, physician
10. liver
11. nerve
12. woman, female

F

1. leukocyte
2. gastritis
3. iatrogenic
4. nephrology
5. erythrocyte
6. hematoma
7. biopsy
8. neuralgia
9. ophthalmoscopy
10. enteritis

G

1. ren/o
2. path/o
3. ophthalm/o
4. sect/o
5. rhin/o
6. sarc/o
7. psych/o
8. ur/o
9. oste/o
10. radi/o
11. thromb/o
12. onc/o

H

1. ophthalmoscopy—process of visual examination of the eye
2. ophthalmoscope—instrument to visually examine the eye
3. oncology—study of tumors
4. osteitis—inflammation of bone
5. psychosis—abnormal condition of the mind
6. thrombocyte—clotting cell (platelet)
7. renal—pertaining to the kidney
8. nephrectomy—removal (excision or resection) of the kidney
9. osteotomy—incision of (process of cutting into) a bone
10. resection—process of cutting back (in the sense of "cutting out" or removal)
11. carcinogenic—pertaining to producing cancer
12. sarcoma—tumor of flesh (cancerous tumor of flesh tissue, such as bone, fat, and muscle)

I

1. pain
2. process
3. blood condition
4. record (image)
5. instrument to visually examine
6. condition, usually abnormal
7. excision, removal (resection)
8. pertaining to producing, produced by, or produced in
9. disease condition
10. process of cutting, incision
11. inflammation
12. cell

J

1. carcinogenic
2. leukocytosis
3. hepatoma (hepatocellular carcinoma)
4. arthralgia
5. endocrine
6. cystitis
7. hematoma
8. leukemia
9. iatrogenic
10. enteropathy

K

1. complete, through
2. before
3. self, own
4. no, not, without
5. excessive, above, more than normal
6. deficient, below, less than normal
7. above, upon
8. within
9. behind
10. across, through
11. surrounding
12. out
13. below, under
14. back

L

1. diagnosis—complete knowledge; a decision about the nature of the patient's condition after the appropriate tests are done
2. prognosis—before knowledge; a prediction about the outcome of treatment, given after the diagnosis
3. subhepatic—pertaining to below the liver. A combining vowel is not needed between the prefix and the root.
4. pericardium—the membrane surrounding the heart
5. hyperglycemia—condition of excessive sugar in the blood
6. hypodermic—pertaining to under the skin
7. epigastric—pertaining to above the stomach
8. resection—process of cutting back (in the sense of cutting out)
9. hypoglycemia—condition of deficient (low) sugar in the blood
10. anemia—condition of low numbers of erythrocytes (red blood cells) or deficient hemoglobin in these cells. Notice that the root in this term is *em*, which is shortened from *hem*, meaning blood.

M

1. urology
2. gynecology
3. hematology
4. oncology
5. nephrology
6. neurology
7. pediatrics (combining vowel o has been dropped between *ped* and *iatr*)
8. radiology
9. ophthalmology
10. gastroenterology
11. endocrinology
12. psychiatry
13. pathology
14. cardiology

N

1. cerebrum (largest part of the brain). A cerebrovascular accident, or stroke, is damage to the blood vessels of the cerebrum, leading to death of brain cells.
2. brain. Encephalitis is inflammation of the brain.
3. urinary bladder. A cystoscope is an instrument used to visually examine the urinary bladder. The cystoscope is inserted into the urethra and urinary bladder.
4. across, through. Transhepatic means pertaining to across or through the liver.
5. treatment. Iatrogenic means pertaining to an adverse side effect produced by treatment.
6. under, below, deficient. Hypogastric means pertaining to below the stomach.
7. within. Endocrine glands secrete hormones within the body. Examples of these are the pituitary, thyroid, and adrenal glands.
8. excision or resection. Nephrectomy is the removal of a kidney.
9. outside. Exocrine glands secrete chemicals to the outside of the body. Examples are the sweat, lacrimal or tear-producing, prostate, and salivary glands.
10. pain. Neuralgia is nerve pain.

O

1. osteoarthritis
2. biopsy
3. urologist (a nephrologist is a medical doctor who treats kidney disorders but does not operate on patients)
4. neuropathy
5. pathogenic
6. anemia
7. oncologist
8. thrombocyte
9. prognosis
10. psychiatrist (a psychologist can treat mentally ill patients but is not a medical doctor and cannot prescribe medications)

P

1. radiology
2. urologist
3. anemia
4. cardiologist
5. arthroscopy

Answers to Practical Applications

1. **D** A **cardiologist** is an internal medicine specialist who takes additional (fellowship) training in the diagnosis and treatment of heart disease.
2. **F** A **gynecologist** specializes in surgery and internal medicine to diagnose and treat disorders of the female reproductive system. Ovarian cysts are sacs of fluid that form on and in the ovaries (female organs that produce eggs and hormones).
3. **J** A **psychiatrist** is a specialist in diagnosing and treating mental illness. In bipolar disorder (manic-depressive illness), the mood switches periodically from excessive mania (excitability) to deep depression (sadness, despair, and discouragement).
4. **E** An **oncologist** is an internal medicine specialist who takes fellowship training in the diagnosis and medical (drug) treatment of cancer.
5. **B** A **hematologist** is an internal medicine specialist who takes fellowship training in the diagnosis and treatment of blood disorders such as anemia and clotting diseases.
6. **H** An **ophthalmologist** trains in both surgery and internal medicine in order to diagnose and treat disorders of the eye. The retina is a sensitive layer of light receptor cells in the back of the eye. Retinopathy can occur as a secondary complication of chronic diabetes (from hyperglycemia).
7. **I** A **neurologist** is an internal medicine specialist who takes fellowship training in the diagnosis and treatment of disorders of nervous tissue (brain, spinal cord, and nerves). A **CVA** causes damage to areas of the brain, resulting in loss of function.
8. **C** A **nephrologist** is an internal medicine specialist who takes fellowship training in the diagnosis and medical treatment of kidney disease. A nephrologist does not perform surgery on the urinary tract, but treats kidney disease with drugs.
9. **A** A **gastroenterologist** is an internal medicine specialist who takes fellowship training in the diagnosis and treatment of disorders of the gastrointestinal tract. Examples of inflammatory bowel disease are ulcerative colitis (inflammation of the large intestine) and Crohn disease (inflammation of the last part of the small intestine).
10. **G** A **urologist** is a surgical specialist who operates on organs of the urinary tract (such as the urinary bladder) and treats the male reproductive system.

I

PRONUNCIATION OF TERMS

The markings ¯ and ˘ above the vowels—a, e, i, o, and u—indicate the proper sounds of the vowels in a term. When ¯ is above a vowel, its sound is long—that is, exactly like its name. The ˘ marking indicates a short vowel sound. The CAPITAL letters indicate the accented syllable.

To test your understanding of the terminology in this chapter, write the meaning of each term in the space provided. In addition, you may wish to cover the terms and write them by looking at your definitions. Make sure your spelling is correct. The page number after each term indicates where it is defined or used in the book, so you can easily check your responses. You will find complete definitions for all of these terms and their audio pronunciations on the Evolve website.

Pronunciation Guide

ā as in āpe	ă as in ăpple
ē as in ēven	ĕ as in ĕvery
ī as in īce	ĭ as in ĭnterest
ō as in ōpen	ŏ as in pŏt
ū as in ūnit	ŭ as in ŭnder

Vocabulary and Terminology

TERM	PRONUNCIATION	MEANING
adenitis (7)	ăd-ĕ-NĪ-tĭs	______
adenoma (7)	ăd-ĕ-NŌ-mă	______
adenopathy (14)	ăd-ĕ-NŎP-ă-thē	______
anemia (14)	ă-NĒ-mē-ă	______
arthralgia (13)	ăr-THRĂL-jă	______
arthritis (7)	ăr-THRĪ-tĭs	______
autopsy (14)	ĂW-tŏp-sē	______
biology (7)	bī-ŎL-ō-jē	______
biopsy (7)	BĪ-ŏp-sē	______
carcinogenic (13)	kăr-sĭ-nō-JĔN-ĭk	______
carcinoma (7)	kăr-sĭ-NŌ-mă	______
cardiac (13)	KĂR-dē-ăk	______
cardiology (7)	kăr-dē-ŎL-ō-jē	______
cephalic (7)	sĕ-FĂL-ĭk	______
cerebral (8)	sĕ-RĒ-brăl *or* SĔR-ĕ-brăl	______
cystitis (13)	sĭs-TĪ-tĭs	______
cystoscopy (8)	sĭs-TŎS-kō-pē	______
cytology (9)	sī-TŎL-ō-jē	______
dermatitis (9)	dĕr-mă-TĪ-tĭs	______

TERM	PRONUNCIATION	MEANING
dermatology (10)	dĕr-mă-TŎL-ō-jē	
diagnosis (10)	dī-ăg-NŌ-sĭs	
electrocardiogram (9)	ē-lĕk-trō-KĂR-dē-ō-grăm	
electroencephalogram (9)	ē-lĕk-trō-ĕn-SĔF-ă-lō-grăm	
endocrine glands (8)	ĔN-dō-krĭn glăndz	
endocrinologist (15)	ĕn-dō-krĭ-NŎL-ō-jĭst	
endocrinology (13)	ĕn-dō-krĭ-NŎL-ō-jē	
endoscope (14)	ĔN-dō-skōp	
endoscopy (14)	ĕn-DŎS-kō-pē	
enteritis (9)	ĕn-tĕ-RĪ-tĭs	
enteropathy (14)	ĕn-tĕ-RŎP-ă-thē	
epidermis (15)	ĕp-ĭ-DĔR-mĭs	
epigastric (15)	ĕp-ĭ-GĂS-trĭk	
erythrocyte (9)	ĕ-RĬTH-rō-sīt	
excision (8)	ĕk-SĬ-zhŭn	
exocrine glands (15)	ĔK-sō-krĭn glăndz	
gastrectomy (9)	găs-TRĔK-tō-mē	
gastric (13)	GĂS-trĭk	
gastroenterology (14)	găs-trō-ĕn-tĕr-ŎL-ō-jē	
gastrotomy (9)	găs-TRŎT-ō-mē	
gynecologist (26)	gī-nĕ-KŎL-ō-jĭst	
gynecology (10)	gī-nĕ-KŎL-ō-jē	
hematology (10)	hē-mă-TŎL-ō-jē	
hematoma (10)	hē-mă-TŌ-mă	
hemoglobin (10)	HĒ-mō-glō-bĭn	
hepatitis (10)	hĕp-ă-TĪ-tĭs	
hepatoma (13)	hĕp-ă-TŌ-mă	
hyperglycemia (10)	hī-pĕr-glī-SĒ-mē-ă	
hyperthyroidism (15)	hī-pĕr-THĪ-rŏyd-ĭsm	
hypodermic (9)	hī-pō-DĔR-mĭk	

TERM	PRONUNCIATION	MEANING
hypogastric (15)	hī-pō-GĂS-trĭk	
hypoglycemia (15)	hī-pō-glī-SĒ-mē-ă	
iatrogenic (10)	ī-ăt-rō-JĔN-ĭk	
incision (8)	ĭn-SĬ-zhŭn	
leukemia (13)	lū-KĒ-mē-ă	
leukocyte (10)	LŪ-kō-sīt	
leukocytosis (14)	lū-kō-sī-TŌ-sĭs	
nephrectomy (13)	nĕ-FRĔK-tō-mē	
nephritis (10)	nĕ-FRĪ-tĭs	
nephrology (10)	nĕ-FRŎL-ō-jē	
nephrosis (14)	nĕ-FRŌ-sĭs	
neural (13)	NŪ-răl	
neuralgia (13)	nū-RĂL-jă	
neurologic (13)	nū-rō-LŎJ-ĭk	
neurology (10)	nū-RŎL-ō-jē	
oncologist (11)	ŏn-KŎL-ō-jĭst	
oncology (11)	ŏn-KŎL-ō-jē	
ophthalmologist (13)	ŏf-thăl-MŎL-ō-jĭst	
ophthalmoscope (11)	ŏf-THĂL-mō-skōp	
osteitis (11)	ŏs-tē-Ī-tĭs	
osteoarthritis (11)	ŏs-tē-ō-ăr-THRĪ-tĭs	
osteotomy (14)	ŏs-tē-ŎT-ō-mē	
pathogenic (13)	păth-ō-JĔN-ĭk	
pathologist (11)	pă-THŎL-ŏ-jĭst	
pathology (11)	pă-THŎL-ō-jē	
pediatric (11)	pē-dē-ĂT-rĭk	
pericardium (15)	pĕr-ĭ-KĂR-dē-ŭm	
prognosis (10)	prŏg-NŌ-sĭs	
prostate gland (15)	PRŎS-tāt glănd	
psychiatrist (12)	sī-KĪ-ă-trĭst	

I

TERM	PRONUNCIATION	MEANING
psychology (12)	sī-KŎL-ō-jē	________________
radiology (12)	rā-dē-ŎL-ō-jē	________________
renal (12)	RĒ-năl	________________
resection (12)	rē-SĔK-shŭn	________________
retrocardiac (15)	rĕ-trō-KĂR-dē-ăc	________________
rhinitis (12)	rī-NĪ-tĭs	________________
sarcoma (12)	săr-KŌ-mă	________________
subhepatic (15)	sŭb-hĕ-PĂT-ĭk	________________
thrombocyte (12)	THRŎM-bō-sīt	________________
transhepatic (15)	trănz-hĕ-PĂT-ĭk	________________
urology (12)	ū-RŎL-ō-jē	________________

REVIEW SHEET

This Review Sheet and the others that follow each chapter are complete lists of the word elements contained in the chapter. They are designed to pull together the terminology and to reinforce your learning by giving you the opportunity to write the meanings of each word part in the spaces provided and to **test yourself.** Check your answers with the information in the chapter or in the Glossary (Medical Word Parts—English), at the end of the book. It's a good idea to tab the Glossary so that you can easily locate it.

Combining Forms

COMBINING FORM	MEANING	COMBINING FORM	MEANING
aden/o	______	hem/o, hemat/o	______
arthr/o	______	hepat/o	______
bi/o	______	iatr/o	______
carcin/o	______	leuk/o	______
cardi/o	______	log/o	______
cephal/o	______	nephr/o	______
cerebr/o	______	neur/o	______
cis/o	______	onc/o	______
crin/o	______	ophthalm/o	______
cyst/o	______	oste/o	______
cyt/o	______	path/o	______
derm/o, dermat/o	______	ped/o	______
electr/o	______	psych/o	______
encephal/o	______	radi/o	______
enter/o	______	ren/o	______
erythr/o	______	rhin/o	______
gastr/o	______	sarc/o	______
glyc/o	______	sect/o	______
gnos/o	______	thromb/o	______
gynec/o	______	ur/o	______

Suffixes

SUFFIX	MEANING	SUFFIX	MEANING
-ac	________	-itis	________
-al	________	-logy	________
-algia	________	-oma	________
-cyte	________	-opsy	________
-ectomy	________	-osis	________
-emia	________	-pathy	________
-genic	________	-scope	________
-globin	________	-scopy	________
-gram	________	-sis	________
-ic, -ical	________	-tomy	________
-ion	________	-y	________
-ist	________		

Prefixes

PREFIX	MEANING	PREFIX	MEANING
a-, an-	________	in-	________
aut-, auto-	________	peri-	________
dia-	________	pro-	________
endo-	________	re-	________
epi-	________	retro-	________
ex-, exo-	________	sub-	________
hyper-	________	trans-	________
hypo-	________		

evolve *Please visit the Evolve website for additional exercises, games, and images related to this chapter.*

CHAPTER 2

Terms Pertaining to the Body as a Whole

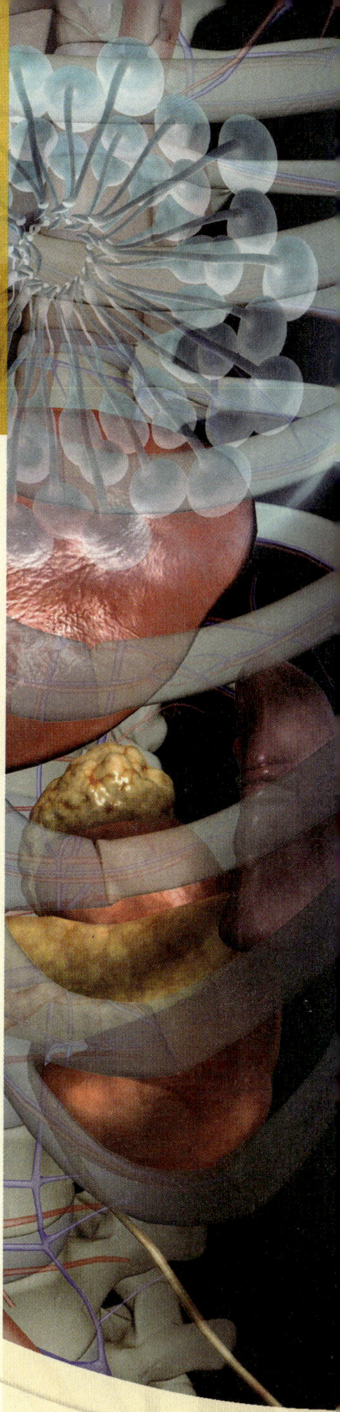

This chapter is divided into the following sections:

CHAPTER GOALS

- Define terms that apply to the structural organization of the body.
- Identify the body cavities and recognize the organs contained within those cavities.
- Locate and identify the anatomic and clinical divisions of the abdomen.
- Locate and name the anatomic divisions of the back.
- Become acquainted with terms that describe positions, directions, and planes of the body.
- Identify the meanings for new word elements and use them to understand medical terms.

STRUCTURAL ORGANIZATION OF THE BODY

This chapter provides you with an orientation to the body as a whole—cells, tissues, organs, systems, and terminology describing positions and directions within the body. We begin with the smallest living unit, the **cell,** and build to an understanding of complex body systems. In order to know how organs function in both health and disease, it is important to appreciate the workings of their individual cellular units.

CELLS

The cell is the fundamental unit of all living things (animal or plant). Cells are everywhere in the human body—every tissue, every organ is made up of these individual units.

Similarity in Cells. All cells are similar in that they contain a gelatinous substance composed of water, protein, sugar, acids, fats, and various minerals. Several parts of a cell, described next, are pictured in Figure 2-1 as they might look when photographed with an electron microscope. Label the structures on Figure 2-1. Throughout the book, numbers or letters in brackets indicate that the boldface term preceding it is to be used in labeling.

The **cell membrane** [1] not only surrounds and protects the cell but also regulates what passes into and out of the cell.

The **nucleus** [2] controls the operations of the cell. It directs cell division and determines the structure and function of the cell.

Chromosomes [3] are rod-like structures within the nucleus. All human body cells—except for the sex cells, the egg and the sperm (short for spermatozoon)—contain 23 pairs of chromosomes. Each sperm and each egg cell have only 23 unpaired chromosomes. After

2

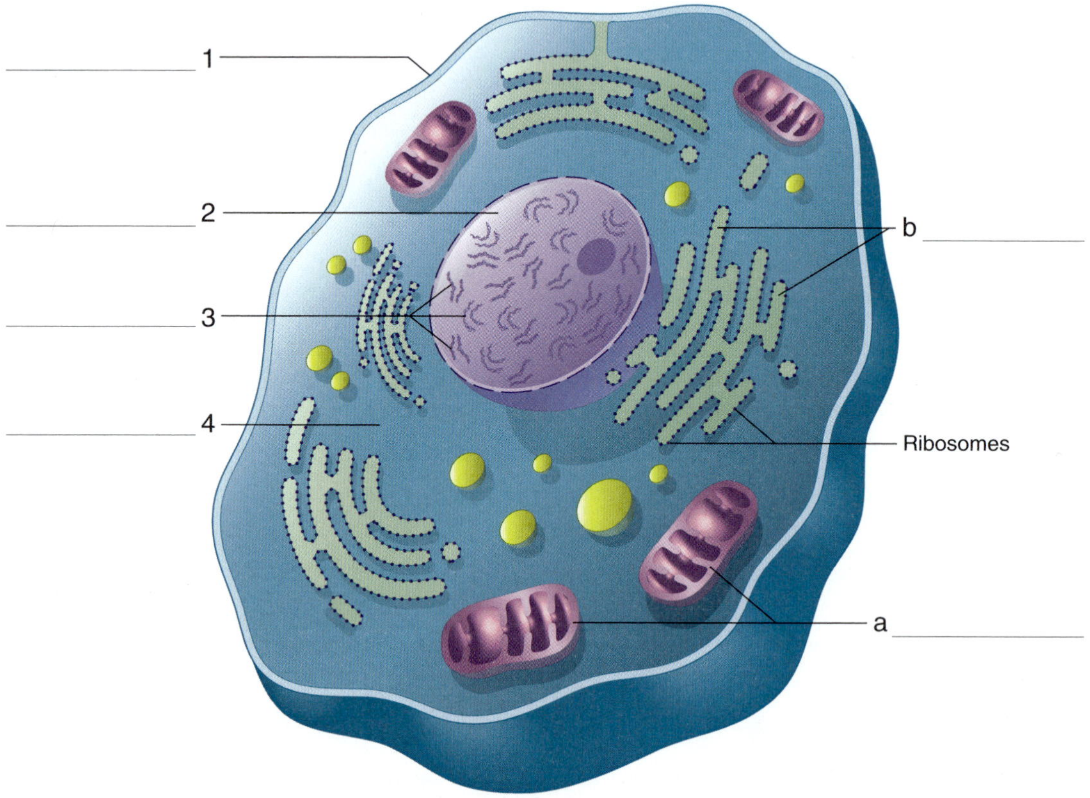

FIGURE 2-1 **Major parts of a cell. Ribosomes** (RĪ-bō-sōmz) are small granules that help the cell make proteins.

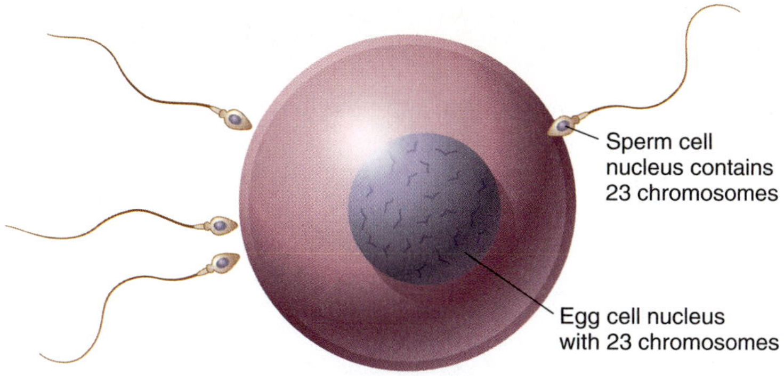

FIGURE 2-2 **Egg and sperm cells,** each containing 23 chromosomes.

an egg and a sperm cell unite to form the embryo, each cell of the embryo then has 46 chromosomes (23 pairs) (Figure 2-2).

Chromosomes contain regions called **genes.** There are several thousand genes, in an orderly sequence, on every chromosome. Each gene contains a chemical called **DNA** (deoxyribonucleic acid). DNA regulates the activities of the cell according to its sequence (arrangement into genes) on each chromosome. The DNA sequence resembles a series of recipes in code. This code, when passed out of the nucleus to the rest of the cell, directs the activities of the cell, such as cell division and synthesis of proteins.

A **karyotype** is a photograph of an individual's chromosomes, arranged by size, shape, and number (Figure 2-3). Karyotyping can determine whether chromosomes are normal. For example, an obstetrician may recommend amniocentesis (puncture of the sac around the

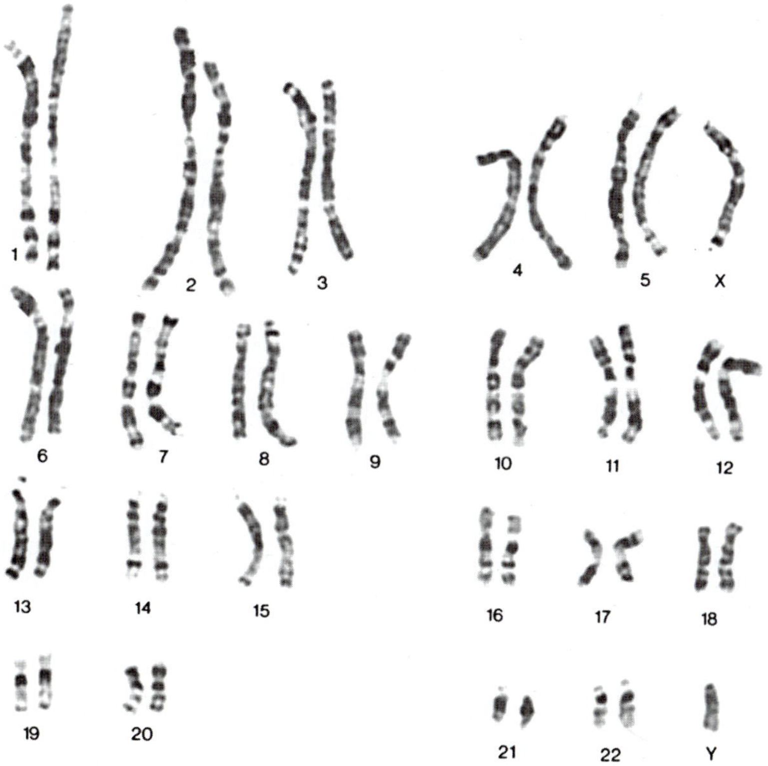

FIGURE 2-3 **Karyotype of a normal male.** Twenty-three pairs of chromosomes are shown. The 23rd pair is the XY pair present in normal males. In normal females, the 23rd pair is XX. For this karyotype, the chromosomes were treated with chemicals so that bands of light and dark areas are seen.

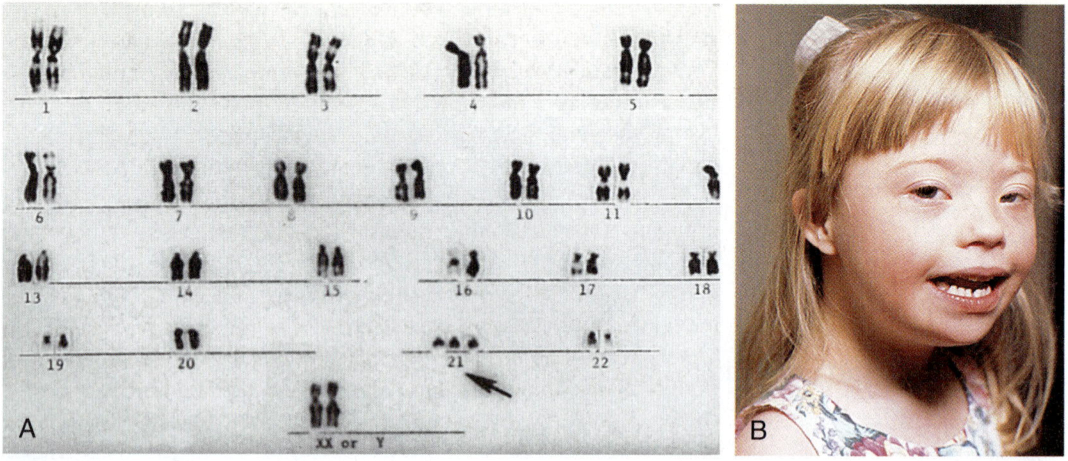

FIGURE 2-4 **A,** Karyotype of a Down syndrome female patient showing trisomy 21. There is an extra copy of chromosome 21, in addition to the usual pair, for a total of three (tri-). **B,** Photograph of a child with the typical facial appearance in Down syndrome. Features include a small, somewhat flat nose and upward slant of the eyes. Other characteristics of Down syndrome patients are mental deficiency and heart defects.

fetus for removal of fluid and cells) for a pregnant woman so that the karyotype of the baby can be examined.

If a baby is born with a chromosomal abnormality, serious problems can result. In Down syndrome, the karyotype shows 47 chroxmosomes instead of the normal number, 46 (Figure 2-4). The extra chromosome 21 results in the development of a child with Down syndrome (also called trisomy 21 syndrome). Its incidence is about 1 in every 750 live births, but as the mother's age increases, the presence of the chromosomal abnormality increases.

Continue labeling Figure 2-1.

The **cytoplasm** [4] (cyt/o = cell, -plasm = formation) includes all of the material outside the nucleus and enclosed by the cell membrane. It carries on the work of the cell (e.g., in a muscle cell, it does the contracting; in a nerve cell, it transmits impulses). The cytoplasm contains specialized apparatus to supply the chemical needs of the cell.

Mitochondria [a] are small sausage-shaped bodies that provide the principal source of energy for the cell. They use nutrients and oxygen to release energy that is stored in food. During the chemical process called **catabolism,** complex foods such as sugar and fat are broken down into simpler substances and energy is released by the mitochondria. Thus, catabolism provides the energy for cells to do the work of the body.

The **endoplasmic reticulum** [b] is a network (reticulum) of canals within the cell. These canals are cellular tunnel systems that manufacture proteins for the cell. Attached to the endoplasmic reticulum are **ribosomes,** which build long chains of proteins. **Anabolism,** occurring on the endoplasmic reticulum, is the process of building large proteins from small protein pieces called amino acids. Examples of important proteins for cell growth are hormones and enzymes.

Together, these two processes—**anabolism** and **catabolism**—make up the cell's **metabolism.** Metabolism, then, is the total of the chemical processes occurring in a cell. If a person has a "fast metabolism," foods such as sugar and fat are used up very quickly, and energy is released. If a person has a "slow metabolism," foods are burned slowly, and fat accumulates in cells.

STUDY SECTION 1

Practice spelling each term, and know its meaning.

anabolism	Process of building up large proteins from small protein pieces called amino acids. Ana- means up, bol means to cast, and -ism is a process.
catabolism	Process whereby complex nutrients are broken down to simpler substances and energy is released. Cata- means down, bol means to cast, and -ism is a process.
cell membrane	Structure surrounding and protecting the cell. It determines what enters and leaves the cell.
chromosomes	Rod-shaped structures in the nucleus that contain regions of DNA called genes. There are 46 chromosomes (23 pairs) in every cell except for the egg and sperm cells, which contain only 23 individual, unpaired chromosomes.
cytoplasm	All the material that is outside the nucleus and yet contained within the cell membrane.
DNA	Chemical found within each chromosome. Arranged like a sequence of recipes in code, it directs the activities of the cell.
endoplasmic reticulum	Network of canals within the cytoplasm of the cell. Here, large proteins are made from smaller protein pieces.
genes	Regions of DNA within each chromosome.
karyotype	Picture of chromosomes in the nucleus of a cell. The chromosomes are arranged in numerical order to determine their number and structure.
metabolism	Total of the chemical processes in a cell. It includes catabolism and anabolism. Meta- means change, bol means to cast, and -ism means a process.
mitochondria	Structures in the cytoplasm that provide the principal source of energy (miniature "power plants") for the cell. **Catabolism** is the process that occurs in mitochondria. (From the Greek *mitos* meaning thread, and *chondrion* meaning granule.)
nucleus	Control center of the cell. It contains chromosomes and directs the activities of the cell.

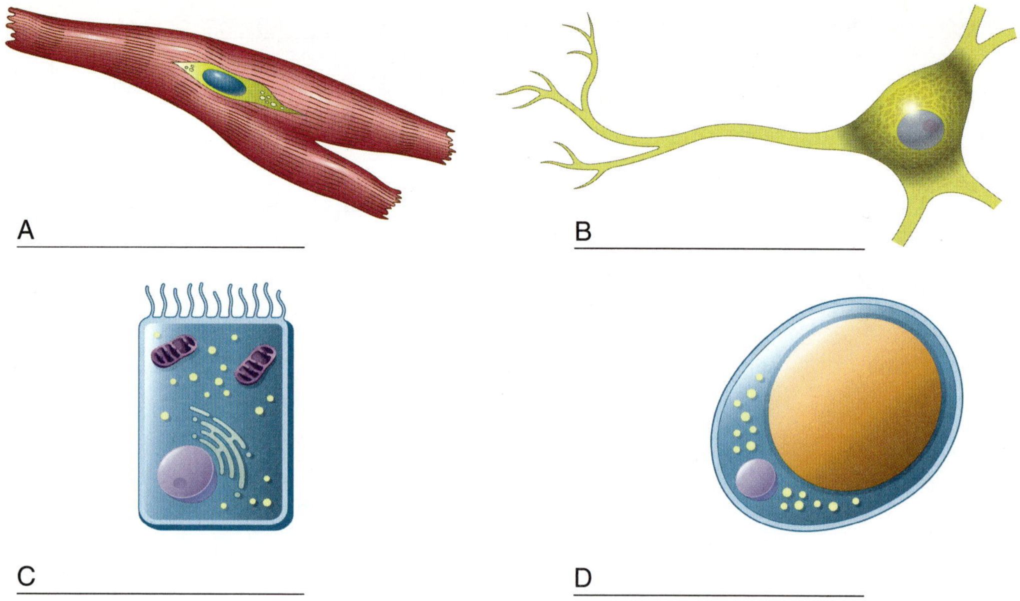

FIGURE 2-5 **Types of cells. A,** muscle cell; **B,** nerve cell; **C,** epithelial cell; and **D,** fat cell.

Differences in Cells. While we have just seen how cells contain similar structures, as they develop in the embryo, cells change to form many different types. Cells are different, or specialized, throughout the body to carry out their individual functions. For example, a **muscle cell** is long and slender and contains fibers that aid in contracting and relaxing; an **epithelial cell** (a lining and skin cell) may be square and flat to provide protection; a **nerve cell** may be long and have various fibrous extensions that aid in its job of carrying impulses; a **fat cell** contains large, empty spaces for fat storage. These are only a few of the many types of cells in the body. Figure 2-5 illustrates the different sizes and shapes of muscle, nerve, fat, and epithelial cells.

TISSUES

A tissue is a group of similar cells working together to do a specific job. A **histologist** (hist/o = tissue) is a scientist who specializes in the study of tissues. Several different types of tissue are recognized. Tissues of the same type may be located in various regions of the body. Figure 2-6 illustrates four types of tissues.

Epithelial Tissue. Epithelial tissue, located all over the body, forms the linings of internal organs, and the outer surface of the skin covering the body. It also lines exocrine and endocrine glands. The term **epithelial** originally referred to the tissue on (epi-) the breast nipple (thel/o). Now it describes all tissue that covers the outside of the body and lines the inner surface of internal organs.

Muscle Tissue. Voluntary muscle is found in arms and legs and parts of the body where movement is under conscious control. Involuntary muscle, found in the heart and digestive system, as well as other organs, allows movement that is not under conscious control. Cardiac muscle is a specialized type of muscle found only in the heart. Contractions of this muscle type can be seen as a beating heart in an ultrasound scan of a 6-week-old fetus.

Connective Tissue. Examples are **adipose** (fat) tissue, **cartilage** (elastic, fibrous tissue attached to bones), bone, and blood.

Nerve Tissue. Nerve tissue conducts impulses all over the body.

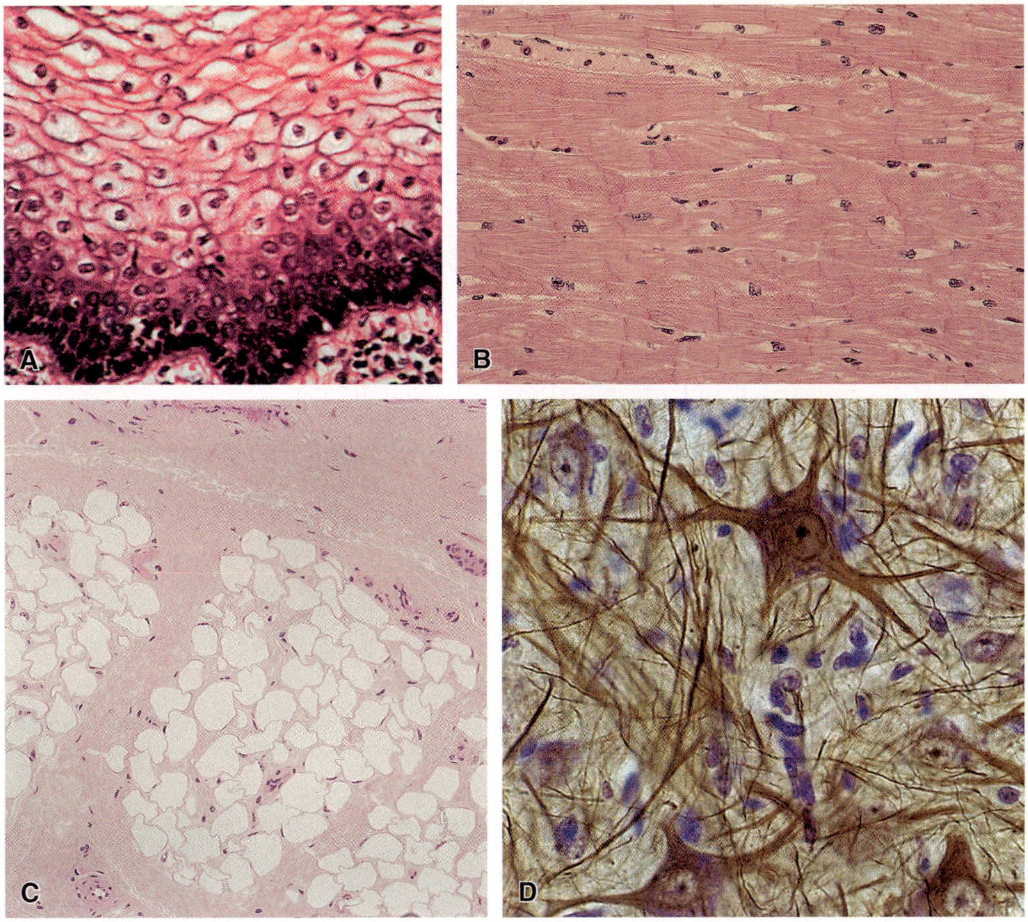

FIGURE 2-6 Types of tissues. A, Epithelial. B, Muscle. C, Fat. D, Nerve.

ORGANS

Different types of tissue combine to form an organ. For example, an organ such as the stomach is composed of muscle tissue, nerve tissue, and glandular epithelial tissue. The medical term for internal organs is **viscera** (singular: **viscus**). Examples of abdominal viscera (organs located in the abdomen) are the liver, stomach, intestines, pancreas, spleen, and gallbladder.

SYSTEMS

Systems are groups of organs working together to perform complex functions. For example, the mouth, esophagus, stomach, and small and large intestines are organs that do the work of the digestive system to digest food and absorb it into the bloodstream.

The body systems with their individual organs are listed next. Learn to spell and identify the organs in **boldface.**

SYSTEM	ORGANS
Digestive	Mouth, **pharynx** (throat), esophagus, stomach, intestines (small and large), liver, gallbladder, pancreas.
Urinary or excretory	Kidneys, **ureters** (tubes from the kidneys to the urinary bladder), urinary bladder, **urethra** (tube from the bladder to the outside of the body).

SYSTEM	ORGANS
Respiratory	Nose, pharynx, **larynx** ("voice box"), **trachea** ("windpipe"), bronchial tubes, lungs (where the exchange of gases takes place).
Reproductive	*Female*: Ovaries, fallopian tubes, **uterus** (womb), vagina, mammary glands. *Male*: Testes and associated tubes, urethra, penis, prostate gland.
Endocrine	**Thyroid gland** (in the neck), **pituitary gland** (at the base of the brain), sex glands (ovaries and testes), adrenal glands, pancreas (islets of Langerhans), parathyroid glands.
Nervous	Brain, spinal cord, nerves, and collections of nerves.
Circulatory	Heart, blood vessels (arteries, veins, and capillaries), lymphatic vessels and nodes, spleen, thymus gland.
Musculoskeletal	Muscles, bones, and joints.
Skin and sense organs	Skin, hair, nails, sweat glands, and sebaceous (oil) glands; eye, ear, nose, and tongue.

2

STUDY SECTION 2

Practice spelling each term, and know its meaning.

adipose tissue	Collection of fat cells.
cartilage	Flexible connective tissue attached to bones at joints. For example, it surrounds the trachea and forms part of the external ear and nose.
epithelial cells	Skin cells that cover the outside of the body and line the internal surfaces of organs.
histologist	Specialist in the study of tissues.
larynx	"Voice box"; located at the upper part of the trachea.
pharynx	Throat. The pharynx serves as the common passageway for food (from the mouth going to the esophagus) and air (from the nose to the trachea).
pituitary gland	Endocrine gland at the base of the brain.
thyroid gland	Endocrine gland that surrounds the trachea in the neck.
trachea	"Windpipe" (tube leading from the throat to the bronchial tubes).
ureter	One of two tubes, each leading from a single kidney to the urinary bladder. *Spelling clue*: Ureter has two e's, and there are two ureters.
urethra	Tube from the urinary bladder to the outside of the body. *Spelling clue*: Urethra has one e, and there is only one urethra.
uterus	The womb. The organ that holds the embryo/fetus as it develops.
viscera	Internal organs.

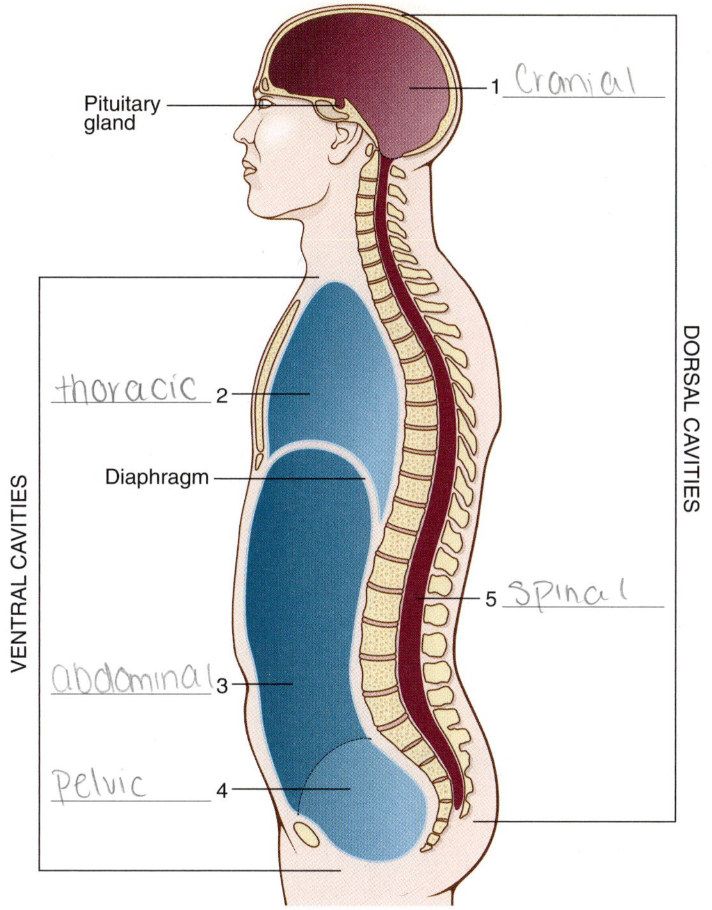

FIGURE 2-7 **Body cavities. Ventral** (anterior) cavities are in the front of the body (blue). **Dorsal** (posterior) cavities are in the back (red).

2

BODY CAVITIES

A body cavity is a space within the body that contains internal organs (viscera). Label Figure 2-7 as you learn the names of the body cavities. Some of the important viscera contained within those cavities are listed as well.

CAVITY	ORGANS
Cranial [1]	Brain, pituitary gland.
Thoracic [2]	Lungs, heart, esophagus, trachea, bronchial tubes, thymus gland, aorta (large artery).

The thoracic cavity is divided into two smaller cavities (Figure 2-8):

a. **Pleural cavity**—space between the folds of the pleura surrounding each lung. The **pleura** is a double-folded membrane that surrounds the lungs and protects them. If the pleura is inflamed (as in pleuritis, also called pleurisy), the pleural cavity may fill with fluid.

b. **Mediastinum**—centrally located space outside of and between the lungs. It contains the heart, aorta, trachea, esophagus, thymus gland, bronchial tubes, and many lymph nodes.

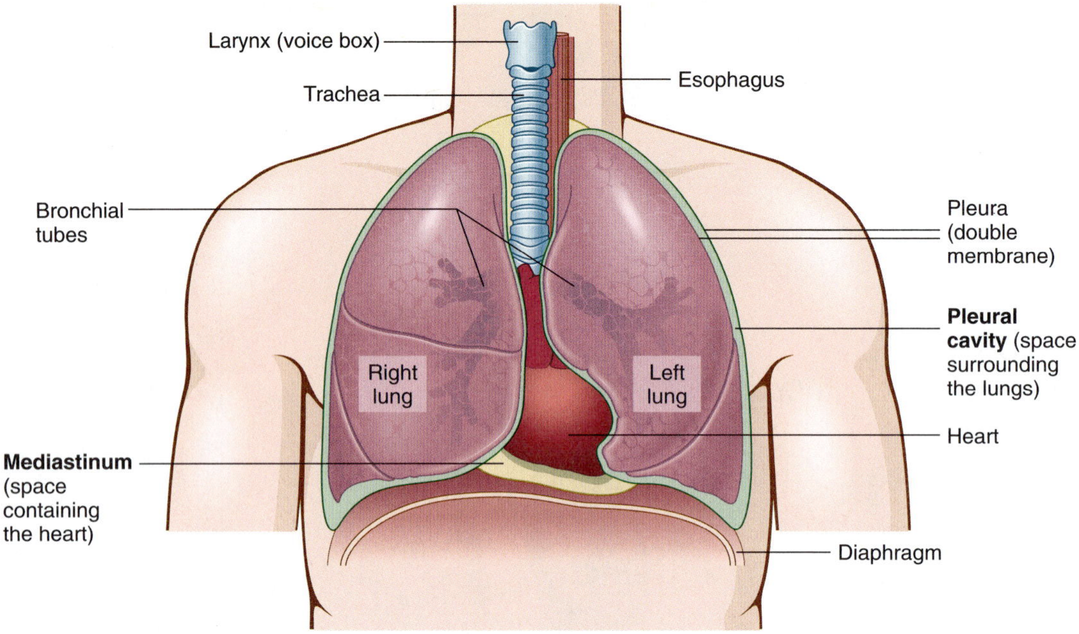

FIGURE 2-8 **Divisions of the thoracic cavity.**

CAVITY	ORGANS
Continue labeling Figure 2-7.	
Abdominal [3]	The **peritoneum** is the double-folded membrane surrounding the abdominal cavity (Figure 2-9). The kidneys are two bean-shaped organs situated behind (retroperitoneal area) the abdominal cavity on either side of the backbone (see Figures 2-9 and 2-11). Also contains the stomach, small and large intestines, spleen, pancreas, liver, and gallbladder. The **diaphragm** (a muscular wall) divides the abdominal and thoracic cavities (see Figure 2-7).
Pelvic [4]	Portions of the small and large intestines, rectum, urinary bladder, urethra, and ureters; uterus and vagina in the female.
Spinal [5]	Nerves of the spinal cord.

The cranial and spinal cavities are the **dorsal** body cavities because of their location on the back (posterior) portion of the body. The thoracic, abdominal, and pelvic cavities are **ventral** body cavities because they are on the front (anterior) portion of the body (see Figure 2-7).

While the thoracic and abdominal cavities are separated by a muscular wall called the **diaphragm,** the abdominal and pelvic cavities are not separated and are referred to together as the **abdominopelvic cavity.** Figures 2-10 and 2-11 show the abdominal and thoracic viscera from anterior (ventral) and posterior (dorsal) views.

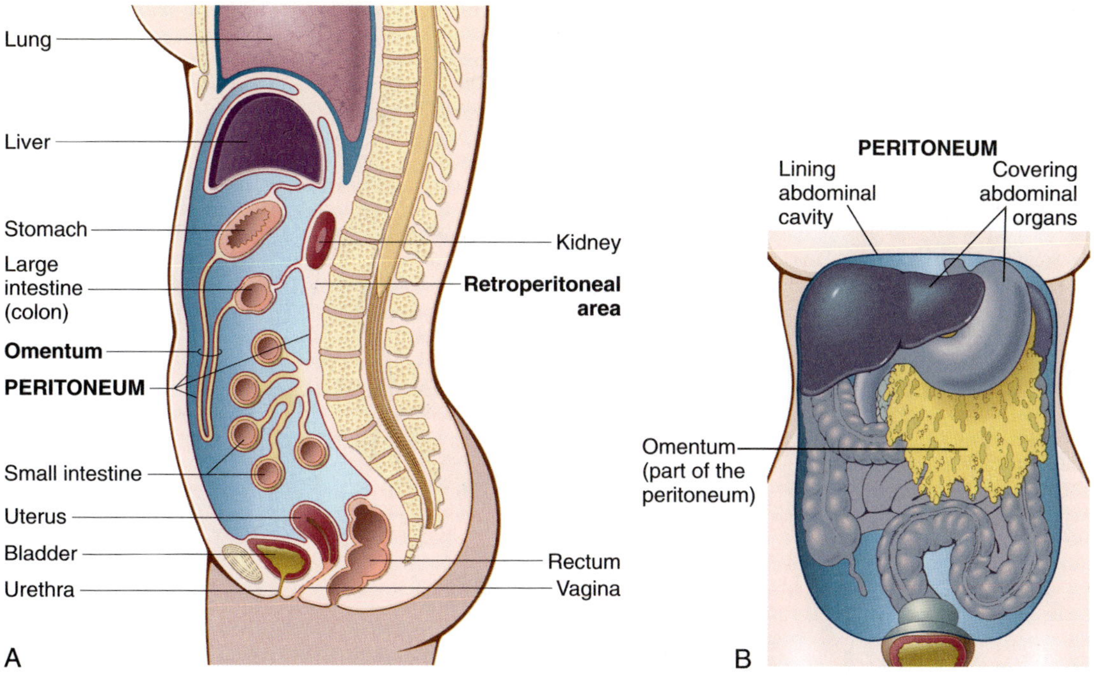

FIGURE 2-9 **A, Abdominal cavity** (*side view* and in *light blue*). Notice the **peritoneum** (outlined in *red*), which is a membrane surrounding the organs in the abdominal cavity. The **retroperitoneal area** is behind the peritoneum. The **omentum** is a part of the peritoneum in the front of the abdomen. It contains fat and hangs down loosely like an apron over the intestines to keep them warm. **B,** Frontal view of the peritoneum.

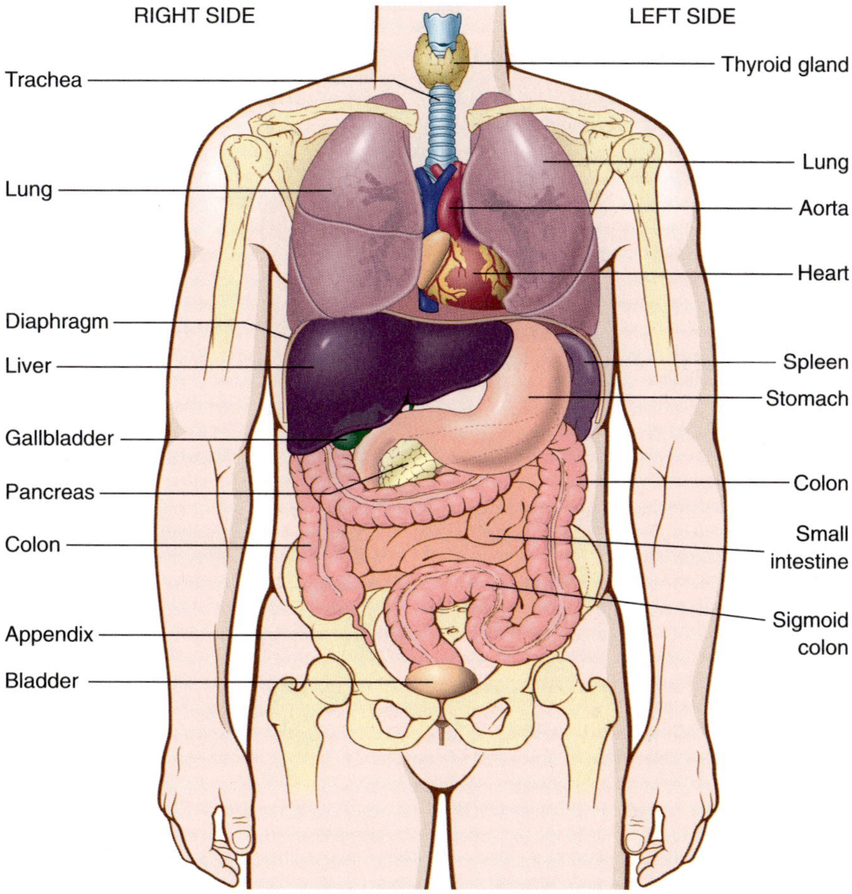

FIGURE 2-10 **Organs of the abdominopelvic and thoracic cavities, anterior view.**

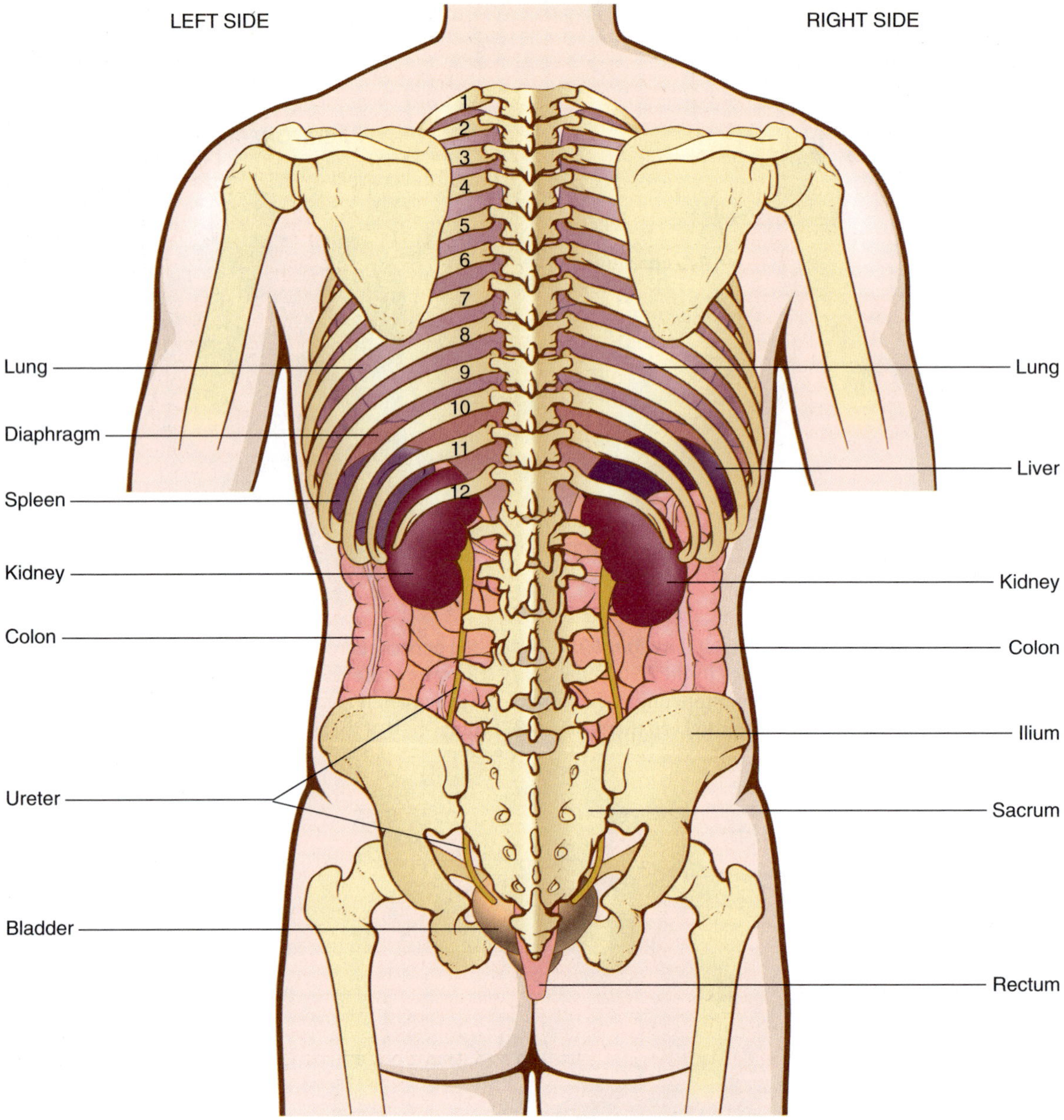

FIGURE 2-11 Organs of the abdominopelvic and thoracic cavities, posterior view.

STUDY SECTION 3

Practice spelling each term, and know its meaning.

abdominal cavity	Space below the chest containing organs such as the liver, stomach, gallbladder, and intestines; also called the **abdomen.**
cranial cavity	Space in the head containing the brain and surrounded by the skull. **Cranial** means **pertaining to the skull.**
diaphragm	Muscle separating the abdominal and thoracic cavities. The diaphragm moves up and down and aids in breathing.
dorsal (posterior)	Pertaining to the back.
mediastinum	Centrally located space outside of and between the lungs.
pelvic cavity	Space below the abdomen containing portions of the intestines, rectum, urinary bladder, and reproductive organs. **Pelvic** means **pertaining to the pelvis,** composed of the hip bones surrounding the pelvic cavity.
peritoneum	Double-folded membrane surrounding the abdominal cavity.
pleura	Double-folded membrane surrounding each lung. Pleural means pertaining to the pleura.
pleural cavity	Space between the pleural layers.
spinal cavity	Space within the spinal column (backbones) containing the spinal cord. Also called the **spinal canal.**
thoracic cavity	Space in the chest containing the heart, lungs, bronchial tubes, trachea, esophagus, and other organs.
ventral (anterior)	Pertaining to the front.

Peritoneum and Other Membranes

Many vital organs are covered and protected by membranes. The **peritoneum** surrounds abdominal viscera (liver, small and large intestines, stomach), the **pleura** covers the lungs, the **periosteum** protects bones, and the **meninges** are membranes surrounding the brain and spinal cord.

Pleural/Plural

Don't confuse ***pleural,*** which refers to the **membranes surrounding the lungs,** with ***plural,*** which means **more than one!**

ABDOMINOPELVIC REGIONS AND QUADRANTS

REGIONS

Doctors divide the abdominopelvic area into nine regions. Label these regions in Figure 2-12.

Right hypochondriac region [1]: right upper region below (hypo-) the cartilage (chondr/o) of the ribs that extend over the abdomen.
Left hypochondriac region [2]: left upper region below the rib cartilage.
Epigastric region [3]: region above the stomach.
Right lumbar region [4]: right middle region near the waist.
Left lumbar region [5]: left middle region near the waist.
Umbilical region [6]: region of the navel or umbilicus.
Right inguinal region [7]: right lower region near the groin (inguin/o = groin), which is the area where the legs join the trunk of the body. This region also is known as the **right iliac region** because it lies near the ilium (the upper portion of the hip bone).
Left inguinal region [8]: left lower region near the groin. Also called the **left iliac region.**
Hypogastric region [9]: middle lower region below the umbilical region.

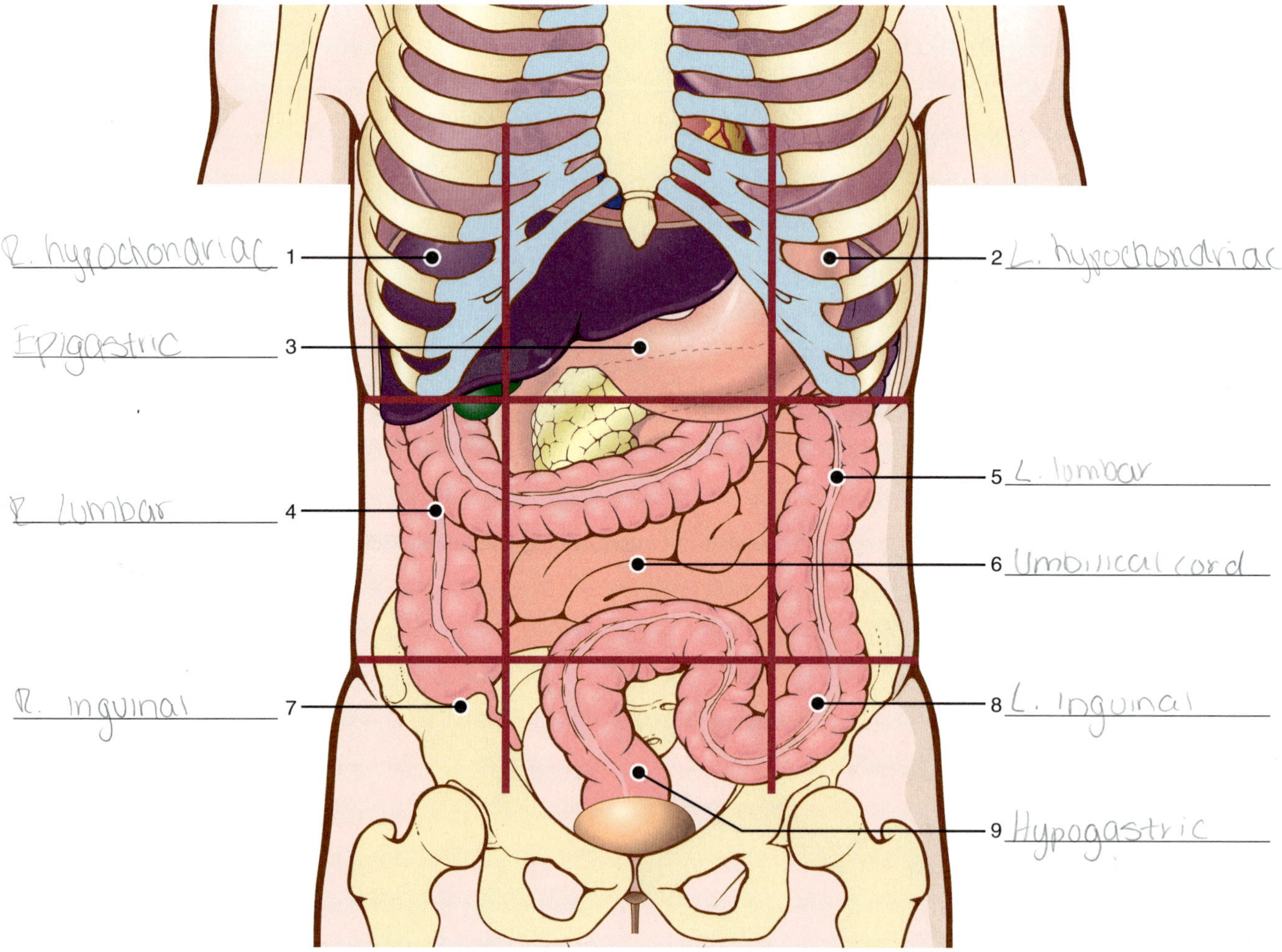

FIGURE 2-12 **Abdominopelvic regions.** These regions can be used clinically to locate internal organs.

QUADRANTS

The abdominopelvic area can be divided into four quadrants by two imaginary lines—one horizontal and one vertical—that cross at the midsection of the body. Figure 2-13 shows the four abdominopelvic quadrants; add the proper abbreviation on the line under each label on the diagram.

Right upper quadrant (RUQ)—contains the liver (right lobe), gallbladder, part of the pancreas, parts of the small and large intestines

Left upper quadrant (LUQ)—contains the liver (left lobe), stomach, spleen, part of the pancreas, parts of the small and large intestines

Right lower quadrant (RLQ)—contains parts of the small and large intestines, right ovary, right fallopian tube, appendix, right ureter

Left lower quadrant (LLQ)—contains parts of the small and large intestines, left ovary, left fallopian tube, left ureter

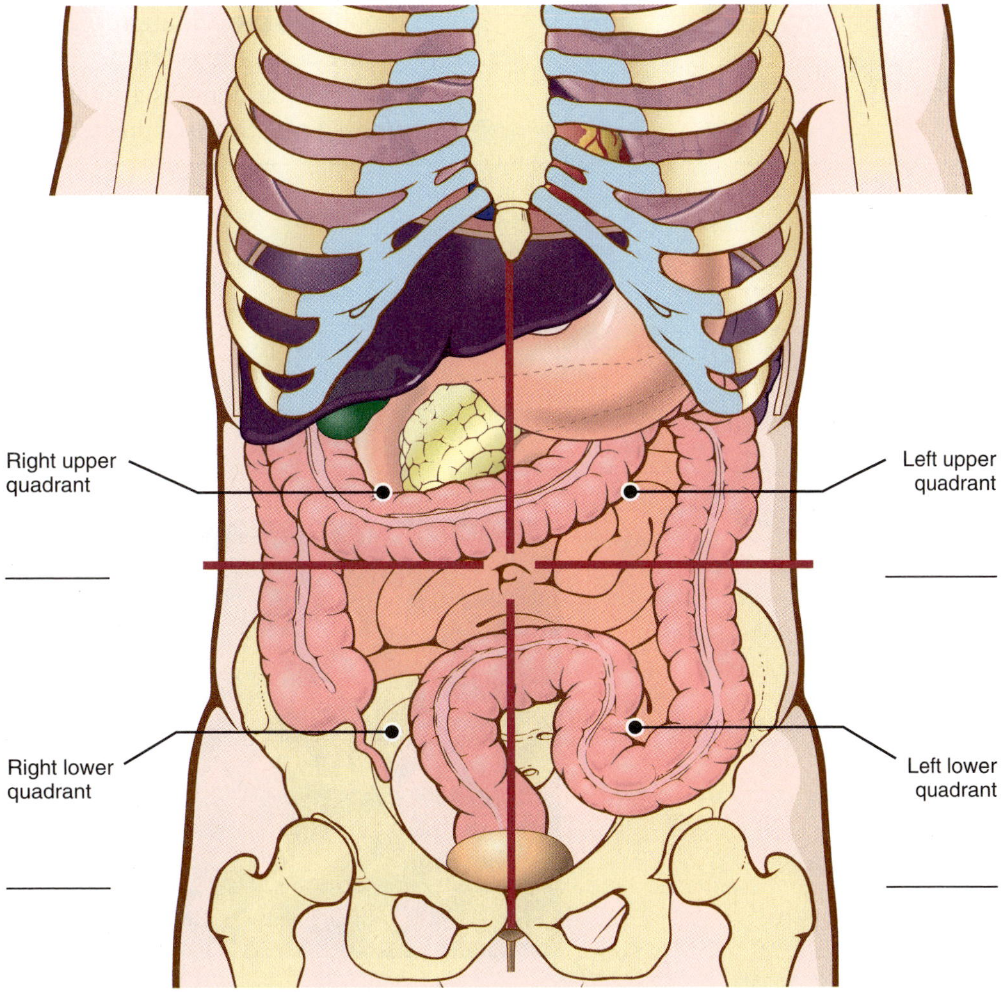

FIGURE 2-13 **Abdominopelvic quadrants.** Write the abbreviation for each quadrant on the line provided.

Divisions of the Back (Spinal Column)

The spinal column is composed of a series of bones that extend from the neck to the tailbone. Each bone is a **vertebra** (plural: **vertebrae**).

Label the divisions of the back on Figure 2-14A as you study the following:

DIVISION OF THE BACK	ABBREVIATION	LOCATION
Cervical [1]	C	Neck region. There are seven cervical vertebrae (C1 to C7).
Thoracic [2]	T	Chest region. There are 12 thoracic vertebrae (T1 to T12). Each bone is joined to a rib.
Lumbar [3]	L	Loin (waist) or flank region (between the ribs and the hipbone). There are five lumbar vertebrae (L1 to L5).
Sacral [4]	S	Five bones (S1 to S5) are fused to form one bone, the **sacrum.**
Coccygeal [5]		The **coccyx** (tailbone) is a small bone composed of four fused pieces.

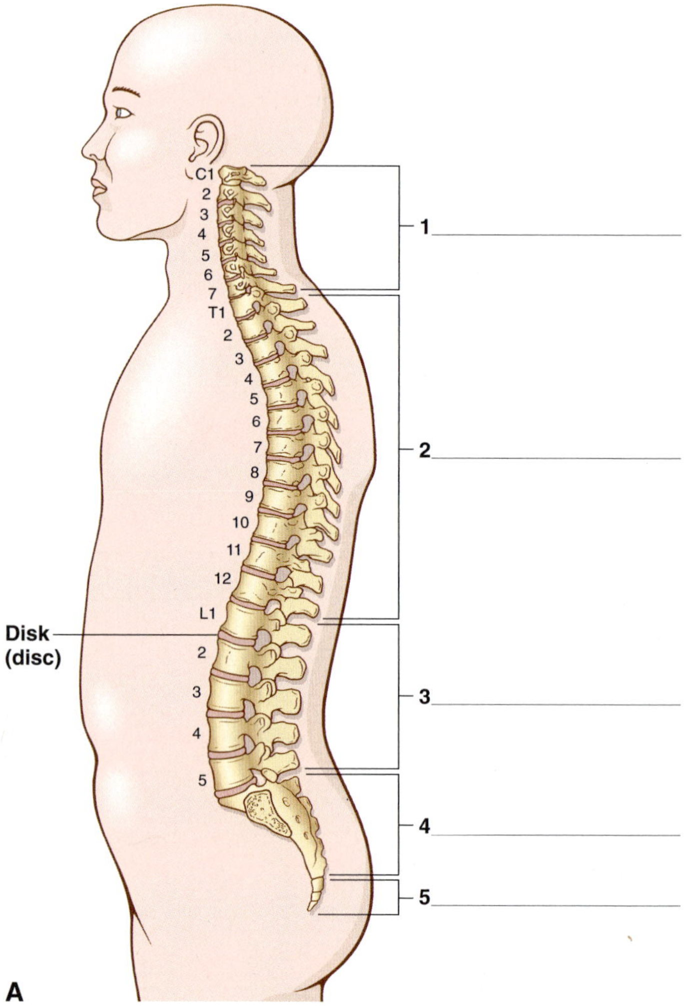

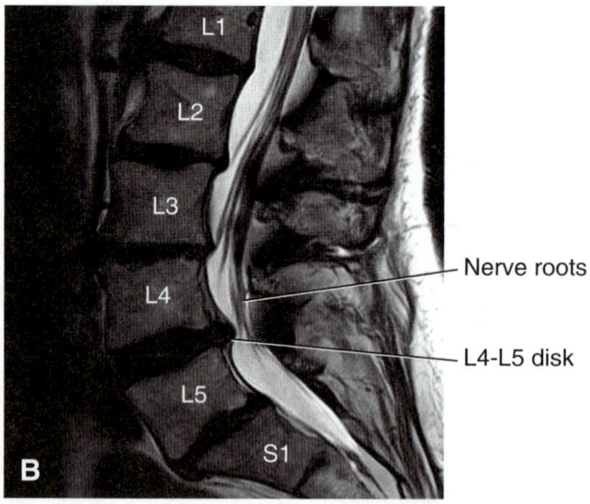

FIGURE 2-14 Anatomic divisions of the back (spinal column). A, A **disk** (disc) is a small pad of cartilage between each backbone. **B, MRI (magnetic resonance image)** of a **herniated disk** at the L4-L5 level of the spinal column.

Do not confuse the **spinal column** (back bones or vertebrae) with the **spinal cord** (nerves surrounded by the column). The column is bone tissue, whereas the cord is nervous tissue.

The spaces between the vertebrae (intervertebral spaces) are identified according to the two vertebrae between which they occur—for example, the L5–S1 space is between the fifth lumbar vertebra and the first sacral vertebra; T2–3 is between the second and third thoracic vertebrae. Within the space and between vertebrae is a small pad called a **disk,** or **disc.** The disk, composed of water and cartilage, is a shock absorber. Occasionally, a disk may move out of place (herniate) and put pressure on a nerve (see Figure 2-14B). This **"slipped disk"** can cause pain in an area of the body affected by the nerve.

STUDY SECTION 4

Practice spelling each term, and know its meaning.

ABDOMINOPELVIC REGIONS	
hypochondriac	Right and left upper regions beneath the ribs.
epigastric	Middle upper region above the stomach.
lumbar	Right and left middle regions near the waist.
umbilical	Central region near the navel.
inguinal	Right and left lower regions near the groin. Also called **iliac regions.**
hypogastric	Middle lower region below the umbilical region.
ABDOMINOPELVIC QUADRANTS	
RUQ	Right upper quadrant.
LUQ	Left upper quadrant.
RLQ	Right lower quadrant.
LLQ	Left lower quadrant.
DIVISIONS OF THE BACK	
cervical	Neck region (C1 to C7).
thoracic	Chest region (T1 to T12).
lumbar	Loin (waist) region (L1 to L5).
sacral	Region of the sacrum (S1 to S5).
coccygeal	Region of the coccyx (tailbone).
RELATED TERMS	
vertebra	Single backbone.
vertebrae	Backbones.
spinal column	Bone tissue surrounding the spinal cavity.
spinal cord	Nervous tissue within the spinal cavity.
disk (disc)	Pad of cartilage between vertebrae.

2

Positional and Directional Terms

Label Figure 2-15 to identify the following positional and directional terms.

Note that the figure is in the anatomic position with the palms of the hands facing outward and the fifth (little) finger in a medial position (closer to the center of the body). The thumb, then, is lateral.

LOCATION	RELATIONSHIP
Anterior (ventral) [1]	Front side of the body. *Example*: The forehead is on the **anterior** side of the body.
Posterior (dorsal) [2]	The back side of the body. *Example*: The back of the head is **posterior (dorsal)** to the face.
Deep [3]	Away from the surface. *Example*: The stab wound penetrated **deep** into the abdomen.
Superficial [4]	On the surface. *Example*: **Superficial** veins can be viewed through the skin.
Proximal [5]	Near the point of attachment to the trunk or near the beginning of a structure. *Example*: The **proximal** end of the thigh bone (femur) joins with the hip socket.
Distal [6]	Far from the point of attachment to the trunk or far from the beginning of a structure. *Example*: At its **distal** end, the femur joins with the knee.
Inferior [7]	Below another structure. *Example*: The feet are at the **inferior** part of the body. They are inferior to the knees. The term **caudal** (pertaining to the tail, or to the lower portion of the body) also means away from the head or below another structure.
Superior [8]	Above another structure. *Example*: The head lies **superior** to the neck. **Cephalic** (pertaining to the head) also means above another structure.
Medial [9]	Pertaining to the middle, or nearer the medial plane of the body. *Example*: When in the anatomic position (palms of the hands facing outward), the fifth (little) finger is **medial**.
Lateral [10]	Pertaining to the side. *Example*: When in the anatomic position (palms of the hands facing outward), the thumb is **lateral.**
Supine [11]	Lying on the back. *Example*: The patient lies **supine** during an examination of the abdomen. (The face is **up** in the s**up**ine position.)
Prone [12]	Lying on the belly. *Example*: The backbones are examined with the patient in a **prone** position. (The patient lies **on** his or her stomach in the pr**on**e position.)

2

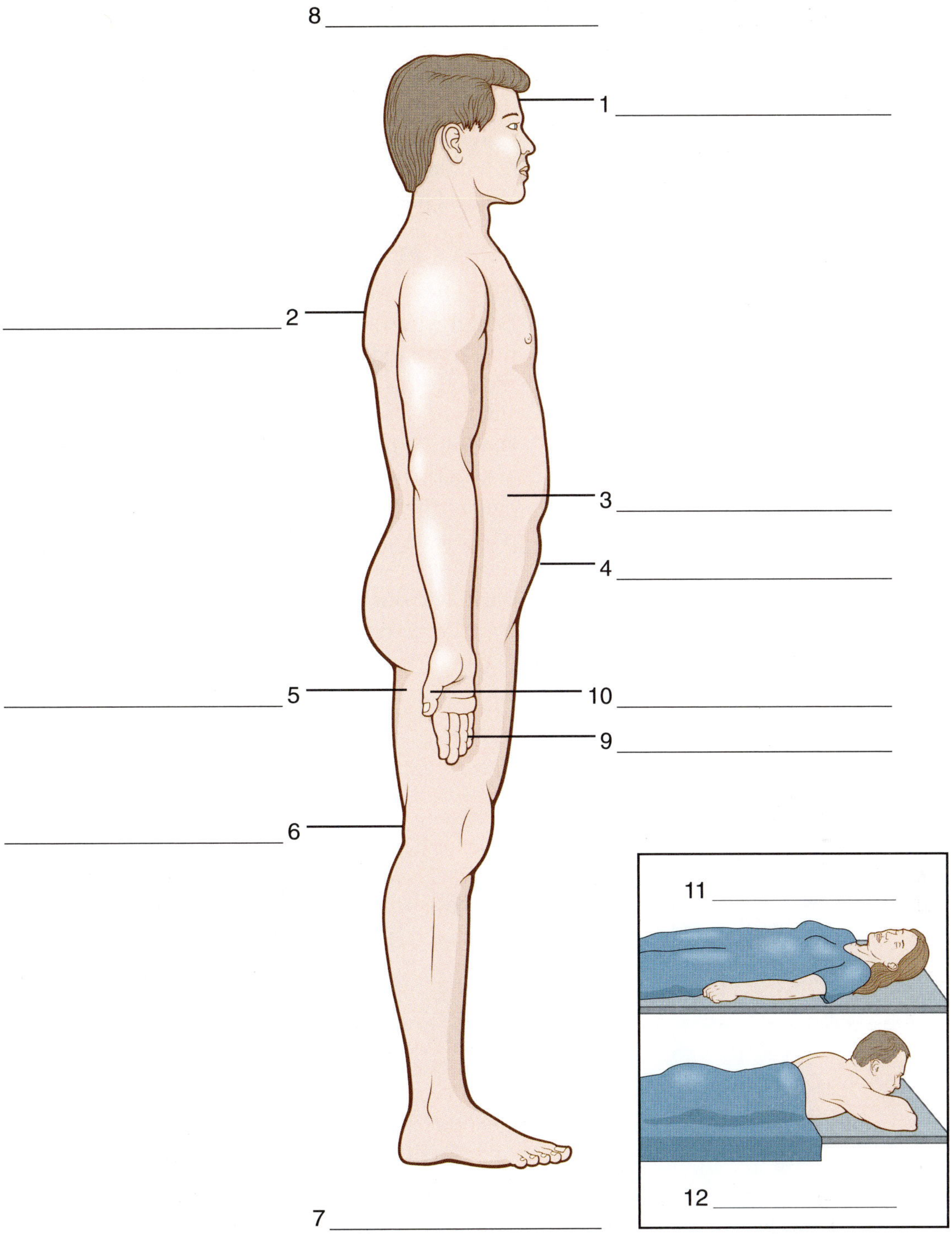

FIGURE 2-15 Positional and directional terms.

Planes of the Body

A plane is an imaginary flat surface. Label Figure 2-16 to identify the following planes of the body:

PLANE	LOCATION
Frontal (coronal) plane [1]	Vertical plane dividing the body or structure into anterior and posterior portions. A common chest x-ray view is a PA (posteroanterior—viewed from back to front) view, which is in the **frontal (coronal)** plane.
Sagittal (lateral) plane [2]	Lengthwise vertical plane dividing the body or structure into right and left sides. The **midsagittal** plane divides the body into right and left halves. A **lateral** (side-to-side) chest x-ray film is taken in the **sagittal** plane.
Transverse (axial) plane [3]	Horizontal (cross-sectional) plane running across the body parallel to the ground. This **cross-sectional** plane divides the body or structure into upper and lower portions. A CT (computed tomography) scan is one of a series of x-ray pictures taken in the transverse (axial or cross-sectional) plane.

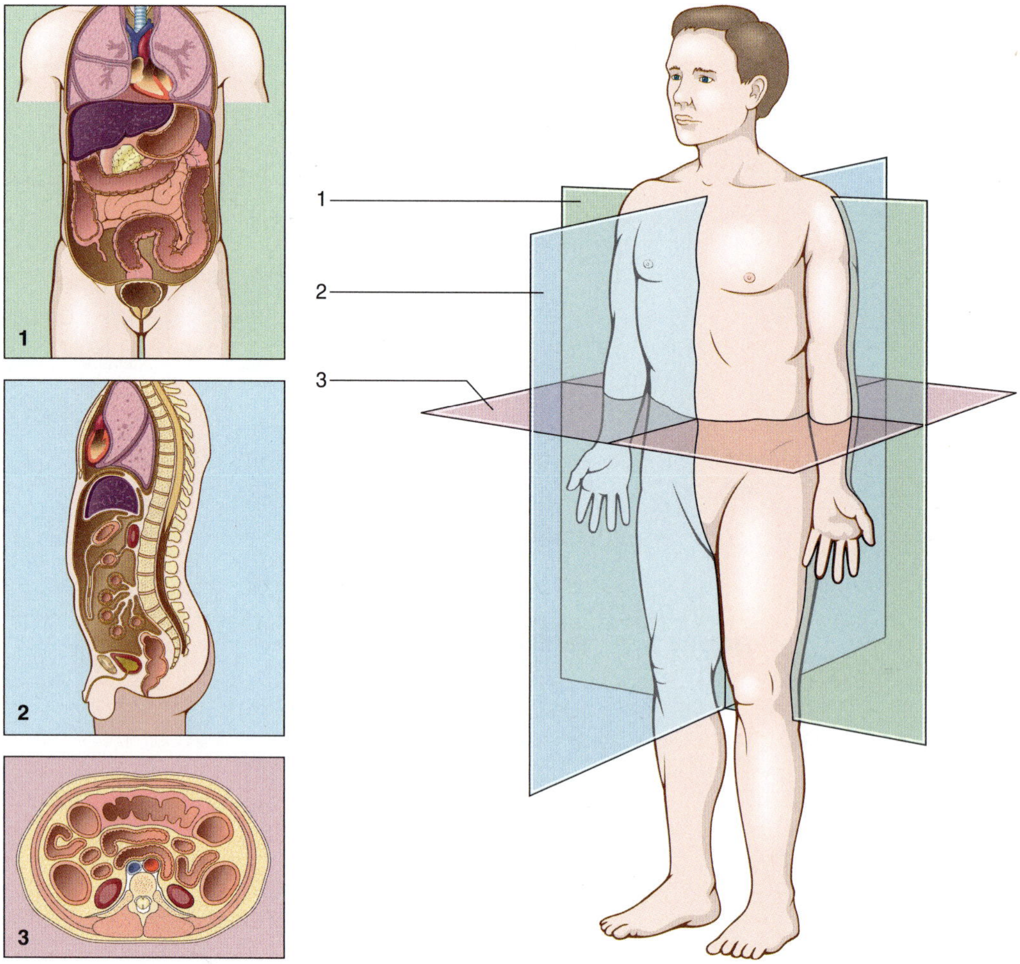

FIGURE 2-16 **Planes of the body.** The figure is in the **anatomic position.** Note the views of the body represented by each plane.

STUDY SECTION 5

Practice spelling each term, and know its meaning.

anterior (ventral)	Front surface of the body.
deep	Away from the surface.
distal	Far from the point of attachment to the trunk or far from the beginning of a structure.
frontal (coronal) plane	Vertical plane dividing the body or structure into anterior and posterior portions.
inferior (caudal)	Below another structure; pertaining to the tail or lower portion of the body.
lateral	Pertaining to the side.
medial	Pertaining to the middle or near the medial plane of the body.
posterior (dorsal)	Back surface of the body.
prone	Lying on the belly (face down, palms down).
proximal	Near the point of attachment to the trunk or near the beginning of a structure.
sagittal (lateral) plane	Lengthwise, vertical plane dividing the body or structure into right and left sides. From the Latin *sagitta*, meaning arrow. As an arrow is shot from a bow it enters the body in the sagittal plane, dividing right from left. The **midsagittal** plane divides the body into right and left halves.
superficial	On the surface.
superior (cephalic)	Above another structure; pertaining to the head.
supine	Lying on the back (face up, palms up).
transverse (axial) plane	Horizontal (cross-sectional) plane dividing the body into upper and lower portions.

2

TERMINOLOGY

Divide each term into its component parts, and write its meaning in the space provided.

COMBINING FORMS

COMBINING FORM	MEANING	TERMINOLOGY	MEANING
abdomin/o	abdomen	abdominal *The abdomen is the region below the chest containing internal organs (such as the liver, intestines, stomach, and gallbladder).*	______________________
adip/o	fat	adipose *The suffix -ose means pertaining to or full of.*	______________________
anter/o	front	anterior *The suffix -ior means pertaining to.*	______________________

COMBINING FORM	MEANING	TERMINOLOGY	MEANING
bol/o	to cast (throw)	anabolism	*The prefix ana- means up. The suffix -ism means process. In this cellular process, proteins are built up (protein synthesis).*
cervic/o	neck (of the body or of the uterus)	cervical	*The **cervix** is the neck of the uterus. The term cervical can mean pertaining to the neck of the body or to the neck (lower part) of the uterus.*
chondr/o	cartilage (type of connective tissue)	chondroma	*This is a benign tumor.*
		chondrosarcoma	*This is a malignant tumor. The root sarc indicates that the malignant tumor arises from a type of flesh or connective tissue.*
chrom/o	color	chromosomes	*These nuclear structures absorb the color of dyes used to stain the cell. The suffix -somes means bodies. Literally, this term means "bodies of color," because this is how they appeared to researchers who first saw them under the microscope.*
coccyg/o	coccyx (tailbone)	coccygeal	
crani/o	skull	craniotomy	
cyt/o	cell	cytoplasm	*The suffix -plasm means formation.*
dist/o	far, distant	distal	
dors/o	back portion of the body	dorsal	*The dorsal fin of a fish is on its back (see Figure 2-17).*
hist/o	tissue	histology	
ili/o	ilium (part of the pelvic bone)	iliac	*See Figure 2-18 for a picture of the ilium.*
inguin/o	groin	inguinal	
kary/o	nucleus	karyotype	*The suffix -type means classification or picture.*

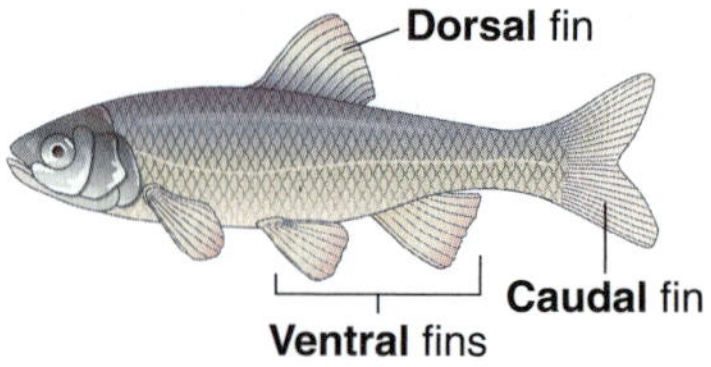

FIGURE 2-17 Notice the **dorsal, caudal,** and **ventral** fins of a fish.

COMBINING FORM	MEANING	TERMINOLOGY	MEANING
later/o	side	lateral	______________
lumb/o	lower back (side and back between the ribs and the pelvis)	lumbosacral	______________
medi/o	middle	medial	______________
nucle/o	nucleus	nucleic	______________
pelv/i	pelvis, hip region	pelvic *The pelvis includes all the bones that surround the pelvic cavity (Figure 2-18).*	______________
poster/o	back, behind	posterior	______________
proxim/o	nearest	proximal	______________
sacr/o	sacrum	sacral	______________
sarc/o	flesh	sarcoma	______________
spin/o	spine, backbone	spinal	______________

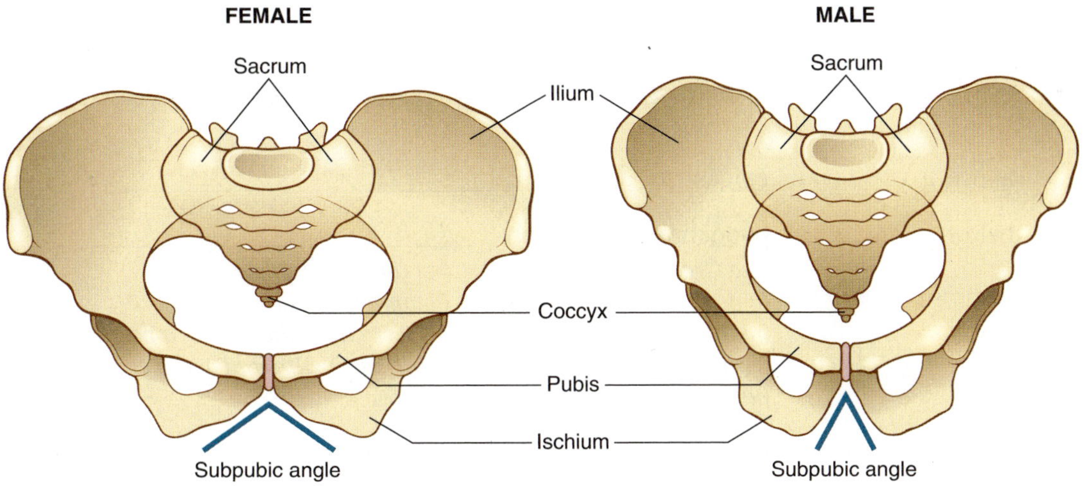

FIGURE 2-18

Pelvis: Comparison of Female and Male

The **female pelvis** is **wider** and **more massive** than the male pelvis. **The female pelvic opening is a larger, rounded, oval shape, whereas the male pelvic opening is deep, narrow, and funnel- or heart-shaped.** Thus, the female pelvis can accommodate the fetus during pregnancy and its downward passage through the pelvic cavity in childbirth.

COMBINING FORM	MEANING	TERMINOLOGY	MEANING
thel/o, theli/o	nipple	epithelial cell *This cell, originally identified in the skin of the nipples, lies on body surfaces, externally (outside the body) and internally (lining cavities and organs).*	
thorac/o	chest	thoracic	
		thoracotomy	
trache/o	trachea, windpipe	tracheal	
umbilic/o	navel, umbilicus	umbilical	
ventr/o	belly side of the body	ventral	
vertebr/o	vertebra(e), backbone(s)	vertebral	
viscer/o	internal organs	visceral	

PREFIXES

PREFIX	MEANING	TERMINOLOGY	MEANING
ana-	up	anabolic	
cata-	down	catabolism *Complex nutrients are broken down into simpler substances and energy is released.*	
epi-	above	epigastric	
hypo-	below	hypochondriac region *The Greeks thought that organs (liver and spleen) in the hypochondriac region of the abdomen were the origin of imaginary illnesses—hence the term hypochondriac, a person with unusual anxiety about his or her health and with symptoms not attributable to any disease process.*	
inter-	between	intervertebral *A disk (disc) is an intervertebral structure.*	
meta-	change	metabolism *Literally, to cast (bol/o) a change (meta-), meaning the chemical changes (processes) that occur in a cell.*	

2

SUFFIXES

The following are some new suffixes introduced in this chapter. See the Glossary at the end of the book, for additional suffixes meaning "pertaining to."

SUFFIX	MEANING	SUFFIX	MEANING
-eal	pertaining to	**-ose**	pertaining to, full of
-iac	pertaining to	**-plasm**	formation
-ior	pertaining to	**-somes**	bodies
-ism	process, condition	**-type**	picture, classification

PRACTICAL APPLICATIONS

Be sure to check your answers with the Answers to Practical Applications on page 65.

SURGICAL PROCEDURES

Match the surgical procedure in Column I with a reason for performing it in Column II. *Note:* You are not looking for the exact meaning of each surgical procedure, but rather why it would be performed.

COLUMN I

Procedures

1. Craniotomy ____
2. Thoracotomy ____
3. Diskectomy ____
4. Mediastinoscopy ____
5. Tracheotomy ____
6. Laryngectomy ____
7. Arthroscopy ____
8. Peritoneoscopy ____

COLUMN II

Indications

A. Emergency effort to remove foreign material from the windpipe
B. Inspection and repair of torn cartilage in the knee
C. Removal of a diseased or injured portion of the brain
D. Inspection of lymph nodes* in the region between the lungs
E. Removal of a squamous cell† carcinoma in the voice box
F. Open heart surgery, or removal of lung tissue
G. Inspection of abdominal organs and removal of diseased tissue
H. Relief of symptoms from a bulging intervertebral disk

*Lymph nodes are collections of tissue containing white blood cells called lymphocytes.
†A squamous cell is a type of epithelial cell.

2

X-RAY VIEWS

Circle the correct answers in the following sentences related to each x-ray view of the chest.

FIGURE A

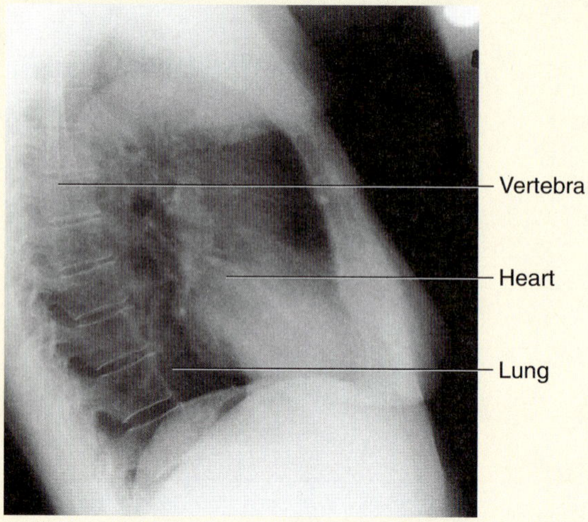

1. This is a/an **(coronal, sagittal, axial)** view. The heart lies **(anterior, posterior, dorsal)** to the vertebrae.

FIGURE B

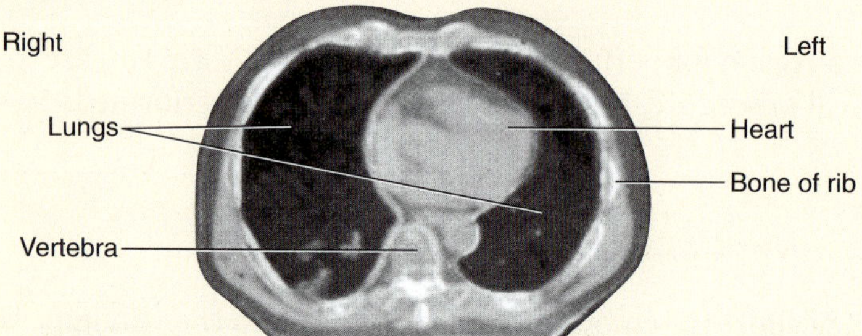

2. This is a/an **(coronal, sagittal, axial)** view. It is a/an **(CT, traditional x-ray)** image.

FIGURE C

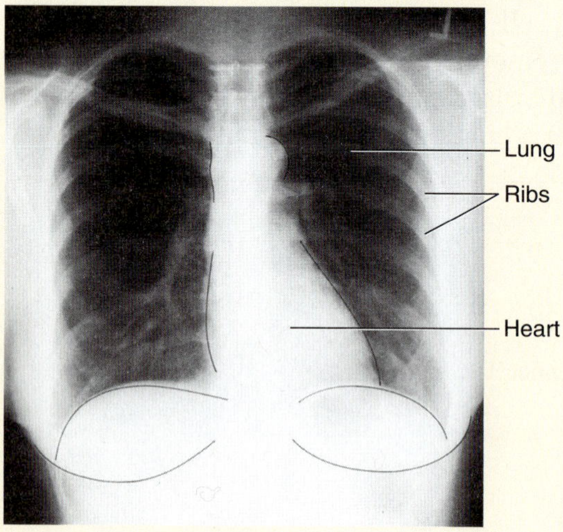

3. This is a/an **(coronal, sagittal, axial)** view. It is a/an **(lateral, transverse, anterior/posterior)** image.

EXERCISES

Remember to check your answers carefully with the Answers to Exercises, page 64.

A The listed terms are parts of a cell. Match each term with its correct meaning.

cell membrane	DNA	mitochondria
chromosomes	endoplasmic reticulum	nucleus
cytoplasm	genes	

1. material of the cell located outside the nucleus and yet enclosed by the cell membrane ________________
2. regions of DNA within each chromosome ________________
3. small sausage-shaped structures that are the principal source of energy for the cell ________________
4. network of canals within the cytoplasm; the site of protein synthesis ________________
5. structure that surrounds and protects the cell ________________
6. control center of the cell, containing chromosomes ________________
7. chemical found within each chromosome ________________
8. rod-shaped structures in the nucleus that contain regions called genes ________________

2

B Use medical terms or numbers to complete the following sentences.

1. A picture of chromosomes in the nucleus of a cell is a/an ________________.
2. The number of chromosomes in a normal male's muscle cell is ________________.
3. The number of chromosomes in a female's egg cell is ________________.
4. The process of building up proteins in a cell is ________________.
5. Complex nutrients are broken down to similar substances and energy is released ________________.
6. The total of the chemical processes in a cell is ________________.
7. A scientist who studies tissues is a/an ________________.
8. The medical term for internal organs is ________________.

C Match each of the listed body parts or tissues with its correct description below.

adipose tissue
cartilage
epithelial tissue
larynx
pharynx
pituitary gland
pleura
thyroid gland
trachea
ureter
urethra
uterus

1. voice box ____________________
2. membrane surrounding the lungs ____________________
3. throat ____________________
4. tube from the kidney to the urinary bladder ____________________
5. collection of fat cells ____________________
6. endocrine organ located at the base of the brain ____________________
7. windpipe ____________________
8. flexible connective tissue attached to bones at joints ____________________
9. skin cells that cover the outside of the body and line internal organs ____________________
10. endocrine gland surrounding the windpipe in the neck ____________________
11. womb ____________________
12. tube leading from the urinary bladder to the outside of the body ____________________

2

D Name the five cavities of the body.

1. cavity surrounded by the skull ____________________
2. cavity in the chest surrounded by the ribs ____________________
3. cavity below the chest containing the stomach, liver, and gallbladder ____________________
4. cavity surrounded by the hip bones ____________________
5. cavity surrounded by the bones of the back ____________________

E Select from the following to define the terms listed on the next page.

space surrounding each lung
space between the lungs
muscle separating the abdominal and thoracic cavities
membrane surrounding the abdominal organs
area below the umbilicus (as well as below the stomach)
area above the stomach
area of the navel
areas near the groin
nervous tissue within the spinal cavity
bony tissue surrounding the spinal cavity
pad of cartilage between two adjoining vertebrae

1. hypogastric region ____________________
2. mediastinum ____________________
3. spinal cord ____________________
4. diaphragm ____________________
5. intervertebral disk ____________________
6. pleural cavity ____________________
7. spinal column ____________________
8. inguinal regions ____________________
9. peritoneum ____________________
10. umbilical region ____________________
11. epigastric region ____________________

F Name the five divisions of the back.

1. region of the neck ____________________
2. region of the chest ____________________
3. region of the waist ____________________
4. region of the sacrum ____________________
5. region of the tailbone ____________________

G Give the meanings of the following abbreviations.

1. LLQ ____________________
2. L5–S1 ____________________
3. RUQ ____________________
4. C3–C4 ____________________
5. RLQ ____________________

H Give the opposites of the following terms.

1. deep ____________________
2. proximal ____________________
3. supine ____________________
4. medial ____________________
5. dorsal ____________________
6. superior ____________________

I **Select from the following medical terms to complete the sentences below.**

distal	midsagittal	transverse (axial)
frontal (coronal)	proximal	vertebra
inferior (caudal)	superior (cephalic)	vertebrae
lateral		

1. The kidney lies ________________ to the spinal cord. (Hint: to the side of)
2. The ________ end of the thigh bone (femur) joins with the kneecap (patella).
3. The ________ plane divides the body into an anterior and a posterior portion.
4. Each backbone is a/an ________________.
5. Several backbones are ________________.
6. The diaphragm lies ________________ to the organs in the thoracic cavity.
7. The ________________ plane divides the body into right and left halves.
8. The ________________ end of the upper arm bone (humerus) is at the shoulder.
9. The ________________ plane divides the body into upper and lower portions.
10. The pharynx is located ________________________ to the esophagus.

J **Use slashes to divide the following terms into component parts, and give meanings for each.**

1. craniotomy ________________________________
2. cervical ________________________________
3. chondroma ________________________________
4. chondrosarcoma ________________________________
5. nucleic ________________________________

K **Give the medical term for the following definitions. Pay attention to spelling!**

1. space below the chest containing the liver, stomach, gallbladder, and intestines

   ____
2. flexible connective tissue attached to bones at joints ________________
3. rod-shaped structures in the cell nucleus, containing regions of DNA ________________
4. muscle separating the abdominal and thoracic cavities ________________
5. voice box ________________________________
6. vertical plane dividing the body into right and left sides ________________
7. pertaining to the neck ________________________________
8. tumor (benign) of cartilage ________________________________
9. control center of the cell; directs the activities of the cell ________________
10. pertaining to the windpipe ________________________________

L Complete each term based on the meaning provided.

1. pertaining to internal organs: ______________________al
2. tumor of flesh tissue (malignant): ______________________oma
3. pertaining to the chest: ______________________ic
4. picture of the chromosomes in the cell nucleus: ______________________type
5. sausage-shaped cellular structures in which catabolism takes place: mito______________________
6. space between the lungs: media______________________
7. endocrine gland at the base of the brain: ______________________ary gland
8. pertaining to skin (surface) cells: epi______________________
9. pertaining to far from the beginning of a structure: ______________________al
10. on the surface of the body: super______________________

M Circle the correct term to complete each sentence.

1. Dr. Curnen said the (**inguinal, superior, superficial**) wound barely scratched the surface.
2. Because the liver and spleen are on opposite sides of the body, the liver is in the (**RUQ, LUQ, LLQ**) of the abdominopelvic cavity and the spleen is in the (**RUQ, LUQ, RLQ**).
3. When a gynecologist performs a pelvic examination, the patient lies on her back in the (**ventral, dorsal, medial**) lithotomy position (Figure 2-19).
4. Sally complained of pain in the area surrounding her navel. The doctor described the pain as (**periumbilical, epigastric, hypogastric**).
5. After sampling the fluid surrounding her 16-week-old fetus and reviewing the chromosomal picture, the doctor explained to Mrs. Jones that the fetus had trisomy 21. The diagnosis was made by analysis of an abnormal (**urine sample, x-ray film, karyotype**).
6. The (**spinal, sagittal, abdominal**) cavity contains digestive organs.
7. The emergency department physician suspected appendicitis when Brandon was admitted with sharp (**LLQ, RLQ, RUQ**) pain.

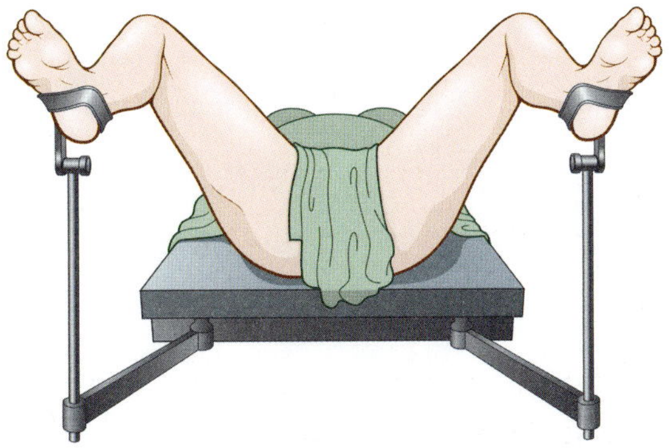

FIGURE 2-19 Dorsal lithotomy position. Lithotomy means incision to remove a stone (lith/o = stone). This position is used for gynecologic examinations and for removal of stones from the urinary tract.

8. Susan had hiccups after rapidly eating spicy Indian food. Her physician explained that the hiccups were involuntary contractions or spasms of the (**umbilicus, diaphragm, mediastinum**) resulting in uncontrolled breathing in of air.

9. Everyone in the society pages was noticeably slimmer this year. Could the popularity of liposuction surgery to remove unwanted (**cartilage, epithelial tissue, adipose tissue**) have something to do with this phenomenon?

10. Maria's coughing and sneezing were a result of an allergy to animal dander that affected her (**respiratory, cardiovascular, urinary**) system.

11. While ice skating, Natalie fell and landed on her buttocks. She had persistent (**cervical, thoracic, coccygeal**) pain for a few weeks but no broken bones on x-ray examination.

ANSWERS TO EXERCISES

A

1. cytoplasm
2. genes
3. mitochondria
4. endoplasmic reticulum
5. cell membrane
6. nucleus
7. DNA
8. chromosomes

B

1. karyotype
2. 46 (23 pairs)
3. 23
4. anabolism
5. catabolism
6. metabolism
7. histologist
8. viscera

C

1. larynx
2. pleura
3. pharynx
4. ureter
5. adipose tissue
6. pituitary gland
7. trachea
8. cartilage
9. epithelial tissue
10. thyroid gland
11. uterus
12. urethra

D

1. cranial
2. thoracic
3. abdominal
4. pelvic
5. spinal

E

1. area below the umbilicus
2. space between the lungs
3. nervous tissue within the spinal cavity
4. muscle separating the abdominal and thoracic cavities
5. pad of cartilage between two adjoining vertebrae
6. space surrounding each lung
7. bony tissue surrounding the spinal cavity
8. areas near the groin
9. membrane surrounding the abdominal organs
10. area of the navel
11. area above the stomach

F

1. cervical
2. thoracic
3. lumbar
4. sacral
5. coccygeal

G

1. left lower quadrant (of the abdominopelvic cavity)
2. between the fifth lumbar vertebra and the first sacral vertebra (a common place for a herniated disk)
3. right upper quadrant (of the abdominopelvic cavity)
4. between the third and fourth cervical vertebrae
5. right lower quadrant (of the abdominopelvic cavity)

H

1. superficial
2. distal
3. prone
4. lateral
5. ventral (anterior)
6. inferior (caudal)

I

1. lateral
2. distal
3. frontal (coronal)
4. vertebra
5. vertebrae
6. inferior (caudal)
7. midsagittal
8. proximal
9. transverse (cross-sectional)
10. superior (cephalic)

J

1. crani/o/tomy—incision of the skull
2. cervic/al—pertaining to the neck (of the body or the cervix of the uterus)
3. chondr/oma—tumor of cartilage (benign or noncancerous tumor)
4. chondr/o/sarc/oma—flesh tumor of cartilage (cancerous, malignant tumor)
5. nucle/ic—pertaining to the nucleus

K

1. abdomen or abdominal cavity
2. cartilage
3. chromosomes
4. diaphragm
5. larynx
6. sagittal—note spelling with two t's
7. cervical
8. chondroma
9. nucleus
10. tracheal

L

1. visceral
2. sarcoma
3. thoracic
4. karyotype
5. mitochondria—memory tip: **cat**abolism and **m**itochondria, **cat** and **mouse**!
6. mediastinum
7. pituitary gland
8. epithelial
9. distal
10. superficial

M

1. superficial
2. RUQ; LUQ
3. dorsal; often called the dorsolithotomy position
4. periumbilical
5. karyotype
6. abdominal
7. RLQ
8. diaphragm
9. adipose tissue
10. respiratory
11. coccygeal

Answers to Practical Applications

Surgical Procedures

1. **C** A trephine is a type of circular saw used for craniotomy.
2. **F**
3. **H** Endoscopic diskectomy is performed through a small incision on the back, lateral to the spine. All or a portion of the disk is removed.
4. **D** A small incision is made above the breastbone and an endoscope is inserted to inspect the lymph nodes around the trachea.
5. **A**
6. **E**
7. **B**
8. **G** A small incision is made near the navel, and a laparoscope is inserted. The procedure, also called laparoscopy (lapar/o means abdomen) or minimally invasive surgery, is used to examine organs and perform less complex surgical operations, such as removal of the gallbladder or appendix or tying off of the fallopian tubes.

X-ray Views

1. sagittal, anterior
2. axial, CT
3. coronal, anterior/posterior

2

PRONUNCIATION OF TERMS

To test your understanding of the terminology in this chapter, write the meaning of each term in the space provided. In addition, you may wish to cover the terms and write them by looking at your definitions. Make sure your spelling is correct. The CAPITAL letters indicate the accented syllable. The page number after each term indicates where it is defined or used in the book, so you can easily check your responses. You will find complete definitions for all of these terms and their audio pronunciations on the Evolve website.

Pronunciation Guide

ā as in āpe	ă as in ăpple
ē as in ēven	ĕ as in ĕvery
ī as in īce	ĭ as in ĭnterest
ō as in ōpen	ŏ as in pŏt
ū as in ūnit	ŭ as in ŭnder

TERM	PRONUNCIATION	MEANING
abdomen (45)	ĂB-dō-mĕn	
abdominal cavity (45)	ăb-DŎM-ĭ-năl KĂ-vĭ-tē	
adipose (40)	ĂD-ĭ-pōs	
anabolism (37)	ă-NĂB-ō-lĭzm	
anterior (50)	an-TĒ-rē-ŏr	
cartilage (40)	KĂR-tĭ-lĭj	
catabolism (37)	kă-TĂB-ō-lĭzm	
caudal (50)	KĂW-dăl	
cell membrane (37)	sĕl MĔM-brān	
cephalic (50)	SĔF-ă-lĭk	
cervical (49)	SĔR-vĭ-kăl	
chondroma (54)	kŏn-DRŌ-mă	
chondrosarcoma (54)	kŏn-drō-săr-KŌ-mă	
chromosome (37)	KRŌ-mō-sōm	
coccygeal (49)	kŏk-sĭ-JĒ-ăl	
coccyx (48)	KŎK-sĭks	
cranial cavity (45)	KRĀ-nē-ăl KĂ-vĭ-tē	
craniotomy (54)	krā-nē-ŎT-ō-mē	
cytoplasm (37)	SĪ-tō-plăzm	
deep (50)	dēp	
diaphragm (45)	DĪ-ă-frăm	
disk (disc) (49)	dĭsk	

TERM	PRONUNCIATION	MEANING
distal (50)	DĬS-tăl	
dorsal (45)	DŎR-săl	
endoplasmic reticulum (37)	ĕn-dō-PLĂZ-mĭk rē-TĬK-ū-lŭm	
epigastric region (49)	ĕp-ĭ-GĂS-trĭk RĒ-jŭn	
epithelial cells (40)	ĕp-ĭ-THĒ-lē-ăl sĕlz	
frontal plane (52)	FRŬN-tăl plān	
genes (37)	jēnz	
histology (54)	hĭs-TŎL-ō-jē	
hypochondriac region (49)	hī-pō-KŎN-drē-ăk RĒ-jŭn	
hypogastric region (49)	hĭ-pō-GĂS-trĭk RĒ-jŭn	
iliac (54)	ĬL-ē-ăk	
inferior (50)	in-FĒR-ē-ŭr	
inguinal region (49)	ĬNG-gwĭ-năl RĒ-jŭn	
intervertebral (56)	ĭn-tĕr-VĔR-tĕ-brăl *or*	
karyotype (37)	KĂR-ē-ō-tīp	
larynx (40)	LĂR-ĭnks	
lateral (50)	LĂT-ĕr-al	
lumbar region (49)	LŬM-băr RĒ-jŭn	
lumbosacral (55)	lŭm-bō-SĀ-krăl	
medial (50)	MĒ-dē-ăl	
mediastinum (45)	mē-dē-ă-STĪ-nŭm	
metabolism (37)	mĕ-TĂB-ō-lĭzm	
mitochondria (37)	mī-tō-KŎN-drē-ă	
nucleic (55)	nū-KLĒ-ĭk	
nucleus (37)	NŪ-klē-ŭs	
pelvic cavity (45)	PĔL-vĭk KĂ-vĭ-tē	
peritoneum (45)	pĕ-rĭ-tō-NĒ-ŭm	
pharynx (40)	FĂR-ĭnks	
pituitary gland (40)	pĭ-TOO-ĭ-tăr-ē glănd	
pleura (45)	PLOO-ră	

2

TERM	PRONUNCIATION	MEANING
pleural cavity (45)	PLOOR-ăl KĂ-vĭ-tē	
posterior (50)	pŏs-TĒR-ē-ŏr	
prone (50)	prōn	
proximal (50)	PRŎKS-ĭ-măl	
sacral (49)	SĀ-krăl	
sacrum (48)	SĀ-krŭm	
sagittal plane (52)	SĂJ-ĭ-tăl plān	
sarcoma (55)	săr-KŌ-mă	
spinal cavity (45)	SPĪ-năl KĂ-vĭ-tē	
spinal column (49)	SPĪ-năl KŎL-ŭm	
spinal cord (49)	SPĪ-năl kŏrd	
superficial (50)	sū-pĕr-FĬSH-ăl	
superior (50)	sū-PĒR-ē-ŭr	
supine (50)	SOO-pīn	
thoracic cavity (45)	thō-RĂS-ĭk KĂ-vĭ-tē	
thoracotomy (56)	thō-ră-KŎT-ō-mē	
thyroid gland (40)	THĪ-royd glănd	
trachea (40)	TRĀ-kē-ă	
tracheal (56)	TRĀ-kē-ăl	
transverse plane (52)	trănz-VĔRS plān	
umbilical region (49)	ŭm-BĬL-ĭ-kăl RĒ-jŭn	
ureter (40)	Ū-rĕ-tĕr *or* ū-RĒ-tĕr	
urethra (40)	ū-RĒ-thră	
uterus (40)	Ū-tĕ-rŭs	
ventral (45)	VĔN-trăl	
vertebra (49)	VĔR-tĕ-bră	
vertebrae (49)	VĔR-tĕ-brā	
vertebral (56)	VĔR-tĕ-brăl *or* vĕr-TĒ-brăl	
viscera (40)	VĬS-ĕr-ă	
visceral (56)	VĬS-ĕr-ăl	

REVIEW SHEET

Write the meaning of each combining form, prefix, or suffix in the space provided, and test yourself. Check your answers with the information in the chapter or in the Glossary (Medical Word Parts—English), at the end of the book.

Combining Forms

COMBINING FORM	MEANING	COMBINING FORM	MEANING
abdomin/o	____________	lumb/o	____________
adip/o	____________	medi/o	____________
anter/o	____________	nucle/o	____________
bol/o	____________	pelv/i	____________
cervic/o	____________	poster/o	____________
chondr/o	____________	proxim/o	____________
chrom/o	____________	sacr/o	____________
coccyg/o	____________	sarc/o	____________
crani/o	____________	spin/o	____________
cyt/o	____________	thel/o, theli/o	____________
dist/o	____________	thorac/o	____________
dors/o	____________	trache/o	____________
hist/o	____________	umbilic/o	____________
ili/o	____________	ventr/o	____________
inguin/o	____________	vertebr/o	____________
kary/o	____________	viscer/o	____________
later/o	____________		

Prefixes

PREFIX	MEANING	PREFIX	MEANING
ana-	____________	hypo-	____________
cata-	____________	inter-	____________
epi-	____________	meta-	____________

Suffixes

SUFFIX	MEANING	SUFFIX	MEANING
-al	________________	-oma	________________
-eal	________________	-ose	________________
-ectomy	________________	-plasm	________________
-iac	________________	-somes	________________
-ior	________________	-tomy	________________
-ism	________________	-type	________________

Label the regions and quadrants (use abbreviations) of the abdominopelvic cavity. Check your answers in the chapter, pages 46 and 47.

REGIONS

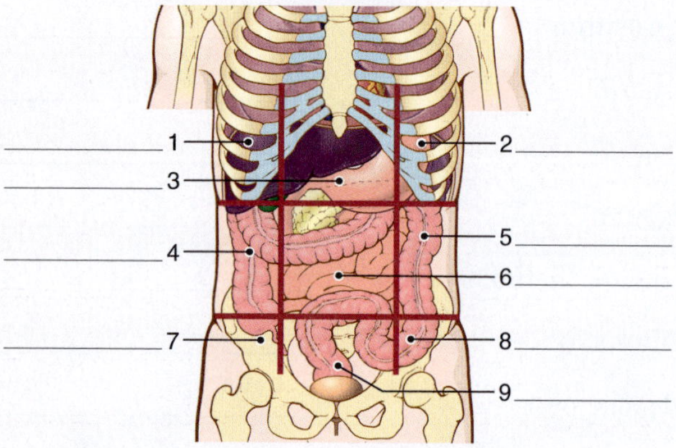

QUADRANTS

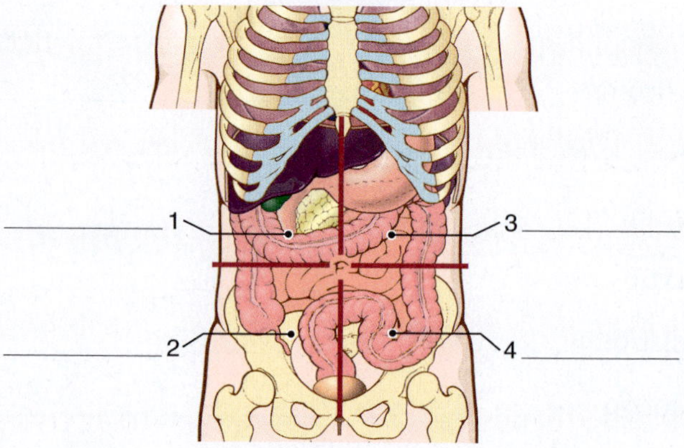

Name the divisions of the spinal column. Check your answers on page 48.

neck region (C1 to C7) ________________________________

chest region (T1 to T12) ________________________________

lower back (loin) region (L1 to L5) ________________________________

region of the sacrum (S1 to S5) ________________________________

tailbone region ________________________________

Name the planes of the head as pictured below. Check your answers on page 52.

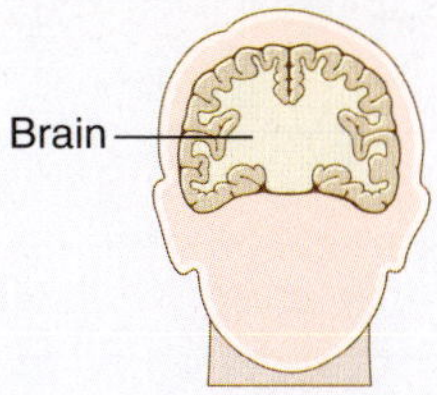

vertical plane that divides the body into anterior and posterior portions

____

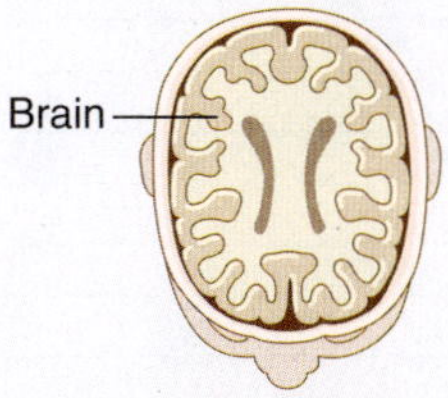

horizontal plane that divides the body into upper and lower portions

____

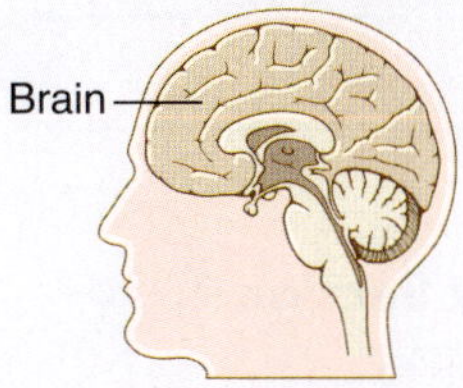

vertical plane that divides the body into right and left portions

____

Name the positional and directional terms. Check your answers on pages 50-51.

front of the body ______________________________

back of the body ______________________________

away from the surface of the body ______________________________

on the surface of the body ______________________________

far from the point of attachment to the trunk or far from the beginning of a structure

____

near the point of attachment to the trunk or near the beginning of a structure

____

below another structure ______________________________

above another structure ______________________________

pertaining to the side ______________________________

pertaining to the middle ______________________________

lying on the belly ______________________________

lying on the back ______________________________

2

Give the meanings of the following terms that pertain to the cell. Check your answers with Study Section 1, page 37.

chromosomes ______________________________

mitochondria ______________________________

nucleus ______________________________

DNA ______________________________

endoplasmic reticulum ______________________________

cell membrane ______________________________

catabolism ______________________________

anabolism ______________________________

metabolism ______________________________

Give the term that suits the meaning provided. Check your answers with Study Section 2, page 40.

membrane surrounding the lungs ______________________________

membrane surrounding the abdominal viscera ______________________________

muscular wall separating the thoracic and abdominal cavities ______________________________

space between the lungs, containing the heart, windpipe, aorta ______________________________

a backbone ______________________________

a pad of cartilage between each backbone and the next ______________________________

2

evolve *Please refer to the Evolve website for additional exercises, games, and images related to this chapter.*

CHAPTER 3

Suffixes

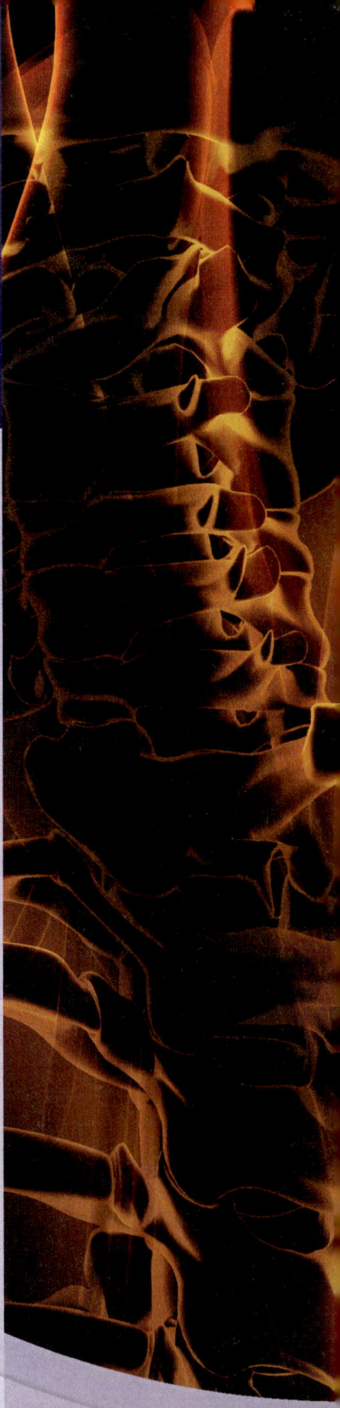

This chapter is divided into the following sections:

CHAPTER GOALS

- Define new suffixes and review those presented in previous chapters.
- Gain practice in word analysis by using these suffixes with combining forms to build and understand terms.
- Identify the functions of the different types of blood cells in the body.

INTRODUCTION

In this chapter you will encounter many of the most common suffixes in the medical language. As you work through the entire book, these suffixes will appear often. An additional group of suffixes is presented in Chapter 6.

Additional combining forms are presented in this chapter to use in making words with suffixes. Your mastery of this material and your analysis of the words in the section on Suffixes and Terminology will increase your medical language vocabulary.

With this new knowledge, you can expect to expand your understanding of terminology beyond basic word analysis. To support this broader understanding, **A Closer Look** beginning of page 84, contains relevant images and gives more detailed explanations of new terms.

COMBINING FORMS

Use the following list of combining forms as you write the meanings of terms starting on page 76.

COMBINING FORMS

COMBINING FORM	MEANING	COMBINING FORM	MEANING
abdomin/o	abdomen	**bronch/o**	bronchial tubes (two tubes, one right and one left, that branch from the trachea to enter the lungs)
acr/o	extremities, top, extreme point	**carcin/o**	cancer
acu/o	sharp, severe, sudden	**cardi/o**	heart
aden/o	gland	**chem/o**	drug, chemical
adip/o	fat	**chondr/o**	cartilage
amni/o	amnion (sac surrounding the embryo in the uterus)	**chron/o**	time
angi/o	vessel	**col/o**	colon (large intestine)
arteri/o	artery	**cyst/o**	urinary bladder
arthr/o	joint	**encephal/o**	brain
axill/o	armpit	**erythr/o**	red
bi/o	life	**hem/o**	blood
blephar/o	eyelid	**hepat/o**	liver

3

COMBINING FORM	MEANING	COMBINING FORM	MEANING
hydr/o	water, fluid	**oste/o**	bone
inguin/o	groin	**ot/o**	ear
isch/o	to hold back	**path/o**	disease
lapar/o	abdomen, abdominal wall	**peritone/o**	peritoneum
laryng/o	larynx	**phag/o**	to eat, swallow
leuk/o	white	**phleb/o**	vein
lymph/o	lymph *Lymph, a clear fluid that bathes tissue spaces, is contained in special lymph vessels and nodes throughout the body.*	**plas/o**	formation, development
		pleur/o	pleura (membrane surrounding lungs and adjacent to chest wall)
mamm/o	breast	**pneumon/o**	lungs
mast/o	breast	**pulmon/o**	lungs
morph/o	shape, form	**radi/o**	x-rays
muc/o	mucus	**rect/o**	rectum
my/o	muscle	**ren/o**	kidney
myel/o	spinal cord, bone marrow *Context of usage indicates the meaning intended.*	**rhin/o**	nose
		sarc/o	flesh
		splen/o	spleen
necr/o	death (of cells or whole body)	**staphyl/o**	clusters
		strept/o	twisted chains
nephr/o	kidney	**thorac/o**	chest
neur/o	nerve	**thromb/o**	clot
neutr/o	neutrophil (a white blood cell)	**tonsill/o**	tonsils
nucle/o	nucleus	**trache/o**	trachea (windpipe)
ophthalm/o	eye	**ven/o**	vein

Larynx and Other Parts of the Body Ending in x

coccy**x** = tailbone
laryn**x** = voice box
pharyn**x** = throat
phalan**x** = finger or toe

To make combining forms for parts of the body that end in x, **substitute g for x:**

coccy**g**/o
laryn**g**/o
pharyn**g**/o
phalan**g**/o

3

SUFFIXES AND TERMINOLOGY

NOUN SUFFIXES

The following list includes common noun suffixes. After the meaning of each suffix, terminology illustrates the use of the suffix in various words. Recall the basic rule for building a medical term: Use a combining vowel, such as o, to connect the root to the suffix. However, drop the combining vowel if the suffix begins with a vowel—for example, **gastr/itis,** *not* "gastr/o/itis."

Beginning on page 84, more detail is given about specific terms. This section, called **A Closer Look,** will give you a fuller understanding of the terminology.

SUFFIX	MEANING	TERMINOLOGY	MEANING
-algia	pain	arthralgia	______
		otalgia	______
		neuralgia	______
		myalgia	______
-cele	hernia *(see **A Closer Look,** page 84)*	rectocele	______
		cystocele	______
-centesis	surgical puncture to remove fluid	thoracentesis *Notice that this term is shortened from thoracocentesis.*	______
		amniocentesis *The amnion is the sac (membrane) surrounding the embryo (fetus after the 8th week) in the uterus. Fluid accumulates within the amnion and may be withdrawn for analysis between the 12th and 18th weeks of pregnancy. See Figure 3-1.*	______
		abdominocentesis *This procedure is more commonly known as abdominal **paracentesis** (para- means beside or near). A tube is placed through an incision in the abdomen and fluid is removed from the peritoneal cavity (beside the abdominal organs).*	______
-coccus (singular) **-cocci** (plural)	berry-shaped bacterium (*plural*: bacteria)	streptococcus *See **A Closer Look: Streptococcus,** page 84.*	______
		staphylococci *(stăf-ĭ-lō-KŎK-sī) Microbiologists often refer to bacteria in clusters as "staph" (staphylococci).*	______

Formation of Plurals

Words ending in **-us** commonly form their plural by dropping **-us** and adding **-i**. Other examples of **-us** plural formation follow:

- nucle**us** → nucle**i**
- bronch**us** → bronch**i**
- thromb**us** → thromb**i**

See Appendix I at the end of the book, page 981, for additional information about plural formation.

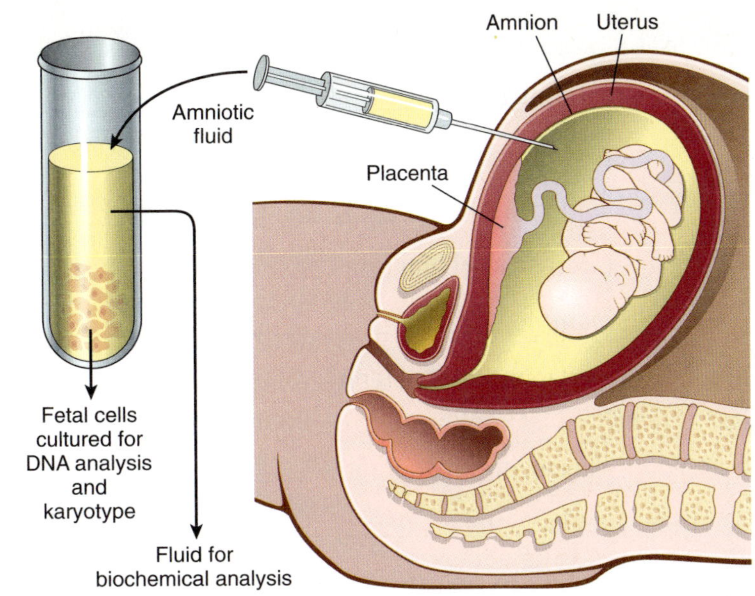

FIGURE 3-1 **Amniocentesis.** Under ultrasound guidance (using imaging based on high-frequency sound waves), the physician inserts a needle through the uterine wall and amnion, into the amniotic cavity. Amniotic fluid, containing fetal cells, is withdrawn and grown (cultured) for microscopic analysis. A karyotype is made to study chromosomes and fluid is examined for high levels of chemicals that indicate defects in the spinal cord of the fetus.

SUFFIX	MEANING	TERMINOLOGY	MEANING
-cyte	cell	erythrocyte	______________ *See **A Closer Look: Blood Cells,** page 85.*
		leukocyte	______________
		thrombocyte	______________
-dynia	pain	pleurodynia	______________ *Pain in the chest wall muscles that is aggravated by breathing.*
-ectomy	excision, removal, resection	laryngectomy	______________
		mastectomy	______________
-emia	blood condition	anemia	______________
		ischemia	______________ *Literally to hold back (isch/o) blood (-emia) from a part of the body or tissue. Because of a decrease in blood supply (blood clot in a vessel or narrowing and closing off of a vessel), tissue becomes **ischemic** and can even die because it becomes deprived of oxygen.*

Anemia

While anemia literally means "no blood," it is actually a condition marked by **reduction** in the number of erythrocytes or in the amount of hemoglobin in blood. Examples of types of anemias are:

- **iron deficiency anemia** (iron is needed to make hemoglobin)
- **sickle cell anemia** (erythrocytes assume an abnormal sickle shape and clog blood vessels)
- **aplastic anemia** (erythrocytes, leukocytes, and thrombocytes are not formed in bone marrow)

SUFFIX	MEANING	TERMINOLOGY	MEANING
-genesis	condition of producing, forming	carcinogenesis	
		pathogenesis	
		angiogenesis	
-gram	record	electroencephalogram	
		mammogram	
-graph	instrument for recording	electroencephalograph	
-graphy	process of recording	electroencephalography	
		angiography	
-itis	inflammation	bronchitis	
		myelitis *Myel/o means spinal cord in this term.*	
		tonsillitis *Tonsils (notice the spelling with one letter, whereas the combining form has a double letter) are lymphatic tissue in the back of the throat. See Figure 3-2.*	
		thrombophlebitis *Also called phlebitis.*	
-logy	study of	ophthalmology	
		morphology	
-lysis	breakdown, destruction, separation	hemolysis *Breakdown of red blood cells with release of hemoglobin.*	
-malacia	softening	osteomalacia	
		chondromalacia	

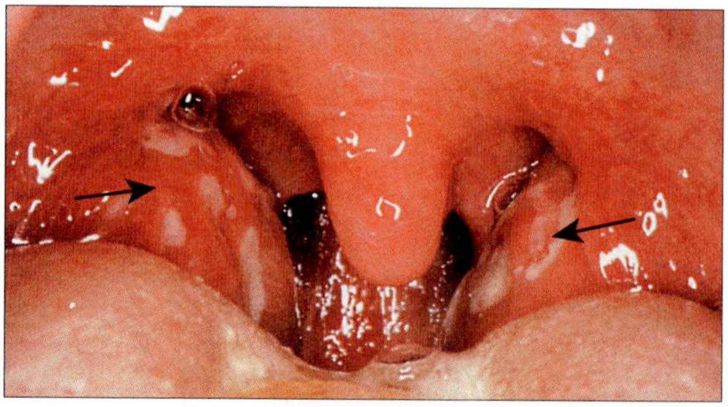

FIGURE 3-2 **Tonsillitis.** This shows streptococcal tonsillitis with intense erythema (redness) of the tonsils (see arrows) and a creamy-yellow exudate (pus containing leukocytes and bacteria). Normally, tonsils contain lymphocytes that fight bacteria. When they become infected and inflamed, **tonsillectomy** may be necessary.

SUFFIX	MEANING	TERMINOLOGY	MEANING
-megaly	enlargement	acromegaly *See **A Closer Look: Acromegaly,** page 86.*	
		splenomegaly *See **A Closer Look: Splenomegaly,** page 86.*	
-oma	tumor, mass, collection of fluid	myoma *A benign tumor.*	
		myosarcoma *A malignant tumor. Muscle is a type of flesh (sarc/o) tissue.*	
		multiple myeloma *Myel/o means bone marrow in this term. This malignant tumor occurs in bone marrow tissue throughout the body.*	
		hematoma	
-opsy	to view	biopsy	
		necropsy *This is an autopsy or postmortem examination.*	
-osis	condition, usually abnormal	necrosis	
		hydronephrosis	
		leukocytosis	
-pathy	disease condition	cardiomyopathy *Primary disease of the heart muscle in the absence of a known underlying etiology (cause).*	
-penia	deficiency	erythropenia	
		neutropenia *In this term, neutr/o indicates neutrophil (a type of white blood cell).*	
		thrombocytopenia	
-phobia	fear	acrophobia *Fear of heights. Acr/o means extremities, in the sense of extreme or far points.*	
		agoraphobia *An anxiety disorder marked by fear of venturing out into a crowded place. Agora means marketplace.*	

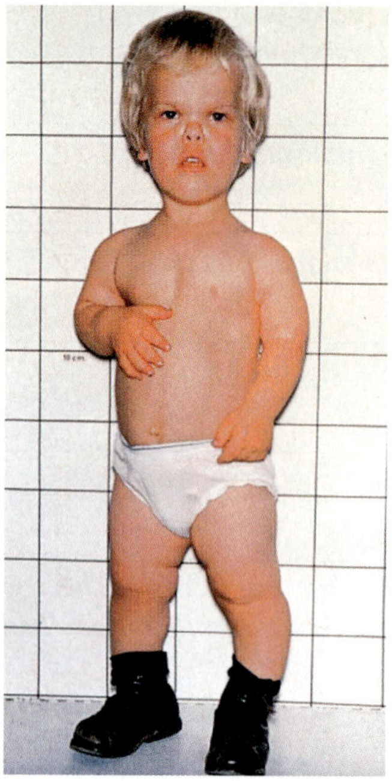

FIGURE 3-3 Achondroplasia. A boy with achondroplasia. His abnormalities include short stature with normal length of the trunk, short limbs and fingers, bowed legs, prominent forehead, and depressed nasal bridge. *(Courtesy of A.E. Chudley, MD, Section of Genetics and Metabolism, Department of Pediatrics and Child Health, Children's Hospital, Winnipeg, Manitoba, Canada.)*

SUFFIX	MEANING	TERMINOLOGY	MEANING
-plasia	development, formation, growth	achondroplasia *This is an inherited disorder or can be the result of a mutation (change) in a specific gene. Bones of the arms and legs do not grow to normal size because of a defect in cartilage and bone formation. Dwarfism results, marked by short limbs, but normal-sized head and trunk and normal intelligence. See Figure 3-3.*	______
-plasty	surgical repair	angioplasty *An interventional cardiologist opens a narrowed blood vessel (artery) using a balloon that is inflated after insertion into the vessel. Stents, or slotted tubes, are then put in place to keep the artery open.*	______
-ptosis	drooping, falling, prolapse	blepharoptosis *Physicians use* ***ptosis*** *(TŌ-sĭs) alone to indicate drooping of the upper eyelids or the breasts. See Figure 3-4.*	______
-sclerosis	hardening	arteriosclerosis *In atherosclerosis (a form of arteriosclerosis), deposits of fat (ather/o means fatty material) collect in an artery.*	______

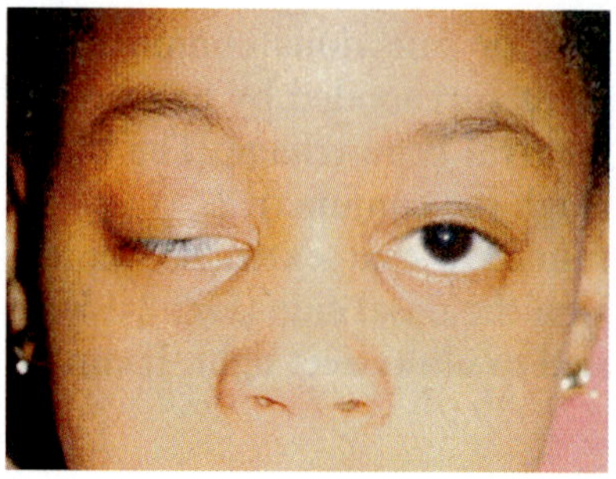

FIGURE 3-4 Ptosis of the upper eyelid (blepharoptosis). This condition may be congenital (appear at birth), can occur with aging, or may be associated with stroke (cerebrovascular accident), cranial nerve damage, and other neurologic disorders. The eyelid droops because of muscle weakness.

SUFFIX	MEANING	TERMINOLOGY	MEANING
-scope	instrument for visual examination	laparoscope	______
-scopy	process of visual examination (with an endoscope)	laparoscopy *See **A Closer Look: Laparoscopy,** page 87.*	______
-stasis	controlling, stopping	metastasis *Meta- means beyond. A metastasis is the spread of a malignant tumor beyond its original site to a secondary organ or location.*	______
		hemostasis *Blood flow is stopped naturally by clotting or artificially by compression or suturing of a wound.*	______
-stomy	opening to form a mouth (stoma)	colostomy	______
		tracheostomy	______
-therapy	treatment	hydrotherapy	______
		chemotherapy	______
		radiotherapy *High-energy radiation is used to treat, not diagnose, illness.*	______
-tomy	incision, cutting into	laparotomy *Also referred to as a "lap," this procedure is creation of a large incision into the peritoneal cavity, often performed on an exploratory basis.*	______
		phlebotomy	______
		tracheotomy *See **A Closer Look: Tracheotomy,** page 88.*	______

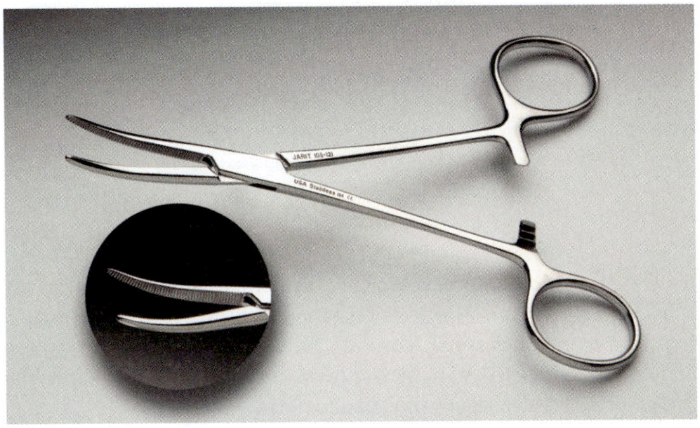

FIGURE 3-5 **Hemostat.**

Hemostasis and Ischemia

Hemostasis is the control of blood loss after injury or during surgery. A **hemostat** is a surgical clamp (Figure 3-5.) **Ischemia** occurs when blood flow to tissues is not sufficient. This condition deprives cells of oxygen and, if not reversed, leads to tissue death.

SUFFIX	MEANING	TERMINOLOGY	MEANING
-trophy	development, nourishment	hypertrophy *Cells increase in size, not number. Muscles of weight lifters often hypertrophy (hī-PĔR-trō-fē).*	
		atrophy *Cells decrease in size. Muscles atrophy when immobilized in a cast and not in use.*	

The following are shorter noun suffixes that usually are attached to roots in words.

SUFFIX	MEANING	TERMINOLOGY	MEANING
-er	one who	radiographer *A technologist who assists in the making of diagnostic x-ray pictures.*	
-ia	condition	leukemia	
		pneumonia	
-ist	specialist	nephrologist	
-ole	little, small	arteriole *See Figure 3-6.*	
-ule	little, small	venule *See Figure 3-6.*	
-um, -ium	structure, tissue	pericardium *This membrane surrounds the heart.*	

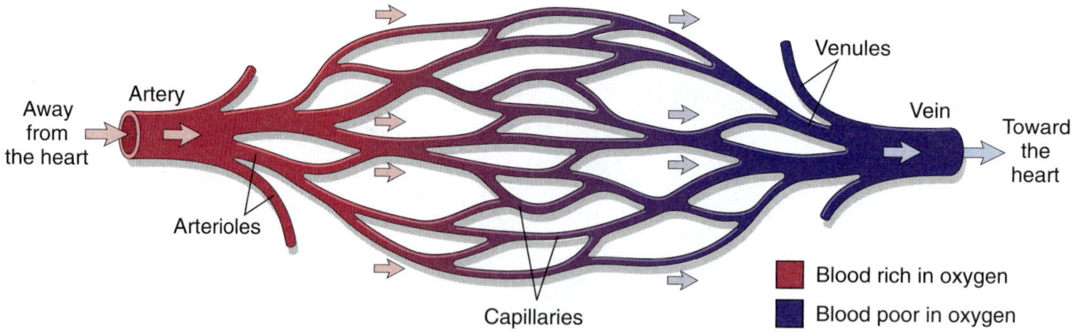

FIGURE 3-6 Relationship of blood vessels. An **artery** carries blood rich in oxygen from the heart to the organs of the body. In the organs, the artery narrows to form **arterioles** (small arteries) that branch into capillaries (the smallest blood vessels). Through the thin walls of capillaries, oxygen leaves the blood and enters cells. Thus, the capillaries branching into **venules** (small veins) carry blood poor in oxygen. Venules lead to a vein that brings oxygen-poor blood back to the heart.

Leukemia and Lymphoma

Leukemia is a malignancy of white blood cells, such as **granulocytes,** that derive from bone marrow **(myeloid)** tissue. An example of a type of leukemia is acute myelogenous leukemia (AML). **Lymphoma** is also a malignancy of white blood cells (**lymphocytes**) that arise in **lymphoid** tissue, such as lymph nodes. Examples of lymphomas are Hodgkin disease and non-Hodgkin lymphoma

SUFFIX	MEANING	TERMINOLOGY	MEANING
-us	structure, substance	mucus	
		esophagus *Eso- means within or inward.*	
-y	condition, process	nephropathy	

ADJECTIVE SUFFIXES

The following are adjective suffixes. No simple rule will explain which suffix meaning "pertaining to" is used with a specific combining form. Concentrate on identifying the suffix in each term, then write the meaning of the term.

SUFFIX	MEANING	TERMINOLOGY	MEANING
-ac, -iac	pertaining to	cardiac	
-al	pertaining to	peritoneal	
		inguinal	
		pleural	
-ar	pertaining to	tonsillar	
-ary	pertaining to	pulmonary	
		axillary	
-eal	pertaining to	laryngeal	
-genic	pertaining to producing, produced by or in	carcinogenic	
		osteogenic *An osteogenic sarcoma is a malignant tumor produced in bone.*	
-ic, -ical	pertaining to	chronic ***Acute** is the opposite of chronic. It describes a disease that is of rapid onset and has severe symptoms and brief duration.*	
		pathologic	
-oid	resembling, derived from	adenoids *See **A Closer Look: Adenoids,** page 88*	
		mucoid	
-ose	pertaining to, full of	adipose	
-ous	pertaining to	mucous membrane ***Mucous** (an adjective) **membranes** produce the sticky secretion called **mucus** (a noun).*	
-tic	pertaining to	necrotic	

A CLOSER LOOK

HERNIA

A **hernia** is protrusion of an organ or the muscular wall of an organ through the cavity that normally contains it. A **hiatal hernia** occurs when the stomach protrudes upward into the mediastinum through the esophageal opening in the diaphragm, and an **inguinal hernia** occurs when part of the intestine protrudes downward into the groin region and commonly into the scrotal sac in the male. A **cystocele** occurs when part of the urinary bladder herniates through the vaginal wall as a result of weakness of the pelvic muscles (Figure 3-7). A **rectocele** is the protrusion of a portion of the rectum toward the vagina (Figure 3-7). An **omphalocele** (omphal/o = umbilicus, navel) is a herniation of the intestines through a weakness in the abdominal wall around the navel occurring in infants at birth.

STREPTOCOCCUS

Streptococcus, a berry-shaped bacterium, grows in twisted chains. One group of **streptococci** causes such conditions as "strep throat," tonsillitis, rheumatic fever, and certain kidney ailments, whereas another group causes infections in teeth, in the sinuses (cavities) of the nose and face, and in the valves of the heart.

Staphylococci, other berry-shaped bacteria, grow in small clusters like grapes. Staphylococcal lesions may be external (skin abscesses, boils, styes) or internal (abscesses in bone and kidney). An **abscess** is a collection of pus, white blood cells, and protein that is present at the site of infection. **MRSA** (methicillin-resistant *Staphylococcus aureus*) is a serious staphylococcal condition that is difficult to treat with antibiotics.

Examples of **diplococci** (berry-shaped bacteria organized in pairs; dipl/o = two) are **pneumococci** (pneum/o = lungs) and **gonococci** (gon/o = seed). Pneumococci cause bacterial pneumonia, and gonococci invade the reproductive organs, causing gonorrhea (a sexually transmitted infection). Figure 3-8 illustrates the different growth patterns of streptococci, staphylococci, and diplococci.

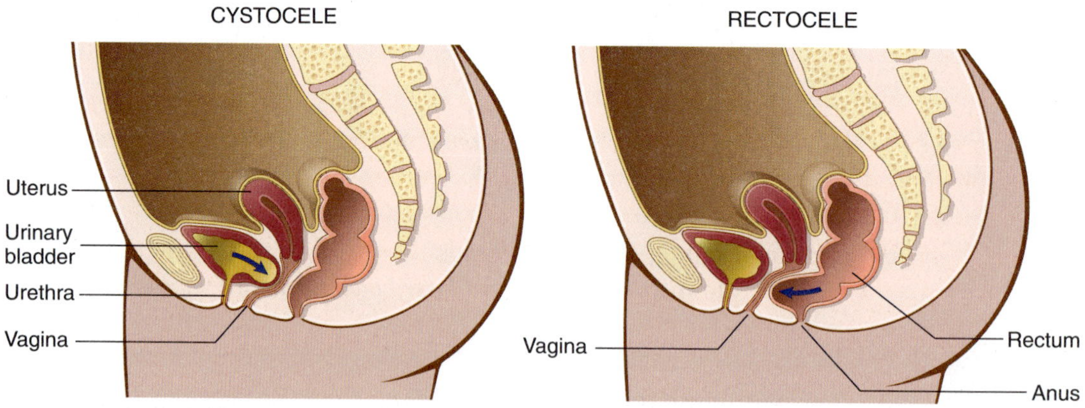

FIGURE 3-7 **Hernias: cystocele and rectocele.** Arrows point to the areas of herniation. In a cystocele a portion of the urinary bladder herniates posteriorly toward the vagina. In a rectocele a portion of the rectum herniates anteriorly toward the vagina.

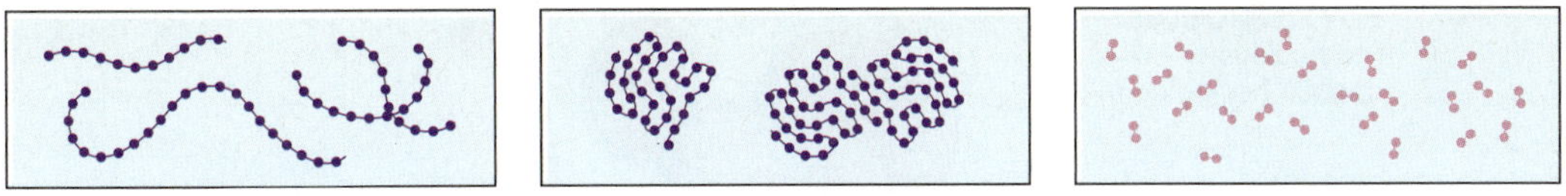

FIGURE 3-8 **Types of coccal bacteria.** Notice the berry or rounded shape of each bacterium. Streptococci and staphylococci are **gram-positive bacteria**, meaning that they retain the light purple color of the stain used in Gram's method (named for Hans C.J. Gram, Danish physician, 1853-1938.) **Gram-negative bacteria (such as diplococci) have the pink color of the counterstain (safranin) used in Gram's method.**

BLOOD CELLS

Study Figure 3-9 as you read the following, to note the differences among the three different types of cells in the blood.

Erythrocytes, or red blood cells, are the first type. These cells are made in the bone marrow (soft tissue in the center of certain bones). They carry oxygen from the lungs through the blood to all body cells. Body cells use oxygen to burn food and release energy (catabolism). **Hemoglobin** (globin = protein), an important protein in erythrocytes, carries the oxygen through the bloodstream.

Leukocytes, or white blood cells, are the second type. There are five different kinds of leukocytes: three granulocytes, or polymorphonuclear cells, and two mononuclear cells.

- **Granulocytes,** or polymorphonuclear cells, contain dark-staining granules in their cytoplasm and have a multilobed nucleus. They are formed in the bone marrow, and there are three types:
  1. **Eosinophils** (granules stain red [eosin/o = rosy] with acidic stain) are active and increased in number in allergic conditions such as asthma. About 3% of leukocytes are eosinophils.
  2. **Basophils** (granules stain blue with basic [bas/o = basic] stain). The function of basophils is not clear, but the number of these cells increases in the healing phase of inflammation. Less than 1% of leukocytes are basophils.
  3. **Neutrophils** (granules stain a pale purple with neutral stain) are important disease-fighting cells. They are **phagocytes** (phag/o = eating, swallowing)—they engulf and digest bacteria. They are the most numerous disease-fighting "soldiers" (50% to 60% of leukocytes are neutrophils) and are referred to as "polys" or **polymorphonuclear leukocytes** (poly = many, morph/o = shape) because of their multilobed nucleus.
- **Mononuclear leukocytes (agranulocytes)** have one large nucleus and only a few granules in their cytoplasm. They are produced in bone marrow as well as in lymph nodes and the spleen. There are two types of mononuclear leukocytes (see Figure 3-9):
  4. **Lymphocytes** (lymph cells) fight disease by producing antibodies, thereby destroying foreign cells. They also may attach directly to foreign cells and destroy them. Two types of lymphocytes are T cells and B cells. About 32% of leukocytes are lymphocytes. In AIDS (acquired immunodeficiency syndrome), patients have a serious depletion of T lymphocytes (T cells).
  5. **Monocytes** (cells with one [mon/o = one] very large nucleus) engulf and destroy cellular debris after neutrophils have attacked foreign cells. Monocytes leave the bloodstream and enter tissues (such as lung and liver) to become **macrophages,** which are large phagocytes. Monocytes make up about 4% of all leukocytes.

Thrombocytes or **platelets** (clotting cells) are the third type of blood cell. These are actually tiny fragments of cells formed in the bone marrow and are necessary for blood clotting.

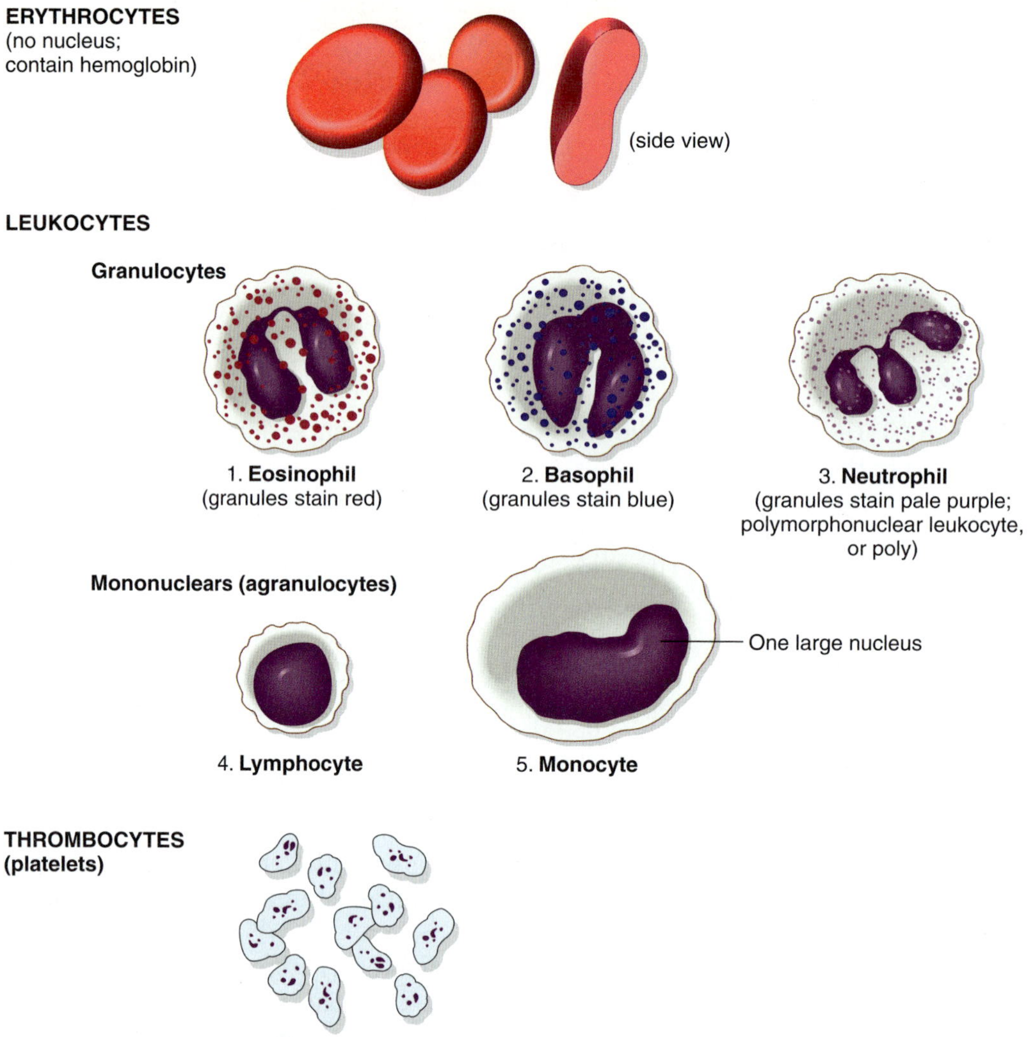

FIGURE 3-9 **Types of blood cells.** Here's an easy way to remember the names of the five leukocytes:
Never (neutrophil)
Let (lymphocyte)
Monkeys (monocyte)
Eat (eosinophil)
Bananas (basophil)

ACROMEGALY

Acromegaly is an endocrine disorder. It occurs when the **pituitary gland,** attached to the base of the brain, produces an excessive amount of growth hormone *after* the completion of puberty. The excess growth hormone most often results from a benign tumor of the pituitary gland. A person with acromegaly typically is of normal height because the long bones have stopped growth after puberty, but bones and soft tissue in the hands, feet, and face grow abnormally (Figure 3-10). Abraham Lincoln was believed to have features of acromegaly. See Chapter 18, Endocrine System, page 747.

SPLENOMEGALY

The spleen is an organ in the left upper quadrant (LUQ) of the abdomen (below the diaphragm and to the side of the stomach). Composed of lymph tissue and blood vessels, it disposes of dying red blood cells and manufactures white blood cells (lymphocytes) to fight

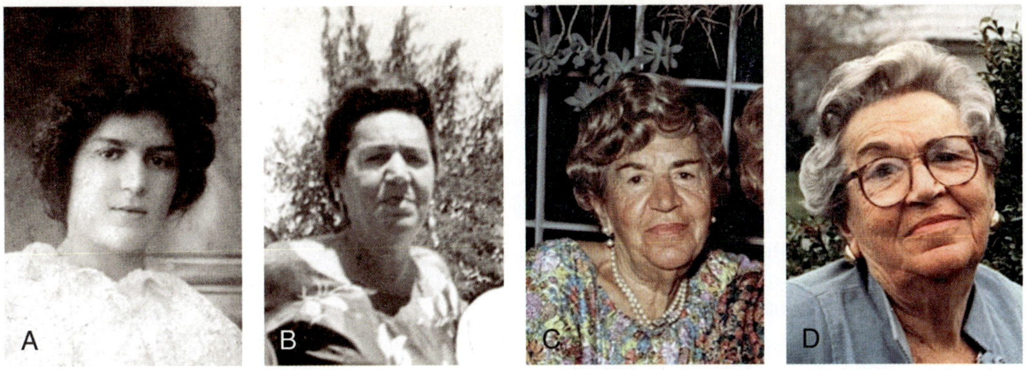

FIGURE 3-10 **Acromegaly.** Notice the changes in facial features (shape of face, protruding nose, jaw and brow) of my grandmother, Bessie Brandwein, at **A,** age 20; **B**, age 40; **C**, age 70; and **D**, age 85.

disease. Splenomegaly occurs with development of high blood pressure in hepatic veins (portal hypertension) and hemolytic blood diseases (anemias involving excessive destruction or lysis of red blood cells). If the spleen is removed **(splenectomy),** other organs carry out its functions.

LAPAROSCOPY

Laparoscopy (a form of **minimally invasive surgery**) is visual examination of the abdominal cavity using a laparoscope. A surgeon inserts the laparoscope, a lighted telescopic instrument, through an incision in the abdomen near the navel. Then, gas (carbon dioxide) is infused into the peritoneal cavity, to separate and prevent injury to abdominal structures during surgery. Surgeons use laparoscopy to examine abdominal viscera for evidence of disease (performing biopsies) or for procedures such as removal of the appendix, gallbladder, adrenal gland, spleen, or ovary, colon resection, and repair of hernias. The laparoscope contains an instrument to clip and collapse the fallopian tubes (tubal ligation), which prevents sperm cells from reaching eggs that leave the ovary (Figure 3-11).

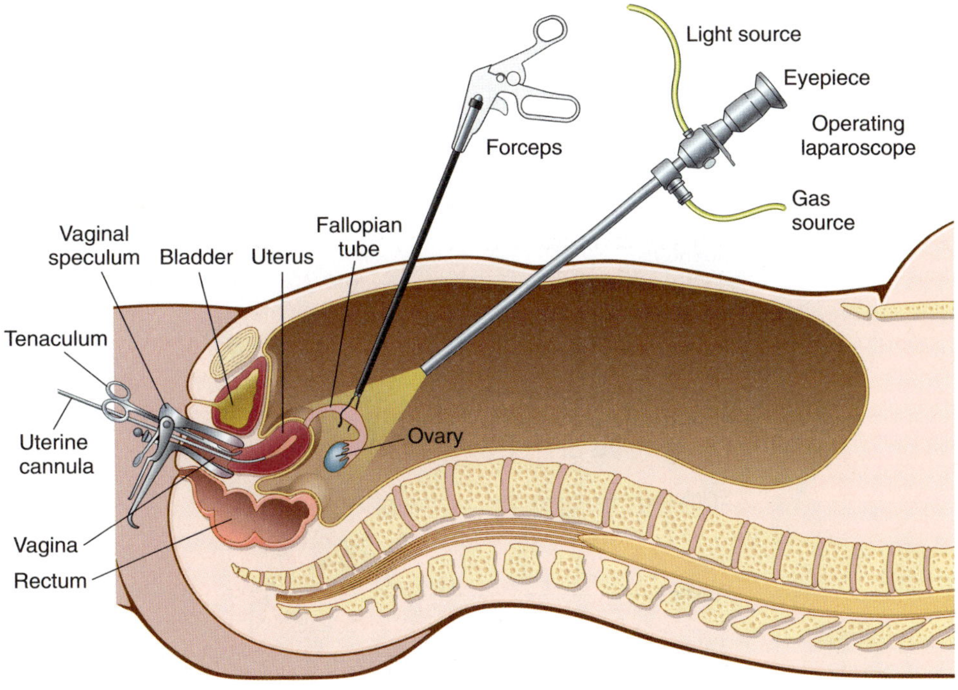

FIGURE 3-11 **Laparoscopy for tubal ligation** (interruption of the continuity of the fallopian tubes) as a means of preventing future pregnancy. The **tenaculum** grasps the cervix. The **vaginal speculum** keeps the vaginal cavity open. The **uterine cannula** is a tube placed into the uterus to manipulate the uterus during the procedure. **Forceps**, placed through the laparoscope, grasp or move tissue.

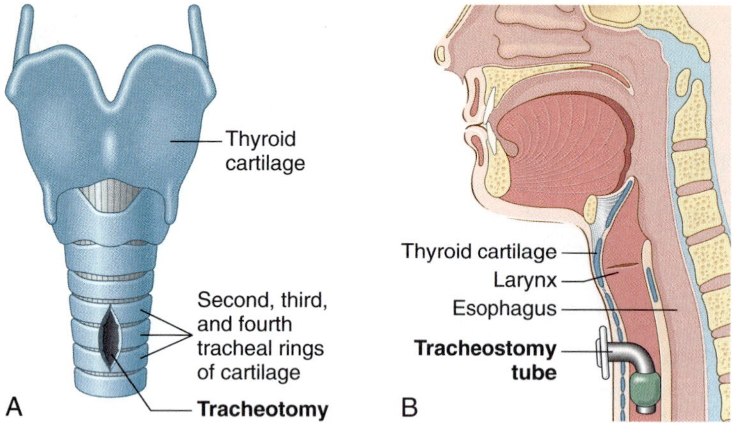

FIGURE 3-12 **A, Tracheotomy. B, Tracheostomy.**

TRACHEOTOMY

A **tracheotomy** is an incision into the trachea to open it below a blockage. Tracheotomy may be performed to remove a foreign body or to obtain a biopsy specimen (Figure 3-12A).

A **tracheostomy** is an opening into the trachea through which an indwelling tube is inserted. The tube is required to allow air to flow into the lungs or to help remove secretions (mucus) from the bronchial tubes. When a temporary tracheostomy is performed, extreme care is used to insert the tracheostomy tube below the larynx so that the vocal cords are not damaged (Figure 3-12B).

ADENOIDS

The **adenoids** are small masses of lymphatic tissue in the part of the pharynx (throat) near the nose and nasal passages. The literal meaning, "resembling glands," is appropriate because they are neither endocrine nor exocrine glands. Enlargement of adenoids may cause blockage of the airway from the nose to the pharynx, and adenoidectomy may be advised. The tonsils also are lymphatic tissue, and their location as well as that of the adenoids is indicated in Figure 3-13.

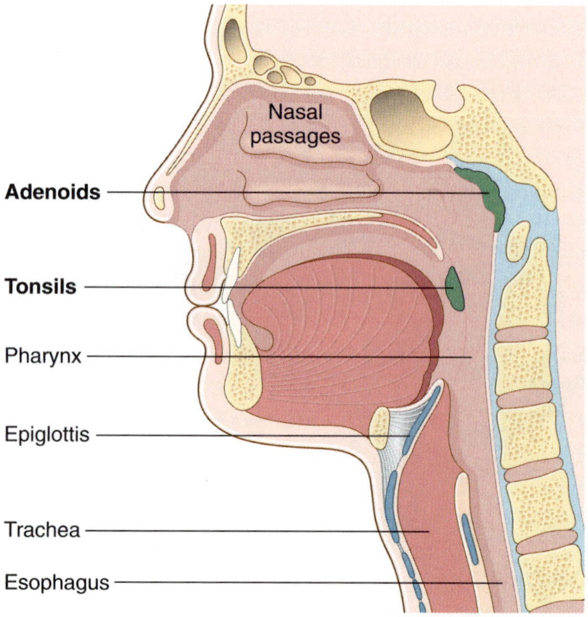

FIGURE 3-13 **Adenoids and tonsils.** The adenoids and tonsils are lymphatic tissue in the pharynx (throat).

PRACTICAL APPLICATIONS

A CASE STUDY: OMPHALOCELE

Baby Joel was born with a giant omphalocele. This is a herniation of intra-abdominal viscera. Usually babies with large omphaloceles have surgery right after birth, but Joel's parents were advised to wait until the abdominal muscles had grown large enough to close over the hernia.

For seven and a half months, Joel's parents covered the omphalocele with bacteriostatic burn cream to protect and toughen the sac. Then they covered it in gauze and foam supports. An ace bandage was wrapped around to push the omphalocele contents back into the abdomen. This procedure is known as "paint and wait."

Surgery was performed at 7.5 months to permanently repair the herniation. Baby Joel has had no further complications.

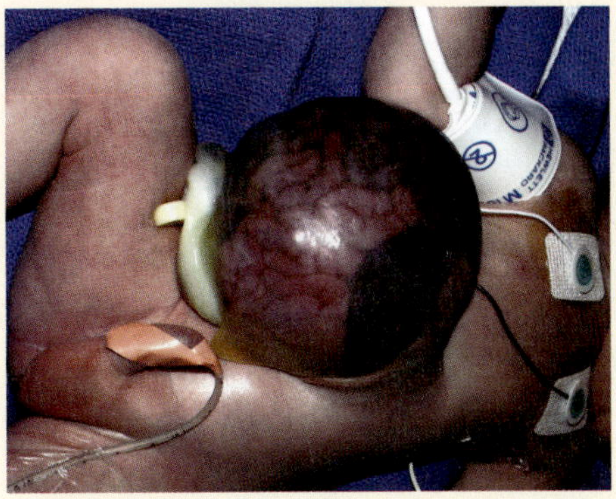

PROCEDURES

Choose the correct diagnostic or treatment procedure for each of the numbered definitions. Answers are on page 99.

amniocentesis	colostomy	mastectomy	thoracentesis
angiography	laparoscopy	paracentesis	tonsillectomy
angioplasty	laparotomy		

1. removal of abdominal fluid from the peritoneal space ____________________
2. large abdominal incision to remove an ovarian adenocarcinoma ____________________
3. removal of the breast ____________________
4. a method used to determine the karyotype of a fetus ____________________
5. surgical procedure to remove pharyngeal lymphatic tissue ____________________
6. surgical procedure to open clogged coronary arteries ____________________
7. method of removing fluid from the chest (pleural effusion) ____________________
8. procedure to drain feces from the body after bowel resection ____________________
9. x-ray procedure used to examine blood vessels before surgery ____________________
10. minimally invasive surgery within the abdomen ____________________

EXERCISES

Remember to check your answers carefully with the Answers to Exercises on pages 98 and 99.

A Give the meanings for the following suffixes.

1. -cele ______________________
2. -emia ______________________
3. -coccus ______________________
4. -gram ______________________
5. -cyte ______________________
6. -algia ______________________
7. -ectomy ______________________
8. -centesis ______________________
9. -genesis ______________________
10. -graph ______________________
11. -itis ______________________
12. -graphy ______________________

B Using the combining forms and your knowledge of suffixes, build medical terms for the following definitions.

amni/o	cyst/o	myel/o
angi/o	isch/o	staphyl/o
arthr/o	laryng/o	strept/o
bronch/o	mast/o	thorac/o
carcin/o	my/o	

3

1. hernia of the urinary bladder ______________________
2. pain of muscle ______________________
3. process of producing cancer ______________________
4. inflammation of the spinal cord ______________________
5. berry-shaped bacteria in twisted chains ______________________
6. surgical puncture to remove fluid from the chest ______________________
7. removal of the breast ______________________
8. inflammation of the tubes leading from the windpipe to the lungs ______________________
9. to hold back blood from cells ______________________
10. process of recording (x-ray) blood vessels ______________________
11. visual examination of joints ______________________
12. berry-shaped bacteria in clusters ______________________
13. resection of the voice box ______________________
14. surgical procedure to remove fluid from the sac around a fetus ______________________

C Match the following terms, which describe blood cells, with their meanings below.

basophil
eosinophil
erythrocyte
lymphocyte
monocyte
neutrophil
thrombocyte

1. granulocytic white blood cell (granules stain purple) that destroys foreign cells by engulfing and digesting them; also called a polymorphonuclear leukocyte ____________________
2. mononuclear white blood cell that destroys foreign cells by making antibodies ____________________
3. clotting cell; also called a platelet ____________________
4. leukocyte with reddish staining granules and numbers elevated in allergic reactions ____________________
5. red blood cell ____________________
6. mononuclear white blood cell that engulfs and digests cellular debris; contains one large nucleus ____________________
7. granulocytic white blood cell that increases during the healing phase of inflammation ____________________

D Give the meanings of the following suffixes.

1. -logy ____________________
2. -lysis ____________________
3. -pathy ____________________
4. -penia ____________________
5. -malacia ____________________
6. -osis ____________________
7. -phobia ____________________
8. -megaly ____________________
9. -oma ____________________
10. -opsy ____________________
11. -plasia ____________________
12. -plasty ____________________
13. -sclerosis ____________________
14. -stasis ____________________

E Using the combining forms below and your knowledge of suffixes, build medical terms for the following definitions.

acr/o	chondr/o	myel/o
arteri/o	hem/o	phleb/o
bi/o	hydr/o	rhin/o
blephar/o	morph/o	sarc/o
cardi/o	my/o	splen/o

1. enlargement of the spleen ____________________
2. study of the shape (of cells) ____________________
3. softening of cartilage ____________________
4. abnormal condition of water (fluid) in the kidney ____________________
5. disease condition of heart muscle ____________________
6. hardening of arteries ____________________
7. tumor (benign) of muscle ____________________
8. flesh tumor (malignant) of muscle ____________________
9. surgical repair of the nose ____________________
10. tumor of bone marrow ____________________
11. fear of heights ____________________
12. view of living tissue under a microscope ____________________
13. stoppage of the flow of blood (by mechanical or natural means) ____________________
14. inflammation of the eyelid ____________________
15. incision of a vein ____________________

F Give the plural formations of the following terms:

1. bacterium ____________________
2. metastasis ____________________
3. vertebra ____________________
4. streptococcus ____________________
5. nucleus ____________________
6. prognosis ____________________

3

G Match the following terms with their meanings.

achondroplasia	colostomy	laparoscopy
acromegaly	hydrotherapy	metastasis
atrophy	hypertrophy	necrosis
chemotherapy	laparoscope	osteomalacia

1. treatment using drugs ______
2. condition of death (of cells) ______
3. softening of bone ______
4. opening of the large intestine to the outside of the body ______
5. no development; shrinkage of cells ______
6. beyond control; spread of a cancerous tumor to another organ ______
7. instrument to visually examine the abdomen ______
8. enlargement of extremities; an endocrine disorder that causes excess growth hormone to be produced by the pituitary gland after puberty ______
9. condition of improper formation of cartilage in the embryo that leads to short bones and dwarfism ______
10. process of viewing the peritoneal (abdominal) cavity ______
11. treatment using water ______
12. excessive development of cells (increase in size of individual cells) ______

3

H Give the meanings of the following suffixes.

1. -ia ______
2. -trophy ______
3. -stasis ______
4. -stomy ______
5. -tomy ______
6. -ole ______
7. -um ______
8. -ule ______
9. -y ______
10. -oid ______
11. -genic ______
12. -ptosis ______

I **Using the lists of combining forms and suffixes below, build medical terms for the following definitions.**

COMBINING FORMS		SUFFIXES		
arteri/o	pleur/o	-dynia	-ole	-therapy
lapar/o	pneumon/o	-ectomy	-pathy	-tomy
mamm/o	radi/o	-gram	-plasty	-ule
nephr/o	ven/o	-ia	-scopy	

1. incision of the abdomen ____________________
2. process of visual examination of the abdomen ____________________
3. a small artery ____________________
4. condition of the lungs ____________________
5. treatment using x-rays ____________________
6. record (x-ray film) of the breast ____________________
7. pain of the chest wall and the membranes surrounding the lungs ____________________
8. a small vein ____________________
9. disease condition of the kidney ____________________
10. surgical repair of the breast ____________________

3

J **Underline the suffix in the following terms, and give the meaning of the entire term.**

1. laryngeal ____________________
2. inguinal ____________________
3. chronic ____________________
4. pulmonary ____________________
5. adipose ____________________
6. peritoneal ____________________
7. axillary ____________________
8. necrotic ____________________
9. mucoid ____________________
10. mucous ____________________
11. agoraphobia ____________________
12. esophagus ____________________

K **Select from the following terms relating to blood and blood vessels to complete the sentences below.**

anemia	hemolysis	leukocytosis
angioplasty	hemostasis	multiple myeloma
arterioles	ischemia	thrombocytopenia
hematoma	leukemia	venules

1. Billy was diagnosed with excessively high numbers of cancerous white blood cells, or ________________. His doctor prescribed chemotherapy and expected an excellent prognosis.
2. Mr. Clark's angiogram showed that he had serious atherosclerosis of one of the arteries supplying blood to his heart. His doctor recommended that ________________ would be helpful to open up his clogged artery by threading a catheter (tube) through his artery and opening a balloon at the end of the catheter to widen the artery.
3. Mrs. Jackson's blood count showed a reduced number of red blood cells, indicating ____________. Her erythrocytes were being destroyed by ________________.
4. Doctors refused to operate on Joe because of his low platelet count, a condition called ________________.
5. Blockage of an artery leading to Mr. Stein's brain led to the holding back of blood flow to nerve tissue in his brain. This condition, called ________________, could lead to necrosis of tissue and a cerebrovascular accident.
6. Small arteries, or ________________, were broken under Ms. Bein's scalp when she was struck on the head with a rock. She soon developed a mass of blood, a/an ________________, under the skin in that region of her head.
7. Sarah Jones had a staphylococcal infection, causing elevation of her white blood cell count, known as ________________. She was treated with antibiotics and her blood count returned to normal.
8. Within the body, the bone marrow (soft tissue within bones) is the "factory" for making blood cells. Mr. Scott developed ________________, a malignant condition of the bone marrow cells in his hip, upper arm, and thigh bones.
9. During operations, surgeons use clamps to close off blood vessels and prevent blood loss. In this way, they maintain ________________ and avoid blood transfusions.
10. Small vessels that carry blood toward the heart from capillaries and tissues are ________________.

3

L Complete the medical term for the following definitions.

DEFINITION	MEDICAL TERM
1. membrane surrounding the heart	peri ______
2. hardening of arteries	arterio ______
3. enlargement of the liver	hepato ______
4. new opening of the windpipe to the outside of the body	tracheo ______
5. inflammation of the tonsils	______ itis
6. surgical puncture to remove fluid from the abdomen	abdomino ______
7. muscle pain	my ______
8. pertaining to the membranes surrounding the lungs	______ al
9. study of the eye	______ logy
10. berry-shaped (spheroidal) bacteria in clusters	______ cocci
11. beyond control (spread of a cancerous tumor)	meta ______
12. pertaining to the voice box	______ eal

M Select from the meanings in Column II to match the suffixes in Column I. Write each meaning in the space provided.

COLUMN I

Suffixes: Conditions

1. -algia or -dynia ______
2. -cele ______
3. -megaly ______
4. -oma ______
5. -penia ______
6. -phobia ______
7. -plasia ______
8. -emia ______
9. -itis ______
10. -trophy ______
11. -stasis ______
12. -sclerosis ______
13. -lysis ______
14. -ptosis ______
15. -malacia ______

COLUMN II

Meanings

blood condition
controlling; stopping
deficiency
destruction; breakdown
development; nourishment
falling; drooping; prolapse
enlargement
fear
formation
hardening
hernia
inflammation
pain
softening
tumor; mass

3

N **Select from the meanings in Column II to match the suffixes in Column I. Write each meaning in the space provided.**

COLUMN I ***Suffixes: Procedures***	COLUMN II ***Meanings***
1. -centesis ____________	excision
2. -opsy ____________	incision
3. -ectomy ____________	instrument to record
4. -tomy ____________	instrument to visually examine
5. -stomy ____________	new opening
6. -therapy ____________	process of recording
7. -plasty ____________	process of visual examination
8. -scopy ____________	record
9. -scope ____________	surgical puncture to remove fluid
10. -graphy ____________	surgical repair
11. -gram ____________	to view
12. -graph ____________	treatment

O **Circle the correct term to complete the following sentences.**

1. Ms. Daley, who has nine children, visited her general practitioner because she was experiencing problems with urination. After examining her, the doctor found that her bladder was protruding into her vagina and told her she had a (**rectocele, cystocele, hiatal hernia**).

2. Susan coughed constantly for a week. Her physician told her that her chest x-ray examination showed evidence of pneumonia. Her sputum (material coughed up from the bronchial tubes) was found to contain (**ischemic, pleuritic, pneumococcal**) bacteria.

3. Mr. Manion went to see his family doctor because he couldn't keep his left upper eyelid from sagging. His doctor told him that he had a neurologic problem called Horner syndrome, characterized by (**necrosis, hydronephrosis, ptosis**) of his eyelid.

4. Jill broke her left arm in a fall while mountain biking. After 6 weeks in a cast to treat the fracture, her left arm was noticeably smaller and weaker than her right arm—the muscles had (**atrophied, hypertrophied, metastasized**). Her physician recommended physical therapy to strengthen the affected arm.

5. Ms. Brody was diagnosed with breast cancer. The first phase of her treatment included a (**nephrectomy, mastectomy, pulmonary resection**) to remove her breast and the tumor. After the surgery, her doctors recommended (**chemotherapy, radiotherapy, hydrotherapy**) using drugs such as doxorubicin (Adriamycin) and paclitaxel (Taxol).

6. At age 29, Kevin's facial features became coarser and his hands and tongue enlarged. After a head CT (computed tomography) scan, doctors diagnosed the cause of these changes as (**hyperglycemia, hyperthyroidism, acromegaly**), a slowly progressive endocrine condition involving the pituitary gland.

7. Each winter during "cold and flu season," Daisy developed (**chondromalacia, bronchitis, cardiomyopathy**). Her doctor prescribed antibiotics and respiratory therapy to help her recover.

8. After undergoing (**arthroscopy, laparotomy, radiotherapy**) on his knee, Alan noticed swelling and inflammation near the small incisions. Dr. Nicholas assured him that this was a common side effect of the procedure that would resolve spontaneously.

9. Under the microscope, Dr. Vance could see grape-like clusters of bacteria called (**eosinophils, streptococci, staphylococci**). She made the diagnosis of (**staphylococcemia, eosinophilia, streptococcemia**), and the patient was started on antibiotic therapy.

10. David enjoyed weight lifting, but he recently noticed a bulge in his right groin region. He visited his doctor, who made the diagnosis of (**hiatal hernia, rectocele, inguinal hernia**) and recommended surgical repair.

ANSWERS TO EXERCISES

A

1. hernia
2. blood condition
3. berry-shaped bacterium
4. record
5. cell
6. pain
7. removal, excision, resection
8. surgical puncture to remove fluid
9. process of producing, forming
10. instrument to record
11. inflammation
12. process of recording

B

1. cystocele
2. myalgia ("myodynia" is not used)
3. carcinogenesis
4. myelitis
5. streptococci (*bacteria* is a plural term)
6. thoracentesis or thoracocentesis
7. mastectomy
8. bronchitis
9. ischemia
10. angiography
11. arthroscopy
12. staphylococci
13. laryngectomy
14. amniocentesis

3

C

1. neutrophil
2. lymphocyte
3. thrombocyte
4. eosinophil
5. erythrocyte
6. monocyte
7. basophil

D

1. process of study
2. breakdown, separation, destruction
3. process of disease
4. deficiency, less than normal
5. softening
6. condition, abnormal condition
7. fear of
8. enlargement
9. tumor, mass
10. process of viewing
11. condition of formation, growth
12. surgical repair
13. hardening, to harden
14. to stop, control

E

1. splenomegaly
2. morphology
3. chondromalacia
4. hydronephrosis
5. cardiomyopathy
6. arteriosclerosis
7. myoma
8. myosarcoma
9. rhinoplasty
10. myeloma (called multiple myeloma)
11. acrophobia
12. biopsy
13. hemostasis
14. blepharitis
15. phlebotomy

F

1. bacteria
2. metastases
3. vertebrae
4. streptococci
5. nuclei
6. prognoses

G

1. chemotherapy
2. necrosis
3. osteomalacia
4. colostomy
5. atrophy
6. metastasis
7. laparoscope
8. acromegaly
9. achondroplasia
10. laparoscopy
11. hydrotherapy
12. hypertrophy

H

1. condition
2. development, nourishment
3. to stop, control
4. new opening
5. incision, cut into
6. small, little
7. structure
8. small, little
9. condition, process
10. resembling
11. pertaining to producing, produced by or in
12. falling, drooping, prolapse

I

1. laparotomy
2. laparoscopy
3. arteriole
4. pneumonia (this condition is actually *pneumonitis*)
5. radiotherapy
6. mammogram
7. pleurodynia
8. venule
9. nephropathy
10. mammoplasty

J

1. laryngeal—pertaining to the voice box
2. inguinal—pertaining to the groin
3. chronic—pertaining to time (over a long period of time)
4. pulmonary—pertaining to the lung
5. adipose—pertaining to (or full of) fat
6. peritoneal—pertaining to the peritoneum (membrane around the abdominal organs)
7. axillary—pertaining to the armpit, under arm
8. necrotic—pertaining to death
9. mucoid—resembling mucus
10. mucous—pertaining to mucus
11. agoraphobia—fear of open spaces (agora means marketplace)
12. esophagus—tube leading from the throat to the stomach

K

1. leukemia
2. angioplasty
3. anemia; hemolysis
4. thrombocytopenia
5. ischemia
6. arterioles; hematoma
7. leukocytosis
8. multiple myeloma
9. hemostasis
10. venules

L

1. pericardium
2. arteriosclerosis
3. hepatomegaly
4. tracheostomy
5. tonsillitis
6. abdominocentesis (this procedure also is known as paracentesis)
7. myalgia
8. pleural
9. ophthalmology
10. staphylococci
11. metastasis
12. laryngeal

M

1. pain
2. hernia
3. enlargement
4. tumor; mass
5. deficiency
6. fear
7. formation
8. blood condition
9. inflammation
10. development; nourishment
11. controlling; stopping
12. hardening
13. destruction; breakdown
14. falling; drooping; prolapse
15. softening

N

1. surgical puncture to remove fluid
2. to view
3. excision
4. incision
5. new opening
6. treatment
7. surgical repair
8. process of visual examination
9. instrument to visually examine
10. process of recording
11. record
12. instrument to record

O

1. cystocele
2. pneumococcal
3. ptosis
4. atrophied
5. mastectomy; chemotherapy
6. acromegaly
7. bronchitis
8. arthroscopy
9. staphylococci; staphylococcemia
10. inguinal hernia

Answers to Practical Applications

1. paracentesis
2. laparotomy
3. mastectomy
4. amniocentesis
5. tonsillectomy
6. angioplasty
7. thoracentesis
8. colostomy
9. angiography
10. laparoscopy

PRONUNCIATION OF TERMS

To test your understanding of the terminology in this chapter, write the meaning of each term in the space provided. In addition, you may wish to cover the terms and write them by looking at your definitions. Make sure your spelling is correct. The CAPITAL letters indicate the accented syllable. The page number after each term indicates where it is defined or used in the text, so you can check your responses. You will find complete definitions for all of these terms and their audio pronunciations on the Evolve site.

Pronunciation Guide

ā as in āpe	ă as in ăpple
ē as in ēven	ĕ as in ĕvery
ī as in īce	ĭ as in ĭnterest
ō as in ōpen	ŏ as in pŏt
ū as in ūnit	ŭ as in ŭnder

3

TERM	PRONUNCIATION	MEANING
abdominocentesis (76)	ăb-dŏm-ĭ-nō-sĕn-TĒ-sĭs	
achondroplasia (80)	ā-kŏn-drō-PLĀ-zē-ă	
acromegaly (79)	ăk-rō-MĔG-ă-lē	
acrophobia (79)	ăk-rō-FŌ-bē-ă	
acute (83)	ă-KŪT	
adenoids (83)	ĂD-ĕ-noydz	
adipose (83)	Ă-dĭ-pōs	
agoraphobia (79)	ă-gŏr-ă-FŌ-bē-ă	
amniocentesis (76)	ăm-nē-ō-sĕn-TĒ-sĭs	
anemia (77)	ă-NĒ-mē-ă	
angiogenesis (78)	ăn-jē-ō-JĔN-ĕ-sĭs	
angiography (78)	ăn-jē-ŎG-ră-fē	
angioplasty (80)	ăn-jē-ō-PLĂS-tē	
arteriole (82)	ăr-TĒR-ē-ōl	
arteriosclerosis (80)	ăr-tē-rē-ō-sklĕ-RŌ-sĭs	
arthralgia (76)	ăr-THRĂL-jă	
atrophy (82)	ĂT-rō-fē	
axillary (83)	ĂK-sĭ-lăr-ē	
basophil (85)	BĀ-sō-fĭl	
biopsy (79)	BĪ-ŏp-sē	
blepharoptosis (80)	blĕf-ă-rŏp-TŌ-sĭs	
bronchitis (78)	brŏng-KĪ-tĭs	
carcinogenesis (78)	kăr-sĭ-nō-JĔN-ĕ-sĭs	

TERM	PRONUNCIATION	MEANING
carcinogenic (83)	kăr-sĭ-nō-JĔN-ik	
cardiac (83)	KĂR-dē-ăk	
cardiomyopathy (79)	kăr-dē-ō-mī-ŎP-ă-thē	
chemotherapy (81)	kē-mō-THĔR-ĕ-pē	
chondromalacia (78)	kŏn-drō-mă-LĀ-shă	
chronic (83)	KRŎN-ĭk	
colostomy (81)	kō-LŎS-tō-mē	
cystocele (76)	SĬS-tō-sēl	
electroencephalogram (78)	ē-lĕk-trō-ĕn-SĔF-ă-lō-grăm	
electroencephalograph (78)	ē-lĕk-trō-ĕn-SĔF-ă-lō-grăf	
electroencephalography (78)	ē-lĕk-trō-ĕn-sĕf-ă-LŎG-ră-fē	
eosinophil (85)	ē-ō-SĬN-ō-fĭl	
erythrocyte (77)	ĕ-RĬTH-rō-sīt	
erythropenia (79)	ĕ-rĭth-rō-PĒ-nē-ă	
esophagus (83)	ĕ-SŎF-ă-gus	
hematoma (79)	hē-mă-TŌ-mă	
hemolysis (78)	hē-MŎL-ĭ-sĭs	
hemostasis (81)	hē-mō-STĀ-sĭs	
hydronephrosis (79)	hī-drō-nĕ-FRŌ-sĭs	
hydrotherapy (81)	hī-drō-THĔR-ă-pē	
hypertrophy (82)	hī-PĔR-trō-fē	
inguinal (83)	ĬNG-wĭ-năl	
ischemia (77)	ĭs-KĒ-mē-ă	
laparoscope (81)	LĂP-ă-rō-skōp	
laparoscopy (81)	lă-pă-RŎS-kō-pē	
laparotomy (81)	lăp-ă-RŎT-ō-mē	
laryngeal (83)	lă-RĬN-jē-ăl *or* lăr-ĭn-JĒ-ăl	
laryngectomy (77)	lăr-ĭn-JĔK-tō-mē	
leukemia (82)	lū-KĒ-mē-ă	
leukocyte (77)	LŪ-kō-sīt	
leukocytosis (79)	lū-kō-sī-TŌ-sĭs	

3

TERM	PRONUNCIATION	MEANING
lymphocyte (85)	LĬM-fō-sīt	
mammogram (78)	MĂM-mō-grăm	
mastectomy (77)	măs-TĔK-tō-mē	
metastasis (81)	mĕ-TĂS-tă-sĭs	
monocyte (85)	MŎN-ō-sīt	
morphology (78)	mŏr-FŎL-ō-jē	
mucoid (83)	MŪ-koyd	
mucous membrane (83)	MŪ-kŭs MĔM-brān	
mucus (83)	MŪ-kŭs	
myalgia (76)	mī-ĂL-jă	
myelitis (78)	MĪ-ĕ-LĪ-tĭs	
myeloma (79)	mī-ĕ-LŌ-mă	
myoma (79)	mī-Ō-mă	
myosarcoma (79)	mī-ō-săr-KŌ-mă	
necropsy (79)	NĔ-krŏp-sē	
necrosis (79)	nĕ-KRŌ-sĭs	
necrotic (83)	nĕ-KRŎT-ĭk	
nephrologist (82)	nĕ-FRŎL-ō-jĭst	
nephropathy (83)	nĕ-FRŎP-ă-thē	
neuralgia (76)	nū-RĂL-jă	
neutropenia (79)	nū-trō-PĒ-nē-ă	
neutrophil (85)	NŪ-trō-fĭl	
ophthalmology (78)	ŏf-thăl-MŎL-ō-jē	
osteogenic (83)	ŏs-tē-ō-JĔN-ĭk	
osteomalacia (78)	ŏs-tē-ō-mă-LĀ-shă	
otalgia (76)	ō-TĂL-jă	
paracentesis (76)	pă-ră-cĕn-TĒ-sĭs	
pathogenesis (78)	păth-ŏ-JĔN-ĕ-sĭs	
pathologic (83)	păth-ō-LŎJ-ĭk	
pericardium (82)	pĕr-ē-KĂR-dē-ŭm	
peritoneal (83)	pĕr-ĭ-tō-NĒ-ăl	

3

TERM	PRONUNCIATION	MEANING
phlebotomy (81)	flĕ-BŎT-ō-mē	______
platelet (85)	PLĀT-lĕt	______
pleural (83)	PLŬR-ăl	______
pleurodynia (77)	plūr-ō-DĬN-ē-ă	______
pneumonia (82)	nū-MŌN-yă	______
polymorphonuclear leukocyte (85)	pŏl-ē-mŏr-fō-NŪ-klē-ăr LŪ-kō-sīt	______
ptosis (80)	TŌ-sĭs	______
pulmonary (83)	PŪL-mō-nā-rē	______
radiographer (82)	rā-dē-ŎG-ră-fĕr	______
radiotherapy (81)	rā-dē-ō-THĔR-ă-pē	______
rectocele (76)	RĔK-tō-sēl	______
splenomegaly (79)	splē-nō-MĔG-ă-lē	______
staphylococci (76)	stăf-ĭ-lō-KŎK-sī	______
streptococcus (76)	strĕp-tō-KŎK-ŭs	______
thoracentesis (76)	thō-ră-sĕn-TĒ-sĭs	______
thrombocyte (77)	THRŌM-bō-sīt	______
thrombocytopenia (79)	thrŏm-bō-sī-tō-PĒ-nē-ă	______
thrombophlebitis (78)	thrŏm-bō-flĕ-BĪ-tĭs	______
tonsillar (83)	TŎN-sĭ-lăr	______
tonsillitis (78)	tŏn-sĭ-LĪ-tĭs	______
tracheostomy (81)	trā-kē-ŎS-tō-mē	______
tracheotomy (81)	trā-kē-ŎT-ō-mē	______
venule (82)	VĔN-ūl	______

3

REVIEW SHEET

Write the meanings of each word part in the space provided and test yourself. Check your answers with the information in the chapter or in the Glossary (Medical Word Parts—English), at the end of this book.

Noun Suffixes

SUFFIX	MEANING	SUFFIX	MEANING
-algia	______	-oma	______
-cele	______	-opsy	______
-centesis	______	-osis	______
-coccus (-cocci)	______	-pathy	______
-cyte	______	-penia	______
-dynia	______	-phobia	______
-ectomy	______	-plasia	______
-emia	______	-plasty	______
-er	______	-ptosis	______
-genesis	______	-sclerosis	______
-gram	______	-scope	______
-graph	______	-scopy	______
-graphy	______	-stasis	______
-ia	______	-stomy	______
-ist	______	-therapy	______
-itis	______	-tomy	______
-logy	______	-trophy	______
-lysis	______	-ule	______
-malacia	______	-um, -ium	______
-megaly	______	-us	______
-ole	______	-y	______

Adjective Suffixes

SUFFIX	MEANING	SUFFIX	MEANING
-ac, -iac	______	-ic, -ical	______
-al	______	-oid	______
-ar	______	-ose	______
-ary	______	-ous	______
-eal	______	-tic	______
-genic	______		

Combining Forms

COMBINING FORM	MEANING	COMBINING FORM	MEANING
abdomin/o	______	cyst/o	______
acr/o	______	encephal/o	______
acu/o	______	erythr/o	______
aden/o	______	hem/o	______
adip/o	______	hepat/o	______
amni/o	______	hydr/o	______
angi/o	______	inguin/o	______
arteri/o	______	isch/o	______
arthr/o	______	lapar/o	______
axill/o	______	laryng/o	______
bi/o	______	leuk/o	______
blephar/o	______	lymph/o	______
bronch/o	______	mamm/o	______
carcin/o	______	mast/o	______
cardi/o	______	morph/o	______
chem/o	______	muc/o	______
chondr/o	______	my/o	______
chron/o	______	myel/o	______
col/o	______	necr/o	______

COMBINING FORM	MEANING	COMBINING FORM	MEANING
nephr/o	______________	pulmon/o	______________
neur/o	______________	radi/o	______________
neutr/o	______________	rect/o	______________
nucle/o	______________	ren/o	______________
ophthalm/o	______________	rhin/o	______________
oste/o	______________	sarc/o	______________
ot/o	______________	splen/o	______________
path/o	______________	staphyl/o	______________
peritone/o	______________	strept/o	______________
phag/o	______________	thorac/o	______________
phleb/o	______________	thromb/o	______________
plas/o	______________	tonsill/o	______________
pleur/o	______________	trache/o	______________
pneumon/o	______________	ven/o	______________

Give the medical term for the following blood cells.

red blood cell ______________________________

clotting cell ______________________________

white blood cell ______________________________

Name 5 different types of white blood cells (the first letter is given).

e ______________________________

b ______________________________

n ______________________________

l ______________________________

m ______________________________

evolve *Please visit the Evolve website for additional exercises, games, and images related to this chapter.*

CHAPTER 4

Prefixes

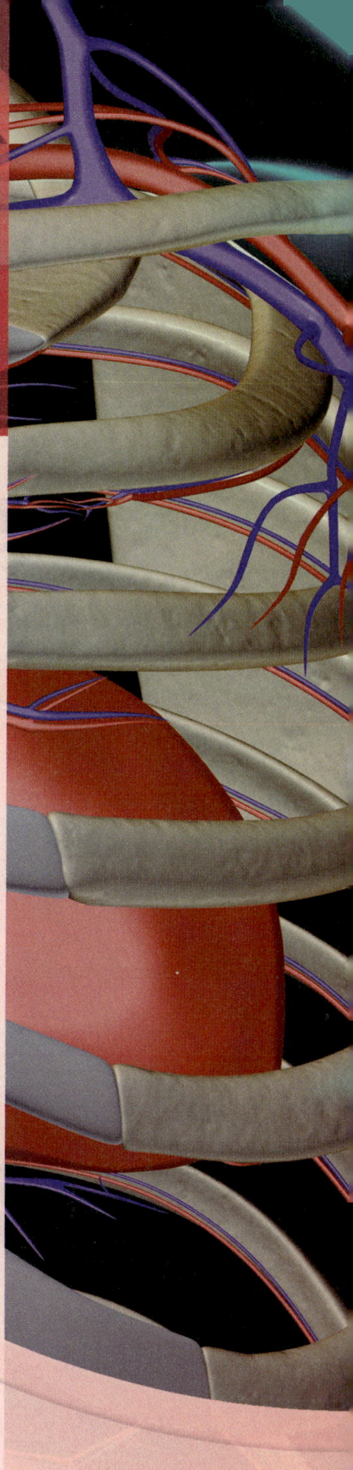

This chapter is divided into the following sections:

CHAPTER GOALS

- Define basic prefixes used in the medical language.
- Analyze medical terms that combine prefixes and other word elements.
- Learn about the Rh condition as an example of an antigen-antibody reaction.

INTRODUCTION

This chapter on prefixes, like the preceding chapter on suffixes, gives you practice in word analysis and provides a foundation for the study of the terminology of body systems that follows.

The list of combining forms, suffixes, and meanings helps you analyze terminology in the rest of the chapter. To support a broader understanding, **A Closer Look,** beginning on page 118, contains more detailed explanation of new terms.

COMBINING FORMS AND SUFFIXES

COMBINING FORMS

COMBINING FORM	MEANING	COMBINING FORM	MEANING
carp/o	wrist bones	**ox/o**	oxygen
cib/o	meals	**pub/o**	pubis (pubic bone); anterior portion of the pelvic or hipbone
cis/o	to cut	**seps/o**	infection
cost/o	rib	**somn/o**	sleep
cutane/o	skin	**son/o**	sound
dactyl/o	fingers, toes	**the/o**	to put, place
duct/o	to lead, carry	**thel/o, theli/o**	nipple
flex/o	to bend	**thyr/o**	thyroid gland; shield (the shape of the thyroid gland resembled [-oid] a shield to those who named it)
furc/o	forking, branching	**top/o**	place, position, location
gloss/o	tongue	**tox/o**	poison
glyc/o	sugar	**trache/o**	windpipe, trachea
immun/o	protection	**urethr/o**	urethra
morph/o	shape, form		
mort/o	death		
nat/i	birth		
nect/o	to bind, tie, connect		
norm/o	rule, order		

SUFFIXES

These suffixes are used in this chapter in combination with prefixes. Some are complex suffixes that contain roots. For example, the suffix -pnea contains a root pne, meaning breathing, and a final suffix -a, meaning condition.

SUFFIX	MEANING
-blast	embryonic, immature
-crine	to secrete
-drome	to run
-fusion	coming together; to pour
-gen	substance that produces
-lapse	to slide, fall, sag
-lysis	breakdown, destruction, separation
-meter	to measure
-mission	to send
-or	one who
-oxia	oxygen
-partum	birth, labor
-phoria	to bear, carry; feeling (mental state)
-physis	to grow
-plasia	development, formation, growth
-plasm	structure or formation
-pnea	breathing
-ptosis	falling, drooping, prolapse
-rrhea	flow, discharge
-stasis	stopping, controlling
-trophy	development, nourishment

PREFIXES AND TERMINOLOGY

Write the meaning of the medical term in the space provided. Remember, the Evolve website contains the definition and pronunciation for each term.

PREFIX	MEANING	TERMINOLOGY	MEANING
a-, an-	no, not, without	apnea	____________
		anoxia	____________
ab-	away from	abnormal	____________
		abductor *A muscle that draws a limb **away** from the body. Memory tip: Notice that in **ab**ductor the **b** faces away from the **a**.*	____________

PREFIX	MEANING	TERMINOLOGY	MEANING
ad-	toward	adductor	______
		*A muscle that draws a limb **toward** the body. Memory tip: Notice that in adductor, the **d** faces toward the **a**.*	
		adrenal glands	______
		These glands actually lie on top of each kidney. See Figure 4-1.	
ana-	up, apart	anabolism	______
		analysis	______
		Urinalysis (urin/o + [an]/alysis) is a laboratory examination of urine that aids in the diagnosis of many medical conditions. In this term, -lysis means separation.	
ante-	before, forward	ante cibum	______
		The notation a.c., seen on prescription orders, means before meals.	
		anteflexion	______
		antepartum	______

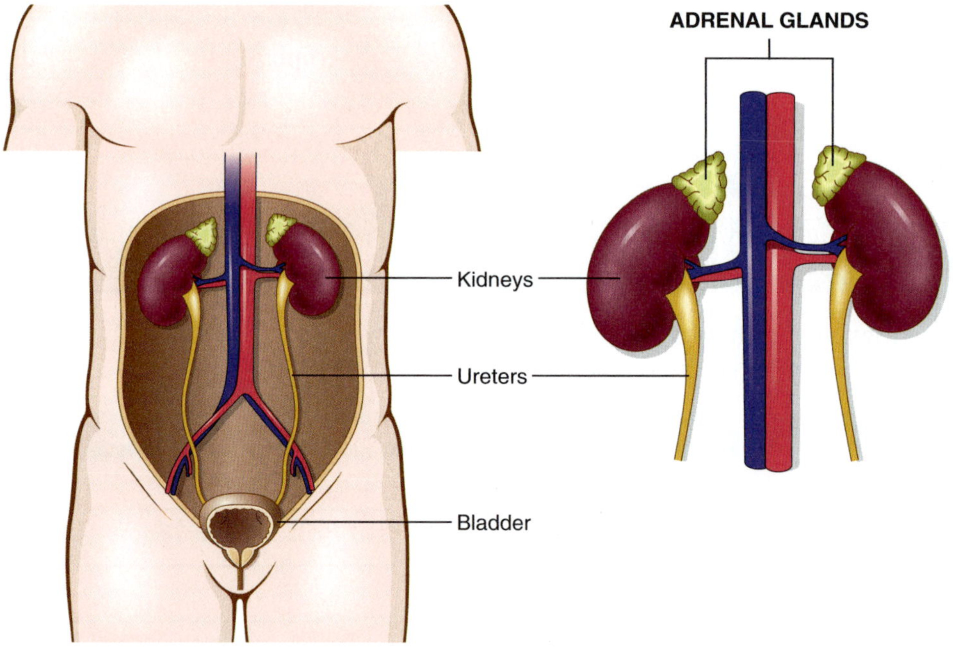

FIGURE 4-1 **Adrenal glands.** These are endocrine glands located above each kidney. One of the hormones they secrete is adrenaline (epinephrine). It causes bronchial tubes to widen, the heart to beat more rapidly and blood pressure to rise.

PREFIX	MEANING	TERMINOLOGY	MEANING
anti-	against	antibiotic *Antibiotics destroy or inhibit the growth of microorganisms such as bacteria. Penicillin was the first antibiotic (discovered in immature plants called molds).*	
		antibody *Protein produced against an antigen (foreign body).*	
		antigen *In this term, anti- is short for antibody. An antigen (bacterium or virus) is a substance that produces (-gen) an antibody.* *See* ***A Closer Look: Antigens and Antibodies,*** *page 118.*	
		antisepsis *An antiseptic (-sis changes to -tic to form an adjective) substance fights infection.*	
		antitoxin *This is an antibody, often from an animal (such as a horse), that acts against a toxin. An example is tetanus antitoxin given against tetanus, an acute bacterial infection of the nervous system.*	
auto-	self, own	autoimmune disease	
bi-	two	bifurcation *Normal splitting into two branches, such as bifurcation of the trachea to form the bronchi.*	
		bilateral	
brady-	slow	bradycardia *Usually, a pulse of less than 60; a slow heart rate.*	
cata-	down	catabolism	
con-	with, together	*congenital anomaly* *See* ***A Closer Look,*** *page 120.*	
		connective *Connective tissue supports and binds other body tissue and parts. Bone, cartilage, and fibrous tissue are connective tissues.*	

Anti- and Ante-

Be careful not to confuse these prefixes. Pay close attention to their different pronunciations. **Ante-** is pronounced ăn-**tē** and **anti-** is pronounced ăn-**tĭ**.

Autoimmune Disease

In an **autoimmune disease**, the body makes antibodies against its own good cells and tissues, causing inflammation and injury. Examples of autoimmune disorders are **rheumatoid arthritis**, affecting joints; **celiac disease,** affecting the intestinal tract; and **Graves disease,** affecting the thyroid gland.

PREFIX	MEANING	TERMINOLOGY	MEANING
contra-	against, opposite	contraindication	______________
		Contra- means against in this term.	
		contralateral	______________
		Contra- means opposite in this term. A stroke affecting the right side of the brain may cause ***contralateral*** *paralysis affecting the left arm and leg. The opposite of contralateral is* ***ipsilateral****. (ipsi- means same).*	
de-	down, lack of	dehydration	______________
dia-	through, complete	diameter	______________
		diarrhea	______________
		dialysis	______________
		Literal meaning is complete (dia-) separation (-lysis). In hemodialysis, waste materials are separated from the blood via a machine (artificial kidney) when the kidneys no longer function. See Figure 7-15, page 234, for an illustration of hemodialysis.	
dys-	bad, painful, difficult, abnormal	dyspnea	______________
		Often caused by respiratory or cardiac conditions, strenuous exercise, or anxiety.	
		dysplasia	______________
ec-, ecto-	out, outside	ectopic pregnancy	______________
		Ectopic means pertaining to out of place and modifies the noun "pregnancy." See Figure 4-2.	

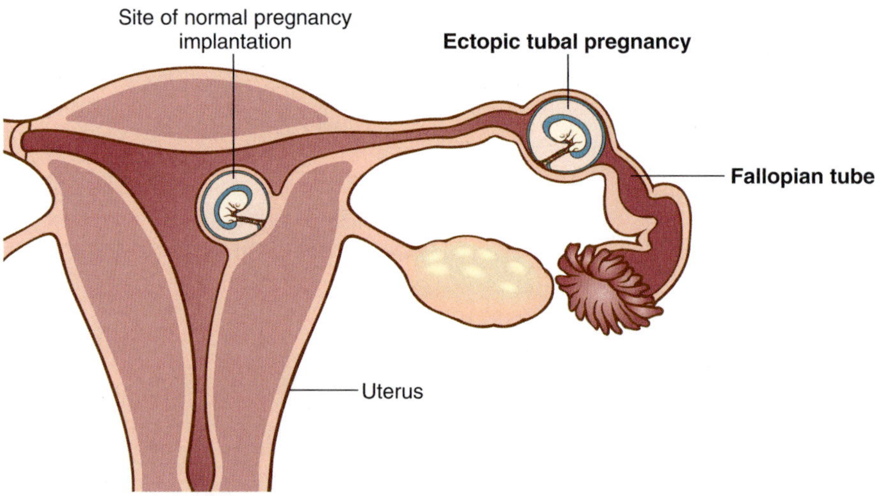

FIGURE 4-2 Ectopic pregnancy. Normal pregnancy implantation is in the upper portion of the uterus. Ectopic pregnancy occurs most commonly in a **fallopian tube** (i.e., tubal pregnancy). Surgery is often necessary to remove an ectopic pregnancy. The fetus is not viable. Tubal surgery may damage a **fallopian tube** and scar tissue can cause future pregnancy problems.

PREFIX	MEANING	TERMINOLOGY	MEANING
endo-	in, within	endocardium	________________
		endoscope	________________
		endotracheal *An endotracheal tube, placed through the mouth into the trachea, is used for giving oxygen and in general anesthesia procedures.*	________________
epi-	upon, on, above	epithelium	________________
eu-	good, normal	euphoria *Feeling of well-being.*	________________
		euthyroid *Normal thyroid function.*	________________
ex-	out, outside, away from	exophthalmos *Protrusion of the eyeball associated with enlargement and overactivity of the thyroid gland; also called proptosis (pro- = forward, -ptosis = prolapse).*	________________
hemi-	half	hemiglossectomy	________________
hyper-	excessive, above	hyperglycemia *This is a sign of diabetes mellitus. Lack of insulin (type 1 diabetes) or ineffective insulin (type 2 diabetes) causes high levels of sugar in the blood.*	________________
		hyperplasia *Increase in cell numbers. Hyperplasia is a characteristic of tumor growth.*	________________
		hypertrophy *Increase in size of individual cells. Muscle, cardiac, and renal cells exhibit hypertrophy when workload is increased.*	________________
hypo-	deficient, under	hypodermic injection	________________
		hypoglycemia	________________
in-	not	insomniac	________________
in-	into, within	incision	________________
infra-	beneath, under	infracostal	________________
inter-	between	intercostal *Intercostal muscles lie between adjacent ribs.*	________________

Signs and Symptoms

A **sign** is **an objective finding that is perceived by an examiner,** such as fever, rash, or abnormal blood cell counts. A **symptom** (from Greek, *symptoma,* meaning that which happens) is **a subjective change in condition as perceived by the patient.** Examples of symptoms are loss of appetite, abdominal pain, and fatigue (tiredness). Both signs and symptoms are useful clues in the diagnosis of a disease, such as diabetes mellitus.

PREFIX	MEANING	TERMINOLOGY	MEANING
intra-	in, within, into	intravenous	
macro-	large	macrocephaly *This is a congenital anomaly.*	
mal-	bad	malaise *This is a French word meaning discomfort. It is a symptom of illness often marking the onset of a disease.*	
		malignant *From the Latin ignis, meaning fire.* ***Benign*** *(ben- = good) is noncancerous, whereas* ***malignant*** *means cancerous.*	
meta-	beyond, change	metacarpal bones *The five hand bones lie beyond the wrist bones but before the finger bones (phalanges).*	
		metamorphosis *Meta- means change in this term. The change in development from the larval (caterpillar) stage to the adult (butterfly) is a form of metamorphosis. Embryonic (immature)* ***stem cells*** *spontaneously change (undergo metamorphosis) to form different types of mature cells.*	
		metastasis *Meta- = beyond and -stasis = controlling, stopping. A metastasis is a malignant tumor that has spread to a secondary location.*	
micro-	small	microscope	
neo-	new	neonatal *The neonatal period is the interval from birth to 28 days.*	
		neoplasm *A neoplasm may be benign or malignant.*	
pan-	all	pancytopenia *Deficiency of erythrocytes, leukocytes, and thrombocytes.*	
para-	abnormal, beside, near	paralysis *Abnormal disruption of the connection between nerve and muscle. Originally from the Greek paralusis, meaning separation or loosening on one side, describing the loss of movement on one side of the body (occurring in stroke patients).*	
		parathyroid glands *Para- means beside. The four parathyroid glands are located behind the thyroid gland. They secrete a hormone that regulates the calcium levels in blood and tissues.*	
per-	through	percutaneous	

Intra-, Inter-, Infra-

Be careful not to confuse these prefixes: **intra-** means in, within, into; **inter-** means between; **infra-** means beneath, under.

PREFIX	MEANING	TERMINOLOGY	MEANING
peri-	surrounding	pericardium	______________
		periosteum	______________
poly-	many, much	polymorphonuclear	______________
		polyneuritis	______________
post-	after, behind	postmortem	______________
		postpartum	______________
pre-	before, in front of	precancerous	______________
		prenatal	______________
pro-	before, forward	prodrome ______________ *__Prodromal__ signs and symptoms (rash, fever) appear before the actual illness (such as chickenpox) and signal its onset. Altered mood, fatigue, flashes of light, or stiff muscles may accompany the prodromal migraine aura that occurs before the actual headache.*	
		prolapse ______________ *The suffix -lapse means to slide, sag, or fall. See Figure 4-3.*	

4

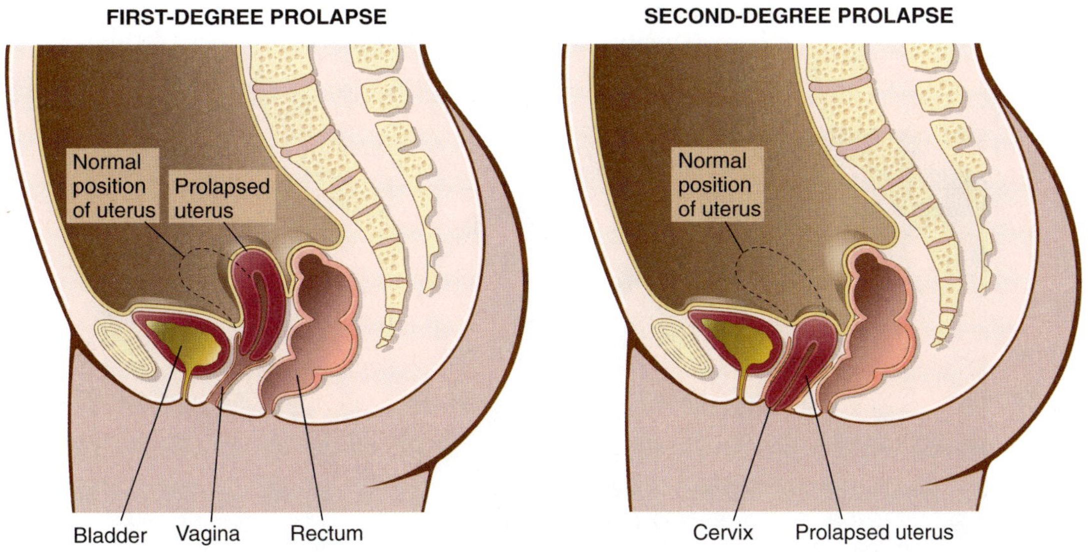

FIGURE 4-3 **Prolapse of the uterus.** In **first-degree prolapse,** the uterus descends into the vaginal canal. In **second-degree prolapse,** the body of the uterus is still within the vagina, but the cervix protrudes from the vaginal orifice (opening). In **third-degree prolapse** (not pictured), the entire uterus projects permanently outside the orifice. As treatment, the uterus may be held in position by a plastic pessary (oval supporting object) that is inserted into the vagina. Some affected women may require hysterectomy (removal of the uterus).

PREFIX	MEANING	TERMINOLOGY	MEANING
pros-	before, forward	prosthesis *An artificial limb is a prosthesis. Figure 4-4 shows Amy Palmiero-Winters running with a prosthetic leg.*	
re-	back, again	relapse *A disease or its signs and symptoms return after an apparent recovery.*	
		remission *Signs and symptoms lessen and the patient feels better. Remission may be spontaneous or the result of treatment. In some cases a permanent remission means the disease is cured.*	
		recombinant DNA *Genetic engineering uses recombinant DNA techniques. See* ***A Closer Look,*** *page 120.*	
retro-	behind, backward	retroperitoneal	
		retroflexion *An abnormal position of an organ, such as the uterus, bent or tilted backward.*	
sub-	under	subcutaneous	
supra-	above, upper	suprapubic *The pubis is one of a pair of pubic bones that forms the anterior part of the pelvic (hip) bone. Pubic bones are pictured in Figure 4-6 on page 117.*	

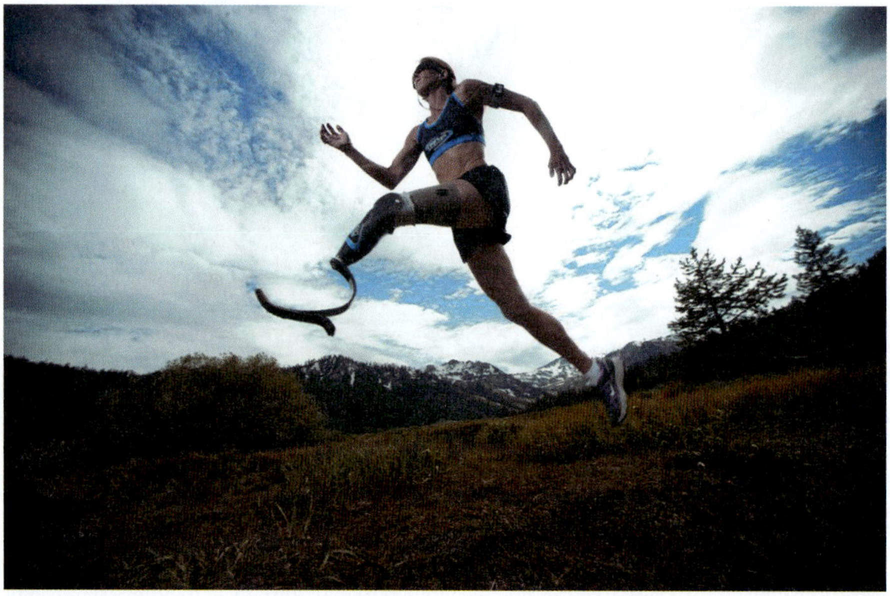

FIGURE 4-4 **Prosthesis.** Amy Palmeiro-Winters is the first female with a prosthetic leg to finish the Badwater 135, a 135-mile race from Badwater in Death Valley to Mount Whitney, California.

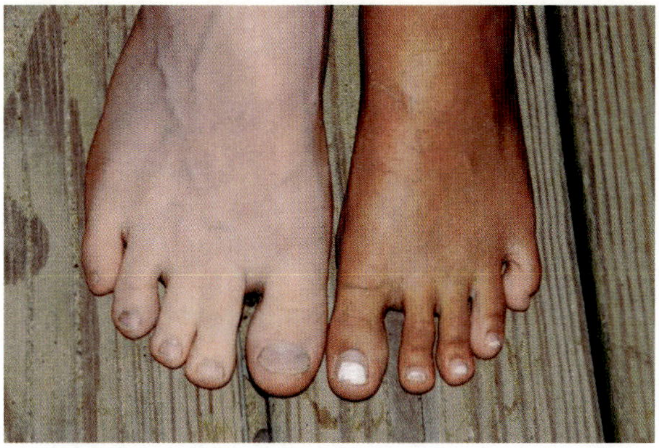

FIGURE 4-5 Syndactyly. The foot on the left (pale) shows syndactyly (webbed toes). The foot on the right (darker) shows normal toes.

PREFIX	MEANING	TERMINOLOGY	MEANING
syn-, sym-	together, with	syndactyly ______ *See Figure 4-5. A hereditary, congenital anomaly of fingers or toes.*	
		synthesis ______ *In protein synthesis, complex proteins are built up from simpler amino acids.*	
		syndrome ______ *See **A Closer Look,** page 121.*	
		symbiosis ______ *Before the letters b, m, and p, **syn-** becomes **sym-.***	
		symmetry ______ *Equality of parts on opposite sides of the body. What is **asymmetry**?*	
		symphysis ______ *A symphysis is a joint in which the bony surfaces are firmly united by a layer of fibrocartilage. See Figure 4-6.*	

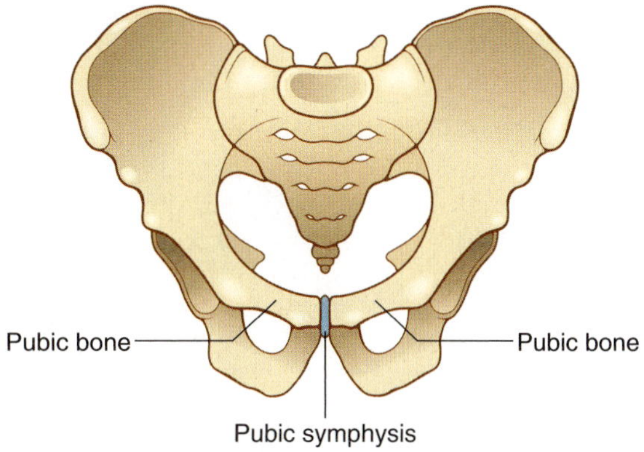

FIGURE 4-6 Pubic symphysis. This is the area in which the pubic bones of the pelvis have grown together. Another example of a symphysis is the two halves of the mandible (lower jawbone), which unite before birth.

Symbiosis

Symbiosis occurs when two organisms live together in close association, either for mutual benefit or not. Examples are:

- bacteria in the intestines and the cells lining the intestines benefit each other.
- parasites (tapeworms and fleas) live off another organism, and are harmful to the host.

In psychiatry, symbiosis is a relationship between two individuals who are emotionally dependent on each other.

PREFIX	MEANING	TERMINOLOGY	MEANING
tachy-	fast	tachypnea (tă-KĬP-nē-ă)	______
trans-	across, through	transfusion *Transfer of blood or blood parts from one person to another.*	______
		transurethral *See **A Closer Look** below.*	______
ultra-	beyond, excess	ultrasonography *See **A Closer Look** below.*	______
uni-	one	unilateral	______

4

A CLOSER LOOK

ANTIGENS AND ANTIBODIES; THE Rh CONDITION

An **antigen**, usually a foreign substance (such as a poison, virus, or bacterium), stimulates the production of **antibodies.** Antibodies are protein substances made by white blood cells in response to the presence of foreign antigens. For example, the flu virus (antigen) enters the body, causing the production of antibodies in the bloodstream. These antibodies then attach to and destroy the antigens (viruses) that produced them. The reaction between an antigen and an antibody is an **immune response** (immun/o means protection). See Figure 4-7. When you receive a **vaccine,** you actually are receiving dead or weakened antigens that stimulate white blood cells (lymphocytes) to make antibodies. These antibodies remain in your blood to protect against those specific antigens when encountered in the future.

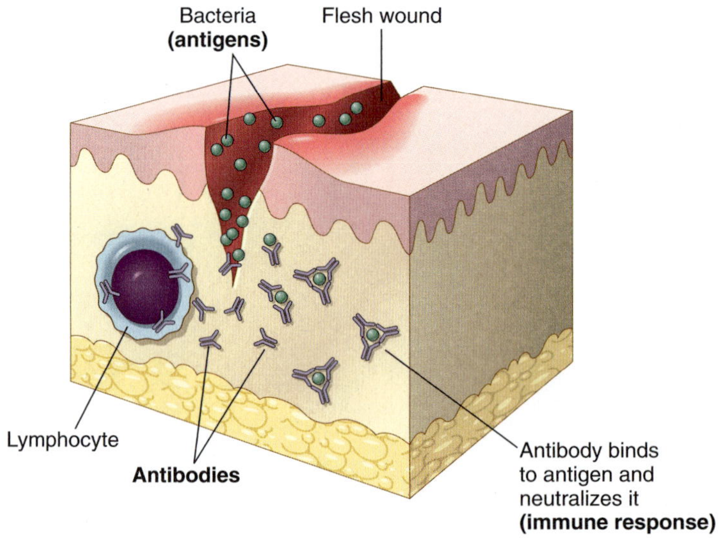

FIGURE 4-7 **Immune response.** When antigens (bacteria) enter the body through a flesh wound, antibodies are produced to destroy the antigens.

Another example of an antigen-antibody reaction is the **Rh condition.** A person who is Rh positive (Rh^+) has a protein coating (antigen) on his or her red blood cells (RBCs). This specific antigen factor is something that the person is born with and is normal. People who are Rh negative (Rh^-) have normal RBCs as well, but their red cells lack the Rh factor antigen.

If an Rh^- woman and an Rh^+ man conceive an embryo, the embryo may be Rh^- or Rh^+. A dangerous condition arises only when the embryo is Rh^+ (because this is different from the Rh^- mother). During delivery of the first Rh^+ baby, some of the baby's blood cells containing Rh^+ antigens can escape into the mother's bloodstream. This sensitizes the mother so that she produces a low level of antibodies to the Rh^+ antigen. Because this occurs at delivery, the first baby is generally not affected and is normal at birth. Sensitization can also occur after a miscarriage, abortion, or blood transfusions (with Rh^+ blood).

Difficulties arise with the second Rh^+ pregnancy. If this embryo also is Rh^+, during pregnancy the mother's acquired antibodies (from the first pregnancy) enter the embryo's bloodstream. These antibodies attack and destroy the embryo's Rh^+ RBCs. The embryo attempts to compensate for this loss by making many new but immature RBCs called erythroblasts (-blast = immature). The affected infant is born with **hemolytic disease of the newborn (HDN)** or **erythroblastosis fetalis.** HDN can occur in the first pregnancy if a mother has had an Rh^+ blood transfusion.

One of the clinical signs of HDN is **jaundice** (yellow skin pigmentation). Jaundice results from excessive destruction of RBCs. When RBCs break down (hemolysis), the hemoglobin within the cells produces **bilirubin** (a chemical pigment). High levels of bilirubin in the bloodstream (hyperbilirubinemia) cause jaundice. To prevent bilirubin from affecting the brain cells of the infant, newborns are treated with exposure to bright lights (phototherapy). The light decomposes the bilirubin, which is excreted from the infant's body.

Physicians administer Rh immunoglobulin to an Rh^- woman within 72 hours after each Rh^+ delivery, abortion, or miscarriage. The globulin binds to Rh^+ cells that escape into the mother's circulation and prevents formation of Rh^+ antibodies. This protects future babies from developing HDN. Figure 4-8 reviews the Rh antigen-antibody reaction.

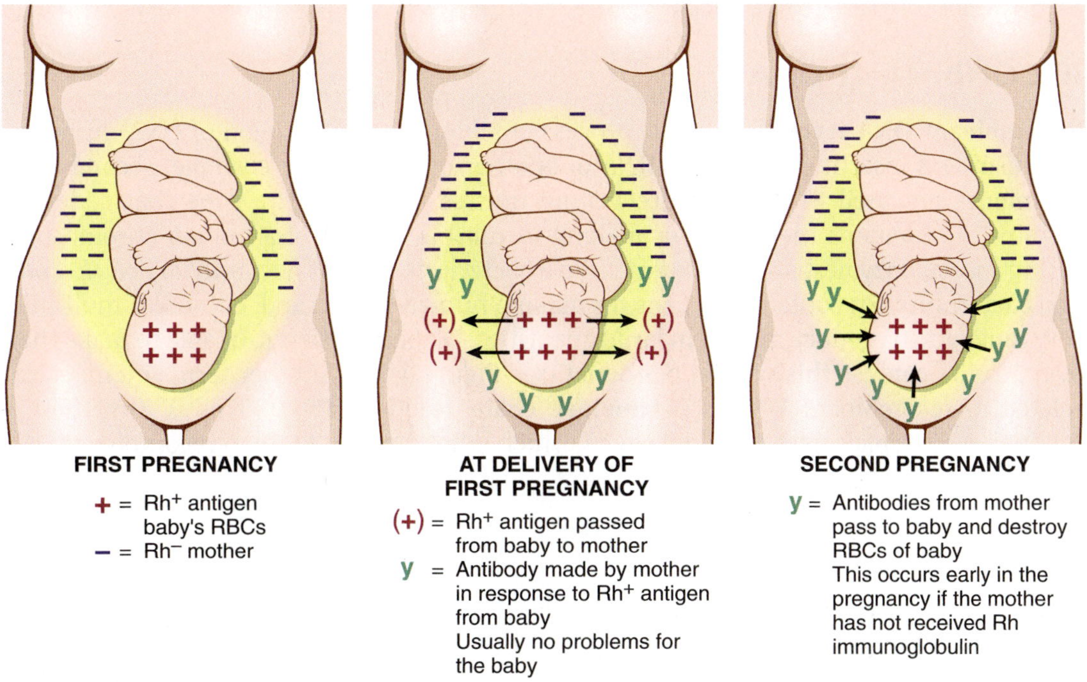

FIGURE 4-8 **Rh condition** as an example of an antigen-antibody reaction.

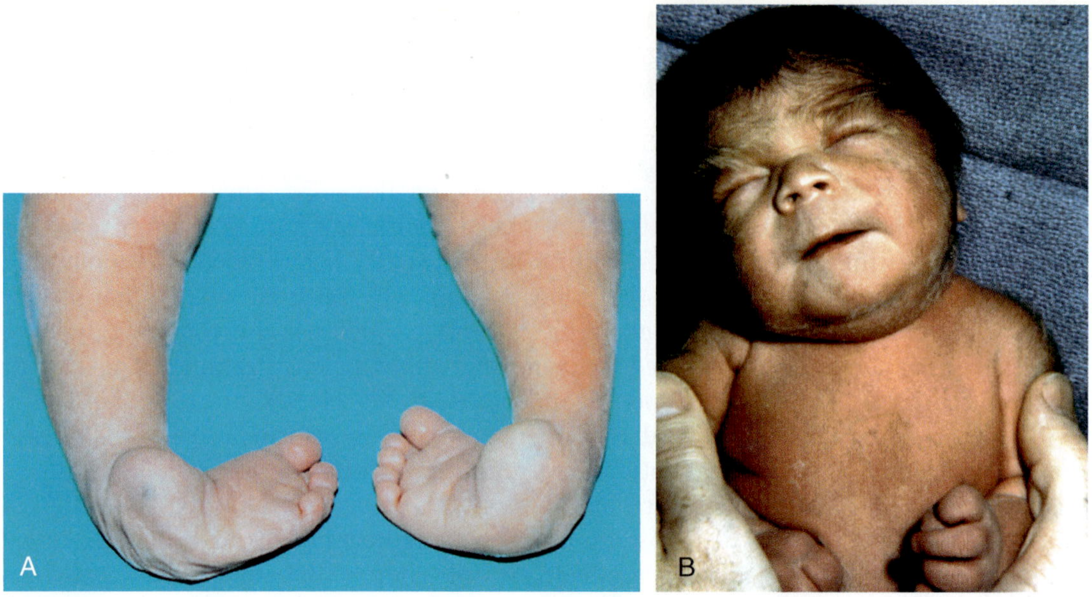

FIGURE 4-9 **Congenital anomalies. (A), Club feet** are a hereditary congenital anomaly. **(B),** Fetal alcohol syndrome (FAS) is a congenital anomaly caused by environmental factors during pregnancy. Note facial features of FAS: skin folds in corners of eyes, long, smooth groove between the nose and upper lip, thin upper lip, and flat nasal bridge.

4

CONGENITAL ANOMALY

An anomaly is an irregularity in a structure or organ. Examples of **congenital anomalies** (those that an infant is born with) include webbed fingers or toes (syndactyly), heart defects, and clubbed feet. See Figure 4-9A. Some congenital anomalies are hereditary (passed to the infant through chromosomes from the father or mother, or both), whereas others are produced by factors present during pregnancy. For example, when a pregnant woman drinks high levels of alcohol during pregnancy, there is a pattern of physical and mental defects in her infant at birth. See Figure 4-9B.

RECOMBINANT DNA

Recombinant DNA technology is the process of taking a gene (a region of DNA) from one organism and inserting it into the DNA of another organism. For example, recombinant techniques are used to manufacture insulin outside the body. The gene that codes for insulin (i.e., contains the recipe for making insulin) is cut out of a human chromosome (using special enzymes) and transferred into a bacterium, such as *Escherichia coli (E. coli).* The bacterium then contains the gene for making human insulin and, because it multiplies very rapidly, can produce insulin in large quantities. Diabetic patients, unable to make their own insulin, can use this synthetic product (see Figure 4-10). Another term you may hear related to recombinant DNA is **polymerase chain reaction** (**PCR**). This is a method of producing multiple copies of a single gene, which is an important tool in recombinant DNA technology.

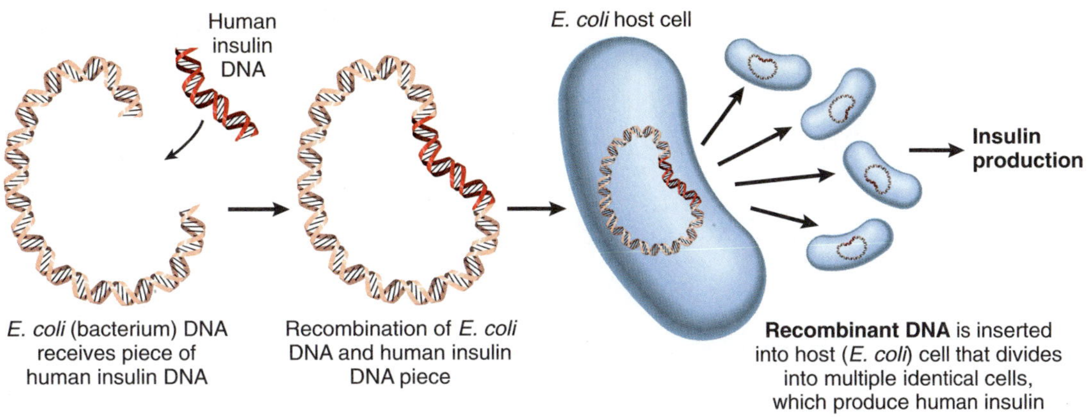

FIGURE 4-10 **Recombinant DNA and insulin production.**

SYNDROME

A **syndrome** (from the Greek *dromos*, meaning a course for running) is a group of signs or symptoms that appear together to produce a typical clinical picture of a disease or inherited abnormality. For example, **Reye syndrome** is characterized by vomiting, swelling of the brain, increased intracranial pressure, hypoglycemia, and dysfunction of the liver. It may occur in children after a viral infection that has been treated with aspirin.

Marfan syndrome is an inherited connective tissue disorder marked by a tall, thin body type with long, "spidery" fingers and toes (arachnodactyly), elongated head, and heart, blood vessel, and ophthalmic abnormalities (see Figure 4-11).

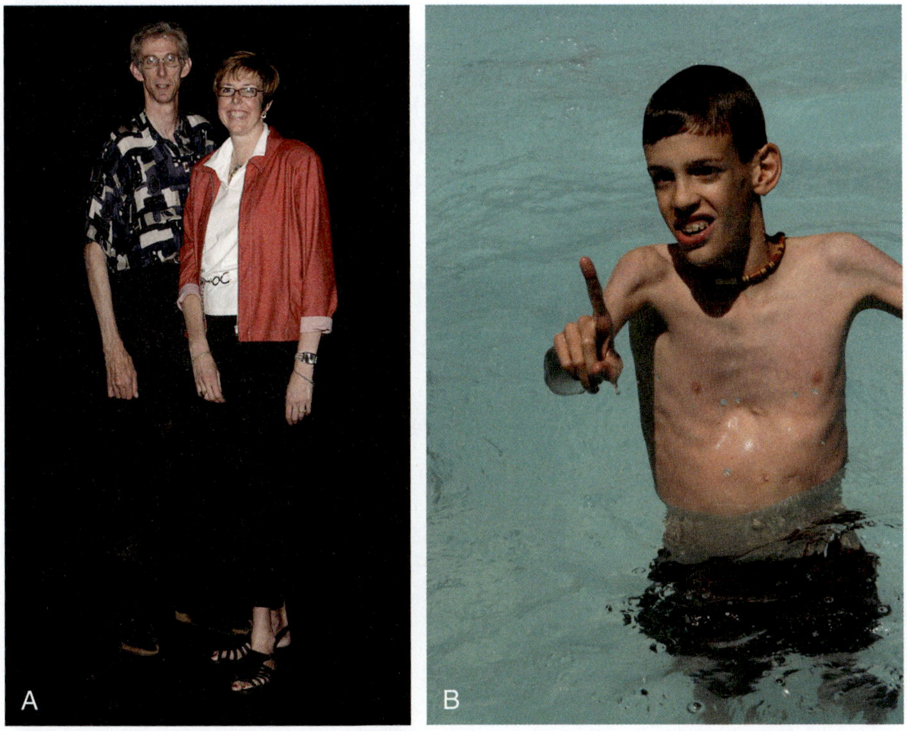

FIGURE 4-11 **Marfan syndrome. A** and **B** show individuals with Marfan's. Note the unusually tall body type (**A**) and long, spidery fingers (**B**). The Olympic swimmer, Michael Phelps, has Marfan syndrome. His height is 6″4′ and his arm span is 6″7′. Go to http://www.clevelandleader.com/node/6446 to read how Michael describes his condition.

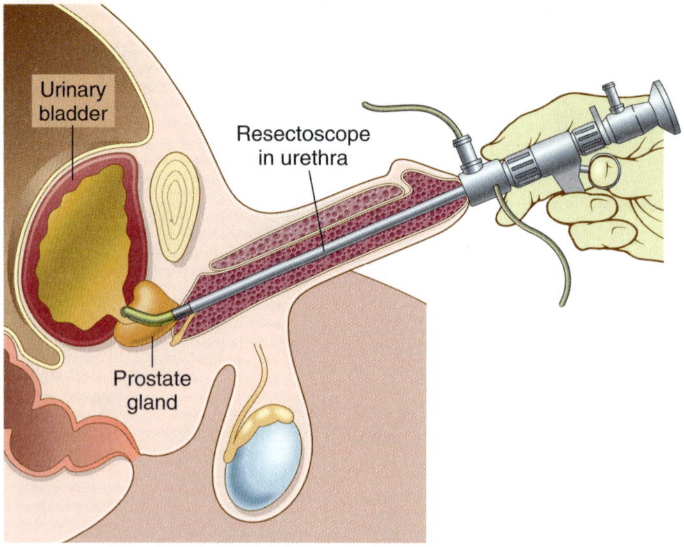

FIGURE 4-12 **Transurethral resection of the prostate (TURP).** The resectoscope contains a light, valves for controlling irrigated fluid, and an electrical loop that cuts tissue and seals blood vessels.

TRANSURETHRAL RESECTION OF THE PROSTATE GLAND

In **transurethral resection of the prostate gland** (**TURP**), a portion of the prostate gland is removed with an instrument (resectoscope) passed through **(trans-)** the urethra. The procedure is indicated when prostatic tissue increases (hyperplasia) and interferes with urination. Figure 4-12 shows TURP.

4

ULTRASONOGRAPHY

Ultrasonography is a diagnostic technique using ultrasound waves (inaudible sound waves) to produce an image of an organ or tissue. A machine records ultrasonic echoes as they pass through different types of tissue. **Echocardiograms** are ultrasound images of the heart. Figure 4-13 shows a fetal ultrasound image **(sonogram).**

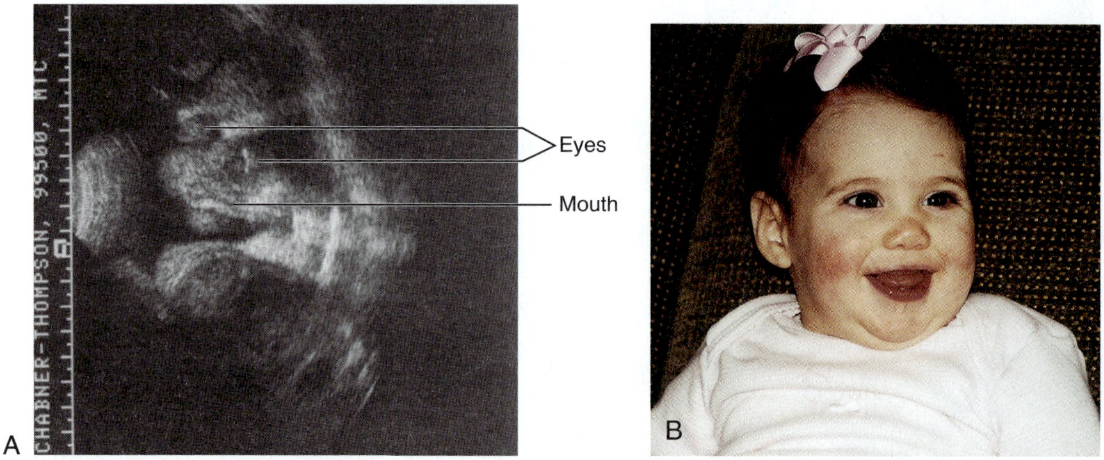

FIGURE 4-13 **Ultrasonography.** **(A)**, Notice the facial features of this beautiful 30-week-old fetus, in a (very) early "baby picture" of my granddaughter, Beatrix Bess Thompson! **(B)**, Bebe, smiling, at 3 months of age. *(Courtesy Dr. Elizabeth Chabner Thompson.)*

PRACTICAL APPLICATIONS

Check your answers with the Answers to Practical Applications on page 131. You should find helpful explanations there.

PROCEDURES

Match the **procedure** or **treatment** in Column I with the best **reason for using it** in Column II. Write the letter of the answer in the space provided.

COLUMN I		COLUMN II
Procedures/Treatments		*Indications*
1. ultrasonography	_____	A. diagnose hepatopathy
2. hemiglossectomy	_____	B. treat renal failure
3. percutaneous liver biopsy	_____	C. obtain prenatal images
4. transfusion of blood cells	_____	D. determine the postmortem status of organs
5. gastric endoscopy	_____	E. treat carcinoma of the tongue
6. autopsy	_____	F. treat benign prostatic hyperplasia
7. endotracheal intubation	_____	G. diagnose disease in the stomach
8. dialysis	_____	H. establish an airway during surgery
9. antibiotics	_____	I. treat pancytopenia
10. transurethral resection	_____	J. treat staphylococcemia

EXERCISES

Remember to check your answers carefully with the Answers to Exercises, pages 130 and 131.

A Give the meanings of the following prefixes.

1. ante- ______________________
2. ab- ______________________
3. ana- ______________________
4. anti- ______________________
5. a-, an- ______________________
6. ad- ______________________
7. auto- ______________________
8. cata- ______________________
9. brady- ______________________
10. contra- ______________________
11. bi- ______________________
12. con- ______________________

B Match the following terms with their meanings below.

adductor	anteflexion	bilateral
adrenal	antepartum	bradycardia
analysis	antisepsis	congenital anomaly
anoxia	apnea	contralateral

1. bending forward ______________________
2. muscle that carries the limb toward the body ______________________
3. before birth ______________________
4. slow heartbeat ______________________
5. gland located near (above) each kidney ______________________
6. absence of breathing ______________________
7. pertaining to the opposite side ______________________
8. against infection ______________________
9. to separate ______________________
10. pertaining to two (both) sides ______________________
11. condition of no oxygen in tissues ______________________
12. irregularity present at birth ______________________

C Select from the following terms to match the descriptions below.

anabolism	antigen	catabolism
antibiotic	antitoxin	congenital anomaly
antibody	autoimmune disease	contraindication

1. chemical substance, such as erythromycin (-mycin = mold), made from molds and used against bacterial life ______________________
2. process of burning food (breaking it down) and releasing the energy stored in the food ______________________
3. reason that a doctor would advise against taking a specific medication ______________________
4. disorder in which the body's own leukocytes make antibodies that damage its own good tissue ______________________
5. a foreign agent (virus or bacterium) that causes production of antibodies ______________________
6. an antibody that acts against poisons that enter the body ______________________
7. process of building up proteins in cells by putting together small pieces of proteins called amino acids ______________________
8. protein made by lymphocytes in response to the presence in the blood of a specific antigen ______________________

D Give the meanings of the following prefixes.

1. ec- ______________________
2. dys- ______________________
3. de- ______________________
4. dia- ______________________
5. hemi- ______________________
6. hypo- ______________________
7. epi- ______________________
8. hyper- ______________________
9. endo- ______________________
10. eu- ______________________
11. in- ______________________
12. inter- ______________________
13. intra- ______________________
14. infra- ______________________
15. macro- ______________________

E **Complete the following terms, based on their meanings as given.**

1. normal thyroid function: ________________________ thyroid
2. painful breathing: ________________________ pnea
3. pregnancy that is out of place (outside the uterus): ________________________ topic
4. instrument to visually examine within the body: endo ________________________
5. removal of half of the tongue: ________________________ glossectomy
6. good (exaggerated) feeling (of well-being): ________________________ phoria
7. pertaining to within the windpipe: endo ________________________
8. blood condition of less than normal sugar: ________________________ glycemia
9. condition (congenital anomaly) of large head: ________________________ cephaly
10. pertaining to between the ribs: ________________________ costal
11. pertaining to within a vein: intra ________________________
12. condition of bad (abnormal) formation (of cells): dys ________________________
13. condition of excessive formation (numbers of cells): ________________________ plasia
14. structure (membrane) that forms the inner lining of the heart: endo ________________________
15. pertaining to below the ribs: infra ________________________
16. blood condition of excessive amount of sugar: hyper ________________________

F **Match the following terms with their meanings below.**

dehydration	incision	metamorphosis
dialysis	insomnia	metastasis
diarrhea	malaise	microscope
exophthalmos (proptosis)	malignant	pancytopenia

1. vague feeling of bodily discomfort ________________________
2. inability to sleep ________________________
3. lack of water ________________________
4. spread of a cancerous tumor to a secondary organ or tissue ________________________
5. instrument used to view small objects ________________________
6. to cut into an organ or tissue ________________________
7. outward bulging of the eyeballs ________________________
8. condition of change in shape or form ________________________
9. watery discharge of wastes from the colon ________________________
10. deficiency of all (blood) cells ________________________
11. separation of wastes from the blood by using a machine that does the job of the kidney

    ____
12. harmful, cancerous ________________________

G Give the meanings of the following prefixes.

1. mal- ______
2. pan- ______
3. per- ______
4. meta- ______
5. para- ______
6. peri- ______
7. poly- ______
8. post- ______
9. pro- ______
10. pre- ______
11. sub- ______
12. supra- ______
13. re- ______
14. retro- ______
15. tachy- ______
16. syn- ______
17. uni- ______
18. trans- ______
19. neo- ______
20. epi- ______

H Underline the prefix in the following terms, and give the meaning of the entire term.

1. periosteum ______
2. percutaneous ______
3. retroperitoneal ______
4. suprapubic ______
5. polyneuritis ______
6. retroflexion ______
7. transurethral ______
8. subcutaneous ______
9. tachypnea ______
10. unilateral ______
11. prosthesis ______

I Match the following terms with their meanings below.

adrenal	prodrome	remission
neoplasm	prolapse	syndactyly
paralysis	recombinant DNA	syndrome
parathyroid	relapse	ultrasonography

1. return of a disease or its symptoms ____________________
2. loss of movement in muscles ____________________
3. congenital anomaly in which fingers or toes are webbed (formed together) ____________________
4. four endocrine glands that are located near (behind) another endocrine gland in the neck ____________________
5. glands that are located above the kidneys ____________________
6. symptoms that come before the actual illness ____________________
7. technique of transferring genetic material from one organism into another ____________________
8. sliding, sagging downward or forward ____________________
9. new growth or tumor ____________________
10. process of using sound waves to create an image of organs and structures in the body ____________________
11. group of symptoms that occur together and indicate a particular disorder ____________________
12. symptoms lessen and a patient feels better ____________________

4

J Complete the following terms, based on their meanings as given.

1. pertaining to new birth: neo____________________
2. after death: post ____________________
3. spread of a cancerous tumor: meta ____________________
4. branching into two: bi ____________________
5. increase in development (size of cells): hyper ____________________
6. pertaining to a chemical that works against bacterial life: ____________________ biotic
7. hand bones (beyond the wrist): ____________________ carpals
8. protein produced by leukocytes to fight foreign organisms: anti ____________________
9. group of symptoms that occur together: ____________________ drome
10. surface or skin tissue of the body: ____________________ thelium

K **Circle the correct term to complete the following sentences.**

1. Dr. Tate felt that Mrs. Snow's condition of thrombocytopenia was a clear (**analysis, contraindication, synthesis**) to performing elective surgery.

2. Medical science was revolutionized by the introduction of (**antigens, antibiotics, antibodies**) in the 1940s. Now some infections can be treated with only one dose.

3. Robert's 82-year-old grandfather complained of (**malaise, dialysis, insomnia**) despite taking the sleeping medication that his doctor prescribed.

4. During her pregnancy, Ms. Payne described pressure on her (**pituitary gland, parathyroid gland, pubic symphysis**), making it difficult for her to find a comfortable position, even when seated.

5. Many times, people with diabetes accidentally take too much insulin. This results in lowering their blood sugar so much that they may be admitted to the emergency department with (**hyperplasia, hypoglycemia, hyperglycemia**).

6. Before his migraine headaches began, John noticed changes in his eyesight, such as bright spots, zigzag lines, and double vision. His physician told him that these were (**symbiotic, exophthalmic, prodromal**) symptoms.

7. After hiking in the Grand Canyon without an adequate water supply, Julie experienced (**hyperglycemia, dehydration, hypothyroidism**).

8. At 65 years of age, Paul Smith often felt fullness in his urinary bladder but had difficulty urinating. He visited his (**cardiologist, nephrologist, urologist**), who examined his prostate gland and diagnosed (**hyperplasia, atrophy, ischemia**). The doctor advised (**intracostal, transurethral, peritoneal**) resection of Paul's prostate.

9. After running the Boston Marathon, Elizabeth felt nauseated and dizzy. She realized that she was experiencing (**malaise, euphoria, hypoglycemia**) and drank a sports drink containing sugar, which made her feel better.

10. While she was taking an antibiotic that reacted with sunlight, Ruth's physician advised her that sunbathing was (**unilateral, contraindicated, contralateral**) and might cause a serious sunburn.

11. Puerperal (pertaining to childbirth) fever was an iatrogenic infection; it was carried from one woman to another by the doctor before the days of (**antigens, antibodies, antisepsis**).

12. Dysplastic nevi (abnormal pigmented lesions or moles) on a patient's skin may be a (**precancerous, metastatic, unilateral**) sign of malignant skin cancer called melanoma.

13. Nerve cells of the brain may (**relapse, hypertrophy, atrophy**) in old age because of ischemia caused by restricted blood flow.

14. Changes in cell growth resulting in cells that differ in size, shape, and appearance are the result of chronic inflammation and irritation. When the condition occurs in the uterine cervix, it is known as cervical (**prolapsed, paralysis, dysplasia**).

ANSWERS TO EXERCISES

A

1. before, forward
2. away from
3. up, apart
4. against
5. no, not, without
6. toward
7. self, own
8. down
9. slow
10. against, opposite
11. two
12. together, with

B

1. anteflexion
2. adductor
3. antepartum
4. bradycardia
5. adrenal
6. apnea
7. contralateral
8. antisepsis
9. analysis
10. bilateral
11. anoxia
12. congenital anomaly

C

1. antibiotic
2. catabolism
3. contraindication
4. autoimmune disease
5. antigen
6. antitoxin
7. anabolism
8. antibody

D

1. out, outside
2. bad, painful, difficult
3. down, lack of
4. through, complete
5. half
6. deficient, under
7. upon, on, above
8. excessive, above, beyond
9. in, within
10. good, well
11. in, not
12. between
13. within
14. below, inferior
15. large

E

1. euthyroid
2. dyspnea
3. ectopic
4. endoscope
5. hemiglossectomy
6. euphoria
7. endotracheal
8. hypoglycemia
9. macrocephaly
10. intercostal
11. intravenous
12. dysplasia
13. hyperplasia
14. endocardium
15. infracostal
16. hyperglycemia

F

1. malaise
2. insomnia
3. dehydration
4. metastasis
5. microscope
6. incision
7. exophthalmos (proptosis)
8. metamorphosis
9. diarrhea
10. pancytopenia
11. dialysis
12. malignant

G

1. bad
2. all
3. through
4. change, beyond
5. near, beside, abnormal
6. surrounding
7. many, much
8. after, behind
9. before, forward
10. before, in front of
11. under
12. above
13. back, again
14. behind, backward
15. fast
16. together, with
17. one
18. across, through
19. new
20. above, upon, on

H

1. periosteum—membrane (structure) surrounding bone
2. percutaneous—pertaining to through the skin
3. retroperitoneal—pertaining to behind the peritoneum
4. suprapubic—above the pubic bone
5. polyneuritis—inflammation of many nerves
6. retroflexion—bending backward
7. transurethral—pertaining to through the urethra
8. subcutaneous—pertaining to below the skin
9. tachypnea—rapid, fast breathing
10. unilateral—pertaining to one side
11. prosthesis—artificial limb or part of the body (literally, to put or place forward)

I

1. relapse
2. paralysis
3. syndactyly
4. parathyroid
5. adrenal
6. prodrome
7. recombinant DNA
8. prolapse
9. neoplasm
10. ultrasonography
11. syndrome
12. remission

J

1. neonatal
2. postmortem
3. metastasis
4. bifurcation
5. hypertrophy
6. antibiotic
7. metacarpals
8. antibody
9. syndrome
10. epithelium

K

1. contraindication
2. antibiotics
3. insomnia
4. pubic symphysis
5. hypoglycemia
6. prodromal
7. dehydration
8. urologist; hypertrophy; transurethral
9. hypoglycemia
10. contraindicated
11. antisepsis
12. precancerous
13. atrophy
14. dysplasia

Answers to Practical Applications

1. **C** Ultrasonography is especially useful to detect fetal structures because no x-rays are used.
2. **E** Malignancies of the oral (mouth) cavity often are treated with surgery to remove the cancerous growth.
3. **A** Diseases such as hepatitis or hepatoma are diagnosed by performing a liver biopsy.
4. **I** Transfusion of leukocytes, erythrocytes, and platelets will increase numbers of these cells in the bloodstream.
5. **G** Placement of an endoscope through the mouth and esophagus and into the stomach is used to diagnose gastric (stomach) disease.
6. **D** A veterinarian performs a postmortem examination of an animal, which is called a necropsy.
7. **H** Endotracheal intubation is necessary during surgery in which general anesthesia is used.
8. **B** Patients experiencing loss of kidney function need dialysis to remove waste materials from the blood.
9. **J** Examples of antibiotics are penicillin, erythromycin, and amoxicillin.
10. **F** A TURP is a transurethral resection of the prostate gland.

PRONUNCIATION OF TERMS

To test your understanding of the terminology in this chapter, write the meaning of each term in the space provided. In addition, you may wish to cover the terms and write them by looking at your definitions. Make sure your spelling is correct. The CAPITAL letters indicate the accented syllable. The page number after each term indicates where it is defined or used in the book, so you can easily check your responses. You will find complete definitions for all of these terms and their audio pronunciations on the Evolve website.

Pronunciation Guide

ā as in āpe	ă as in ăpple
ē as in ēven	ĕ as in ĕvery
ī as in īce	ĭ as in ĭnterest
ō as in ōpen	ŏ as in pŏt
ū as in ūnit	ŭ as in ŭnder

TERM	PRONUNCIATION	MEANING
abductor (109)	ăb-DŬK-tŏr	
abnormal (109)	ăb-NŌR-măl	
adductor (110)	ă-DŬK-tŏr	
adrenal glands (110)	ă-DRĒ-năl glăndz	
anabolism (110)	ă-NĂ-bō-lĭzm	
analysis (110)	ă-NĂL-ĭ-sĭs	
anoxia (109)	ă-NŎK-sē-ă	
ante cibum (110)	ĂN-tē SĒ-bŭm	
anteflexion (110)	ăn-tē-FLĔK-shŭn	
antepartum (110)	ăn-tē-PĂR-tŭm	
antibiotic (111)	ăn-tĭ-bī-ŎT-ĭk	
antibody (111)	ĂN-tĭ-bŏd-ē	
antigen (111)	ĂN-tĭ-jĕn	
antisepsis (111)	ăn-tĭ-SĔP-sĭs	
antitoxin (111)	ăn-tĭ-TŎK-sĭn	
apnea (109)	ĂP-nē-ă *or* ăp-NĒ-ă	
autoimmune disease (111)	ăw-tō-ĭ-MŪN dĭ-ZĒZ	
benign (114)	bē-NĪN	
bifurcation (111)	bī-fŭr-KĀ-shŭn	
bilateral (111)	bī-LĂT-ĕr-ăl	
bradycardia (111)	brăd-ē-KĂR-dē-ă	
catabolism (111)	kă-TĂB-ō-lĭzm	
congenital anomaly (111)	kŏn-JĔN-ĭ-tăl ă-NŎM-ă-lē	
connective tissue (111)	kŏn-NĔK-tĭv TĬ-shū	
contraindication (112)	kŏn-tră-ĭn-dĭ-KĀ-shŭn	
contralateral (112)	kŏn-tră-LĂT-ĕr-ăl	

4

TERM	PRONUNCIATION	MEANING
dehydration (112)	dē-hī-DRĀ-shŭn	________
dialysis (112)	dī-ĂL-ĭ-sĭs	________
diameter (112)	dī-ĂM-ĭ-tĕr	________
diarrhea (112)	dī-ă-RĒ-ă	________
dysplasia (112)	dĭs-PLĀ-zē-ă	________
dyspnea (112)	DĬSP-nē-ă *or* dĭsp-NĒ-ă	________
ectopic pregnancy (112)	ĕk-TŎP-ĭk PRĔG-năn-sē	________
endocardium (113)	ĕn-dō-KĂR-dē-ŭm	________
endoscope (113)	ĔN-dō-skōp	________
endotracheal (113)	ĕn-dō-TRĀ-kē-ăl	________
epithelium (113)	ĕp-ĭ-THĒ-lē-ŭm	________
euphoria (113)	ū-FŎR-ē-ă	________
euthyroid (113)	ū-THĪ-royd	________
exophthalmos (113)	ĕk-sŏf-THĂL-mŏs	________
hemiglossectomy (113)	hĕm-ē-glŏs-SĔK-tō-mē	________
hyperglycemia (113)	hī-pĕr-glī-SĒ-mē-ă	________
hyperplasia (113)	hī-pĕr-PLĀ-zē-ă	________
hypertrophy (113)	hī-PĔR-trō-fē	________
hypodermic injection (113)	hī-pō-DĔR-mĭk ĭn-JĔK-shŭn	________
hypoglycemia (113)	hī-pō-glī-SĒ-mē-ă	________
incision (113)	ĭn-SĬZ-ŏn	________
infracostal (114)	ĭn-fră-KŎS-tăl	________
insomniac (113)	ĭn-SŎM-nē-ăk	________
intercostal (114)	ĭn-tĕr-KŎS-tăl	________
intravenous (114)	ĭn-tră-VĒ-nŭs	________
macrocephaly (114)	măk-rō-SĔF-ă-lē	________
malaise (114)	măl-ĀZ	________
malignant (114)	mă-LĬG-nănt	________
metacarpal bones (114)	mĕ-tă-KĂR-păl bōnz	________
metamorphosis (114)	mĕt-ă-MŎR-fŏ-sĭs	________
metastasis (114)	mĕ-TĂS-tă-sĭs	________
microscope (114)	MĪ-krō-skōp	________
neonatal (114)	nē-ō-NĀ-tăl	________
neoplasm (114)	NĒ-ō-plăzm	________

4

TERM	PRONUNCIATION	MEANING
pancytopenia (114)	păn-sī-tō-PĒ-nē-ă	______________
paralysis (114)	pă-RĂL-ĭ-sĭs	______________
parathyroid glands (114)	păr-ă-THĪ-royd glănz	______________
percutaneous (115)	pĕr-kū-TĀ-nē-ŭs	______________
pericardium (115)	pĕ-rē-KĂR-dē-ŭm	______________
periosteum (115)	pĕr-ē-ŎS-tē-ŭm	______________
polymorphonuclear (115)	pŏl-ē-mŏr-fō-NŪ-klē-ăr	______________
polyneuritis (115)	pŏl-ē-nū-RĪ-tĭs	______________
postmortem (115)	pōst-MŎR-tĕm	______________
postpartum (115)	pōst-PĂR-tŭm	______________
precancerous (115)	prē-KĂN-sĕr-ŭs	______________
prenatal (115)	prē-NĀ-tăl	______________
prodrome (115)	PRŌ-drōm	______________
prolapse (115)	PRŌ-lăps	______________
prosthesis (116)	prŏs-THĒ-sĭs	______________
recombinant DNA (116)	rē-KŎM-bĭ-nănt DNA	______________
relapse (116)	RĒ-lăps	______________
remission (116)	rē-MĬ-shŭn	______________
retroflexion (116)	rĕt-rō-FLĔK-shŭn	______________
retroperitoneal (116)	rĕt-rō-pĕr-ĭ-tō-NĒ-ăl	______________
subcutaneous (116)	sŭb-kū-TĀ-nē-ŭs	______________
suprapubic (116)	sū-pră-PŪ-bĭk	______________
symbiosis (117)	sĭm-bē-Ō-sĭs	______________
symmetry (117)	SĬM-mĕ-trē	______________
symphysis (117)	SĬM-fĭ-sĭs	______________
syndactyly (117)	sĭn-DĂK-tĭ-lē	______________
syndrome (117)	SĬN-drōm	______________
synthesis (117)	SĬN-thĕ-sĭs	______________
tachypnea (118)	tă-KĬP-nē-ă *or* tăk-ĭp-NĒ-ă	______________
transfusion (118)	trăns-FŪ-zhŭn	______________
transurethral (118)	trăns-ū-RĒ-thrăl	______________
ultrasonography (118)	ŭl-tră-sŏ-NŎG-ră-fē	______________
unilateral (118)	ū-nē-LĂT-ĕr-ăl	______________

4

REVIEW SHEET

Write the meanings of each word part in the space provided, and test yourself. Check your answers with the information in the chapter or in the Glossary (Medical Word Parts—English) at the end of the book.

Prefixes

PREFIX	MEANING	PREFIX	MEANING
a-, an-		inter-	
ab-		intra-	
ad-		macro-	
ana-		mal-	
ante-		meta-	
anti-		micro-	
auto-		neo-	
bi-		pan-	
brady-		para-	
cata-		per-	
con-		peri-	
contra-		poly-	
de-		post-	
dia-		pre-	
dys-		pro-	
ec-, ecto-		pros-	
en-, endo-		re-	
epi-		retro-	
eu-		sub-	
ex-		supra-	
hemi-		syn-, sym-	
hyper-		tachy-	
hypo-		trans-	
in-		ultra-	
infra-		uni-	

Combining Forms

COMBINING FORM	MEANING	COMBINING FORM	MEANING
carp/o	______	nect/o	______
cib/o	______	norm/o	______
cost/o	______	ophthalm/o	______
cutane/o	______	ox/o	______
dactyl/o	______	pub/o	______
duct/o	______	ren/o	______
flex/o	______	seps/o	______
furc/o	______	somn/o	______
gloss/o	______	son/o	______
glyc/o	______	the/o	______
immun/o	______	thyr/o	______
later/o	______	top/o	______
morph/o	______	tox/o	______
mort/o	______	trache/o	______
nat/i	______	urethr/o	______
necr/o	______	ven/o	______

Suffixes

SUFFIX	MEANING	SUFFIX	MEANING
-blast	____________	-partum	____________
-crine	____________	-phoria	____________
-drome	____________	-physis	____________
-fusion	____________	-plasia	____________
-gen	____________	-plasm	____________
-lapse	____________	-pnea	____________
-lysis	____________	-ptosis	____________
-meter	____________	-rrhea	____________
-mission	____________	-stasis	____________
-or	____________	-trophy	____________

Prefixes with Similar Meanings

PREFIX	MEANING	PREFIX	MEANING
a-, an-, in-	____________	ec-, ecto-, ex-	____________
ante-, pre-, pro-	____________	endo-, in-, intra-	____________
anti-, contra-	____________	epi-, hyper-, supra-	____________
con-, syn-, sym-	____________	hypo-, infra-, sub-	____________
de-, cata-	____________	re-, retro-, post-	____________
dia-, per-, trans-	____________	ultra-, meta-	____________
dys-, mal-	____________		

evolve *Please visit the Evolve website for additional exercises, games, and images related to this chapter.*

CHAPTER 5

Digestive System

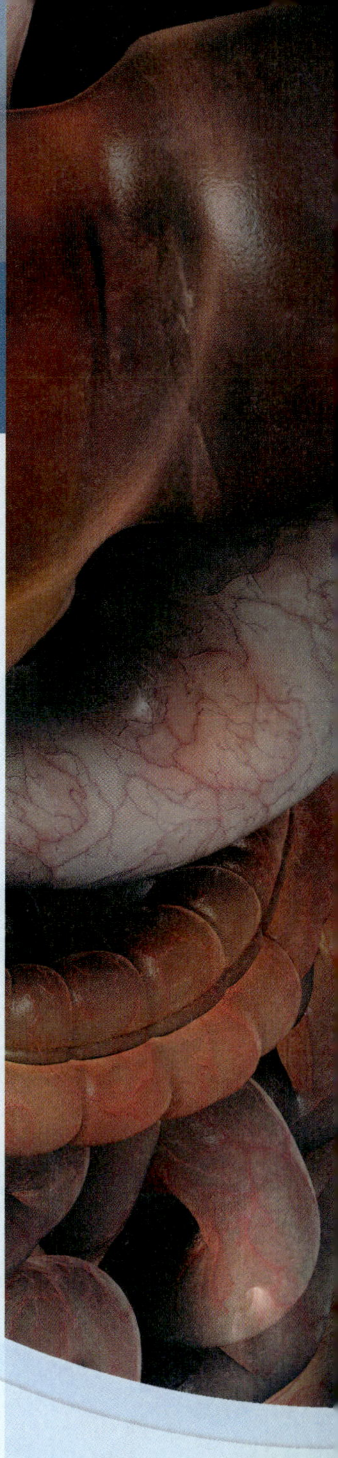

This chapter is divided into the following sections:

CHAPTER GOALS

- Name the organs of the digestive system and describe their locations and functions.
- Define combining forms for organs and know the meaning of related terminology.
- Describe signs, symptoms, and disease conditions affecting the digestive system.

INTRODUCTION

The digestive system is divided between Chapters 5 and 6. Chapter 5 covers the anatomy, physiology, pathology, and basic terminology of the system. Chapter 6 introduces additional terminology and review of digestive system terms, plus laboratory tests, clinical procedures, and abbreviations. My reason for not combining the chapters is that I did not want to overwhelm you with an extraordinarily long chapter so early in your study. In my own teaching, I find that my students are grateful for this separation, and especially for the breather and review of terminology in Chapter 6.

My choice to begin with the digestive system is based on a perception that this body system (resembling a long conveyor belt with the mouth at the entrance and anus at the exit) is one of the more straightforward and easiest to teach and understand. Keep in mind, however, that the book is organized so that you may begin study of the body systems with any chapter to create the order that best reflects your interests.

The digestive or **gastrointestinal tract** begins with the mouth, where food enters, and ends with the anus, where solid waste material leaves the body. The four functions of the system are **ingestion, digestion, absorption,** and **elimination.**

First, complex food material taken into the mouth is **ingested**. Second, it is **digested,** or broken down, mechanically and chemically, as it travels through the gastrointestinal tract. Digestive **enzymes** speed up chemical reactions and aid the breakdown (digestion) of complex nutrients. Complex proteins are digested to simpler **amino acids**; complicated sugars are reduced to simple sugars, such as **glucose**; and large fat or lipid molecules are broken down to simpler substances such as **fatty acids** and **triglycerides** (three parts fatty acids and one part glycerol). Digestion occurs in the mouth, stomach, and small intestine.

Third, via **absorption,** digested food passes through the lining cells or epithelium of the small intestine and into the bloodstream. Nutrients thus travel to all cells of the body. Cells then break down nutrients in the presence of oxygen to release energy. Cells also use amino acid nutrients to build up large protein molecules needed for growth and development. In addition, fat molecules are absorbed into lymphatic vessels from the intestine.

The fourth function of the digestive system is **elimination** of the solid waste materials that cannot be absorbed into the bloodstream. The large intestine concentrates these solid wastes, called **feces,** and the wastes finally pass out of the body through the anus.

ANATOMY AND PHYSIOLOGY

ORAL CAVITY

The gastrointestinal tract begins with the oral cavity. Oral means pertaining to the mouth (or/o). Label Figure 5-1 as you learn the major parts of the oral cavity.

The **cheeks** [1] form the walls of the oval-shaped oral cavity, and the **lips** [2] surround the opening to the cavity.

The **hard palate** [3] forms the anterior portion of the roof of the mouth, and the muscular **soft palate** [4] lies posterior to it. **Rugae** are irregular ridges in the mucous membrane covering the anterior portion of the hard palate. The **uvula** [5], a small soft tissue projection, hangs from the soft palate. It aids production of sounds and speech.

The **tongue** [6] extends across the floor of the oral cavity, and muscles attach it to the lower jawbone. It moves food around during **mastication** (chewing) and **deglutition** (swallowing). **Papillae,** small raised areas on the tongue, contain taste buds that are sensitive to the chemical nature of foods and allow discrimination of different tastes as food moves across the tongue.

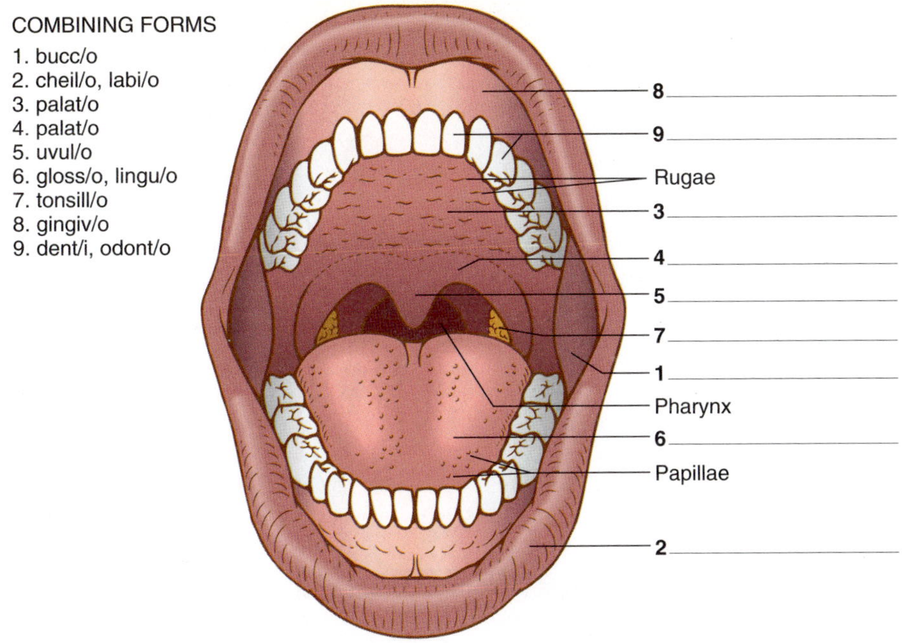

FIGURE 5-1 **Oral cavity.**

The **tonsils** [7], masses of lymphatic tissue located in depressions of the mucous membranes, lie on both sides of the oropharynx (part of the throat near the mouth). They are filters to protect the body from the invasion of microorganisms and produce lymphocytes, disease-fighting white blood cells.

The **gums** [8] are the fleshy tissue surrounding the sockets of the **teeth** [9]. Figure 5-2 shows a dental arch with 16 permanent teeth (there are 32 permanent teeth in the entire oral cavity). The names of the teeth are labeled in Figure 5-2.

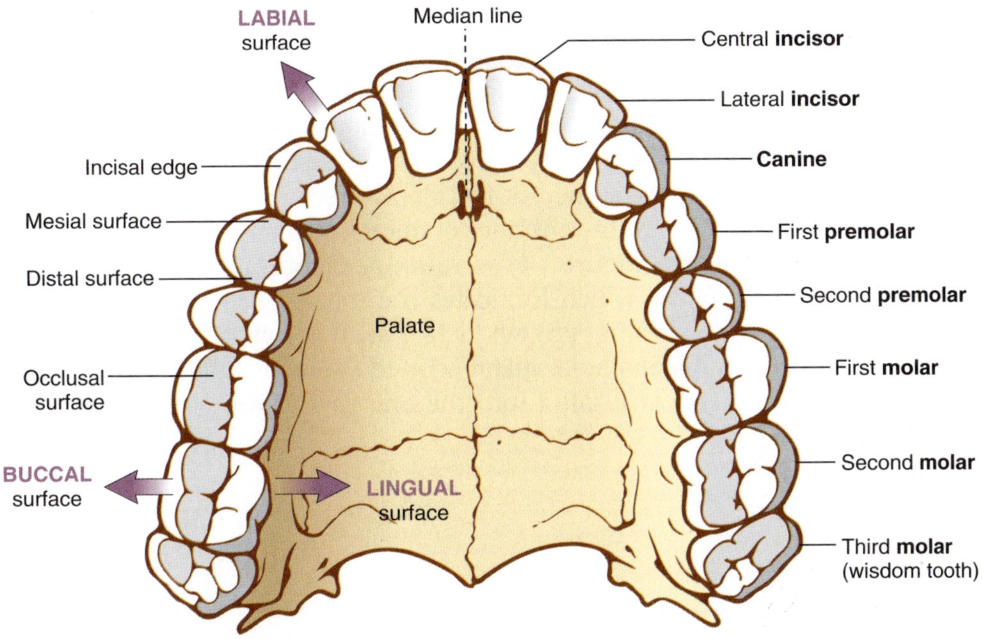

FIGURE 5-2 **Upper permanent teeth within the dental arch.** The **buccal** surface faces the cheek, whereas the **lingual** surface faces the tongue. The **labial** surface faces the lips. Dentists refer to the labial and buccal surfaces as the **facial** (faci/o = face) surface.

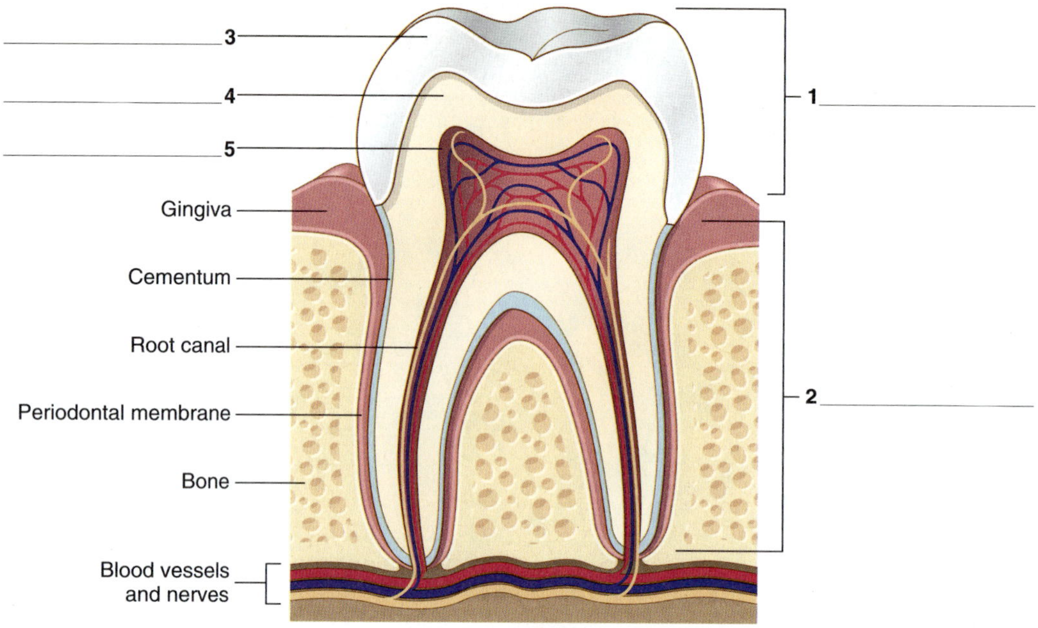

FIGURE 5-3 **Anatomy of a tooth.**

Figure 5-3 shows the inner anatomy of a tooth. Label it as you read the following description:

A tooth consists of a **crown** [1], which shows above the gum line, and a **root** [2], which lies within the bony tooth socket. The outermost protective layer of the crown, the **enamel** [3], protects the tooth. Enamel is a dense, hard, white substance—the hardest substance in the body. **Dentin** [4], the main substance of the tooth, lies beneath the enamel and extends throughout the crown. Dentin is yellow and composed of bony tissue that is softer than enamel. The **cementum** covers, protects, and supports the dentin in the root. A **periodontal membrane** surrounds the cementum and holds the tooth in place in the tooth socket.

The **pulp** [5] lies underneath the dentin. This soft and delicate tissue fills the center of the tooth. Blood vessels, nerve endings, connective tissue, and lymphatic vessels are within the pulp canal (also called the **root canal**). Root canal therapy often is necessary when disease or abscess (pus collection) occurs in the pulp canal. A dentist opens the tooth from above and cleans the canal of infected tissue, nerves, and blood vessels. The canal is then disinfected and filled with material to prevent the entrance of microorganisms that could cause decay.

Three pairs of **salivary glands** (Figure 5-4) surround and empty into the oral cavity. These exocrine glands produce **saliva,** which lubricates the mouth. Saliva contains important digestive **enzymes** as well as healing growth factors such as cytokines. Saliva is released from a **parotid gland** [1], **submandibular gland** [2], and **sublingual gland** [3] on both sides of the mouth. Narrow ducts carry saliva into the oral cavity. The glands produce about 1.5 liters of saliva daily.

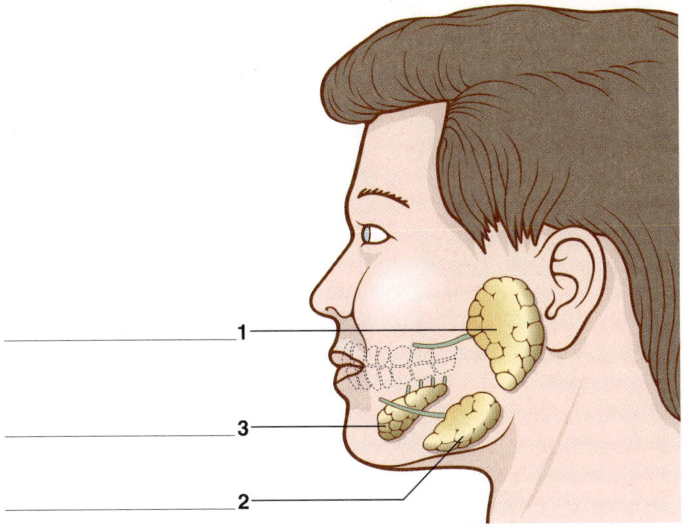

FIGURE 5-4 **Salivary glands.**

PHARYNX

Refer to Figure 5-5. The **pharynx** or **throat** is a muscular tube, about 5 inches long, lined with a mucous membrane. It serves as a passageway both for air traveling from the nose (nasal cavity) to the windpipe (trachea) and for food traveling from the oral cavity to the **esophagus.** When swallowing **(deglutition)** occurs, a cartilaginous flap of tissue, the epiglottis, covers the trachea so that food cannot enter and become lodged there. See Figure 5-5A and B.

5

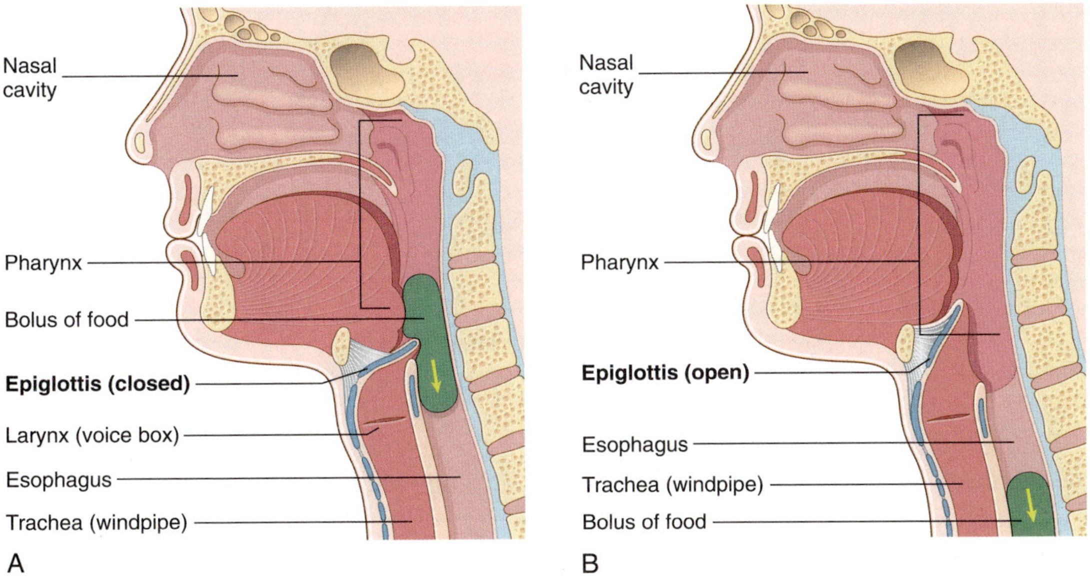

FIGURE 5-5 **Deglutition (swallowing). A, Epiglottis closes** over the trachea as the bolus of food passes down the pharynx toward the esophagus. **B, Epiglottis opens** as the bolus moves down the esophagus.

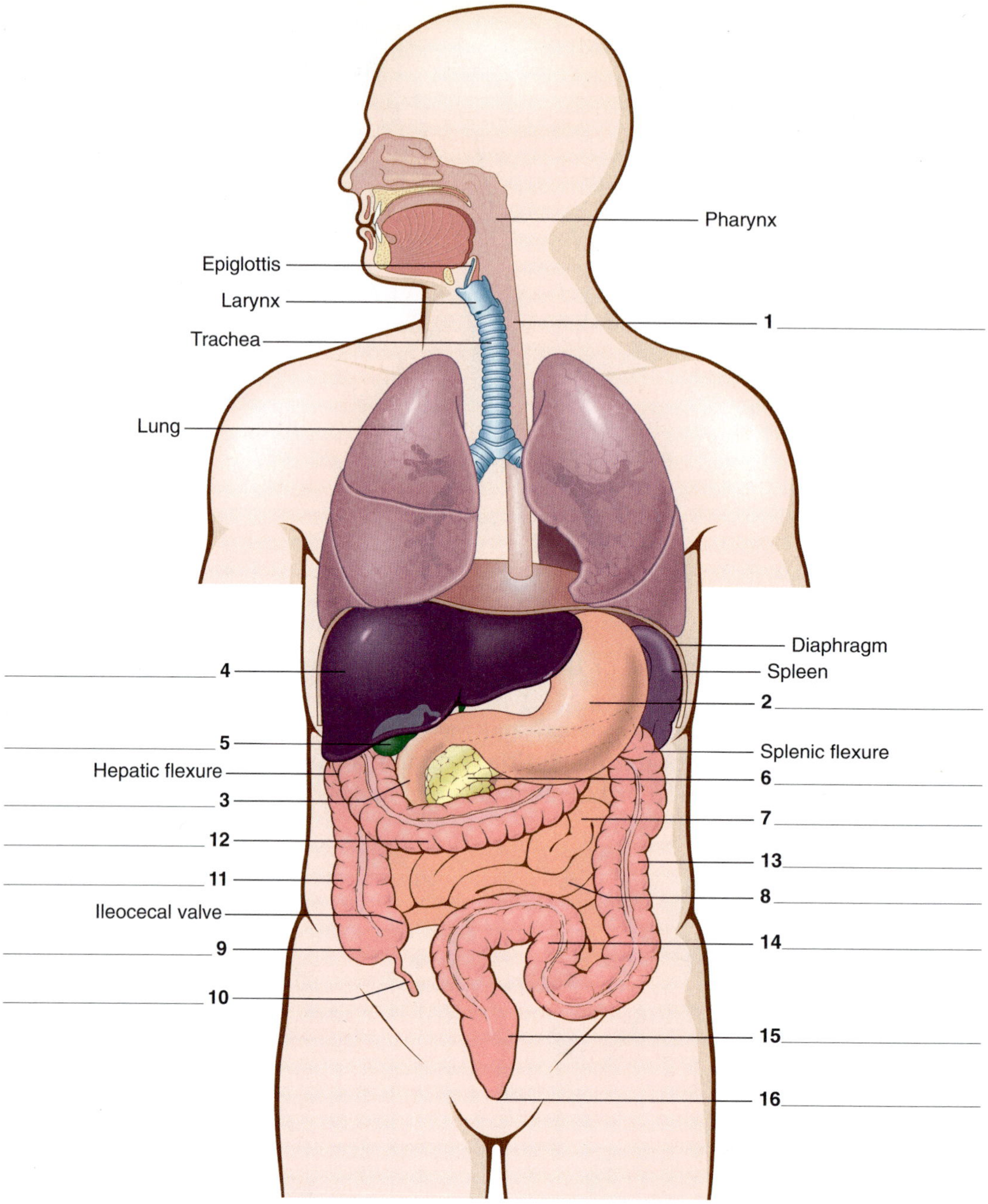

FIGURE 5-6 **The gastrointestinal tract.**

Figure 5-6 shows the passageway for food as it travels from the esophagus through the gastrointestinal tract. Label it as you read the following paragraphs.

ESOPHAGUS

The **esophagus** [1] is a 9- to 10-inch muscular tube extending from the pharynx to the stomach. **Peristalsis** is the involuntary, progressive, rhythmic contraction of muscles in the wall of the esophagus (and other gastrointestinal organs) propelling a **bolus** (mass of food) down toward the stomach. The process is like squeezing a marble through a rubber tube.

STOMACH

Food passes from the esophagus into the **stomach** [2]. The stomach (Figure 5-7) has three main parts: **fundus** (upper portion), **body** (middle section), and **antrum** (lower portion). Rings of muscle called **sphincters** control the openings into and leading out of the stomach. They prevent food from regurgitating (flowing backward from the normal direction). The **lower esophageal sphincter** relaxes and contracts to move food from the esophagus into the stomach; the **pyloric sphincter** allows food to leave the stomach when it is ready. Folds in the mucous membrane **(mucosa)** lining the stomach are called **rugae.** The rugae increase surface area for digestion and contain digestive glands that produce the enzyme **pepsin** (to begin digestion of proteins) and **hydrochloric acid.**

Besides beginning the digestion of proteins, the stomach prepares food for the small intestine, where further digestion and absorption into the bloodstream take place. The stomach controls passage of foods into the first part of the small intestine so that it proceeds only when it is chemically ready and in small amounts. Food leaves the stomach in 1 to 4 hours or longer, depending on the amount and type of food eaten.

SMALL INTESTINE (SMALL BOWEL)

(Continue labeling Figure 5-6 on page 144.)

The **small intestine (small bowel)** extends for 20 feet from the pyloric sphincter to the first part of the large intestine. It has three parts. The first section, the **duodenum** [3], is only 1 foot long. It receives food from the stomach as well as **bile** from the **liver** [4] and **gallbladder** [5] and pancreatic juice from the **pancreas** [6]. Enzymes and bile help digest food before it passes into the second part of the small intestine, the **jejunum** [7], about 8 feet long. The jejunum connects with the third section, the **ileum** [8], about 11 feet long. The ileum attaches to the first part of the large intestine.

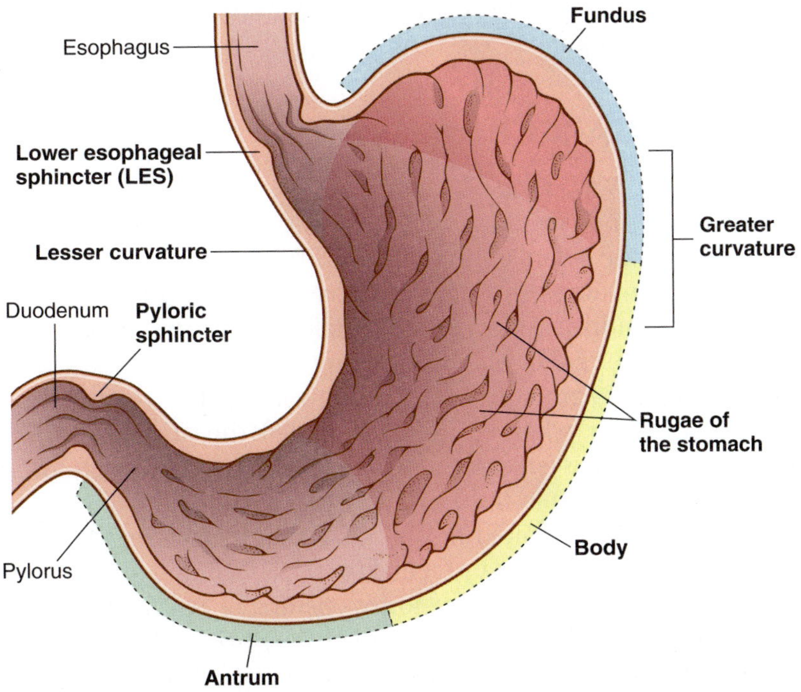

FIGURE 5-7 Parts of the stomach. The **fundus** and **body** (often referred to collectively as the fundus) are a reservoir for ingested food and an area for action by acid and pepsin (gastric enzyme). The **antrum** is a muscular grinding chamber that breaks up food and feeds it gradually into the duodenum.

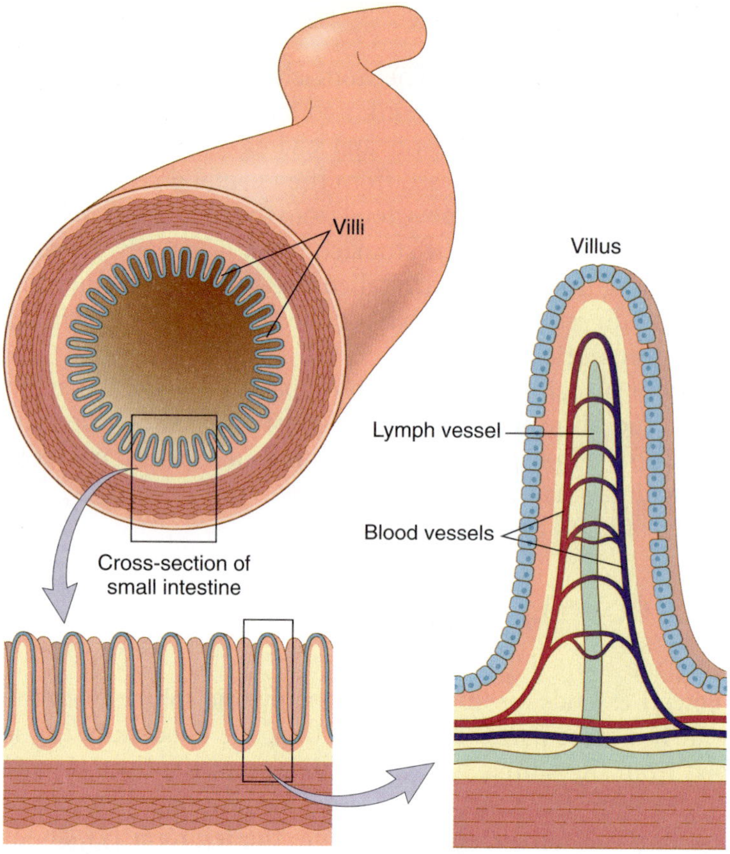

FIGURE 5-8 Villi in the lining of the small intestine. Villi increase the surface area for absorption of nutrients.

5

Millions of tiny, microscopic projections called **villi** line the walls of the small intestine. The tiny capillaries (microscopic blood vessels) in the villi absorb the digested nutrients into the bloodstream and lymph vessels. Figure 5-8 shows several different views of villi in the lining of the small intestine.

LARGE INTESTINE (LARGE BOWEL)

(Continue labeling Figure 5-6 on page 144.)

The **large intestine** extends from the end of the ileum to the anus. It has three main components: the cecum, the colon, and the rectum. The **cecum** [9] is a pouch on the right side that connects to the ileum at the ileocecal valve (sphincter). The **appendix** [10] hangs from the cecum. The appendix has no clear function and can become inflamed and infected when clogged or blocked. The **colon**, about 5 feet long, has four named segments: ascending, descending, transverse, and sigmoid. The **ascending colon** [11] extends from the cecum to the undersurface of the liver, where it turns to the left (hepatic flexure) to become the **transverse colon** [12]. The transverse colon passes horizontally to the left toward the spleen and then turns downward (splenic flexure) into the **descending colon** [13]. The **sigmoid colon** [14], shaped like an S (sigmoid means resembling the Greek letter sigma, which curves like the letter S), begins at the distal end of the descending colon and leads into the **rectum** [15]. The rectum terminates in the lower opening of the gastrointestinal tract, the **anus** [16].

The large intestine receives the fluid waste products of digestion (the material unable to pass into the bloodstream) and stores these wastes until they can be released from the body. Because the large intestine absorbs most of the water within the waste material, the body can expel solid **feces** (stools). **Defecation** is the expulsion or passage of feces from the body through the anus. Diarrhea, or passage of watery stools, results from reduced water absorption into the bloodstream through the walls of the large intestine.

LIVER, GALLBLADDER, AND PANCREAS

Three important additional organs of the digestive system—the liver, gallbladder, and pancreas—play crucial roles in the proper digestion and absorption of nutrients. Label Figure 5-9 as you study the following:

The **liver** [1], located in the right upper quadrant (RUQ) of the abdomen, manufactures a thick, orange-black, sometimes greenish, fluid called **bile.** Bile contains cholesterol (a fatty substance), bile acids, and several bile pigments. One of these pigments, **bilirubin,** is produced from the breakdown of hemoglobin during normal red blood cell destruction. Bilirubin travels via the bloodstream to the liver, where it is conjugated or converted into a water-soluble form. Conjugated bilirubin is then added to bile and enters the intestine (duodenum). Bacteria in the colon degrade bilirubin into a variety of pigments that give feces a brownish color. Bilirubin and bile leave the body in feces.

If the bile duct is blocked or the liver is damaged and unable to excrete bilirubin into bile, the bilirubin remains in the bloodstream, causing **jaundice** (**hyperbilirubinemia**)—yellow discoloration of the skin, whites of the eyes, and mucous membranes. Figure 5-10 reviews the path of bilirubin from red blood cell destruction (hemolysis) to elimination with bile in the feces.

(Continue labeling Figure 5-9.)

The liver continuously releases bile, which then travels through the **hepatic duct** to the **cystic duct.** The cystic duct leads to the **gallbladder** [2], a pear-shaped sac under the liver, which stores and concentrates the bile for later use. After meals, in response to the presence of food in the stomach and duodenum, the gallbladder contracts, forcing the bile out the cystic duct into the **common bile duct** [3]. Meanwhile, the **pancreas** [4] secretes pancreatic juices (enzymes) that are released into the **pancreatic duct** [5], which joins with the common bile duct just as it enters the **duodenum** [6]. The duodenum thus receives a mixture of bile and pancreatic juices.

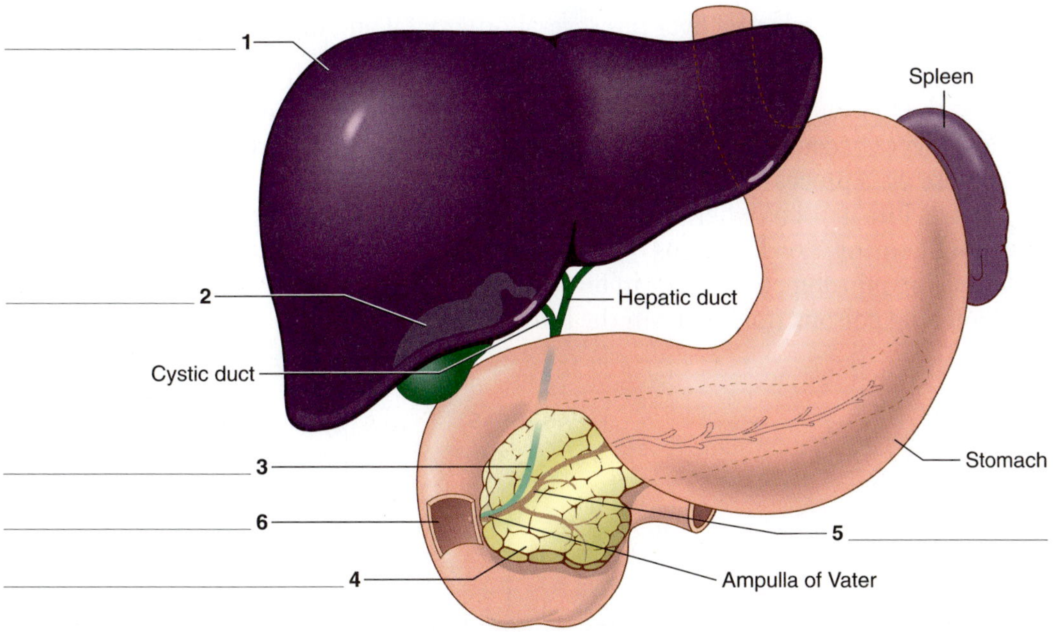

FIGURE 5-9 Liver, gallbladder, and pancreas. The **ampulla of Vater** is at the junction of the pancreatic duct and common bile duct entering the duodenum.

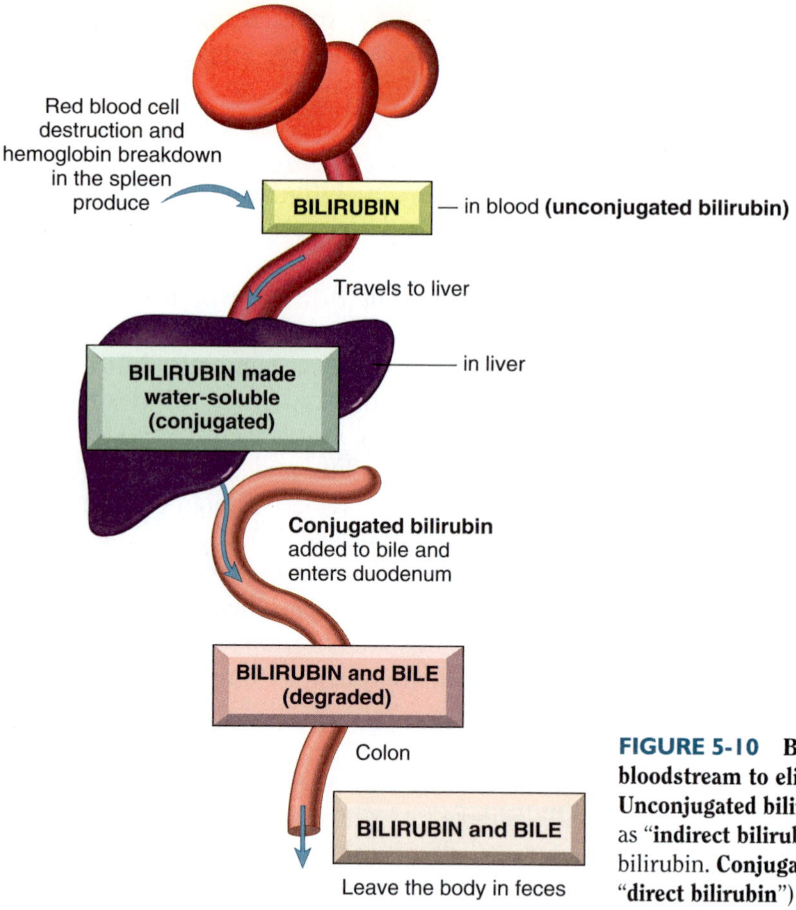

FIGURE 5-10 Bilirubin pathway from bloodstream to elimination in feces. Unconjugated bilirubin (measured in lab tests as "**indirect bilirubin**") is prehepatic, free bilirubin. **Conjugated bilirubin** (measured as "**direct bilirubin**") is posthepatic bilirubin.

Bile has a detergent-like effect on fats in the duodenum. In the process of **emulsification,** bile breaks apart large fat globules, creating more surface area so that enzymes from the pancreas can digest the fats. Without bile, most of the fat taken into the body remains undigested.

Besides producing bile, the liver has several other vital and important functions:

- Maintaining normal blood **glucose** (sugar) levels. The liver removes excess glucose from the bloodstream and stores it as **glycogen** (starch) in liver cells. When the blood sugar level becomes dangerously low, the liver converts stored glycogen back into glucose via a process called **glycogenolysis.** In addition, the liver can convert proteins and fats into glucose, when the body needs sugar, by a process called **gluconeogenesis.**
- Manufacturing blood proteins, particularly those necessary for blood clotting
- Releasing bilirubin, a pigment in bile
- Removing poisons (toxins) from the blood

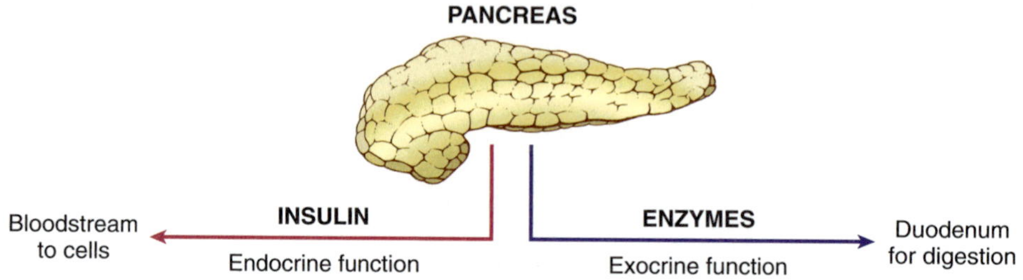

FIGURE 5-11 The pancreas and its functions.

The **portal vein** brings blood to the liver from the intestines. Digested foods pass into the portal vein directly after being absorbed into the capillaries of the small intestine, thus giving the liver the first chance to use the nutrients.

The **pancreas** (Figure 5-11) is both an exocrine and an endocrine organ. As an exocrine gland, it produces enzymes to digest starch, such as **amylase** (amyl/o = starch, -ase = enzyme), to digest fat, such as **lipase** (lip/o = fat), and to digest proteins, such as **protease** (prote/o = protein). These pass into the duodenum through the pancreatic duct.

As an endocrine gland (secreting into the bloodstream), the pancreas secretes **insulin.** This hormone, needed to help release sugar from the blood, acts as a carrier to bring glucose into cells of the body to be used for energy.

Figure 5-12 is a flow chart that traces the pathway of food through the gastrointestinal tract.

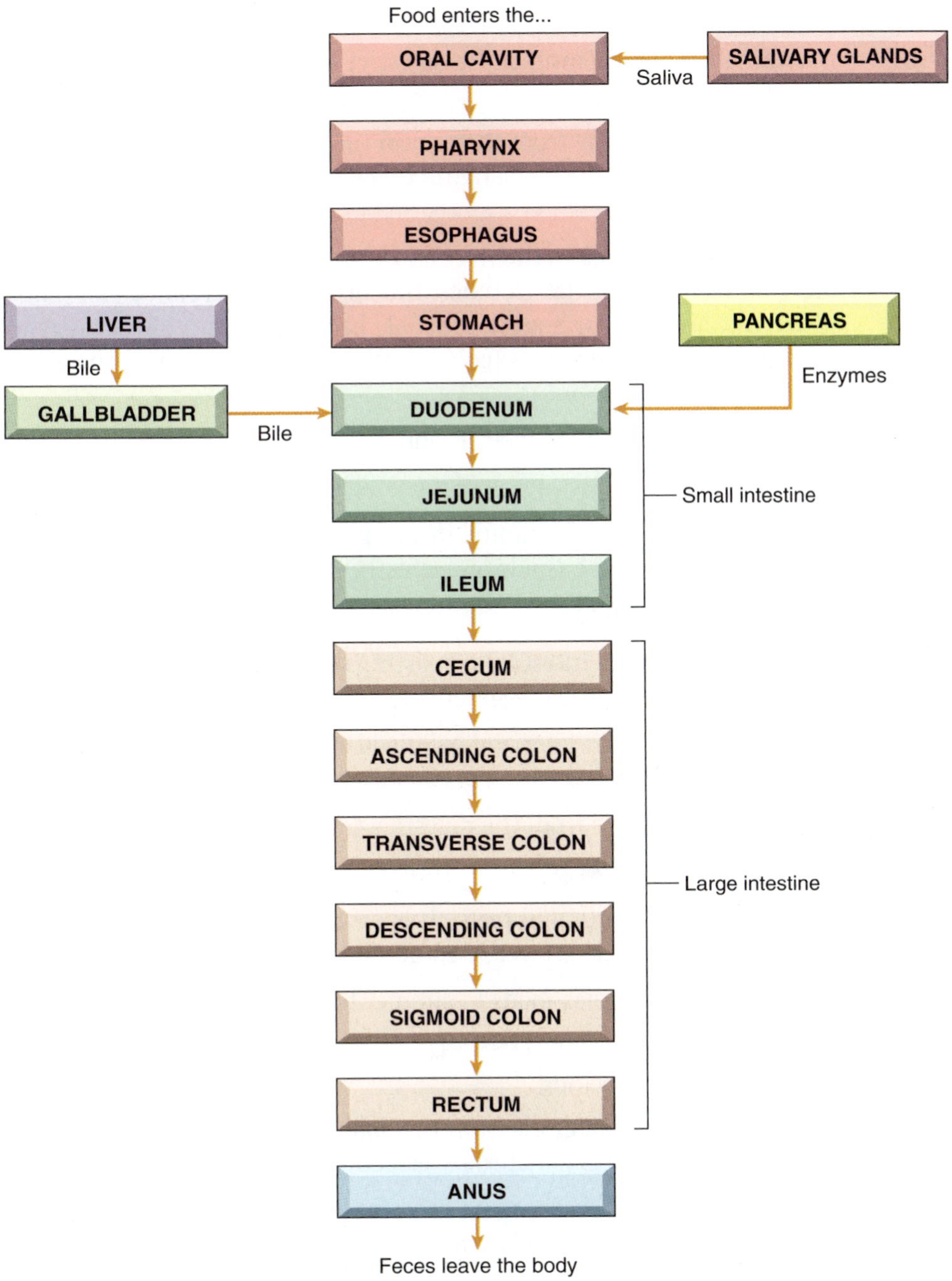

FIGURE 5-12 **Pathway of food through the gastrointestinal tract.**

VOCABULARY

The following list reviews many of the terms introduced in this chapter. Short definitions and additional information reinforce your understanding of the terms. All of the terms are included in the "Pronunciation of Terms" section later in the chapter.

absorption	Passage of materials through the walls of the small intestine into the bloodstream.
amino acids	Small building blocks of proteins (like links in a chain), released when proteins are digested.
amylase	Enzyme (-ase) secreted by the pancreas and salivary glands to digest starch (amyl/o).
anus	Terminal end or opening of the digestive tract to the outside of the body.
appendix	Blind pouch hanging from the cecum (in the right lower quadrant [RLQ]). It literally means hanging (pend/o) onto (ap-, which is a form of ad-).
bile	Digestive juice made in the liver and stored in the gallbladder. It breaks up (emulsifies) large fat globules. Bile originally was called gall (Latin *bilis*, meaning gall or anger), probably because it has a bitter taste. It is composed of bile pigments (colored materials), cholesterol, and bile salts.
bilirubin	Pigment released by the liver in bile.
bowel	Intestine.
canine teeth	Pointed, dog-like teeth (canine means pertaining to dog) next to the incisors. Also called cuspids or eyeteeth.
cecum	First part of the large intestine.
colon	Portion of the large intestine consisting of the ascending, transverse, descending, and sigmoid segments.
common bile duct	Carries bile from the liver and gallbladder to the duodenum. Also called the choledochus.
defecation	Elimination of feces from the digestive tract through the anus.
deglutition	Swallowing.
dentin	Primary material found in teeth. It is covered by the enamel in the crown and a protective layer of cementum in the root.
digestion	Breakdown of complex foods to simpler forms.
duodenum	First part of the small intestine. Duo = 2, den = 10; the duodenum measures 12 inches long.
elimination	Act of removal of materials from the body; in the digestive system, the removal of indigestible materials as feces.
emulsification	Physical process of breaking up large fat globules into smaller globules, thereby increasing the surface area that enzymes can use to digest the fat.

enamel	Hard, outermost layer of a tooth.
enzyme	Chemical that speeds up a reaction between substances. Digestive enzymes break down complex foods to simpler substances. Enzymes are given names that end in -ase.
esophagus	Tube connecting the throat to the stomach. Eso- means inward; phag/o means swallowing.
fatty acids	Substances produced when fats are digested. Fatty acids are a category of lipids.
feces	Solid wastes; stool.
gallbladder	Small sac under the liver; stores bile. *Remember*: gallbladder is one word!
glucose	Simple sugar.
glycogen	Starch; glucose is stored in the form of glycogen in liver cells.
hydrochloric acid	Substance produced by the stomach; necessary for digestion of food.
ileum	Third part of the small intestine; from the Greek *eilos*, meaning twisted. When the abdomen was viewed at autopsy, the intestine appeared twisted, and the ileum often was an area of obstruction.
incisor	Any one of four front teeth in the dental arch.
insulin	Hormone produced by the endocrine cells of the pancreas. It transports sugar from the blood into cells and stimulates glycogen formation by the liver.
jejunum	Second part of the small intestine. The Latin *jejunus* means empty; this part of the intestine was always empty when a body was examined after death.
lipase	Pancreatic enzyme necessary to digest fats.
liver	Large organ located in the RUQ of the abdomen. The liver secretes bile; stores sugar, iron, and vitamins; produces blood proteins; destroys worn-out red blood cells; and filters out toxins. The normal adult liver weighs about 2½ to 3 pounds.
lower esophageal sphincter (LES)	Ring of muscles between the esophagus and the stomach. Also called **cardiac sphincter.**
mastication	Chewing.
molar teeth	Sixth, seventh, and eighth teeth from the middle on either side of the dental arch. **Premolar teeth** are the fourth and fifth teeth, before the molars.
palate	Roof of the mouth. The hard palate lies anterior to the soft palate and is supported by the upper jawbone (maxilla). The soft palate is the posterior fleshy part between the mouth and the throat.
pancreas	Organ under the stomach; produces insulin (for transport of sugar into cells) and enzymes (for digestion of foods).
papillae (*singular*: papilla)	Small elevations on the tongue. A papilla is a nipple-like elevation.
parotid gland	Salivary gland within the cheek, just anterior to the ear. Note the literal meaning of parotid (par- = near; ot/o = ear).

peristalsis	Rhythmic contractions of the tubular organs. In the gastrointestinal tract, peristalsis moves the contents through at different rates: stomach, 0.5 to 2 hours; small intestine, 2 to 6 hours; and colon, 6 to 72 hours. Peri- means surrounding; -stalsis is constriction.
pharynx	Throat, the common passageway for food from the mouth and for air from the nose.
portal vein	Large vein bringing blood to the liver from the intestines.
protease	Enzyme that digests protein.
pulp	Soft tissue within a tooth, containing nerves and blood vessels.
pyloric sphincter	Ring of muscle at the end of the stomach, near the duodenum. From the Greek *pyloros*, meaning gatekeeper. It is normally closed, but opens when a wave of peristalsis passes over it.
pylorus	Distal region of the stomach, opening to the duodenum.
rectum	Last section of the large intestine, connecting the end of the colon and the anus.
rugae	Ridges on the hard palate and the wall of the stomach.
saliva	Digestive juice produced by salivary glands. Saliva contains the enzyme amylase, which begins the digestion of starch to sugar.
salivary glands	Parotid, sublingual, and submandibular glands.
sigmoid colon	Fourth and last, S-shaped segment of the colon, just before the rectum; empties into the rectum.
sphincter	Circular ring of muscle that constricts a passage or closes a natural opening.
stomach	Muscular organ that receives food from the esophagus. The stomach's parts are the fundus (proximal section), body (middle section), and antrum (distal section).

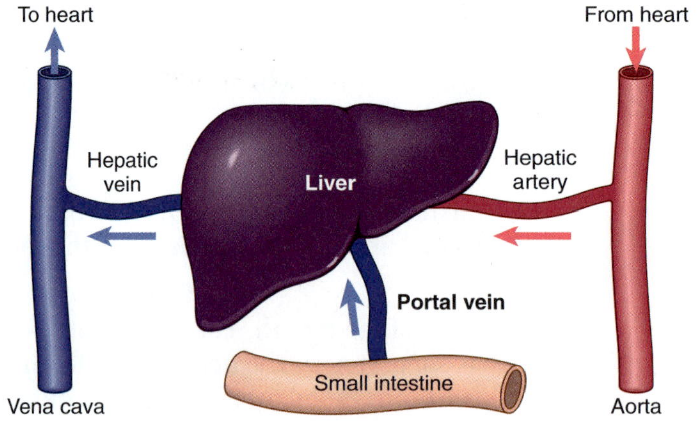

FIGURE 5-13 **Portal vein** and its relationship to the liver and small intestine.

Portal Vein

Notice the relationship of the **portal vein** (also called **hepatic portal vein**) between the intestines and the liver (Figure 5-13). This vein is not a true vein because it doesn't conduct blood directly to the heart as do other veins. In liver disease, blood backs up into the portal vein, causing **portal hypertension** (high blood pressure) and **esophageal varices.** See page 162.

triglycerides	Fat molecules composed of three parts fatty acids and one part glycerol. Triglycerides (fats) are a subgroup of **lipids**. Another type of lipid is cholesterol.
uvula	Soft tissue hanging from the middle of the soft palate. The Latin *uva* means bunch of grapes.
villi (*singular*: villus)	Microscopic projections in the wall of the small intestine that absorb nutrients into the bloodstream.

TERMINOLOGY

Write the meaning of the medical term in the space provided. Check the "Pronunciation of Terms" on pages 181 to 186 for any unfamiliar words.

PARTS OF THE BODY

COMBINING FORM	MEANING	TERMINOLOGY	MEANING
an/o	anus	perianal	______________
append/o	appendix	appendectomy	______________
appendic/o		appendicitis *See Figure 5-14.*	______________
bucc/o	cheek	buccal mucosa *A mucosa is a* ***mucous membrane*** *lining cavities or canals that open to the outside of the body.*	______________
cec/o	cecum	cecal	______________
celi/o	belly, abdomen	celiac *Abdomin/o and lapar/o also mean abdomen. With combining forms that have the same basic meaning, no rule exists for the proper usage of one or the other. You will learn to recognize each in its proper context.*	______________

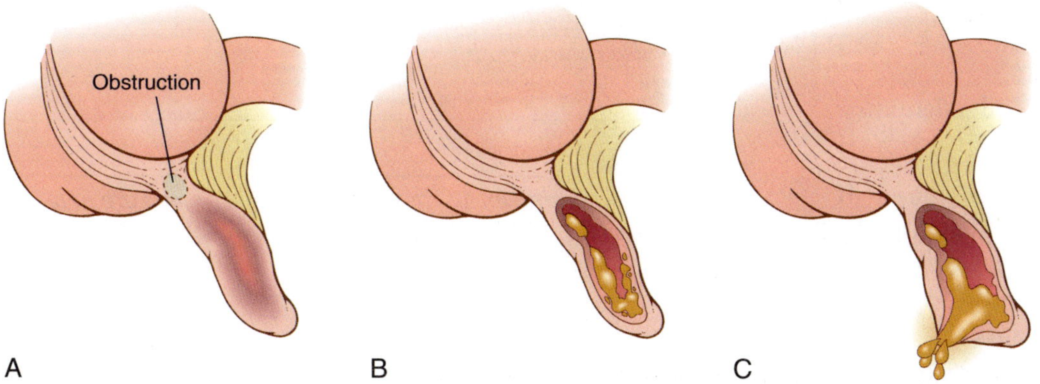

FIGURE 5-14 **Stages of appendicitis. A,** Obstruction and bacterial infection cause red, swollen, and inflamed appendix. **B,** Pus and bacteria invade the wall of the appendix. **C,** Pus perforates (ruptures through) the wall of the appendix into the abdomen, leading to peritonitis (inflammation of the peritoneum).

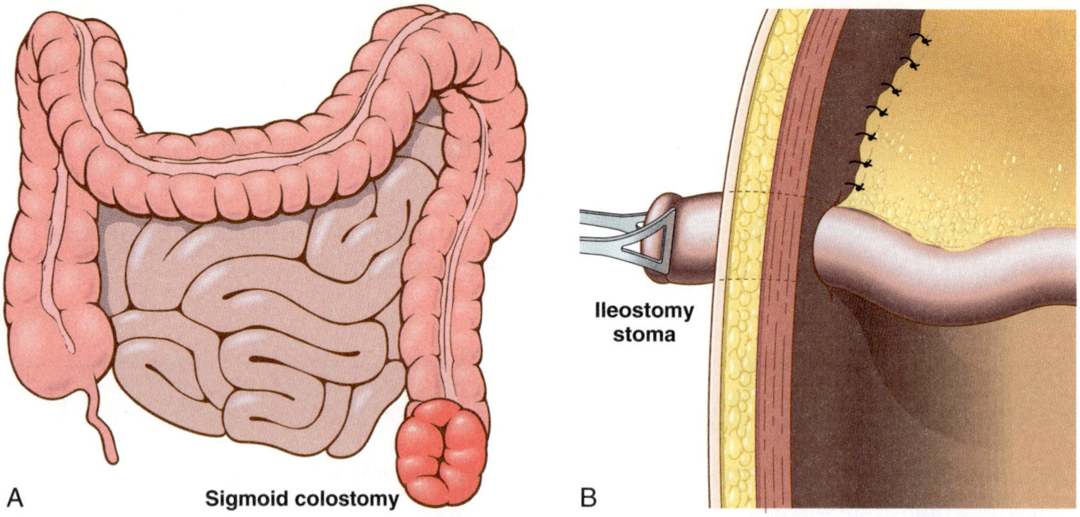

FIGURE 5-15 **Different types of stomas. A, Sigmoid colostomy** after resection of the rectum and part of the sigmoid colon. The stoma is at the end of the colon and attached to the abdominal wall. **B, Ileostomy** after resection of the entire colon. The ileum is drawn through the abdominal wall to form an **ileostomy stoma.**

COMBINING FORM	MEANING	TERMINOLOGY	MEANING
cheil/o	lip	cheilosis *Labi/o also means lip.*	
cholecyst/o	gallbladder	cholecystectomy *Chol/e = gall, bile.*	
choledoch/o	common bile duct	choledochotomy	
col/o	colon	colostomy *The suffix -stomy, when used with a combining form for an organ, means an opening to the outside of the body. A* ***stoma*** *is an opening between an organ and the surface of the body (Figure 5-15).*	
colon/o	colon	colonic	
		colonoscopy	
dent/i	tooth	dentibuccal *Odont/o also means tooth.*	
duoden/o	duodenum	duodenal	
enter/o	intestines, usually small intestine	enterocolitis *When two combining forms for gastrointestinal organs are in a term, the one for the organ closer to the mouth appears first.*	

Cholecyst/o and cyst/o

Don't confuse **cholecyst/o (gallbladder)** with **cyst/o**, which is the **urinary bladder.**

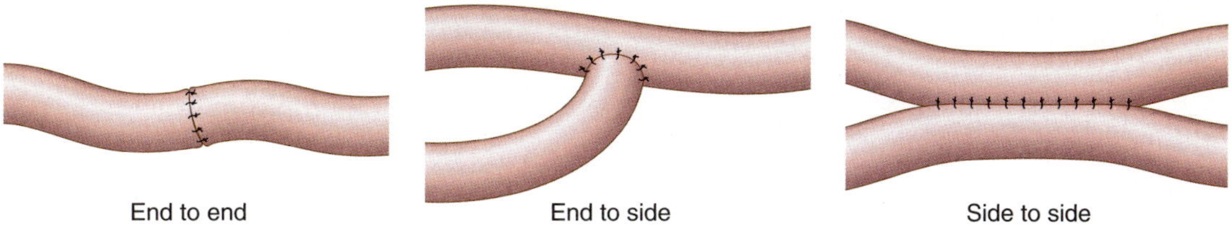

FIGURE 5-16 Three types of anastomoses. These are examples of an enteroenterostomy. The suffix -stomy, when used with two or more combining forms (enter/o and enter/o) indicates the surgical creation of a new opening between those parts of the body.

COMBINING FORM	MEANING	TERMINOLOGY	MEANING
		enteroenterostomy	______________ *New opening between two previously unconnected parts of the small intestine. This is an* ***anastomosis,*** *which is any surgical connection between two parts, such as vessels, ducts, or bowel segments (ana = up, stom = opening, -sis = state of) (Figure 5-16).*
		mesentery	______________ *Part of the double fold of peritoneum that stretches around the organs in the abdomen, the mesentery holds the organs in place. Literally, it lies in the middle (mes-) of the intestines, a membrane attaching the intestines to the muscle wall at the back of the abdomen (Figure 5-17).*
		parenteral	______________ *Par (from para-) means apart from in this term. An intravenous line brings* ***parenteral nutrition*** *directly into the bloodstream, bypassing the intestinal tract (****enteral*** *nutrition). Parenteral injections may be subcutaneous or intramuscular as well.*

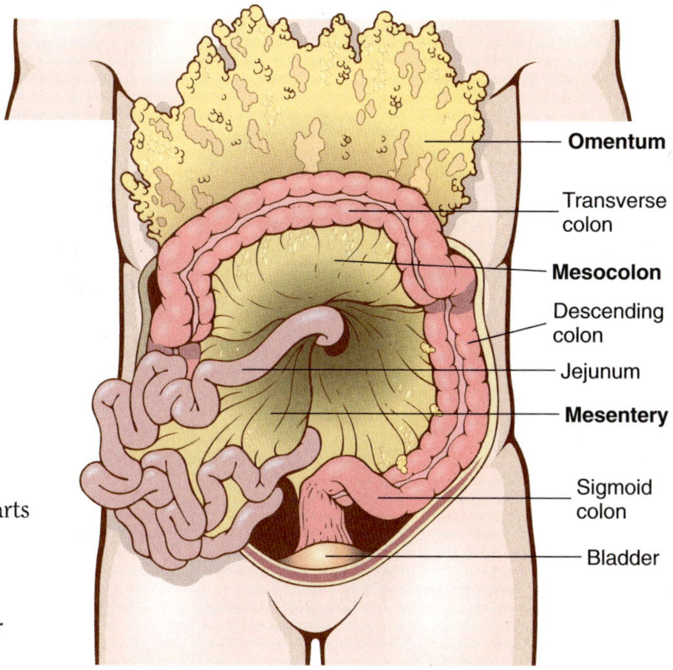

FIGURE 5-17 Mesentery. The **omentum** and **mesocolon** are parts of the mesentery. The omentum (raised in this figure) actually hangs down like an apron over the intestines. The mesentery contains blood and lymph vessels. The lymph nodes in the mesentery are important indicators in the spread of colon cancer (staging of colon cancer).

COMBINING FORM	MEANING	TERMINOLOGY	MEANING
esophag/o	esophagus	esophageal *Note: Changing the suffix from -al to -eal softens the final g (ĕ-sŏf-ă-JĒ-ăl).*	
faci/o	face	facial	
gastr/o	stomach	gastrostomy	
gingiv/o	gums	gingivitis	
gloss/o	tongue	hypoglossal *Lingu/o also means tongue.*	
hepat/o	liver	hepatoma *Also called **hepatocellular carcinoma.***	
		hepatomegaly	
ile/o	ileum	ileocecal sphincter *Also called the ileocecal valve.*	
		ileitis	
		ileostomy *See Figure 5-15B, page 154.*	
jejun/o	jejunum	choledochojejunostomy *An anastomosis.*	
		gastrojejunostomy *This is part of a **gastric bypass** procedure. See Figure 6-7, page 197.*	
labi/o	lip	labial	
lapar/o	abdomen	laparoscopy *A form of **minimally invasive surgery (MIS).** Examples are laparoscopic cholecystectomy (Figure 5-28, page 168) and laparoscopic appendectomy.*	
lingu/o	tongue	sublingual	
mandibul/o	lower jaw, mandible	submandibular	
odont/o	tooth	orthodontist *Orth/o means straight.*	
		periodontist	
		endodontist *Performs root canal therapy.*	

Ileum and Ilium

Don't confuse the **ileum,** which is the third part of the small intestine with the **ilium,** uppermost and largest part of the pelvis (hip bone).

COMBINING FORM	MEANING	TERMINOLOGY	MEANING
or/o	mouth	oral *Stomat/o also means mouth.*	______________
palat/o	palate	palatoplasty *Procedure to repair cleft palate and cleft lip; repair of a cleft palate.*	______________
pancreat/o	pancreas	pancreatitis	______________
peritone/o	peritoneum	peritonitis *The e of the root has been dropped in this term.*	______________
pharyng/o	throat	pharyngeal	______________
		palatopharyngoplasty *Used to treat cases of snoring or sleep apnea caused by obstructions in the throat or nose.*	______________
proct/o	anus and rectum	proctologist	______________
pylor/o	pyloric sphincter	pyloroplasty	______________
rect/o	rectum	rectocele	______________
sialaden/o	salivary gland	sialadenitis	______________
sigmoid/o	sigmoid colon	sigmoidoscopy	______________
stomat/o	mouth	stomatitis	______________
uvul/o	uvula	uvulectomy	______________

SUBSTANCES

COMBINING FORM	MEANING	TERMINOLOGY	MEANING
amyl/o	starch	amylase *The suffix -ase means enzyme.*	______________
bil/i	gall, bile	biliary *The **biliary tract** includes the organs (liver and gallbladder) and ducts (hepatic, cystic, and common bile ducts) that secrete, store, and empty bile into the duodenum.*	______________
bilirubin/o	bilirubin (bile pigment)	hyperbilirubinemia	______________
chol/e	gall, bile	cholelithiasis *Lith/o means stone or calculus; -iasis means abnormal condition.*	______________

Chol/e and Col/o

Don't confuse **chol/e,** which means gall, bile with **col/o,** which is the colon! The context of the term will help you determine the correct spelling.

COMBINING FORM	MEANING	TERMINOLOGY	MEANING
chlorhydr/o	hydrochloric acid	achlorhydria ____ *Absence of gastric juice is associated with gastric carcinoma.*	
gluc/o	sugar	gluconeogenesis ____ *Liver cells make new sugar from fats and proteins.*	
glyc/o	sugar	hyperglycemia ____	
glycogen/o	glycogen, animal starch	glycogenolysis ____ *Liver cells change glycogen back to glucose when blood sugar levels drop.*	
lip/o	fat, lipid	lipoma ____	
lith/o	stone	lithogenesis ____	
prote/o	protein	protease ____	
py/o	pus	pyorrhea ____ *Periodontitis; an advanced stage of periodontal disease (gingivitis).*	
sial/o	saliva, salivary	sialolith ____	
steat/o	fat	steatorrhea ____ *Improperly digested (malabsorbed) fats will appear in the feces.*	

5

SUFFIXES

SUFFIX	MEANING	TERMINOLOGY	MEANING
-ase	enzyme	lipase ____ *Enzymes speed up chemical reactions. Lipase aids in the digestion of fats. In all types of liver disease, liver enzyme levels may be elevated, indicating damage to liver cells. Signs and symptoms include malaise, anorexia, hepatomegaly, jaundice, and abdominal pain.*	
-chezia	defecation, elimination of wastes	hematochezia ____ *(hē-mă-tō-KĒ-zē-ă) Bright red blood is found in the feces.*	
-iasis	abnormal condition	choledocholithiasis ____	
-prandial	meal	postprandial ____ ***Post cibum*** *(p.c.), seen on written prescriptions, also means after meals.*	

Pyorrhea and Pyuria

Pyorrhea is discharge (-rrhea) of pus from gums, and **pyuria** is urine containing pus (sign of a urinary tract infection).

PATHOLOGY OF THE DIGESTIVE SYSTEM

This section presents medical terms that describe **signs and symptoms** (clinical indications of illness) and pathologic conditions of the gastrointestinal tract. Sentences following each definition describe the **etiology** (eti/o = cause) of the illness and treatment. When the etiology (cause) is not understood, the condition is **idiopathic** (idi/o = unknown). You can find a list of drugs prescribed to treat gastrointestinal signs and symptoms and conditions on pages 894-895 in Chapter 21, Pharmacology.

SIGNS AND SYMPTOMS

anorexia

Lack of appetite.

Anorexia (-orexia = appetite) often is a sign of malignancy or liver disease. **Anorexia nervosa** is loss of appetite associated with emotional problems such as anger, anxiety, and irrational fear of weight gain. It is an eating disorder and is discussed along with a similar eating disorder, bulimia nervosa, in Chapter 22.

ascites

Abnormal accumulation of fluid in the abdomen.

This condition occurs when fluid passes from the bloodstream and collects in the peritoneal cavity. It can be a sign of neoplasm or inflammatory disorders in the abdomen, venous hypertension (high blood pressure) caused by liver disease (cirrhosis), or heart failure (Figure 5-18). Treatment for ascites includes administration of diuretic drugs and paracentesis to remove abdominal fluid.

borborygmus (*plural:* borborygmi)

Rumbling or gurgling noise produced by the movement of gas, fluid, or both in the gastrointestinal tract.

A sign of hyperactive intestinal peristalsis, borborygmi (bowel sounds) often are present in cases of gastroenteritis and diarrhea.

constipation

Difficulty in passing stools (feces).

When peristalsis is slow, stools are dry and hard. A diet of fruit, vegetables, and water is helpful. **Laxatives** and **cathartics** are medications to promote movement of stools.

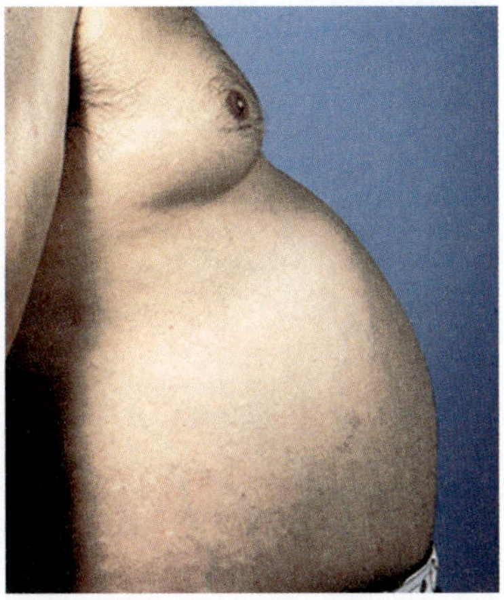

FIGURE 5-18 Ascites in a male patient. The photograph was taken after **paracentesis** (puncture to remove fluid from the abdomen) was performed. Notice the gynecomastia (condition of female-type breasts) in this patient due to an excess of estrogen, which can accompany cirrhosis, especially in persons with alcoholism.

Signs and Symptoms

A **sign** is an **objective** finding—such as an increase in body temperature, a rash, or a sound heard on listening to the chest—indicating the presence of disease as **perceived by an examiner.** However, a **symptom** is a **subjective** sensation or change in health—such as itching, pain, fatigue, or nausea—as **experienced by the patient.** Clearly, the same feature may be noticed by both doctor and patient, which makes it at once both a sign and a symptom!

diarrhea **Frequent passage of loose, watery stools.**

Abrupt onset of diarrhea immediately after eating suggests acute infection or toxin in the gastrointestinal tract. Untreated, severe diarrhea may lead to dehydration. Antidiarrheal drugs are helpful.

dysphagia **Difficulty in swallowing.**

This sensation feels like a "lump in the throat" when a swallowed bolus fails to progress, either because of a physical obstruction (obstructive dysphagia) or because of a motor disorder in which esophageal peristalsis is not coordinated (motor dysphagia).

eructation **Gas expelled from the stomach through the mouth.**

Eructation produces a characteristic sound and also is called **belching.**

flatus **Gas expelled through the anus.**

Flatulence is the presence of excessive gas in the stomach and the intestines.

hematochezia **Passage of fresh, bright red blood from the rectum.**

The cause of hematochezia usually is bleeding due to colitis or from ulcers or polyps in the colon or rectum.

jaundice (icterus) **Yellow-orange coloration of the skin and whites of the eyes caused by high levels of bilirubin in the blood (hyperbilirubinemia).** See Figure 5-19.

Jaundice can occur when (1) excessive destruction of erythrocytes, as in **hemolysis,** causes excess bilirubin in the blood; (2) malfunction of liver cells (hepatocytes) due to **liver disease** prevents the liver from excreting bilirubin with bile; or (3) **obstruction of bile flow,** such as from choledocholithiasis or tumor, prevents bilirubin in bile from being excreted into the duodenum.

5

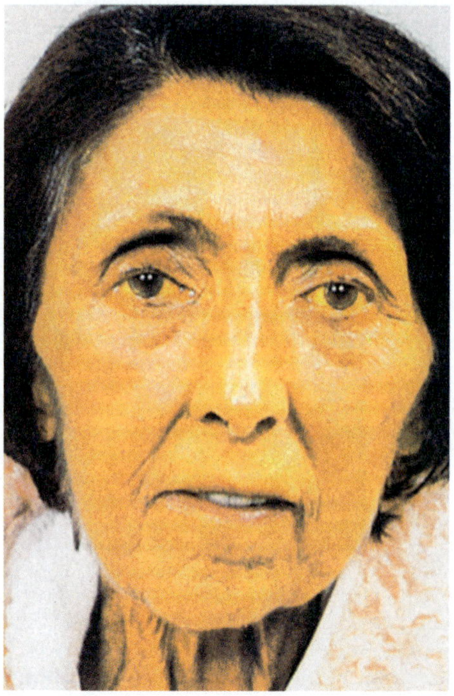

FIGURE 5-19 Jaundice due to liver disease.

melena — **Black, tarry stools; feces containing digested blood.**

This clinical sign usually reflects a condition in which blood has had time to be digested (acted on by intestinal juices) and results from bleeding in the upper gastrointestinal tract (duodenal ulcer). A positive result on **stool guaiac testing** (see page 193) indicates blood in the stool.

nausea — **Unpleasant sensation in the stomach associated with a tendency to vomit.**

Common causes are sea and motion sickness and early pregnancy. Nausea and vomiting may be symptomatic of a perforation (hole in the wall) of an abdominal organ; obstruction of a bile duct, stomach, or intestine; or exposure to toxins (poisons).

steatorrhea — **Fat in the feces; frothy, foul-smelling fecal matter.**

Improper digestion or absorption of fat can cause fat to remain in the intestine. This may occur with disease of the pancreas (pancreatitis) when pancreatic enzymes are not excreted. It also is a sign of intestinal disease that involves malabsorption of fat.

PATHOLOGIC CONDITIONS

ORAL CAVITY AND TEETH

aphthous stomatitis — **Inflammation of the mouth with small, painful ulcers.**

The ulcers associated with this condition are commonly called **canker** (KĂNK-ĕr) **sores**; the cause is unknown (Figure 5-20B).

dental caries — **Tooth decay.**

Dental plaque results from the accumulation of foods, proteins from saliva, and necrotic debris on the tooth enamel. Bacteria grow in the plaque and cause production of acid that dissolves the tooth enamel, resulting in a cavity (area of decay) (Figure 5-20C). If the bacterial infection reaches the pulp of the tooth, root canal therapy may be necessary.

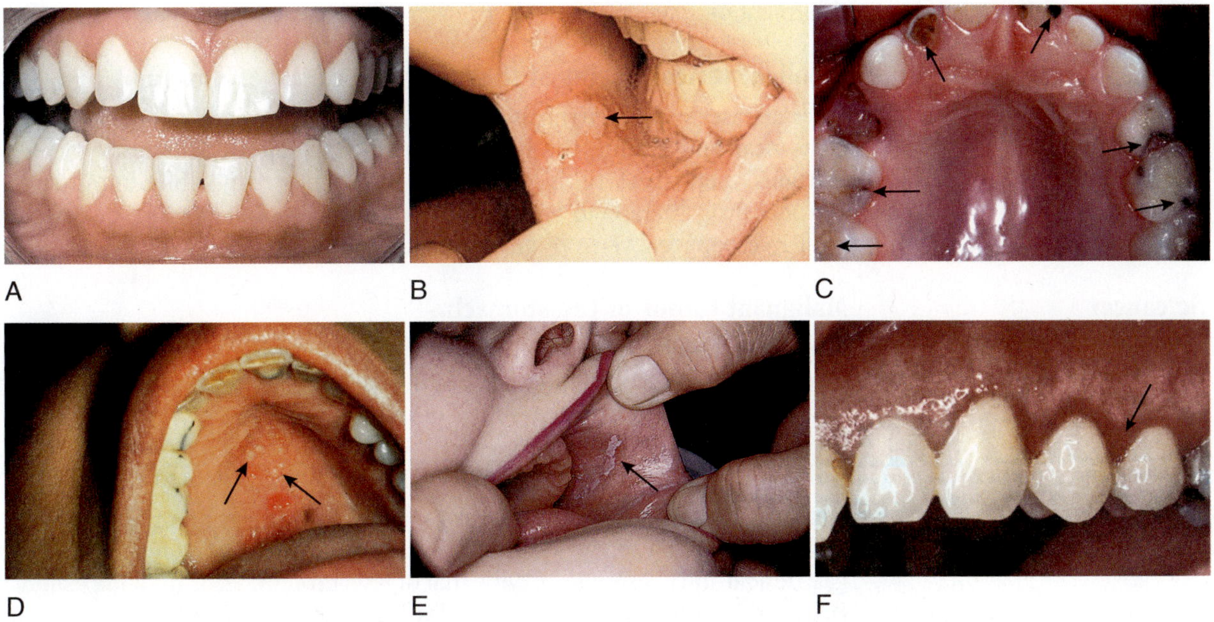

FIGURE 5-20 Normal teeth and gums and pathologic conditions. A, Normal teeth and gums. B, Aphthous stomatitis. C, Dental caries. D, Herpetic stomatitis. E, Oral leukoplakia. F, Gingivitis.

5

herpetic stomatitis

Inflammation of the mouth caused by infection with the herpesvirus.

Painful fluid-filled blisters on the lips, palate, gums, and tongue, commonly called **fever blisters** or **cold sores** (Figure 5-20D). It is caused by herpes simplex virus type 1 (HSV1). Treatment is with medication to relieve symptoms. Herpes genitalis (due to HSV2) occurs on the reproductive organs. Both conditions are highly contagious.

oral leukoplakia

White plaques or patches on the mucosa of the mouth.

This precancerous lesion (Figure 5-20E) can result from chronic tobacco use (pipe smoking or chewing tobacco). Malignant potential is assessed by microscopic study of biopsied tissue.

periodontal disease

Inflammation and degeneration of gums, teeth, and surrounding bone.

Gingivitis (Figure 5-20F) occurs as a result of accumulation of **dental plaque** and **dental calculus** or **tartar** (a yellow-brown calcified deposit on teeth). In **gingivectomy**, a periodontist uses a metal instrument to scrape away plaque and tartar from teeth; any pockets of pus (pyorrhea) are then drained and removed to allow new tissue to form. Localized infections are treated with systemic antibiotics.

UPPER GASTROINTESTINAL TRACT

achalasia

Failure of the lower esophagus sphincter (LES) muscle to relax.

Achalasia (-chalasia = relaxation) results from the loss of peristalsis so that food cannot pass easily through the esophagus. Both failure of the LES to relax and the loss of peristalsis cause dilatation (widening) of the esophagus above the constriction. Physicians recommend a bland diet low in bulk and mechanical stretching of the LES to relieve symptoms.

5

esophageal cancer

Malignant tumor of the esophagus.

The most common symptom of esophageal cancer is difficulty swallowing (dysphagia). Smoking and chronic alcohol use are major risk factors. Long-term irritation of the esophagus caused by gastric reflux is a premalignant condition called **Barrett esophagus.** Surgery, radiation therapy, and chemotherapy are treatment options.

esophageal varices

Swollen, varicose veins at the lower end of the esophagus.

Liver disease (such as cirrhosis and chronic hepatitis) causes increased pressure in veins near and around the liver **(portal hypertension).** This leads to enlarged, tortuous esophageal veins with danger of hemorrhage (bleeding). Treatment includes drug therapy to lower portal hypertension and banding or tying off the swollen esophageal veins (Figure 5-21A and B).

gastric cancer

Malignant tumor of the stomach.

Chronic gastritis associated with bacterial infection is a major risk factor for gastric carcinoma. Gastric endoscopy and biopsy diagnose the condition. Cure depends on early detection and surgical removal of the cancerous tissue.

gastroesophageal reflux disease (GERD)

Solids and fluids return to the mouth from the stomach.

Heartburn is the burning sensation caused by regurgitation of hydrochloric acid from the stomach to the esophagus. Chronic exposure of esophageal mucosa to gastric acid and pepsin (an enzyme that digests protein) leads to **reflux esophagitis.** Drug treatment for GERD includes antacid (acid-suppressive) agents and medication to increase the tone of the LES.

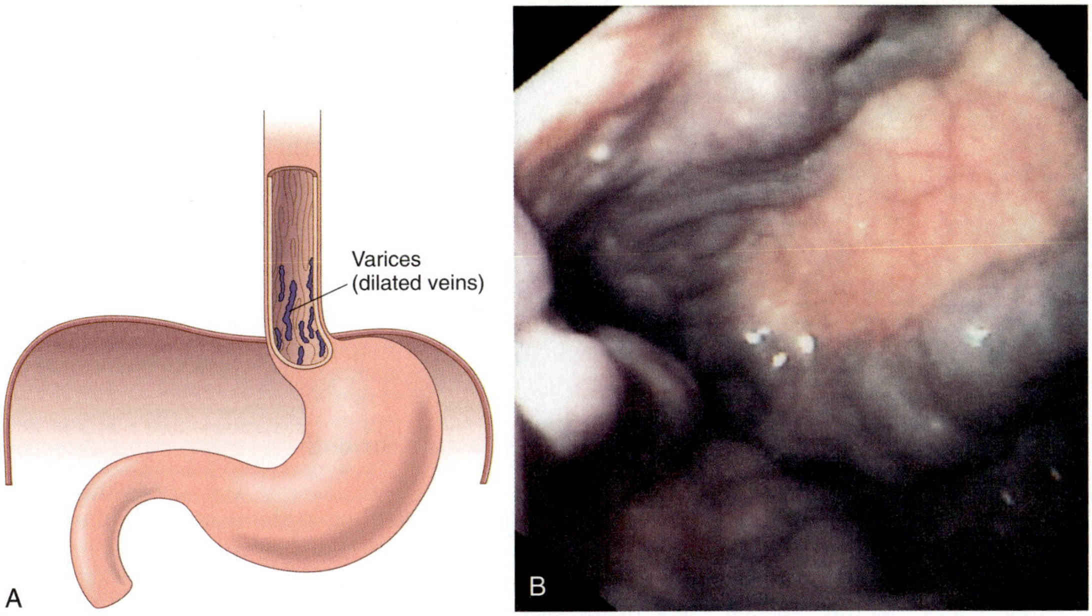

FIGURE 5-21 **A, Esophageal varices. B, Endoscopic view of esophageal varices.**

hernia

Protrusion of an organ or part through the tissues and muscles normally containing it.

A **hiatal hernia** occurs when the upper part of the stomach protrudes upward through the diaphragm (Figure 5-22A). This condition can lead to GERD. An **inguinal hernia** occurs when a small loop of bowel protrudes through a weak lower abdominal wall tissue (fascia) surrounding muscles (Figure 5-22B). Surgical repair of inguinal hernias is known as herniorrhaphy (-rrhaphy means suture).

peptic ulcer

Open sore in the lining of the stomach or duodenum.

A bacterium, *Helicobacter pylori* (*H. pylori*), is responsible for peptic ulcer disease. The combination of bacteria, hyperacidity, and gastric juice damages epithelial linings. Drug treatment includes antibiotics, antacids, and agents to protect the lining of the stomach and intestine.

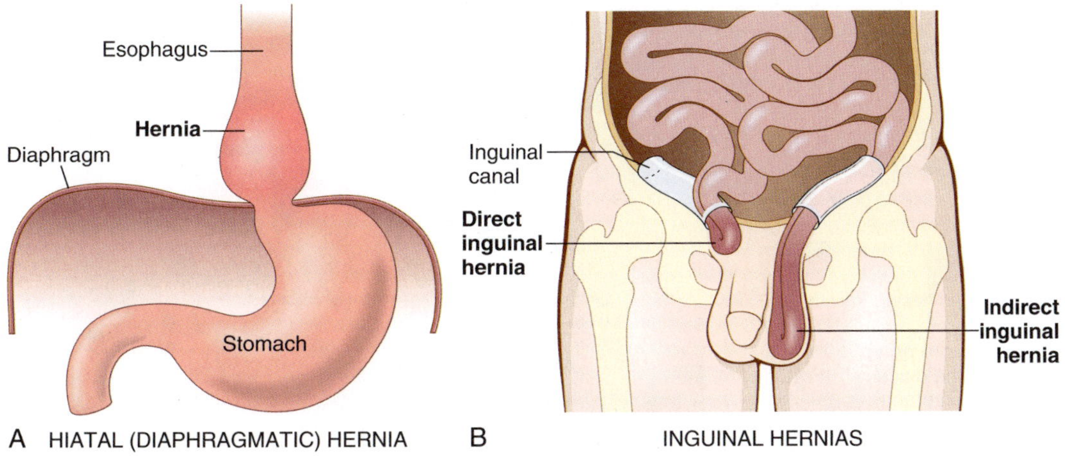

FIGURE 5-22 **Hernias. A, Hiatal hernia. B, Inguinal hernias.** A **direct inguinal hernia** occurs through the abdominal wall in an area of muscular weakness. An **indirect inguinal hernia** occurs through the inguinal canal (passageway in the lower abdomen), where the herniated tissue/bowel descends into the scrotal sac.

LOWER GASTROINTESTINAL TRACT (SMALL AND LARGE INTESTINES)

anal fistula

Abnormal tube-like passageway near the anus.

The fistula often results from a break or **fissure** in the wall of the anus or rectum, or from an **abscess** (infected area) there (Figure 5-23A).

colonic polyps

Polyps (benign growths) protrude from the mucous membrane of the colon.

Figure 5-23A illustrates two types of polyps: **pedunculated** (attached to the membrane by a stalk) and **sessile** (sitting directly on the mucous membrane). Figure 5-23B shows multiple polyps of the colon. Many polyps are premalignant (adenomatous polyps) and are often removed (polypectomy) for biopsy.

colorectal cancer

Adenocarcinoma of the colon or rectum, or both.

Colorectal cancer (Figure 5-24) can arise from polyps in the colon or rectal region. Diagnosis is determined by detecting melena (blood in stool) and by colonoscopy. Prognosis depends on the stage (extent of spread) of the tumor, including size, depth of invasion, and involvement of lymph nodes. Surgical treatment may require excision of a major section of colon with rejoining of the cut ends (anastomosis). Chemotherapy and radiotherapy are administered as needed.

Crohn disease ("Crohn's")

Chronic inflammation of the intestinal tract.

Crohn's can occur anywhere from mouth to anus but most commonly in the ileum (ileitis) and colon. Signs and symptoms include diarrhea, severe abdominal pain, fever, anorexia, weakness, and weight loss. Both Crohn disease and ulcerative colitis are forms of **inflammatory bowel disease (IBD).** Treatment is with drugs that control inflammation and other symptoms or by surgical removal of diseased portions of the intestine, with anastomosis of remaining parts. Read the ***In Person*** story about Crohn's on page 170.

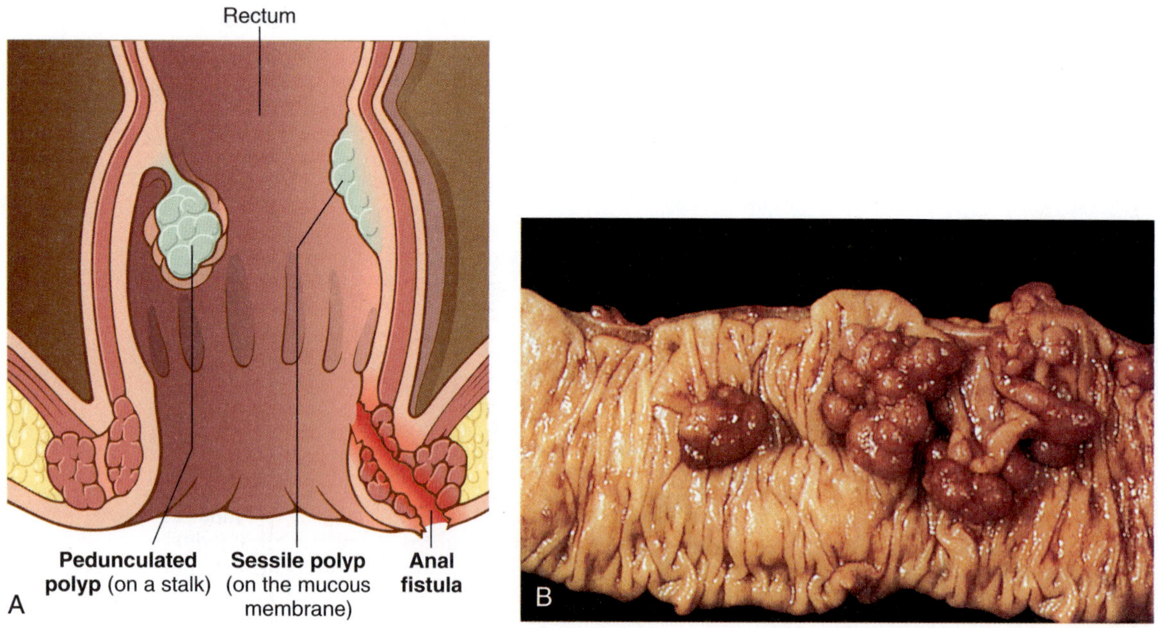

FIGURE 5-23 **Anal fistula and colonic polyps. A,** Anal fistula and two types of polyps. **B,** Multiple polyps of the colon.

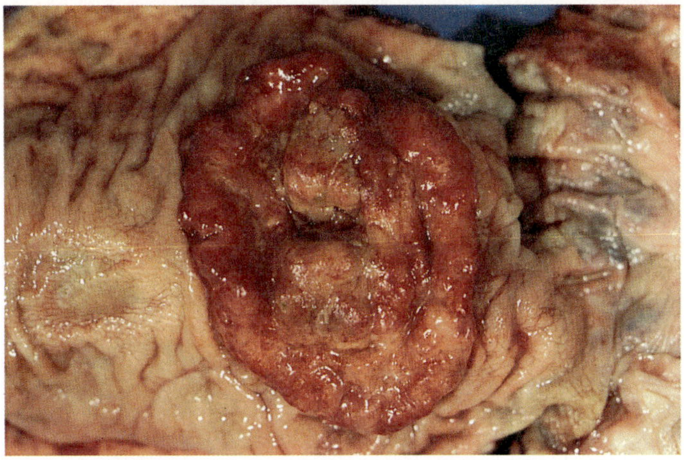

FIGURE 5-24 **Adenocarcinoma of the colon.** This tumor has "heaped-up" edges and an ulcerated central portion.

diverticulosis

Abnormal outpouchings (diverticula) in the intestinal wall of the colon. See Figure 5-25A.

Diverticulitis is a complication of diverticulosis. When fecal matter becomes trapped in diverticula, **diverticulitis** can occur. Pain and rectal bleeding are symptoms. Figure 5-25B and C show diverticulitis in a section through the sigmoid colon. Initial treatment for an attack of diverticulitis includes a liquid diet and oral antibiotics. In severe cases, patients may need hospitalization, IV antibiotics, and surgery to remove the affected area of the colon with anastomosis of the cut ends.

dysentery

Painful, inflamed intestines commonly caused by bacterial infection.

Often occurring in the colon, dysentery results from ingestion of food or water containing bacteria (salmonellae or shigellae), amebae (one-celled organisms), or viruses. Symptoms are bloody stools and abdominal pain.

hemorrhoids

Swollen, twisted, varicose veins in the rectal region.

Varicose veins can be internal (within the rectum) or external (outside the anal sphincter). Pregnancy and chronic constipation, which put pressure on anal veins, often cause hemorrhoids.

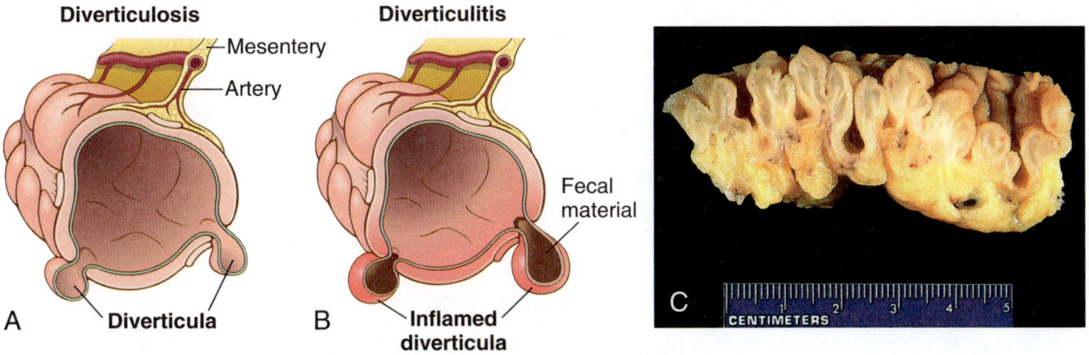

FIGURE 5-25 **A, Diverticula (diverticulosis)** form when the mucous membrane lining of the colon bulges through the weakened muscular wall. **B and C, Diverticulitis** can result when fecal material lodges in diverticula. Avoidance of foods with seeds and nuts decreases the risk of this condition.

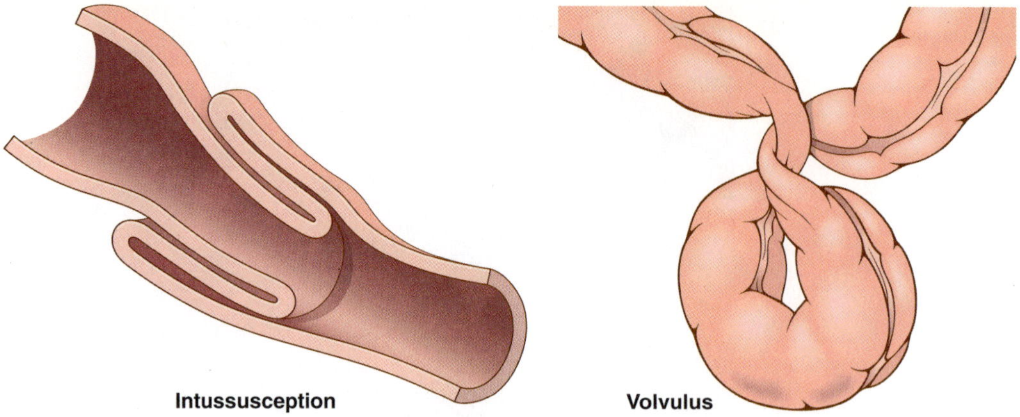

FIGURE 5-26 **Intussusception and volvulus.**

ileus — **Loss of peristalsis with resulting obstruction of the intestines.**

Surgery, trauma, or bacterial injury to the peritoneum can lead to a **paralytic ileus** (acute, transient loss of peristalsis).

inflammatory bowel disease (IBD) — **Inflammation of the colon and small intestine.** See **Crohn disease** and **ulcerative colitis.**

intussusception — **Telescoping of the intestines.**

In this condition, one segment of the bowel collapses into the opening of another segment (Figure 5-26). It often occurs in children and at the ileocecal region. Intestinal obstruction with pain and vomiting can occur. A barium enema can diagnose and may successfully reduce the intussusception. Otherwise, surgery to remove the affected segment of bowel (followed by anastomosis) may be necessary.

irritable bowel syndrome (IBS) — **Group of GI symptoms (abdominal pain, bloating, diarrhea, constipation), but without abnormalities in the intestines.**

IBS may be associated with stress or occur after infection. Treatment is symptomatic, with a diet high in bran and fiber to soften stools and establish regular bowel habits. Other names for IBS are **irritable colon** and **spastic colon.** IBS is a type of **functional gastrointestinal disorder (FGID)**. These are disorders of how the GI tract functions, but without structural or biochemical abnormalities.

ulcerative colitis — **Chronic inflammation of the colon with presence of ulcers.**

This idiopathic, chronic, recurrent diarrheal disease (an **inflammatory bowel disease**) presents with rectal bleeding and pain. Often beginning in the colon, the inflammation spreads proximally, involving the entire colon. Drug treatment and careful attention to diet are recommended. Resection of diseased bowel with ileostomy may be necessary. In some cases it is cured by total colectomy. Patients with ulcerative colitis have a higher risk of colon cancer.

Irritable Bowel Syndrome (IBS) and Inflammatory Bowel Disease (IBD)

While **IBS** is a condition with no structural abnormalities of the intestines, **IBD** (**Crohn's** and **ulcerative colitis**) involves structural abnormalities.

volvulus

Twisting of the intestine on itself.

Volvulus causes intestinal obstruction. Severe pain, nausea and vomiting, and absence of bowel sounds are clinical features. Surgical correction is necessary to prevent necrosis of the affected segment of the bowel (see Figure 5-26).

LIVER, GALLBLADDER, AND PANCREAS

cholelithiasis

Gallstones in the gallbladder.

Calculi (stones) prevent bile from leaving the gallbladder and bile ducts (Figure 5-27). Many patients remain asymptomatic and do not require treatment; symptoms related to gallbladder stones are either **biliary colic** (pain from blocked ducts) or **cholecystitis** (inflammation and infection of the gallbladder), both of which require treatment. Currently, **laparoscopic** or **minimally invasive surgery (laparoscopic cholecystectomy)** is performed to remove the gallbladder and stones (Figure 5-28A and B).

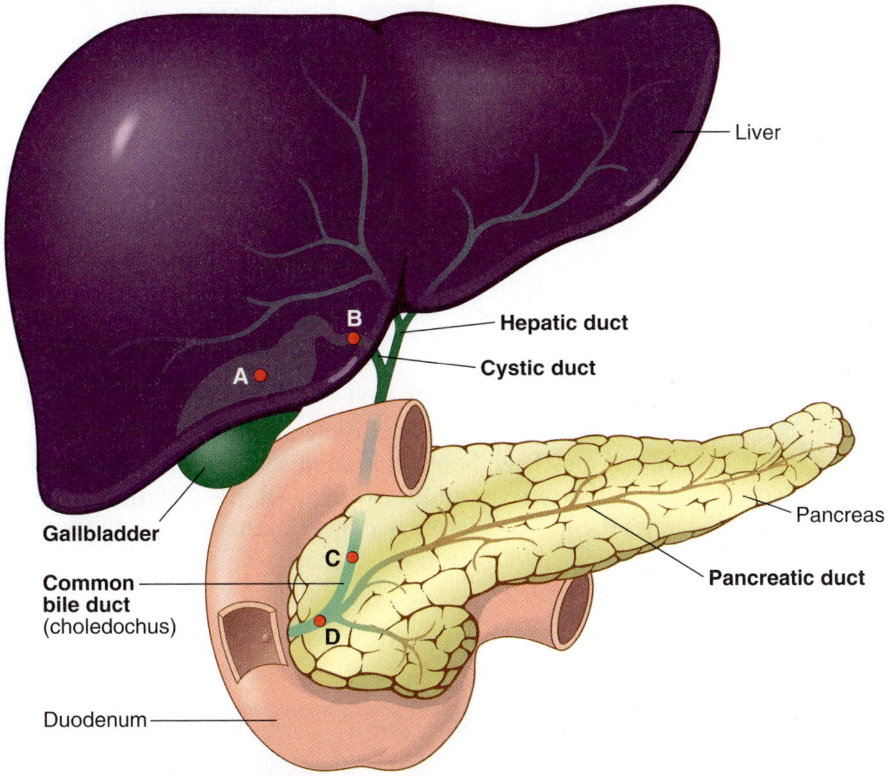

FIGURE 5-27 Gallstone positions in the gallbladder and bile ducts. A, Stone in the gallbladder causing mild or no symptoms. **B,** Stone obstructing the cystic duct, causing pain. **C,** Stone obstructing the common bile duct, causing pain and jaundice. **D,** Stone at the lower end of the common bile duct and pancreatic duct, causing pain, jaundice, and pancreatitis.

What's "in" Gallstones?

Gallstones are composed of cholesterol, bilirubin (pigment in bile) and calcium salts. They can vary in size and shape from as small as a grain of sand to as large as a golf ball!

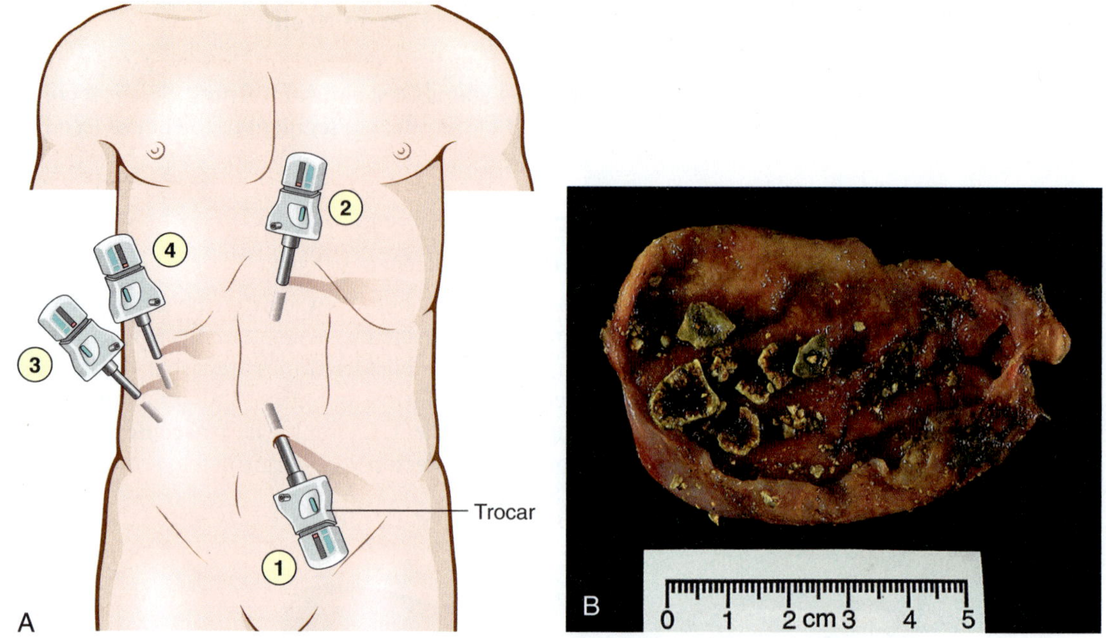

FIGURE 5-28 **A, Trocars in place for laparoscopic cholecystectomy.** Trocars are used to puncture and enter the abdomen. These devices are metal sleeves consisting of a hollow metal tube (cannula) into which fits an obturator (a solid, removable metal instrument with a sharp, three-cornered tip) used to puncture the wall. *Circled numbers* show common positions for trocar insertion: **1** is an umbilical 10/11-mm trocar (the largest trocar diameter is 15). **2** is a 10/11-mm trocar at the midline. **3** and **4** are 5-mm trocars placed in the right upper quadrant of the abdomen. **B, Gallstones.** Mechanical manipulation during laparoscopic cholecystectomy has caused fragmentation of several cholesterol gallstones, revealing interiors that are pigmented because of entrapped bile pigments. The gallbladder mucosa is reddened and irregular as a result.

cirrhosis

Chronic degenerative disease of the liver.

Cirrhosis is commonly the result of chronic alcoholism, viral hepatitis, or other causes. Lobes of the liver become scarred with fibrous tissue, hepatic cells degenerate, and the liver is infiltrated with fat. Cirrh/o means yellow-orange, which describes the liver's color caused by fat accumulation. Figure 5-29 shows a normal liver and a liver with alcoholic cirrhosis.

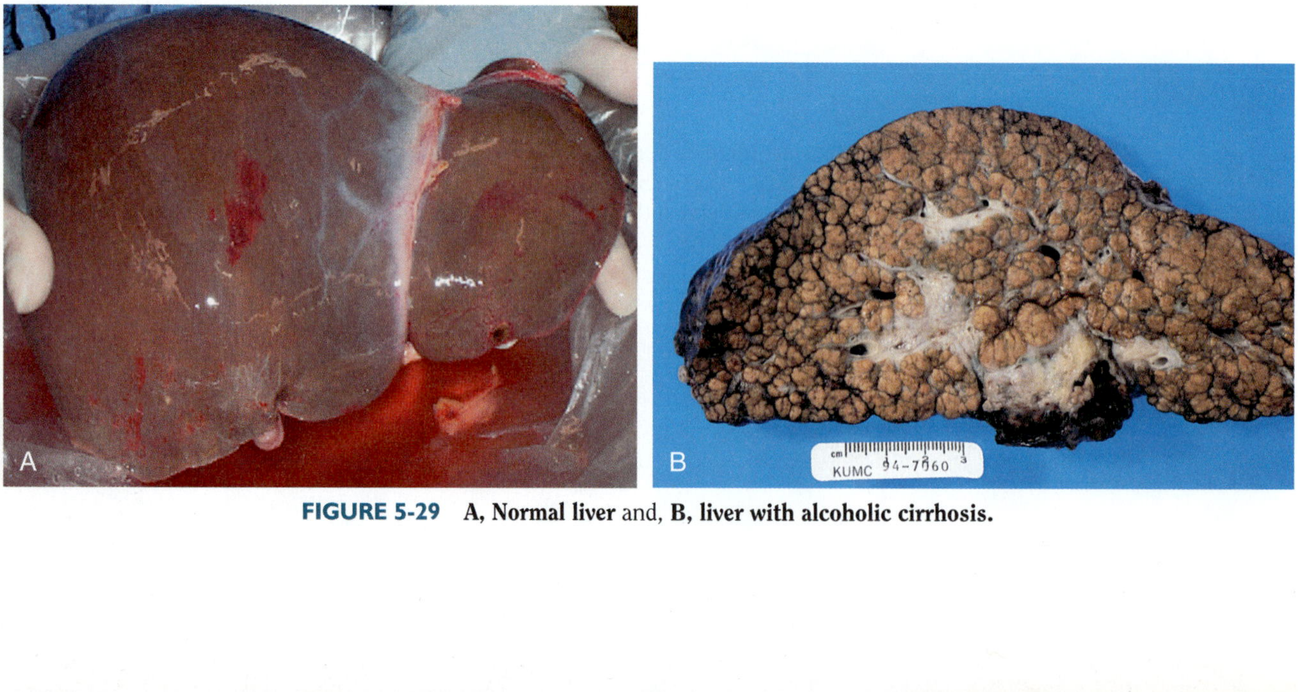

FIGURE 5-29 **A, Normal liver** and, **B, liver with alcoholic cirrhosis.**

pancreatic cancer

Malignant tumor of the pancreas.

It often occurs in the head of the pancreas (closer to the duodenum), where it can block ducts. Although the cause is unknown, pancreatic cancer is more common in smokers and people with diabetes and chronic pancreatitis. Symptoms and signs are abdominal pain, fatigue, jaundice, anorexia, and weight loss. The standard surgical treatment is a **pancreatoduodenectomy (Whipple procedure).**

pancreatitis

Inflammation of the pancreas.

Digestive enzymes attack pancreatic tissue and damage the gland. Other etiologic factors include chronic alcoholism, drug toxicity, gallstone obstruction of the common bile duct, and viral infections. Treatment includes medications to relieve epigastric pain, intravenous fluids, bowel rest, and subtotal pancreatectomy if necessary.

viral hepatitis

Inflammation of the liver caused by a virus.

Hepatitis A is viral hepatitis caused by the hepatitis A virus (HAV). It is a benign disorder spread by contaminated food or water and characterized by slow onset of symptoms. **Hepatitis B** is caused by the hepatitis B virus (HBV) and is transmitted by blood transfusion, sexual contact, or the use of contaminated needles or instruments. Severe infection can cause destruction of liver cells, cirrhosis, or death. A vaccine that provides immunity is available and recommended for persons at risk for exposure. **Hepatitis C** is caused by the hepatitis C virus (HCV) and is transmitted by blood transfusions or needle inoculation (such as among intravenous drug users sharing needles). The acute illness may progress to chronic hepatitis and hepatocellular carcinoma.

In all types, liver enzyme levels may be elevated, indicating damage to liver cells. Signs and symptoms include malaise, anorexia, hepatomegaly, jaundice, and abdominal pain.

Whipple Procedure for Pancreatic Cancer

This surgery consists of:
- removal of the distal half of the stomach (antrectomy)
- removal of gallbladder and common bile duct (cholecystectomy and choledochectomy)
- removal of part of the pancreas and duodenum, (pancreatoduodenectomy)
- reconstruction consists of pancreatojejunostomy, hepaticojejunostomy, and gastrojejunostomy

Steve Jobs, co-founder of Apple Inc, and Luciano Pavarotti, opera singer, had this surgery.

IN PERSON

This first-person narrative was written by a woman living with Crohn disease ("Crohn's").

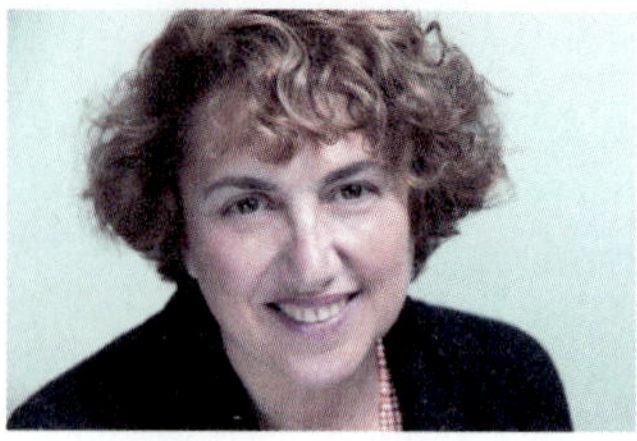

When a friend told me she was felled by the flu yesterday, I was jealous. To someone with a chronic illness, like me, having something acute always seems luxurious. Lie in bed, read glossy magazines, take over-the-counter meds, sleep it off, and in a matter of days you're okay. I have Crohn disease, a chronic inflammation of the small intestine, which is characterized by flare-ups and remission. During flare-ups, I've experienced fever, diarrhea, vomiting, pain, and intestinal obstruction. Even in remission I am never "okay."

Right now I have been in remission two years after a third surgery to remove yet another portion of my small bowel. This time internal bleeding, a rather rare symptom of Crohn's, necessitated the surgery. I was enduring weekly iron infusions, which turned into bimonthly blood transfusions, as my hemoglobin plummeted to 6 (12 is normal). It was no way to live. After the surgery, the bleeding stopped, but I had bouts of urgent, watery diarrhea for a year. That was no way to live either, and unfortunately, as wonderful as my doctor is, I've found that few GIs want to address after-effects of small bowel surgery. After visiting several doctors and by trial-and-error, I finally got these symptoms under control with codeine, Lomotil, and Metamucil, but I will never be able to absorb vitamin B_{12}, so I must inject it monthly for the rest of my life. In addition to taking medicine to cope with having less and less small bowel, I take medicine in the hopes of preventing the next flare-up. Every few weeks, I inject myself with a biologic medicine, Humira, but I must eventually be weaned off this drug because it has possible long-term side effects, the scariest of which is lymphoma. At 52 and with two school-age children, however, I have learned to think of valuing my present quality of life the most, over possible unknown dangers lurking in the future.

I do often think about the past. What would my life be like if our family doctor hadn't told my parents that my constant episodes of diarrhea—which occurred since I was a child—were caused by "nerves?" By the time I was 21, my weight had dropped below 100 pounds, and I was twisted in pain after every meal. My dad arranged for me to visit his own doctor, who gave me a small bowel series that showed I had Crohn's and that a portion of my small intestine was "as narrow as a pencil." By then it was too late for even prednisone (then the drug of choice despite side effects ranging from puffy face to psychosis) to open up the inflamed passage, and I had my first surgery just months after I was diagnosed. Thinking of those times—as well as all the other flare-up times—makes me flinch. While you can never relive pain, you can remember what it felt like. In my case, it was as if a large metal bike lock chain was being forced through my tender gut.

Before that first surgery, I was just out of college and longing to make my mark on the world, but I spent most of my evenings curled up in my small bedroom, listening to the soothing strains of "Make Believe Ballroom Hour" on the radio. Or, because vomiting and diarrhea usually accompanied the pain, I lay with my back pressed against the cold tiles of the bathroom floor. Later on, as a mom with two young children, I would lie on the couch watching life swirl around me, feeling guilty that I could not take part.

There was a silver lining to those flare-ups, and that is the tender affection of those around me: husband, family, and friends. When you have Crohn's, no one knows you have it until things get unbearable. It's not the kind of illness you discuss, but when you have pain and fever, you can kind of approximate those times of being felled by the flu. Yet you know that it will take more than a dose of Nyquil or a night's sleep to get "better." You know you'll face another course of medications—often untried ones—or that you will likely end up in the hospital undergoing yet another surgery.

Nancy J. Brandwein is a writer, editor, and food columnist.

EXERCISES

Remember to check your answers carefully with the "Answers to Exercises", pages 179 and 180.

A Match the following digestive system structures with their meanings below.

anus	esophagus	liver
cecum	gallbladder	pancreas
colon	ileum	pharynx
duodenum	jejunum	sigmoid colon

1. consists of ascending, transverse, descending, and sigmoid sections ____________
2. small sac under the liver; stores bile ____________
3. first part of the large intestine ____________
4. end of the digestive tract opening to the outside of the body ____________
5. second part of the small intestine ____________
6. tube connecting the throat to the stomach ____________
7. third part of the small intestine ____________
8. large organ in the RUQ; secretes bile, stores sugar, produces blood proteins ____________
9. throat ____________
10. lowest part of the colon ____________
11. first part of the small intestine ____________
12. organ under the stomach; produces insulin and digestive enzymes ____________

5

B **Label the following flow chart of the pathway of food through the gastrointestinal tract. The terms you will need are listed below:**

anus	gallbladder	rectum
ascending colon	ileum	salivary glands
cecum	jejunum	sigmoid colon
descending colon	liver	stomach
duodenum	pancreas	transverse colorn
esophagus	pharynx	

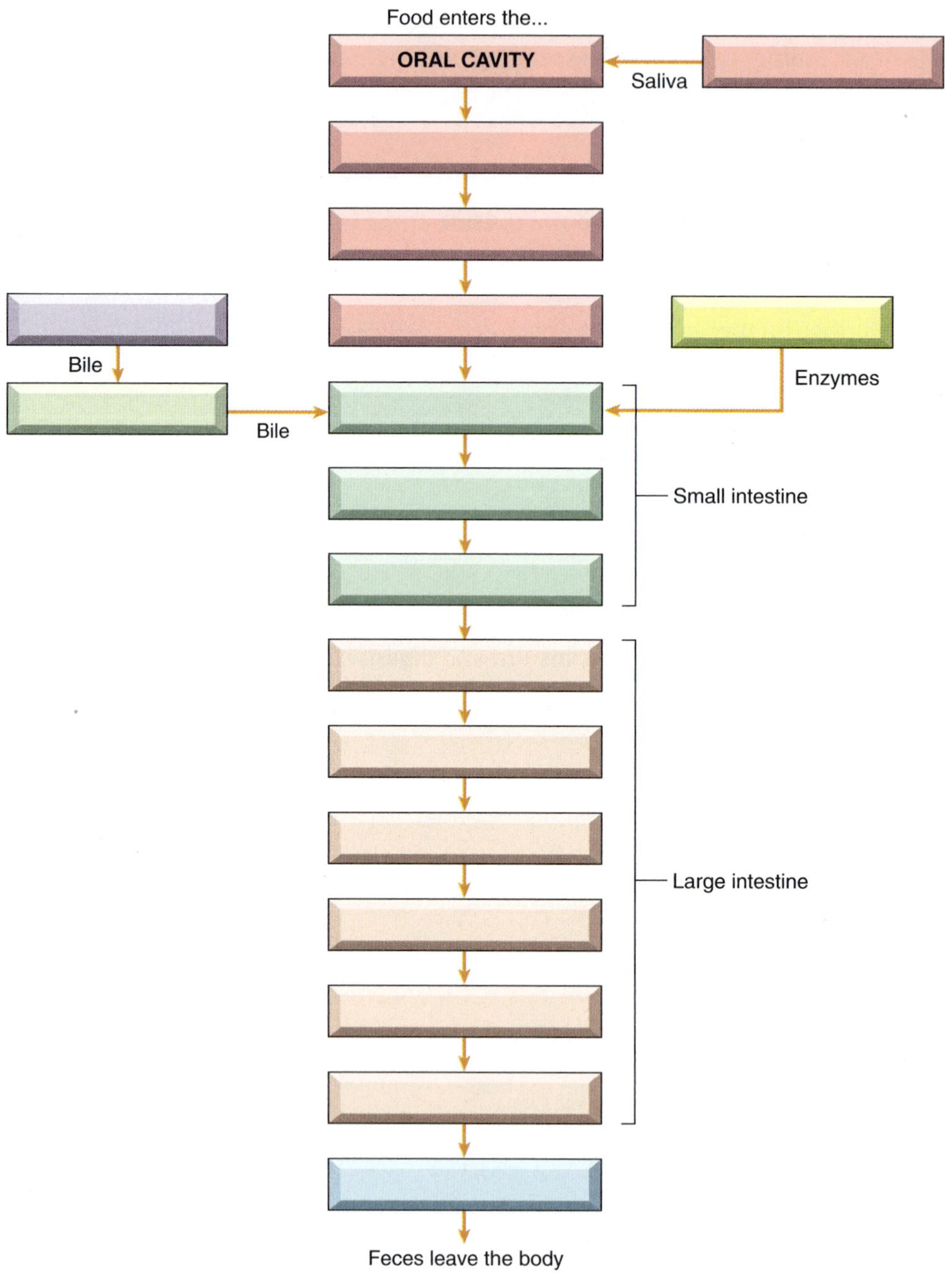

C Circle the term that fits the given definition. You should be able to define the other terms as well!

1. microscopic projections in the walls of the small intestine:
   papillae villi rugae
2. salivary gland near the ear:
   submandibular sublingual parotid
3. ring of muscle at the end of the stomach:
   pyloric sphincter uvula lower esophageal sphincter
4. soft, inner section of a tooth:
   dentin enamel pulp
5. chemical that speeds up reactions and helps digest foods:
   triglyceride amino acid enzyme
6. pigment released with bile:
   glycogen bilirubin melena
7. hormone produced by endocrine cells of the pancreas:
   insulin amylase lipase
8. rhythm-like contraction of the muscles in the walls of the gastrointestinal tract:
   deglutition mastication peristalsis
9. breakdown of large fat globules:
   absorption emulsification anabolism
10. pointed, dog-like tooth medial to premolars:
    incisor canine molar

D Complete the following.

1. Labi/o and cheil/o mean ______________________________
2. Gloss/o and lingu/o mean ______________________________
3. Or/o and stomat/o mean ______________________________
4. Dent/i and odont/o mean ______________________________
5. Lapar/o and celi/o mean ______________________________
6. Gluc/o and glyc/o mean ______________________________
7. Lip/o, steat/o, and adip/o mean ______________________________
8. The suffixes -iasis and -osis mean ______________________________
9. Chol/e and bil/i mean ______________________________
10. Resection and -ectomy mean ______________________________

5

E **Build medical terms based on the given definitions.**

1. removal of a salivary gland ______________________________
2. pertaining to the throat ______________________________
3. hernia of the rectum ______________________________
4. enlargement of the liver ______________________________
5. surgical repair of the roof of the mouth ______________________________
6. after meals ______________________________
7. visual examination of the anal and rectal region ______________________________
8. study of the cause (of disease) ______________________________
9. incision of the common bile duct ______________________________
10. pertaining to teeth and cheek ______________________________
11. disease condition of the small intestine ______________________________
12. new opening between the common bile duct and the jejunum ______________________________
13. pertaining to surrounding the anus ______________________________
14. new opening from the colon to the outside of the body ______________________________
15. under the lower jaw ______________________________
16. pertaining to the face ______________________________

5

F **Match the following doctors or dentists with their specialties.**

colorectal surgeon	nephrologist	periodontist
endodontist	oral surgeon	proctologist
gastroenterologist	orthodontist	urologist

1. treats disorders of the anus and rectum ______________________________
2. operates on the organs of the urinary tract ______________________________
3. straightens teeth ______________________________
4. performs root canal therapy ______________________________
5. operates on the mouth and teeth ______________________________
6. treats kidney disorders ______________________________
7. diagnoses and treats gastrointestinal disorders ______________________________
8. treats gum disease ______________________________
9. operates on the intestinal tract ______________________________

G **Build medical terms to describe the following inflammations.**

1. inflammation of the appendix ____________________
2. inflammation of the large intestine ____________________
3. inflammation of the passageway from the throat to the stomach ____________________
4. inflammation of the membrane surrounding the abdomen ____________________
5. inflammation of the gallbladder ____________________
6. inflammation of the third part of the small intestine ____________________
7. inflammation of the pancreas ____________________
8. inflammation of the gums ____________________
9. inflammation of the liver ____________________
10. inflammation of the mouth ____________________
11. inflammation of the salivary gland ____________________
12. inflammation of the small and large intestines ____________________

H **Match the following terms with their meanings below.**

anastomosis	gluconeogenesis	mesentery
biliary	glycogenolysis	mucosa
defecation	hyperbilirubinemia	parenteral
cheilitis	hyperglycemia	portal vein

1. high level of blood sugar ____________________
2. inflammation of the lip ____________________
3. pertaining to administration of medicines and fluid other than by mouth ____________________
4. mucous membrane ____________________
5. expulsion of feces from the body through the anus ____________________
6. breakdown (conversion) of starch to sugar ____________________
7. fan-like membrane that connects the small intestine to the abdominal wall ____________________
8. large vessel that takes blood to the liver from the intestines ____________________
9. new surgical connection between structures or organs ____________________
10. pertaining to bile ducts ____________________
11. process of forming new sugar from proteins and fats ____________________
12. high levels of a bile pigment in the bloodstream ____________________

I Give the names of the following gastrointestinal signs or symptoms based on their descriptions.

1. passage of bright red blood from the rectum ______________________
2. lack of appetite ______________________
3. fat in the feces ______________________
4. black, tarry stools; feces containing digested blood ______________________
5. abnormal accumulation of fluid in the abdomen ______________________
6. rumbling noise produced by gas in the GI tract ______________________
7. gas expelled through the anus ______________________
8. an unpleasant sensation in the stomach and a tendency to vomit ______________________
9. loose, watery stools ______________________
10. difficulty in passing stools (feces) ______________________
11. difficulty in swallowing ______________________
12. gas expelled from the stomach through the mouth ______________________

J Write short answers for the following questions.

1. What is jaundice? ______________________
2. List three ways in which a patient can become jaundiced
   a. ______________________
   b. ______________________
   c. ______________________
3. What does it mean when a disease is described as *idiopathic*? ______________________

K Select from the list of pathologic conditions to make a diagnosis.

achalasia	colorectal cancer	herpetic stomatitis
anal fistula	Crohn disease (Crohn's)	oral leukoplakia
aphthous stomatitis	dental caries	pancreatic cancer
colonic polyps	esophageal cancer	periodontal disease

1. Mr. Jones, a smoker and heavy drinker, complained of dysphagia in recent months. A longstanding condition of Barrett esophagus resulted in his malignant condition.

   Diagnosis: ______________________.
2. An abnormal tube-like passageway near his anus caused Mr. Rosen's proctalgia. His doctor performed surgery to close off the abnormality. Diagnosis: ______________________.
3. Carol's dentist informed her that the enamel of three teeth was damaged by bacteria-producing acid. Diagnosis: ______________________.

4. Paola's symptoms of chronic diarrhea, abdominal cramps, and fever led her doctor to suspect that she suffered from an inflammatory bowel disease affecting the distal portion of her ileum. The doctor prescribed steroid drugs to heal her condition. Diagnosis: ________________________.
5. Mr. Hart learned that his colonoscopy showed the presence of small benign growths protruding from the mucous membrane of his large intestine. Diagnosis: ________________________.
6. During a routine dental checkup, Dr. Friedman discovered white plaques on Mr. Longo's buccal mucosa. He advised Mr. Longo, who was a chronic smoker and heavy drinker, to have these precancerous lesions removed. Diagnosis: ________________________.
7. Every time Carl had a stressful time at work, he developed a fever blister (cold sore) on his lip, resulting from reactivation of a previous viral infection. His doctor told him that there was no treatment 100% effective in preventing the reappearance of these lesions.

   Diagnosis: ________________________.
8. Mr. Green had a biopsy of a neoplastic lesion in his descending colon. The pathology report indicated a malignancy. A partial colectomy was necessary. Diagnosis: ________________________.
9. Small ulcers (canker sores) appeared on Diane's gums. They were painful and annoying.

   Diagnosis: ________________________.
10. Sharon's failure to floss her teeth and remove dental plaque regularly led to development of gingivitis and pyorrhea. Her dentist advised consulting a specialist who could treat her condition.

    Diagnosis: ________________________.
11. Imaging tests revealed a tumor in a section of Mr. Smith's pancreas. His physician told him that since it had not spread, he could hope for a cure with surgery. He had a pancreatoduodenectomy (Whipple procedure), which was successful. Diagnosis: ________________________.
12. Mr. Clark complained of pain during swallowing. His physician explained that the pain was caused by a failure of muscles in his lower esophagus to relax during swallowing.

    Diagnosis: ________________________.

L Match the following pathologic diagnoses with their definitions.

cholecystolithiasis (gallstones)	hemorrhoids	pancreatitis
cirrhosis	hiatal hernia	peptic ulcer
diverticulosis	ileus	ulcerative colitis
dysentery	intussusception	viral hepatitis
esophageal varices	irritable bowel syndrome	volvulus

1. protrusion of the upper part of the stomach through the diaphragm ____________________
2. painful, inflamed intestines caused by bacterial infection ____________________
3. swollen, twisted veins in the rectal region ____________________
4. open sore or lesion of the mucous membrane of the stomach or duodenum ____________________
5. loss of peristalsis ____________________
6. twisting of the intestine on itself ____________________
7. swollen, varicose veins on the surface of the distal portion of the esophagus ____________________
8. abnormal outpouchings in the intestinal wall ____________________
9. chronic inflammation of the colon with destruction of its inner surface ____________________
10. telescoping of the intestines ____________________
11. inflammation of the liver caused by type A, type B, or type C virus ____________________
12. inflammation of the pancreas ____________________
13. calculi in the sac that stores bile ____________________
14. chronic degenerative liver disease with scarring resulting from alcoholism or infectious hepatitis

    ____
15. gastrointestinal symptoms (diarrhea or constipation, abdominal pain, bloating) with no evidence of structural abnormalities ____________________

M Complete the following terms from their meanings given below.

1. membrane (peritoneal fold) that holds the intestines together: mes ____________________
2. removal of the gallbladder: ____________________ ectomy
3. black or dark brown, tarry stools containing blood: mel ____________________
4. high levels of pigment in the blood (jaundice): hyper ____________________
5. pertaining to under the tongue: sub ____________________
6. twisting of the intestine on itself: vol ____________________
7. organ under the stomach that produces insulin and digestive enzymes:

   pan ____________________
8. lack of appetite: an ____________________
9. swollen, twisted veins in the rectal region: ____________________ oids

10. new connection between two previously unconnected tubes: ana ______________________
11. absence of acid in the stomach: a ______________________
12. return of solids and fluids to the mouth from the stomach: gastro re ______________________ disease
13. removal of soft tissue hanging from the roof of the mouth: ______________________ ectomy
14. formation of stones: ______________________ genesis.

ANSWERS TO EXERCISES

A

1. colon
2. gallbladder
3. cecum
4. anus
5. jejunum
6. esophagus
7. ileum
8. liver
9. pharynx
10. sigmoid colon
11. duodenum
12. pancreas

B

See Figure 5-12 on page 149.

C

1. Villi. Papillae are nipple-like projections in the tongue where taste buds are located, and rugae are folds in the mucous membrane of the stomach and hard palate.
2. Parotid. The submandibular gland is under the lower jaw, and the sublingual gland is under the tongue.
3. Pyloric sphincter. The uvula is soft tissue hanging from the soft palate, and the lower esophageal sphincter is a ring of muscle between the esophagus and stomach.
4. Pulp. Dentin is the hard part of the tooth directly under the enamel and in the root, and enamel is the hard, outermost part of the tooth composing the crown.
5. Enzyme. A triglyceride is a large fat molecule, and an amino acid is a substance produced when proteins are digested.
6. Bilirubin. Glycogen is animal starch that is produced in liver cells from sugar, and melena is dark, tarry stools.
7. Insulin. Amylase and lipase are digestive enzymes produced by the exocrine cells of the pancreas.
8. Peristalsis. Deglutition is swallowing, and mastication is chewing.
9. Emulsification. Absorption is the passage of materials through the walls of the small intestine into the bloodstream, and anabolism is the process of building up proteins in a cell (protein synthesis).
10. Canine. An incisor is one of the four front teeth in the dental arch (not pointed or like a dog's tooth), and a molar is any of three large teeth just behind (distal to) the two premolar teeth.

D

1. lip
2. tongue
3. mouth
4. tooth
5. abdomen
6. sugar
7. fat
8. abnormal condition
9. gall, bile
10. removal, excision

E

1. sialadenectomy
2. pharyngeal
3. rectocele
4. hepatomegaly
5. palatoplasty
6. postprandial (post cibum—cib/o refers to meals or feeding)
7. proctoscopy
8. etiology
9. choledochotomy
10. dentibuccal
11. enteropathy
12. choledochojejunostomy
13. perianal
14. colostomy
15. submandibular
16. facial

F

1. proctologist
2. urologist
3. orthodontist
4. endodontist
5. oral surgeon
6. nephrologist
7. gastroenterologist
8. periodontist
9. colorectal surgeon

5

G

1. appendicitis
2. colitis
3. esophagitis
4. peritonitis (note that the e is dropped)
5. cholecystitis
6. ileitis
7. pancreatitis
8. gingivitis
9. hepatitis
10. stomatitis
11. sialadenitis
12. enterocolitis (when two combining forms for gastrointestinal organs are in a term, use the one that is closest to the mouth first)

H

1. hyperglycemia
2. cheilitis
3. parenteral
4. mucosa
5. defecation
6. glycogenolysis
7. mesentery
8. portal vein
9. anastomosis
10. biliary
11. gluconeogenesis
12. hyperbilirubinemia

I

1. hematochezia
2. anorexia
3. steatorrhea
4. melena
5. ascites
6. borborygmus
7. flatus
8. nausea
9. diarrhea
10. constipation
11. dysphagia
12. eructation

J

1. yellow-orange coloration of the skin and other tissues (hyperbilirubinemia)
2. a. any liver disease (hepatopathy—such as cirrhosis, hepatoma, or hepatitis), so that bilirubin is not processed into bile and cannot be excreted in feces
   b. obstruction of bile flow, so that bile and bilirubin are not excreted and accumulate in the bloodstream
   c. excessive hemolysis leading to overproduction of bilirubin and high levels in the bloodstream
3. cause is not known

K

1. esophageal cancer
2. anal fistula
3. dental caries
4. Crohn disease (Crohn's)
5. colonic polyps
6. oral leukoplakia
7. herpetic stomatitis
8. colorectal cancer
9. aphthous stomatitis
10. periodontal disease
11. pancreatic cancer
12. achalasia

L

1. hiatal hernia
2. dysentery
3. hemorrhoids
4. peptic ulcer
5. ileus
6. volvulus
7. esophageal varices
8. diverticulosis
9. ulcerative colitis
10. intussusception
11. viral hepatitis
12. pancreatitis
13. cholecystolithiasis (gallstones)
14. cirrhosis
15. irritable bowel syndrome

M

1. mesentery
2. cholecystectomy
3. melena
4. hyperbilirubinemia
5. sublingual
6. volvulus
7. pancreas
8. anorexia
9. hemorrhoids
10. anastomosis
11. achlorhydria
12. gastroesophageal reflux
13. uvulectomy
14. lithogenesis

PRONUNCIATION OF TERMS

To test your understanding of the terminology in this chapter, write the meaning of each term in the space provided. In addition, you may wish to cover the terms and write them by looking at your definitions. Make sure your spelling is correct. The page number after each term indicates where it is defined or used in the book, so you can easily check your responses. You will find complete definitions for all of these terms and their audio pronunciations on the Evolve website.

Pronunciation Guide

ā as in āpe	ă as in ăpple
ē as in ēven	ĕ as in ĕvery
ī as in īce	ĭ as in ĭnterest
ō as in ōpen	ŏ as in pŏt
ū as in ūnit	ŭ as in ŭnder

Vocabulary and Terminology

TERM	PRONUNCIATION	MEANING
absorption (150)	ăb-SŎRP-shŭn	______
achlorhydria (158)	ā-chlōr-HĪD-rē-ă	______
amino acids (150)	ă-MĒ-nō ĂS-ĭdz	______
amylase (150)	ĂM-ĭ-lās	______
anastomosis (155)	ă-năs-tō-MŌ-sĭs	______
anus (150)	Ā-nŭs	______
appendectomy (153)	ăp-ĕn-DĔK-tō-mĒ	______
appendicitis (153)	ă-pĕn-dĭ-SĪ-tĭs	______
appendix (150)	ă-PĔN-dĭks	______
bile (150)	bīl	______
biliary (157)	BĬL-ē-ăr-ē	______
bilirubin (150)	bĭl-ĭ-ROO-bĭn	______
bowel (150)	BŎW-ĕl	______
buccal mucosa (153)	BŬK-ăl mū-KŌ-să	______
canine teeth (150)	KĀ-nīn tēth	______
cecal (153)	SĒ-kăl	______
cecum (150)	SĒ-kŭm	______
celiac (153)	SĒ-lē-ăk	______
cheilosis (154)	kī-LŌ-sĭs	______
cholecystectomy (154)	kō-lĕ-sĭs-TĔK-tō-mē	______
choledocholithiasis (158)	kō-lĕ-dō-kō-lĭ-THĪ-ă-sĭs	______
choledochojejunostomy (156)	kō-lĕ-dō-kō-jĭ-jū-NŎS-tō-mē	______
choledochotomy (154)	kō-lĕ-dō-KŎT-ō-mē	______

TERM	PRONUNCIATION	MEANING
cholelithiasis (157)	kō-lē-lĭ-THĪ-ă-sĭs	
colon (150)	KŌ-lŏn	
colonic (154)	kō-LŎN-ĭk	
colonoscopy (154)	kō-lŏn-ŎS-kō-pē	
colostomy (154)	kŏ-LŎS-tō-mē	
common bile duct (150)	KŎM-ŏn bīl dŭkt	
defecation (150)	dĕf-ĕ-KĀ-shŭn	
deglutition (150)	dē-gloo-TĬSH-ŭn	
dentibuccal (155)	dĕn-tĭ-BŬK-ăl	
dentin (150)	DĔN-tĭn	
digestion (150)	dī-JĔST-yŭn	
duodenal (155)	dū-ō-DĒ-năl *or* dū-ŎD-ĕ-năl	
duodenum (150)	dū-ō-DĒ-nŭm *or* dū-ŎD-ĕ-nŭm	
elimination (150)	ē-lĭm-ĭ-NĀ-shŭn	
emulsification (150)	ē-mŭl-sĭ-fĭ-KĀ-shŭn	
enamel (151)	ē-NĂM-ĕl	
endodontist (156)	ĕn-dō-DŎN-tĭst	
enterocolitis (155)	ĕn-tĕr-ō-kō-LĪ-tĭs	
enteroenterostomy (155)	ĕn-tĕr-ō-ĕn-tĕr-ŎS-tō-mē	
enzyme (151)	ĔN-zīm	
esophageal (156)	ĕ-sŏf-ă-JĒ-ăl	
esophagus (151)	ĕ-SŎF-ă-gŭs	
fatty acids (151)	FĂT-tē Ă-sĭdz	
facial (156)	FĀ-shŭl	
feces (151)	FĒ-sēz	
gallbladder (151)	GAWL-blă-dĕr	
gastrointestinal tract (140)	găs-trō-ĭn-TĔS-tĭn-ăl trăct	
gastrojejunostomy (156)	găs-trō-jĕ-jū-NŎS-tō-mē	
gastrostomy (156)	găs-TRŎS-tō-mē	
gingivitis (156)	jĭn-jĭ-VĪ-tĭs	
gluconeogenesis (158)	gloo-kō-nē-ō-JĔN-ĕ-sĭs	

TERM	PRONUNCIATION	MEANING
glucose (151)	GLOO-kōs	______
glycogen (151)	GLĪ-kō-jĕn	______
glycogenolysis (158)	glī-kō-jĕ-NŎL-ĭ-sĭs	______
hepatoma (156)	hĕ-pă-TŌ-mă	______
hepatomegaly (156)	hĕ-pă-tō-MĔG-ă-lĒ	______
hydrochloric acid (151)	hī-drō-KLŎR-ĭk Ă-sĭd	______
hyperbilirubinemia (157)	hī-pĕr-bĭl-ĭ-roo-bĭ-NĒ-mē-ă	______
hyperglycemia (158)	hī-pĕr-glī-SĒ-mē-ă	______
hypoglossal (156)	hī-pō-GLŎ-săl	______
ileitis (156)	ĭl-ē-Ī-tĭs	______
ileocecal sphincter (156)	ĭl-ē-ō-SĒ-kăl SFĬNK-tĕr	______
ileostomy (156)	ĭl-ē-ŎS-tō-mē	______
ileum (151)	ĬL-ē-ŭm	______
incisor (151)	ĭn-SĪ-zŏr	______
insulin (151)	ĬN-sŭ-lĭn	______
jejunum (151)	jĕ-JOO-nŭm	______
labial (156)	LĀ-bē-ăl	______
laparoscopy (156)	lă-pă-RŎS-kō-pē	______
lipase (151)	LĪ-pās	______
lithogenesis (158)	lĭth-ō-JĔN-ĕ-sĭs	______
liver (151)	LĬ-vĕr	______
lower esophageal sphincter (151)	LŌW-ĕr ĕ-sŏf-ă-JĒ-ăl SFĬNK-tĕr	______
mastication (151)	măs-tĭ-KĀ-shŭn	______
mesentery (155)	MĔS-ĕn-tĕr-ē	______
molar teeth (151)	MŌ-lăr tēth	______
oral (157)	ŎR-ăl	______
orthodontist (156)	ŏr-thō-DŎN-tĭst	______
palate (151)	PĂL-ăt	______
palatopharyngoplasty (157)	păl-ă-tō-fă-RĬNG-gō-plăs-tē	______
palatoplasty (157)	PĂL-ă-tō-plăs-tē	______
pancreas (151)	PĂN-krē-ăs	______
pancreatitis (157)	păn-krē-ă-TĪ-tĭs	______
papillae (151)	pă-PĬL-ē	______

5

TERM	PRONUNCIATION	MEANING
parenteral (155)	pă-RĔN-tĕr-ăl	
parotid gland (151)	pă-RŎT-ĭd glănd	
perianal (153)	pĕ-rē-Ā-năl	
periodontist (156)	pĕr-ē-ō-DŎN-tĭst	
peritonitis (157)	pĕr-ĭ-tō-NĪ-tĭs	
peristalsis (152)	pĕr-ĭ-STĂL-sĭs	
pharyngeal (157)	făr-ăn-JĒ-ăl *or* fă-RĬN-jē-ăl	
pharynx (152)	FĂR-ĭnks	
portal vein (152)	PŎR-tăl vān	
postprandial (158)	pōst-PRĂN-dē-ăl	
premolar teeth (141)	prē-MŌ-lăr tēth	
proctologist (157)	prŏk-TŎL-ō-jĭst	
protease (152)	PRŌ-tē-āse	
pulp (152)	pŭlp	
pyloric sphincter (152)	pī-LŎR-ĭk SFĬNK-tĕr	
pyloroplasty (157)	pī-LŎR-ō-plăs-tē	
pylorus (152)	pī-LŎR-ŭs	
rectocele (157)	RĔK-tō-sēl	
rectum (152)	RĔK-tŭm	
rugae (152)	ROO-gē	
saliva (152)	să-LĪ-vă	
salivary glands (152)	SĂL-ĭ-vār-ē glăndz	
sialadenitis (157)	sī-ăl-ă-dĕ-NĪ-tĭs	
sialolith (158)	sī-ĂL-ō-lĭth	
sigmoid colon (152)	SĬG-moyd KŌ-lŏn	
sigmoidoscopy (157)	sĭg-moyd-ŎS-kō-pē	
sphincter (152)	SFĬNK-tĕr	
steatorrhea (158)	stē-ă-tō-RĒ-ă	
stomach (152)	STŎM-ak	
stomatitis (157)	stō-mă-TĪ-tĭs	
sublingual (156)	sŭb-LĬNG-wăl	
submandibular (156)	sŭb-măn-DĬB-ū-lăr	

TERM	PRONUNCIATION	MEANING
triglycerides (153)	trī-GLĬ-sĕ-rīdz	____________
uvula (153)	Ū-vū-lă	____________
uvulectomy (157)	ū-vū-LĔK-tō-mē	____________
villi (153)	VĬL-ī	____________

Pathologic Terminology

TERM	PRONUNCIATION	MEANING
achalasia (162)	ăk-ăh-LĀ-zē-ă	____________
anal fistula (164)	Ā-năl FĬS-tū-lă	____________
anorexia (159)	ăn-ō-RĔK-sē-ă	____________
aphthous stomatitis (161)	ĂF-thŭs stō-mă-TĪ-tĭs	____________
ascites (159)	ă-SĪ-tēz	____________
borborygmus (159)	bŏr-bō-RĬG-mŭs	____________
cholelithiasis (167)	kō-lĕ-lĭ-THĪ-ă-sĭs	____________
cirrhosis (167)	sĭr-RŌ-sĭs	____________
colonic polyps (164)	kō-LŎN-ĭk pŏlĭps	____________
colorectal cancer (164)	kō-lō-RĔK-tăl KĂN-sĕr	____________
constipation (159)	cŏn-stĭ-PĀ-shŭn	____________
Crohn disease (164)	krōn dĭ-ZĒZ	____________
dental caries (161)	DĔN-tăl KĂR-ēz	____________
diarrhea (160)	dī-ăh-RĒ-ă	____________
diverticula (165)	dī-vĕr-TĬK-ū-lă	____________
diverticulitis (165)	dī-vĕr-tĭk-ū-LĪ-tĭs	____________
diverticulosis (165)	dī-vĕr-tĭk-ū-LŌ-sĭs	____________
dysentery (165)	DĬS-ĕn-tĕr-ē	____________
dysphagia (160)	dĭs-PHĀ-jē-ă	____________
eructation (160)	ē-rŭk-TĀ-shŭn	____________
esophageal cancer (162)	ĕ-sŏf-ă-JĒ-ăl KăN-sĕr	____________
esophageal varices (162)	ĕ-sŏf-ă-JĒ-ăl VĂR-ĭ-sēz	____________
etiology (159)	ē-tē-ŎL-ō-jē	____________
flatus (160)	FLĀ-tŭs	____________

TERM	PRONUNCIATION	MEANING
gastric cancer (162)	GĂS-trĭk KĂN-sĕr	
gastroesophageal reflux disease (162)	găs-trō-ĕ-sŏf-ă-JĒ-ăl RĒ-flŭx dĭ-ZĒZ	
hematochezia (160)	hē-mă-tō-KĒ-zē-ă	
hemorrhoids (165)	HĔM-ō-roydz	
herpetic stomatitis (162)	hĕr-PĔT-ĭk stō-mă-TĪ-tĭs	
hiatal hernia (163)	hī-Ā-tăl HĔR-nē-ă	
icterus (160)	ĬK-tĕr-ŭs	
idiopathic (159)	ĭd-ē-ō-PĂTH-ĭk	
ileus (166)	ĬL-ē-ŭs	
inflammatory bowel disease (166)	ĭn-FLĂ-mă-tō-rē BŎW-ĕl dĭ-ZĒZ	
inguinal hernia (163)	ĬNG-wĭ-năl HĔR-nē-ă	
intussusception (166)	ĭn-tŭs-sŭs-SĔP-shŭn	
irritable bowel syndrome (166)	ĬR-ĭ-tă-bl BŎW-ĕl SĬN-drōm	
jaundice (160)	JĂWN-dĭs	
lipoma (158)	lī-PŌ-mă	
melena (161)	MĔL-ĕ-nă *or* mĕ-LĒ-nă	
nausea (161)	NĂW-zē-ă	
oral leukoplakia (162)	ŎR-ăl lū-kō-PLĀ-kē-ă	
pancreatic cancer (169)	păn-krē-Ă-tĭc KĂN-sĕr	
pancreatitis (169)	păn-krē-ă-TĪ-tĭs	
peptic ulcer (163)	PĔP-tĭc ŬL-sĕr	
periodontal disease (162)	pĕr-ē-ō-DŎN-tăl dĭ-ZĒZ	
pyorrhea (158)	pī-ŏr-RĒ-ă	
ulcerative colitis (166)	ŬL-sĕr-ă-tĭv kō-LĪ-tĭs	
viral hepatitis (169)	VĪ-răl hĕp-ă-TĪ-tĭs	
volvulus (167)	VŌL-vū-lŭs	

Note: The "Review Sheet" for this chapter is combined with the "Review Sheet" for Chapter 6 on page 213.

evolve *Please visit the Evolve site for additional exercises, games, and images related to this chapter.*

CHAPTER 6

Additional Suffixes and Digestive System Terminology

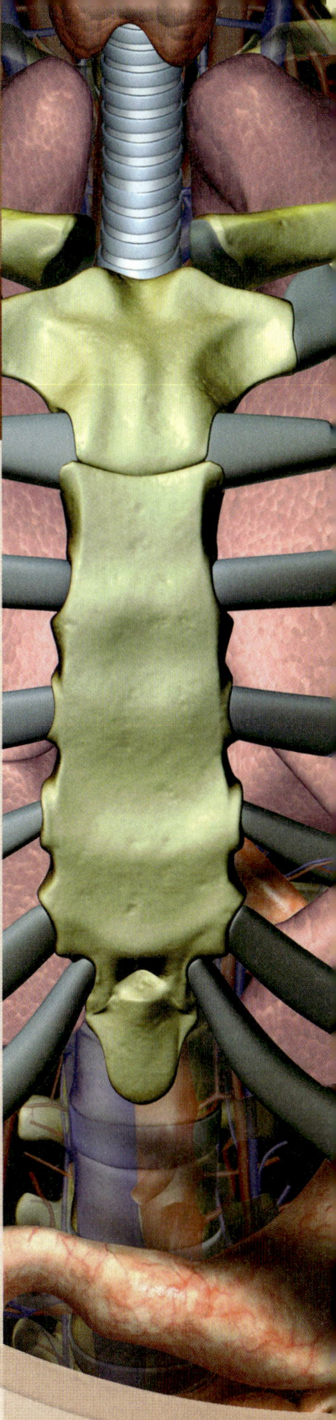

This chapter is divided into the following sections:

CHAPTER GOALS

- Define new suffixes and use them to form terms related to the digestive system.
- List and explain laboratory tests, clinical procedures, and abbreviations relevant to the digestive system.
- Apply your new knowledge to understanding medical terms in their proper context, such as in medical reports and records and in personal vignettes.

INTRODUCTION

This chapter gives you practice in word building, while not introducing a large number of new terms. It uses many familiar terms from Chapter 5, which should give you a breather after your hard work.

Study the suffixes below and complete the meanings of the terms. Checking the meanings of the terms with a dictionary may prove helpful and add another dimension to your understanding.

The information included under Laboratory Tests and Clinical Procedures and in the Abbreviations section relates to the gastrointestinal system and will be useful for work in clinical or laboratory medical settings.

The Practical Applications section gives you examples of medical language in context. Congratulate yourself as you decipher medical sentences, operative reports, and case studies.

SUFFIXES

Write the meaning of the medical term in the space provided.

SUFFIX	MEANING	TERMINOLOGY	MEANING
-ectasis, -ectasia	dilation, (dilatation), widening	cholangiectasis *Cholangi/o means bile duct (vessel). This condition is secondary to bile duct obstruction.*	________
-emesis	vomiting	hematemesis *Bright red blood is vomited, often associated with esophageal varices or peptic ulcer.*	________
-pepsia	digestion	dyspepsia	________
-phagia	eating, swallowing	polyphagia *Excessive appetite and uncontrolled eating.*	________
		dysphagia	________
-plasty	surgical repair	abdominoplasty *This is commonly referred to as a "tummy tuck." Other surgical repairs are rhinoplasty and blepharoplasty.*	________

-ectasis, -ectasia

These suffixes are commonly used in respiratory system terminology in Chapter 12. Examples are bronchiectasis and atelectasis (a- = not, tel = complete), which is a collapsed lung.

Dysphagia/Dysplasia/Dysphasia

Don't confuse **dysphagia** , which is difficulty in swallowing, with **dysplasia**, which is abnormal formation (plas/o = formation), or **dysphasia**, which is abnormal speech (phas/o = speech).

SUFFIX	MEANING	TERMINOLOGY	MEANING
-ptysis	spitting	hemoptysis *From the respiratory tract and lungs.*	_______
-rrhage, -rrhagia	bursting forth (of blood)	hemorrhage *Loss of a large amount of blood in a short period.*	_______
		gastrorrhagia	_______
-rrhaphy	suture	herniorrhaphy *Repair (as in stitching or suturing) of a hernia. Hernioplasty is a synonym. Tenorrhaphy (ten = tendon) is another common use of this suffix.*	_______
-rrhea	flow, discharge	diarrhea *The embedded root rrh means flow or discharge.*	_______
-spasm	involuntary contraction of muscles	pylorospasm	_______
		bronchospasm *A chief characteristic of bronchitis and asthma.*	_______
-stasis	stopping, controlling	cholestasis *Flow of bile from the liver to the duodenum is interrupted.*	_______
-stenosis	narrowing, tightening	pyloric stenosis *This is a congenital defect in newborns blocking the flow of food into the small intestine.*	_______

6

Hemoptysis and Hematemesis

Hemoptysis is spitting up blood from the respiratory tract, a sign of bleeding and disease within the bronchial tubes and lungs. **Hematemesis** is vomiting blood, a sign of bleeding from the upper part of the gastrointestinal tract.

-rrhea

The suffix –rrhea is used to indicate flow or discharge of various substances:

- rhinorrhea – mucus from the nose
- pyorrhea – pus from the gums
- menorrhea – menstrual (men/o) blood from the uterine lining
- leukorrhea – white, yellowish fluid from the vagina

Stenosis

Stenosis comes from the Greek meaning "narrowing." It is sometimes called a **stricture**. While it is used in the gastrointestinal system to describe narrowing, as in bowel obstruction, biliary tract stenosis, and pyloric stenosis, there are other stenoses as well. These include:

- arterial stenosis
- heart valve stenosis
- spinal stenosis
- tracheal stenosis

SUFFIX	MEANING	TERMINOLOGY	MEANING
-tresia	opening	atresia ______ *Absence of a normal opening.* esophageal atresia ______ *A congenital anomaly in which the esophagus does not connect with the stomach. A tracheoesophageal fistula often accompanies this abnormality (Figure 6-1).* biliary atresia ______ *Congenital hypoplasia or nonformation of bile ducts causes neonatal cholestasis and jaundice.*	

Examples of suffixes that are used alone as separate terms are:

emesis (emetic) If a child swallows poison, the physician may prescribe a drug to induce **emesis.** An example of an **emetic** is a strong solution of salt or ipecac syrup.

lysis The disease caused **lysis** of liver cells.

spasm Eating spicy foods can lead to **spasm** of gastric sphincters.

stasis Overgrowth of bacteria within the small intestine can cause **stasis** of the intestinal contents.

stenosis Projectile vomiting in an infant during feeding is a clinical sign of pyloric **stenosis.**

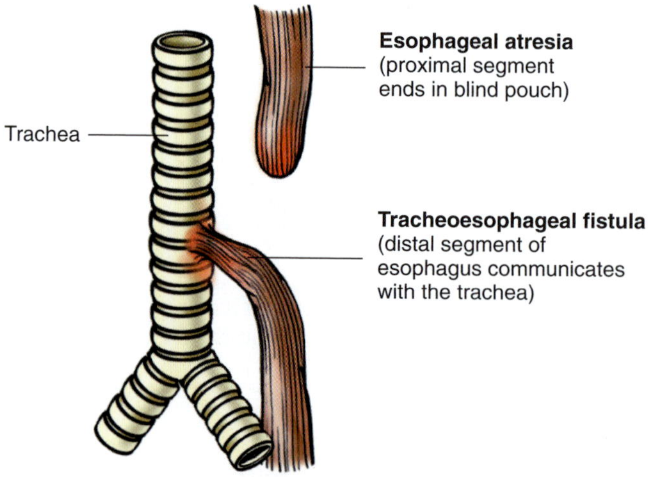

FIGURE 6-1 Esophageal atresia with tracheoesophageal fistula.

TERMINOLOGY

Write the meaning of the terms in the spaces provided.

COMBINING FORM	MEANING	TERMINOLOGY	MEANING
bucc/o	______	buccal	______
cec/o	______	cecal volvulus	______
celi/o	______	celiac disease *Damage to the lining of the small intestine as a reaction to eating* ***gluten*** *(protein found in wheat, barley, and rye). Malabsorption and malnutrition occur. Treatment consists of a lifelong gluten-free diet. It is also called* ***celiac sprue.***	______
cheil/o	______	cheilosis *Characterized by scales and fissures on the lips and resulting from a deficiency of vitamin B_2 (thiamine) in the diet.*	______
chol/e	______	cholelithiasis	______
cholangi/o	______	cholangitis *In this term, one i is dropped. The most common cause of this condition is bacterial infection.*	______
		cholangiocarcinoma	______
cholecyst/o	______	cholecystectomy	______
choledoch/o	______	choledochal	______
		choledochectasia	______
col/o	______	colectomy *Surgeons perform* ***laparoscopic-assisted colectomy (LAC)*** *as an alternative to open colectomy to remove nonmetastatic colorectal carcinomas.*	______
colon/o	______	colonoscopy	______
dent/i	______	dentalgia	______
duoden/o	______	duodenal	______
enter/o	______	gastroenteritis	______
esophag/o	______	esophageal atresia *This congenital anomaly must be corrected surgically.*	______
gastr/o	______	gastrojejunostomy	______
		gastrostomy *Also called a* ***G tube*** *or "button". One type is a PEG (percutaneous endoscopic gastrostomy) tube, which is inserted (laparoscopically) through the abdomen into the stomach to deliver food and liquids when swallowing is impossible.*	______

6

COMBINING FORM	MEANING	TERMINOLOGY	MEANING
gingiv/o		gingivectomy	
gloss/o		glossectomy	
gluc/o		gluconeogenesis	
glyc/o		glycogen *A form of sugar stored in the liver.*	
hepat/o		hepatomegaly	
herni/o		herniorrhaphy	
ile/o		ileostomy	
jejun/o		cholecystojejunostomy	
labi/o		labiodental	
lingu/o		sublingual	
lip/o		lipase	
lith/o		cholecystolithiasis	
odont/o		periodontal membrane	
or/o		oropharynx *The tonsils are located in the oropharynx.*	
palat/o		palatoplasty *Also called palatorrhaphy, this procedure corrects cleft (split) palate, a congenital anomaly.*	
pancreat/o		pancreatic	
		pancreatoduodenectomy *Sometimes called a pancreaticoduodenectomy. This is a* ***Whipple procedure,*** *a surgical treatment for pancreatic cancer. See page 200.*	
proct/o		proctosigmoidoscopy	
pylor/o		pyloric stenosis	
rect/o		rectal carcinoma	
sialaden/o		sialadenectomy	
splen/o		splenic flexure *The downward bend in the transverse colon near the spleen. The* ***hepatic flexure*** *is the bend in the transverse colon near the liver.*	
steat/o		steatorrhea	
stomat/o		aphthous stomatitis	

LABORATORY TESTS AND CLINICAL PROCEDURES

Concentrate on learning the meanings in **bold** opposite the laboratory test or procedure. Additional information is provided to increase your understanding of terms.

LABORATORY TESTS

amylase and lipase tests

Tests for the levels of amylase and lipase enzymes in the blood.
Increased levels are associated with pancreatitis.

liver function tests (LFTs)

Tests for the presence of enzymes and bilirubin in blood.
LFTs are performed on blood serum (clear fluid that remains after blood has clotted). Examples of LFTs are tests for **ALT** (alanine transaminase) and **AST** (aspartate transaminase). ALT and AST are enzymes present in many tissues. **Levels are elevated in the serum of patients with liver disease.** High ALT and AST levels indicate damage to liver cells (as in hepatitis).

Alkaline phosphatase (alk phos) is another enzyme that may be elevated in patients with liver, bone, and other diseases.

Serum bilirubin levels are elevated in patients with liver disease and jaundice. A **direct bilirubin test** measures conjugated bilirubin. High levels indicate liver disease or biliary obstruction. An **indirect bilirubin test** measures unconjugated bilirubin. Increased levels mean excessive hemolysis, as may occur in a newborn.

stool culture

Test for microorganisms present in feces.
Feces are placed in a growth medium and examined microscopically. See Figure 6-2A.

stool guaiac test or Hemoccult test

Test to detect occult (hidden) blood in feces.
This is an important screening test for colon cancer. **Guaiac** (GWĪ-ăk) is a chemical from the wood of trees. When added to a stool sample, it reacts with any blood present in the feces. See Figure 6-2B.

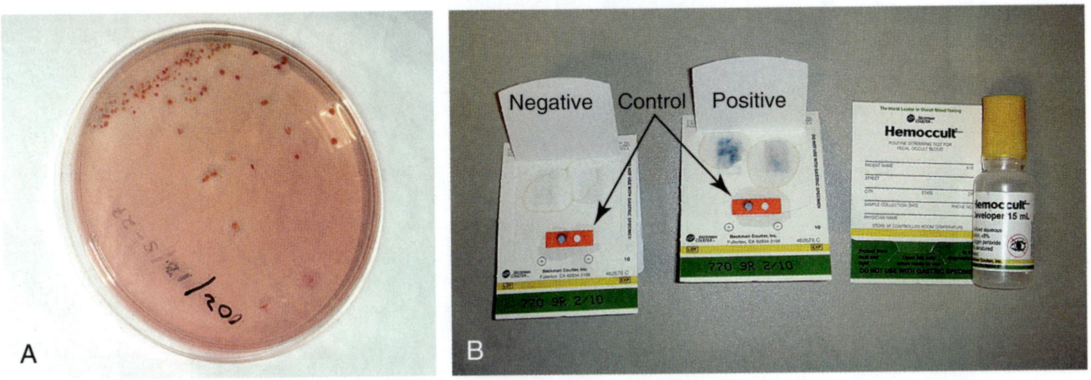

FIGURE 6-2 **A, Stool culture. B, Stool guaiac test.**

CLINICAL PROCEDURES

X-Ray Tests

X-ray imaging is used in many ways to detect pathologic conditions. In dental practice, x-ray images are commonly used to locate cavities (caries). Many of the x-ray tests listed here use a **contrast medium** (substance that x-rays cannot penetrate) to visualize a specific area of the digestive system. The contrast, because of its increased density relative to body tissue, allows organs and parts to be distinguished from one another on the film or screen.

lower gastrointestinal series (barium enema)

X-ray images of the colon and rectum obtained after injection of barium into the rectum.

Radiologists inject barium (a contrast medium) by enema into the rectum. Figure 6-3A shows a barium enema study of a colon with diverticulosis.

upper gastrointestinal series

X-ray images of the esophagus, stomach, and small intestine obtained after administering barium by mouth.

Often performed immediately after an upper gastrointestinal series, a **small bowel follow-through** study shows sequential x-ray pictures of the small intestine as barium passes through (Figure 6-3B). A **barium swallow** is a study of the esophagus.

cholangiography

X-ray examination of the biliary system performed after injection of contrast into the bile ducts.

In **percutaneous transhepatic cholangiography,** the contrast medium is injected using a needle placed through the abdominal wall into the liver. In **endoscopic retrograde cholangiopancreatography (ERCP)** (Figure 6-4A), contrast medium is administered through an oral catheter (tube) and then passes through the esophagus, stomach, and duodenum and into bile ducts. This procedure helps diagnose problems involving the bile ducts, gallbladder, and pancreas.

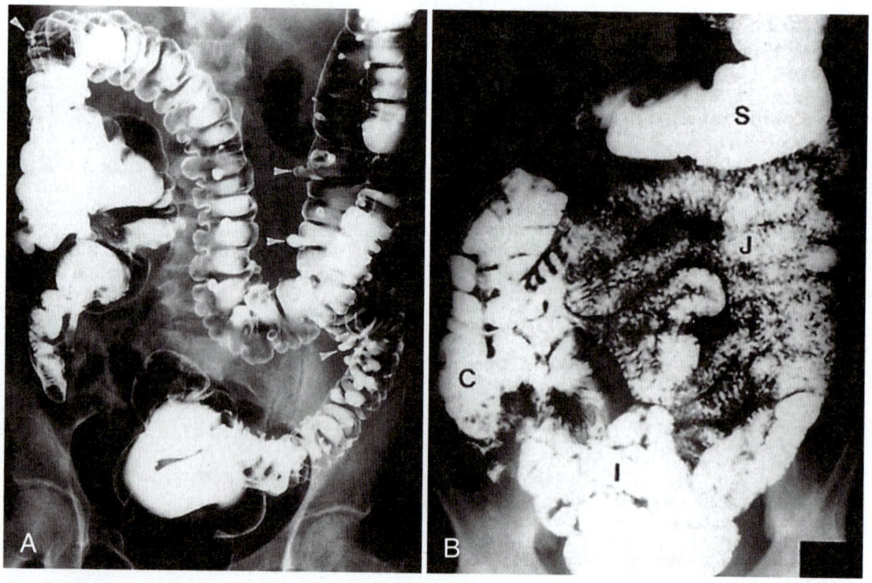

FIGURE 6-3 **A, Barium enema.** This x-ray image of a barium enema demonstrates diverticulosis. The *arrowheads* point to the diverticula throughout the colon. Most patients with diverticula are asymptomatic, but complications (diverticulitis, perforated diverticulum, obstruction, or hemorrhage) may occur. **B,** An x-ray image of a **small-bowel follow-through** study demonstrating the normal appearance of the jejunum (J) in the upper left abdomen and of the ileum (I) in the right lower abdomen. Notice the contrast material within the stomach (S) and cecum (C).

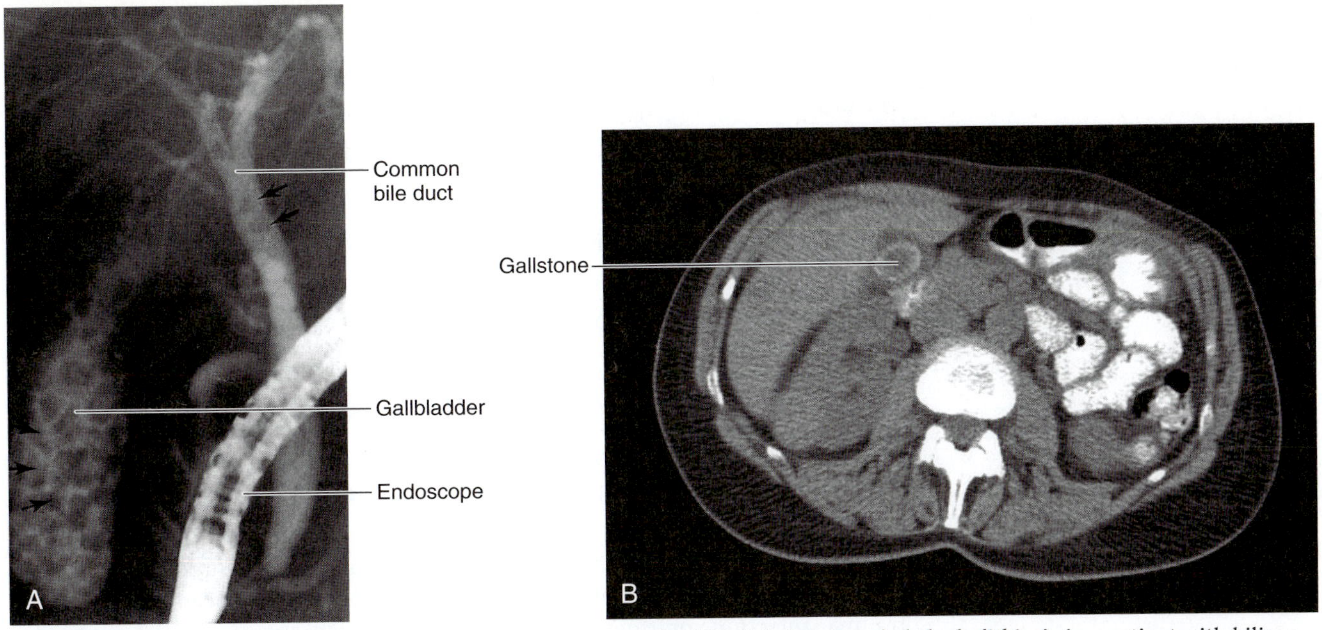

FIGURE 6-4 A, **Endoscopic retrograde cholangiopancreatography (ERCP) showing choledocholithiasis** in a patient with biliary colic (pain). Multiple stones are visible in the gallbladder and common bile duct. The stones (*arrows*) are seen as filling defects in the contrast-opacified gallbladder and duct. This patient was treated with open (performed via laparotomy) cholecystectomy and choledocholithotomy. **B, Computed tomography scan** with contrast showing large "porcelain stone" in the gallbladder. The patient was asymptomatic, but a therapeutic option with this type of stone is removal of the gallbladder (using laparoscopy) to prevent any future problems (cholecystitis or carcinoma of the gallbladder). *(B, Courtesy Radiology Department, Massachusetts General Hospital, Boston.)*

6

computed tomography (CT)

A series of x-ray images are taken in multiple views (especially cross section).

A **CT scan** uses a circular array of x-ray beams to produce the cross-sectional image based on differences in tissue densities. Use of contrast material allows visualization of organs and blood vessels and highlights differences in blood flow between normal and diseased tissues (Figure 6-4B and Figures 6-5A and B). **Tomography** (tom/o means cutting) produces a series of x-ray pictures showing multiple views of an organ. An earlier name for a CT scan is "CAT scan" (computerized axial tomography scan).

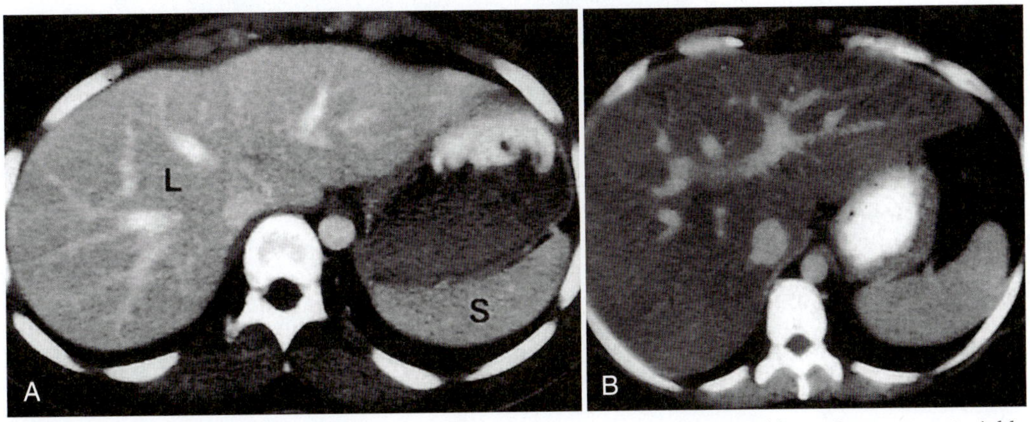

FIGURE 6-5 **Computed tomography (CT) images** of normal and diseased liver. **A, Normal liver.** Contrast material has been injected intravenously, making blood vessels appear bright. The liver (L) and spleen (S) are the same density on this CT image. **B, Fatty liver.** The radiodensity of the liver tissue is reduced because of the large volume of fat contained in the tissue, making it appear darker than normal. Excess fat can lead to inflammation of the liver and cirrhosis.

ULTRASOUND EXAMINATIONS

abdominal ultrasonography

Sound waves beamed into the abdomen produce an image of abdominal viscera.

Ultrasonography is especially useful for examination of fluid-filled structures such as the gallbladder.

endoscopic ultrasonography (EUS)

Use of an endoscope combined with ultrasound to examine the organs of the gastrointestinal tract.

An endoscope is inserted through the mouth or rectum, and ultrasound images are obtained. This test is often used in assessing pancreatic cancer.

MAGNETIC RESONANCE

magnetic resonance imaging (MRI)

Magnetic waves produce images of organs and tissues in all three planes of the body.

This technique does not use x-rays. It detects subtle differences in tissue composition, water content, and blood vessel density, and can show sites of trauma, infection, or cancer. See Figure 6-6, which shows an MRI study of a patient with rectosigmoid carcinoma and polyps in the rectum. CT scanning would not have shown these lesions as clearly.

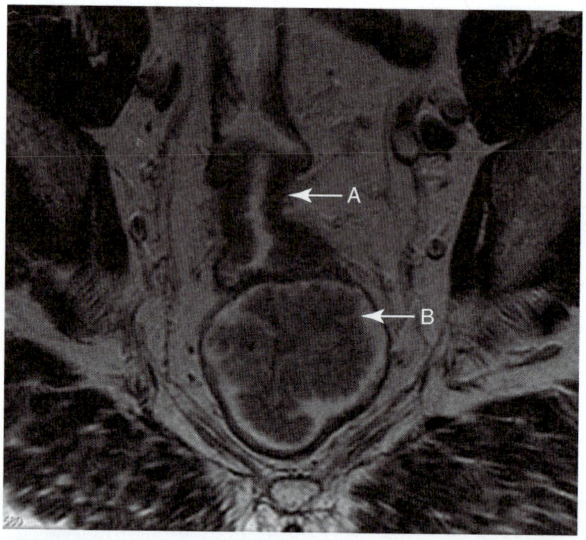

FIGURE 6-6 **Rectal MRI.** A 68-year-old male presents with rectal bleeding. MRI demonstrates a **colonic adenocarcinoma** in the rectosigmoid area (**A**) as well as a **villous adenoma** in the rectum (**B**).

NUCLEAR MEDICINE TEST

HIDA scan

Radioactive imaging procedure that tracks the production and flow of bile from the liver and gallbladder to the intestine.

HIDA stands for hepatobiliary iminodiacetic acid. **Cholescintigraphy** is another name for this test, which determines if the gallbladder is functioning properly.

OTHER PROCEDURES

gastric bypass or bariatric surgery

Reducing the size of the stomach and diverting food to the jejunum (gastrojejunostomy).

This is **bariatric** (bar/o = weight; iatr/o = treatment) **surgery** for severe obesity. The **Roux-en-Y gastric bypass procedure** reduces the size of the stomach to a volume of 2 tablespoons and bypasses much of the small intestine (Figure 6-7). The name Roux-en-Y comes from the surgeon who first described it (César Roux) and the anastomosis of the duodenum and jejunum, which looks like the letter Y.

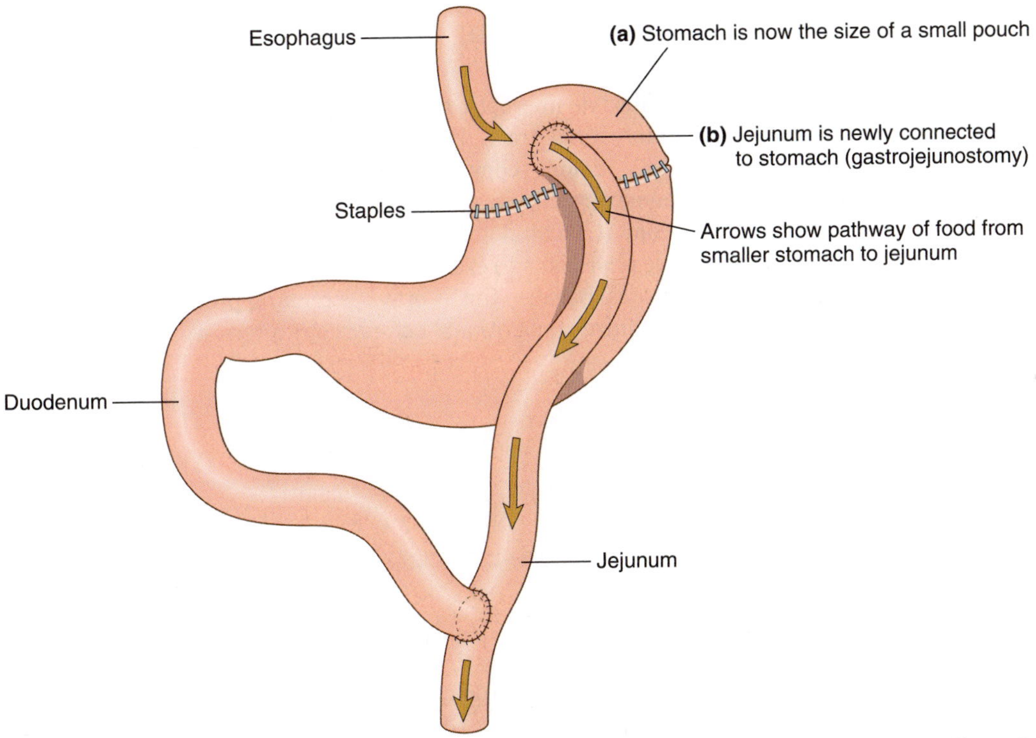

FIGURE 6-7 Gastric bypass. First **(a)** the stomach is stapled so that it is reduced in size to a small pouch. Next **(b)** a shortened jejunum is brought up to connect with the smaller stomach. This diverts food so that it has a shorter travel time through the intestine and less food is absorbed into the bloodstream.

6

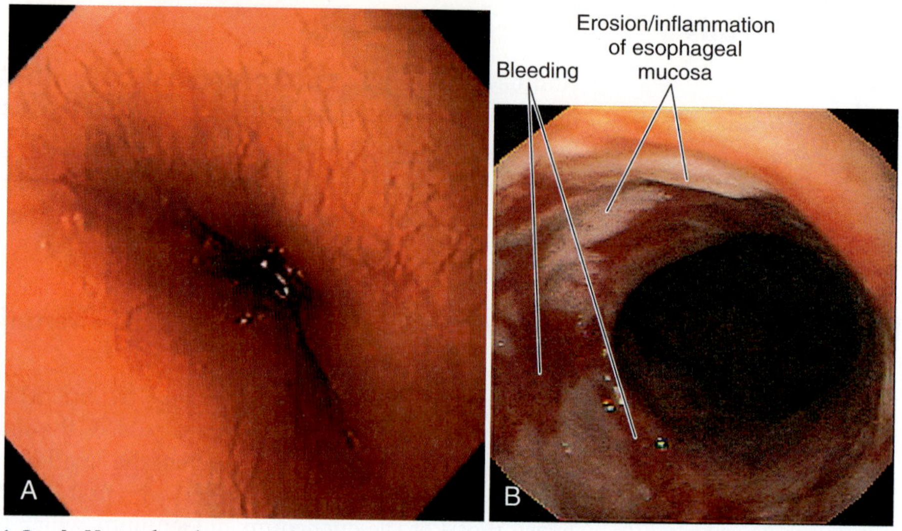

FIGURE 6-8 **A, Normal endoscopy of the esophagus. B, Esophagogastroduodenoscopy.** This endoscopic view shows severe esophagitis in a patient who had gastroesophageal reflux disease (GERD).

gastrointestinal endoscopy

Visual examination of the gastrointestinal tract using an endoscope.

A physician places a flexible fiberoptic tube through the mouth or the anus to view parts of the gastrointestinal tract. Examples are **esophagogastroduodenoscopy (EGD)** (Figure 6-8), **colonoscopy** (Figures 6-9 and 6-10), **sigmoidoscopy**, **proctoscopy**, and **anoscopy**.

Virtual colonoscopy (CT colonography) combines CT scanning and computer technology to enable physicians to examine the entire length of the colon by x-ray imaging in just minutes. Because this is only a screening procedure, patients with abnormal findings require conventional colonoscopy afterward.

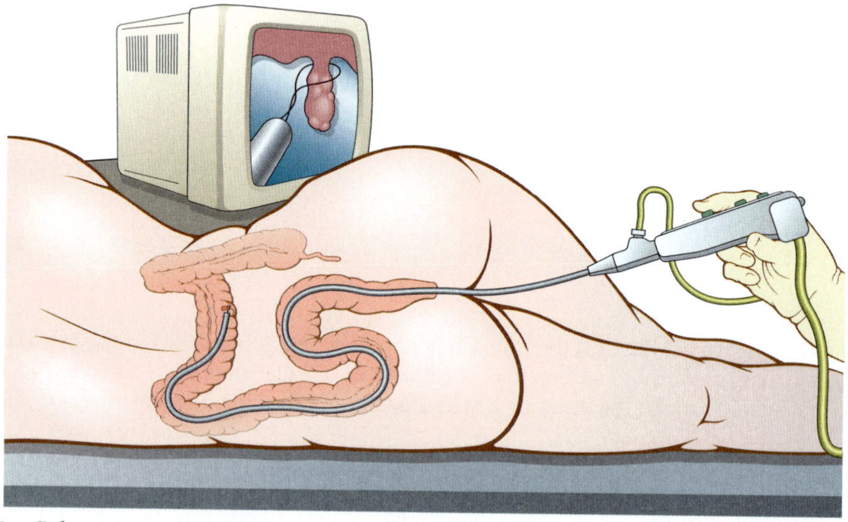

FIGURE 6-9 **Colonoscopy with polypectomy.** Before the procedure, the patient ingests agents to clean the bowel of feces. The patient is sedated and the gastroenterologist advances the instrument in retrograde fashion, guided by images from a video camera on the tip of the colonoscope. When a polyp is located, a wire snare is passed through the endoscope and looped around the stalk. After the loop is gently tightened, an electrical current is applied to cut through the stalk. The polyp is removed for microscopic tissue examination (biopsy).

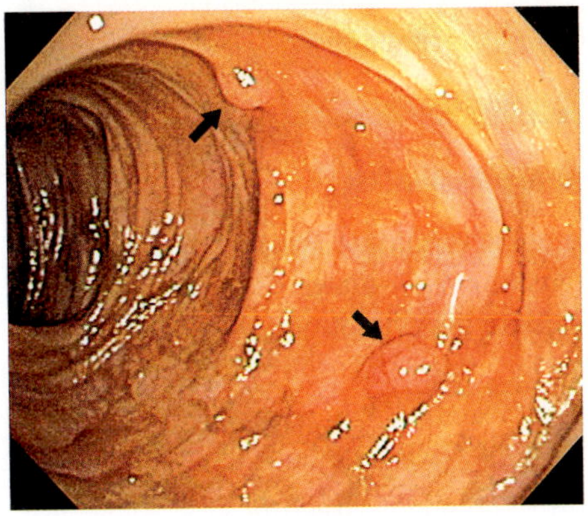

FIGURE 6-10 **Colonoscopy case report.** A 60-year-old man with a history of multiple and prominent colon adenomas (with some areas of high-grade dysplasia) underwent colonoscopy. The endoscope was passed through the anus and advanced to the cecum. Two pedunculated polyps (arrows) were found at the hepatic flexure. Polypectomy was performed using a hot snare. Resection and retrieval were complete.

laparoscopy

Visual (endoscopic) examination of the abdomen with a laparoscope inserted through small incisions in the abdomen.

Laparoscopic cholecystectomy (see Figure 5-28, page 168) and laparoscopic appendectomy are performed by gastrointestinal and general surgeons. See the ***In Person*** story of a woman who underwent laparoscopic cholecystectomy (see page 201).

liver biopsy

Removal of liver tissue for microscopic examination.

A physician inserts a needle through the skin to remove a small piece of tissue for microscopic examination. The average sample is less than 1 inch long. The procedure helps doctors diagnose cirrhosis, chronic hepatitis, and tumors of the liver.

nasogastric intubation

Insertion of a tube through the nose into the stomach.

Physicians use a nasogastric (NG) tube to remove fluid postoperatively and to obtain gastric or intestinal contents for analysis (Figure 6-11).

paracentesis (abdominocentesis)

Surgical puncture to remove fluid from the abdomen.

This procedure is necessary to drain fluid (accumulated in ascites) from the peritoneal (abdominal) cavity.

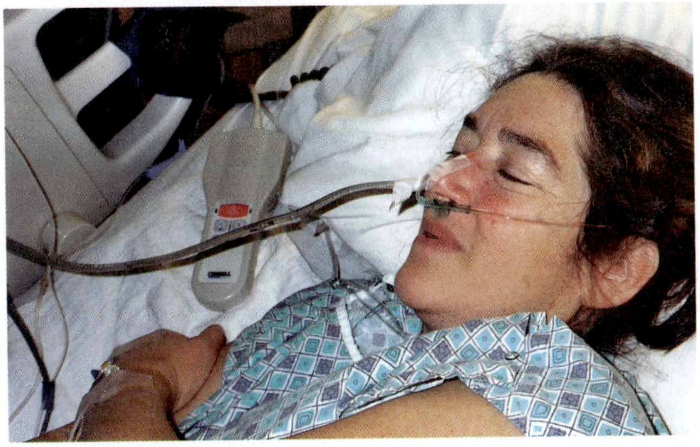

FIGURE 6-11 **Nasogastric intubation.** This patient is recovering from surgery and the nasogastric tube is suctioning secretions from the stomach postoperatively.

ABBREVIATIONS

alk phos	alkaline phosphatase
ALT, AST	alanine transaminase, aspartate transaminase—enzymes measured to evaluate liver function
BE	barium enema
BM	bowel movement
BRBPR	bright red blood per rectum—hematochezia (Latin *per* means through)
CD	celiac disease
CT	computed tomography
EGD	esophagogastroduodenoscopy
ERCP	endoscopic retrograde cholangiopancreatography
EUS	endoscopic ultrasonography
FOBT	fecal occult blood test
G tube	gastrostomy tube; also called stomach tube and PEG tube—used to introduce nutrients into the stomach after insertion through the abdominal wall with laparoscopic instruments
GB	gallbladder
GERD	gastroesophageal reflux disease
GI	gastrointestinal
HBV	hepatitis B virus
IBD	inflammatory bowel disease (Crohn disease and ulcerative colitis)
LAC	laparoscopic-assisted colectomy
LFTs	liver function tests—alk phos, bilirubin, AST, ALT
MRI	magnetic resonance imaging
NG tube	nasogastric tube
NPO	nothing by mouth (Latin nil per os)
PEG tube	percutaneous endoscopic gastrostomy tube—feeding tube
PEJ tube	percutaneous endoscopic jejunostomy tube—feeding tube
PTHC	percutaneous transhepatic cholangiography
PUD	peptic ulcer disease
TPN	total parenteral nutrition Intravenous TPN solutions typically contain sugar (dextrose), proteins (amino acids), electrolytes (sodium, potassium, chloride), and vitamins.
T tube	tube placed in the bile duct for drainage into a small pouch (bile bag) on the outside of the body

6

PRACTICAL APPLICATIONS

Answers to the questions about the case report are on page 209.

CASE REPORT: PANCREATIC CANCER AND WHIPPLE PROCEDURE

A 62-year-old man came to the ED [emergency department] with complaints of fatigue, weight loss, jaundice, and anorexia. Diagnostic studies including abdominal CT with contrast, ERCP, and EUS were performed. The CT scan showed a 4-cm mass at the head of the pancreas, and ERCP revealed evidence of bile duct obstruction; a stent was placed to open the duct. Examination of a tissue biopsy specimen obtained under US guidance confirmed a localized adenocarcinoma of the head of the pancreas.

Additional studies showed no evidence of hepatic or other metastases. Surgical treatment with a Whipple procedure was recommended. This procedure was performed and included pancreatoduodenectomy, choledochojejunostomy, and gastrojejunostomy. Lymph node removal and cholecystectomy were part of the operative procedure. During surgery, it was determined that the tumor was confined to the head of the pancreas. Despite removal of the tumor, the chance of recurrence is high, with a cure rate of only about 20%.

Questions about the Case Report

1. What caused the patient's jaundice?
   a. Excessive hemolysis
   b. Viral hepatitis
   c. Bile duct obstruction
   d. Cholelithiasis

2. What test identified mass as adenocarcinoma?
   a. Whipple procedure
   b. Biopsy with endoscopic ultrasonography
   c. CT scan with contrast
   d. ERCP

3. Which is included in a Whipple procedure?
   a. Removal of the pancreas (malignant area) and duodenum
   b. Removal of the gallbladder
   c. Removal of lymph nodes
   d. All of the above

4. What anastomosis was performed?
   a. Gallbladder and duodenum united.
   b. Common bile duct, pancreatic duct, and small intestine were connected together.
   c. Stomach and pancreas reconnected.
   d. Liver and pancreas connected to the stomach.

IN PERSON

This first-person narrative describes the symptoms and treatment of a 42-year-old woman with gallbladder stones.

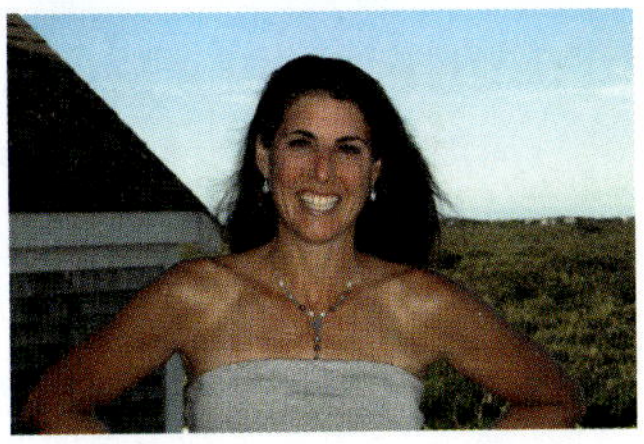

Everyone enjoys a little dessert after dinner, but when the ice cream or a creamy tart leads to pain, most would avoid it. I loved sweets, and despite the revenge they took on my waistline, I still would not pass up an ice cream cone—until my gallbladder decided it had had enough. After several late nights spent doubled over in pain, I tried to steer clear of fatty foods but could not resist the temptation of frozen yogurt.

With one hand, I pushed my cart through the supermarket; with the other hand, I fed myself some delicious low-fat (not non-fat) frozen yogurt. I never dreamed that the attendant at the quick service window actually gave me soft-serve ice cream. Within 10 minutes of eating the questionable yogurt, I broke out into a sweat; a wave of nausea took me, and a knifelike pain stabbed me in my right upper quadrant. It hurt even more when I pressed my hand on the area in an attempt to brace the pain.

Several months earlier, after a similar painful episode, I had undergone an ultrasound of my gallbladder, and the surgeon then recommended cholecystectomy. The U/S showed multiple stones in my gallbladder. Most of the stones were just the right size to lodge in the common bile duct and cause blockage of the outflow of bile that occurs after a fatty meal. When I heard the ultrasound results, I swore off all fatty foods.

I just did not imagine that ice cream masquarading as "low-fat yogurt"would be the straw that broke the camel's back! Soon enough, I abandoned my shopping cart and apologized to the manager of the store for vomiting all over aisle 4. The unrelenting pain did not cease when I vomited—it only intensified. I have no idea how I made it home and into bed, but my husband found me several hours later in a deep sweat. I managed to call my surgeon and arrange for "semi-emergent" surgery the next morning.

Dr. Fernandez and his team performed a laparoscopic cholecystectomy and relayed to me as I came out of anesthesia that I no longer had a "bag of marbles" for a gallbladder. I had a gassy, distended feeling in my abdomen over the two weeks after surgery (carbon dioxide gas was injected into the abdomen before surgery to allow space between abdominal organs). I felt "tight as a drum" for the first few days and the day by day it went away. My four tiny incisions healed just fine, and in about 2 weeks I was feeling back to "normal." Now I can eat ice cream to my heart's content, only suffering the padding on my waistline, not the stabbing pain just above. Without missing a beat, my liver now delivers the bile into my small intestine right after I eat a fatty meal. The bile emulsifies (breaks down) the fat. I just don't have a storage bag to hold bile in reserve.

I've had an appendectomy, my wisdom teeth removed, and now I gave up my gallbladder! How many more "useless" body parts are there to go?

Elizabeth Chabner Thompson is the CEO/Founder of BFFL Co, a company devoted to improving the patient experience. She is also a physician, ultra-marathoner, wife, and the proud mother of four children ages 9-15.

6

EXERCISES

Remember to check your answers carefully with the Answers to Exercises, pages 208 and 209.

A Give the meanings of the following suffixes.

1. -pepsia ______
2. -ptysis ______
3. -emesis ______
4. -phagia ______
5. -rrhea ______
6. -rrhage, -rrhagia ______
7. -rrhaphy ______
8. -plasty ______
9. -ectasis, -ectasia ______
10. -stenosis ______
11. -stasis ______
12. -spasm ______
13. -tresia ______

B Give medical terms for the definitions that follow. Use the listed combining forms as appropriate to create terms.

chol/e	gastr/o	herni/o
cholangi/o	hemat/o	palat/o
choledoch/o	hem/o	pylor/o

6

1. stoppage of bile (flow) ______
2. suture of a hernia ______
3. dilation of bile ducts ______
4. spitting up blood (from the respiratory tract) ______
5. vomiting blood (from the digestive tract) ______
6. surgical repair of roof of the mouth ______
7. narrowing of the pyloric sphincter ______
8. bursting forth of blood from the stomach ______
9. sudden, involuntary contraction of muscles at the distal region of the stomach

   ______
10. bursting forth of blood ______
11. incision of the common bile duct ______

C **Give the meanings of the following terms.**

1. dysphagia ______
2. polyphagia ______
3. dyspepsia ______
4. biliary atresia ______
5. pyorrhea ______
6. cholestasis ______
7. esophageal atresia ______
8. pyloroplasty ______
9. splenorrhagia ______
10. proctosigmoidoscopy ______
11. hemorrhage ______
12. cholangitis ______

D **Match the following surgical procedures with their meanings below.**

abdominoplasty	colectomy	palatoplasty
cecostomy	gingivectomy	pancreatoduodenectomy
cholecystectomy	herniorrhaphy	paracentesis
cholecystojejunostomy	ileostomy	sphincterotomy

1. removal of the gallbladder ______
2. large bowel resection ______
3. suture of a weakened muscular wall (hernia) ______
4. new opening of the first part of the colon to the outside of the body ______
5. surgical repair of the abdomen ______
6. incision of a ring of muscles ______
7. removal of the pancreas and duodenum ______
8. opening of the third part of the small intestine to the outside of the body ______
9. removal of gum tissue ______
10. Anastomosis between the gallbladder and second part of the small intestine ______
11. surgical puncture of the abdomen for withdrawal of fluid ______
12. surgical repair of the roof of the mouth ______

E **Use the given meanings to complete the following terms.**

1. discharge of fat: steat__________________________
2. difficulty in swallowing: dys__________________________
3. abnormal condition of gallstones: chole__________________________
4. pertaining to the cheek: __________________________al
5. pertaining to lips and teeth: __________________________dental
6. vomiting blood: hemat__________________________
7. enlargement of the liver: hepato__________________________
8. pertaining to under the tongue: sub__________________________
9. removal of the gallbladder: __________________________ectomy
10. pertaining to the common bile duct: chole__________________________
11. hemorrhage from the stomach: gastro__________________________

F **Give the meanings of the following terms.**

1. cecal volvulus ____
2. aphthous stomatitis ____
3. celiac disease ____
4. lipase ____
5. cheilosis ____
6. oropharynx ____
7. glycogen ____
8. glossectomy ____
9. sialadenectomy ____
10. periodontal membrane ____
11. choledochectasia ____
12. cholangiocarcinoma ____

G **Match the name of the laboratory test or clinical procedure with its description.**

abdominal ultrasonography
barium enema
CT scan of the abdomen
endoscopic retrograde cholangiopancreatography
endoscopic ultrasonography
gastric bypass (bariatric surgery)
gastrostomy (G tube)
HIDA scan
laparoscopy
liver biopsy
nasogastric intubation
percutaneous transhepatic cholangiography
serum bilirubin
small bowel follow-through
stool culture
stool guaiac (Hemoccult)

1. measurement of bile pigment in the blood ______________________________
2. placement of feces in a growth medium for bacterial analysis ______________________________
3. x-ray examination of the lower gastrointestinal tract ______________________________
4. imaging of abdominal viscera via sound waves ______________________________
5. test to reveal hidden blood in feces ______________________________
6. sequential x-ray images of the small intestine ______________________________
7. injection of contrast material through the skin into the liver, to obtain x-ray images of bile vessels ______________________________
8. insertion of a tube through the nose into the stomach ______________________________
9. transverse x-ray pictures of the abdominal organs ______________________________
10. injection of contrast material via endoscope to obtain x-ray images of the pancreas and bile ducts ______________________________
11. reduction of stomach size and gastrojejunostomy ______________________________
12. insertion of an endoscope and use of ultrasound imaging to visualize the organs of the gastrointestinal tract ______________________________
13. percutaneous removal of liver tissue followed by microscopic examination ______________________________
14. visual examination (endoscopic) of abdominal viscera through small abdominal incisions ______________________________
15. new opening of the stomach to the outside of the body for feeding ______________________________
16. radioactive imaging of the liver, gallbladder, and intestine ______________________________

H Give the meanings of the abbreviations in Column I. Then select the letter of the correct description from Column II.

COLUMN I

1. TPN ____________ ______
2. PUD ____________ ______
3. EGD ____________ ______
4. IBD ____________ ______
5. BE ____________ ______
6. BRBPR ____________ ______
7. LFTs ____________ ______
8. GERD ____________ ______
9. HBV ____________ ______
10. CT ____________ ______

COLUMN II

A. Tests such as measurement of ALT, AST, alk phos, and serum bilirubin.
B. Heartburn is a symptom of this condition.
C. This general condition includes Crohn disease and ulcerative colitis.
D. *H. pylori* causes this condition.
E. Intravenous injection of nutrition.
F. This is a lower gastrointestinal series.
G. X-ray procedure that produces a series of cross-sectional images.
H. This infectious agent causes chronic inflammation of the liver.
I. Hematochezia describes this gastrointestinal symptom.
J. Endoscopic visualization of the upper gastrointestinal tract.

I Give the suffixes for the following terms.

1. bursting forth (of blood) ____________
2. flow, discharge ____________
3. suture ____________
4. dilation ____________
5. narrowing (stricture) ____________
6. vomiting ____________
7. spitting ____________
8. excision ____________
9. digestion ____________
10. eating, swallowing ____________
11. hardening ____________
12. stopping, controlling ____________
13. surgical repair ____________
14. opening ____________
15. surgical puncture ____________
16. involuntary contraction ____________
17. new opening ____________
18. incision ____________

6

J **Circle the correct term in parentheses to complete each sentence.**

1. When Mrs. Smith began to have diarrhea and crampy abdominal pain, she consulted a **(urologist, nephrologist, gastroenterologist)** and worried that the cause of her symptoms might be **(inflammatory bowel disease, esophageal varices, achalasia).**
2. After taking a careful history and performing a thorough physical examination, Dr. Blakemore diagnosed Mr. Bean, a long-time drinker, with **(hemorrhoids, pancreatitis, appendicitis).** Mr. Bean had complained of sharp midepigastric pain and a change in bowel habits.
3. Many pregnant women cannot lie flat after eating without experiencing a burning sensation in their chest and throat. The usual cause of this symptom is **(volvulus, dysentery, gastroesophageal reflux).**
4. Mr. and Mrs. Cho brought their young infant son to the clinic after he had several bouts of projectile vomiting. The pediatric surgeon suspected a diagnosis of **(inguinal hernia, pyloric stenosis, ascites).**
5. Boris had terrible problems with his teeth. He needed not only a periodontist for his **(aphthous stomatitis, oral leukoplakia, gingivitis)** but also an **(endodontist, oral surgeon, orthodontist)** to straighten his teeth.
6. After 6 weeks of radiation therapy to her throat, Betty experienced severe esophageal irritation and inflammation. She complained to her doctor about her resulting **(dyspepsia, dysphagia, hematemesis).**
7. Steven, age 7 years, is brought to the clinic because of recurrent abdominal pain, occasional constipation and diarrhea, and weight loss. His pediatrician's diagnosis is (**lipase deficiency, dysentery, celiac disease**) and recommends a (**fat, gluten, sugar**)-free diet.
8. Chris had been a heavy alcohol drinker all of his adult life. His wife noticed worsening yellow discoloration of the whites of his eyes and skin. After a physical examination and blood tests, his family physician told him his **(colon, skin, liver)** was diseased. The yellow discoloration was **(jaundice, melena, flatus),** and his condition was **(cheilosis, cirrhosis, steatorrhea).**
9. When Carol was working as a phlebotomist, she accidentally cut her finger while drawing a patient's blood. Unfortunately the patient had **(pancreatitis, hemoptysis, hepatitis),** and HBV was transmitted to Carol. Blood tests and **(liver biopsy, gastrointestinal endoscopy, stool culture)** confirmed Carol's unfortunate diagnosis. Her doctor told her that her condition was chronic and that she might be a candidate for a **(bone marrow, liver, kidney)** transplant procedure in the future.
10. Operation Smile is a rescue project that performs **(herniorrhaphy, oral gingivectomy, palatoplasty)** on children with a congenital cleft in the roof of the mouth.

ANSWERS TO EXERCISES

A

1. digestion
2. spitting (from the respiratory tract)
3. vomiting
4. eating, swallowing
5. flow, discharge
6. bursting forth of blood
7. suture
8. surgical repair
9. dilation (dilatation), widening
10. narrowing, tightening
11. to stop; control
12. sudden, involuntary contraction of muscles
13. opening

B

1. cholestasis
2. herniorrhaphy
3. cholangiectasia
4. hemoptysis
5. hematemesis
6. palatoplasty
7. pyloric stenosis
8. gastrorrhagia
9. pylorospasm
10. hemorrhage
11. choledochotomy

C

1. difficulty in swallowing
2. excessive (much) eating
3. difficult digestion
4. biliary ducts are not open (congenital anomaly)
5. discharge of pus from the gums
6. stoppage of flow of bile
7. esophagus is not open (closed off) at birth (congenital anomaly)
8. surgical repair of the pyloric sphincter
9. bursting forth of blood (hemorrhage) from the spleen
10. visual (endoscopic) examination of the rectum and sigmoid colon
11. bursting forth of blood
12. inflammation of bile duct (vessel)

D

1. cholecystectomy
2. colectomy
3. herniorrhaphy
4. cecostomy
5. abdominoplasty
6. sphincterotomy
7. pancreatoduodenectomy
8. ileostomy
9. gingivectomy
10. cholecystojejunostomy
11. paracentesis (abdominocentesis)
12. palatoplasty

6

E

1. steatorrhea
2. dysphagia
3. cholelithiasis
4. buccal
5. labiodental
6. hematemesis
7. hepatomegaly
8. sublingual
9. cholecystectomy
10. choledochal
11. gastrorrhagia

F

1. twisted intestine in the area of the cecum
2. inflammation of the mouth with small ulcers
3. autoimmune disorder in which villi in the lining of the small intestine are damaged, resulting from dietary glutens, such as wheat, barley, and rye.
4. enzyme to digest fat
5. abnormal condition of lips
6. the part of the throat near the mouth
7. storage form of sugar
8. removal of part or all of the tongue
9. removal of a salivary gland
10. membrane surrounding a tooth
11. dilation of the common bile duct
12. malignant tumor of bile vessels

G

1. serum bilirubin
2. stool culture
3. barium enema
4. abdominal ultrasonography
5. stool guaiac (Hemoccult)
6. small bowel follow-through
7. percutaneous transhepatic cholangiography (PTHC)
8. nasogastric intubation
9. CT scan of the abdomen
10. endoscopic retrograde cholangiopancreatography (ERCP)
11. gastric bypass (bariatric surgery)
12. endoscopic ultrasonography (EUS)
13. liver biopsy
14. laparoscopy (form of minimally invasive surgery)
15. gastrostomy (G tube)
16. HIDA scan

H

1. total parenteral nutrition: E
2. peptic ulcer disease: D
3. esophagoduodenoscopy: J
4. inflammatory bowel disease: C
5. barium enema: F
6. bright red blood per rectum: I
7. liver function tests: A
8. gastroesophageal reflux disease: B
9. hepatitis B virus: H
10. computed tomography: G

I

1. -rrhagia, -rrhage
2. -rrhea
3. -rrhaphy
4. -ectasis, -ectasia
5. -stenosis
6. -emesis
7. -ptysis
8. -ectomy
9. -pepsia
10. -phagia
11. -sclerosis
12. -stasis
13. -plasty
14. -tresia
15. -centesis
16. -spasm
17. -stomy
18. -tomy

J

1. gastroenterologist; inflammatory bowel disease
2. pancreatitis
3. gastroesophageal reflux
4. pyloric stenosis
5. gingivitis; orthodontist
6. dysphagia
7. celiac disease; gluten
8. liver; jaundice; cirrhosis
9. hepatitis; liver biopsy; liver
10. palatoplasty

Answers to Practical Applications

Case Report: Pancreatic Cancer and Whipple Procedure

1. c
2. b
3. d
4. b

PRONUNCIATION OF TERMS

To test your understanding of the terminology in this chapter, write the meaning of each term in the space provided. In addition, you may wish to cover the terms and write them by looking at your definitions. Make sure your spelling is correct. The page number after each term indicates where it is defined in the text, so you can easily check your responses. You will find complete definitions for all of these terms and their audio pronunciations on the Evolve website.

Pronunciation Guide

ā as in āpe	ă as in ăpple
ē as in ēven	ĕ as in ĕvery
ī as in īce	ĭ as in ĭnterest
ō as in ōpen	ŏ as in pŏt
ū as in ūnit	ŭ as in ŭnder

TERM	PRONUNCIATION	MEANING
abdominal ultrasonography (196)	ăb-DŎM-ĭn-ăl ŭl-tră-sō-NŎG-ră-fē	
abdominoplasty (188)	ăb-DŎM-ĭn-ō-plăs-tē	
amylase and lipase tests (193)	ă-mĭ-LĀS and LĪ-pās tests	
aphthous stomatitis (192)	ĂF-thŭs stō-mă-TĪ-tĭs	
atresia (190)	ā-TRĒ-zē-ă	
bariatric surgery (197)	bă-rē-Ă-trĭk SŬR-gĕr-ē	
biliary atresia (190)	BĬL-ē-ăr-ē ā-TRĒ-zē-ă	
bronchospasm (189)	BRŎN-kō-spăsm	
buccal (191)	BŬK-ăl	
cecal volvulus (191)	SĒ-kăl VŎL-vū-lŭs	
celiac disease (191)	SĒ-lē-ăk dĭ-ZĒZ	
cheilosis (191)	kī-LŌ-sĭs	
cholangiectasis (188)	kō-lăn-jē-ĔK-tă-sĭs	
cholangiocarcinoma (191)	kō-lăn-jē-ō-kăr-sĭ-NŌ-mă	
cholangitis (191)	kōl-ăn-JĪ-tĭs	
cholangiography (194)	kōl-ăn-jē-ŎG-ră-fē	
cholangiopancreatography (194)	kōl-ăn-jē-ō-păn-krē-ă-TŎG-ră-fē	
cholecystectomy (191)	kō-lē-sĭs-TĔK-tō-mē	
cholecystojejunostomy (192)	kō-lē-sĭs-tō-jĕ-jŭ-NŎS-tō-mē	
cholecystolithiasis (192)	kō-lē-sĭs-tō-lĭ-THĪ-ă-sĭs	
choledochal (191)	kō-lē-DŌK-ăl	
choledochectasia (191)	kō-lē-dō-kĕk-TĀ-zē-ă	

TERM	PRONUNCIATION	MEANING
cholelithiasis (191)	kō-lē-lĭ-THĪ-ă-sĭs	______
cholestasis (189)	kō-lē-STĀ-sĭs	______
colectomy (191)	kō-LĔK-tō-mē	______
colonoscopy (191)	kō-lŏn-ŎS-kō-pē	______
computed tomography (195)	kŏm-PŪ-tĕd tō-MŎG-ră-FĒ	______
dentalgia (191)	dĕn-TĂL-jă	______
diarrhea (189)	dī-ă-RĒ-ă	______
duodenal (191)	dōō-ō-DĒ-năl	______
dyspepsia (188)	dĭs-PĔP-sē-ă	______
dysphagia (188)	dĭs-FĀ-jē-ă	______
endoscopic ultrasonography (196)	ĕn-dō-SKŎP-ĭk ŭl-tră-sō-NŎG-ră-fē	______
esophageal atresia (190)	ĕ-sŏf-ă-JĒ-ăl ā-TRĒ-zē-ă	______
gastric bypass (197)	GĂS-trĭk BĪ-păs	______
gastroenteritis (191)	găs-trō-ĕn-tĕ-RĪ-tĭs	______
gastrointestinal endoscopy (197)	găs-trō-ĭn-TĔS-tĭn-ăl ĕn-DŎS-kō-pē	______
gastrojejunostomy (191)	găs-trō-jĕ-jōō-NŎS-tō-mē	______
gastrorrhagia (189)	găs-trō-RĂ-jă	______
gastrostomy (191)	găs-TRŎS-tō-mē	______
gingivectomy (192)	gĭn-gĭ-VĔK-tō-mē	______
glossectomy (192)	glŏs-ĔK-tō-mē	______
gluconeogenesis (192)	glū-kō-nē-ō-JĔN-ĕ-sĭs	______
glycogen (192)	GLĪ-kō-jĕn	______
hematemesis (188)	hē-mă-TĔM-ĕ-sĭs	______
hemoptysis (189)	hē-MŎP-tĭ-sĭs	______
hemorrhage (189)	HĔM-ŏr-ĭj	______
hepatomegaly (192)	hĕp-ă-tō-MĔG-ă-lē	______
herniorrhaphy (189)	hĕr-nē-ŎR-ă-fē	______
HIDA scan (197)	HĬ-dă scăn	______
ileostomy (192)	ĭl-ē-ŎS-tō-mē	______

6

TERM	PRONUNCIATION	MEANING
labiodental (192)	lā-bē-ō-DĔN-tăl	
laparoscopy (197)	lă-păr-ŎS-kō-pē	
lipase (192)	LĪ-pās	
liver biopsy (197)	LĬ-vĕr BĪ-ŏp-sē	
liver function tests (193)	LĬ-vĕr FŬNG-shŭn tests	
lower gastrointestinal series (194)	LŎW-ĕr găs-trō-ĭn-TĔS-tĭ-năl SĒR-ēz	
magnetic resonance imaging (196)	măg-NĔT-ĭk RĔ-zō-năns ĬM-ă-gĭng	
nasogastric intubation (197)	nā-zō-GĂS-trĭk ĭn-tōō-BĀ-shŭn	
oropharynx (192)	ŏr-ō-FĂR-ĭnks	
palatoplasty (192)	PĂL-ă-tō-plăs-tē	
pancreatic (192)	păn-krē-ĂH-tĭk	
pancreatoduodenectomy (192)	păn-krē-ăh-tō-dōō-ō-dĕ-NĔK-tō-mē	
paracentesis (197)	păr-ă-sĕn-TĒ-sĭs	
periodontal membrane (192)	pĕr-ē-ō-DŎN-tăl MĔM-brān	
polyphagia (188)	pŏl-ē-FĀ-jē-ă	
proctosigmoidoscopy (192)	prŏk-tō-sĭg-moyd-ŎS-kō-pē	
pyloric stenosis (189)	pī-LŎR-ĭk stĕ-NŌ-sĭs	
pylorospasm (189)	pī-LŎR-ō-spăzm	
rectal carcinoma (192)	RĔK-tăl kăr-sĭ-NŌ-mă	
sialadenectomy (192)	sī-ăl-ă-dĕ-NĔK-tō-mē	
splenic flexure (192)	SPLĔN-ĭk FLĔK-shŭr	
steatorrhea (192)	stē-ă-tō-RĒ-ă	
stool culture (193)	stool KŬL-chŭr	
stool guaiac (193)	stool GWĪ-ăk	
sublingual (192)	sŭb-LĬNG-wăl	
upper gastrointestinal series (194)	ŬP-ĕr găs-trō-ĭn-TĔS-tĭ-năl SĔR-ēz	

REVIEW SHEET

Write meanings for combining forms and suffixes in the spaces provided. Check your -answers with information in Chapters 5 and 6 or in the Glossary (Medical Word Parts—English) at the end of this book.

Combining Forms

COMBINING FORM	MEANING	COMBINING FORM	MEANING
abdomin/o	________	gastr/o	________
amyl/o	________	gingiv/o	________
an/o	________	gloss/o	________
append/o, appendic/o	________	gluc/o, glyc/o	________
bil/i	________	glycogen/o	________
bilirubin/o	________	hem/o, hemat/o	________
bucc/o	________	hepat/o	________
cec/o	________	herni/o	________
celi/o	________	idi/o	________
cervic/o	________	ile/o	________
cheil/o	________	pancreat/o	________
chlorhydr/o	________	peritone/o	________
chol/e	________	pharyng/o	________
cholangi/o	________	proct/o	________
cholecyst/o	________	prote/o	________
choledoch/o	________	py/o	________
cib/o	________	pylor/o	________
cirrh/o	________	rect/o	________
col/o, colon/o	________	sialaden/o	________
dent/i	________	splen/o	________
duoden/o	________	steat/o	________
enter/o	________	stomat/o	________
esophag/o	________	tonsill/o	________
eti/o	________		

6

Suffixes

SUFFIX	MEANING	SUFFIX	MEANING
-ase	______________	-orexia	______________
-centesis	______________	-rrhage	______________
-chezia	______________	-rrhagia	______________
-ectasia	______________	-rrhaphy	______________
-ectasis	______________	-rrhea	______________
-ectomy	______________	-scopy	______________
-emesis	______________	-spasm	______________
-emia	______________	-stasis	______________
-genesis	______________	-stenosis	______________
-graphy	______________	-stomy	______________
-iasis	______________	-tomy	______________
-megaly	______________	-tresia	______________

6

evolve *Please visit the Evolve website for additional exercises, games, and images related to this chapter.*

CHAPTER 7

Urinary System

This chapter is divided into the following sections:

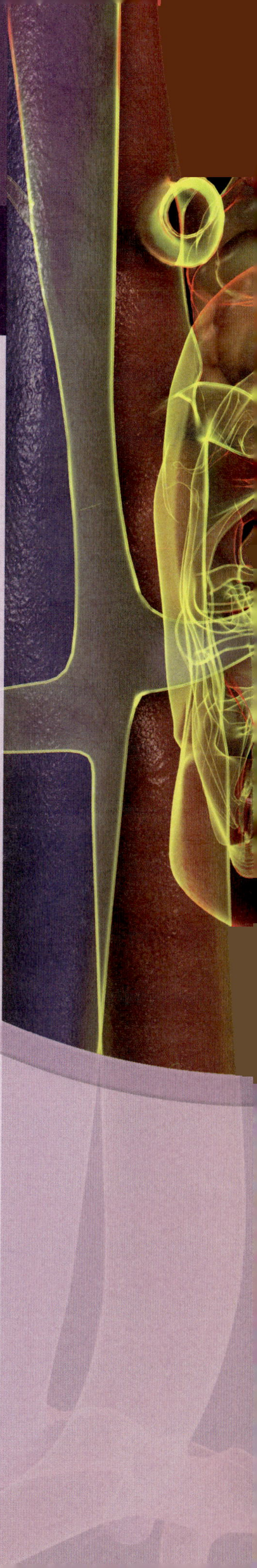

CHAPTER GOALS

- Name essential organs of the urinary system and describe their locations and functions.
- Identify common pathologic conditions affecting the urinary system.
- Recognize how urinalysis is used and interpreted as a diagnostic test.
- Define urinary system–related combining forms, prefixes, and suffixes.
- List and explain laboratory tests, clinical procedures, and abbreviations that pertain to the urinary system.
- Understand medical terms in their proper contexts, such as medical reports and records.

INTRODUCTION

When foods containing proteins are used by cells in the body, nitrogenous waste products **(urea, creatinine,** and **uric acid)** are released into the bloodstream. The urinary system removes these nitrogenous wastes from the blood so that they do not accumulate and become harmful. As blood passes through the kidneys, the kidneys filter nitrogenous wastes to form **urine** (composed of water, salts, and acids). Urine leaves the body through the ureters, urinary bladder, and urethra. Every day, the kidneys process about 200 quarts of blood to filter out 2 quarts of urine.

Besides removing urea and other nitrogenous wastes from the blood, the kidneys maintain the proper balance of water, electrolytes, and acids in body fluids. **Electrolytes** such as **sodium (Na^+)** and **potassium (K^+)** are small molecules that conduct an electrical charge. Electrolytes are necessary for proper functioning of muscle and nerve cells. The kidney adjusts the amounts of water and electrolytes by secreting some substances into the urine and holding back others in the bloodstream for use in the body.

In addition to forming and excreting (eliminating) urine from the body, the kidneys secrete hormones such as **renin** (RĒ-nĭn) and **erythropoietin** (ĕ-rĭth-rō-PŌY-ĕ-tĭn). **Renin** raises blood pressure (to keep blood moving through the kidney). **Erythropoietin (EPO)** is a hormone that stimulates red blood cell production in the bone marrow.

The kidneys also secrete **calciferol**, an active form of vitamin D, necessary for the absorption of calcium from the intestine. In addition, the kidneys degrade and eliminate hormones such as insulin and parathyroid hormone from the bloodstream. Box 7-1 reviews the functions of the kidneys.

ANATOMY OF THE MAJOR ORGANS

The following paragraphs describe the organs of the urinary system. Label Figure 7-1 as you identify each organ.

The **kidney** [1] is one of two bean-shaped organs behind the abdominal cavity (retroperitoneal) on either side of the spine in the lumbar region. A cushion of adipose (fatty) tissue and fibrous connective tissue surrounds each kidney for protection. Each kidney (about the size of a fist) weighs about 4 to 6 ounces.

The kidneys consist of an outer **cortex** region (cortex means bark, as the bark of a tree) and an inner **medulla** region (medulla means marrow). The **hilum** is a depression on the medial border of the kidney. Blood vessels and nerves pass through the hilum.

The **ureter** [2] is one of two muscular tubes (16 to 18 inches long) lined with mucous membrane. Ureters carry urine in peristaltic waves from the kidneys to the urinary bladder.

The **urinary bladder** [3], a hollow, muscular sac, is a temporary reservoir for urine. The **trigone** is a triangular region at the base of the bladder where the ureters enter and the urethra exits.

BOX 7-1 FUNCTIONS OF THE KIDNEYS

- **Remove nitrogenous wastes**: urea, creatinine, uric acid
- **Balance water and electrolytes** (sodium, potassium)
- **Release hormones**: renin, erythropoietin, calciferol
- **Degrade and eliminate hormones** from bloodstream

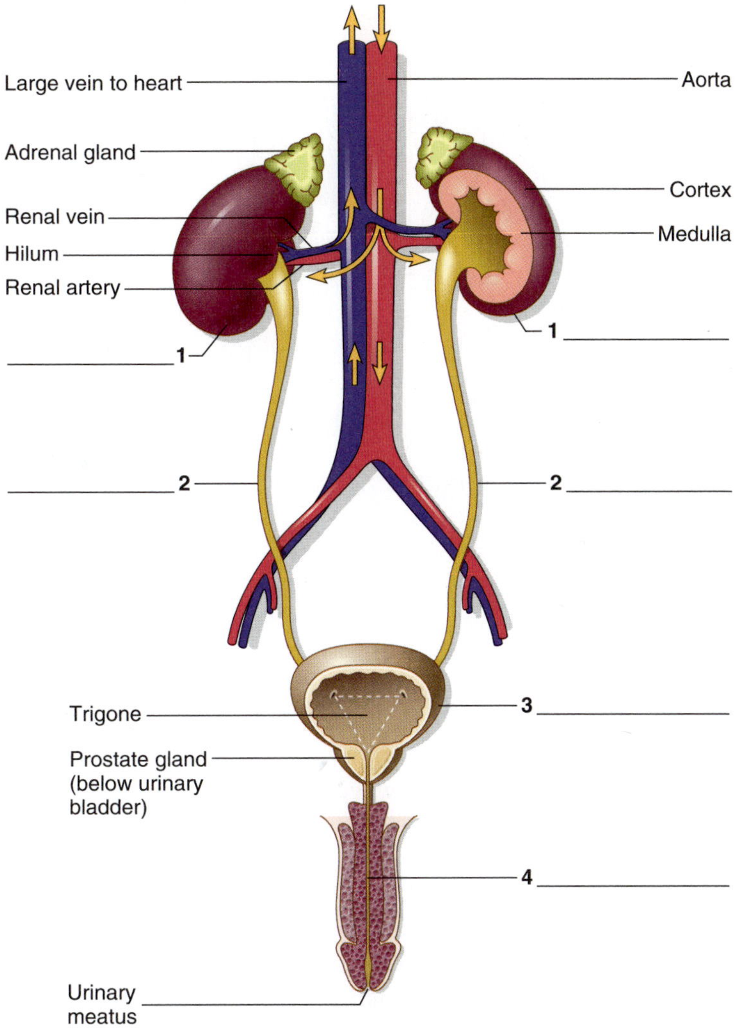

FIGURE 7-1 Male urinary system.

The **urethra** [4] is a tube that carries urine from the urinary bladder to the outside of the body. The process of expelling urine through the urethra is called **urination** or **voiding.** The external opening of the urethra is the **urinary meatus.** The female urethra, about 1½ inches long, lies anterior to the vagina and vaginal meatus. The male urethra, about 8 inches long, extends downward through the prostate gland to the urinary meatus at the tip of the penis. Figure 7-2 illustrates the female urinary system. Compare it with Figure 7-1, which shows the male urinary system.

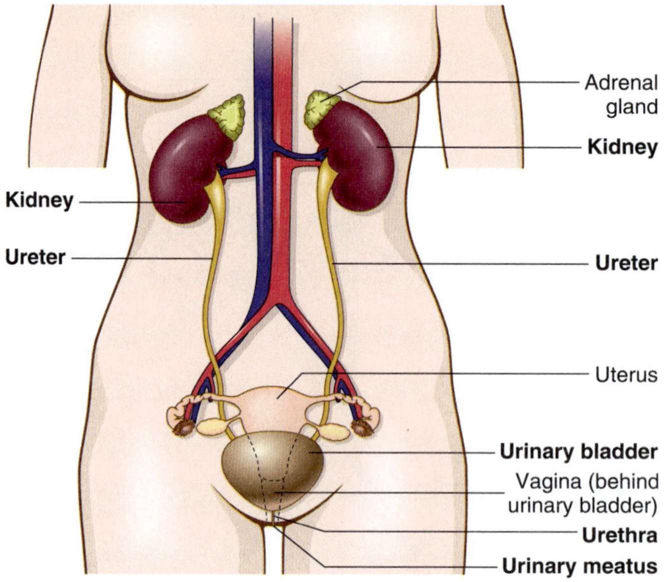

FIGURE 7-2 **Female urinary system.**

PHYSIOLOGY: HOW THE KIDNEYS PRODUCE URINE

Blood enters each kidney from the aorta by way of the right and left **renal arteries.** After the renal artery enters the kidney (at the hilum), it branches into smaller and smaller arteries. The smallest arteries are called **arterioles** (Figure 7-3A).

Because the arterioles are small, blood passes through them slowly but constantly. Blood flow through the kidney is so essential that the kidneys have their own special device for maintaining blood flow. If blood pressure falls in the vessels of the kidney, so that blood flow diminishes, the kidney produces **renin** and discharges it into the blood. Renin promotes the formation of a substance that stimulates the contraction of arterioles. This increases blood pressure and restores blood flow in the kidneys to normal.

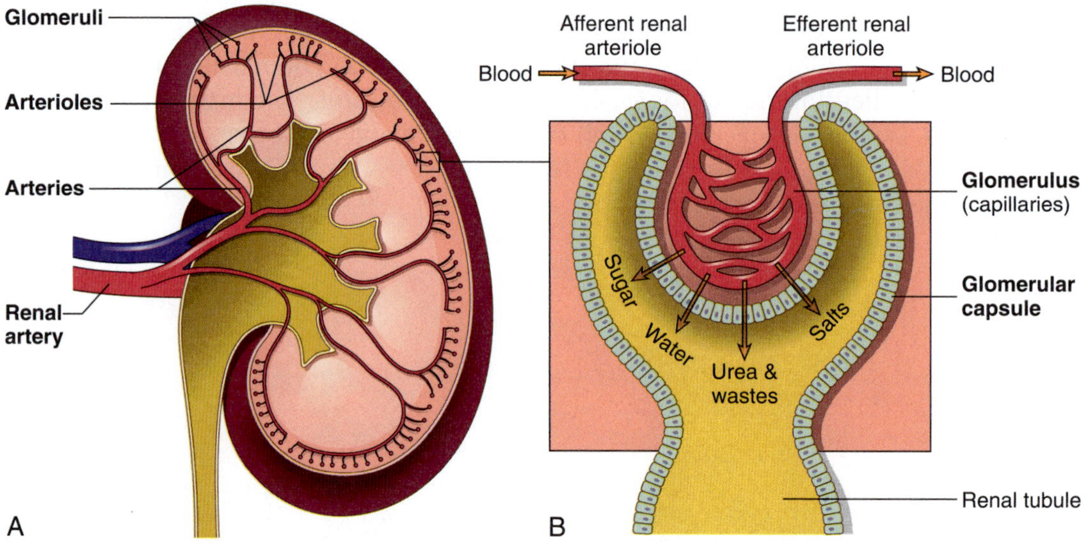

FIGURE 7-3 **A, Renal artery** branching to form smaller arteries and arterioles, and glomeruli. **B, Glomerulus** and **glomerular capsule.** Afferent arteriole carries blood toward (in this term, af- is a form of ad-) the glomerulus. Efferent arteriole carries blood away (ef- is a form of ex-) from the glomerulus.

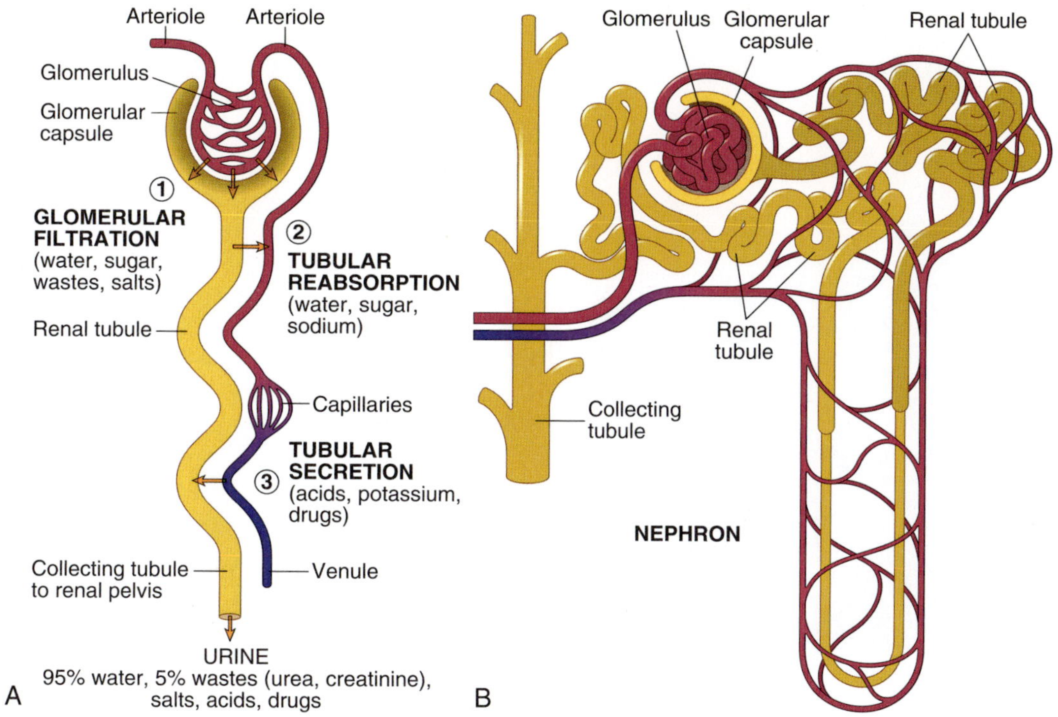

FIGURE 7-4 **A, Three steps in the formation of urine: (1) Glomerular filtration** of water, sugar, wastes (urea and creatinine), and sodium. **(2) Tubular reabsorption** of water, sugar, and sodium. **(3) Tubular secretion** of acids, potassium, and drugs. **B, Nephron.**

Each arteriole in the cortex of the kidney leads into a mass of very tiny, coiled, and intertwined smaller blood vessels called **glomeruli** (see Figure 7-3A). Each **glomerulus** (singular) is a collection of tiny capillaries formed in the shape of a small ball. There are about 1 million glomeruli in the cortex region of each kidney.

The kidneys produce urine by **filtration.** As blood passes through the many glomeruli, the thin walls of each glomerulus (the filter) permit water, salts, sugar, and **urea** (with other nitrogenous wastes such as **creatinine** and **uric acid**) to leave the bloodstream. These materials collect in a tiny, cup-like structure, a **glomerular (Bowman) capsule,** that surrounds each glomerulus (Figure 7-3B). The walls of the glomeruli prevent large substances, such as proteins and blood cells, from filtering into the capsule. These substances remain in the blood and normally do not appear in urine.

Attached to each glomerular capsule is a long, twisted tube called a **renal tubule** (see Figures 7-3B and 7-4). As water, sugar, salts, urea, and other wastes pass through the renal tubule, most of the water, all of the sugar, and almost all of the sodium return to the bloodstream through tiny capillaries surrounding each tubule. This active process of **reabsorption** ensures that the body retains essential substances such as sugar (glucose), water, and sodium. The final process in the formation of urine is **secretion** of some substances from the bloodstream into the renal tubule. These waste products of metabolism become toxic if allowed to accumulate in the body. Thus, acids, drugs (such as penicillin), and potassium (as a salt) leave the body in urine.

Only wastes, water, salts, acids, and some drugs (often as metabolites—partially broken-down forms of the original drug) remain in the renal tubule. Each renal tubule, now containing urine (95% water and 5% urea, creatinine, salts, acids, and drugs), ends in a larger collecting tubule. See Figure 7-4A, which reviews the steps involved in urine formation. The combination of a glomerulus and a renal tubule forms a unit called a **nephron** (Figure 7-4B). Each kidney contains about 1 million nephrons.

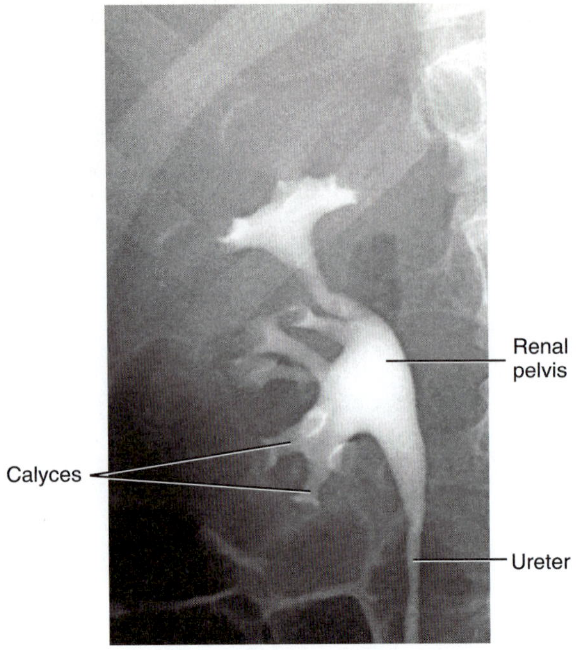

FIGURE 7-5 Renal pelvis, calyces, and ureter as seen on CT urogram (intravenous dye was used).

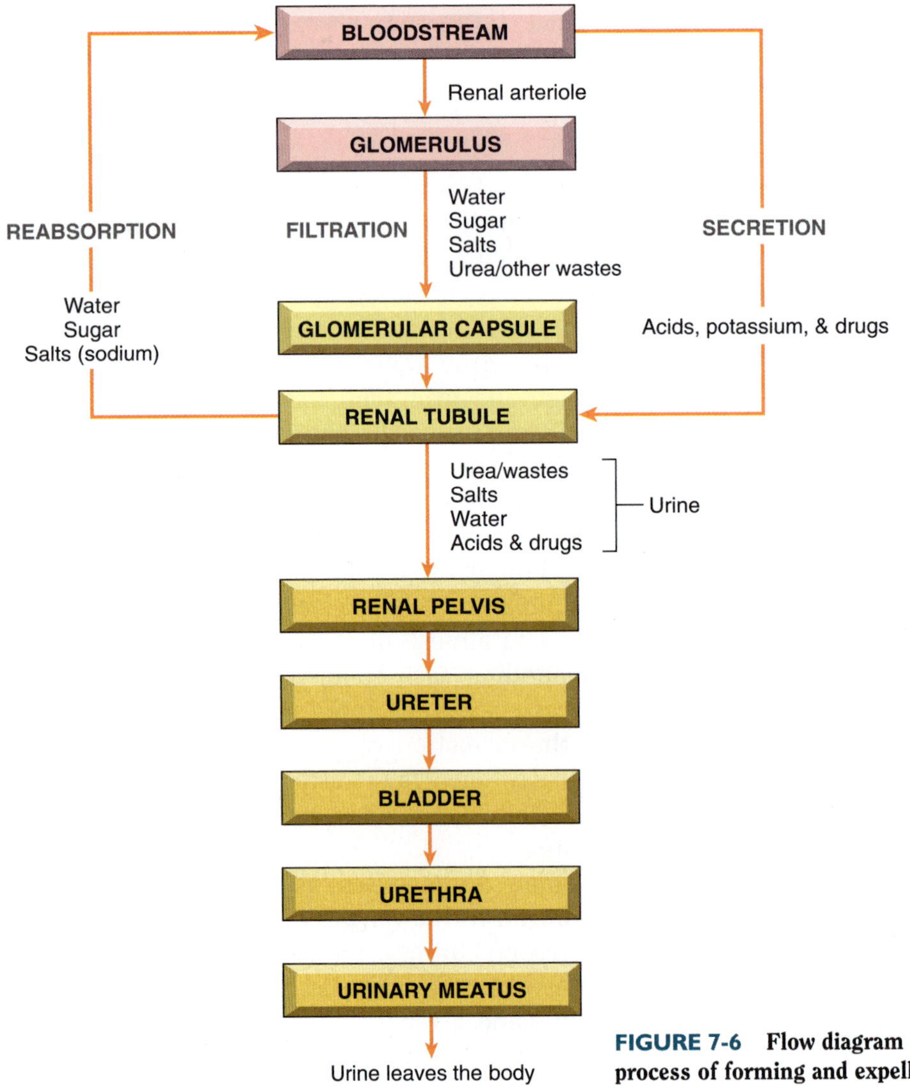

FIGURE 7-6 Flow diagram illustrating the process of forming and expelling urine.

All collecting tubules lead to the **renal pelvis,** a basin-like area in the central part of the kidney. Small, cup-like regions of the renal pelvis are called **calyces** or **calices** (singular: **calyx** or **calix**). Figure 7-5 is an x-ray image of a kidney showing the renal pelvis, calyces, and ureter.

The renal pelvis narrows into the **ureter,** which carries the urine to the **urinary bladder.** The bladder, a muscular sac, temporarily stores urine. Sphincter muscles control the exit area of the bladder to the **urethra.** As the bladder fills and pressure increases at the base of the bladder, an individual notices a need to urinate and voluntarily relaxes sphincter muscles.

Study the flow diagram in Figure 7-6 to trace the process of forming urine and expelling it from the body.

VOCABULARY

arteriole	Small artery.
calciferol	Active form of Vitamin D, secreted by the kidney.
calyx *or* **calix** (*plural:* **calyces** or **calices**)	Cup-like collecting region of the renal pelvis. The term comes from Greek, *kalux* meaning a cup or case surrounding a flower bud.
catheter	Tube for injecting or removing fluids.
cortex	Outer region of an organ; the renal cortex is the outer region of the kidney (**cortical** means pertaining to the cortex).
creatinine	Nitrogenous waste excreted in urine. **Creatinine clearance** is a measure of the efficiency of the kidneys in removing (clearing) creatinine from the blood.
electrolyte	Chemical element that carries an electrical charge when dissolved in water. Electrolytes are necessary for functioning of muscles and nerves. The kidneys maintain the proper balance of electrolytes and water in the blood. Potassium (K^+) and sodium (Na^+) are electrolytes.
erythropoietin (EPO)	Hormone secreted by the kidney to stimulate the production of red blood cells by bone marrow. –Poietin means a substance that forms.
filtration	Process whereby some substances, but not all, pass through a filter.
glomerular capsule	Enclosing structure surrounding each glomerulus. The glomerular capsule is also known as Bowman's capsule and it collects the material that is filtered from the blood through the walls of the glomerulus.
glomerulus (*plural:* **glomeruli**)	Tiny ball of capillaries (microscopic blood vessels) in the kidney.
hilum	Depression in an organ where blood vessels and nerves enter and leave. Hilum comes from the Latin meaning a small thing. It is also used in the respiratory system to mark the depression in the lung where blood vessels, bronchus, and lymphatic vessels enter and leave.

Filtration of blood through the kidney.

This process is maintained by output from the heart (25% of cardiac output goes to the kidneys) and adequate blood pressure to force blood through the glomerulus (filter). About 200 quarts (189L) of fluid are filtered daily but 98% to 99% of water and salts are returned to the blood. Only about 2 quarts (1500 mL) of urine are excreted daily.

kidney	One of two bean-shaped organs on either side of the backbone in the lumbar region; it filters nitrogenous wastes from the bloodstream to form urine.
meatus	Opening or canal.
medulla	Inner region of an organ. The renal medulla is the inner region of the kidney. The term comes from the Latin *medulla,* meaning marrow (inner part). The **medullary cavity** in long bones is the innermost part containing red and yellow marrow.
nephron	Combination of glomerulus and renal tubule where filtration, reabsorption, and secretion take place in the kidney. It is the functional unit of the kidney, each capable of forming urine by itself. There are about 1 million nephrons in a kidney.
nitrogenous waste	Substance containing nitrogen and excreted in urine. Examples of nitrogenous wastes are urea, uric acid, and creatinine.
potassium (K^+)	Electrolyte regulated by the kidney so that a proper concentration is maintained within the blood. Potassium is essential for allowing muscle contraction and conduction of nervous impulses.
reabsorption	Process whereby renal tubules return materials necessary to the body back into the bloodstream.
renal artery	Blood vessel that carries blood to the kidney.
renal pelvis	Central collecting region in the kidney.
renal tubule	Microscopic tube in the kidney where urine is formed after filtration.
renal vein	Blood vessel that carries blood away from the kidney and toward the heart.
renin	Hormone secreted by the kidney; it raises blood pressure by influencing vasoconstriction (narrowing of blood vessels).
sodium (Na^+)	Electrolyte regulated in the blood and urine by the kidneys; needed for proper transmission of nerve impulses, heart activity, and other metabolic functions. A common form of sodium is sodium chloride (table salt).
trigone	Triangular area in the urinary bladder.
urea	Major nitrogenous waste excreted in urine.
ureter	One of the two tubes leading from the kidneys to the urinary bladder.
urethra	Tube leading from the urinary bladder to the outside of the body.
uric acid	Nitrogenous waste excreted in the urine.
urinary bladder	Hollow, muscular sac that holds and stores urine.
urination (voiding)	Process of expelling urine; also called micturition.

TERMINOLOGY: STRUCTURES, SUBSTANCES, AND URINARY SIGNS AND SYMPTOMS

Write the meanings of the medical terms in the spaces provided.

STRUCTURES

COMBINING FORM	MEANING	TERMINOLOGY	MEANING
cali/o, calic/o	calyx (calix); cup-shaped	caliectasis	______
		caliceal	______
cyst/o	urinary bladder	cystitis *Bacterial infections often cause acute or chronic cystitis. In acute cystitis, the bladder contains blood as a result of mucosal hemorrhage (Figure 7-7).*	______
		cystectomy	______
		cystostomy *An opening is made into the urinary bladder from the outside of the body. A catheter is placed into the bladder for drainage.*	______
glomerul/o	glomerulus	glomerular capsule	______
meat/o	meatus	meatal stenosis	______

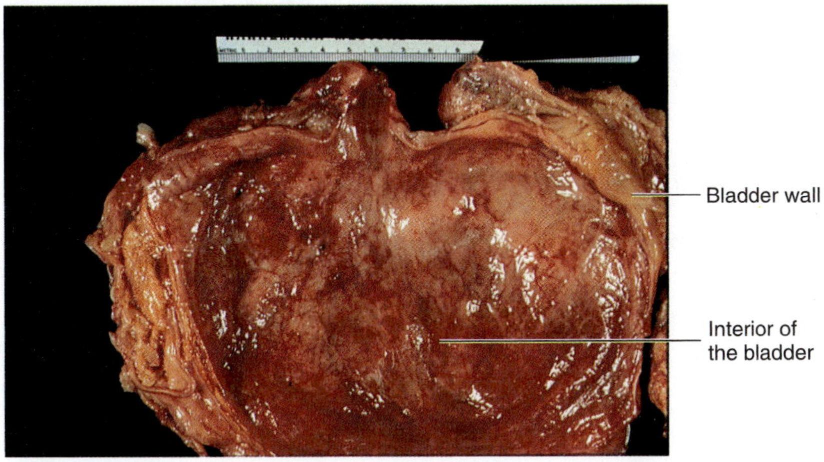

FIGURE 7-7 Acute cystitis. Notice that the mucosa of the bladder is red and swollen. Bladder and urinary tract infections are more common in women because of the shorter urethra, which allows easier bacterial colonization of the urinary bladder. They usually occur without a known cause but may be acquired during sexual intercourse ("honeymoon cystitis") or after surgical procedures and urinary catheterization.

COMBINING FORM	MEANING	TERMINOLOGY	MEANING
nephr/o	kidney	paranephric	_______________
		nephropathy *(nĕ-FRŎ-pă-thē)*	_______________
		nephroptosis *Downward displacement or dropping of a kidney when its anatomic supports are weakened.* ***Nephropexy*** *(-pexy means fixation) is an operation to put a "floating" kidney in place.*	_______________
		nephrolithotomy *Incision (percutaneous) into the kidney to remove a stone.*	_______________
		hydronephrosis *Obstruction of urine flow may be caused by renal calculi (Figure 7-8), compression of the ureter by tumor, or hyperplasia of the prostate gland at the base of the bladder in males.*	_______________
		nephrostomy *Surgical opening to the outside of the body (from the renal pelvis). This is necessary when a ureter becomes obstructed and the obstruction cannot be removed easily. The renal pelvis becomes distended with urine (hydronephrosis), making nephrostomy necessary.*	_______________

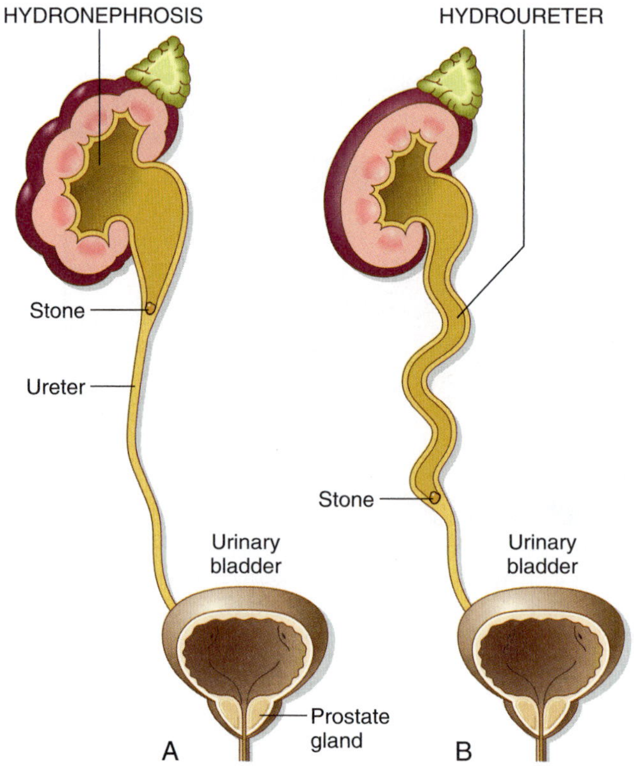

FIGURE 7-8 **A, Hydronephrosis** caused by a stone (obstruction) in the proximal part of a ureter. Notice the buildup of excess fluid in the kidney. **B, Hydroureter** with hydronephrosis caused by a stone in the distal part of the ureter.

COMBINING FORM	MEANING	TERMINOLOGY	MEANING
pyel/o	renal pelvis	pyelolithotomy *Removal of a large calculus (stone) contributing to blockage of urine flow and development of infection. The renal pelvis is surgically opened.*	______
ren/o	kidney	renal ischemia	______
		renal colic ***Colic** is intermittent spasms of pain caused by inflammation and distention of an organ. In renal colic, pain results from calculi in the kidney or ureter.*	______
trigon/o	trigone (region of the bladder)	trigonitis	______
ureter/o	ureter	ureteroplasty	______
		ureteroileostomy *After cystectomy, the urologic surgeon forms a pouch from a segment of the ileum, used in place of the bladder to carry urine from the ureters out of the body (Figure 7-9). It is an **ileal conduit.***	______
urethr/o	urethra	urethritis	______
		urethroplasty	______
		urethral stricture *A **stricture** is an abnormal narrowing of an opening or passageway.*	______

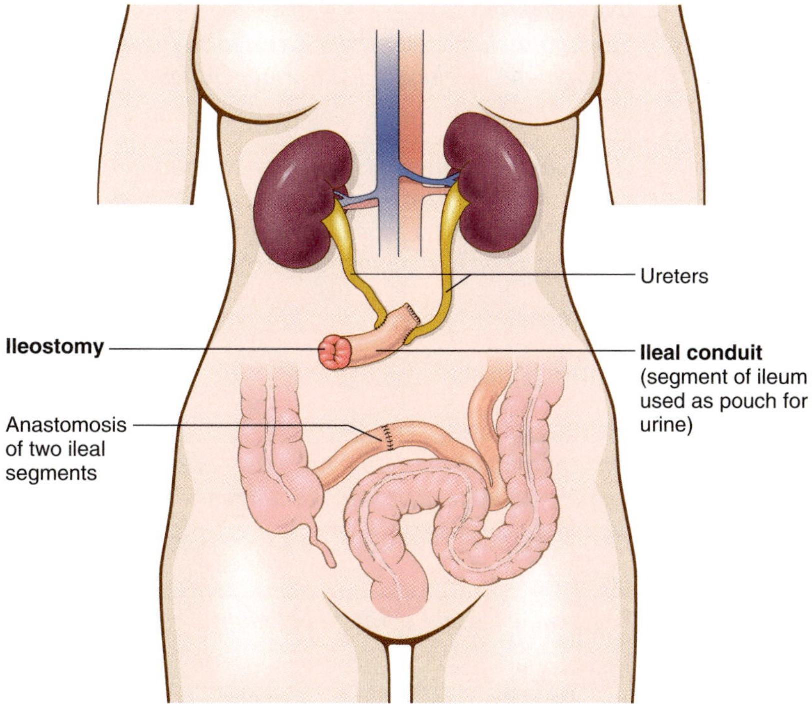

FIGURE 7-9 Ileostomy and ileal conduit after cystectomy.

COMBINING FORM	MEANING	TERMINOLOGY	MEANING
vesic/o	urinary bladder	intravesical ______ *Do not confuse the term **vesical** with the term **vesicle,** which is a small blister on the skin.*	
		vesicoureteral reflux ______	

SUBSTANCES AND URINARY SIGNS AND SYMPTOMS

COMBINING FORM OR SUFFIX	MEANING	TERMINOLOGY	MEANING
albumin/o	albumin (a protein in the blood)	albuminuria ______ *The suffix -uria means urine condition. This finding can indicate malfunction of the kidney as protein leaks out of damaged glomeruli. **Microalbuminuria** is leakage of very small amounts of albumin through the glomeruli.*	
azot/o	nitrogen	azotemia ______ *This toxic condition is characteristic of uremia. It is indicated by an elevated **BUN (blood urea nitrogen)** test.*	
bacteri/o	bacteria	bacteriuria ______ *Usually a sign of **urinary tract infection (UTI).** The bacteria in the urine are cultured (grown in a special nutrient environment) and then tested with antibiotics to determine which will inhibit growth. This is known as **culture and sensitivity testing (C&S).***	
dips/o	thirst	polydipsia ______ *Commonly, a sign of diabetes insipidus or diabetes mellitus.*	
kal/o	potassium	hyperkalemia ______ *Since potassium is normally excreted by the kidneys, it accumulates in blood when the kidneys fail.*	
ket/o, keton/o	ketone bodies (ketoacids and **acetone**)	ketosis ______ *Often called **ketoacidosis,** because acids accumulate in the blood and tissues. The breath of a patient with ketosis has a sweet or "fruity" odor. This is produced by **acetone** (a ketone body) released from the blood in the lungs and exhaled through the mouth.*	
		ketonuria ______	
lith/o	stone	nephrolithiasis ______	
natr/o	sodium	hyponatremia ______ *This condition can occur when water intake is excessive—primary polydipsia, or when athletes drink too much water in high-endurance events.*	
noct/o	night	nocturia ______ *Frequent, excessive urination at night.*	
olig/o	scanty	oliguria ______	

7

COMBINING FORM OR SUFFIX	MEANING	TERMINOLOGY	MEANING
-poietin	substance that forms	erythropoietin	____________
py/o	pus	pyuria	____________
-tripsy	crushing	lithotripsy	____________
ur/o	urine (urea)	uremia *This toxic state results when nitrogenous waste accumulates abnormally in the blood.*	____________
		enuresis *Literally, a condition of being "in urine"; bed-wetting.*	____________
		diuresis *Di- (from dia-) means complete. Caffeine and alcohol are well-known* ***diuretics****—they induce increased excretion of urine (diuresis).*	____________
		antidiuretic hormone *This hormone from the pituitary gland normally acts on the renal tubules to promote water reabsorption. It is also called* ***vasopressin*** *and is abbreviated* ***ADH****.*	____________
urin/o	urine	urinary incontinence *Incontinence literally means not (in-) able to hold (tin) together (con-). This is loss of control of the passage of urine from the bladder.* ***Stress incontinence*** *occurs with strain on the bladder opening during coughing or sneezing.* ***Urgency incontinence*** *occurs with the inability to hold back urination when feeling the urge to void.*	____________
		urinary retention *This symptom results when the outflow of urine from the bladder is blocked.*	____________
-uria	urination; urine condition	dysuria	____________
		anuria *Commonly caused by renal failure or urinary tract obstruction.*	____________
		hematuria ***Microhematuria*** *is hematuria that is visible only under a microscope, as opposed to* ***gross hematuria,*** *which can be seen with the naked eye.*	____________
		glycosuria *A sign of diabetes mellitus.*	____________
		polyuria *A symptom of both diabetes insipidus and diabetes mellitus.*	____________

Enuresis/Nocturia

Enuresis is the *involuntary* discharge of urine or bed-wetting, whereas **nocturia** is *voluntary*, frequent urination at night.

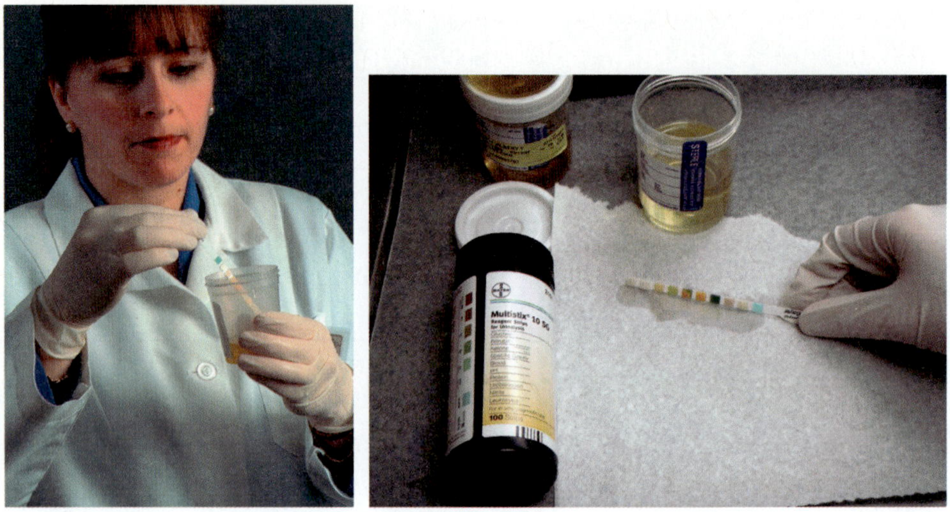

FIGURE 7-10 Dipstick testing and urinalysis.

URINALYSIS

Urinalysis is an examination of urine to determine the presence of abnormal elements that may indicate various pathologic conditions. See Figure 7-10.

The following are some of the tests included in a urinalysis:

1. **Color**—Normal urine color is yellow (amber) or straw-colored. A colorless, pale urine indicates a large amount of water in the urine, whereas a smoky-red or brown color of urine indicates the presence of large amounts of blood. Foods such as beets and certain drugs also can produce a red coloration of urine.
2. **Appearance**—Normally, urine should be clear. Cloudy or **turbid** urine indicates a urinary tract infection with **pus (pyuria)** and **bacteria (bacteriuria).**
3. **pH**—Determination of pH reveals the chemical nature of urine. It indicates to what degree a solution is **acid** or **alkaline (basic)** (Figure 7-11). Normal urine is slightly acidic pH of 6.5. However, in some infections of the bladder, the urine pH may be alkaline, owing to the actions of bacteria in the urine that break down urea and release ammonia (an alkaline substance).
4. **Protein**—Small amounts of protein are normally found in the urine but not in sufficient quantity to produce a positive result by ordinary methods of testing. When urinary tests for protein become positive, **albumin** is usually responsible. Albumin is the major protein in blood plasma. If it is detected in urine **(albuminuria),** it may indicate a leak in the glomerular membrane, which allows albumin to enter the renal tubule and pass into the urine.

   Through more sensitive testing, smaller abnormal amounts of albumin may be detected **(microalbuminuria)** when ordinary tests are negative. Microalbuminuria is recognized as the earliest sign of renal involvement in diabetes mellitus.

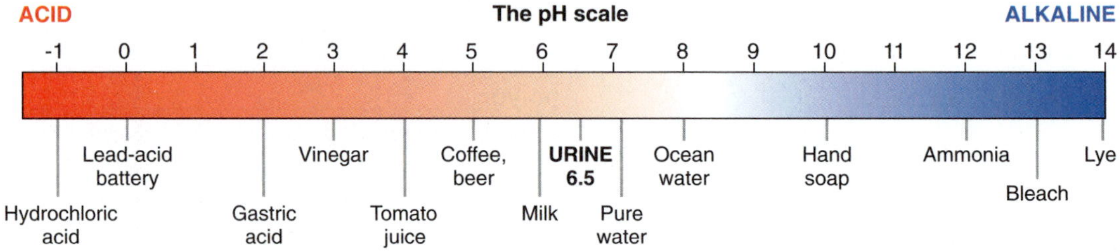

FIGURE 7-11 The pH scale. Pure water has a neutral pH.

5. **Glucose**—Sugar is not normally found in the urine. In most cases, when it does appear **(glycosuria),** it indicates **diabetes mellitus.** In diabetes mellitus, there is excess sugar in the bloodstream (hyperglycemia), which leads to the "spilling over" of sugar into the urine. The renal tubules cannot reabsorb all the sugar that filters out through the glomerular membrane.
6. **Specific gravity**—The specific gravity of urine reflects the amounts of wastes, minerals, and solids in the urine. It is a comparison of the density of urine with that of water. The urine of patients with diabetes mellitus has a higher-than-normal specific gravity because of the presence of sugar.
7. **Ketone bodies**—Ketones (or **acetones,** a type of ketone body) are formed when fatty acids are broken down in the liver. Ketones accumulate in blood and urine when the body breaks down fat, instead of sugar, for fuel. **Ketonuria** occurs in diabetes mellitus when cells deprived of sugar must use up their available fat for energy. In starvation, when sugar is not available, ketonuria and ketosis (ketones in the blood) occur as fat is catabolized abnormally.

   Ketones in the blood are dangerous because they increase the acidity of the blood **(ketoacidosis).** This can lead to coma (unconsciousness) and death.
8. **Sediment and casts**—The presence of abnormal particles in the urine is a sign of a pathologic condition. Such particles, which may settle to the bottom of a urine sample as sediment, may include cells (epithelial cells, white blood cells, or red blood cells), bacteria, crystals, and casts (cylindrical structures of protein often containing cellular elements).
9. **Phenylketonuria (PKU)**—This is a rare condition in which a baby is born unable to break down an amino acid, phenylalanine. Resulting high levels of phenylalanine (phenylketones are detected in urine) can lead to mental retardation. While the PKU test was originally performed on urine samples, now it is done via blood sample by pricking the newborn's heel. If phenylalanine is detected, the infant is fed a low-protein diet excluding phenylalanine. Affected children remain on this diet until adulthood.
10. **Bilirubin**—This pigment substance, which results from hemoglobin breakdown, may be present in the urine (bilirubinuria) of patients with liver disease. Urobilinogen, a breakdown product of bilirubin, may also be found in the urine.

PATHOLOGIC TERMINOLOGY: KIDNEY, BLADDER, AND ASSOCIATED CONDITIONS

KIDNEY

glomerulonephritis

Inflammation of the glomeruli within the kidney.

This condition can follow a streptococcal infection. It results in leaky glomeruli, hematuria, red blood cell casts, albuminuria, renal failure, and uremia. Drugs may be useful to control inflammation, and dialysis or renal transplantation may be necessary if uremia occurs.

interstitial nephritis

Inflammation of the connective tissue that lies between the renal tubules.

The connective tissue lying between the renal tubules is called the renal interstitium. Acute interstitial nephritis, an increasingly common disorder, may develop after use of NSAIDS (nonsteroidal anti-inflammatory drugs, such as ibuprofen) and other drugs. It may be marked by fever, skin rash, and eosinophils in the blood and urine.

nephrolithiasis

Kidney stones (renal calculi).

Kidney stones usually are composed of uric acid or calcium salts. Stones often lodge in the ureter or bladder, as well as in the renal pelvis, and may require removal by **lithotripsy** (see page 234) or surgery.

nephrotic syndrome (nephrosis)

Group of clinical signs and symptoms caused by excessive protein loss in urine.

Nephrotic syndrome may follow glomerulonephritis or exposure to toxins or certain drugs, immune diseases, and other pathologic conditions, such as diabetes mellitus and cancer. Two important signs of nephrotic syndrome are **edema** (swelling caused by fluid in tissue spaces) and **hypoalbuminemia.** Both of these signs are caused by massive leakage of protein into urine.

polycystic kidney disease (PKD)

Multiple fluid-filled sacs (cysts) within and on the kidney.

There are two types of hereditary PKD. One type is usually **asymptomatic** (without symptoms) until middle age and then is marked by hematuria, urinary tract infections, nephrolithiasis, and renal failure. The other type of PKD occurs in infants or children and results in renal failure. Figure 7-12A shows polycystic kidney disease.

pyelonephritis

Inflammation of the lining of the renal pelvis and renal parenchyma.

The **parenchyma** of an organ is its essential and distinctive tissue. Nephrons are the renal parenchyma. Bacterial infection in the urinary tract causes collections of pus to form in the kidney, often associated with bacteria spilling into the bloodstream. Urinalysis reveals pyuria. Treatment consists of antibiotics and surgical correction of any obstruction to urine flow.

7

renal cell carcinoma (hypernephroma)

Cancerous tumor of the kidney in adulthood.

This tumor (see Figure 7-12B) accounts for 2% of all cancers in adults. Hematuria is the primary abnormal finding, and the tumor often metastasizes to bones and lungs. Nephrectomy or partial nephrectomy is the primary treatment.

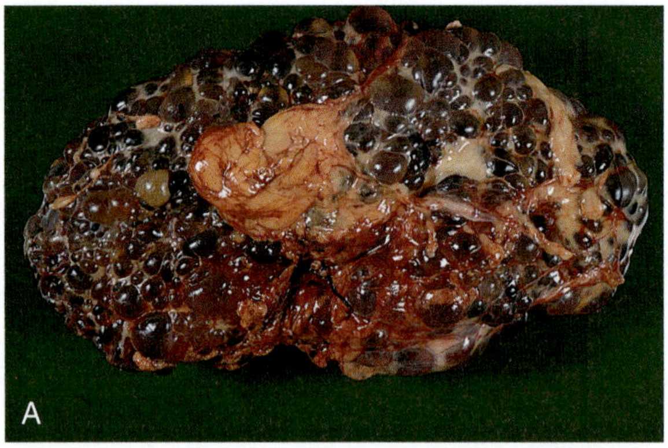

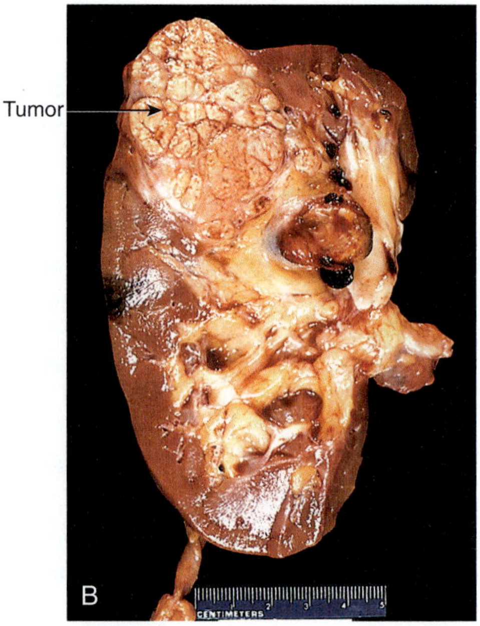

FIGURE 7-12 **A, Polycystic kidney disease.** The kidneys contain masses of cysts. Typically, polycystic kidneys weigh 20 times more than their usual weight (150 to 200 grams). **B, Renal cell carcinoma.**

renal failure

Decrease in excretion of wastes results from impaired filtration function.

A large number of conditions, including high blood pressure, infection, and diabetes, can lead to renal failure, which may be acute (ARF) or chronic (CRF), reversible or progressive, mild or severe. A newer classification of **chronic kidney disease (CKD)** stages patients according to the level of creatinine clearance and glomerular filtration rate (GFR), ranging from normal (stage 1) to end-stage renal failure (stage 5). See page 237 under CKD stages.

renal hypertension

High blood pressure resulting from kidney disease.

Renal hypertension is the most common type of **secondary hypertension** (high blood pressure caused by an abnormal condition such as glomerulonephritis). If the cause of high blood pressure is not known, the condition is called **essential hypertension**. Chronic **essential hypertension** causes arterial and arteriolar damage, potentially resulting in stroke, myocardial infarction (heart attack), heart failure, or renal failure.

Wilms tumor

Malignant tumor of the kidney occurring in childhood.

This tumor may be treated with surgery, radiation therapy, and chemotherapy.

URINARY BLADDER

bladder cancer

Malignant tumor of the urinary bladder.

Bladder cancer occurs more frequently in men (often smokers) and in persons older than 50 years of age, especially industrial workers exposed to dyes and leather tanning agents. Signs and symptoms include gross (visible to the naked eye) or microscopic hematuria and dysuria. Cystoscopy with biopsy is the most common diagnostic procedure. Staging of the tumor is based on the depth to which the tumor invades the bladder wall and presence of metastasis. Superficial tumors are removed by electrocauterization (burning). Cystectomy, chemotherapy, and radiation therapy are treatments for disease that has spread deeply into the bladder wall, to regional lymph nodes, or to distant organs.

ASSOCIATED CONDITIONS

diabetes insipidus (DI)

Antidiuretic hormone (ADH) is not secreted, or there is a resistance of the kidney to ADH.

In DI, the kidney produces large amounts of dilute urine (polyuria). Lack of ADH prevents water from being reabsorbed into the blood through the renal tubules. Insipidus means tasteless, reflecting very dilute and watery urine, not sweet as in diabetes mellitus. The term **diabetes** comes from the Greek *diabainein*, meaning to pass through. Both types of diabetes (insipidus and mellitus) are marked by polyuria and polydipsia.

diabetes mellitus (DM)

Insulin is not secreted adequately or tissues are resistant to its effects.

The major signs and symptoms of diabetes mellitus are glycosuria, hyperglycemia, polyuria, and polydipsia. Without insulin, sugar cannot leave the bloodstream and is not available to body cells for energy. Sugar remains in the blood (hyperglycemia) and spills over into the urine (glycosuria). Mellitus means sweet, reflecting the content of the urine. The term diabetes, when used alone, refers to diabetes mellitus. See Chapter 18 for more information about diabetes mellitus.

LABORATORY TESTS AND CLINICAL PROCEDURES

LABORATORY TESTS

blood urea nitrogen (BUN)

Measurement of urea levels in blood.

Normally, the blood urea level is low because urea is excreted in the urine continuously. However, when the kidney is diseased or fails, urea accumulates in the blood (uremia), leading to unconsciousness and death.

creatinine clearance

Measurement of the rate at which creatinine is cleared from the blood by the kidney.

This is an important test to assess the functioning of the kidney. A blood sample is drawn and the creatinine concentration in blood is compared with the amount of creatinine excreted in the urine during a fixed time period. If the kidney is not functioning well in its job of clearing creatinine from the blood, the amount of creatinine in the blood will be high relative to the amount in urine. Creatinine clearance is a useful indicator of the **glomerular filtration rate (GFR)**, which normally is 90 to 120 mL/minute.

CLINICAL PROCEDURES

X-Ray Studies

CT urography

X-ray images obtained using computed tomography show multiple cross-sectional and other views of the kidney.

CT scanners show multiple views of the kidney, taken with or without contrast material. Two main indications are to detect kidney stones and to evaluate patients with hematuria. (Figure 7-13A).

kidneys, ureters, and bladder (KUB)

X-ray examination (without contrast) of the kidneys, ureters, and bladder.

A KUB study demonstrates the size and location of the kidneys in relation to other organs in the abdominopelvic region.

renal angiography

X-ray examination (with contrast) of the blood vessels of the kidney.

This procedure helps diagnose obstruction or constriction of blood vessels leading to the kidney. The same changes can be seen on CT and MRI urography.

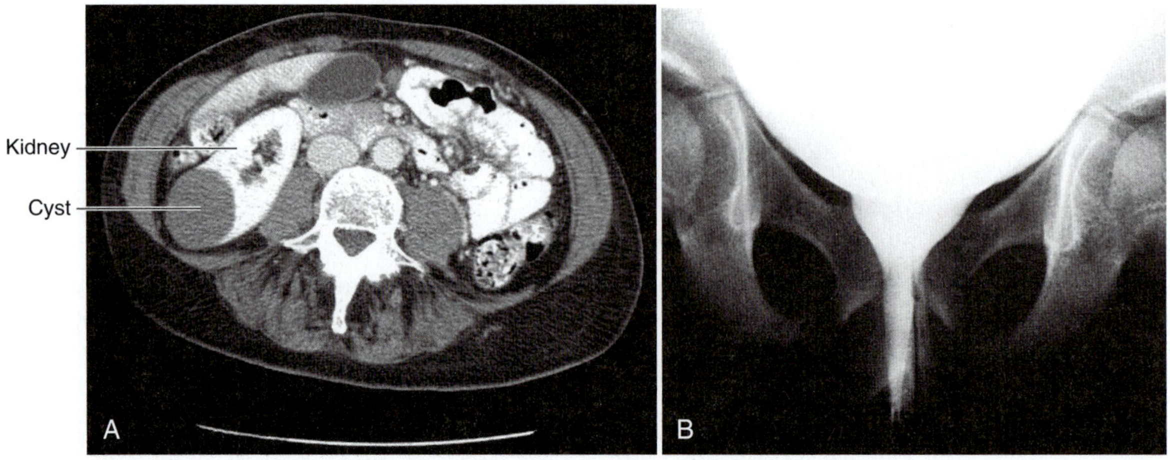

FIGURE 7-13 **A, CT urography with contrast** (axial view) shows a benign cyst on the kidney. It does not take up the contrast and is smooth and round. **B, Voiding cystourethrogram** showing a normal female urethra. *(Courtesy William H. Bush, Jr., MD, University of Washington, Seattle.)*

retrograde pyelogram (RP)

X-ray image of the renal pelvis and ureters after injection of contrast through a urinary catheter into the ureters from the bladder.

This technique is useful in locating urinary stones and obstructions.

voiding cystourethrogram (VCUG)

X-ray image (with contrast) of the urinary bladder and urethra obtained while the patient is voiding. See Figure 7-13B.

The bladder is filled with contrast material, followed by fluoroscopy (real-time x-ray imaging). Reflux of contrast into the ureters is abnormal and may occur with recurrent urinary tract infections.

Ultrasound Examination

ultrasonography

Imaging of urinary tract structures using high-frequency sound waves.

Kidney size, tumors, hydronephrosis, polycystic kidney disease, and ureteral and bladder obstruction can be diagnosed using ultrasound techniques.

Radioactive Study

radioisotope scan

Image of the kidney obtained after injecting a radioactive substance (radioisotope) into the bloodstream.

Pictures show the size and shape of the kidney **(renal scan)** and its functioning **(renogram).** These studies can indicate narrowing of blood vessels, diagnose obstruction, and determine the individual functioning of each kidney.

Magnetic Resonance Imaging

MRI urography

Changing magnetic field produces images of the kidney and surrounding structures in three planes of the body.

The patient lies within a cylindrical magnetic resonance machine, and images are made of the pelvic and retroperitoneal regions using magnetic waves. This test is useful in visualizing tumor invasion of blood vessels, lymph nodes, and adjacent tissues.

OTHER PROCEDURES

cystoscopy

Direct visualization of the urethra and urinary bladder with an endoscope (cystoscope).

The procedure can be performed in two ways. **Flexible cystoscopy** uses a thin fiberoptic cystoscope and is used for diagnosis and check-ups of the urinary bladder. **Rigid cystoscopy** uses a hollow metal tube, passed through the urethra and into the bladder. It is used to take biopsy samples, remove polyps, or perform laser treatments. (Figure 7-14A and B).

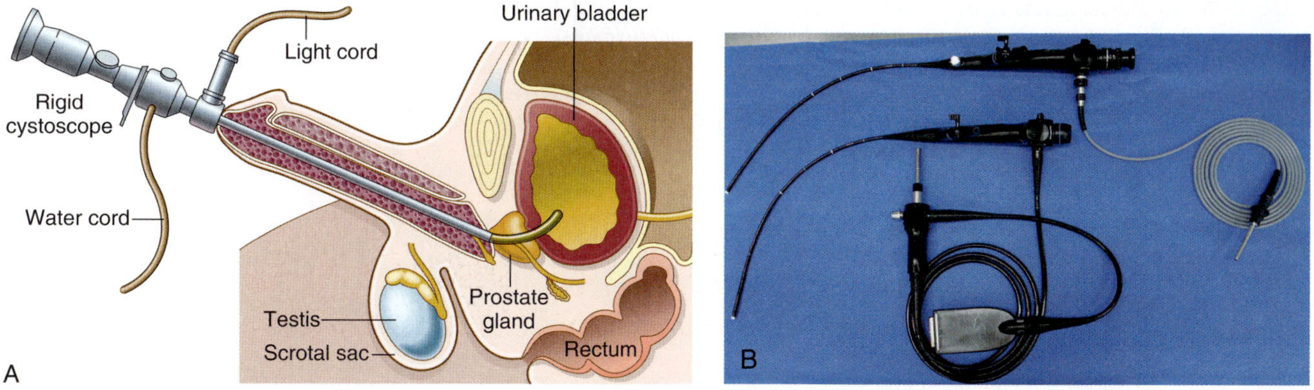

FIGURE 7-14 **Cystoscopy. A,** Shows a **rigid cystoscope** in place. **B,** Shows a **flexible cystoscope.**

dialysis

Process of separating nitrogenous waste materials from the blood.

Dialysis is used to treat acute or chronic renal failure and some cases of drug use. There are two methods:

1. **Hemodialysis (HD)** uses an artificial kidney machine that receives waste-filled blood from the patient's bloodstream, filters it through an artificial porous membrane (dialyzer), and returns the dialyzed blood to the patient's body (Figure 7-15A). An **arteriovenous fistula** (communication between an artery and vein) is created surgically to provide easy access for hemodialysis (Figure 7-15B).
2. **Peritoneal dialysis (PD)** uses a **catheter** to introduce fluid into the peritoneal (abdominal) cavity. Waste materials, such as urea, in the capillaries of the peritoneum pass out of the bloodstream and into the fluid. The fluid (with wastes) is then removed by catheter. When used to treat patients with chronic kidney disease, PD may be performed continuously by the patient without mechanical support (CAPD—continuous ambulatory PD; Figure 7-16) or with the aid of a mechanical apparatus used at night during sleep.

lithotripsy

Urinary tract stones are crushed.

The **extracorporeal** method uses shock waves directed toward the stone from the outside of the body (extra = outside, corpor/o = body). The patient receives light sedation or an anesthetic. Stones pass from the body in urine after the procedure. Abbreviation is **ESWL (extracorporeal shock wave lithotripsy).**

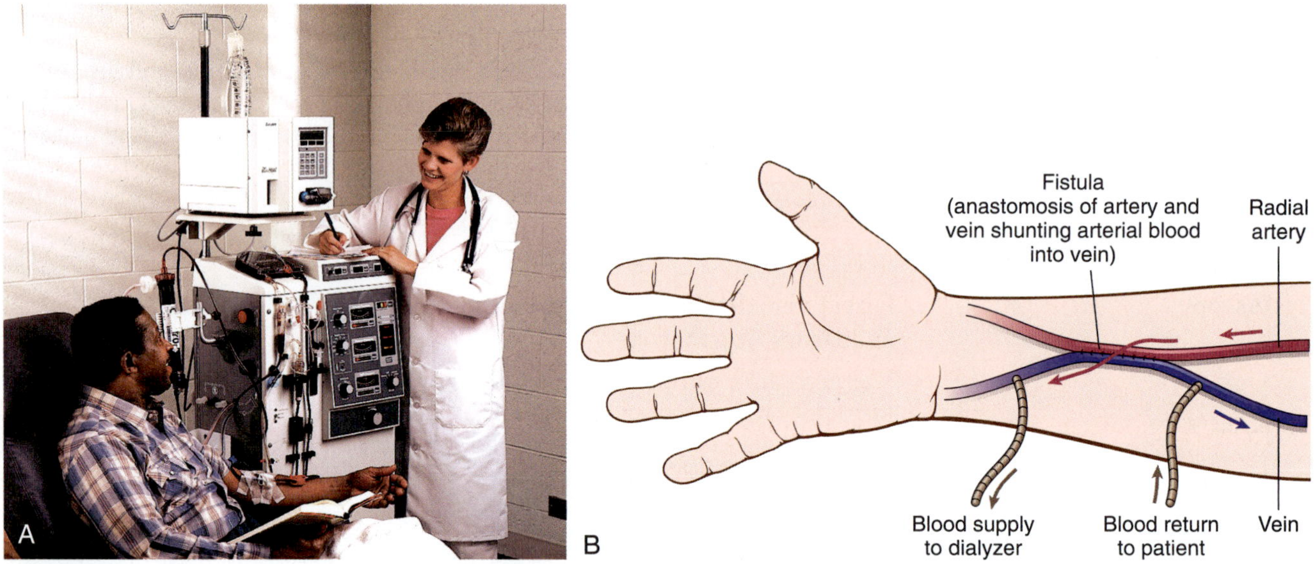

FIGURE 7-15 **Hemodialysis (HD). A,** Patient receiving HD. Conventional HD involves 3 to 4 hours of dialysis three times weekly. Newer alternative modalities include slower and longer dialysis, nocturnal HD, and daily short HD. **B, Arteriovenous fistula** for hemodialysis.

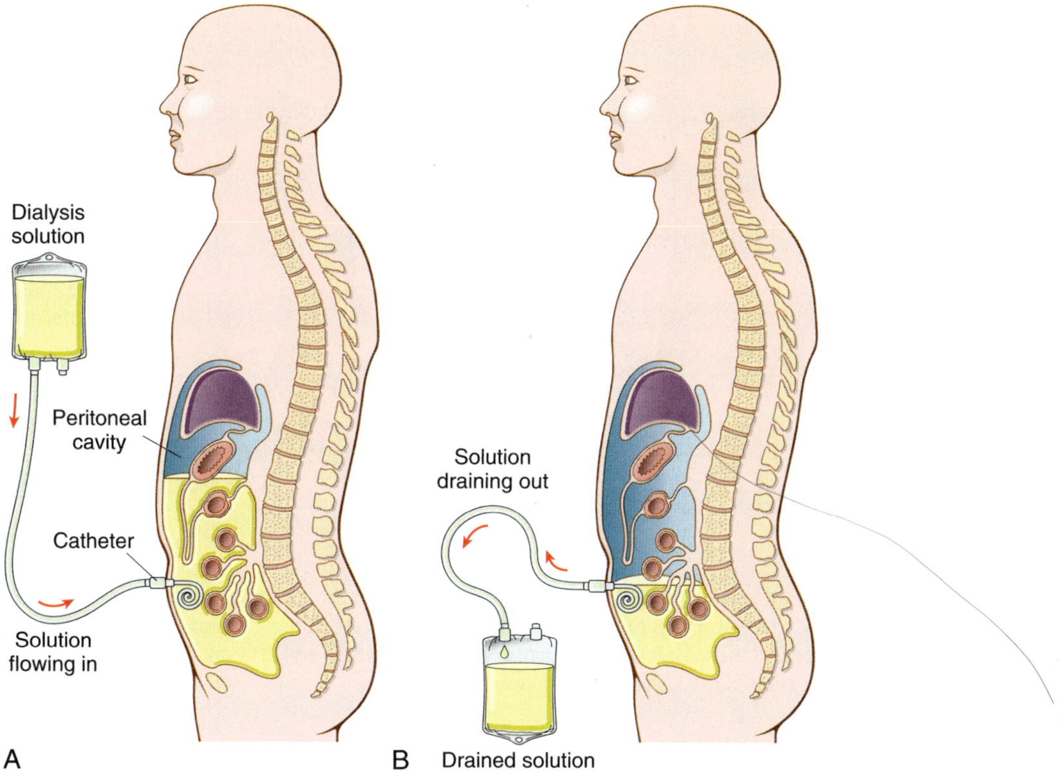

FIGURE 7-16 Continuous ambulatory peritoneal dialysis (CAPD). (A) The dialysis solution (dialysate) flows from a collapsible plastic bag through a catheter (Tenckhoff peritoneal catheter) into the patient's peritoneal cavity. The empty bag is then folded and inserted into undergarments. **(B)** After 4 to 8 hours, the bag is unfolded, and the fluid is allowed to drain into it by gravity. The full bag is discarded, and a new bag of fresh dialysate is attached.

renal angioplasty

Dilation of narrowed areas in renal arteries.

A balloon attached to a catheter is inserted into the artery and then inflated to enlarge the vessel diameter. Afterward, stents (metal-mesh tubes) may be inserted to keep the vessel open. This procedure is used to treat renal hypertension and to preserve renal function.

renal biopsy

Removal of kidney tissue for microscopic examination.

Biopsy may be performed at the time of surgery (open) or through the skin (percutaneous, or closed). When the latter technique is used, the patient lies in the prone position; then, after administration of local anesthesia to the overlying skin and muscles of the back, the physician inserts a biopsy needle downward into the kidney. Several specimens are obtained for examination by a pathologist.

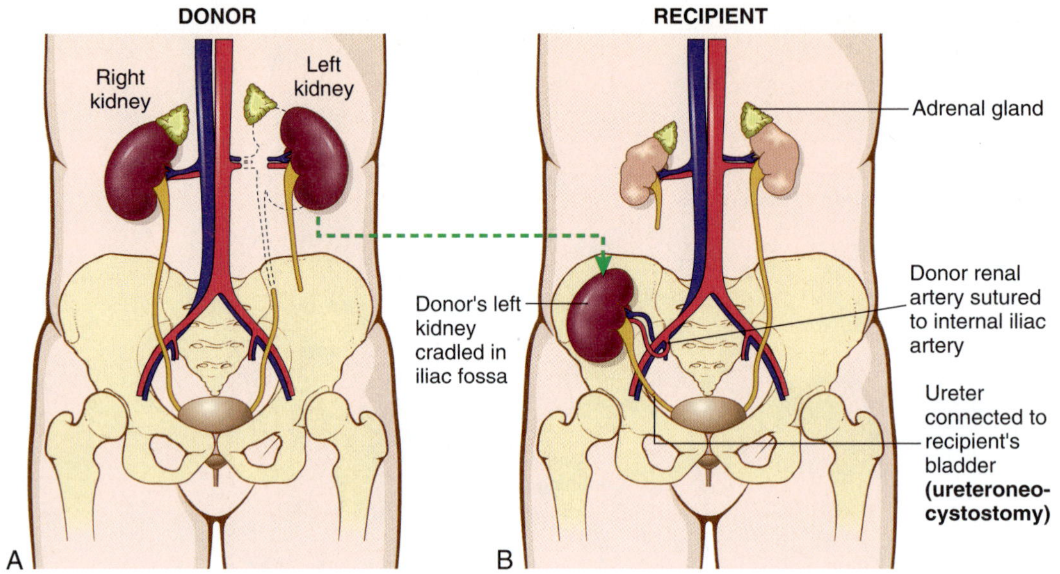

FIGURE 7-17 **Renal (kidney) transplantation. A,** Left kidney of donor is removed for transplantation. **B,** Kidney is transplanted to right pelvis of the recipient. The renal artery and vein of the donor kidney are joined to the recipient kidney's artery and vein, and the end of the donor ureter is connected to the recipient's bladder **(ureteroneocystostomy)**. The health of the donor is not affected by losing one kidney. In fact, the remaining kidney is able to take over full function.

7

renal transplantation

Surgical transfer of a kidney from a donor to a recipient.

Patients with renal failure may receive a kidney from a living donor, such as an identical twin (isograft) or other person (allograft), or from a patient at the time of death (cadaver transplant). Best results occur when the donor is closely related to the recipient—98% of transplanted kidneys survive for 1 year or longer (Figure 7-17). See ***In Person*** account, page 240, of a kidney transplant donor.

urinary catheterization

Passage of a flexible, tubular instrument through the urethra into the urinary bladder.

Catheters are used primarily for short- or long-term drainage of urine. A **Foley catheter** is an indwelling (left in the bladder) catheter held in place by a balloon inflated with liquid (Figure 7-18).

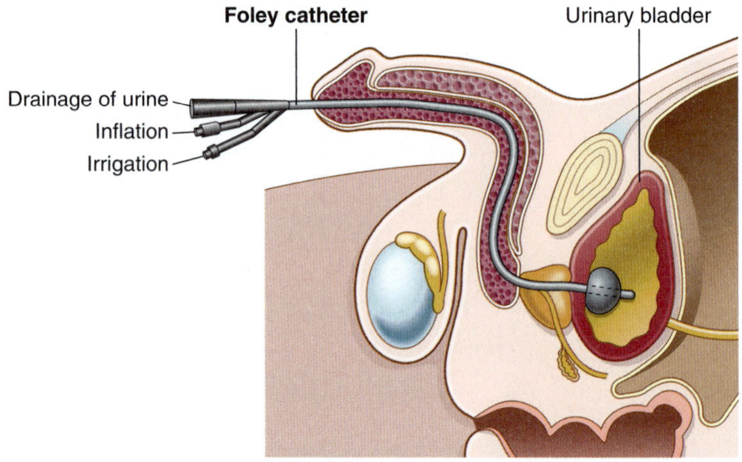

FIGURE 7-18 **Foley catheter** in place in the urinary bladder. The three-way catheter has three separate lumens: for drainage of urine, for inflation of balloons in the bladder, and for introduction of irrigating solutions into the bladder.

ABBREVIATIONS

ADH	antidiuretic hormone—vasopressin	**HD**	hemodialysis
AKI	acute renal injury	**IC**	interstitial cystitis—chronic inflammation of the bladder wall; not caused by bacterial infection and not responsive to conventional antibiotic therapy
BUN	blood urea nitrogen	**IVP**	intravenous pyelogram
CAPD	continuous ambulatory peritoneal dialysis	**K^+**	potassium—an electrolyte
CKD	chronic kidney disease—a condition during which serum creatinine and BUN levels rise, which may result in impairment of all body systems	**KUB**	kidney, ureter, and bladder
Cl^-	chloride—an electrolyte excreted by the kidney	**Na^+**	sodium—an electrolyte
CrCl	creatinine clearance	**PD**	peritoneal dialysis
CRF	chronic renal failure—progressive loss of kidney function	**pH**	potential hydrogen; scale to indicate degree of acidity or alkalinity
C&S	culture and sensitivity testing—to determine antibiotic effectiveness against bacteria grown from a patient's urine specimen	**PKD**	polycystic kidney disease
cysto	cystoscopic examination	**PUL**	percutaneous ultrasound lithotripsy
eGFR	estimated glomerular filtration rate	**RP**	retrograde pyelography
ESWL	extracorporeal shock wave lithotripsy	**sp gr**	specific gravity
HCO_3^-	bicarbonate—an electrolyte conserved by the kidney	**UA**	urinalysis
		UTI	urinary tract infection
		VCUG	voiding cystourethrogram

CKD Stages

There are 5 stages that reflect increasing severity of kidney disease:

Stage 1 = eGFR >90
Stage 2 = eGFR 60-90
Stage 3 = eGFR 30-60
Stage 4 = eGFR 15-30
Stage 5 = eGFR <15

PRACTICAL APPLICATIONS

Answers to the questions about the case report and the urinalysis findings are on page 248.

UROLOGIC CASE REPORT

The patient, a 50-year-old woman, presented to the clinic complaining of painless hematuria and clots. There had been no history of urolithiasis, pyuria, or previous hematuria. Nocturia had been present about 5 years earlier. Endoscopy revealed a carcinoma located about 2 cm from the left ureteral orifice. A metastatic workup was negative. Partial cystectomy was carried out and the lesion cleared. Bilateral pelvic lymphadenectomy revealed no positive nodes. No ileal conduit was necessary.

Questions about the Case Report

1. Urologic refers to which system of the body?
   a. Digestive
   b. Endocrine
   c. Excretory
2. What was the patient's reason for appearing at the clinic?
   a. Scanty urination
   b. Inability to urinate
   c. Blood in urine
3. Which of the following was a previous symptom?
   a. Excessive urination at night
   b. Blood in the urine
   c. Pus in the urine
4. What diagnostic procedure was carried out?
   a. Lithotripsy
   b. Cystoscopy
   c. Urinalysis
5. The patient's diagnosis was
   a. Malignant tumor of the bladder
   b. Tumor in the proximal ureter
   c. Lymph nodes affected by tumor
6. Treatment was
   a. Ureteroileostomy
   b. Removal of tumor and subtotal removal of the bladder
   c. Not necessary because of negative lymph nodes

URINALYSIS FINDINGS

TEST	NORMAL	ABNORMAL
Color	Amber-yellow	Smoky-red (blood in urine): renal calculi; tumor; kidney disease; cystitis; urinary obstruction
Appearance	Clear	Cloudy (pyuria): urinary tract infection (UTI)
pH	4.6-8.0	Alkaline: UTI
Protein	None or small amount	Proteinuria: nephritis; renal failure
Glucose	None	Glycosuria: diabetes mellitus
Ketones	None	Ketonuria: diabetes mellitus
Bilirubin	None	Bilirubinuria: hepatitis or gallbladder disease
Specific gravity	1.003-1.030	High: renal calculi; diabetes mellitus Low: diabetes insipidus
Sediment	None	Casts: nephritis; renal disease

Name the appropriate test for detecting or evaluating each of the following.

1. Sugar in urine ____________________
2. Level of bile pigment in urine ____________________
3. Hematuria ____________________
4. Albumin in urine ____________________
5. Structures in the shape of renal tubules in urine ____________________
6. Chemical reaction of urine ____________________
7. Dilution or concentration of urine ____________________
8. Acetones in urine ____________________
9. Pus in urine ____________________

UROLOGIC CASE STUDY

A 22-year-old Brazilian fashion model comes to the ED with a history of fever, dysuria, and shaking chills. Results of her UA, with normal findings for comparison, are as follows:

	URINALYSIS (UA) RESULTS	NORMAL FINDINGS
Color	amber yellow	amber yellow
Appearance	turbid	clear
Specific gravity	1.040	1.003-1.030
pH	8.4	6.5 (range, 4.6-8.0)
Protein	neg	neg
Glucose	neg	neg
Ketones	neg	neg
Bili	neg	neg
WBC count	>100 units	0
Bacteria	bacilli (rods)	0
Sediment	WBC casts	none

What's the probable diagnosis?

a. Diabetes mellitus with glycosuria
b. Glomerulonephritis with staphylococcal infection
c. Nephrotic syndrome with albuminuria
d. Urinary tract infection with pyelonephritis

7

IN PERSON

This first-person narrative was written by a kidney donor.

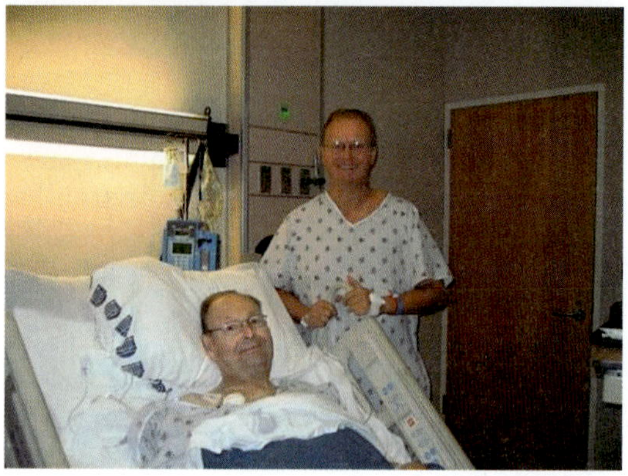

When my 64 year-old father-in-law announced to my wife and me that his kidney function was failing, it didn't really enter our minds that one of us might ultimately have a part to play in his survival. Five years later, dialysis was taking its toll on his organ systems, and there had been no success in obtaining a cadaveric kidney. Things had reached the point where he needed a kidney in short order, before his health deteriorated to the point where he would no longer be a candidate for transplantation.

My wife's blood type ruled out the possibility of her being a direct donor, so I volunteered to be tested. Turns out that we were a match on 5 of the 7 key traits—a really good fit! The next round of testing—blood work and my kidney function—was able to be done locally. I remember carrying around a specimen container (on ice), having to provide a full liter of urine in 24 hours!

The results of those tests were favorable, and two weeks later I made the 3½-hour drive to the transplant center at the University of Virginia in Charlottesville. While a transplant is really a team of two—donor and recipient—the entire process at UVA was very much individualized. A transplant coordinator (an experienced RN) was assigned specifically to our case, and I had a team of doctors and support staff dedicated exclusively to me, the donor. Similarly, there was a team that dealt only with my father-in-law as the recipient.

My visit involved some more in-depth blood tests and cardiac studies largely to determine that I was healthy enough for major surgery. My transplant team and I spent an entire afternoon discussing the implications of being a donor—the inherent risk in any surgery, potential implications for me and my family, the likely recovery time, and the possibility that, despite all of the up-front testing, the transplant might not be successful. The discussions that afternoon only reaffirmed that I was making the right decision. I had an opportunity to positively impact someone else's life, with relatively little risk to my own health.

The events around the surgery itself were pretty straightforward. We drove up from Greensboro on Wednesday evening, with the surgery scheduled for 8:00 AM Thursday morning. I didn't get much sleep that night—I watched my favorite "comfort" movie, "Love Actually," at 3:00 AM—but was excited and ready to go in the morning. As you might imagine, the moments immediately before going into pre-op were very emotional for all of us. We shed a lot of tears—of apprehension for the surgeries and of joy at the prospect of a new beginning for my father-in-law. The surgery is a more involved procedure for the donor than for the recipient, so I was taken back first. A nurse started an IV and pushed a mild sedative. From that point, my only memory is of one last hug for my wife and children, and then being shifted from the stretcher onto the operating table.

When I woke up in recovery, the news was all good. My surgery had gone well—four laparoscopic incisions through which the surgeons did most all of their work, and a lateral incision in my lower abdomen through which the kidney was removed. Equally important, my father-in-law had come through his surgery well and the kidney had immediately begun to function! I was discharged from the hospital on Sunday, and cleared to return home the next Friday, 8 days post-op.

All told, I was out of work for 12 days—2 days the week of the surgery and the following 2 weeks. As is typical following a major surgery, it took about 6 weeks for me to feel "normal" again. During those 6 weeks, I had weekly blood tests to chart the progress of my kidney function. I went back to UVA for a routine follow-up visit at the 6 week mark. I was recovering as expected, and my remaining kidney was actually growing in size and capacity. Blood tests continued on a monthly basis until I was officially "discharged" from the transplant center's care six months after the surgery.

Now, 5 years after the transplant, both my father-in-law and I continue to do well. As my mother-in-law likes to say, I donated a "rock star" kidney that has allowed our family to enjoy many visits and create many cherished memories that will last a lifetime. My two children, now 17 and 14, have enjoyed their grandfather's love and guidance during some very important years in their lives. This is especially meaningful to me, as I lost my father before my wife and I started our family, and our children missed out on an opportunity to know and love a wonderful man.

John Melson lives in Greensboro, North Carolina, with his wife and two wonderful children. He is a finance and marketing executive with a global textile firm, and enjoys golf, tennis, and traveling. He is pictured with his father-in-law, Rod Beckwith.

EXERCISES

Remember to check your answers carefully with the Answers to Exercises, pages 247 and 248.

A Using the following terms, trace the path of urine from the renal arterioles (bloodstream) to the point at which urine leaves the body. The first answer is provided.

glomerular capsule	renal pelvis	ureter	urinary bladder
glomerulus	renal tubule	urethra	urinary meatus

1. *glomerulus* ____________
2. ____________
3. ____________
4. ____________
5. ____________
6. ____________
7. ____________
8. ____________

B Match the term in Column I with its definition or a term of similar meaning in Column II. Write the correct letter in the spaces provided.

COLUMN I		COLUMN II
1. voiding	______	A. hormone secreted by the kidney that stimulates formation of red blood cells
2. trigone	______	B. notch on the surface of the kidney where blood vessels and nerves enter
3. renal cortex	______	C. urination; micturition
4. renal medulla	______	D. nitrogenous waste
5. urea	______	E. cup-like collecting region of the renal pelvis
6. erythropoietin	______	F. small molecule that carries an electric charge in solution
7. renin	______	G. inner region of the kidney
8. electrolyte	______	H. hormone made by the kidney; increases blood pressure
9. hilum	______	I. triangular area in the bladder
10. calyx (calix)	______	J. outer section of the kidney

C **Give the meanings of the following medical terms.**

1. caliceal ______
2. uric acid ______
3. urinary meatal stenosis ______
4. cystocele ______
5. pyelolithotomy ______
6. trigonitis ______
7. ureteroileostomy ______
8. urethrostenosis ______
9. vesicoureteral reflux ______
10. creatinine ______
11. medullary ______
12. cortical ______
13. calciferol ______

D **The following terms all contain the suffix -uria, meaning urination. Write their meanings in the spaces provided.**

1. nocturia ______
2. dysuria ______
3. oliguria ______
4. polyuria ______
5. anuria ______

E **In the following terms, -uria means urine condition (substance in the urine). What's in the urine?**

1. pyuria ______
2. albuminuria ______
3. hematuria ______
4. glycosuria ______
5. ketonuria ______
6. bacteriuria ______

F **Give the meanings of the following terms that relate to urinary signs and symptoms.**

1. azotemia ______
2. polydipsia ______
3. urinary incontinence ______
4. enuresis ______
5. urinary retention ______
6. ketosis ______

G **Give short answers for the following.**

1. What is the difference between hematuria and uremia? ____________________
2. What is diuresis? ____________________
3. What is a diuretic? ____________________
4. What is antidiuretic hormone? ____________________
5. What is hyponatremia? ____________________
6. What is hyperkalemia? ____________________
7. What is PKU? ____________________

H **Match the following terms that pertain to urinalysis with their meanings below.**

albuminuria	hematuria	pyuria
bilirubinuria	ketonuria	sediment
glycosuria	pH	specific gravity

1. Abnormal particles present in the urine—cells, bacteria, casts, and crystals

   ____
2. Smoky-red color of urine caused by the presence of blood ____________________
3. Turbid (cloudy) urine caused by the presence of polymorphonuclear leukocytes and pus

   ____
4. Sugar in the urine; a sign of diabetes mellitus and a result of hyperglycemia

   ____
5. Urine test that reflects the acidity or alkalinity of the urine ____________________
6. High levels of acids and acetones accumulate in the urine as a result of abnormal fat breakdown

   ____
7. Dark pigment that accumulates in urine as a result of liver or gallbladder disease

   ____
8. Urine test that reflects the concentration of the urine ____________________
9. Leaky glomeruli can produce accumulation of protein in the urine ____________________

I Describe the following abnormal conditions that affect the kidney.

1. renal failure ______
2. polycystic kidney ______
3. interstitial nephritis ______
4. glomerulonephritis ______
5. nephrolithiasis ______
6. renal cell carcinoma ______
7. pyelonephritis ______
8. Wilms tumor ______
9. nephrotic syndrome ______
10. renal hypertension ______

J Match the following terms with their meanings below.

abscess	edema	renal colic
catheter	essential hypertension	secondary hypertension
diabetes insipidus	nephroptosis	stricture
diabetes mellitus		

1. idiopathic high blood pressure ______
2. swelling, fluid in tissues ______
3. narrowed area in a tube ______
4. collection of pus ______
5. inadequate secretion of insulin or improper utilization of insulin leads to this condition

   ______
6. high blood pressure caused by kidney disease or another disease ______
7. tube for withdrawing or giving fluid ______
8. inadequate secretion or resistance of the kidney to the action of antidiuretic hormone

   ______
9. prolapse of a kidney ______
10. severe pain resulting from a stone that is blocking a ureter or a kidney

    ______

K **Give the meanings of the following abbreviations. Then select the letter of the sentence that is the best association for each.**

COLUMN I

1. CAPD ____________________ ________
2. BUN ____________________ ________
3. RP ____________________ ________
4. cysto ____________________ ________
5. UA ____________________ ________
6. UTI ____________________ ________
7. CKD ____________________ ________
8. K^+ ____________________ ________
9. VCUG ____________________ ________
10. HD ____________________ ________

COLUMN II

A. Bacterial invasion leads to this condition; acute cystitis is an example.
B. This electrolyte is secreted by renal tubules into the urine.
C. A machine removes nitrogenous wastes from the patient's blood.
D. High levels measured on this test lead to the suspicion of renal disease.
E. This endoscopic procedure is used to examine the interior of the urinary bladder.
F. Dialysate (fluid) is injected into the peritoneal cavity and then drained out.
G. Contrast is injected into the urinary bladder and ureters and x-ray pictures of the urinary tract are taken.
H. X-ray pictures of the urinary bladder and urethra are taken while the patient urinates.
I. The parts of this test include specific gravity, color, protein, glucose, and pH.
J. This condition includes mild to severe kidney failure.

L **Match the following procedures with their meanings below.**

cystectomy	nephrectomy	ureterolithotomy
cystoscopy	nephrolithotomy	urethroplasty
cystostomy	nephrostomy	ureteroileostomy
lithotripsy		

1. Excision of a kidney ____________________
2. Surgical incision into the kidney to remove a stone ____________________
3. Visual examination of the urinary bladder via endoscope ____________________
4. Crushing of stones ____________________
5. New opening of the ureters to a segment of ileum (in place of the bladder)

   ____
6. Surgical repair of the urethra ____________________
7. Creation of an artificial opening into the kidney (via catheter) from the outside of the body

   ____
8. Surgical formation of an opening from the bladder to the outside of the body

   ____
9. Removal of the urinary bladder ____________________
10. Incision of a ureter to remove a stone ____________________

M Circle the correct term to complete the following sentences.

1. After diagnosis of renal cell carcinoma (made by renal biopsy), Dr. Davis advised Donna that **(nephrostomy, meatotomy, nephrectomy)** would be necessary.
2. Ever since Bill's condition of gout was diagnosed, he has been warned that uric acid crystals could accumulate in his blood and tissues, leading to **(pyuria, renal calculi, cystocele).**
3. The voiding cystourethrogram demonstrated blockage of urine flow from Jim's bladder and **(hydronephrosis, renal ischemia, azotemia).**
4. Narrowed arterioles in the kidney increase blood pressure, so **(urinary incontinence, urinary retention, nephrosclerosis)** is often associated with hypertension.
5. Eight-year-old Willy continually wet his bed at night while sleeping. His pediatrician instructed his mother to limit Willy's intake of fluids in the evening to discourage his **(nocturia, oliguria, enuresis).**
6. David's chronic type 1 diabetes eventually resulted in **(nephropathy, meatal stenosis, urolithiasis),** which led to renal failure.
7. After Sue's bilateral renal failure, her doctor advised dialysis and possible **(cystostomy, nephrolithotomy, renal transplantation).**
8. When Maria's left kidney stopped functioning, her contralateral kidney overdeveloped or **(metastasized, atrophied, hypertrophied)** to meet the increased workload.
9. A popular diet program recommends eating foods high in fats and protein. People on this diet check their urine for the presence of **(ketones, glucose, amino acids).**
10. Andrea's urinalysis revealed proteinuria, and her ankles began to swell, demonstrating pitting, a condition known as **(ascites, edema, stricture).** Her **(gastroenterologist, urologist, nephrologist)** diagnosed Andrea's condition as **(polycystic kidneys, nephrotic syndrome, bladder carcinoma)** and recommended drugs to heal leaky glomeruli and diuretics to reduce swelling.

ANSWERS TO EXERCISES

A

1. glomerulus
2. glomerular capsule
3. renal tubule
4. renal pelvis
5. ureter
6. urinary bladder
7. urethra
8. urinary meatus

B

1. C
2. I
3. J
4. G
5. D
6. A
7. H
8. F
9. B
10. E

C

1. pertaining to a calix (collecting cup of renal pelvis)
2. nitrogenous waste excreted in urine; high levels of uric acid in the blood are associated with gouty arthritis
3. narrowing of the urinary meatus
4. hernia of the urinary bladder
5. incision to remove a stone from the renal pelvis
6. inflammation of the trigone (triangular area in the bladder in which the ureters enter and urethra exits)
7. new opening between the ureter and the ileum (an anastomosis); urine then leaves the body through an ileostomy; this surgery (ileal conduit) is performed when the bladder has been removed
8. narrowing (narrowed portion) of the urethra
9. backflow of urine from the bladder into the ureter
10. nitrogenous waste produced as a result of muscle metabolism and excreted in the urine
11. pertaining to the inner, middle section (of the kidney)
12. pertaining to the outer section (of the kidney)
13. active form of vitamin D secreted by the kidneys

D

1. frequent urination at night
2. painful urination
3. scanty urination
4. excessive urination
5. no urination

E

1. pus
2. protein
3. blood
4. sugar
5. ketones or acetones
6. bacteria

F

1. excess nitrogenous waste in the bloodstream
2. condition of much thirst
3. inability to hold urine in the bladder
4. bed-wetting
5. inability to release urine from the bladder
6. abnormal condition of ketone bodies (acids and acetones) in the blood and body tissues

G

1. Hematuria is the presence of blood in the urine, and uremia is a toxic condition of excess urea (nitrogenous waste) in the bloodstream. Hematuria is a symptomatic condition of the urine (-uria), and uremia is an abnormal condition of the blood (-emia).
2. Diuresis is the excessive production of urine (polyuria).
3. A diuretic is a drug or chemical (caffeine or alcohol) that causes diuresis to occur.
4. Antidiuretic hormone is a hormone produced by the pituitary gland that normally helps the renal tubules to reabsorb water back into the bloodstream. It works against diuresis to help retain water in the blood.
5. Hyponatremia is abnormally low levels of sodium in the bloodstream.
6. Hyperkalemia is abnormally high concentration of potassium in the blood. The major cause is chronic renal failure.
7. PKU is phenylketonuria. This occurs when there are high levels of phenylketones in urine and phenylalanine in the blood. The condition causes mental retardation in infants.

H

1. sediment
2. hematuria (blood in the urine)
3. pyuria (pus in the urine)
4. glycosuria (sugar in the urine)
5. pH
6. ketonuria (ketone bodies in the urine)
7. bilirubinuria (high levels of bilirubin in the urine)
8. specific gravity
9. albuminuria

I

1. kidney does not excrete wastes
2. multiple fluid-filled sacs form in and on the kidney
3. inflammation of the connective tissue (interstitium) lying between the renal tubules
4. inflammation of the glomerulus of the kidney (may be a complication after a streptococcal infection)
5. condition of kidney stones (renal calculi)
6. malignant tumor of the kidney in adults
7. inflammation of the renal pelvis and parenchyma of the kidney (caused by a bacterial infection, such as with *Escherichia coli,* that spreads to the urinary tract from the gastrointestinal tract)
8. malignant tumor of the kidney in children
9. group of symptoms (proteinuria, edema, hypoalbuminemia) that appears when the kidney is damaged by disease; also called nephrosis
10. high blood pressure caused by kidney disease

J

1. essential hypertension
2. edema
3. stricture
4. abscess
5. diabetes mellitus
6. secondary hypertension
7. catheter
8. diabetes insipidus
9. nephroptosis
10. renal colic

K

1. continuous ambulatory peritoneal dialysis: F
2. blood urea nitrogen: D
3. retrograde pyelogram: G
4. cystoscopy: E
5. urinalysis: I
6. urinary tract infection: A
7. chronic kidney disease: J
8. potassium: B
9. voiding cystourethrogram: H
10. hemodialysis: C

7

L

1. nephrectomy
2. nephrolithotomy
3. cystoscopy
4. lithotripsy
5. ureteroileostomy
6. urethroplasty
7. nephrostomy
8. cystostomy
9. cystectomy
10. ureterolithotomy

M

1. nephrectomy
2. renal calculi—don't confuse a calculus (stone) with dental calculus, which is an accumulation of dental plaque that has hardened
3. hydronephrosis
4. nephrosclerosis
5. enuresis
6. nephropathy
7. renal transplantation
8. hypertrophied
9. ketones
10. edema, nephrologist, nephrotic syndrome

Answers to Practical Applications

Urologic Case Report

1. c
2. c
3. a
4. b
5. a
6. b

Urinalysis Findings

1. glucose
2. bilirubin
3. color
4. protein
5. sediment
6. pH
7. specific gravity
8. ketones
9. appearance

Urologic Case Study

Correct diagnosis is d.

PRONUNCIATION OF TERMS

To test your understanding of the terminology in this chapter, write the meaning of each term in the space provided. In addition, you may wish to cover the terms and write them by looking at your definitions. Make sure your spelling is correct. The page number after each term indicates where it is defined or used in the book, so you can easily check your responses. You will find complete definitions for all of these terms and audio pronunciations on the Evolve website.

Pronunciation Guide

ā as in āpe	ă as in ăpple
ē as in ēven	ĕ as in ĕvery
ī as in īce	ĭ as in ĭnterest
ō as in ōpen	ŏ as in pŏt
ū as in ūnit	ŭ as in ŭnder

TERM	PRONUNCIATION	MEANING
acetone (229)	ĂS-ĕ-tōn	
albuminuria (226)	ăl-bū-mĭn-Ū-rē-ă	
antidiuretic hormone (227)	ăn-tĭ-dī-ū-RĔ-tĭk HŎR-mōn	
anuria (227)	ăn-Ū-rē-ă	
arteriole (221)	ăr-TĔR-ē-ōl	
azotemia (226)	ă-zō-TĒ-mē-ă	
bacteriuria (226)	băk-tē-rē-Ū-rē-ă	
calciferol (221)	căl-SĬ-fĕr-ŏl	
caliceal (223)	kā-lĭ-SĒ-ăl	
caliectasis (223)	kā-lē-ĔK-tă-sĭs	
calyx (calix); *plural*: calyces (calices) (221)	KĀ-lĭks; KĀ-lĭ-sēz	
catheter (221)	KĂ-thĕ-tĕr	
cortex (221)	KŎR-tĕks	
cortical (221)	KŎR-tĭ-kăl	
creatinine (221)	krē-ĂT-ĭ-nēn	
creatinine clearance (232)	krē-ĂT-ĭ-nēn KLĒR-ăns	
CT urography (232)	CT ū-RŎG-ră-fē	
cystectomy (223)	sĭs-TĔK-tō-mē	
cystitis (223)	sĭs-TĪ-tĭs	
cystoscopy (233)	sĭs-TŎS-kō-pē	
cystostomy (223)	sĭs-TŎS-tō-mē	
diabetes insipidus (231)	dī-ă-BĒ-tēz ĭn-SĬP-ĭ-dŭs	
diabetes mellitus (231)	dī-ă-BĒ-tēz MĔL-ĭ-tŭs	

7

TERM	PRONUNCIATION	MEANING
diuresis (227)	dī-ūr-RĒ-sĭs	
dysuria (227)	dĭs-Ū-rē-ă	
edema (230)	ĕ-DĒ-mă	
electrolyte (221)	ē-LĔK-trō-līt	
enuresis (227)	ĕn-ū-RĒ-sĭs	
erythropoietin (221)	ĕ-rĭth-rō-PŌY-ĕ-tĭn	
essential hypertension (231)	ē-SĔN-shŭl hī-pĕr-TĔN-shŭn	
filtration (221)	fĭl-TRĀ-shŭn	
glomerular capsule (221)	glō-MĔR-ū-lăr KĂP-sŭl	
glomerulonephritis (229)	glō-mĕr-ū-lō-nĕ-FRĪ-tĭs	
glomerulus; *plural*: glomeruli (221)	glō-MĔR-ū-lŭs; glō-MĔR-ū-lī	
glycosuria (227)	glī-kōs-Ū-rē-ă	
hematuria (227)	hēm-ă-TŪ-rē-ă	
hemodialysis (234)	hē-mō-dī-ĂL-ĭ-sĭs	
hilum (221)	HĪ-lŭm	
hydronephrosis (224)	hī-drō-nĕ-FRŌ-sĭs	
hyperkalemia (226)	hī-pĕr-kă-LĒ-mē-ă	
hyponatremia (226)	hī-pō-nă-TRĒ-mē-ă	
interstitial nephritis (229)	ĭn-tĕr-STĬ-shŭl nĕ-FRĪ-tĭs	
intravesical (226)	ĭn-tră-VĔS-ĭ-kăl	
ketonuria (226)	kē-tōn-Ū-rē-ă	
ketosis (226)	kē-TŌ-sĭs	
kidney (222)	KĬD-nē	
lithotripsy (234)	LĬTH-ō-trĭp-sē	
meatal stenosis (223)	mē-Ā-tăl stĕ-NŌ-sĭs	
meatus (222)	mē-Ā-tŭs	
medulla (222)	mĕ-DŪL-ă *or* mĕ-DŬL-ă	
medullary (222)	MĔD-ū-lăr-ē	
MRI urography (233)	MRI ū-RŎG-ră-fē	
nephrolithiasis (230)	nĕf-rō-lĭ-THĪ-ă-sĭs	

7

TERM	PRONUNCIATION	MEANING
nephrolithotomy (224)	nĕf-rō-lĭ-THŎT-ō-mē	________
nephron (222)	NĔF-rŏn	________
nephropathy (223)	nĕ-FRŎ-pă-thē	________
nephroptosis (224)	nĕf-rŏp-TŌ-sĭs	________
nephrostomy (224)	nĕ-FRŎS-tō-mē	________
nephrotic syndrome (230)	nĕ-FRŎT-ĭk SĬN-drōm	________
nitrogenous waste (222)	nī-TRŎJ-ĕ-nŭs wāst	________
nocturia (226)	nŏk-TŪ-rē-ă	________
oliguria (226)	ŏl-ĭ-GŪ-rē-ă	________
parenchyma (230)	păr-ĔN-kĭ-mă	________
paranephric (224)	pă-ră-NĔF-rĭk	________
peritoneal dialysis (234)	pĕr-ĭ-tō-NĒ-ăl dī-ĂL-ĭ-sĭs	________
phenylketonuria (229)	fē-nĭl-kē-tōn-ŪR-ē-ă	________
polycystic kidney disease (230)	pŏl-ē-SĬS-tĭk KĬD-nē dĭ-ZĒZ	________
polydipsia (226)	pŏl-ē-DĬP-sē-ā	________
polyuria (227)	pŏl-ē-Ū-rē-ă	________
potassium (222)	pō-TĂ-sē-ŭm	________
pyelolithotomy (225)	pī-ĕ-lō-lĭ-THŎT-ō-mē	________
pyelonephritis (230)	pī-ĕ-lō-nĕf-RĪ-tĭs	________
pyuria (227)	pī-Ū-rē-ă	________
reabsorption (222)	rē-ăb-SŎRP-shŭn	________
renal angiography (232)	RĒ-năl ăn-jē-ŎG-ră-fē	________
renal angioplasty (235)	RĒ-năl ĂN-jē-ō-plăs-tē	________
renal artery (222)	RĒ-năl ĂR-tĕ-rē	________
renal calculi (230)	RĒ-năl KĂL-kū-lī	________
renal cell carcinoma (230)	RĒ-năl sĕl kăr-sĭ-NŌ-mă	________
renal colic (225)	RĒ-năl KŎL-ĭk	________
renal failure (231)	RĒ-năl FĀL-ūr	________
renal hypertension (231)	RĒ-năl hī-pĕr-TĔN-shŭn	________
renal ischemia (225)	RĒ-năl ĭs-KĒ-mē-ă	________
renal pelvis (222)	RĒ-năl PĔL-vĭs	________

7

TERM	PRONUNCIATION	MEANING
renal transplantation (236)	RĒ-năl trăns-plăn-TĀ-shŭn	
renal tubule (222)	RĒ-năl Tōō-būl	
renal vein (222)	RĒ-năl vān	
renin (222)	RĒ-nĭn	
retrograde pyelogram (233)	RĔ-trō-grād PĪ-ĕ-lō-grăm	
secondary hypertension (231)	SĔ-kŏn-dă-rē hī-pĕr-TĔN-shŭn	
sodium (222)	SŌ-dē-ŭm	
stricture (225)	STRĬK-shŭr	
trigone (222)	TRĪ-gōn	
trigonitis (225)	trī-gō-NĪ-tĭs	
urea (222)	ū-RĒ-ă	
uremia (227)	ū-RĒ-mē-ă	
ureter (222)	ū-RĒ-tĕr *or* ŪR-ĕ-tĕr	
ureteroileostomy (225)	ū-rē-tĕr-ō-ĭl-ē-ŎS-tō-mē	
ureteroneocystostomy (236)	ū-rē-tĕr-ō-nē-ō-sĭs-TŎS-tō-mē	
ureteroplasty (225)	ū-rē-tĕr-ō-PLĂS-tē	
urethra (222)	ū-RĒ-thră	
urethral stricture (225)	ū-RĒ-thrăl STRĬK-shŭr	
urethritis (225)	ū-rē-THRĪ-tĭs	
urethroplasty (225)	ū-rē-thrō-PLĂS-tē	
uric acid (222)	Ū-rĭk ĂS-ĭd	
urinalysis (228)	ū-rĭn-ĂL-ĭ-sĭs	
urinary bladder (222)	ŪR-ĭ-năr-ē BLĂ-dĕr	
urinary catheterization (236)	ŪR-ĭ-năr-ē kă-thĕ-tĕr-ĭ-ZĀ-shŭn	
urinary incontinence (227)	ŪR-ĭ-năr-ē ĭn-KŎN-tĭ-nĕns	
urinary retention (227)	ŪR-ĭ-năr-ē rē-TĔN-shŭn	
urination (222)	ūr-ĭ-NĀ-shŭn	
vesicoureteral reflux (226)	vĕs-ĭ-kō-ū-RĒ-tĕr-ăl RĒ-flŭks	
voiding (222)	VOY-dĭng	
voiding cystourethrogram (233)	VOY-dĭng sĭs-tō-ū-RĒ-thrō-grăm	
Wilms tumor (231)	wĭlmz Tōō-mŭr	

7

REVIEW SHEET

Write the meanings of the combining forms, suffixes, and prefixes in the spaces provided. Check your answers with the information in the chapter or in the Glossary (Medical Word Parts—English) at the end of this book.

Combining Forms

COMBINING FORM	MEANING	COMBINING FORM	MEANING
albumin/o	______	meat/o	______
angi/o	______	natr/o	______
azot/o	______	necr/o	______
bacteri/o	______	nephr/o	______
cali/o	______	noct/o	______
calic/o	______	olig/o	______
cyst/o	______	py/o	______
dips/o	______	pyel/o	______
glomerul/o	______	ren/o	______
glycos/o	______	trigon/o	______
hydr/o	______	ur/o	______
isch/o	______	ureter/o	______
kal/o	______	urethr/o	______
ket/o	______	urin/o	______
keton/o	______	vesic/o	______
lith/o	______		

Suffixes

SUFFIX	MEANING	SUFFIX	MEANING
-ectasis	______	-pathy	______
-ectomy	______	-plasty	______
-emia	______	-poietin	______
-esis	______	-ptosis	______
-gram	______	-rrhea	______
-lithiasis	______	-sclerosis	______
-lithotomy	______	-stenosis	______
-lysis	______	-stomy	______
-megaly	______	-tomy	______
-ole	______	-tripsy	______
-osis	______	-uria	______

7

Prefixes

PREFIX	MEANING	PREFIX	MEANING
a-, an-	______________	hypo-	______________
anti-	______________	peri-	______________
dia-	______________	poly-	______________
dys-	______________	retro-	______________
en-	______________		

Anatomic Terms

Match the locations/functions in Column I with the urinary system structures in Column II. Write the number of the correct structure in the blanks provided.

COLUMN I		COLUMN II
Tiny structure surrounding each glomerulus; receives filtered materials from blood.	_____	1. urethra
Tubes carrying urine from kidney to urinary bladder.	_____	2. cortex
Tubules leading from the glomerular capsule. Urine is formed there as water, sugar, and salts are reabsorbed into the bloodstream.	_____	3. glomerular capsule
Inner (middle) region of the kidney.	_____	4. calices
Muscular sac that serves as a reservoir for urine.	_____	5. renal pelvis
Cup-like divisions of the renal pelvis that receive urine from the renal tubules.	_____	6. glomerulus
Tube carrying urine from the bladder to the outside of the body.	_____	7. medulla
Central urine-collecting basin in the kidney that narrows into the ureter.	_____	8. renal tubules
Collection of capillaries through which materials from the blood are filtered into the glomerular capsule.	_____	9. urinary bladder
Outer region of the kidney.	_____	10. ureters

7

Give the medical terms for the following conditions related to urine or substances in urine.

1. sugar in urine ____________________
2. protein in urine ____________________
3. painful urination ____________________
4. scanty urination ____________________
5. bacteria in urine ____________________
6. excessive urination ____________________
7. blood in urine ____________________
8. ketones in urine ____________________
9. absence of urination ____________________
10. pus in urine ____________________
11. excessive urination at night ____________________

evolve *Please visit the Evolve website for additional exercises, games, and images related to this chapter.*

7

CHAPTER 8

Female Reproductive System

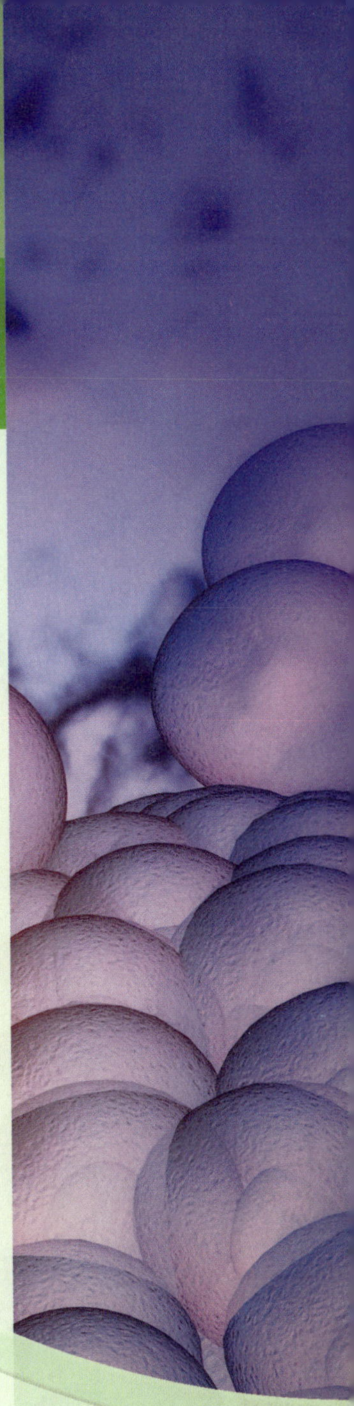

This chapter is divided into the following sections:

CHAPTER GOALS

- Name and locate female reproductive organs and learn their combining forms.
- Explain how these organs and their hormones function in the normal processes of ovulation, menstruation, and pregnancy.
- Identify abnormal conditions of the female reproductive system and of the newborn.
- Describe important laboratory tests and clinical procedures used in gynecology and obstetrics, and recognize related abbreviations.
- Apply your new knowledge to understanding medical terms in their proper contexts, such as medical reports and records.

INTRODUCTION

Sexual reproduction is the union of the nuclei of the **ovum** (the female sex cell) and the **sperm** cell (the male sex cell) that results in the creation of an embryo. The ovum and the sperm cell are specialized cells that differ from normal body cells. Each sex cell, known as a **gamete,** contains exactly half the number of chromosomes of a normal body cell. When the nuclei of ovum and sperm cell unite, the cell produced receives half of its genetic material from its female parent and half from its male parent; thus, it contains a full, normal complement of hereditary material.

Special organs called **gonads** in males and females produce the egg and sperm cells. The female gonads are the **ovaries,** and the male gonads are the **testes.** After an ovum leaves the ovary, it travels down one of two **fallopian tubes** leading to the **uterus** (womb). If **coitus** (copulation, sexual intercourse) has occurred and sperm cells travel into the fallopian tube, they can penetrate the ovum. This is **fertilization.** The fertilized ovum is then known as a **zygote.** After many cell divisions, a ball of cells forms, and the zygote is called an **embryo** (2 to 8 weeks) and finally a **fetus** (8 to 38 or 40 weeks). The period of development within the uterus is **gestation,** or **pregnancy.**

The female reproductive system consists of organs that produce **ova** and provide a place for the growth of the embryo. In addition, the female reproductive organs supply important hormones that contribute to the development of female secondary sex characteristics (body hair, breast development, structural changes in bones and fat).

The eggs, or ova, are present from birth in the female ovary but begin to mature and are released from the ovary in a 21- to 28-day cycle when secondary sex characteristics develop. The occurrence of the first cycle is called **menarche.** Menstrual cycles continue until **menopause,** when all eggs have been released, hormone production diminishes, and menstruation ends. If fertilization occurs during the years between menarche and menopause, the fertilized egg may grow and develop within the uterus. A new, blood vessel–rich **organ** called a **placenta** (connected to the embryo by the umbilical cord) develops to nourish the embryo, which implants in the uterine lining. Various hormones are secreted from the ovary and from the placenta to stimulate the expansion of the placenta. If fertilization does not occur, hormone changes result in shedding of the uterine lining, and bleeding, or **menstruation,** occurs.

The hormones of the ovaries, **estrogen** and **progesterone,** play important roles in the processes of menstruation and pregnancy, and in the development of secondary sex characteristics. The **pituitary gland,** located at the base of the brain, secretes other hormones that govern the reproductive functions of the ovaries, breasts, and uterus.

Gynecology is the study of the female reproductive system (organs, hormones, and diseases); **obstetrics** (Latin *obstetrix* means midwife) is a specialty concerned with pregnancy and the delivery of the fetus; and **neonatology** is the study of the care and treatment of the newborn.

ORGANS OF THE FEMALE REPRODUCTIVE SYSTEM

UTERUS, OVARIES, AND ASSOCIATED ORGANS

Label Figures 8-1 and 8-3 as you read the following description of the female reproductive system.

Figure 8-1 shows a side view of the female reproductive organs and their relationship to the other organs in the pelvic cavity. The **ovaries** [1] (only one ovary is shown in this lateral view) are a pair of small almond-shaped organs located in the pelvis. The **fallopian tubes** [2] (only one is shown in this view) lead from each ovary to the **uterus** [3], which is a

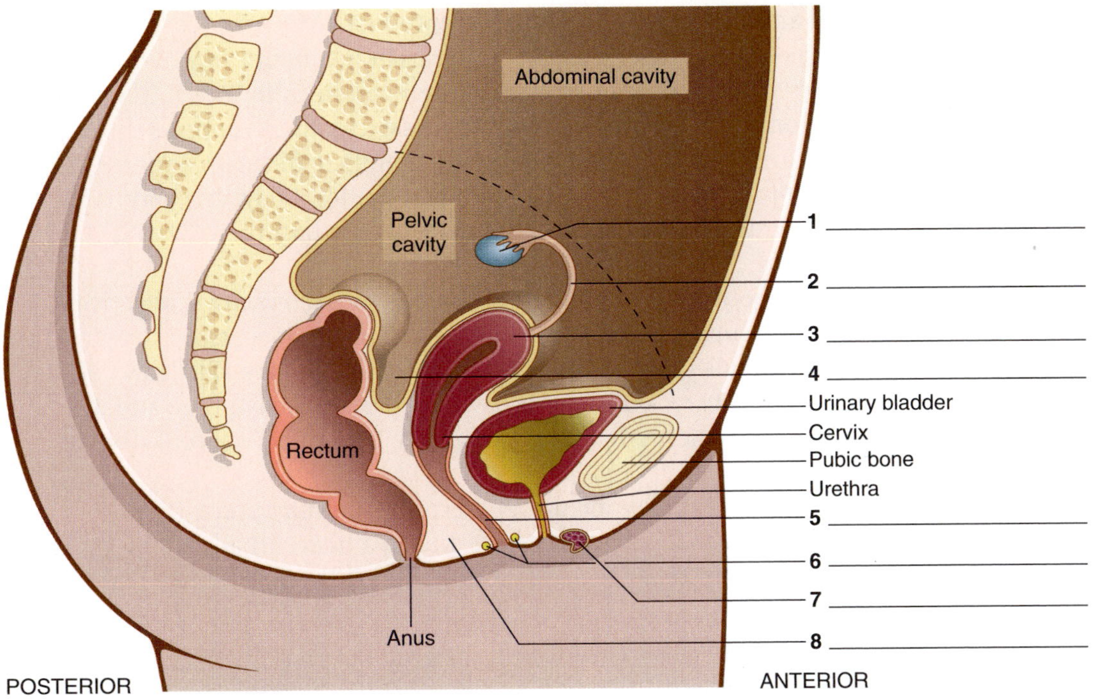

FIGURE 8-1 **Organs of the female reproductive system,** lateral view.

fibromuscular organ situated between the urinary bladder and the rectum. The uterus (womb) normally is the size and shape of a pear and is about 3 inches long in a nonpregnant woman. Midway between the uterus and the rectum is a region in the abdominal cavity known as the **cul-de-sac** [4].

The **vagina** [5], a tubular structure, extends from the uterus to the exterior of the body. **Bartholin glands** [6] are two small, rounded glands on either side of the vaginal orifice. These glands produce a mucous secretion that lubricates the vagina. The **clitoris** [7] is an organ of sensitive, erectile tissue located anterior to the vaginal orifice and in front of the urethral meatus. The region between the vaginal orifice and the anus is the **perineum** [8].

The external genitalia of the female are collectively called the **vulva.** Figure 8-2 shows the various structures that are part of the vulva. The **labia majora,** the outer lips of the vagina, surround the smaller, inner lips, the **labia minora.** The **hymen,** a thin membrane partially covering the entrance to the vagina, is broken apart during the first episode of intercourse. The clitoris and Bartholin glands also are parts of the vulva.

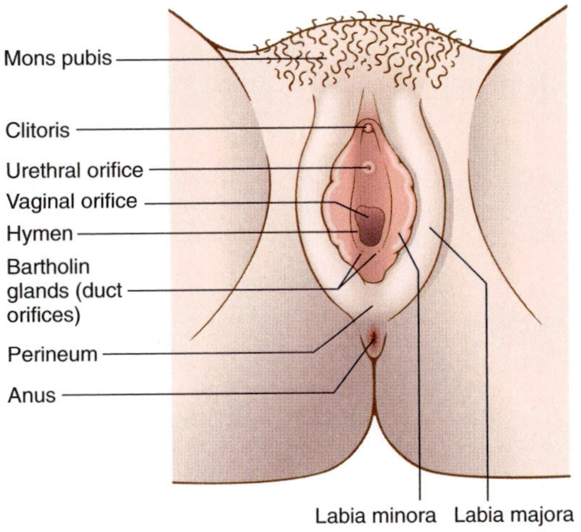

FIGURE 8-2 **Female external genitalia (vulva).** The mons pubis (Latin *mons*, mountain) is a pad of tissue overlying the pubic symphysis. After puberty it is covered with pubic hair.

8

Figure 8-3 shows an anterior view of the female reproductive system. Each **ovary** [1] is held in place on either side of the uterus by a **utero-ovarian ligament** [2].

Within each ovary are thousands of small sacs—the **ovarian follicles** [3]. Each follicle contains an **ovum** [4]. During **ovulation**, an ovum matures; its follicle ruptures through the surface and releases the ovum from the ovary. A ruptured follicle fills with a yellow, fat-like material. It is then called the **corpus luteum** [5], meaning yellow body. The corpus luteum secretes hormones (both estrogen and progesterone) that maintain the very first stages of pregnancy.

A **fallopian tube** [6] is about 5½ inches long and lies near each ovary. Collectively, the fallopian tubes, ovaries, and supporting ligaments are the **adnexae** (accessory structures) of the uterus. The finger-like ends of the fallopian tube are the **fimbriae** [7]. They catch the egg after its release from the ovary. **Cilia** (small hairs) line the fallopian tube and, through their motion, sweep the ovum along. It usually takes the ovum about 2 to 3 days to pass through the fallopian tube.

If sperm cells are present in the fallopian tube, fertilization may occur (Figure 8-4). If sperm cells are not present, the ovum remains unfertilized and eventually disintegrates.

The fallopian tubes, one on each side, lead into the **uterus** [8], a pear-shaped organ with muscular walls and a mucous membrane lining filled with a rich supply of blood vessels. The rounded upper portion of the uterus is the **fundus,** and the larger, central section is the **corpus** (body of the organ). The inner layer, a specialized epithelial mucosa of the uterus is the **endometrium** [9]; the middle, muscular layer of the uterine wall is the **myometrium** [10]; and the outer, membranous tissue layer is the **uterine serosa** [11], a lining that produces a watery, serum-like secretion. The outermost layer of an organ in the abdomen or thorax is known as a serosa.

The narrow, lowermost portion of the uterus is the **cervix** [12] (Latin *cervix* means neck). The cervical opening leads into a 3-inch-long muscular, mucosa-lined canal called the **vagina** [13], which opens to the outside of the body.

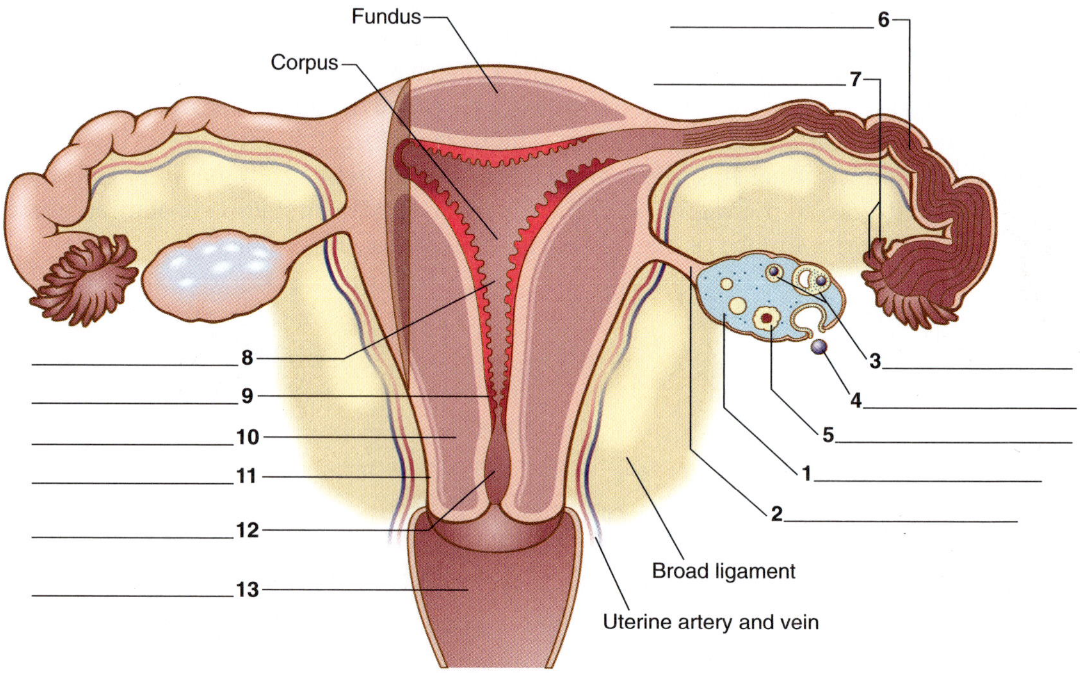

FIGURE 8-3 Organs of the female reproductive system, anterior view.

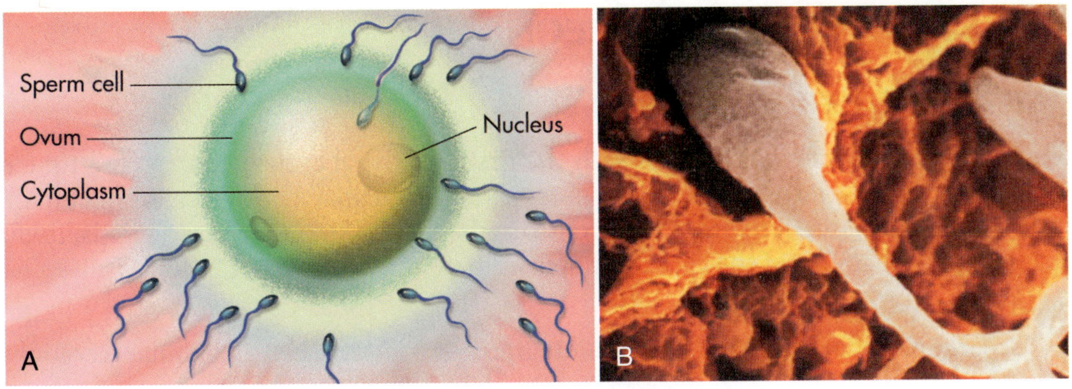

FIGURE 8-4 Fertilization.

THE BREAST (ACCESSORY ORGAN OF REPRODUCTION)

Label Figure 8-5 as you read the following description of breast structures.

The breasts, located on the upper anterior region of the chest, are composed mostly of **mammary glands.** The **glandular tissue** [1] contains milk glands or lobules that develop in response to hormones from the ovaries during puberty. The breasts also contain **fibrous** and **fatty tissue** [2], special **lactiferous** (milk-carrying) **ducts** [3], and **sinuses** (cavities) [4] that carry milk to the nipple, which has small openings for the ducts to release their milk. The breast nipple is the **mammary papilla** [5], and the dark pigmented area around the mammary papilla is the **areola** [6].

During pregnancy the hormones from the ovaries and the placenta stimulate glandular and other tissues in the breasts to their full development. After **parturition** (giving birth), hormones from the pituitary gland stimulate the normal secretion of milk **(lactation).**

8

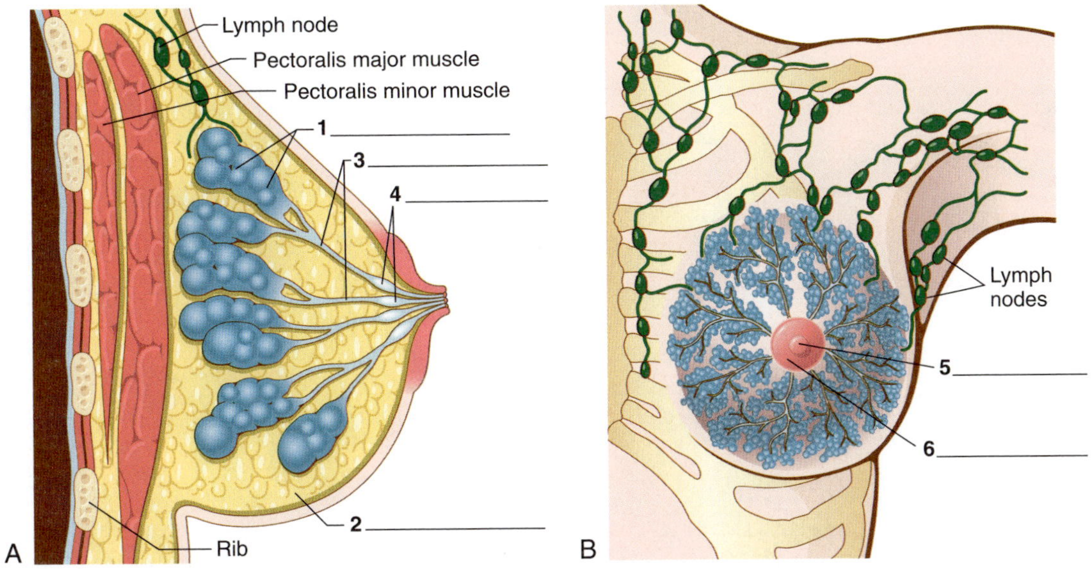

FIGURE 8-5 **Views of the breast. A,** Sagittal. **B,** Frontal. Notice the numerous lymph nodes.

MENSTRUATION AND PREGNANCY

MENSTRUAL CYCLE (FIGURE 8-6)

Menarche, or onset of menstruation with the first menstrual cycle, occurs at the time of puberty. An average menstrual cycle lasts for 28 days but may be shorter or longer, and cycles may be irregular in length. These days can be divided into four time periods, useful in describing the events of the cycle. The approximate time periods are as follows:

Days 1 to 5 (menstrual period)
Discharge of bloody fluid containing disintegrated endometrial cells, glandular secretions, and blood cells.

Days 6 to 12
After bleeding ceases, the endometrium begins to repair itself. The maturing follicle in the ovary releases **estrogen,** which aids in the repair. The ovum grows in the follicle during this period.

Days 13 and 14 (ovulatory period)
On about the 14th day of the cycle, the follicle ruptures and the egg leaves the ovary **(ovulation),** passing through the fallopian tube.

Days 15 to 28
The empty follicle fills with a yellow material and becomes the **corpus luteum.** The corpus luteum functions as an endocrine organ and secretes the hormone **progesterone** into the bloodstream. This hormone stimulates the building up of the lining of the uterus in anticipation of fertilization of the egg and pregnancy.

If fertilization does *not* occur, the corpus luteum in the ovary stops producing progesterone and regresses. At this time, lowered levels of progesterone and estrogen probably are responsible for some women's symptoms of depression, breast tenderness, and irritability before menstruation. The combination of these symptoms is known as **premenstrual syndrome (PMS).** After 2 days of decrease in hormones, the uterine endometrium breaks down, and the menstrual period begins (days 1 to 5).

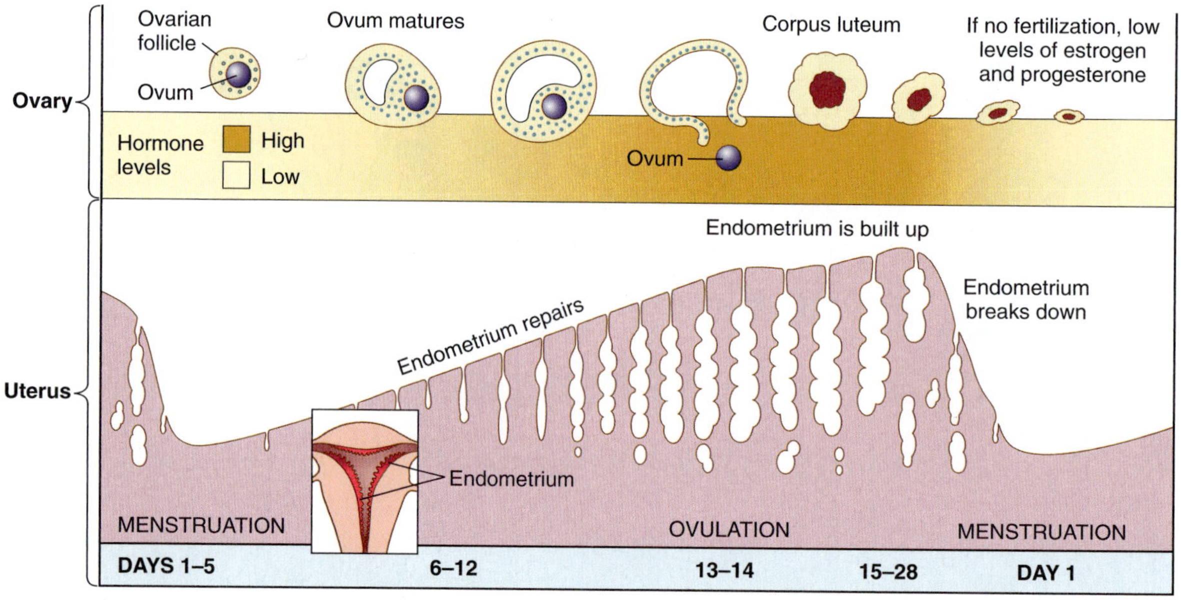

FIGURE 8-6 **The menstrual cycle.** *Tip*: Don't try to memorize this figure. Just get the big picture! In the **ovary,** as the ovum matures, hormone levels rise, culminating in ovulation (days 13 and 14). At the same time, in the **uterus** the endometrium is building up in anticipation of pregnancy. If pregnancy does not occur, hormone levels drop and **menstruation** begins.

Note: Cycles vary in length, ranging from 21 to 42 days or longer. Ovulation typically occurs 14 days before the end of the cycle. A woman with a 42-day cycle ovulates on day 28, whereas a woman with a 21-day cycle ovulates on day 7.

PREGNANCY

If fertilization does occur in the fallopian tube, the fertilized egg travels to the uterus and implants in the uterine endometrium. The corpus luteum in the ovary continues to produce progesterone and estrogen. These hormones support the vascular and glandular development of the uterine lining.

The **placenta,** a vascular organ, now forms, attached to the uterine wall. The placenta is derived from maternal endometrium and from the **chorion,** the outermost membrane that surrounds the developing embryo. The **amnion,** the innermost of the embryonic membranes, holds the fetus suspended in an amniotic cavity surrounded by a fluid called the **amniotic fluid.** The amnion with its fluid is also known as the "bag of waters" or amniotic sac, which ruptures (breaks) during labor.

The maternal blood and the fetal blood never mix during pregnancy, but important nutrients, oxygen, and wastes are exchanged as the blood vessels of the fetus (coming from the umbilical cord) lie side by side with the mother's blood vessels in the placenta. Figure 8-7A and B shows implantation in the uterus and the embryo's relationship to the placenta and enveloping membranes (chorion and amnion).

As the placenta develops in the uterus, it produces its own hormone, **human chorionic gonadotropin (hCG).** When women test their urine with a pregnancy test kit, presence or absence of hCG confirms or rules out that they are pregnant. This hormone stimulates the corpus luteum to continue producing hormones until about the third month of pregnancy, when the placenta takes over the endocrine function and releases estrogen and progesterone. Progesterone maintains the development of the placenta. Low levels of progesterone can lead to spontaneous abortion in pregnant women and menstrual irregularities in nonpregnant women.

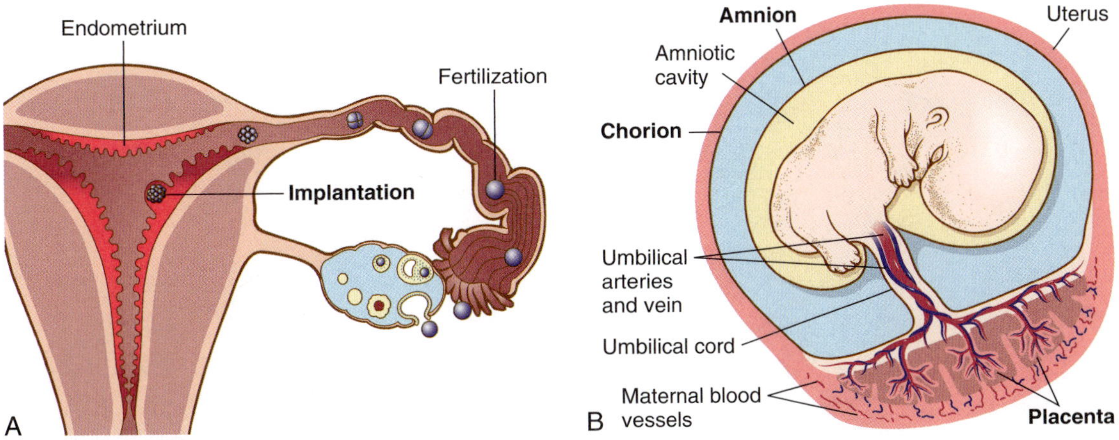

FIGURE 8-7 **A, Implantation of the embryo** in the endometrium. **B,** The **placenta, chorion,** and **amnion** membranes.

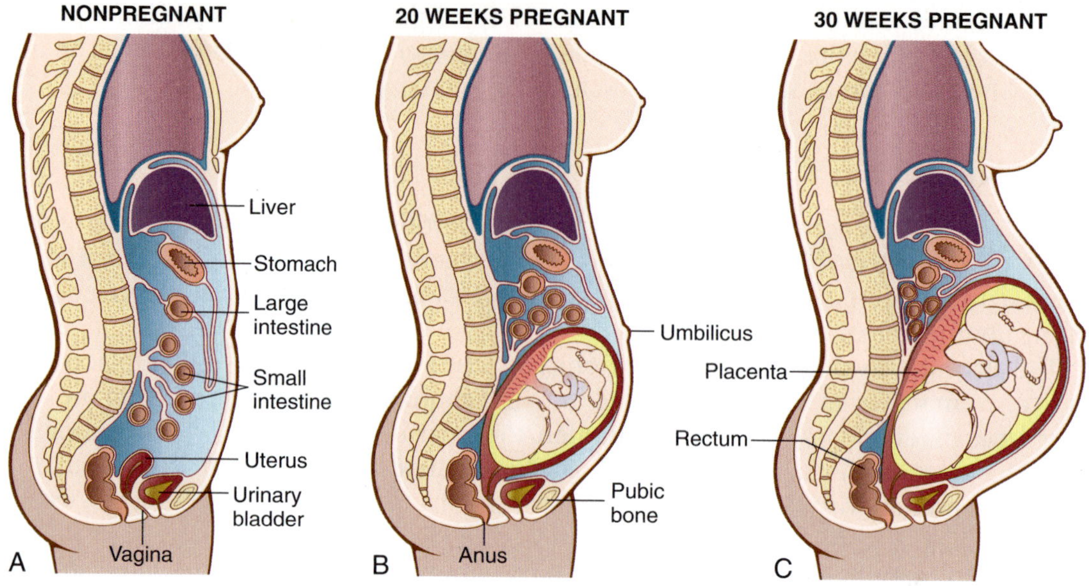

FIGURE 8-8 **The growing uterus changes the pelvic anatomy during pregnancy,** as shown here in sagittal section: **A,** nonpregnant woman, **B,** 20 weeks pregnant, **C,** 30 weeks pregnant.

The uterus normally lies within the pelvis. During pregnancy the uterus expands as the fetus grows, and the superior part rises out of the pelvic cavity to become an abdominal organ. By about 28 to 30 weeks, it occupies a large part of the abdominopelvic cavity and reaches the epigastric region (Figure 8-8).

The onset of true labor is marked by rhythmic contractions, dilation and thinning (effacement) of the cervix, and a discharge of bloody mucus from the cervix and vagina (the "show"). In a normal delivery position, the baby's head appears first (cephalic presentation). After vaginal delivery of the baby, the placenta follows, and the umbilical cord is cut (Figure 8-9). Figures 8-10A and B are photographs of a newborn and the placenta with attached cord, minutes after birth. The expelled placenta is the **afterbirth.**

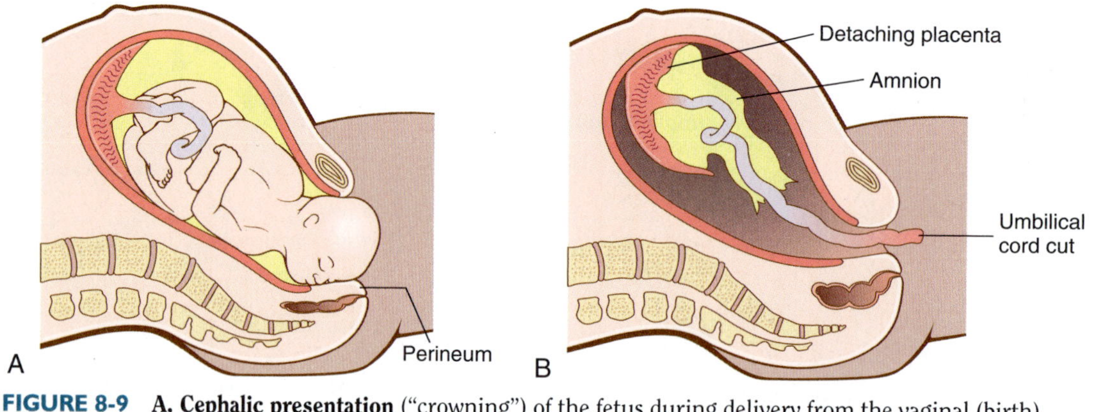

FIGURE 8-9 **A, Cephalic presentation** ("crowning") of the fetus during delivery from the vaginal (birth) canal. **B,** Usually within 15 minutes after parturition (birth), the placenta separates from the uterine wall. Forceful contractions expel the placenta and attached membranes, now called the **afterbirth.** The three phases of labor are (1) dilation of the cervix, (2) expulsion or birth of the infant, and (3) delivery of the placenta.

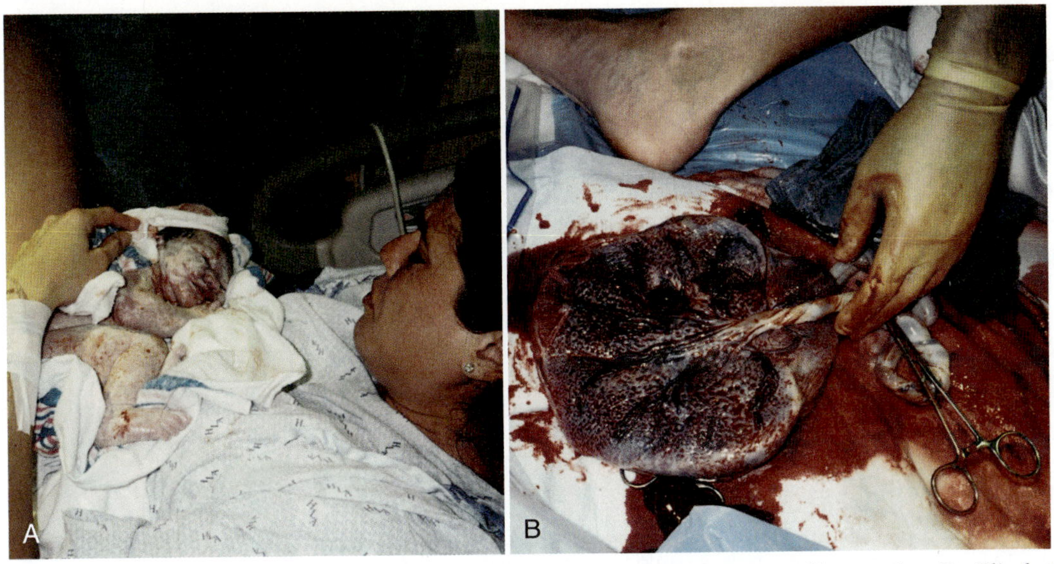

FIGURE 8-10 **A,** My newborn granddaughter, Beatrix Bess (Bebe) Thompson, and her mother, Dr. Elizabeth Chabner Thompson, minutes after Bebe's birth. Notice that Bebe's skin is covered with **vernix caseosa,** a mixture of a fatty secretion from fetal sebaceous (oil) glands and dead skin. The vernix protects the fetus's delicate skin from abrasions, chapping, and hardening as a result of being bathed in amniotic fluid.
B, The **placenta and umbilical cord** just after expulsion from the uterus.

HORMONAL INTERACTIONS

The events of menstruation and pregnancy depend on hormones not only from the ovaries (estrogen and progesterone) but also from the **pituitary gland.** The pituitary gland secretes **follicle-stimulating hormone (FSH)** and **luteinizing hormone (LH)** after the onset of menstruation. As their levels rise in the bloodstream, FSH and LH stimulate maturation of the ovum and ovulation. After ovulation, LH in particular influences the maintenance of the corpus luteum and its production of estrogen and progesterone.

During pregnancy, the high levels of estrogen and progesterone from the ovary and placenta cause the pituitary gland to stop producing FSH and LH. Therefore, while a woman is pregnant, additional eggs do not mature and ovulation cannot occur. Oral contraceptives (birth control pills) work in the same way.

Another female birth control method is an **IUD (intrauterine device).** A physician inserts the IUD, a small device designed to remain inside the uterus. It works by preventing implantation of the embryo. Birth control pills and an IUD do not protect a woman against sexually transmitted disease or HIV infection. See page 290 for a table of contraceptive choices and their features.

When all of the ova are released and secretion of estrogen from the ovaries lessens, **menopause** begins. Menopause signals the gradual ending of the menstrual cycle. Premature menopause occurs before age 45, whereas delayed menopause occurs after age 55. Artificial menopause occurs if the ovaries are removed by surgery or made nonfunctional as a result of radiation therapy or some forms of chemotherapy.

How do birth control pills work?

Birth control pills contain a combination of estrogen and progesterone. When taken as directed, they increase the levels of these hormones in your bloodstream. High levels of estrogen and progesterone send a signal to the pituitary gland to shut down its secretion of follicle-stimulating hormone (FSH) and luteinizing hormone (LH). When these hormones are blocked, the ovaries will NOT release eggs and pregnancy cannot occur! During pregnancy, levels of estrogen and progesterone are ALSO high, and the ovaries will not release eggs then either! So, birth control pills effectively fool the body into "thinking" that you are pregnant and your ovaries stop producing eggs.

During menopause, when estrogen levels fall, the most common signs and symptoms are hot flashes (temperature regulation in the brain is disturbed), insomnia, and vaginal atrophy (lining of the vagina dries and thins, predisposing the affected woman to irritation and discomfort during sexual intercourse). **Hormone replacement therapy (HRT),** given orally or as a transdermal patch or vaginal ring, relieves these symptoms of menopause and delays the development of weak bones (osteoporosis). HRT use may be associated with an increased risk of breast cancer, endometrial cancer, stroke, or heart attack. This therapy should be used only after careful consideration of potential risks and benefits.

VOCABULARY

The following list reviews many of the new terms introduced in the text. Short definitions reinforce your understanding of the terms.

adnexae uteri	Fallopian tubes, ovaries, and supporting ligaments.
amnion	Innermost membranous sac surrounding the developing fetus.
areola	Dark-pigmented area surrounding the breast nipple.
Bartholin glands	Small mucus-secreting exocrine glands at the vaginal orifice (opening to outside of the body). Caspar Bartholin was a Danish anatomist, who described the glands in 1637.
cervix	Lower, neck-like portion of the uterus.
chorion	Outermost layer of the two membranes surrounding the embryo; it forms the fetal part of the placenta.
clitoris	Organ of sensitive erectile tissue anterior to the opening of the female urethra.
coitus	Sexual intercourse; copulation. Pronunciation is KŌ-ĭ-tus.
corpus luteum	Empty ovarian follicle that secretes progesterone after release of the egg cell; literally means yellow (luteum) body (corpus).
cul-de-sac	Region in the lower abdomen, midway between the rectum and the uterus.
embryo	Stage in prenatal development from 2 to 8 weeks.
endometrium	Inner, mucous membrane lining of the uterus.
estrogen	Hormone produced by the ovaries; promotes female secondary sex characteristics.
fallopian tube	One of a pair of ducts through which the ovum travels to the uterus; also called an **oviduct.** The tubes were named for Gabriello Fallopia, an Italian anatomist.
fertilization	Union of the sperm cell and ovum from which the embryo develops.
fetus	Stage in prenatal development from 8 to 39 or 40 weeks.
fimbriae (*singular:* fimbria)	Finger- or fringe-like projections at the end of the fallopian tubes.
follicle-stimulating hormone (FSH)	Secreted by the pituitary gland to stimulate maturation of the egg cell (ovum).
gamete	Male or female sexual reproductive cell; sperm cell or ovum.

genitalia	Reproductive organs; also called genitals.
gestation	Period from fertilization of the ovum to birth.
gonad	Female or male reproductive organ that produces sex cells and hormones; ovary or testis.
gynecology	Study of the female reproductive organs including the breasts.
human chorionic gonadotropin (hCG)	Hormone produced by the placenta to sustain pregnancy by stimulating (-tropin) the ovaries to produce estrogen and progesterone.
hymen	Mucous membrane partially or completely covering the opening to the vagina.
labia	Lips of the vagina; labia majora are the larger, outermost lips, and labia minora are the smaller, innermost lips.
lactiferous ducts	Tubes that carry milk within the breast.
luteinizing hormone (LH)	Secreted by the pituitary gland to promote ovulation.
mammary papilla	Nipple of the breast. A **papilla** is any small nipple-shaped projection.
menarche	Beginning of the first menstrual period and ability to reproduce.
menopause	Gradual ending of menstruation.
menstruation	Monthly shedding of the uterine lining. The flow of blood and tissue normally discharged during menstruation is called the **menses** (Latin *mensis* means month).
myometrium	Muscle layer of the uterus.
neonatology	Branch of medicine that studies the disorders and care of the newborn (neonate).
obstetrics	Branch of medicine concerned with pregnancy and childbirth.
orifice	An opening.
ovarian follicle	Developing sac enclosing each ovum within the ovary. Only about 400 of these sacs mature in a woman's lifetime.
ovary	One of a pair of female organs (gonads) on each side of the pelvis. Ovaries are almond-shaped, about the size of large walnuts, and produce egg cells (ova) and hormones.
ovulation	Release of the ovum from the ovary.
ovum (*plural:* **ova**)	Mature egg cell (female gamete). Ova develop from immature egg cells called oocytes.
parturition	Act of giving birth.
perineum	In females, the area between the anus and the vagina.
pituitary gland	Endocrine gland at the base of the brain. It produces hormones that stimulate the ovaries. The pituitary gland also regulates other endocrine organs.
placenta	Vascular organ attached to the uterine wall during pregnancy. It permits the exchange of oxygen, nutrients, and fetal waste products between mother and fetus.
pregnancy	Condition in a female of having a developing embryo and fetus in her uterus for about 40 weeks.

progesterone	Hormone produced by the corpus luteum in the ovary and the placenta of pregnant women.
puberty	Point in the life cycle at which secondary sex characteristics appear and gametes are produced.
uterine serosa	Outermost layer surrounding the uterus.
uterus	Hollow, pear-shaped muscular female organ in which the embryo and fetus develop, and from which menstruation occurs. The upper portion is the fundus; the middle portion is the corpus; and the lowermost, neck-like portion is the cervix (see Figure 8-3, page 260).
vagina	Muscular, mucosa-lined canal extending from the uterus to the exterior of the body.
vulva	External female genitalia; includes the labia, hymen, clitoris, and vaginal orifice.
zygote	Stage in prenatal development from fertilization and implantation up to 2 weeks.

TERMINOLOGY

Write the meanings of the medical terms in the spaces provided.

COMBINING FORMS

COMBINING FORM	MEANING	TERMINOLOGY	MEANING
amni/o	amnion	amniocentesis	______________________
		amniotic fluid *Produced by fetal membranes and the fetus.*	______________________
bartholin/o	Bartholin gland	bartholinitis *A Bartholin cyst is a fluid-filled sac caused by blockage of a duct from the Bartholin gland. If bacterial infection occurs, an abscess may form.*	______________________
cervic/o	cervix, neck	endocervicitis	______________________
chori/o, chorion/o	chorion	chorionic	______________________
colp/o	vagina	colposcopy	______________________
culd/o	cul-de-sac	culdocentesis *A needle is placed through the posterior wall of the vagina and fluid is withdrawn for diagnostic purposes.*	______________________
episi/o	vulva	episiotomy *An incision through the skin of the perineum enlarges the vaginal orifice for delivery. The incision is repaired by* ***perineorrhaphy.***	______________________
galact/o	milk	galactorrhea *Abnormal, persistent discharge of milk, commonly seen with pituitary gland tumors.*	______________________

COMBINING FORM	MEANING	TERMINOLOGY	MEANING
gynec/o	woman, female	gynecomastia ______ *Enlargement of breasts in a male. It often occurs with puberty or aging, or the condition can be drug-related.*	
hyster/o	uterus, womb	hysterectomy ______ ***Total abdominal hysterectomy (TAH)*** *is removal of the entire uterus (including the cervix) through an abdominal incision (Figure 8-11).* ***Vaginal hysterectomy (VH)*** *is removal through the vagina.* ***Laparoscopic supracervical hysterectomy*** *(see Figure 8-11) is a partial hysterectomy that preserves the cervix.*	
		hysteroscopy ______ *A gynecologist uses an endoscope (passed through the vagina and cervix) to view the uterine cavity.*	
lact/o	milk	lactation ______ *The normal secretion of milk.*	
mamm/o	breast	inframammary ______ *Infra- means below.*	
		mammoplasty ______ *Includes reduction and augmentation (enlargement) operations.*	

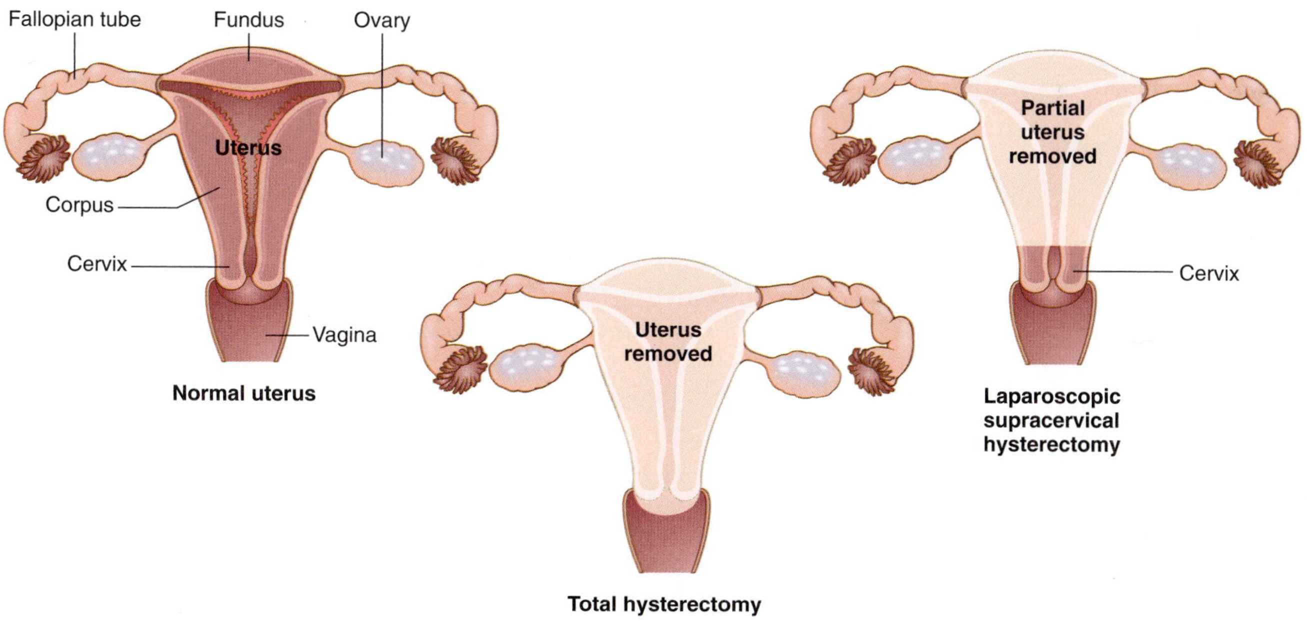

FIGURE 8-11 **Normal uterus and hysterectomies. Total hysterectomy** is removal of the entire uterus—fundus, corpus, and cervix. This may be performed via an abdominal incision or vaginally. **Laparoscopic supracervical hysterectomy** is removal of the top portion of the uterus (above the cervix), leaving the cervix intact. Three to five small incisions are made in the abdomen and the uterus is removed via laparoscope. Robotic hysterectomy (da Vinci surgery) is another option using small incisions, three-dimensional vision, and a magnified view of the surgical site.

COMBINING FORM	MEANING	TERMINOLOGY	MEANING
mast/o	breast	mastitis *Usually caused by streptococcal or staphylococcal infection.*	
		mastectomy *Mastectomy procedures are discussed under carcinoma of the breast (see page 278).*	
men/o	menses, menstruation	amenorrhea *Absence of menses for 6 months or for longer than three of the patient's normal menstrual cycles.*	
		dysmenorrhea	
		oligomenorrhea *Infrequent menstrual periods or scanty menses.*	
		menorrhagia *Abnormally heavy or long menstrual periods.* ***Fibroids*** *(see page 276) are a leading cause of menorrhagia.*	
metr/o, metri/o	uterus	metrorrhagia *Bleeding between menses. Possible causes of metrorrhagia include ectopic pregnancy, cervical polyps, and ovarian and uterine tumors.*	
		menometrorrhagia *Excessive uterine bleeding during and between menstrual periods.*	
my/o, myom/o	muscle, muscle tumor	myometrium	
		myomectomy *Removal of fibroids (myomas) from the uterus.*	
nat/i	birth	neonatal	
obstetr/o	pregnancy and childbirth	obstetrics *From the Latin obstetrix, midwife.*	
o/o	egg	oogenesis	
		oocyte *Immature ovum.*	
oophor/o	ovary	oophorectomy *Oophor/o means to bear (phor/o) eggs (o/o). In a bilateral oophorectomy, both ovaries are removed.*	
ov/o	egg	ovum *Mature egg cell.*	
ovari/o	ovary	ovarian	
ovul/o	egg	anovulatory	
perine/o	perineum	perineorrhaphy	

COMBINING FORM	MEANING	TERMINOLOGY	MEANING
phor/o	to bear	oophoritis	______
salping/o	fallopian tubes	salpingectomy *Figure 8-12 shows a total hysterectomy with bilateral salpingo-oophorectomy (BSO).*	______
uter/o	uterus	uterine prolapse	______
vagin/o	vagina	vaginal orifice *An orifice is an opening.*	______
		vaginitis *Bacteria and yeasts (usually* Candida*) commonly cause this infection. Use of antibiotic therapy may cause loss of normal vaginal bacteria, resulting in an environment allowing yeast to grow.*	______
vulv/o	vulva	vulvovaginitis	______
		vulvodynia *Chronic pain (with no identifiable cause) that affects the vulvar area (labia, clitoris, and vaginal opening).*	______

SUFFIXES

SUFFIX	MEANING	TERMINOLOGY	MEANING
-arche	beginning	menarche	______
-cyesis	pregnancy	pseudocyesis *Pseudo- means false. No pregnancy exists, but physical changes such as weight gain and amenorrhea occur.*	______
-gravida	pregnant	primigravida *A woman during her first pregnancy (primi- means first). Gravida also is used to designate a pregnant woman, often followed by a number to indicate the number of pregnancies (gravida 1, 2, 3).*	______

8

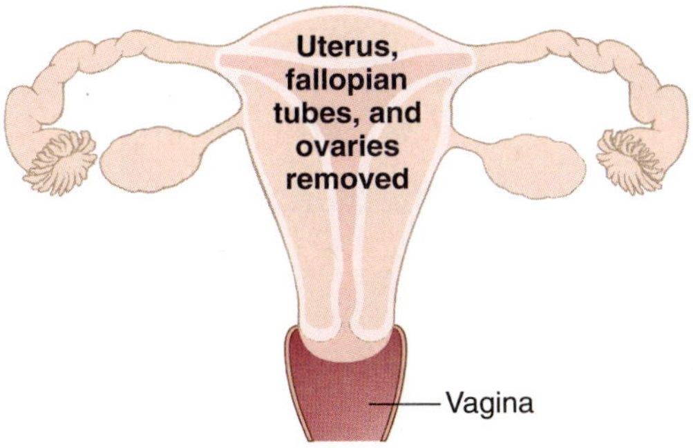

FIGURE 8-12 **Total hysterectomy with bilateral salpingo-oophorectomy.**

SUFFIX	MEANING	TERMINOLOGY	MEANING
-parous	bearing, bringing forth	primiparous *An adjective describing a woman who has given birth to at least one child.* ***Para*** *also is used as a noun, often followed by a number to indicate the number of deliveries after the 20th week of gestation (para 1, para 2, para 3). When a woman arrives in the birthing facility, her gravidity and parity are important facts to include in the medical and surgical history. For example, G2P2 is medical shorthand for a woman who has had 2 pregnancies and 2 deliveries.*	
-rrhea	discharge	leukorrhea *This vaginal discharge is normal or becomes more yellow (purulent or pus-containing) as a sign of infection.*	
		menorrhea	
-salpinx	fallopian (uterine) tube	pyosalpinx	
-tocia	labor, birth	dystocia	
		oxytocia *Oxy- means rapid. The pituitary gland releases* ***oxytocin,*** *which stimulates the pregnant uterus to contract (labor begins). It also stimulates milk secretion from mammary glands.*	
-version	act of turning	cephalic version *The fetus turns so that the head is the body part closest to the cervix (version can occur spontaneously or can be performed by the obstetrician).* ***Fetal presentation*** *is the manner in which the fetus appears to the examiner during delivery. A* ***breech presentation*** *is buttocks first, or feet first in a footling breech; a* ***cephalic presentation*** *is head first.*	

8

PREFIXES

PREFIX	MEANING	TERMINOLOGY	MEANING
dys-	painful	dyspareunia *(dĭs-pă-ROO-nē-ă.) Pareunia means sexual intercourse.*	
endo-	within	endometritis *Usually caused by a bacterial infection.*	
in-	in	involution of the uterus *Vol- means to roll. The uterus returns to its normal nonpregnant size.*	
intra-	within	intrauterine device *Figure 8-13A shows an IUD.*	

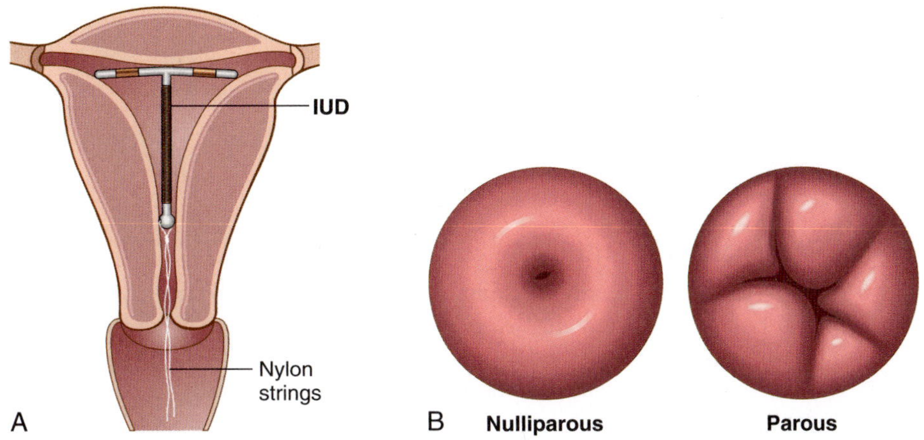

FIGURE 8-13 **A, Intrauterine device (IUD)** in place to prevent implantation of a fertilized egg. **B,** The cervix of a **nulliparous** woman (the os, or opening, is small and perfectly round) and the cervix of a **parous** woman (the os is wide and irregular). These views would be visible under **colposcopic examination**.

PREFIX	MEANING	TERMINOLOGY	MEANING
multi-	many	multipara	_______________
		multigravida	_______________
		A woman who has been pregnant more than once.	
nulli-	no, not, none	nulligravida	_______________
		nullipara	_______________
		Para 0. Figure 8-13B shows the cervix of a nulliparous woman and the cervix of a parous woman (who has had a vaginal delivery).	
pre-	before	prenatal	_______________
primi-	first	primipara	_______________
retro-	backward	retroversion	_______________
		The uterus is abnormally tilted backward. This occurs in 30% of women.	

8

PATHOLOGY: GYNECOLOGIC, BREAST, PREGNANCY, AND NEONATAL

GYNECOLOGIC

Uterus

carcinoma of the cervix

Malignant cells within the cervix (cervical cancer).

Infection with **human papillomavirus (HPV)** is the most important cause of and risk factor for cervical cancer. Other factors that may act together with HPV to increase the risk of developing cervical cancer include cigarette smoking, having multiple sexual partners, and having a weakened immune system (e.g., patients with AIDS). HPV infection is one of the most common sexually transmitted infections in the world. Some types of HPV cause **genital warts** (benign growths on the vulva, cervix, vagina, or anus), whereas others cause cancer, especially HPV types 16 and 18.

Although most HPV infections do not progress to cervical cancer, the risk of developing cancer increases as Pap tests (see page 282) become abnormal and biopsies reveal **dysplasia** (abnormal cell growth), or more seriously, **carcinoma in situ (CIS),** a localized form of cancer (Figure 8-14). Local resection **(conization)** may be necessary to treat CIS and prevent development of invasive cancer. Figure 8-15 shows a normal cervix and one with cervical cancer.

Surgical treatment for cervical cancer requires **radical (complete) hysterectomy,** in which the entire uterus with ligaments, supportive tissues, and the top one third of the vagina are removed. Radiation therapy and chemotherapy are used to treat disease that has spread beyond the uterus, into the pelvis, and to distant organs.

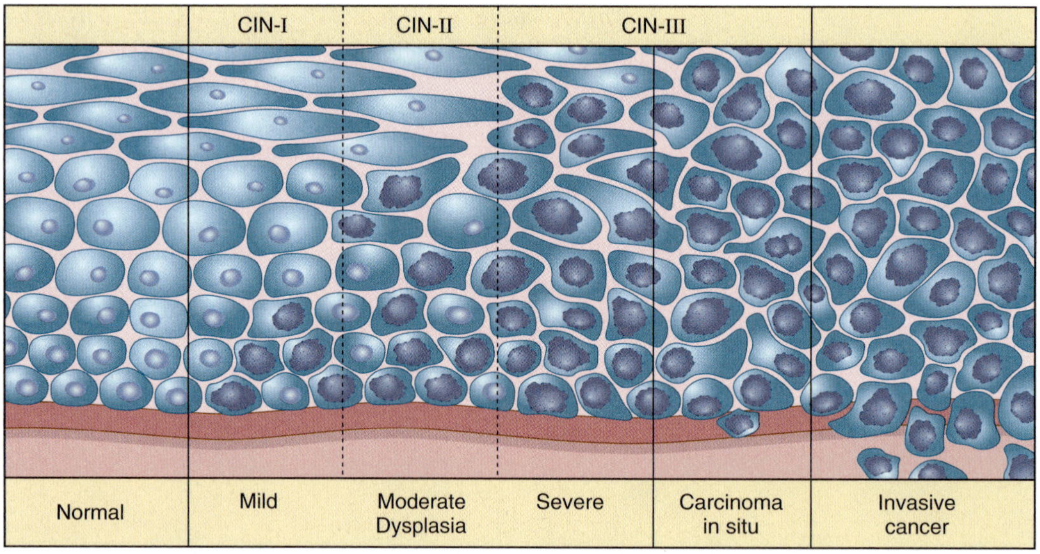

FIGURE 8-14 Preinvasive neoplastic lesions are called **cervical intraepithelial neoplasia (CIN).** Pathologists diagnose such lesions from a **Pap test** (microscopic examination of cells scraped from cervical epithelium) and grade them as CIN I to CIN III.

HPV Vaccine

In 2006, the U.S. Food and Drug Administration (FDA) approved Gardasil, the first vaccine developed to prevent cervical cancer, precancerous genital lesions, and genital warts due to human papillomavirus (HPV) types 6, 11, 16, and 18. **HPV vaccine** is recommended for girls 11 to 12 years of age. The vaccine is also recommended for females aged 13 to 26 years who have not been previously vaccinated. It is important for girls to get HPV vaccine before their first sexual contact. For these girls, the vaccine can prevent almost 100% of disease caused by the four types of HPV targeted by the vaccine. Papillomavirus also causes cancer of the throat (oropharynx) and nasal passages and cancer of the penis. The FDA has licensed two HPV vaccines for use in young males.

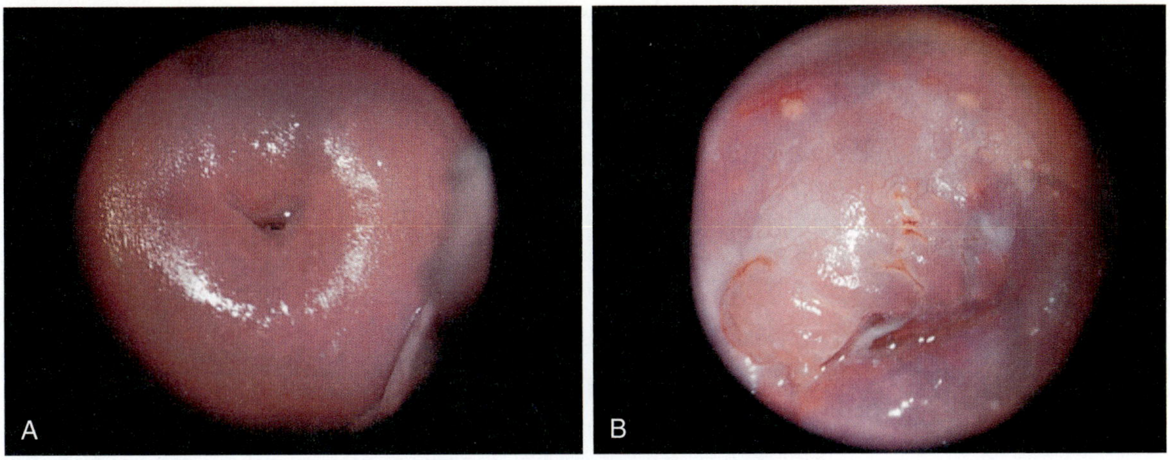

FIGURE 8-15 **Normal cervix (A)** and **cervix with cervical cancer (B)** as seen via **colposcopy.**

cervicitis

Inflammation of the cervix.

This condition can become chronic because the lining of the cervix is not renewed each month as is the uterine lining during menstruation.

Bacteria such as *Chlamydia trachomatis* and *Neisseria gonorrhoeae* commonly cause cervicitis. Acute cervicitis, marked by **cervical erosions** or ulcerations, appears as raw, red patches on the cervical mucosa. **Leukorrhea** (clear, white, or yellow pus-filled vaginal discharge) also is a sign of cervical erosion.

After the presence of malignancy has been excluded (by Pap test or biopsy), **cryocauterization** (destroying tissue by freezing) of the eroded area and treatment with antibiotics may be indicated.

carcinoma of the endometrium (endometrial cancer)

Malignant tumor of the uterine lining (adenocarcinoma).

The most common sign of endometrial cancer is postmenopausal bleeding. This malignancy occurs more often in women exposed to high levels of estrogen, either from exogenous estrogen (pills) or estrogen-producing tumors or with obesity (estrogen is produced by fat tissue) and in nulliparous women. Physicians perform endometrial biopsy, hysteroscopy, and **dilation** or **dilatation** (widening the cervical canal) and **curettage** (scraping the inner lining of the uterus) for diagnosis. When the cancer is confined to the uterus, surgery (hysterectomy and bilateral salpingo-oophorectomy) is curative. Radiation oncologists administer radiation therapy as additional treatment.

endometriosis

Endometrial tissue located outside the uterus.

Endometrial tissue may be found in ovaries, fallopian tubes, supporting ligaments or small intestine, causing inflammation and scar tissue. When the endometrium sheds and bleeds in its monthly cycle, it may cause dysmenorrhea and pelvic pain. Infertility (inability to become pregnant) and dyspareunia may also occur. Most cases are the result of growth of bits of menstrual endometrium that have passed backward through the **lumen** (opening) of the fallopian tube and into the peritoneal cavity. Often, when disease affects the ovaries, large blood-filled cysts (endometriomas, or "**chocolate cysts**") develop. Treatment ranges from symptomatic relief of pain and hormonal drugs that suppress the menstrual cycle to surgical removal of ectopic endometrial tissue and hysterectomy.

8

fibroids

Benign tumors in the uterus.

Fibroids, also called **leiomyomata** or **leiomyomas** (lei/o = smooth, my/o = muscle, and -oma = tumor), are composed of fibrous tissue and muscle. If fibroids grow too large and cause symptoms such as metrorrhagia, pelvic pain, or menorrhagia, hysterectomy or myomectomy is indicated. Fibroid ablation (destruction) without surgery may be accomplished by **uterine artery embolization (UAE),** in which tiny pellets (acting as emboli) are injected into a uterine artery, blocking the blood supply to fibroids, causing them to shrink. Figure 8-16, A and B, show the location of uterine fibroids.

Ovaries

ovarian carcinoma (cancer)

Malignant tumor of the ovary (adenocarcinoma).

Each year, about 22,000 women in the United States are diagnosed with ovarian cancer. Two types of ovarian cancer are most common: **serous** (clear fluid) and **mucinous** (thick, pasty fluid) **cystic adenocarcinomas.** The tumor usually is discovered in an advanced stage as an abdominal mass and may produce few symptoms in its early stages. In most patients, the disease metastasizes beyond the ovary before diagnosis and often causes **ascites** (accumulation of fluid in the abdominal cavity). Treatment consists of total abdominal hysterectomy, bilateral salpingo-oophorectomy, and removal of the omentum, which often contains deposits of tumor, followed by chemotherapy. A protein marker produced by tumor cells, CA 125, can be measured in the bloodstream to assess effectiveness of treatment.

Inherited mutations (changes) in genes greatly increase the risk of developing ovarian and breast cancer. These mutations are ***BRCA1*** and ***BRCA2*** (short for breast cancer 1 and breast cancer 2). Women with a strong family history of ovarian cancer (with multiple members of the family affected) may seek genetic counseling to determine if they should be tested for these inherited defects. **Prophylactic** (preventive) **oophorectomy** significantly reduces the odds of developing ovarian cancer if a woman is at high risk.

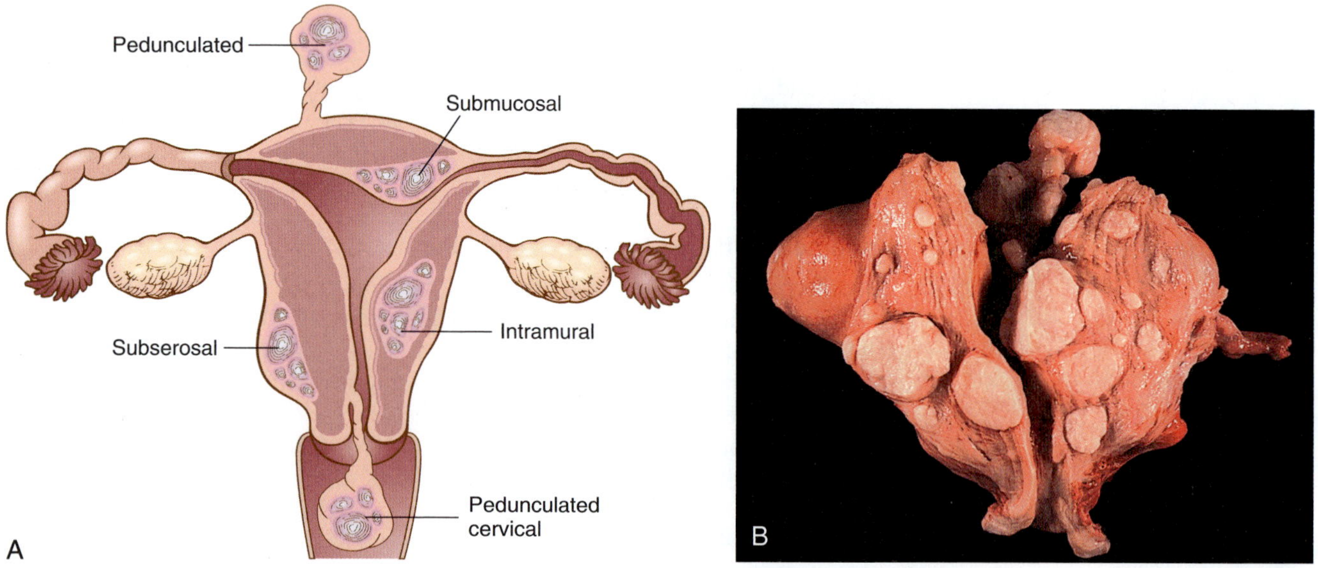

FIGURE 8-16 **A, Location of uterine fibroids (leiomyomas). Pedunculated** growths protrude on stalks. A **subserosal** mass lies under the serosal (outermost) layer of the uterus. A **submucosal** leiomyoma grows under the mucosal (innermost) layer. **Intramural** (mural means wall) masses arise within the muscular uterine wall. **B, Fibroids** shown after hysterectomy.

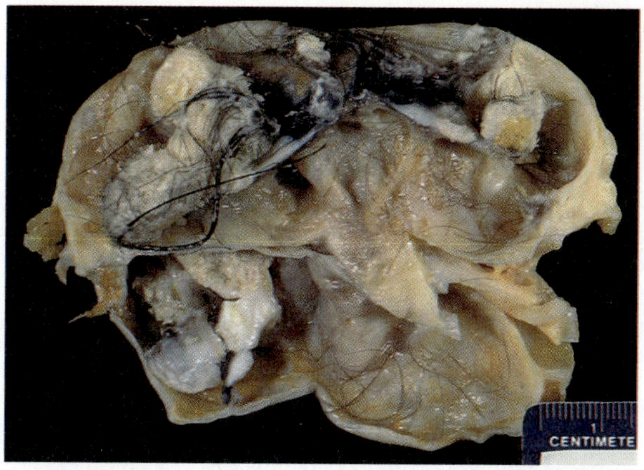

FIGURE 8-17 **Dermoid cyst of the ovary** with hair, skin, and teeth. *(Courtesy Dr. Elizabeth Chabner Thompson.)*

ovarian cysts

Collections of fluid within a sacs (cysts) in the ovary.

Some cysts are benign and lined by typical cells of the ovary. These cysts originate in unruptured ovarian follicles (follicular cysts) or in follicles that have ruptured and have immediately been sealed (luteal cysts). Other cysts are malignant and lined with atypical or tumor cells (**cystadenocarcinomas**). Physicians decide to remove these cysts to distinguish between benign and malignant tumors.

Dermoid cysts contain a variety of cell types, including skin, hair, teeth, and cartilage, and arise from immature egg cells in the ovary. Because of the strange assortment of tissue types in the tumor (Figure 8-17), this tumor often is called a benign cystic **teratoma** (terat/o = monster) or a **mature teratoma.** Surgical removal of the cyst cures the condition. Cysts are bilateral 15% of the time.

Fallopian Tubes

pelvic inflammatory disease (PID)

Inflammation and infection of organs in the pelvic region; salpingitis, oophoritis, endometritis, endocervicitis.

The leading causes of PID are **sexually transmitted diseases (STDs).** Repetitive episodes of these infections lead to formation of adhesions and scarring within the fallopian tubes. After PID, women have an increased risk of ectopic pregnancy and infertility. Signs and symptoms include fever, vaginal discharge, abdominal pain in the left and right lower quadrants (LLQ and RLQ), and tenderness to **palpation** (examining by touch) of the cervix. Antibiotics treat PID.

Sexually Transmitted Diseases (STDs) or Infections (STIs)

Examples of bacterial and viral STDs in women are:

- **gonorrhea** (gonococcal bacteria)
- **chlamydial infection** (chlamydial bacteria)
- **syphilis** (spirochete bacteria)
- **genital herpes** (herpes simplex virus - HSV)
- **HPV infection and genital warts** (human papillomavirus)

More information on STDs in women and men is on page 322.

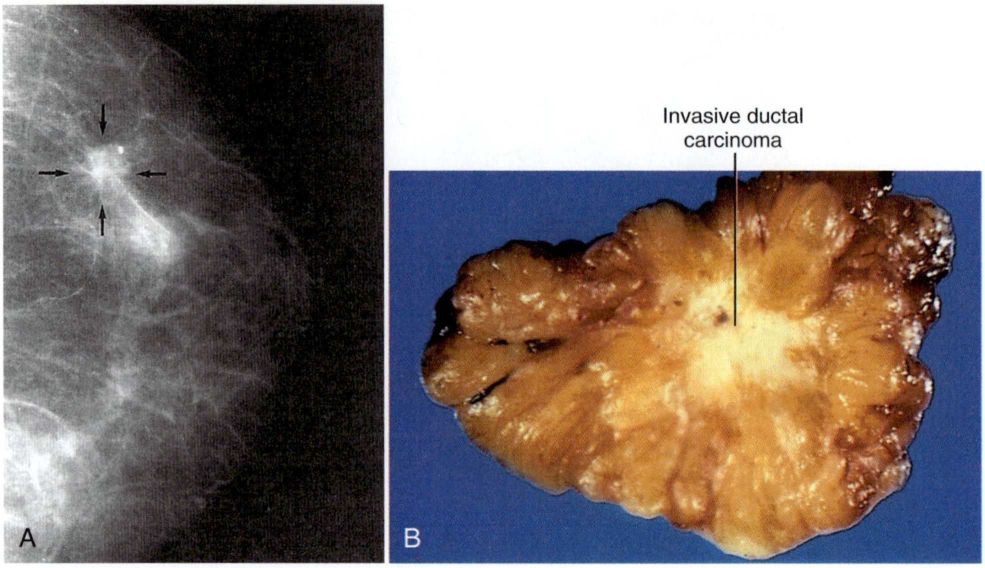

FIGURE 8-18 **A,** *Arrows* in **mammogram** point to invasive carcinoma of the breast. A dense white fragment of calcium is seen at 2 o'clock in the mass; calcifications like this are frequently a sign of cancer. **B,** Cut section of **invasive ductal carcinoma** of the breast.

BREAST

8

carcinoma of the breast (breast cancer)

Malignant tumor of the breast (arising from milk glands and ducts).

The most common type of breast cancer is **invasive ductal carcinoma.** Figure 8-18A shows the tumor on a mammogram. Figure 8-18B shows a cut section of an invasive ductal carcinoma. Other histopathologic (histo- means tissue) types are **lobular** and **medullary carcinoma** of the breast.

Breast cancer spreads first to lymph nodes in the axilla (armpit) adjacent to the affected breast and then to the skin and chest wall. From the lymph nodes it also may metastasize to other body organs, including bone, liver, lung, and brain. The diagnosis is first established by biopsy, either needle aspiration, or surgical removal of the specimen. A **stereotactic core needle biopsy** uses mammography to guide a biopsy needle into an area of concern. See the **"In Person"** account of stereotactic needle core biopsy on page 291.

For small primary tumors, the lump with immediately surrounding tissue can be removed **(lumpectomy).** To determine whether the tumor has spread to lymph nodes, a **sentinel node biopsy (SNB)** is performed. For this procedure, a blue dye or a radioisotope is injected into the tumor site and tracks to the axillary (underarm) lymph nodes. See Figure 8-19. After lumpectomy, radiation therapy to the breast and to any involved lymph nodes then follows, to kill remaining tumor cells.

An alternative surgical procedure is **mastectomy** (Figure 8-20A), which is removal of the breast. After either lumpectomy or mastectomy if lymph nodes are involved with cancer, adjuvant (aiding) chemotherapy is given to prevent recurrence of the tumor. Breast reconstruction is an option after mastectomy. See Figure 8-20B.

After surgery, further treatment may be indicated to prevent recurrence. To determine which treatment is best, it is important to test the breast cancer tumor for the presence of **estrogen receptors (ERs).** These receptor proteins indicate that the tumor will respond to hormonal therapy. If metastases should subsequently develop, this information will be valuable in selecting further treatment. There are two types of drugs that block the effects of estrogen and thereby kill ER-positive

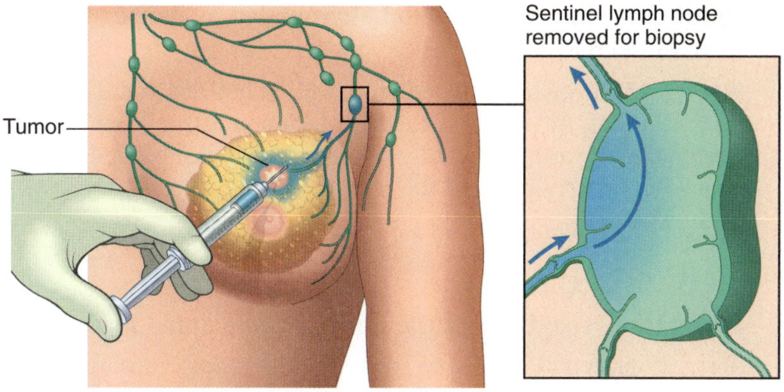

FIGURE 8-19 Sentinel node biopsy. After injection of dye or radioisotope, its path is visualized and the sentinel (first) lymph node is identified. It is the one most likely to contain a tumor if cells have left the breast. The sentinel node is removed and biopsied. If it is negative for tumor cells, the breast cancer has not spread.

breast cancer cells. Drugs of the first type directly block the ER reception. An example is **tamoxifen.** Drugs of the second type block the production of estrogen by inhibiting the enzyme, aromatase. These **aromatase inhibitors** are particularly useful in treating postmenopausal women. Examples are anastrozole (Arimidex) and letrozole (Femara).

A second receptor protein, **her-2/neu,** is found in some breast cancers and signals a high risk of tumor recurrence. **Herceptin,** an antibody that binds to and blocks her-2/neu, is effective in stopping growth when used with chemotherapy. **Triple-negative tumors** lack estrogen, progesterone, and her-2/neu and are highly aggressive.

Testing for hereditary mutations, ***BRCA1*** and ***BRCA2***, is advised for women with a strong family history of breast cancer. Some women who test positively for the breast cancer genes elect to have prophylactic (preventive) bilateral mastectomy with reconstruction, to eliminate risk of developing a new breast cancer.

8

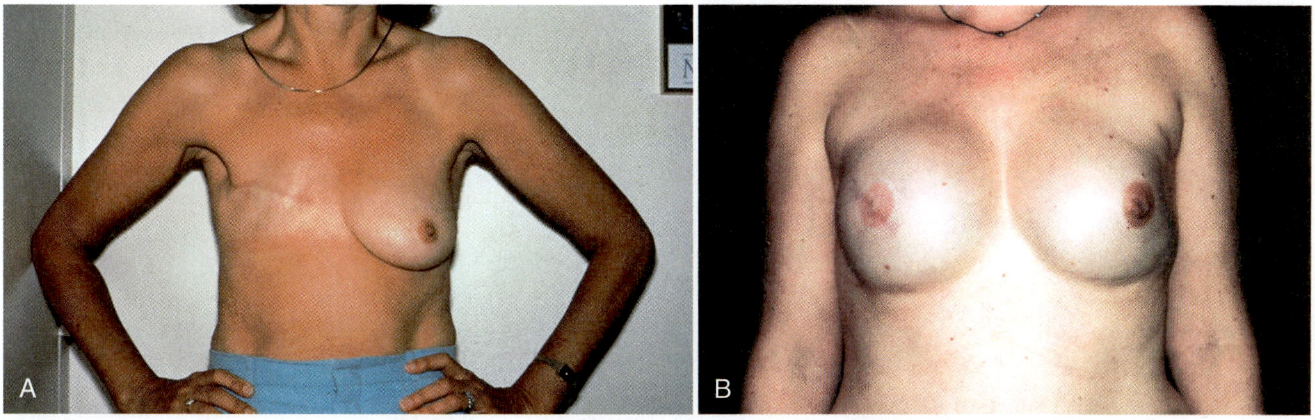

FIGURE 8-20 A, Surgical scar, mastectomy, right breast. A **modified radical mastectomy** removes the breast and axillary lymph nodes (usually 20 to 30 nodes). *(Courtesy Dr. Elizabeth Chabner Thompson.)* **B, Reconstruction of right breast after skin-sparing mastectomy.** A gel silicone implant was used. At a second operation, local tissue was manipulated to create the semblance of a nipple/areola complex. The procedure was completed by tattooing color around the nipple. In this patient, the left breast tissue was removed prophylactically and a silicone implant was inserted via an inframammary incision.

fibrocystic breast disease

Numerous small sacs of fluid surrounded by dense strands of fibrous tissue in the breast.

Women with this common benign condition notice a nodular (lumpy) consistency of the breast, often associated with premenstrual tenderness and fullness. Mammography and surgical biopsy are often indicated to differentiate fibrocystic changes from carcinoma of the breast.

PREGNANCY

abruptio placentae

Premature separation of the normally implanted placenta.

Abruptio placentae (Latin *ab*, away from; *ruptus*, ruptured) occurs because of trauma, such as a fall, or may be secondary to vascular insufficiency resulting from hypertension or preeclampsia (see page 281). Signs and symptoms of acute abruption include sudden searing (burning) abdominal pain and bleeding. It is an obstetric emergency.

ectopic pregnancy

Implantation of the fertilized egg in any site other than the normal uterine location.

The condition occurs in 15% of pregnancies, and 90% of these occur in the fallopian tubes **(tubal pregnancy).** Rupture of the ectopic implant within the fallopian tube can lead to massive abdominal bleeding and death. Surgeons can remove the implant, or treatment with medication (methotrexate) can destroy it, thereby preserving the fallopian tube before rupture occurs. Other sites of ectopic pregnancy include the ovaries and abdominal cavity; whatever the location, ectopic pregnancy often constitutes a surgical emergency.

8

multiple gestations

More than one fetus inside the uterus.

Multiple births are increasing in the United States (often because of in vitro fertilization procedures; see page 287). These pregnancies are at higher risk for preterm delivery, growth restriction, high blood pressure, and diabetes.

placenta previa

Implantation of the placenta over the cervical opening or in the lower region of the uterus (Figure 8-21).

Maternal signs and symptoms include painless bleeding, hemorrhage, and premature labor. Cesarean delivery usually is recommended.

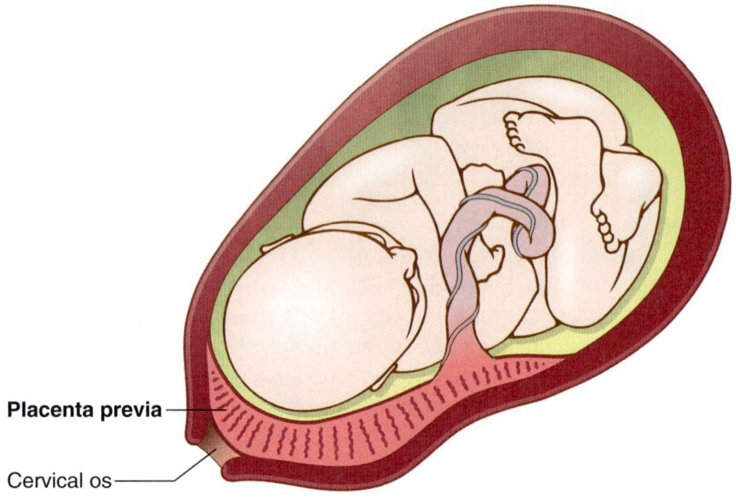

FIGURE 8-21 Placenta previa. Previa means before or in the front of. Three forms of this abnormal implantation of the placenta are: **placenta accreta** (on the wall but not in muscle), **placenta increta** (in uterine muscle), and **placenta percreta** (attaching to another organ).

preeclampsia

Abnormal condition associated with pregnancy, marked by high blood pressure, proteinuria, edema, and headache.

Mild preeclampsia can be managed by bed rest and close monitoring of blood pressure. Women with severe preeclampsia need treatment with medications such as magnesium sulfate to prevent seizures, and the baby is delivered as quickly as possible. The Greek word *eklampein* means to shine forth, referring to the convulsions and hypertension—typically with visual symptoms of flashing lights—that accompany the condition. **Eclampsia** is the final and most severe phase of untreated preeclampsia. It often causes seizures and even death of the mother and baby.

NEONATAL

The following terms describe conditions or symptoms that can affect the newborn. The **Apgar score** (Figure 8-22) is a system of scoring an infant's physical condition 1 and 5 minutes after birth. **Heart rate, respiration, color, muscle tone,** and **response to stimuli** each are rated 0, 1, or 2. The maximum total score is 10. Infants with Apgar scores below 7 require special immediate medical attention such as suctioning of the airways or oxygen to help breathing.

Down syndrome

Chromosomal abnormality (trisomy 21) results in mental retardation, retarded growth, a flat face with a short nose, low-set ears, and slanted eyes.

erythroblastosis fetalis

Hemolytic disease in the newborn (HDN) caused by a blood group (Rh factor) incompatibility between the mother and the fetus. See explanation in Chapter 4, page 119.

8

hyaline membrane disease

Acute lung disease commonly seen in the premature newborn.

This condition, also called **respiratory distress syndrome of the newborn (RDS),** is caused by deficiency of **surfactant,** a protein necessary for proper lung function. Surfactant can be administered to the newborn to cure the condition. Hyaline refers to the shiny (hyaline means glassy) membrane that forms in the lung sacs.

SIGN	SCORE		
	0	1	2
Heart rate	Absent	Below 100	Over 100
Respiratory effort	Absent	Slow, irregular	Good, crying
Muscle tone	Limp	Some flexion of extremities	Active motion
Response to catheter in nostril (tested after oropharynx is clear)	No response	Grimace	Cough or sneeze
Color	Blue, pale	Body pink, extremities blue	Completely pink

FIGURE 8-22 Apgar scoring chart. This test is named for anesthesiologist Virginia Apgar (1909-1974), who devised it in 1953. Dr. Joseph Butterfield, in 1963, introduced an "APGAR" acronym as a mnemonic (memory device): Appearance (color), Pulse (heart rate), Grimace (response to catheter in nostril), Activity (muscle tone), and Respiration (respiratory effort).

hydrocephalus

Accumulation of fluid in the spaces of the brain.

In an infant, the entire head can enlarge because the bones of the skull do not completely fuse together at birth. Infants normally have a soft spot or **fontanelle** between the cranial bones that allows for some swelling during the birth of the baby. Hydrocephalus occurs because of a problem in the circulation of fluid within the brain and spinal cord, resulting in fluid accumulation.

meconium aspiration syndrome

Abnormal inhalation of meconium (first stool) produced by a fetus or newborn.

Meconium, a thick, sticky, greenish to black substance, is actually the first stool of the fetus and newborn. If it is inhaled during birth, meconium can block air passages and cause respiratory distress as the lungs fail to expand. **Meconium ileus** is obstruction of the small intestine in the newborn caused by impaction of thick, dry meconium near the ileocecal valve.

pyloric stenosis

Narrowing of the opening of the stomach to the duodenum.

Present at birth; surgical repair of the pyloric opening may be necessary.

CLINICAL TESTS AND PROCEDURES

CLINICAL TESTS

Pap test (Pap smear)

Microscopic examination of stained cells removed from the vagina and cervix.

After inserting a vaginal **speculum** (instrument to hold apart the vaginal walls), the physician uses a small spatula to remove exfoliated (peeling and sloughing off) cells from the cervix and vagina (Figure 8-23). Microscopic analysis of the cell smear detects cervical or vaginal cellular abnormalities.

pregnancy test

Blood or urine test to detect the presence of hCG.

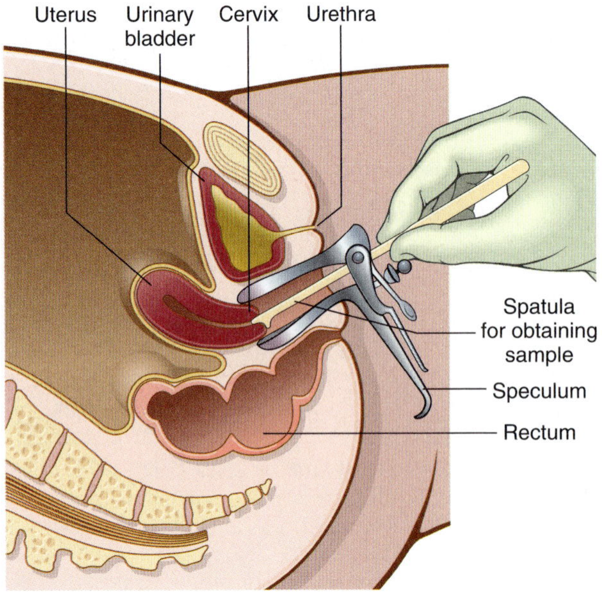

FIGURE 8-23 Method of obtaining a sample for a **Pap test.** The test is 95% accurate in diagnosing early carcinoma of the cervix. It was invented by and named for a Greek physician, Georgios Papanikolaou.

PROCEDURES

X-Ray Studies

hysterosalpingography (HSG) — **X-ray imaging of the uterus and fallopian tubes after injection of contrast material.**

This radiologic procedure is used to evaluate tubal patency (adequate opening) and uterine cavity abnormalities.

mammography — **X-ray imaging of the breast.**

Women are advised to have a baseline mammogram at 40 years of age for later comparison if needed. A mammogram every year is recommended for women older than 40, to screen for breast cancer. Figure 8-24 illustrates mammography.

A new method of mammography is **digital tomosynthesis.** In this procedure, an x-ray tube moves in an arc around the breast as several images are taken. These images are sent to a computer and clear, highly focused three-dimensional pictures are produced. In addition to being less painful, this procedure makes breast cancer easier to find in dense breast tissue.

Ultrasound Examination and Magnetic Resonance Imaging (MRI)

breast ultrasound imaging and breast MRI — **Technologies using sound waves and magnetic waves to create images of breast tissue.**

These imaging techniques confirm the presence of a mass and can distinguish a cystic from a solid mass. MRI is very useful in detecting masses in young women with dense breasts or in women with a strong family history of breast cancer and at high risk for this condition. Breast ultrasound imaging is useful to evaluate a specific area of cancer on a mammogram.

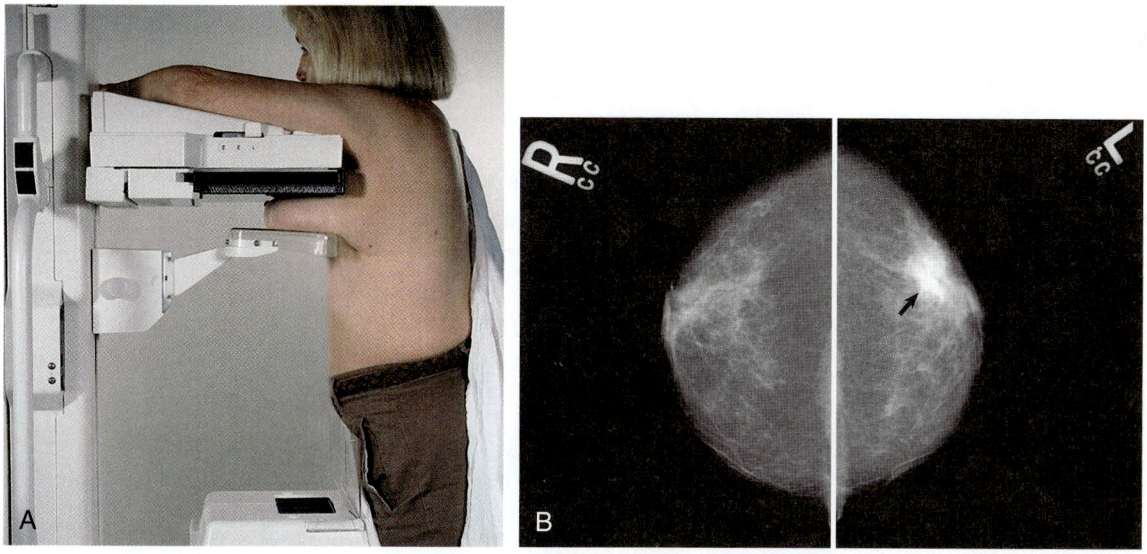

FIGURE 8-24 **A, Mammography.** The machine compresses the breast and x-ray pictures (top to bottom and lateral) are taken. **B, Mammograms** from a 63-year-old woman. The right breast is normal, and the left breast contains a carcinoma.

pelvic ultrasonography

Recording images of sound waves as they bounce off organs in the pelvic region.

This technique can evaluate fetal size, fetal maturity, and organ development, as well as fetal and placental position. Uterine tumors and other pelvic masses, including abscesses, also are diagnosed by ultrasonography. **Transvaginal ultrasound** allows the radiologist a closer, sharper look at organs within the pelvis. The sound probe is placed in the vagina instead of over the pelvis or abdomen; this method is best used to evaluate fluid-filled cysts.

Gynecologic Procedures

aspiration

Withdrawal of fluid from a cavity or sac with an instrument using suction.

Aspiration needle biopsy is a valuable evaluation technique for patients with breast disease.

cauterization

Destruction of tissue by burning.

Destruction of abnormal tissue with chemicals (silver nitrate), or an electrically heated instrument. Cauterization is used to treat cervical dysplasia or cervical erosion. The **loop electrocautery excision procedure (LEEP)** (see Figure 8-26A) is used to further assess and often treat abnormal cervical tissue.

colposcopy

Visual examination of the vagina and cervix using a colposcope.

A colposcope is a lighted magnifying instrument resembling a small, mounted pair of binoculars. Gynecologists prefer colposcopy for pelvic examination when cervical dysplasia is present because it identifies the specific areas of abnormal cells. A biopsy specimen can then be taken for more accurate diagnosis (Figure 8-25).

conization

Removal of a cone-shaped section (cone biopsy) of the cervix.

The physician resects the tissue using a **LEEP (loop electrocautery excision procedure),** or with a carbon dioxide laser or surgical knife (scalpel). Figure 8-26A shows conization with LEEP, and Figure 8-26B shows the cone biopsy specimen removed surgically.

cryosurgery

Use of cold temperatures to destroy tissue.

A liquid nitrogen probe produces the freezing (cry/o means cold) temperature. Also called **cryocauterization.**

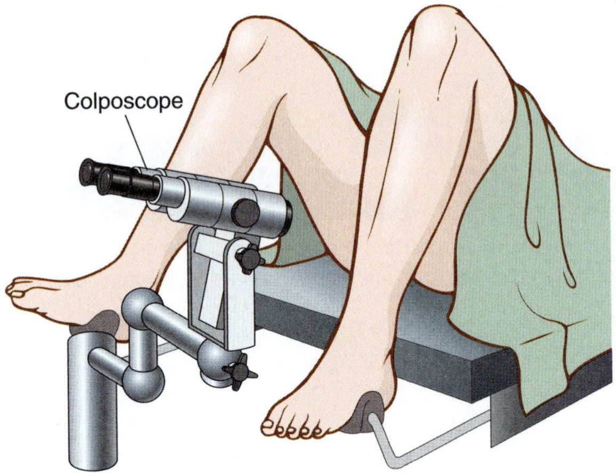

FIGURE 8-25 **Colposcopy** is used to evaluate a patient with an abnormal Pap test. For this examination, the woman lies in the dorsal lithotomy position. This is the same position used to remove a urinary tract stone (lithotomy means incision to remove a stone).

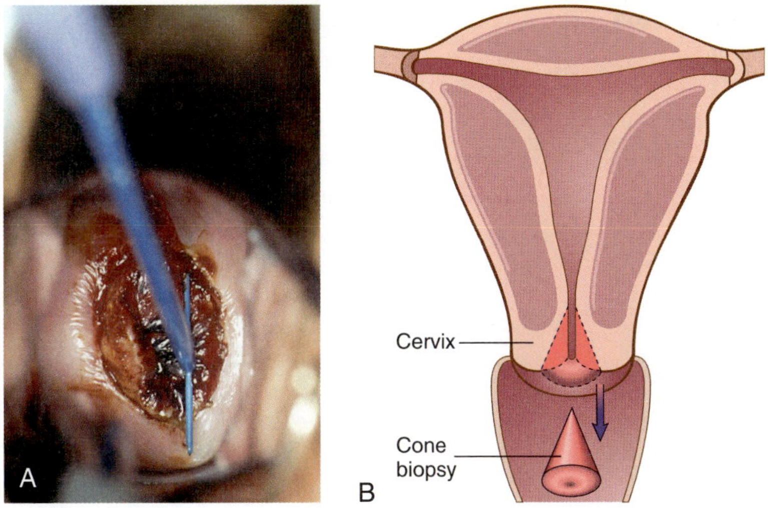

FIGURE 8-26 **A, Cervical loop electrocautery excision procedure (LEEP)** for cone biopsy. **B,** Surgical removal of **cone biopsy** specimen. *(**A,** Courtesy Dr. A. K. Goodman, Massachusetts General Hospital, Boston.)*

culdocentesis

Needle aspiration of fluid from the cul-de-sac.

The physician inserts a needle through the vagina into the cul-de-sac. The presence of blood may indicate a ruptured ectopic pregnancy or ruptured ovarian cyst.

dilation (dilatation) and curettage (D&C)

Widening the cervix and scraping off the endometrial lining of the uterus.

Dilation is accomplished by inserting a series of dilators of increasing diameter. A **curet** (metal loop at the end of a long, thin handle) is then used to sample the uterine lining. This procedure helps diagnose uterine disease and can temporarily halt prolonged or heavy uterine bleeding. When necessary, a D&C is used to remove the tissue during a spontaneous or therapeutic abortion (Figure 8-27).

8

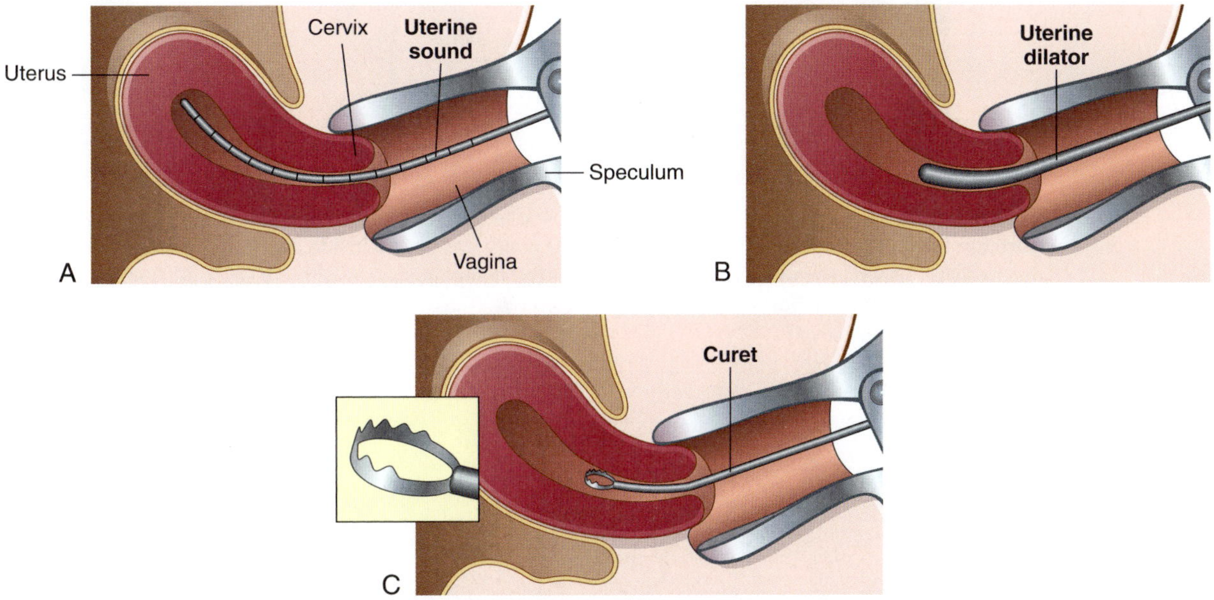

FIGURE 8-27 **Dilation and curettage (D&C) of the uterus. A,** The uterine cavity is explored with a **uterine sound** (a slender instrument used to measure the depth of the uterus) to prevent perforation during dilation. **B, Uterine dilators** (Hanks or Hagar) in graduated sizes are used to gradually dilate the cervix. **C,** The uterus is gently curetted and specimens are collected.

exenteration

Removal of internal organs within a cavity.

Pelvic exenteration is removal of the organs and adjacent structures of the pelvis.

laparoscopy

Visual examination of the abdominal cavity using an endoscope (laparoscope).

In this procedure, a form of **minimally invasive surgery (MIS),** small incisions (5 to 10 mm long) are made near the woman's navel for introduction of the laparoscope and other instruments. Uses of laparoscopy include inspection and removal of ovaries and fallopian tubes, diagnosis and treatment of endometriosis, and removal of fibroids. Laparoscopy also is used to perform subtotal (cervix is left in place) and total hysterectomies (Figure 8-28).

tubal ligation

Blocking the fallopian tubes to prevent fertilization from occurring.

This **sterilization** procedure (making an individual incapable of reproduction) is performed using laparoscopy or through a hysteroscope inserted via the cervical os (opening). **Ligation** means tying off and does not pertain solely to the fallopian tubes—which may be "tied" using clips or bands, or by surgically cutting or burning through the tissue.

Procedures Related to Pregnancy

abortion (AB)

Termination of pregnancy before the embryo or fetus can exist on its own.

Abortions are **spontaneous** or **induced**. Spontaneous abortions, commonly called "miscarriages," occur without apparent cause. Induced abortions can be **therapeutic** or **elective**. A therapeutic abortion is performed when the health of the pregnant woman is endangered. An elective abortion is performed at the request of the woman. Major methods for abortion include vaginal evacuation by D&C or vacuum aspiration (suction) and stimulation of uterine contractions by injection of saline (salt solution) into the amniotic cavity (in second-trimester pregnancies).

8

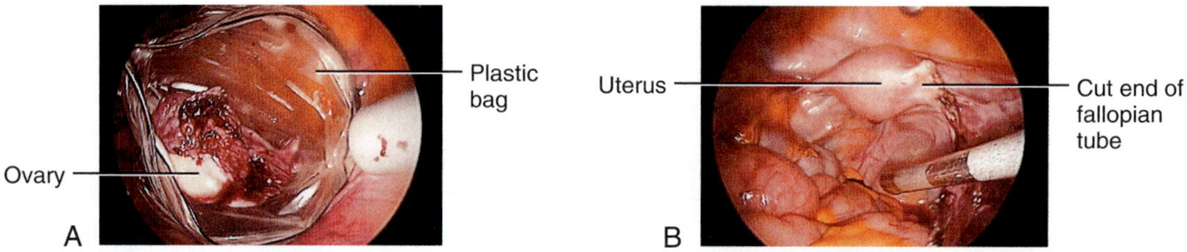

FIGURE 8-28 **Laparoscopic oophorectomy. A,** Notice the ovary placed in a plastic bag. The bag was inserted through the laparoscope and then opened, and the ovary was placed inside. **B,** Both are extracted through the laparoscope, leaving the uterus and the cut end of the fallopian tube. *(Courtesy Dr. A. K. Goodman, Massachusetts General Hospital, Boston.)*

amniocentesis

Needle puncture of the amniotic sac to withdraw amniotic fluid for analysis (Figure 8-29).

The cells of the fetus, found in the fluid, are cultured (grown), and cytologic and biochemical studies are performed to check fetal chromosomes, concentrations of proteins and bilirubin, and fetal maturation.

cesarean section

Surgical incision of the abdominal wall and uterus to deliver a fetus.

Indications for cesarean section include cephalopelvic disproportion (the baby's head is too big for the mother's birth canal), abruptio placentae or placenta previa, fetal distress (fetal hypoxia), and breech or shoulder presentation. The name comes from a law during the time of Julius Caesar requiring removal of a fetus before a deceased pregnant woman could be buried.

chorionic villus sampling (CVS)

Sampling of placental tissues (chorionic villi) for prenatal diagnosis.

The sample of tissue is removed with a catheter inserted into the uterus. The procedure can be performed earlier than amniocentesis, at about 9 to 12 weeks of gestation.

fetal monitoring

Continuous recording of the fetal heart rate and maternal uterine contractions to assess fetal status and the progress of labor.

in vitro fertilization (IVF)

Egg and sperm cells are combined outside the body in a laboratory dish (in vitro) to facilitate fertilization.

After an incubation period of 48 to 72 hours, the fertilized ova are injected into the uterus through the cervix. (Latin *in vitro* means in glass, as used for laboratory containers.) From 30% to 50% of all IVF procedures are now associated with **intracytoplasmic sperm injection** (**ICSI**). This is the direct injection of sperm into harvested ova.

pelvimetry

Measurement of the dimensions of the maternal pelvis.

Pelvimetry helps determine if the mother's pelvis will allow passage of the fetus through the birth canal. This examination is important during protracted labor or with breech presentation.

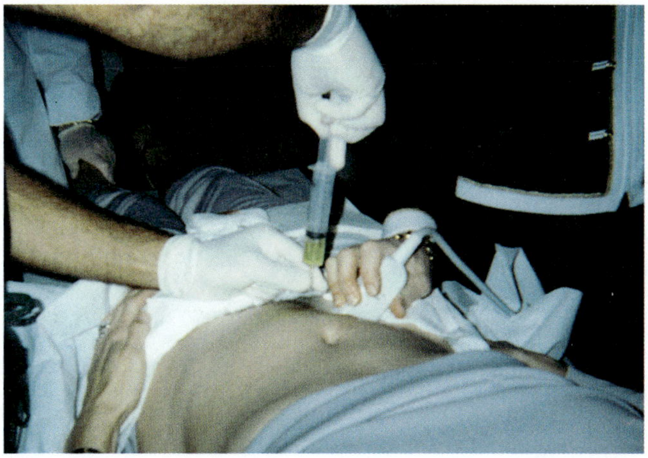

FIGURE 8-29 Amniocentesis. The obstetrician places a long needle through the pregnant woman's abdominal wall into the amniotic cavity. Needle placement (avoiding the fetus and the placenta) is guided by concurrent ultrasound imaging, performed using the transducer in the radiologist's hand. The yellow amniotic fluid is aspirated into the syringe attached to the needle. This procedure took place in the 16th week of pregnancy. The indication for the amniocentesis was a low alpha-fetoprotein (AFP) level. This suggested a higher risk of Down syndrome in the baby. Karyotype analysis (received 10 days later) showed normal chromosome configuration.

8

ABBREVIATIONS

AB	abortion
AFP	alpha-fetoprotein—high levels in amniotic fluid of fetus or maternal serum indicate increased risk of neurologic birth defects in the infant.
BRCA1 BRCA2	breast cancer *1* and *2*—genetic mutations associated with increased risk for breast cancer
BSE	breast self-examination
CA-125	protein marker elevated in ovarian cancer (normal range of values is 0 to 35 U/mL)
C-section, CS	cesarean section
CIN	cervical intraepithelial neoplasia
CIS	carcinoma in situ
CVS	chorionic villus sampling
Cx	cervix
D&C	dilation (dilatation) and curettage
DCIS	ductal carcinoma in situ; a precancerous breast lesion that indicates a higher risk for invasive ductal breast cancer
DUB	dysfunctional uterine bleeding
FHR	fetal heart rate
FSH	follicle-stimulating hormone
G	gravida (pregnant)
GnRH	gonadotropin-releasing hormone—secreted by the hypothalamus to stimulate release of FSH and LH from the pituitary gland
GYN	gynecology
hCG *or* HCG	human chorionic gonadotropin
HDN	hemolytic disease of the newborn
HPV	human papillomavirus
HRT	hormone replacement therapy
HSG	hysterosalpingography
IUD	intrauterine device; contraceptive
IVF	in vitro fertilization
LEEP	loop electrocautery excision procedure
LH	luteinizing hormone
LMP	last menstrual period
multip	multipara; multiparous
OB	obstetrics
para 2-0-1-2	a woman's reproductive history: 2 full-term infants, 0 preterm, 1 abortion, and 2 living children
Pap test	test for cervical or vaginal cancer
PID	pelvic inflammatory disease
PMS	premenstrual syndrome
primip	primipara; primiparous
SLN biopsy *or* SNB	sentinel lymph node biopsy—blue dye or a radioisotope (or both) identifies the first lymph node draining the breast lymphatics
TAH-BSO	total abdominal hysterectomy with bilateral salpingo-oophorectomy
UAE	uterine artery embolization
VH	vaginal hysterectomy

PRACTICAL APPLICATIONS

This section contains an actual operative report and brief excerpts from other medical records using words that you have studied in this and previous chapters. Explanations of more difficult terms are added in brackets.

OPERATIVE REPORT

Preoperative diagnosis: Menorrhagia, leiomyomata

Anesthetic: General

Material forwarded to laboratory for examination:

A. Endocervical curettings
B. Endometrial curettings

Operation performed: Dilation and curettage of the uterus

With the patient in the dorsal lithotomy position [legs are flexed on the thighs, thighs flexed on the abdomen and abducted] and sterilely prepped and draped, manual examination of the uterus revealed it to be 6- to 8-week size, retroflexed; no adnexal masses noted. The anterior lip of the cervix was then grasped with a tenaculum [a hook-like surgical instrument for grasping and holding parts]. The cervix was dilated up to a #20 Hank's dilator. The uterus was sounded [depth measured] up to 4 inches. A sharp curettage of the endocervix showed only a scant amount of tissue. With a sharp curet, the uterus was curetted in a clockwise fashion with an irregularity noted in the posterior floor. A large amount of endometrial tissue was removed. The patient tolerated the procedure well.

Operative diagnosis: Leiomyomata uteri

Recommendation: Hysterectomy for myomectomy

8

SENTENCES USING MEDICAL TERMINOLOGY

1. *Mammogram report:* The breast parenchyma [essential tissue] is symmetrical bilaterally. There are no abnormal masses or calcifications in either breast. The axillae are normal.

2. This is a 43-year-old gravida 3, para 2 with premature ovarian failure and now on HRT. She has history of endocervical atypia [cells are not normal or typical] secondary to chlamydial infection, which is now being treated.

3. The patient is a 40-year-old gravida 3, para 2 admitted for exploratory laparotomy to remove and evaluate a 10-cm left adnexal mass. Discharge diagnosis: (1) endometriosis, left ovary; (2) benign cystic teratoma [dermoid cyst], left ovary.

4. *History:* 51-year-old G3 P3; LMP early 40s; on HRT until age 49 when diagnosed with carcinoma of breast; treated with mastectomy and tamoxifen. Followed by ultrasounds showing slightly thickened 9-10 mm endometrium. No bleeding.
   Operative findings: office endometrial biopsy, scant tissue
   Clinical diagnosis: rule out hyperplasia

OPERATING ROOM SCHEDULE

The operating room schedule for one day in a large general hospital listed six different gynecologic procedures. Match the surgical procedures in Column I with the indications for surgery in Column II. Write the letter of the indication in the blanks provided. Answers are on page 302.

COLUMN I

1. Left oophorectomy ______
2. Vaginal hysterectomy with colporrhaphy ______
3. TAH-BSO, pelvic and periaortic lymphadenectomy ______
4. Exploratory laparotomy for uterine myomectomy ______
5. Conization of the cervix ______
6. Lumpectomy with SLN biopsy ______

COLUMN II

A. LLQ pain; ovarian mass on pelvic ultrasound
B. Fibroids
C. Endometrial carcinoma
D. Small invasive ductal carcinoma of the breast
E. Suspected cervical cancer
F. Uterine prolapse

CONTRACEPTIVE CHOICES

Review and compare the various birth control options available today.

METHOD	UNINTENDED PREGNANCY RATES: TYPICAL USE / PERFECT USE	PROTECTION AGAINST STDs AND HIV INFECTION
1. Abstinence—no sexual intercourse	0% / 0%	100%
2. Cervical cap—inserted by doctor or nurse	16% / 9%	none
3. Condom—male	15% / 2%	some
4. Condom—female	21% / 5%	some
5. Diaphragm (with spermicide)	16% / 6%	none
6. Film and foam (with spermicide)	29% / 18%	none
7. Implant—inserted into upper arm; releases hormones; effective for 3 years	0.05% / 0.05%	none
8. Injectable—Depo-Provera given every 3 months	3% / 3%	none
9. Intrauterine (IUD)	less than 1%	none
10. Oral contraceptives (birth control pills)	8% / 3%	none
11. Patch—applied to skin weekly	8% / 3%	none
12. Ring—inserted in vagina; effective for 1 month	8% / less than 1%	none
13. Sponge—used by women who have never given birth	16% / 9%	none
14. Suppositories—inserted in vagina (with spermicide)	29% / 15%	none
15. Withdrawal	27% / 4%	none

8

IN PERSON

This first-person narrative describes a woman experiencing a stereotactic needle biopsy.

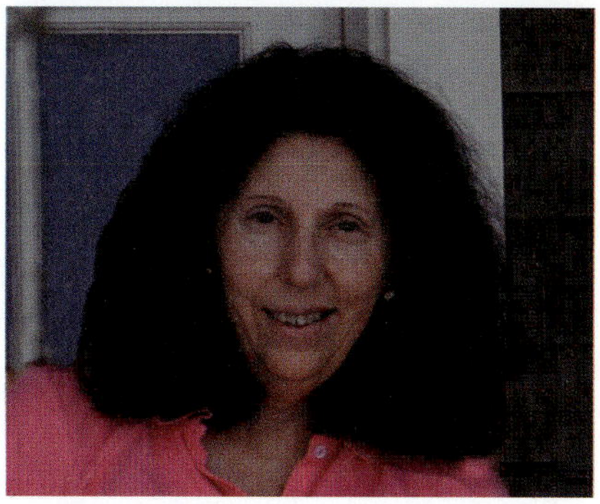

MARY BRAUN: STEREOTACTIC NEEDLE BIOPSY

After three mammograms and one ultrasound all performed within 13 months, I was told that I needed to have a stereotactic biopsy. The mammograms and ultrasounds showed calcifications in my breast that were suspicious. Once you get that letter in the mail with the horrible word, "suspicious," all sorts of negative thoughts begin to seep into your brain. With a family history of breast cancer (my mother died from it at age 50), I was extremely anxious to get this done right away.

As I arrived at the hospital, full of trepidation, I reminded myself of a saying I had read many years ago. It went something like this: "In my life I have known many troubles, most of them never realized." And, with that thought in mind, I walked into the procedure room wearing my lovely orange gown that never seems to tie easily.

The technician was extremely nice and began a long recital of all the procedures that were to follow. (As they say, sometimes ignorance is bliss.) First, they applied a numbing substance to the exterior of my breast, and then injected lidocaine as a local anesthetic. After taking some additional x-ray views, they placed me on the table, face down. The appropriate breast was positioned downward into a chamber so that the radiologist could make a small incision and insert the needle to take samples.

This is a vacuum-assisted biopsy taken using a vacuum-powered instrument to collect multiple tissue samples during one needle insertion. A small titanium marker was left in my breast. (In case of a negative prognosis, the titanium marker serves as a beacon for the surgeon who will remove cancerous tissue in the area.)

The radiologist was very nice, making some small talk with me, and telling me that if anything hurt too much, he would stop. I could tell he was a very kind soul and resigned myself to getting through the next hour. Apart from mild discomfort of the lidocaine injection, the rest of the procedure was relatively pain free. I think that one of the hard parts for patients is trying to lie as still as possible for 30-40 minutes. After they were satisfied that the samples were sufficient, the needle was removed and another technician came to apply pressure to the area for about 10 minutes.

An antiseptic, gauze, and bandage were applied to the wound and instructions given on how to proceed for the next few days. After 24 hours, I was permitted to shower and could change the gauze and bandage. For a day or two, no strenuous exercise was allowed. An additional mammogram was taken before I left the hospital and I was given an ice pack for my breast.

The worst part of this procedure was the anticipation. Who wants to be lying on a table with your boob hanging through a small hole waiting to be punctured with a metal object? To all the women who are reading this and wondering what it will be like, take my word for it, get it done, the worst part is in your head anticipating it.

Mary Braun is Vice President, Investments, at Chapin Davis, Baltimore, Maryland.

8

EXERCISES

Remember to check your answers carefully with the Answers to Exercises, page 300.

A Match the following terms for structures or tissues with their meanings below.

amnion	fallopian tubes	perineum
areola	fimbriae	placenta
cervix	labia	uterine serosa
chorion	mammary papilla	vagina
clitoris	ovaries	vulva
endometrium		

1. inner lining of the uterus ________________
2. area between the anus and the vagina in females ________________
3. dark-pigmented area around the breast nipple ________________
4. finger-like ends of the fallopian tube ________________
5. ducts through which the egg travels into the uterus from the ovary ________________
6. organ of sensitive erectile tissue in females; anterior to urethral orifice ________________
7. nipple of the breast ________________
8. vascular organ that attaches to the uterine wall during pregnancy ________________
9. lower, neck-like portion of the uterus ________________
10. innermost membrane around the developing embryo ________________
11. outermost layer of the membranes around the developing embryo and forming part of the placenta ________________
12. outermost layer surrounding the uterus ________________
13. lips of the vulva ________________
14. female gonads; producing ova and hormones ________________
15. includes the perineum, labia and clitoris, and hymen; external genitalia ________________
16. muscular, mucosa-lined canal extending from the uterus to the exterior of the body

____

B Identify the following terms.

1. fetus ______
2. lactiferous ducts ______
3. gametes ______
4. gonads ______
5. adnexa uteri ______
6. cul-de-sac ______
7. genitalia ______
8. Bartholin glands ______
9. ovarian follicle ______
10. corpus luteum ______

C Match the terms below with their descriptions.

coitus	human chorionic gonadotropin	myometrium
estrogen	luteinizing hormone	prenatal
fertilization	menarche	progesterone
follicle-stimulating hormone		

1. hormone produced by the ovaries; promotes female secondary sex characteristics ______
2. hormone secreted by the pituitary gland to stimulate maturation of the egg cell (ovum) ______
3. sexual intercourse ______
4. before birth ______
5. beginning of the first menstrual period ______
6. hormone produced by the placenta to sustain pregnancy by stimulating the ovaries to produce estrogen and progesterone ______
7. muscle layer of the uterus ______
8. hormone produced by the corpus luteum in the ovary and the placenta of a pregnant woman ______
9. hormone produced by the pituitary gland to promote ovulation ______
10. union of the sperm cell and ovum from which the embryo develops ______

D Supply definitions to complete the following sentences.

1. galact/o and lact/o both mean ______________________________.
2. colp/o and vagin/o both mean ______________________________.
3. mamm/o and mast/o both mean ______________________________.
4. metr/o, uter/o, and hyster/o all mean ______________________________.
5. oophor/o and ovari/o both mean ______________________________.
6. o/o, ov/o, and ovul/o all mean ______________________________.
7. in- and endo- both mean ______________________________.
8. -cyesis and -gravida both mean ______________________________.
9. salping/o and -salpinx both mean ______________________________.
10. episi/o and vulv/o both mean ______________________________.

E Match the following terms with their meanings below.

bilateral salpingo-oophorectomy	lactation	oxytocin
cervicitis	neonatology	total hysterectomy
chorion	obstetrics	vulvovaginitis
culdocentesis		

1. study of the newborn ______________________
2. hormone that stimulates the pregnant uterus to contract ______________________
3. secretion of milk ______________________
4. removal of the entire uterus ______________________
5. inflammation of the neck of the uterus ______________________
6. branch of medicine concerned with pregnancy and childbirth ______________________
7. outermost membrane surrounding the fetus ______________________
8. removal of both fallopian tubes and both ovaries ______________________
9. inflammation of the external female genitalia and vagina ______________________
10. needle puncture to remove fluid from the cul-de-sac ______________________

F Give the meanings of the following signs and symptoms.

1. amenorrhea ______________________________
2. dysmenorrhea ______________________________
3. leukorrhea ______________________________
4. metrorrhagia ______________________________
5. galactorrhea ______________________________
6. menorrhagia ______________________________

7. pyosalpinx ______
8. dyspareunia ______
9. menometrorrhagia ______
10. oligomenorrhea ______

G State whether the following sentences are true or false, and explain your answers.

1. After a total (complete) hysterectomy, a woman still has regular menstrual periods. ______
2. After a total hysterectomy, a woman may still produce estrogen and progesterone. ______
3. Birth control pills prevent pregnancy by keeping levels of estrogen and progesterone high. ______
4. After a total hysterectomy with bilateral salpingo-oophorectomy, a doctor may advise hormone replacement therapy. ______
5. Human papillomavirus can cause genital warts and ovarian cancer. ______
6. A Pap test can detect cervical dysplasia. ______
7. Human chorionic gonadotropin is produced by the ovaries during pregnancy. ______
8. Gynecomastia is a common condition in pregnant women. ______
9. Treatment for endometriosis is uterine myomectomy. ______
10. A gravida 3 para 2 is a woman who has given birth 3 times. ______
11. A nulligravida is a woman who has had several pregnancies. ______
12. Pseudocyesis is the same condition as a tubal pregnancy. ______
13. Fibrocystic changes in the breast are a malignant condition. ______
14. Cystadenomas occur in the ovaries. ______
15. FSH and LH are ovarian hormones. ______

H Give the meanings of the following terms.

1. parturition ______________________________
2. menopause ______________________________
3. menarche ______________________________
4. ovulation ______________________________
5. gestation ______________________________
6. anovulatory ______________________________
7. dilatation ______________________________
8. lactation ______________________________
9. nulliparous ______________________________
10. oophoritis ______________________________
11. bartholinitis ______________________________
12. vulvodynia ______________________________

I Match the following terms with their meanings as given below.

abruptio placentae
cervical carcinoma
cervicitis
cystadenocarcinoma
endometrial carcinoma
endometriosis
leiomyoma
multiple gestations
placenta previa
preeclampsia

1. malignant tumor of the ovary ______________________________
2. chlamydial infection causing inflammation in the lower, neck-like portion of the uterus ______________________________
3. condition during pregnancy or shortly thereafter, marked by hypertension, proteinuria, and edema ______________________________
4. uterine tissue located outside the uterus—for example, in the ovaries, cul-de-sac, fallopian tubes, or peritoneum ______________________________
5. premature separation of a normally implanted placenta ______________________________
6. placenta implantation over the cervical opening ______________________________
7. more than one fetus inside the uterus ______________________________
8. malignant condition that can be diagnosed by a Pap test, revealing dysplastic changes in cells ______________________________
9. malignant condition of the inner lining of the uterus ______________________________
10. benign muscle tumor in the uterus ______________________________

J **Name the appropriate test or procedure for each of the following descriptions.**

1. burning of abnormal tissue with chemicals or an electrically heated instrument ______________________
2. contrast material is injected into the uterus and fallopian tubes, and x-ray images are obtained ______________________
3. cold temperature is used to destroy tissue ______________________
4. visual examination of the vagina and cervix ______________________
5. widening the cervical opening and scraping the lining of the uterus ______________________
6. withdrawal of fluid by suction with a needle ______________________
7. process of recording x-ray images of the breast ______________________
8. removal of a cone-shaped section of the cervix for diagnosis or treatment of cervical dysplasia ______________________
9. surgical puncture to remove fluid from the cul-de-sac ______________________
10. echoes from sound waves create an image of structures in the pelvic region ______________________
11. blocking the fallopian tubes to prevent fertilization from occurring ______________________
12. visual examination of the abdominal cavity with an endoscope ______________________
13. hCG is measured in the urine or blood ______________________
14. cells are scraped from the cervix or vagina for microscopic analysis ______________________
15. removal of internal gynecologic organs and adjacent structures in the pelvis ______________________

K Match the obstetrical and neonatal terms with the descriptions given below.

abortion	fetal monitoring	in vitro fertilization
Apgar score	fetal presentation	meconium aspiration syndrome
cephalic version	fontanelle	pelvimetry
cesarean section	hyaline membrane disease	pyloric stenosis
erythroblastosis fetalis	hydrocephalus	

1. Turning the fetus so that the head presents during birth ____________________
2. Measurement of the dimensions of the maternal pelvic bone ____________________
3. The soft spot between the newborn's cranial bones ____________________
4. The evaluation of the newborn's physical condition ____________________
5. Premature termination of pregnancy ____________________
6. Removal of the fetus by abdominal incision of the uterus ____________________
7. Acute lung disease in the premature newborn: surfactant deficiency ____________________
8. Use of a machine to electronically record fetal heart rate during labor ____________________
9. Narrowing of the opening of the stomach to the small intestine in the infant

   ____
10. Hemolytic disease of the newborn ____________________
11. Accumulation of fluid in the spaces of a neonate's brain ____________________
12. Manner in which the fetus appears to the examiner during delivery ____________________
13. Condition resulting from inhalation of a thick, sticky black substance by the newborn

    ____
14. Union of the egg and sperm cell in a laboratory dish ____________________

8

L Give medical terms for the following definitions. Pay careful attention to spelling.

1. benign muscle tumors in the uterus ____________________
2. no menses ____________________
3. removal of an ovary ____________________
4. condition of female breasts (in a male) ____________________
5. ovarian hormone that sustains pregnancy ____________________
6. nipple-shaped elevation on the breast ____________________

M **Give the meanings of the abbreviations in Column I. Then select the letter of the correct description from Column II.**

COLUMN I		COLUMN II
1. CIS ____________________	________	A. This woman has given birth to more than one infant.
2. FSH ____________________	________	B. Egg and sperm cells are combined outside the body.
3. D&C ____________________	________	C. This woman has given birth for the first time.
4. multip ____________________	________	D. Secretion from the pituitary gland stimulates the ovaries.
5. C-section ____________________	________	E. This procedure helps diagnose uterine disease.
6. IVF ____________________	________	F. Localized cancer growth.
7. Cx ____________________	________	G. Surgical procedure to remove the uterus, fallopian tubes, and ovaries.
8. TAH-BSO ____________________	________	H. Surgical delivery of an infant through an abdominal incision.
9. primip ____________________	________	I. Branch of medicine dealing with pregnancy and delivery of infants.
10. OB ____________________	________	J. Lower, neck-like region of the uterus.

N **Match the following abbreviations in Column I with the best description in Column II.**

COLUMN I		COLUMN II
1. Pap test	________	A. Precancerous lesion in the breast.
2. HSG	________	B. X-ray record of the uterus and fallopian tubes.
3. AB	________	C. Hormones given to menopausal women.
4. HPV	________	D. Diagnoses cervical and vaginal cancer.
5. DCIS	________	E. Termination of pregnancy; spontaneous or induced.
6. HRT	________	F. Cause of cervical cancer.

O **Circle the term in parentheses that best completes the meaning of each sentence.**

1. Dr. Hanson felt that it was important to do a **(culdocentesis, Pap test, amniocentesis)** once yearly on each of her GYN patients to screen for abnormal cells.

2. When Doris missed her period, her doctor checked for the presence of **(LH, IUD, hCG)** in Doris's urine to see if she was pregnant.

3. Ellen was 34 weeks pregnant and experiencing bad headaches and blurry vision, with a 10-pound weight gain in 2 days. Dr. Murphy told her to go to the obstetric emergency department because she suspected **(preeclampsia, pelvic inflammatory disease, fibroids).**

4. Fifty-two-year-old Sally noticed increasing pain, fullness, and swelling in her abdomen. She had a history of ovarian cancer, so her physician recommended (**sentinel node biopsy, pelvic ultrasonography, colposcopy**).

8

5. Clara knew that she should not ignore her fevers and yellow vaginal discharge and the pain in her side. She had previous episodes of **(PMS, PID, HRT)** treated with IV antibiotics. She worried that she might have a recurrence.

6. After years of trying to become pregnant, Jill decided to speak to her **(hematologist, gynecologist, urologist)** about in vitro **(gestation, parturition, fertilization).**

7. To harvest her ova, Jill's physician prescribed hormones to stimulate egg maturation and **(coitus, lactation, ovulation).** Ova were surgically removed and fertilized with sperm cells in a Petri dish.

8. Next, multiple embryos were implanted into Jill's **(fallopian tube, vagina, uterus),** and she received hormones to ensure the survival of at least one embryo.

9. The IVF was successful and after **(abdominal CT, ultrasound examination, pelvimetry),** Jill was told that she would have twins in 8½ months.

10. At 37 weeks, Jill went into labor. Under continuous **(chorionic villus sampling, culdocentesis, fetal monitoring),** two healthy infants were delivered vaginally.

11. At age 41, Carol had a screening (**hysterosalpingogram, mammogram, conization**) of her breasts. The results showed tiny calcium deposits or calcifications, behind her (**areola, chorion, adnexae uteri**). A core needle (**laparoscopy, colposcopy, biopsy**) was performed and showed cells that were an early sign of cancer called (**CIN, DCIS, DUB**). Her surgical oncologist recommended (**lumpectomy, TAH-BSO, chorionic villus sampling**) to remove the calcifications and surrounding tissue as treatment.

8

ANSWERS TO EXERCISES

A

1. endometrium
2. perineum
3. areola
4. fimbriae
5. fallopian tubes
6. clitoris
7. mammary papilla
8. placenta
9. cervix
10. amnion
11. chorion
12. uterine serosa
13. labia
14. ovaries
15. vulva
16. vagina

B

1. embryo from the third month (after 8 weeks) to birth
2. tubes that carry milk within the breast
3. sex cells; the egg and sperm cells
4. organs (ovaries and testes) in the female and male that produce gametes
5. ovaries, fallopian tubes, and supporting ligaments (accessory parts of the uterus)
6. region of the abdomen between the rectum and the uterus
7. reproductive organs (genitals)
8. small exocrine glands at the vaginal orifice that secrete a lubricating fluid
9. developing sac in the ovary that encloses the ovum
10. empty follicle that secretes progesterone after ovulation

C

1. estrogen
2. follicle-stimulating hormone
3. coitus
4. prenatal
5. menarche
6. human chorionic gonadotropin
7. myometrium
8. progesterone
9. luteinizing hormone
10. fertilization

D

1. milk
2. vagina
3. breast
4. uterus
5. ovary
6. egg
7. in, within
8. pregnancy
9. fallopian tube
10. vulva (external female genitalia)

E

1. neonatology
2. oxytocin
3. lactation
4. total hysterectomy
5. cervicitis
6. obstetrics
7. chorion
8. bilateral salpingo-oophorectomy
9. vulvovaginitis
10. culdocentesis

F

1. no menstrual flow
2. painful menstrual flow
3. white discharge (normally from the vagina and also associated with cervicitis)
4. bleeding from the uterus at irregular intervals
5. abnormal discharge of milk from the breasts
6. profuse or prolonged menstrual periods occurring at regular intervals
7. pus in the fallopian (uterine) tubes
8. painful sexual intercourse
9. heavy bleeding at and between menstrual periods
10. scanty menstrual flow

G

1. False. Total hysterectomy means removal of the entire uterus so that menstruation does not occur.
2. True. Total hysterectomy does not mean that the ovaries have been removed.
3. True. Birth control pills contain estrogen and progesterone; high levels prevent ovulation and pregnancy.
4. True. This may be necessary to treat symptoms of estrogen loss (vaginal atrophy, hot flashes) and to prevent bone deterioration (osteoporosis).
5. False. HPV does produce genital warts but not ovarian cancer. In some cases, HPV infection may lead to cervical cancer.
6. True. A Pap test can detect abnormal changes in the cervix from cervical dysplasia to cervical intraepithelial neoplasia (CIN) and CIS (carcinoma in situ).
7. False. The hormone hCG is produced by the *placenta* during pregnancy.
8. False. Gynecomastia is a condition of increased breast development in *males*.
9. False. Myomectomy means removal of muscle tumors (fibroids). Endometriosis is abnormal location of uterine tissue outside the uterine lining.
10. False. A gravida 3 para 2 is a woman who has had two children but is pregnant with her third.
11. False. A nulligravida has had no pregnancies. A multigravida has had many pregnancies.
12. False. A pseudocyesis is a false pregnancy (no pregnancy occurs), and a tubal pregnancy is an example of ectopic pregnancy (pregnancy occurs in the fallopian tube, not in the uterus).
13. False. Fibrocystic changes in the breast are a benign condition.
14. True. Cystadenomas are glandular sacs lined with tumor cells; they occur in the ovaries.
15. False. FSH and LH are pituitary gland hormones. Estrogen and progesterone are secreted by the ovaries.

H

1. act of giving birth
2. gradual ending of menstrual function
3. beginning of the first menstrual period at puberty
4. release of the ovum from the ovary
5. pregnancy
6. pertaining to no ovulation (egg is not released from the ovary)
7. widening
8. natural secretion of milk
9. a woman who has never given birth
10. inflammation of the ovaries
11. inflammation of Bartholin glands
12. pain in the vulva

I

1. cystadenocarcinoma
2. cervicitis
3. preeclampsia
4. endometriosis
5. abruptio placentae
6. placenta previa
7. multiple gestations
8. cervical carcinoma
9. endometrial carcinoma
10. leiomyoma

J

1. cauterization
2. hysterosalpingography
3. cryosurgery or cryocauterization
4. colposcopy
5. dilation (dilatation) and curettage
6. aspiration
7. mammography
8. conization
9. culdocentesis
10. pelvic ultrasonography
11. tubal ligation
12. laparoscopy
13. pregnancy test
14. Pap test
15. pelvic exenteration

K

1. cephalic version
2. pelvimetry
3. fontanelle
4. Apgar score
5. abortion
6. cesarean section
7. hyaline membrane disease (respiratory distress syndrome of the newborn)
8. fetal monitoring
9. pyloric stenosis
10. erythroblastosis fetalis
11. hydrocephalus
12. fetal presentation
13. meconium aspiration syndrome
14. in vitro fertilization

L

1. fibroids or leiomyomata
2. amenorrhea
3. oophorectomy
4. gynecomastia
5. progesterone
6. mammary papilla

M

1. carcinoma in situ: F
2. follicle-stimulating hormone: D
3. dilation (dilatation) and curettage: E
4. multipara: A
5. cesarean section: H
6. in vitro fertilization: B
7. cervix: J
8. total abdominal hysterectomy with bilateral salpingo-oophorectomy: G
9. primipara: C
10. obstetrics: I

N

1. D
2. B
3. E
4. F
5. A
6. C

O

1. Pap test
2. hCG
3. preeclampsia
4. pelvic ultrasonography
5. PID
6. gynecologist; fertilization
7. ovulation
8. uterus
9. ultrasound examination
10. fetal monitoring
11. mammogram; areola; biopsy; DCIS; lumpectomy

Answers to Practical Applications

Operating Room Schedule

1. A
2. F
3. C
4. B
5. E
6. D

8

PRONUNCIATION OF TERMS

To test your understanding of the terminology in this chapter, write the meaning of each term in the space provided. In addition, you may wish to cover the terms and write them by looking at your definitions. Make sure your spelling is correct. The page number after each term indicates where it is defined or used in the book, so you can easily check your responses. You will find complete definitions for all of these terms and audio pronunciations on the Evolve website.

Pronunciation Guide

ā as in āpe	ă as in ăpple
ē as in ēven	ĕ as in ĕvery
ī as in īce	ĭ as in ĭnterest
ō as in ōpen	ŏ as in pŏt
ū as in ūnit	ŭ as in ŭnder

Vocabulary and Terminology

TERM	PRONUNCIATION	MEANING
adnexa uteri (266)	ăd-NĔK-să Ū-tĕ-rī	
amenorrhea (270)	āmĕn-ō-RĒ-ă	
amniocentesis (268)	ăm-nē-ō-sĕn-TĒ-sĭs	
amnion (266)	ĂM-nē-ŏn	
amniotic fluid (268)	ăm-nē-ŎT-ĭk FLOO-ĭd	
anovulatory (270)	ăn-ŎV-ū-lă-tōr-ē	
areola (266)	ă-RĒ-ō-lă	
Bartholin glands (266)	BĂR-thō-lĭn glăndz	
bartholinitis (268)	băr-thō-lĭ-NĪ-tĭs	
cephalic version (272)	sē-FĂL-lĭk VĔR-shŭn	
cervix (266)	SĔR-vĭkz	
chorion (268)	KŎ-rē-ŏn	
chorionic (268)	kŏ-rē-ŎN-ĭk	
clitoris (266)	KLĬ-tō-rĭs	
coitus (266)	KŌ-ĭ-tŭs	
colposcopy (268)	kŏl-PŎS-kō-pē	
corpus luteum (266)	KŎR-pŭs LOO-tē-ŭm	
cul-de-sac (266)	KŬL-dē-săk	
culdocentesis (268)	kŭl-dō-sĕn-TĒ-sĭs	
dysmenorrhea (270)	dĭs-mĕn-ō-RĒ-ă	
dyspareunia (272)	dĭs-pă-ROO-nē-ă	

8

TERM	PRONUNCIATION	MEANING
dystocia (272)	dĭs-TŌ-sē-ă	
embryo (266)	ĔM-brē-ō	
endocervicitis (268)	ĕn-dō-sĕr-vĭs-SĪ-tĭs	
endometritis (272)	ĕn-dō-mĕ-TRĪ-tis	
endometrium (266)	ĕn-dō-MĒ-trē-ŭm	
episiotomy (268)	ĕ-pĭs-ē-ŎT-ō-mē	
estrogen (266)	ĔS-trō-jĕn	
fallopian tube (266)	fă-LŌ-pē-ăn tūb	
fertilization (266)	fĕr-tĭl-ĭ-ZĀ-shŭn	
fetal presentation (272)	FĒ-tăl prĕ-sĕn-TĀ-shŭn	
fetus (266)	FĒ-tŭs	
fimbriae (266)	FĬM-brē-ē	
follicle-stimulating hormone (266)	FŎL-lĭ-kl STĬM-ū-lā-tĭng HŌR-mōn	
galactorrhea (268)	gă-lăk-tō-RĒ-ă	
gamete (266)	GĂM-ēt	
genitalia (267)	jĕn-ĭ-TĀ-lē-ă	
gestation (267)	jĕs-TĀ-shŭn	
gonad (267)	GŌ-năd	
gynecology (267)	gī-nĕ-KŎL-ō-jē	
gynecomastia (269)	gī-nĕ-kō-MĂS-tē-ă	
human chorionic gonadotropin (267)	HŪ-măn kō-rē-ŎN-ĭk gō-nă-dō-TRŌ-pĭn	
hymen (267)	HĪ-mĕn	
hysterectomy (269)	hĭs-tĕr-ĔK-tō-mē	
hysteroscopy (269)	hĭs-tĕr-ŎS-kō-pē	
inframammary (269)	ĭn-fră-MĂM-ăr-ē	
intrauterine device (272)	ĭn-tră-Ū-tĕ-rĭn dĕ-VĪS	
involution (272)	ĭn-vō-LOO-shŭn	
labia (267)	LĀ-bē-ă	
lactation (269)	lăk-TĀ-shŭn	

8

TERM	PRONUNCIATION	MEANING
lactiferous ducts (267)	lăk-TĬ-fĕ-rŭs dŭkts	______
leukorrhea (272)	loo-kō-RĒ-ă	______
luteinizing hormone (267)	LOO-tē-nī-zĭng HŎR-mōn	______
mammary papilla (267)	MĂM-ăr-ē pă-PĬL-ă	______
mammoplasty (269)	MĂM-ō-plăs-tē	______
mastectomy (270)	măs-TĔK-tō-mē	______
mastitis (270)	măs-TĪ-tĭs	______
menarche (267)	mĕ-NĂR-kē	______
menometrorrhagia (270)	mĕn-ō-mĕt-rō-RĀ-jă	______
menopause (267)	MĔN-ō-păwz	______
menorrhea (272)	mĕn-ō-RĒ-ă	______
menorrhagia (270)	mĕn-ō-RĀ-jă	______
menstruation (267)	mĕn-strū-Ā-shŭn	______
metrorrhagia (270)	mĕ-trō-RĀ-jă	______
multigravida (273)	mŭl-tĭ-GRĂV-ĭ-dă	______
multipara (273)	mŭl-TĬP-ă-ră	______
myomectomy (270)	mī-ō-MĔK-tō-mē	______
myometrium (267)	mī-ō-MĒ-trē-ŭm	______
neonatal (270)	nē-ō-NĀ-tăl	______
neonatology (267)	nē-ō-nā-TŎL-ō-jē	______
nulligravida (273)	nŭl-lē-GRĂ-vĭ-dă	______
nullipara (273)	nŭl-LĬP-ă-ră	______
obstetrics (267)	ŏb-STĔT-rĭks	______
oligomenorrhea (270)	ŏl-ĭ-gō-mĕn-ō-RĒ-ă	______
oocyte (270)	ō-ō-SĪT	______
oogenesis (270)	ō-ō-JĔN-ĕ-sĭs	______
oophorectomy (270)	oo-fō-RĔK-tō-mē *or* ō-ŏf-ō-RĔK-tō-mē	______
oophoritis (271)	ō-ŏf-ōr-Ī-tĭs	______
orifice (267)	ŎR-ĭ-fĭs	______
ovarian (270)	ō-VĀ-rē-ăn	______

8

TERM	PRONUNCIATION	MEANING
ovarian follicle (267)	ō-VĀ-rē-ăn FŎL-lĭ-kl	
ovary (267)	Ō-vă-rē	
ovulation (267)	ŏv-ū-LĀ-shŭn	
ovum; ova (267)	Ō-vŭm; Ō-vă	
oxytocia (272)	ŏks-ē-TŌ-sē-ă	
oxytocin (272)	ŏks-ē-TŌ-sĭn	
parturition (267)	păr-tū-RĬSH-ŭn	
perineorrhaphy (270)	pĕ-rĭ-nē-ŎR-ră-fē	
perineum (267)	pĕ-rĭ-NĒ-ŭm	
pituitary gland (267)	pĭ-TOO-ĭ-tăr-ē glănd	
placenta (267)	plă-SĔN-tă	
pregnancy (267)	PRĔG-năn-sē	
prenatal (273)	prē-NĀ-tăl	
primigravida (271)	prī-mĭ-GRĂV-ĭ-dă	
primipara (273)	prī-MĬP-ă-ră	
primiparous (272)	prī-MĬP-ă-rŭs	
progesterone (268)	prō-JĔS-tĕ-rōn	
pseudocyesis (271)	sū-dō-sī-Ē-sĭs	
puberty (268)	PŪ-bĕr-tē	
pyosalpinx (272)	pī-ō-SĂL-pĭnks	
retroversion (273)	rĕ-trō-VĔR-zhŭn	
salpingectomy (271)	săl-pĭn-JĔK-tō-mē	
salpingitis (277)	săl-pĭn-JĪ-tĭs	
uterine prolapse (271)	Ū-tĕr-ĭn PRŌ-lăps	
uterine serosa (268)	Ū-tĕr-ĭn sē-RŌ-să	
uterus (268)	Ū-tĕr-ŭs	
vagina (268)	vă-JĪ-nă	
vaginal orifice (271)	VĂ-jĭ-năl ŎR-ĭ-fĭs	
vaginitis (271)	vă-jĭ-NĪ-tĭs	
vulva (268)	VŬL-vă	

8

TERM	PRONUNCIATION	MEANING
vulvodynia (271)	vŭl-vō-DĬ-nē-ă	____________
vulvovaginitis (271)	vŭl-vō-vă-jĭ-NĪ-tĭs	____________
zygote (268)	ZĪ-gōt	____________

Pathologic Conditions, Clinical Tests, and Procedures

TERM	PRONUNCIATION	MEANING
abortion (286)	ă-BŎR-shŭn	____________
abruptio placentae (280)	ă-BRŬP-shē-ō plă-SĔN-tā	____________
Apgar score (281)	ĂP-găr skōr	____________
aspiration (284)	ăs-pĭ-RĀ-shŭn	____________
carcinoma in situ (274)	kăr-sĭ-NŌ-mă ĭn SĪ-tū	____________
carcinoma of the breast (278)	kăr-sĭ-NŌ-mă of the brĕst	____________
carcinoma of the cervix (274)	kăr-sĭ-NŌ-mă of the SĔR-vĭks	____________
carcinoma of the endometrium (275)	kăr-sĭ-NŌ-mă of the ĕn-dō-MĒ-trē-ŭm	____________
cauterization (284)	kaw-tĕr-ĭ-ZĀ-shŭn	____________
cervical dysplasia (274)	SĔR-vĭ-kăl dĭs-PLĀ-zē-ă	____________
cervicitis (275)	sĕr-vĭ-SĪ-tĭs	____________
cesarean section (287)	sē-ZĀ-rē-ăn SĔK-shŭn	____________
chorionic villus sampling (287)	kō-rē-ŎN-ik VĬL-us SĂMP-lĭng	____________
colposcopy (284)	kōl-PŎS-kō-pē	____________
conization (284)	kō-nĭ-ZĀ-shŭn	____________
cryocauterization (284)	krī-ō-kaw-tĕr-ĭ-ZĀ-shŭn	____________
culdocentesis (285)	kŭl-dō-sĕn-TĒ-sĭs	____________
dermoid cysts (277)	DĔR-moyd sĭsts	____________
dilatation (285)	dĭ-lă-TĀ-shŭn	____________
dilation and curettage (285)	dī-LĀ-shŭn and kŭr-ĕ-TĂZH	____________
Down syndrome (281)	Dŏwn SĬN-drōm	____________
ectopic pregnancy (280)	ĕk-TŎP-ĭk PRĔG-năn-sē	____________
endometriosis (275)	ĕn-dō-mē-trē-Ō-sĭs	____________

TERM	PRONUNCIATION	MEANING
erythroblastosis fetalis (281)	ĕ-rĭth-rō-blăs-TŌ-sĭs fē-TĂ-lĭs	
exenteration (286)	ĕks-ĕn-tĕ-RĀ-shŭn	
fetal monitoring (287)	FĒ-tăl MŎN-ĭ-tŏ-rĭng	
fibrocystic breast disease (280)	fī-brō-SĬS-tĭk brĕst dĭ-ZĒZ	
fibroids (277)	FĪ-broydz	
hyaline membrane disease (281)	HĪ-ă-lĭn MĔM-brān dĭ-ZĒZ	
hydrocephalus (282)	hī-drō-SĔF-ă-lŭs	
hysterosalpingography (283)	hĭs-tĕr-ō-săl-pĭng-ŎG-ră-fē	
in vitro fertilization (287)	ĭn VĒ-trō fĕr-tĭl-ĭ-ZĀ-shŭn	
laparoscopy (286)	lă-pă-RŎS-kō-pē	
leiomyomas (276)	lī-ō-mī-Ō-măz	
mammography (283)	măm-MŎG-ră-fē	
meconium aspiration syndrome (282)	mĕ-KŌ-nē-ŭm ăs-pĭ-RĀ-shŭn SĬN-drōm	
multiple gestation (280)	MŬL-tĭ-pl jĕs-TĀ-shŭn	
ovarian carcinoma (276)	ō-VĀR-ē-an kăr-sĭ-NŌ-mă	
ovarian cysts (277)	ō-VĀR-ē-an sĭsts	
palpation (277)	păl-PĀ-shŭn	
Pap test (282)	păp tĕst	
pelvic inflammatory disease (277)	PĔL-vĭk ĭn-FLĂM-mă-tō-rē dĭ-ZĒZ	
pelvic ultrasonography (284)	PĔL-vĭk ŭl-tră-sŏn-ŎG-ră-fē	
pelvimetry (287)	pĕl-VĬM-ĭ-trē	
placenta previa (280)	plă-SĔN-tă PRĒ-vē-ă	
preeclampsia (281)	prē-ē-KLĂMP-sē-ă	
pregnancy test (282)	PRĔG-năn-sē tĕst	
pyloric stenosis (282)	pī-LŎR-ĭk stĕ-NŌ-sĭs	
respiratory distress syndrome (281)	RĔS-pĭr-ă-tō-rē dĭs-STRĔS SĬN-drōm	
tubal ligation (286)	TOO-băl lī-GĀ-shŭn	

REVIEW SHEET

Write the meanings of the word parts in the spaces provided, and test yourself. Check your answers with the information in the chapter or in the Glossary (Medical Word Parts—English) at the end of the book.

Combining Forms

COMBINING FORM	MEANING	COMBINING FORM	MEANING
amni/o	________	myom/o	________
bartholin/o	________	nat/i	________
cephal/o	________	obstetr/o	________
cervic/o	________	olig/o	________
chori/o, chorion/o	________	o/o	________
colp/o	________	oophor/o	________
culd/o	________	ov/o	________
episi/o	________	ovari/o	________
galact/o	________	ovul/o	________
gynec/o	________	perine/o	________
hyster/o	________	phor/o	________
lact/o	________	py/o	________
mamm/o	________	salping/o	________
mast/o	________	uter/o	________
men/o	________	vagin/o	________
metr/o, metri/o	________	vulv/o	________
my/o	________		

Prefixes

PREFIX	MEANING	PREFIX	MEANING
bi-	________	oxy-	________
dys-	________	peri-	________
endo-	________	pre-	________
in-	________	primi-	________
intra-	________	pseudo-	________
multi-	________	retro-	________
nulli-	________	uni-	________

8

Suffixes

SUFFIX	MEANING	SUFFIX	MEANING
-arche	______________	-plasty	______________
-cyesis	______________	-rrhagia	______________
-dynia	______________	-rrhaphy	______________
-ectomy	______________	-rrhea	______________
-flexion	______________	-salpinx	______________
-genesis	______________	-scopy	______________
-gravida	______________	-stenosis	______________
-itis	______________	-stomy	______________
-pareunia	______________	-tocia	______________
-parous	______________	-tomy	______________
-plasia	______________	-version	______________

Match the following diagnostic procedures with their descriptions. Check your answers with the information in the chapter.

DIAGNOSTIC PROCEDURES	DESCRIPTIONS
1. aspiration ______________	A. Uterus and fallopian tubes are imaged (x-rays)
2. colposcopy ______________	B. hCG is measured
3. culdocentesis ______________	C. X-rays are taken of the breast
4. hysterosalpingography ______________	D. Useful procedure to biopsy breast tissue (using a needle)
5. mammography ______________	E. Removal and analysis of cervical and vaginal cells
6. Pap test ______________	F. Fluid is obtained from the region between the rectum and uterus
7. pregnancy test ______________	G. Images of ovarian masses may be seen
8. pelvic ultrasonography ______________	H. Process of microscopic visual examination of the vagina and cervix

8

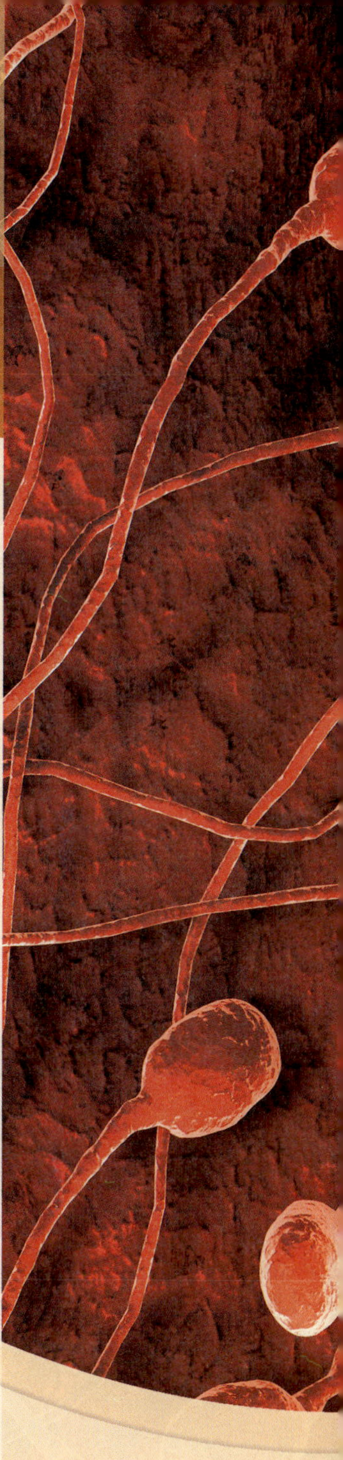

CHAPTER 9

Male Reproductive System

This chapter is divided into the following sections:

CHAPTER GOALS

- Name, locate, and describe the functions of the organs of the male reproductive system.
- Define abnormal conditions and infectious diseases that affect the male reproductive system.
- Differentiate among several types of sexually transmitted diseases.
- Define combining forms used to describe the structures of this system.
- Describe various laboratory tests and clinical procedures pertinent to disorders of the male reproductive system, and recognize related abbreviations.
- Apply your new knowledge to understanding medical terms in their proper contexts, such as medical reports and records.

INTRODUCTION

The male sex cell, the **spermatozoon** (sperm cell), is microscopic—in volume, only one third the size of a red blood cell and less than 1/100,000 the size of the female ovum. A relatively uncomplicated cell, the sperm is composed of a head region, containing nuclear hereditary material (chromosomes), and a tail region, consisting of a **flagellum** (hair-like process). The flagellum makes the sperm motile and makes it look somewhat like a tadpole. The spermatozoon cell contains relatively little food and cytoplasm, because it lives only long enough (3 to 5 days) to travel from its point of release from the male to where the egg cell lies within the female reproductive tract (fallopian tube). Only one spermatozoon out of approximately 300 million sperm cells released during a single **ejaculation** (ejection of sperm and fluid from the male urethra) can penetrate a single ovum and result in fertilization of the ovum. Figure 9-1 shows a diagram of a **sperm cell** and a photograph of **spermatozoa**.

If more than one egg is passing down the fallopian tube when sperm are present, multiple fertilizations are possible, and twins, triplets, quadruplets, and so on may occur. Twins resulting from the fertilization of separate ova by separate sperm cells are called **fraternal twins.** Fraternal twins, developing with separate placentas, can be of the same sex or different sexes and resemble each other no more than ordinary brothers and sisters. Fraternal twinning is hereditary; the daughters of mothers of twins can carry the gene.

Identical twins result from fertilization of a single egg cell by a single sperm. As the fertilized egg cell divides and forms many cells, it somehow splits, and each part continues separately to undergo further division, each producing an embryo. Most identical twins have one placenta and two amniotic sacs. Identical twins are always of the same sex and are very similar in form and feature.

The organs of the male reproductive system are designed to produce and release billions of spermatozoa throughout the lifetime of a male from puberty onward. In addition, the male reproductive system secretes a hormone called **testosterone.** Testosterone is responsible for the production of the bodily characteristics of the male (such as beard, pubic hair, and deeper voice) and for the proper development of male gonads **(testes)** and accessory organs **(prostate gland** and **seminal vesicles)** that secrete fluids to ensure the lubrication and viability of sperm.

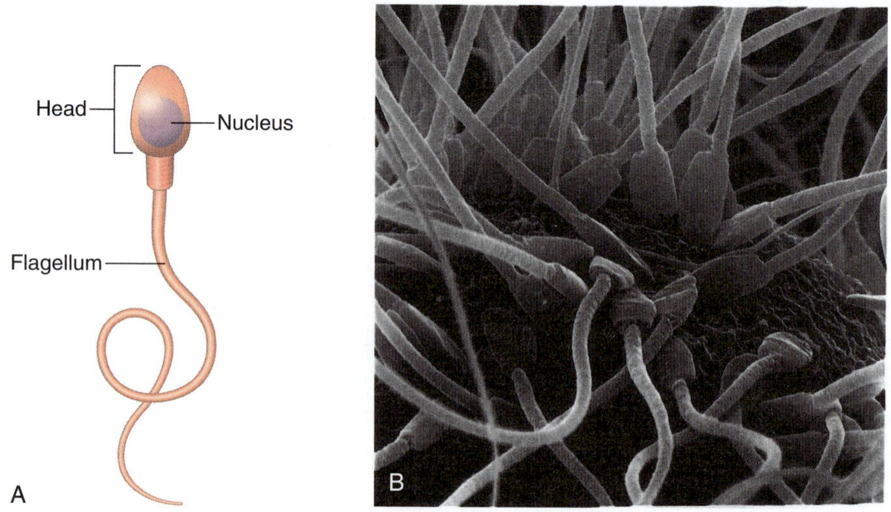

FIGURE 9-1 **A, Sperm cell. B,** Photograph of spermatozoa.

ANATOMY

Label Figure 9-2 as you study the following description of the anatomy of the male reproductive system.

Each male gonad is a **testis** [1]. There are two **testes** (plural) or **testicles** that develop in the abdomen at about the level of the kidneys before descending during embryonic development into the **scrotum** [2], a sac enclosing the testes on the outside of the body.

The scrotum, lying between the thighs, exposes the testes to a lower temperature than that of the rest of the body. This lower temperature is necessary for the adequate maturation and development of sperm **(spermatogenesis).** Located between the anus and the scrotum, at the floor of the pelvic cavity in the male, the **perineum** [3] is analogous to the perineal region in the female.

The interior of a testis is composed of a large mass of narrow, coiled tubules called the **seminiferous tubules** [4]. These tubules contain cells that manufacture spermatozoa. The seminiferous tubules are the **parenchymal tissue** of the testis, which means that they perform the essential work of the organ (formation of sperm). Other cells in the testis, lying adjacent to seminiferous tubules, are **interstitial cells.** They manufacture an important male hormone, **testosterone.**

All body organs contain **parenchyma,** which perform the essential functions of the organ. Organs also contain supportive, connective, and framework tissue, such as blood vessels, connective tissues, and sometimes muscle as well. This supportive tissue is called **stroma (stromal tissue).**

After formation, sperm cells move through the seminiferous tubules and collect in ducts that lead to a large tube, the **epididymis** [5], at the upper part of each testis. The spermatozoa

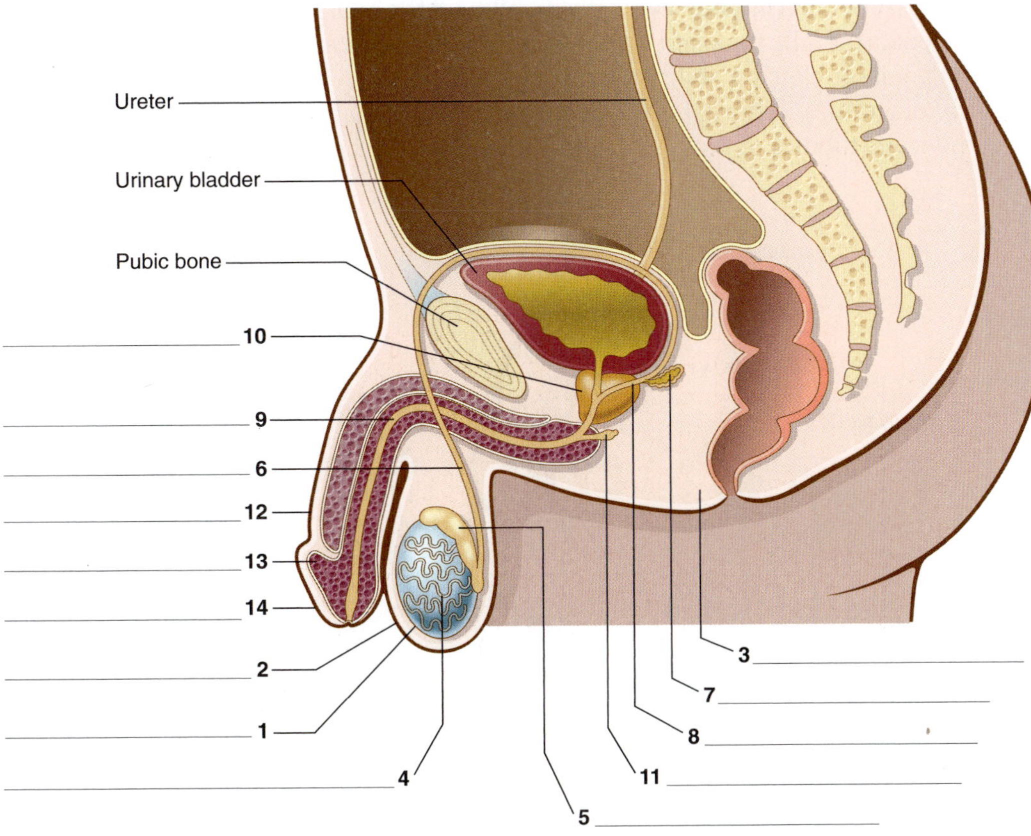

FIGURE 9-2 **Male reproductive system,** sagittal view.

mature, become motile in the epididymis, and are temporarily stored there. An epididymis runs down the length of each testicle (the coiled tube is about 16 feet long) and then turns upward again and becomes a narrow, straight tube called the **vas deferens** [6] or **ductus deferens.** Figure 9-3 shows the internal structure of a testis and the epididymis. The vas deferens is about 2 feet long and carries the sperm up into the pelvic region, at the level of the urinary bladder, merging with ducts from the **seminal vesicles** [7] to form the **ejaculatory duct** [8] leading toward the urethra. During a **vasectomy** or **sterilization** procedure, the urologist cuts and ties off each vas deferens by making an incision in the scrotum.

The seminal vesicles, two glands (only one is shown in Figure 9-2) located at the base of the bladder, open into the ejaculatory duct as it joins the **urethra** [9]. They secrete a thick, sugary, yellowish substance that nourishes the sperm cells and forms a portion of ejaculated semen. **Semen,** a combination of fluid (seminal fluid) and spermatozoa (sperm cells account for less than 1% of the semen volume), is ejected from the body through the urethra. In the male, as opposed to that in the female, the genital orifice combines with the urinary (urethral) opening.

The **prostate gland** [10] lies at the region where the vas deferens enters the urethra, almost encircling the upper end of the urethra. It secretes a thick fluid that, as part of semen, aids the motility of the sperm. The muscular tissue of the prostate aids in the expulsion of fluid during ejaculation. About 60% of ejaculate comes from seminal vesicles and 40% from the prostate. **Bulbourethral glands** [11], lying below the prostate gland, also secrete fluid into the urethra.

The urethra passes through the **penis** [12] to the outside of the body. The penis is composed of erectile tissue and at its tip expands to form a soft, sensitive region called the **glans penis** [13]. Ordinarily, a fold of skin called the **prepuce,** or **foreskin** [14], covers the glans penis. During a circumcision the foreskin is removed, leaving the glans penis visible at all times.

9

Erectile dysfunction (impotence) is the inability of the adult male to achieve an erection. Viagra (sildenafil), Cialis (tadalafil), and Levitra (vardenafil) are drugs that increase blood flow to the penis, enhancing ability to have an erection.

The flow diagram in Figure 9-4 traces the path of spermatozoa from their formation in the seminiferous tubules of the testes to the outside of the body.

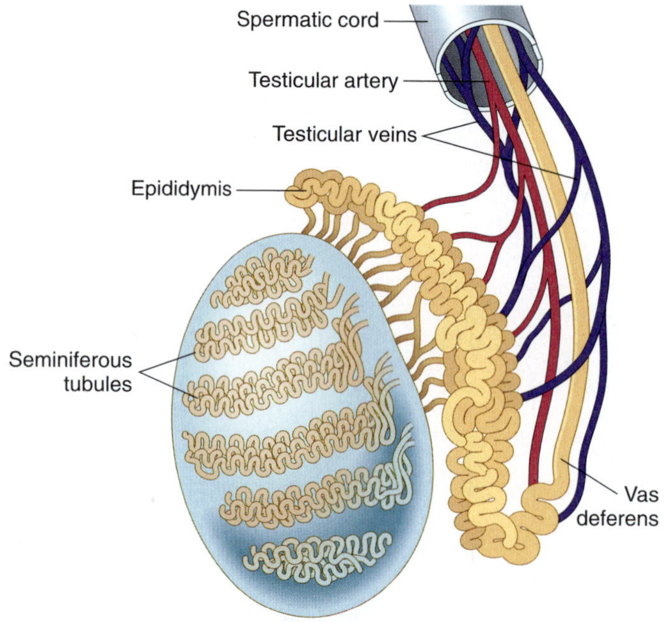

FIGURE 9-3 Internal structure of a testis and the epididymis.

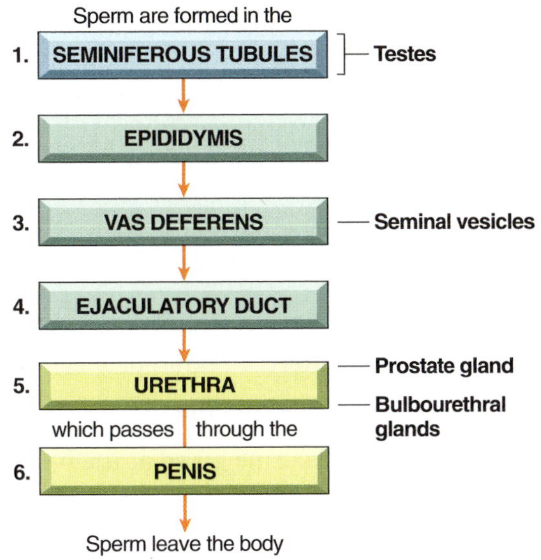

FIGURE 9-4 The **passage of sperm** from the seminiferous tubules in the testes to the outside of the body.

VOCABULARY

This list reviews new terms introduced in the text. Short definitions reinforce your understanding.

bulbourethral glands	Pair of exocrine glands near the male urethra. They secrete fluid into the urethra. Also called **Cowper glands**.
ejaculation	Ejection of sperm and fluid from the male urethra.
ejaculatory duct	Tube through which semen enters the male urethra.
epididymis (*plural:* **epididymides**)	One of a pair of long, tightly coiled tubes above each testis. It stores and carries sperm from seminiferous tubules to the vas deferens.
erectile dysfunction	Inability of an adult male to achieve an erection; impotence.
flagellum	Hair-like projection on a sperm cell that makes it motile (able to move).
fraternal twins	Two infants resulting from fertilization of two separate ova by two separate sperm cells (Figure 9-5).
glans penis	Sensitive tip of the penis; comparable to the clitoris in the female.

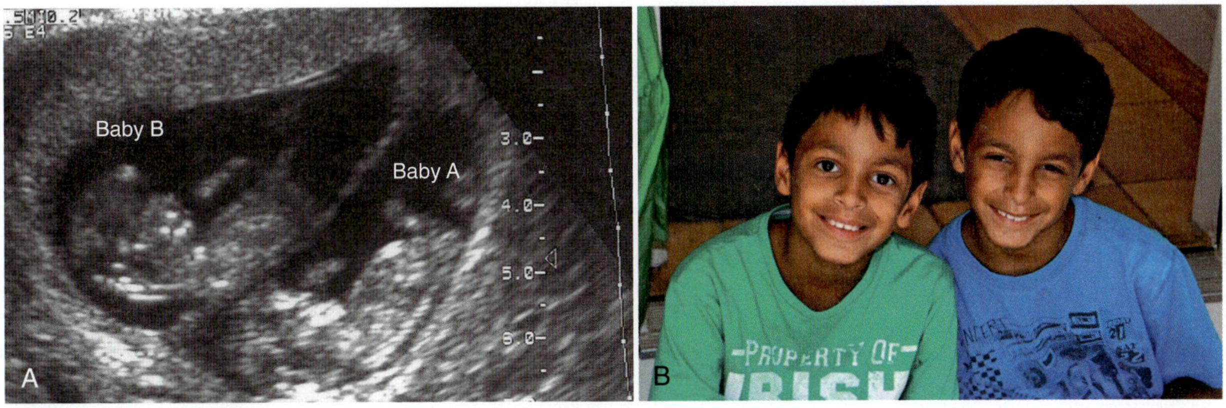

FIGURE 9-5 **Fraternal twins. A,** Notice the 6-week-old embryos in two separate amniotic sacs. **B,** Twins Marcos and Matheus De Como are 10 years old. *(Courtesy Juliana Do Carmo.)*

identical twins	Two infants resulting from division of one fertilized egg into two distinct embryos. **Conjoined** ("**Siamese**") **twins** are incompletely separated identical twins.
interstitial cells of the testes	Specialized cells that lie adjacent to the seminiferous tubules in the testes. These cells produce testosterone and are also called **Leydig cells.**
parenchymal tissue	Essential distinctive cells of an organ. In the testis, the seminiferous tubules that produce sperm are parenchymal.
penis	Male external organ of reproduction.
perineum	External region between the anus and scrotum in the male.
prepuce	Foreskin; fold of skin covering the tip of the penis.
prostate gland	Exocrine gland at the base of the male urinary bladder. The prostate secretes one of the fluid parts of semen into the urethra during ejaculation.
scrotum	External sac that contains the testes.
semen	Spermatozoa (sperm cells) and seminal fluid (prostatic and seminal vesicle secretions), discharged from the urethra during ejaculation.
seminal vesicles	Paired sac-like exocrine glands that secrete fluid (a major component of semen) into the vas deferens.
seminiferous tubules	Narrow, coiled tubules that produce sperm in the testes.
spermatozoon (*plural:* **spermatozoa**)	Sperm cell.
sterilization	Procedure that removes a person's ability to produce or release reproductive cells; removal of testicles, vasectomy, and oophorectomy are sterilization procedures.
stromal tissue	Supportive, connective tissue of an organ, as distinguished from its parenchyma. Also called **stroma.**
testis (*plural:* **testes**)	Male gonad (**testicle**) that produces spermatozoa and the hormone testosterone. *Remember:* Testis means one testicle, and testes are two testicles.
testosterone	Hormone secreted by the interstitial tissue of the testes; responsible for male sex characteristics.
vas deferens	Narrow tube (one on each side) carrying sperm from the epididymis toward the urethra. Also called **ductus deferens.**

Perineum/Peritoneum

Don't confuse *perineum*, which is the area between the anus and scrotum in the male and the anus and vagina in females, with the *peritoneum*, which is the membrane surrounding the abdominal cavity!

Prostate/Prostrate

Don't confuse *prostate* with *prostrate*, which means lying down.

Semen/Sperm

Don't confuse *semen* with *sperm*. *Semen* is the thick, whitish secretion discharged from the urethra during ejaculation. **Sperm (spermatozoa)** are cells that develop in the testes. Semen contains sperm.

Sterilization/Impotence

Don't confuse *sterilization*, which can be performed in men and women, with *impotence*, which is the inability of a male to sustain an erection or achieve ejaculation.

TERMINOLOGY

Write the meanings of the medical terms in the spaces provided.

COMBINING FORMS

COMBINING FORM	MEANING	TERMINOLOGY	MEANING
andr/o	male	androgen *Testosterone is an androgen. The testes in males and the adrenal glands in both men and women produce androgens.*	______
balan/o	glans penis (Greek *balanos*, means acorn)	balanitis *An inflammation usually caused by overgrowth of organisms (bacteria and yeast) (Figure 9-6A).*	______
cry/o	cold	cryogenic surgery *Technique for prostate cancer treatment using freezing temperatures to destroy cancer cells.*	______
crypt/o	hidden	cryptorchidism *In this congenital condition, one or both testicles do not descend, by the time of birth, into the scrotal sac from the abdominal cavity (Figure 9-6B).*	______
epididym/o	epididymis	epididymitis *This is an inflammation usually caused by bacteria. Signs and symptoms are fever, chills, pain in the groin, and tender, swollen epididymis.*	______
gon/o	seed (Greek *gone*, seed)	gonorrhea *See page 322.*	______
hydr/o	water, fluid	hydrocele *See page 320.*	______

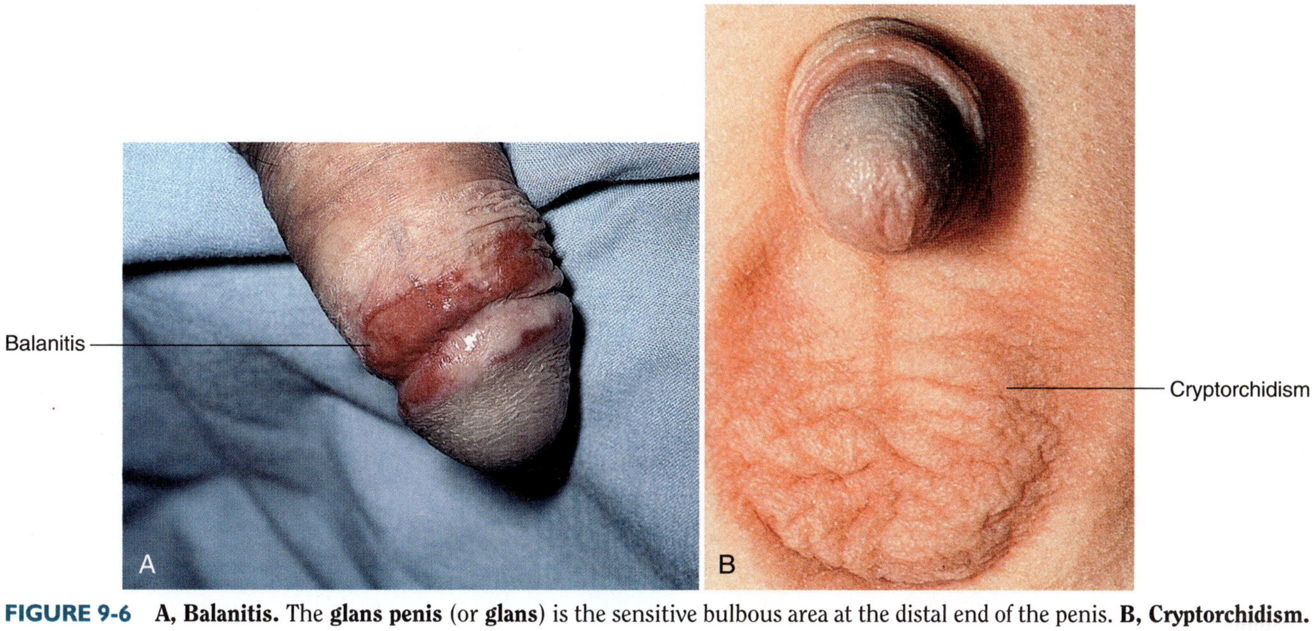

FIGURE 9-6 **A, Balanitis.** The **glans penis** (or **glans**) is the sensitive bulbous area at the distal end of the penis. **B, Cryptorchidism.**

COMBINING FORM	MEANING	TERMINOLOGY	MEANING
orch/o, orchi/o, orchid/o	testis, testicle	orchiectomy *Castration in males. (Also called orchidectomy.)*	
		orchitis *Caused by injury or by the mumps virus, which also infects the salivary glands.*	
pen/o	penis	penile *-ile means pertaining to.*	
		penoscrotal	
prostat/o	prostate gland	prostatitis *Bacterial* (E. coli) *prostatitis often is associated with urethritis and infection of the lower urinary tract.*	
		prostatectomy	
semin/i	semen, seed	seminiferous tubules *The suffix -ferous means pertaining to bearing, or bearing or carrying.*	
sperm/o, spermat/o	spermatozoa, semen	spermolytic *Noun suffixes ending in -sis, like -lysis, form adjectives by dropping the -sis and adding -tic.*	
		oligospermia	
		aspermia *Lack of semen (sperm and fluid). One cause of aspermia is retrograde ejaculation (sperm flows backward into the urinary bladder) as a result of prostate surgery.*	
terat/o	monster (Greek *teras*, monster)	teratoma *This tumor occurs in the testes or ovaries and is composed of different types of tissue, such as bone, hair, cartilage, and skin cells. Teratomas in the testes are malignant.*	
test/o	testis, testicle	testicular *The term testis originates from a Latin term meaning witness. In ancient times men would take an oath with one hand on their testes, swearing by their manhood to tell the truth.*	
varic/o	varicose veins	varicocele *A collection of varicose (swollen, twisted) veins above the testis. See page 320.*	
vas/o	vessel, duct; vas deferens	vasectomy *See page 326. Remember: in this term, vas/o refers to the vas deferens, and not to any other vessel or duct.*	

Derivation of orchid/o

This combining form is derived from the Greek word *orchis* (testicle). The botanical name for orchid, the flower, is also derived from the same Greek word because of the fleshy tubers of the plant.

COMBINING FORM	MEANING	TERMINOLOGY	MEANING
zo/o	animal life	azoospermia ______ *Lack of spermatozoa in the semen. Causes include testicular dysfunction, chemotherapy, blockage of the epididymis, and vasectomy.*	

SUFFIXES

SUFFIX	MEANING	TERMINOLOGY	MEANING
-genesis	formation	spermatogenesis ______	
-one	hormone	testosterone ______ *Ster/o indicates that this is a type of steroid compound. Examples of other steroids are estrogen, cortisol, and progesterone.*	
-pexy	fixation, put in place	orchiopexy ______ *A surgical procedure to correct cryptorchidism.*	
-stomy	new opening	vasovasostomy ______ *Reversal of vasectomy; a urologist rejoins the cut ends of the vas deferens.*	

9

Pathologic Conditions; Sexually Transmitted Diseases

TUMORS AND ANATOMIC/STRUCTURAL DISORDERS

Testes

carcinoma of the testes (testicular cancer)

Malignant tumor of the testicles.

Testicular tumors are rare except in the 15- to 35-year-old age group. The most common tumor, a **seminoma,** arises from embryonic cells in the testes (Figure 9-7A). Nonseminomatous tumors are **embryonal carcinoma** (Figure 9-7B), **teratoma, choriocarcinoma,** and **yolk sac tumor.** Teratomas are composed of tissue such as bone, hair, cartilage, and skin cells (terat/o means monster).

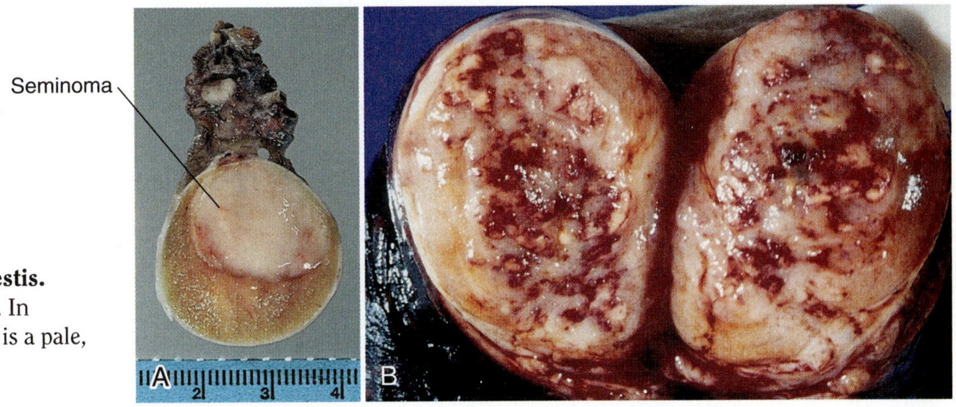

FIGURE 9-7 **A, Seminoma of a testis. B, Embryonal carcinoma** of a testis. In contrast with the seminoma, which is a pale, homogeneous mass, the embryonal carcinoma is a hemorrhagic mass.

Azoospermia/Aspermia

Azoospermia is semen without sperm cells while *aspermia* is no semen at all.

If detected early, testicular cancers can be treated and cured with surgery (orchiectomy), radiotherapy, and chemotherapy. Tumors produce the proteins **human chorionic gonadotropin (hCG)** and **alpha-fetoprotein (AFP).** Serum levels of these proteins are used as **tumor markers** to determine success of treatment.

cryptorchidism; cryptorchism — **Undescended testicles.**

Orchiopexy is performed to bring the testes into the scrotum, if they do not descend on their own by the age of 1 or 2 years. Undescended testicles are associated with a high risk for sterility and increased risk of developing testicular cancer.

hydrocele — **Sac of clear fluid in the scrotum.**

Hydroceles (Figure 9-8) may be congenital or occur as a response to infection or tumors. Often idiopathic, they can be differentiated from testicular masses by ultrasound imaging. If the hydrocele does not resolve on its own, the sac fluid is aspirated using a needle and syringe, or hydrocelectomy may be necessary. In this procedure, the sac is surgically removed through an incision in the scrotum.

testicular torsion — **Twisting of the spermatic cord** (see Figure 9-8).

The rotation of the spermatic cord cuts off blood supply to the testis. Torsion occurs most frequently in childhood. Surgical correction within hours of onset of symptoms can save the testis.

varicocele — **Enlarged, dilated veins near the testicle.**

Varicocele (see Figure 9-8) may be associated with oligospermia and azoospermia. Oligospermic men with varicocele and scrotal pain should have a varicocelectomy. In this procedure, the internal spermatic vein is ligated (the affected segment is cut out and the ends are tied off). On occasion, this leads to an increase in fertility.

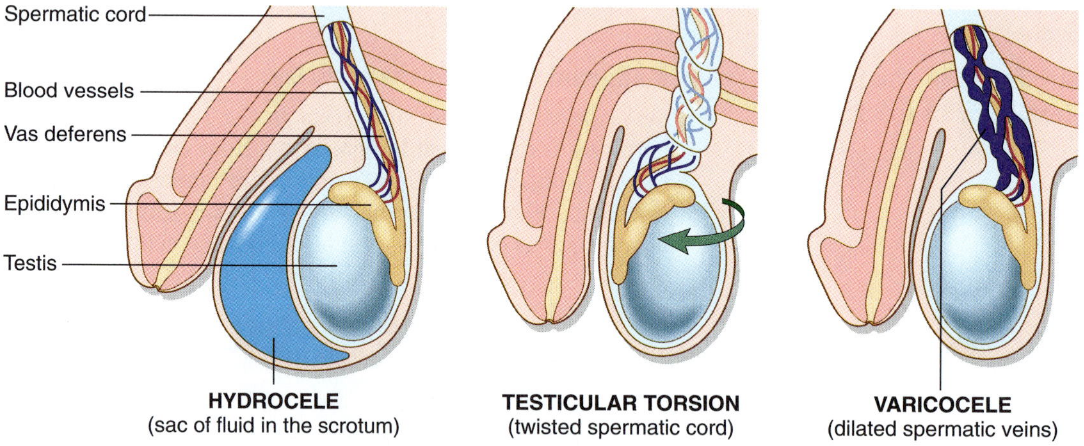

FIGURE 9-8 **Hydrocele, testicular torsion, and varicocele.**

Testicular Cancer Detection

There may be no signs or symptoms of testicular cancer. Regular testicular self-examinations, however, can help identify growths earlier, when the chance for successful treatment is highest. A man should see a doctor if he detects any mass, pain, or swelling in his scrotum.

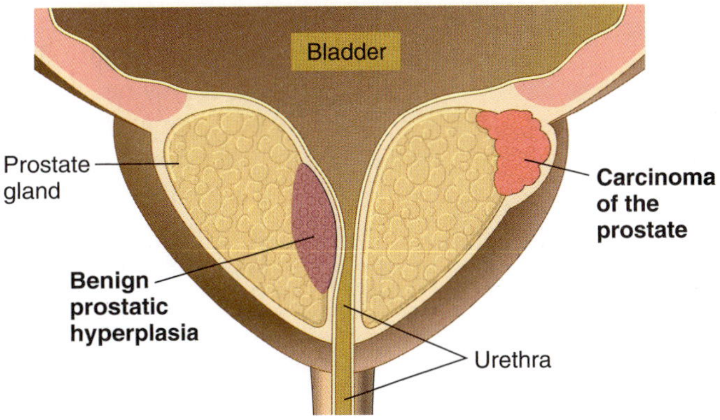

FIGURE 9-9 **The prostate gland with carcinoma and benign prostatic hyperplasia (BPH).** Carcinoma usually arises around the sides of the gland, whereas BPH occurs in the center of the gland. Because prostate cancers are located more peripherally, they can be palpated on digital rectal exam (DRE).

Prostate Gland

benign prostatic hyperplasia (BPH)

Benign growth of cells within the prostate gland.

BPH is a common condition in men older than 60 years of age. Urinary obstruction and inability to empty the bladder completely are symptoms. Figure 9-9 shows the prostate gland with BPH and with carcinoma. Surgical treatment by **transurethral resection of the prostate (TURP)** relieves the obstruction, but overgrowth of cells may recur over several years. In this procedure, an endoscope (resectoscope) is inserted into the penis and through the urethra. Prostatic tissue is removed by an electrical hot loop attached to the resectoscope (see page 325).

Several drugs to relieve BPH symptoms have been approved by the FDA. Finasteride (Proscar) inhibits production of a potent testosterone that promotes enlargement of the prostate. Other drugs, alpha-blockers such as tamsulosin (Flomax), act by relaxing the smooth muscle of the prostate and the neck of the bladder.

Lasers also may be used to destroy prostatic tissue and relieve obstruction. A **laser TURP** or **GreenLight PVP** procedure uses a green light laser at the end of an endoscope (see page 325).

carcinoma of the prostate (prostate cancer)

Malignant tumor (adenocarcinoma) of the prostate gland.

This cancer commonly occurs in men who are older than 50 years. **Digital rectal examination (DRE)** (Figure 9-10) can detect the tumor at a later stage, but early detection depends on a **prostate-specific antigen (PSA) test.** PSA is a protein that is secreted by tumor cells into the bloodstream. PSA levels are elevated in prostate cancer patients even at an early stage of tumor growth. The normal PSA level is 4.0 ng/mL or less.

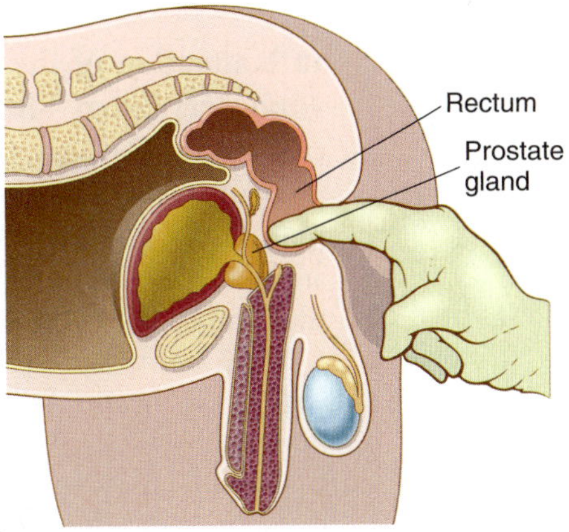

FIGURE 9-10 **Digital rectal examination (DRE) of the prostate gland.**

Diagnosis requires identification by a pathologist of abnormal prostate tissue in a prostate biopsy. **Transrectal ultrasound (TRUS)** guides the precise placement of the biopsy needle. Multiple needle biopsy specimens are taken through the rectal wall. Computed tomography (CT) detects lymph node metastases.

Treatment consists of surgery (prostatectomy), radiation therapy, and/or hormonal chemotherapy. Because prostatic cells are stimulated to grow in the presence of androgens, antiandrogen hormones slow tumor growth by depriving the cells of testosterone. Prostate cancer also is treated with leupron, a hormone that blocks pituitary stimulation of the testes and reduces the level of androgens in the bloodstream. Tumor cells can also be destroyed by brachytherapy (brachy = near), which means that radioactive seeds are implanted directly into the prostate gland. See the ***"In Person"*** account, page 329, describing one man's experience with prostate cancer.

Penis

hypospadias

Congenital abnormality in which the male urethral opening is on the undersurface of the penis, instead of at its tip.

Hypospadias (-spadias means the condition of tearing or cutting) occurs in 1 in every 300 live male births and can be corrected surgically (Figure 9-11A).

phimosis

Narrowing (stricture) of the opening of the prepuce over the glans penis.

This condition (phim/o = muzzle) can interfere with urination and cause secretions to accumulate under the prepuce, leading to infection. Treatment is by circumcision (cutting around the prepuce to remove it) (Figure 9-11B).

9

SEXUALLY TRANSMITTED DISEASES

Sexually transmitted diseases (STDs) are infections transmitted by sexual or other genital contact. Also known as **sexually transmitted infections (STIs)** and venereal diseases (from Latin *Venus*, the goddess of love), they occur in both men and women and are some of the most prevalent communicable diseases in the world.

chlamydial infection

Bacterial invasion (by *Chlamydia trachomatis*) of the urethra and reproductive tract.

Within 3 weeks after becoming infected, men may experience a burning sensation on urination and notice a white or clear discharge from the penis.

Infected women may notice a yellowish vaginal discharge (from the endocervix), but often the disease is asymptomatic. Antibiotics cure the infection, but if untreated, this STD can cause salpingitis (pelvic inflammatory disease [PID]) and infertility in women.

gonorrhea

Inflammation of the genital tract mucosa, caused by infection with gonococci (berry-shaped bacteria).

Other areas of the body, such as the eye, oral mucosa, rectum, and joints, may be affected as well. Signs and symptoms include dysuria and a yellow, mucopurulent (**purulent** means pus-filled) discharge from the male urethra (Figure 9-12A). The ancient Greeks mistakenly thought that this discharge was a leakage of semen, so they named the condition gonorrhea, meaning discharge of seed (gon/o = seed).

Many women carry the disease asymptomatically, whereas others have pain, vaginal and urethral discharge, and salpingitis (PID). As a result of sexual activity, men and women can acquire anorectal and pharyngeal gonococcal infections as well. Chlamydial infection and gonorrhea often occur together. When treating these infections, doctors give antibiotics for both and treat both partners.

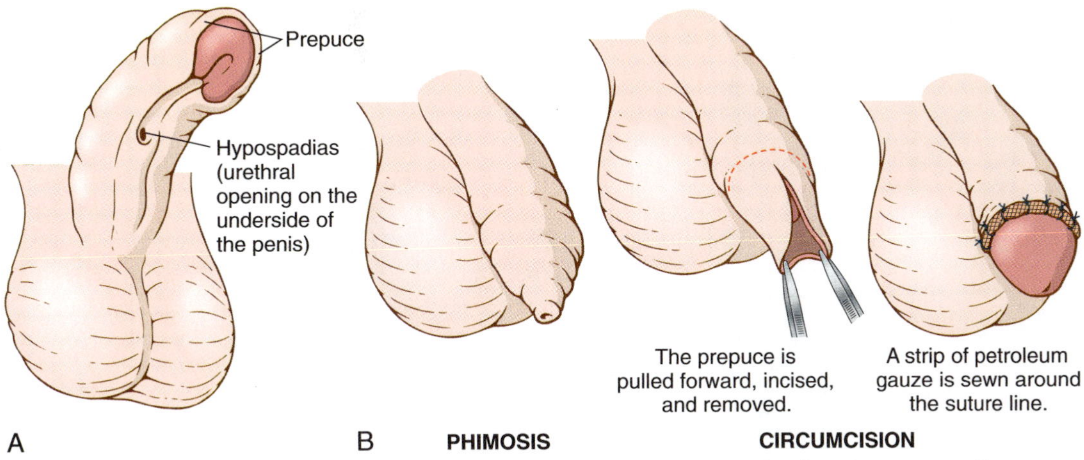

FIGURE 9-11 **A, Hypospadias.** Surgical repair involves elongating the urethra by using surrounding tissue or using a graft from tissue elsewhere in the body and bringing it to the exit at the tip of the penis. **B, Phimosis** and **circumcision** to correct the condition.

herpes genitalis

Infection of skin and genital mucosa, caused by the herpes simplex virus (HSV).

Most cases of herpes genitalis are caused by HSV type 2 (although some are caused by HSV type 1, which commonly is associated with oral infections such as cold sores or fever blisters). The usual clinical presentation is reddening of skin with formation of small, **fluid-filled blisters** and ulcers (Figure 9-12B). Initial episodes also may involve inguinal lymphadenopathy, fever, headache, and malaise. Remissions and relapse periods occur; no drug is known to be effective as a cure. Neonatal herpes affects infants born to women with active infection near the time of delivery. Gynecologists may deliver infants by cesarean section to prevent infection of these babies by HSV. Studies suggest that women with herpes genitalis are at a higher risk for developing vulvar and cervical cancer.

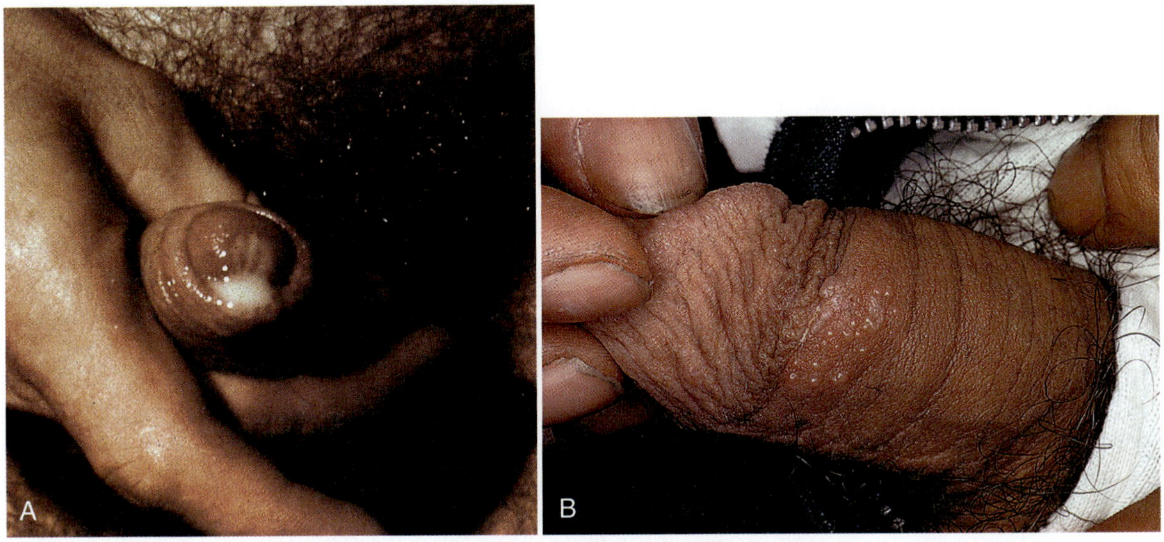

FIGURE 9-12 **A, Gonorrhea.** Discharge from the penis can be seen. **B, Herpes genitalis.** The classic blisters (vesicles) are evident.

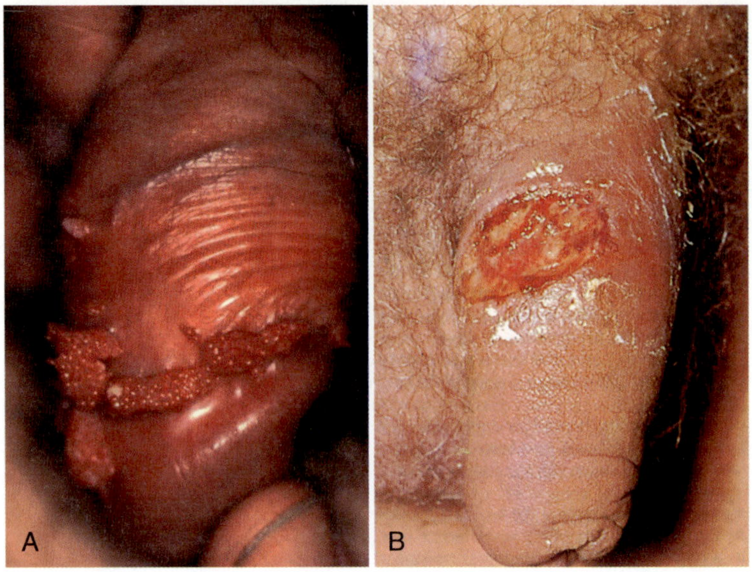

FIGURE 9-13 **A, Genital warts. B, Primary syphilis** with **chancre** on penis.

human papillomavirus (HPV) infection

Infection of the skin and mucous membranes in the anogenital region by the human papillomavirus.

Some types of HPV cause **genital warts** (see Figure 9-13A) and lead to cancer of the cervix as well as cancer in men. A vaccine is available for young girls and women (and under evaluation for men) that protects against four types of HPV.

9

syphilis

Chronic STD caused by a spirochete (spiral-shaped bacterium).

A **chancre** (hard ulcer or sore) usually appears on the external genitalia a few weeks after bacterial infection (Figure 9-13B). Two to six months after the chancre disappears, secondary syphilis begins. Tertiary syphilis includes damage to the brain, spinal cord, and heart, which may appear years after the earlier symptoms disappear. Syphilis (which was so often fatal in early times that it was known as the "great pox"—versus the more familiar smallpox) can be congenital in the fetus if it is transmitted from the mother during pregnancy. Penicillin is effective for treatment in most cases.

LABORATORY TESTS AND CLINICAL PROCEDURES

LABORATORY TESTS

PSA test

Measurement of levels of prostate-specific antigen (PSA) in the blood.

PSA is produced by cells within the prostate gland. Elevated levels of PSA are associated with enlargement of the prostate gland and may be a sign of prostate cancer.

semen analysis

Microscopic examination of ejaculated fluid.

Sperm cells are counted and examined for motility and shape. The test is part of fertility studies and is required to establish the effectiveness of vasectomy. Men with sperm counts of less than 20 million/mL of semen usually are sterile (not fertile). Sterility can result in an adult male who becomes ill with mumps, an infectious disease affecting the testes (inflammation leads to deterioration of spermatozoa).

CLINICAL PROCEDURES

castration

Surgical excision of testicles or ovaries.

Castration may be performed to reduce production and secretion of hormones that stimulate growth of malignant cells (in breast cancer and prostate cancer). When a boy is castrated before puberty, he becomes a eunuch (Greek, *eune*, couch; *echein*, to guard). Male secondary sex characteristics fail to develop.

circumcision

Surgical procedure to remove the prepuce of the penis.

See Figure 9-11B, page 323.

digital rectal examination (DRE)

Finger palpation through the anal canal and rectum to examine the prostate gland.

See Figure 9-10, page 321.

photoselective vaporization of the prostate (GreenLight PVP)

Removal of tissue to treat benign prostatic hyperplasia (BPH) using a green light laser (laser TURP).

This minimally invasive procedure in selected cases replaces TURP for treatment of BPH.

transurethral resection of the prostate (TURP)

Excision of benign prostatic hyperplasia using a resectoscope through the urethra.

This procedure treats benign prostatic hyperplasia (BPH). An electrical hot loop cuts the prostatic tissue; the bits of tissue (chips) are removed through the resectoscope (Figure 9-14).

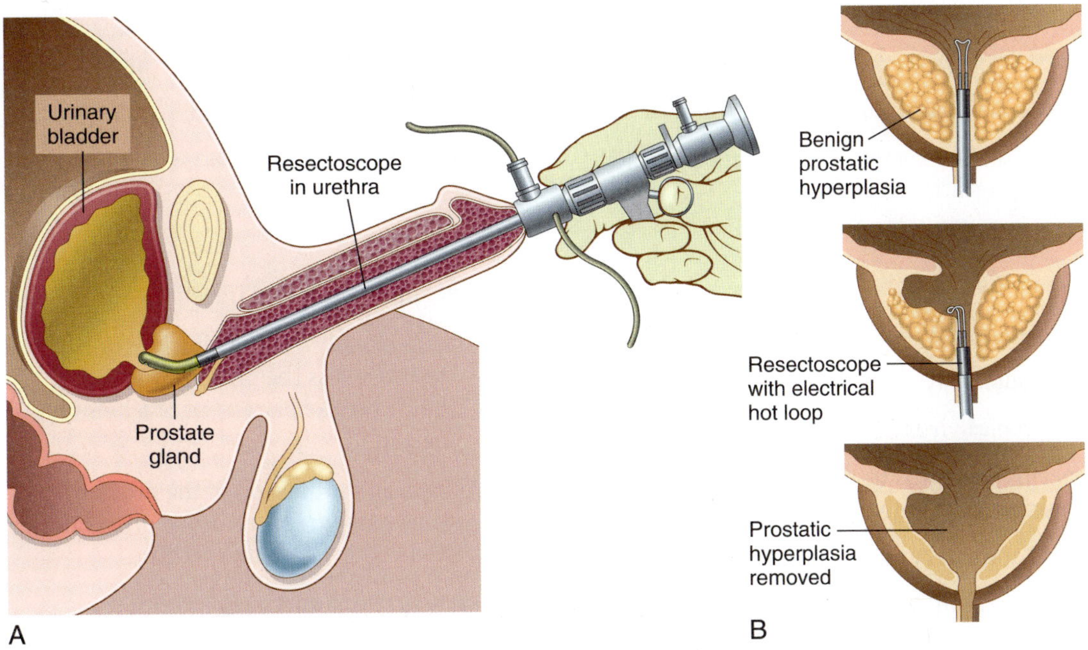

FIGURE 9-14 **Transurethral resection of the prostate (TURP). A,** The resectoscope contains a light, valves for controlling irrigating fluid, and an electrical loop that cuts tissue and seals blood vessels. **B,** The urologist uses a wire loop through the resectoscope to remove obstructing tissue one piece at a time. The pieces are carried by the fluid into the bladder and flushed out at the end of the operation.

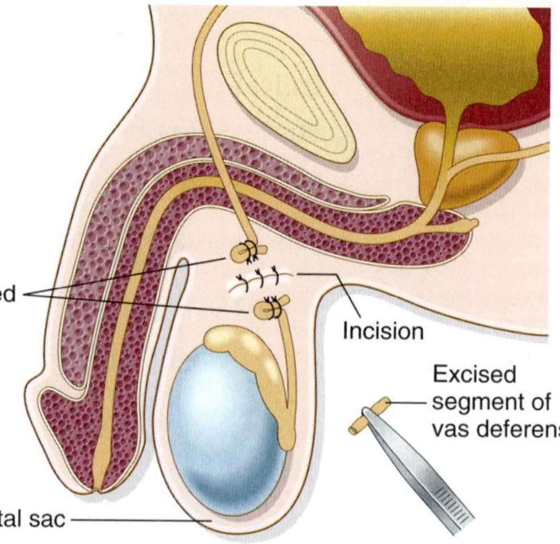

FIGURE 9-15 **Vasectomy.**

vasectomy

Bilateral surgical removal of a part of the vas deferens.

A urologist cuts the vas deferens on each side, removes a piece, and performs a **ligation** (tying and binding off) of the free ends with sutures (Figure 9-15). The procedure is performed using local anesthesia and through an incision in the scrotal sac. Because spermatozoa cannot leave the body, the vasectomized male is sterile, but not castrated. Normal hormone secretion, sex drive, and potency (ability to have an erection) are intact. The body reabsorbs unexpelled sperm. In a small number of cases, a vasovasostomy can successfully reverse vasectomy.

ABBREVIATIONS

BPH	benign prostatic hyperplasia (also called benign prostatic hypertrophy)
DRE	digital rectal examination
ED	erectile dysfunction
GU	genitourinary
HPV	human papillomavirus
HSV	herpes simplex virus
NSU	nonspecific urethritis (not due to gonorrhea or chlamydial infection)
PID	pelvic inflammatory disease
PIN	prostatic intraepithelial neoplasia; a precursor of prostate cancer
PSA	prostate-specific antigen
PVP	photoselective vaporization of the prostate; GreenLight PVP
RPR	rapid plasma reagin [test]; a test for syphilis
STD	sexually transmitted disease
STI	sexually transmitted infection
TRUS	transrectal ultrasound [examination]; test to assess the prostate and guide precise placement of a biopsy needle
TUIP	transurethral incision of the prostate; successful in less enlarged prostates and less invasive than TURP
TUMT	transurethral microwave thermotherapy
TUNA	transurethral needle ablation; radiofrequency energy destroys prostate tissue
TURP	transurethral resection of the prostate

PRACTICAL APPLICATIONS

Reproduced here from actual medical records is a case report on a patient with post-TURP complaints. Background data and explanations of more difficult terms are added in brackets. Answers to the questions are on page 337.

Also presented for your review is an actual surgical pathology report for a man diagnosed with prostate cancer, as well as a summary of current knowledge on anabolic steroids.

CASE REPORT: A MAN WITH POST-TURP COMPLAINTS

The patient is a 70-year-old man who underwent a TURP for BPH 5 years ago and now has severe obstructive urinary symptoms with a large postvoid residual.

On DRE, his prostate was found to be large, bulky, and nodular, with palpable extension to the left seminal vesicle. His PSA level was 15 ng/mL [normal is 0 to 4 ng/mL] and a bone scan was negative. A CT scan revealed bilateral external iliac adenopathy with lymph nodes measuring 1.5 cm on average [normal lymph node size is less than 1 cm]. A prostatic biopsy revealed a poorly differentiated adenocarcinoma.

This patient most likely has at least stage T3 N+ disease [extension into seminal vesicles and nodal metastases]. Recommendation is anti-testosterone hormonal drug treatment.

Questions about the Case Report

1. Five years previously, the patient had which type of surgery?
   a. Removal of testicles
   b. Perineal prostatectomy
   c. Partial prostatectomy (transurethral)
2. What was the reason for the surgery then?
   a. Cryptorchidism
   b. Benign overgrowth of the prostate gland
   c. Testicular cancer
3. What symptom does he have now?
   a. Burning pain on urination
   b. Urinary retention
   c. Premature ejaculation
4. What examination allowed the physician to feel the tumor?
   a. Palpation by a finger inserted into the rectum
   b. CT scan
   c. Prostate-specific antigen test
5. Where had the tumor spread?
   a. Testes
   b. Pelvic lymph nodes and left seminal vesicle
   c. Pelvic bone
6. What is likely to stimulate prostatic adenocarcinoma growth?
   a. Hormonal drug treatment
   b. Prostatic biopsy
   c. Testosterone secretion

7. Stage T3 N+ means that the tumor
   a. Is localized to the hip area
   b. Is confined to the prostate gland
   c. Has spread locally and beyond lymph nodes

8. Why is staging of tumors important?
   a. To classify the extent of spread of the tumor and to plan treatment
   b. To make the initial diagnosis
   c. To make an adequate biopsy of the tumor

SURGICAL PATHOLOGY REPORT: PROSTATE CANCER/HYPERPLASIA

Patient name: Bill Scott
DOB: 9/14/1942 (Age: 69)
Gender: M
Clinical Data: ?Nodule, right side of prostate; PSA 7.1
Specimen(s):
A. Right prostate biopsy
B. Left prostate biopsy

FINAL PATHOLOGIC DIAGNOSIS

A. Needle biopsy of right prostate gland (six cores)
ADENOCARCINOMA, MODERATELY TO POORLY DIFFERENTIATED
Gleason score 4 + 3 = 7
Estimated tumor load,10% of prostatic tissue
Represented in both specimens A and B

B. Needle biopsy of left prostate gland
BENIGN HYPERPLASIA

ABOUT ANABOLIC STEROIDS

Anabolic steroids are male hormones (androgens) that increase body weight and muscle size and may be used by doctors to increase growth in boys who do not mature physically as expected for their age. Steroids also may be used by athletes in an effort to increase strength and enhance performance; however, significant detrimental side effects of these drugs have been recognized:

- High levels of anabolic steroids cause acne, hepatic tumors, and sterility (testicular atrophy and oligospermia).
- In women, the androgenic effect of anabolic steroids leads to male hair distribution, deepening of the voice, amenorrhea, and clitoral enlargement.
- Anabolic steroid use also causes hypercholesterolemia, hypertension, jaundice (liver abnormalities), and salt and water retention (edema).

Gleason Score

The Gleason score (named after Dr. Donald Gleason, a pathologist who developed it in the 1960s) is based on the microscopic appearance of the prostate biopsy specimen. Cancers with a higher Gleason score are more aggressive and carry a worse prognosis. The pathologist assigns a grade (number) to the most common tumor cells and another to the next most common tumor cells. Adding these numbers together gives the Gleason score. The score is based on a scale from 1 to 5. More well-differentiated (closer to normal) cells are given a lower grade, and poorly differentiated (malignant) cells are given a higher grade.

IN PERSON

This is a first-person narrative of a man diagnosed with prostate cancer.

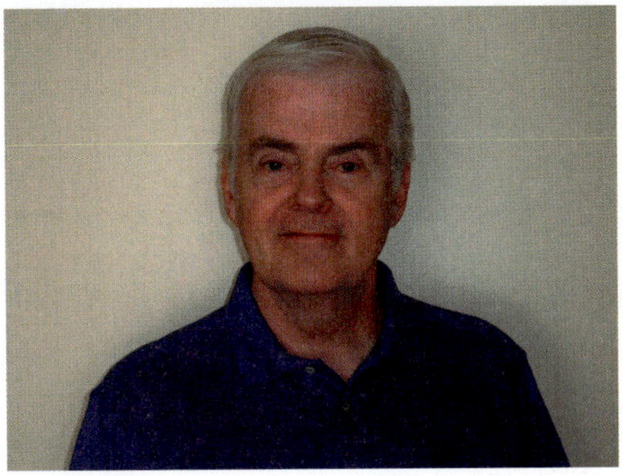

As with many men in their late 50s, the PSA prostate-related lab test was the first item I would always look at when having my annual physical. Over a few years, the PSA had been going up gradually, but nothing that seemed to indicate anything unusual. So it was a bit of a surprise when my primary care doctor suggested that it might be time to have a further medical review of the slowly increasing results. The PSA was 4.37 (4.0 or less is considered normal).

Being in good overall health, I expected the follow-up prostate exam and biopsy to be of a routine nature. It was with great surprise that the prostate biopsy showed that 3 of 12 samples were positive for cancerous cells. My Gleason score was 6 (3 + 3). This situation was described to me as favorable, an early-stage cancer. Nevertheless, I had no idea of the treatment options available.

I decided that the best way to reach a decision for a treatment plan was to get together with the doctors at the Mass General Cancer Center in the genitourinary area, have my situation reviewed and to learn more about my options. I realized that the possibilities ranged widely, including watchful waiting, external radiation, internal radiation, and prostate surgery (prostatectomy). In the end, the decision becomes your own in early-stage prostate cancer, and that, in itself, can leave you second guessing the choice numerous times.

After careful thought and review of the information with my physicians and family, I decided to pursue the internal radiation option, or brachytherapy, often referred to as implantation of radiation seeds. Even up to the time of the procedure, the question remained with me as to whether I was making the right choice: should I wait a while and just see how things go, and would there be any of the unlikely side effects that are noted for this procedure? When the time came, I decided to go forward and had the procedure done at MGH. The entire medical team there made the process from start to completion as successful an event as one could hope for. The best news was that after the procedure, my PSA dropped to 2.5.

Now a year has passed, and I am happy to see that the PSA has continued downward. The long-term side effects of the brachytherapy procedure were related to urination and erectile dysfunction. While urination post-procedure was painful, discomfort dissipated within a week or so. Long term, managing the control of urination was an issue, but after a year it has definitely improved. Erectile dysfunction after any type of prostate procedure is an issue. I found it to be a major effect early on, but less as time progressed. There is still the required monitoring and checkups needed to see that nothing further develops from here on, but taking warning signs seriously, educating yourself, and making an informed decision with the help of the best medical team possible will make you feel good about your choices.

Kevin Mahoney is a U.S. Veteran, now working as a Program Manager. He enjoys spending time with his family, including his wife, children and grandchildren.

9

EXERCISES

Remember to check your answers carefully with those given in the Answers to Exercises, page 336.

A Using the terms below, fill in the flow chart showing the passage of sperm.

epididymis	penis	urethra
ejaculatory duct	seminiferous tubules	vas deferens

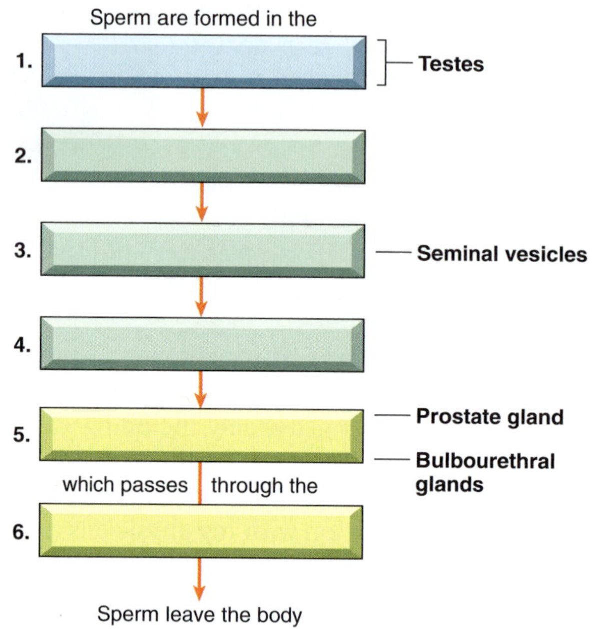

B Select from the following terms to match the descriptions below.

bulbourethral glands	scrotum	spermatozoon
epididymis	seminal vesicles	testis
prepuce	seminiferous tubules	vas deferens
prostate gland		

1. one of a pair of long, tightly coiled tubes above each testis; carries and stores sperm ______________
2. exocrine gland at the base of the male urinary bladder ______________
3. narrow coiled tubules that produce sperm in the testes ______________
4. sperm cell ______________
5. foreskin ______________
6. male gonad; produces testosterone and sperm cells ______________
7. paired sac-like exocrine glands that secrete fluid into the vas deferens ______________
8. external sac that contains the testes ______________
9. narrow tube carrying sperm from the epididymis toward the urethra ______________
10. pair of exocrine glands near the male urethra; Cowper glands ______________

C Select from the following terms to match the descriptions below.

ejaculation
ejaculatory duct
erectile dysfunction
flagellum
fraternal twins
glans penis
identical twins
interstitial cells
parenchymal tissue
perineum

1. hair-like projection on a sperm cell that makes it motile ______
2. sensitive tip of the penis ______
3. tube through which semen enters the urethra ______
4. two infants resulting from division of one fertilized egg into separate embryos ______
5. external region between the anus and scrotum ______
6. essential distinctive cells of an organ ______
7. two infants resulting from fertilization of two ova by two sperm cells ______
8. inability of an adult male to achieve erection; impotence ______
9. specialized cells that lie adjacent to the seminiferous tubules ______
10. ejection of sperm and fluid from the urethra ______

D Match the following terms with their descriptions.

aspermia
azoospermia
impotence
oligospermia
penis
semen
sterilization
stromal tissue
testicle
testosterone

1. male external organ of reproduction ______
2. sperm cells and seminal fluid ______
3. hormone secreted by interstitial cells of the testes ______
4. supportive connective tissue of an organ ______
5. lack of semen ______
6. lack of sperm cells in semen ______
7. procedure that removes a person's ability to produce or release reproductive cells ______
8. semen with a low concentration of sperm ______
9. male gonad ______
10. inability of a male to sustain or achieve an erection ______

E Build medical terms for the following definitions. Parts of words are given.

1. inflammation of the testes: ____________________________itis
2. inflammation of the tube that carries the spermatozoa to the vas deferens:

   ________________________________itis
3. resection of the prostate gland: ____________________________ectomy
4. inflammation of the prostate gland: ____________________________itis
5. process of producing (the formation of) sperm cells: ________________________genesis
6. fixation of undescended testicle: orchio______________________________
7. inflammation of the glans penis: ____________________________itis
8. condition of scanty sperm: ____________________________spermia
9. lack of semen: a______________________________
10. pertaining to a testicle: ____________________________ar

F Answer true or false

1. _______________ Cryogenic surgery uses cold temperatures to destroy tissue.
2. _______________ Estrogen is an example of an androgen.
3. _______________ Castration (orchiectomy or oophorectomy) is an example of sterilization.
4. _______________ A teratoma is a benign tumor of the prostate gland.
5. _______________ Spermolytic means formation of sperm.
6. _______________ Balanitis is inflammation of a testicle.
7. _______________ Azoospermia causes infertility.
8. _______________ Aspermia can result from retrograde ejaculation.
9. _______________ Seminiferous tubules are the interstitial cells of the testes.
10. _______________ Testosterone is produced by the parenchymal tissue of the testes.
11. _______________ Vasectomy produces impotence.
12. _______________ Vasovasostomy is an anastomosis that can restore fertility (ability to reproduce offspring).

9

G **Match the term in Column I with its meaning in Column II. Write the correct letter in the space provided.**

COLUMN I		COLUMN II
1. castration	_______	A. to tie off or bind
2. semen analysis	_______	B. removal of a piece of the vas deferens
3. ejaculation	_______	C. orchiectomy
4. purulent	_______	D. removal of the prepuce
5. vasectomy	_______	E. destruction of tissue by freezing
6. circumcision	_______	F. pus-filled
7. ligation	_______	G. test of fertility (reproductive ability)
8. cryosurgery	_______	H. ejection of sperm and fluid from the urethra
9. seminoma	_______	I. narrowing (stricture) of the opening of the prepuce over the glans penis
10. phimosis	_______	J. malignant tumor of the testis

H **Select from the following terms to fit the descriptions below.**

adenocarcinoma of the prostate	herpes genitalis	hypospadias
benign prostatic hyperplasia	human HPV infection	syphilis
cryptorchidism	hydrocele	varicocele
gonorrhea		

1. prostatic enlargement, nonmalignant ______________________
2. opening of the urethra on the undersurface of the penis ______________________
3. infection of skin and genital mucosa with HSV ______________________
4. malignant tumor of the prostate gland ______________________
5. enlarged, swollen veins near the testes ______________________
6. sexually transmitted disease with primary stage marked by formation of a chancre ____________
7. infection of the skin and mucous membranes in the anogenital region by human papillomavirus

   ____
8. STD caused by berry-shaped bacteria and marked by inflammation of genital mucosa and mucopurulent discharge ______________________
9. undescended testicles ______________________
10. sac of clear fluid in the scrotum ______________________

9

I **Spell out the abbreviations in Column I. Then match each abbreviation with its correct meaning from Column II.**

COLUMN I

1. PSA ________________________ ______
2. BPH ________________________ ______
3. TURP ________________________ ______
4. TRUS ________________________ ______
5. DRE ________________________ ______
6. HSV ________________________ ______
7. STD ________________________ ______

COLUMN II

A. Manual diagnostic procedure to examine the prostate gland
B. Relieves symptoms of prostate gland enlargement
C. Etiologic agent of a sexually transmitted disease characterized by blister formation
D. Noncancerous enlargement of the prostate gland
E. Chlamydial infection, gonorrhea, and syphilis are examples of this general category of infections
F. Helpful procedure in guiding a prostatic biopsy needle
G. High serum levels of this protein indicate prostatic carcinoma

J **Give the meanings of the following word parts.**

1. -one ________________________
2. -stomy ________________________
3. semin/i ________________________
4. -cele ________________________
5. -pexy ________________________
6. -genesis ________________________
7. -plasia ________________________
8. prostat/o ________________________
9. orch/o ________________________
10. terat/o ________________________
11. gon/o ________________________
12. hydr/o ________________________
13. pen/o ________________________
14. balan/o ________________________
15. varic/o ________________________
16. vas/o ________________________
17. test/o ________________________
18. zo/o ________________________
19. crypt/o ________________________
20. andr/o ________________________

K **Match the following surgical procedures with the reasons they would be performed.**

circumcision	photoselective vaporization of the prostate	varicocelectomy
hydrocelectomy	radical (complete) prostatectomy	vasectomy
orchiectomy		vasovasostomy
orchiopexy		

1. carcinoma of the prostate gland ____________________
2. cryptorchidism ____________________
3. sterilization (hormones remain and potency is not impaired) ____________________
4. benign prostatic hyperplasia ____________________
5. abnormal collection of fluid in a scrotal sac ____________________
6. reversal of sterilization procedure ____________________
7. embryonal carcinoma of the testes ____________________
8. phimosis ____________________
9. ligation of swollen, twisted veins above the testes ____________________

L **Use the given definitions to complete the terms. Check your answers carefully.**

1. gland at the base of the urinary bladder in males: pro____________________ gland
2. coiled tube on top of each testis: epi____________________
3. essential tissue of an organ: par____________________ tissue
4. foreskin: pre____________________
5. bacterial infection that invades the urethra and reproductive tract of men and women and is the major cause of nonspecific urethritis in males and cervicitis in females:

   ch____________________
6. ulcer that forms on genital organs after infection with syphilis: ch____________________
7. androgen produced by the interstitial cells of the testis: test____________________
8. fluid secreted by male reproductive glands and ejaculated with sperm: se____________________
9. malignant tumor of the testis: sem____________________
10. pertaining to the penis: pen____________________

M **Circle the correct term(s) to complete the following sentences.**

1. When Fred was a newborn infant, his doctors could feel only one testicle within the scrotum and suggested close monitoring of his condition of **(gonorrhea, cryptorchidism, benign prostatic hyperplasia)**.
2. Bob had many sexual partners, one of whom had been diagnosed with **(testosterone, phimosis, chlamydial infection)**, a highly communicable STD.
3. At age 65, Mike had some difficulty with urgency and discomfort when urinating. His doctor did a digital rectal examination to examine his **(prostate gland, urinary bladder, vas deferens)**.

4. Just after Nick's birth, his parents had a difficult time deciding whether to have their infant son undergo **(TURP, castration, circumcision)**.
5. Ted noticed a hard ulcer on his penis and made an appointment with his doctor, a **(gastroenterologist, gynecologist, urologist)**. The doctor viewed a specimen of the ulcer under the microscope and did a blood test, which revealed that Ted had contracted **(gonorrhea, herpes genitalis, syphilis)**, so the ulcer was a **(blister, chancre, seminoma)**.
6. After his fifth child was born, Art decided to have a **(vasovasostomy, hydrocelectomy, vasectomy)** to prevent conception of another child. A/an **(nephrologist, urologist, abdominal surgeon)** performed the procedure to cut and ligate the **(urethra, epididymis, vas deferens)**.
7. Twenty-six-year-old Lance noticed a hard testicular mass. His physician prescribed a brief trial with **(antibodies, antibiotics, pain killers)** to rule out **(epididymitis, testicular cancer, varicocele)**. The mass remained and Lance underwent **(epididymectomy, orchiectomy, prostatectomy)**. The mass was a **(seminoma, prostate cancer, hydrocele)**.
8. Sarah and Steve had been trying to conceive a child for 7 years. Steve had a **(digital rectal examination, TURP, semen analysis)**, which revealed 25% normal sperm count with 10% motility. He was told he had **(phimosis, azoospermia, oligospermia)**.
9. To boost his sperm count, Steve was given **(estrogen, testosterone, progesterone)**. As a side effect, this **(androgen, progestin, enzyme)** gave him a case of acne lasting several months.
10. Sarah eventually became pregnant. An ultrasound examination showed two embryos with two separate placentas and in separate **(peritoneal, scrotal, amniotic)** sacs. Sarah gave birth to two healthy **(identical, fraternal, perineal)** twin girls.

9

ANSWERS TO EXERCISES

A

1. seminiferous tubules
2. epididymis
3. vas deferens
4. ejaculatory duct
5. urethra
6. penis

B

1. epididymis
2. prostate gland
3. seminiferous tubules
4. spermatozoon
5. prepuce
6. testis
7. seminal vesicles
8. scrotum
9. vas deferens
10. bulbourethral (Cowper) glands

C

1. flagellum
2. glans penis
3. ejaculatory duct
4. identical twins
5. perineum
6. parenchymal tissue
7. fraternal twins
8. erectile dysfunction
9. interstitial cells
10. ejaculation

D

1. penis
2. semen
3. testosterone
4. stromal tissue
5. aspermia
6. azoospermia
7. sterilization
8. oligospermia
9. testicle
10. impotence

E

1. orchitis
2. epididymitis
3. prostatectomy
4. prostatitis
5. spermatogenesis
6. orchiopexy
7. balanitis
8. oligospermia
9. aspermia
10. testicular

F

1. True.
2. False. Estrogen is a female hormone. Androgens are male hormones. Testosterone is an androgen.
3. True.
4. False. Teratoma is a malignant tumor in the testis.
5. False. Spermolytic is destruction of sperm. Spermatogenesis is formation of sperm.
6. False. Balanitis is inflammation of the glans penis. Orchitis is inflammation of a testicle.
7. True.
8. True. Semen is discharged backward into the urinary bladder and not ejaculated.
9. False. Seminiferous tubules are the parenchymal tissue of the testes. The interstitial cells of the testis are the Leydig cells that secrete testosterone.
10. False. Testosterone is produced by the interstitial cells of the testis.
11. False. Vasectomy results in the inability of sperm to leave the body in semen. It does not affect erectile dysfunction and does not produce impotence.
12. True.

G

1. C
2. G
3. H
4. F
5. B
6. D
7. A
8. E
9. J
10. I

H

1. benign prostatic hyperplasia
2. hypospadias
3. herpes genitalis
4. adenocarcinoma of the prostate
5. varicocele
6. syphilis
7. HPV infection
8. gonorrhea
9. cryptorchidism
10. hydrocele

I

1. prostate-specific antigen: G
2. benign prostatic hyperplasia: D
3. transurethral resection of the prostate: B
4. transrectal ultrasound: F
5. digital rectal examination: A
6. herpes simplex virus: C
7. sexually transmitted disease: E

J

1. hormone
2. opening
3. semen, seed
4. hernia, swelling
5. fixation
6. formation
7. formation
8. prostate gland
9. testis
10. monster
11. seed
12. water
13. penis
14. glans penis
15. varicose veins
16. vessel, duct, vas deferens
17. testis, testicle
18. animal life
19. hidden
20. male

K

1. radical (complete) prostatectomy
2. orchiopexy
3. vasectomy
4. photoselective vaporization of the prostate
5. hydrocelectomy
6. vasovasostomy
7. orchiectomy
8. circumcision
9. varicocelectomy

L

1. prostate
2. epididymis
3. parenchymal
4. prepuce
5. chlamydia
6. chancre
7. testosterone
8. semen or seminal fluid
9. seminoma
10. penile

M

1. cryptorchidism
2. chlamydial infection
3. prostate gland
4. circumcision
5. urologist; syphilis; chancre
6. vasectomy; urologist; vas deferens
7. antibiotics; epididymitis; orchiectomy; seminoma
8. semen analysis; oligospermia
9. testosterone; androgen
10. amniotic; fraternal

Answers to Practical Applications

Case Report: A Man with Post-TURP Complaints

1. c
2. b
3. b
4. a
5. b
6. c
7. c
8. a

PRONUNCIATION OF TERMS

To test your understanding of the terminology in this chapter, write the meaning of each term in the space provided. In addition, you may wish to cover the terms and write them by looking at your definitions. Make sure your spelling is correct. The page number after each term indicates where it is defined or used in the book, so you can easily check your responses. You will find complete definitions for all of these terms and their audio pronunciations on the Evolve website.

Pronunciation Guide

ā as in āpe	ă as in ăpple
ē as in ēven	ĕ as in ĕvery
ī as in īce	ĭ as in ĭnterest
ō as in ōpen	ŏ as in pŏt
ū as in ūnit	ŭ as in ŭnder

TERM	PRONUNCIATION	MEANING
androgen (317)	ĂN-drō-jĕn	
aspermia (318)	ā-SPĔR-mē-ă	
azoospermia (319)	ā-zō-ō-SPĔR-mē-ă	
balanitis (317)	băl-ă-NĪ-tĭs	
benign prostatic hyperplasia (321)	bē-NĪN-prŏs-TĂT-ĭk hī-pĕr-PLĀ-zē-ă	
bulbourethral glands (315)	bŭl-bō-ū-RĒ-thrăl glăndz	
carcinoma of the prostate (321)	kăr-sĭ-NŌ-mă of the PRŎS-tāt	
carcinoma of the testes (319)	kăr-sĭ-NŌ-mă of the TĔS-tēz	
castration (325)	kăs-TRĀ-shŭn	
chancre (324)	SHĂNG-kĕr	
chlamydial infection (322)	klă-MĬD-ē-ăl ĭn-FEK-shŭn	
circumcision (325)	sĭr-kŭm-SĬZH-ŭn	
cryogenic surgery (317)	krī-ō-GĔN-ĭk SŬR-jĕr-ē	
cryptorchidism (317)	krĭp-TŎR-kĭdĭzm	
digital rectal exam (325)	DĬJ-ĕ-tăl RĔK-tăl ĕk-ZĂM	
ejaculation (315)	ē-jăk-ū-LĀ-shŭn	
ejaculatory duct (315)	ē-JĂK-ū-lă-tōr-ē dŭkt	
embryonal carcinoma (319)	ĕm-brē-ŌN-ăl kăr-sĭ-NŌ-mă	
epididymis (315)	ĕp-ĭ-DĬD-ĭ-mĭs	
epididymitis (317)	ĕp-ĭ-dĭd-ĭ-MĪ-tĭs	
erectile dysfunction (315)	ē-RĔK-tīl dĭs-FŬNK-shŭn	
flagellum (315)	flă-JĔL-ŭm	

TERM	PRONUNCIATION	MEANING
fraternal twins (315)	fră-TĔR-năl twĭnz	________
glans penis (315)	glănz PĒ-nĭs	________
gonorrhea (322)	gŏn-ō-RĒ-ă	________
herpes genitalis (323)	HĔR-pēz jĕn-ĭ-TĂL-ĭs	________
human papillomavirus (324)	HŪ-măn păp-ĭ-LŌ-mă VĪ-rŭs	________
hydrocele (317)	HĪ-drō-sēl	________
hypospadias (322)	hī-pō-SPĀ-dē-ăs	________
identical twins (316)	ī-DĔN-tĭ-kăl twĭnz	________
impotence (316)	ĬM-pō-tĕns	________
interstitial cells of the testes (316)	ĭn-tĕr-STĬ-shŭl sĕlz of the TĔS-tĭs	________
ligation (326)	lī-GĀ-shŭn	________
oligospermia (318)	ŏl-ĭ-gō-SPĔR-mē-ă	________
orchiectomy (318)	ŏr-kē-ĔK-tō-mē	________
orchiopexy (319)	ŏr-kē-ō-PĔK-sē	________
orchitis (318)	ŏr-KĪ-tĭs	________
parenchymal tissue (316)	pă-RĔNG-kĭ-măl TĬS-ū	________
penile (318)	PĒ-nīl	________
penis (316)	PĒ-nĭs	________
penoscrotal (318)	pē-nō-SKRŌ-tăl	________
perineum (316)	pĕr-ĭ-NĒ-ŭm	________
phimosis (322)	fi-MŌ-sĭs	________
photoselective vaporization of the prostate (325)	fō-tō-sĕ-LĔK-tĭv vā-pŏr-ĭ-ZĀ-shŭn of the PRŎS-tāt	________
prepuce (316)	PRĒ-pŭs	________
prostatectomy (318)	prŏs-tă-TĔK-tō-mē	________
prostate gland (316)	PRŎS-tāt glănd	________
prostatitis (318)	prŏs-tă-TĪ-tĭs	________
purulent (322)	PŪR-ū-lĕnt	________
scrotum (316)	SKRŌ-tŭm	________
semen (316)	SĒ-mĕn	________

9

TERM	PRONUNCIATION	MEANING
semen analysis (324)	SĒ-mĕn ă-NĂL-ĭ-sĭs	
seminal vesicles (316)	SĔM-ĭn-ăl VĔS-ĭ-klz	
seminiferous tubules (316)	sĕ-mĭ-NĬF-ĕr-ŭs TOOB-ūlz	
seminoma (319)	sĕ-mĭ-NŌ-mă	
spermatogenesis (319)	spĕr-mă-tō-JĔN-ĕ-sĭs	
spermatozoa (316)	spĕr-mă-tō-ZŌ-ă	
spermatozoon (316)	spĕr-mă-tō-ZŌ-ĕn	
spermolytic (318)	spĕr-mō-LĬT-ĭk	
sterilization (316)	stĕr-ĭ-lĭ-ZĀ-shŭn	
stromal tissue (316)	STRŌ-măl TĬS-ū	
syphilis (324)	SĬF-ĭ-lĭs	
teratoma (318)	tĕr-ă-TŌ-mă	
testicular (318)	tĕs-TĬK-ū-lăr	
testicular torsion (320)	tĕs-TĬK-ū-lăr TŎR-shŭn	
testis (316)	TĔS-tĭs	
testosterone (316)	tĕs-TŎS-tĕ-rōn	
transurethral resection of the prostate (325)	trănz-ū-RĒ-trăl rē-SĔK-shun of the PRŎS-tāt	
varicocele (318)	VĂR-ĭ-kō-sēl	
vas deferens (316)	văs DĔF-ĕr-ĕnz	
vasectomy (326)	vă-SĔK-tō-mē	
vasovasostomy (319)	vă-zō-vă-ZŎS-tō-mē	

9

REVIEW SHEET

Write the meanings of the word parts in the spaces provided. Check your answers with the information in the chapter or in the Glossary (Medical Word Parts—English) at the end of the book.

Combining Forms

COMBINING FORM	MEANING	COMBINING FORM	MEANING
andr/o	______________	pen/o	______________
balan/o	______________	prostat/o	______________
cry/o	______________	semin/i	______________
crypt/o	______________	sperm/o	______________
epididym/o	______________	spermat/o	______________
gon/o	______________	terat/o	______________
hydr/o	______________	test/o	______________
orch/o	______________	varic/o	______________
orchi/o	______________	vas/o	______________
orchid/o	______________	zo/o	______________

Suffixes

SUFFIX	MEANING	SUFFIX	MEANING
-cele	______________	-one	______________
-ectomy	______________	-pexy	______________
-gen	______________	-plasia	______________
-genesis	______________	-rrhea	______________
-genic	______________	-stomy	______________
-lysis	______________	-tomy	______________
-lytic	______________	-trophy	______________

evolve *Please visit the Evolve website for additional exercises, games, and images related to this chapter.*

9

CHAPTER 10

Nervous System

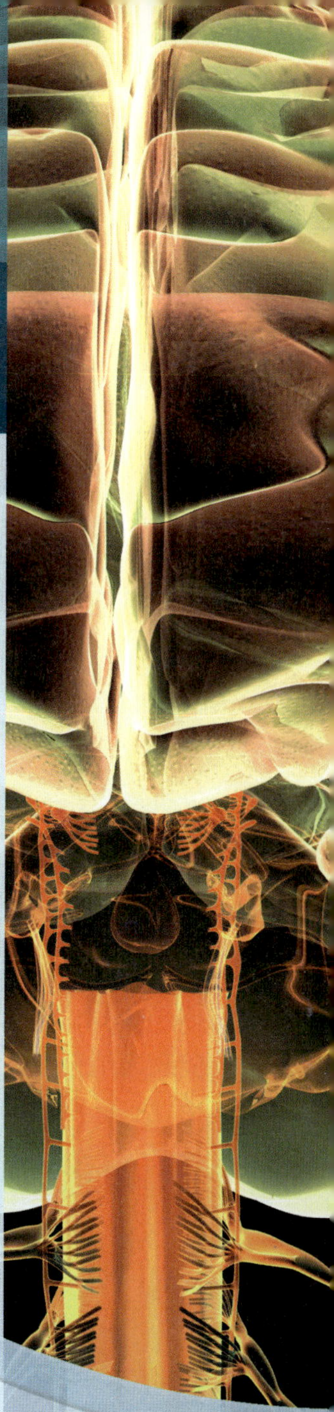

This chapter is divided into the following sections:

CHAPTER GOALS

- Name, locate, and describe the major organs of the nervous system and their functions.
- Learn nervous system combining forms and use them with suffixes and prefixes.
- Define pathologic conditions affecting the nervous system.
- Describe nervous system–related laboratory tests, clinical procedures, and abbreviations.
- Apply your new knowledge to understanding medical terms in their proper contexts, such as medical reports and records.

INTRODUCTION

The nervous system is one of the most complex of all human body systems. More than 100 billion nerve cells operate constantly all over the body to coordinate the activities we do consciously and voluntarily, as well as those that occur unconsciously or involuntarily. We speak, move muscles, hear, taste, see, and think. Our glands secrete hormones, and we respond to danger, pain, temperature, and touch. All of these functions comprise only a small number of the many activities controlled by the nervous system.

Fibers exiting from microscopic **nerve cells** (**neurons**) are collected into macroscopic bundles called **nerves,** which carry electrical messages all over the body. External stimuli, as well as internal chemicals such as **acetylcholine,** activate the cell membranes of nerve cells, which results in electrical discharges of these cells. These electrical discharges, **nervous impulses**, may then traverse the length of the associated nerves. External **receptors** (sense organs) as well as internal receptors in muscles and blood vessels receive these impulses and may in turn transmit impulses to the complex network of nerve cells in the brain and spinal cord. Within this central part of the nervous system, impulses are recognized, interpreted, and finally relayed to other nerve cells that extend out to all parts of the body, such as muscles, glands, and internal organs.

GENERAL STRUCTURE OF THE NERVOUS SYSTEM

10

The nervous system is classified into two major divisions: the **central nervous system (CNS)** and the **peripheral nervous system (PNS).** The central nervous system consists of the **brain** and **spinal cord.** The peripheral nervous system consists of **cranial nerves** and **spinal nerves, plexuses,** and **peripheral nerves** throughout the body (Figure 10-1). Cranial nerves carry impulses between the brain and the head and neck. The one exception is the 10th cranial nerve, called the **vagus nerve.** It carries messages to and from the neck, chest, and abdomen. Figure 10-2 shows cranial nerves, their functions, and the parts of the body that they carry messages to and from. Spinal nerves carry messages between the spinal cord and the chest, abdomen, and extremities.

A **plexus** is a large network of nerves in the peripheral nervous system. The cervical, brachial (brachi/o means arm), and lumbosacral plexuses are examples that include cervical, lumbar, and sacral nerves. Figure 10-1 illustrates the relationship of the brain and spinal cord to the spinal nerves and plexuses.

The spinal and cranial nerves are composed of nerves that help the body respond to changes in the outside world. They include sense **receptors** for sight (eye), hearing and balance (ear), smell (olfactory), and touch (skin sensation) and **sensory (afferent) nerves** that carry messages related to changes in the environment *toward* the spinal cord and brain. In addition, **motor (efferent) nerves** travel *from* the spinal cord and brain to muscles of the body, telling them how to respond. For example, when you touch a hot stove, temperature and pain receptors in the skin stimulate afferent nerves, which carry messages toward the spinal cord and brain. Instantaneously, the message is conveyed to efferent nerve cells in the spinal cord, which then activate voluntary muscles to pull your hand away from the stove.

Plexus

There are other **plexuses** in the body—networks of intersecting blood vessels (vascular) and lymphatic vessels.
- Lymphatic plexus is an interconnecting network of lymph vessels.
- Rectal plexus is a plexus of veins in the rectal region.
- Vertebral plexus is a plexus of veins related to the backbone.

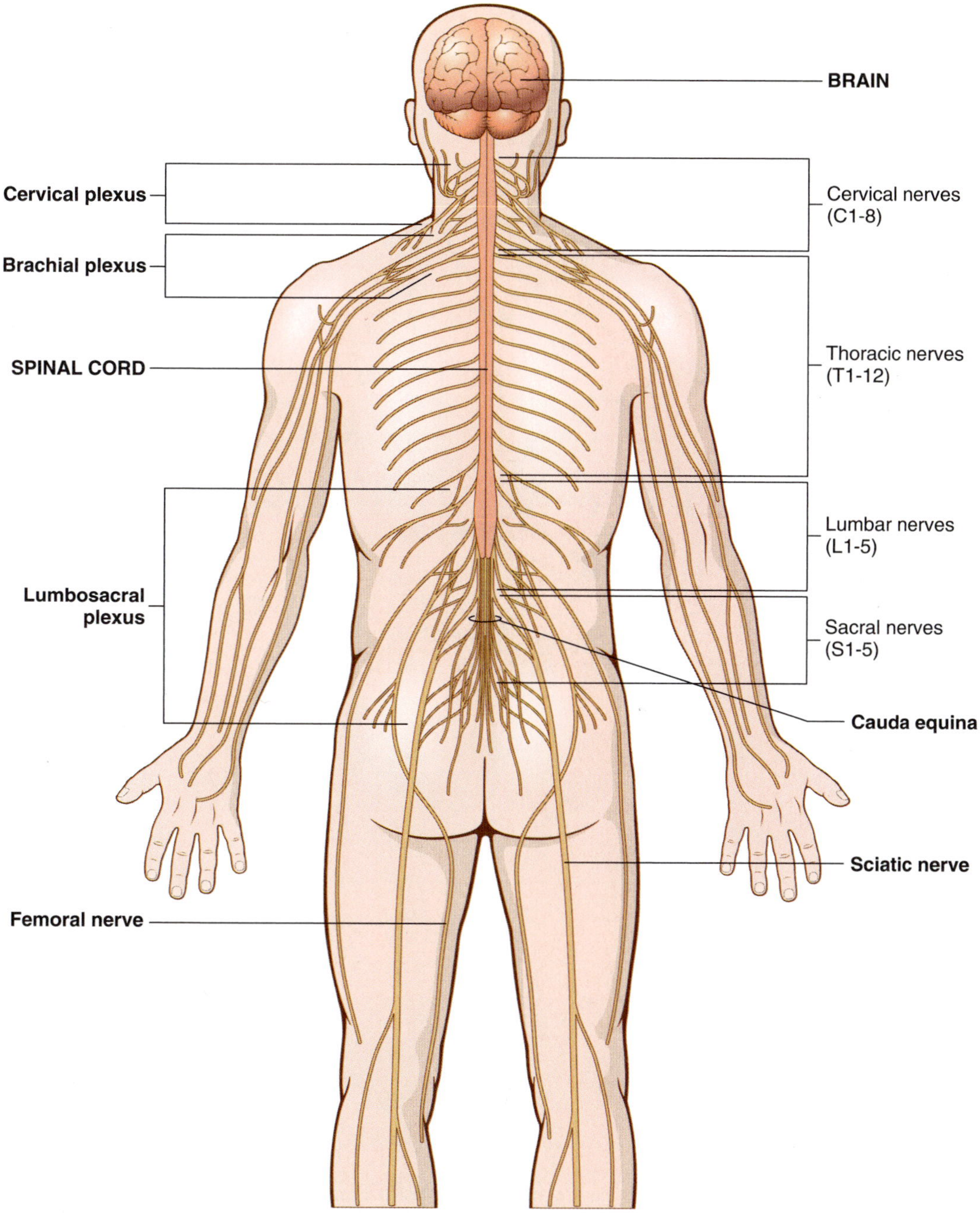

FIGURE 10-1 **The brain and the spinal cord, spinal nerves, and spinal plexuses.** The **femoral nerve** is a lumbar nerve leading to and from the thigh (femur). The **sciatic nerve** is a nerve beginning in a region of the hip. The **cauda equina** (Latin for "horse's tail") is a bundle of spinal nerves below the end of the spinal cord.

In addition to the spinal and cranial nerves (whose functions are mainly voluntary and involved with sensations of smell, taste, sight, hearing, and muscle movements), the peripheral nervous system also contains a large group of nerves that function involuntarily or automatically, without conscious control. These peripheral nerves belong to the **autonomic nervous system.** This system of nerve fibers carries impulses *away from* the CNS to the glands, heart, blood vessels, and involuntary muscles found in the walls of tubes like the intestines and hollow organs like the stomach and urinary bladder.

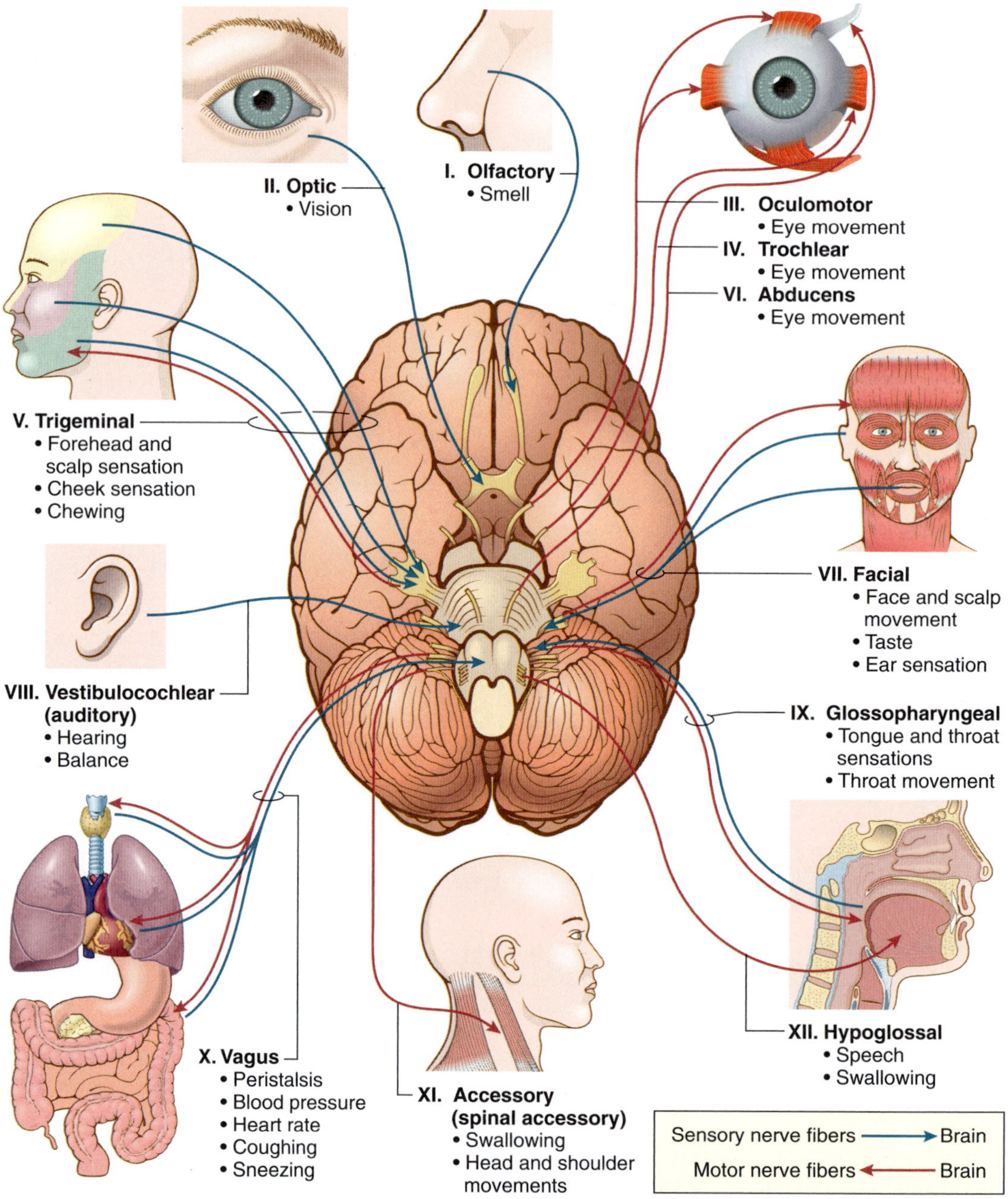

FIGURE 10-2 **Cranial nerves** (I to XII) leading from the base of the brain and showing the parts of the body they affect. **Sensory** or **afferent** nerves are colored *blue* and carry messages *toward* the brain. **Motor** or **efferent** nerves are colored *red* and carry messages *from* the brain to muscles and organs. Some nerves (mixed) carry both sensory and motor fibers. Don't try to memorize this figure! Just get the big picture: Cranial nerves carry messages to and from the brain to all parts of head and neck and also (in the case of the vagus nerve) to other parts of the body.

Some autonomic nerves are **sympathetic** nerves and others are **parasympathetic** nerves. The sympathetic nerves stimulate the body in times of stress and crisis. They increase heart rate and forcefulness, dilate (relax) airways so more oxygen can enter, and increase blood pressure. In addition, sympathetic neurons stimulate the adrenal glands to secrete epinephrine (adrenaline), while also inhibiting intestinal contractions to slow digestion. The parasympathetic nerves normally act as a balance for the sympathetic nerves.

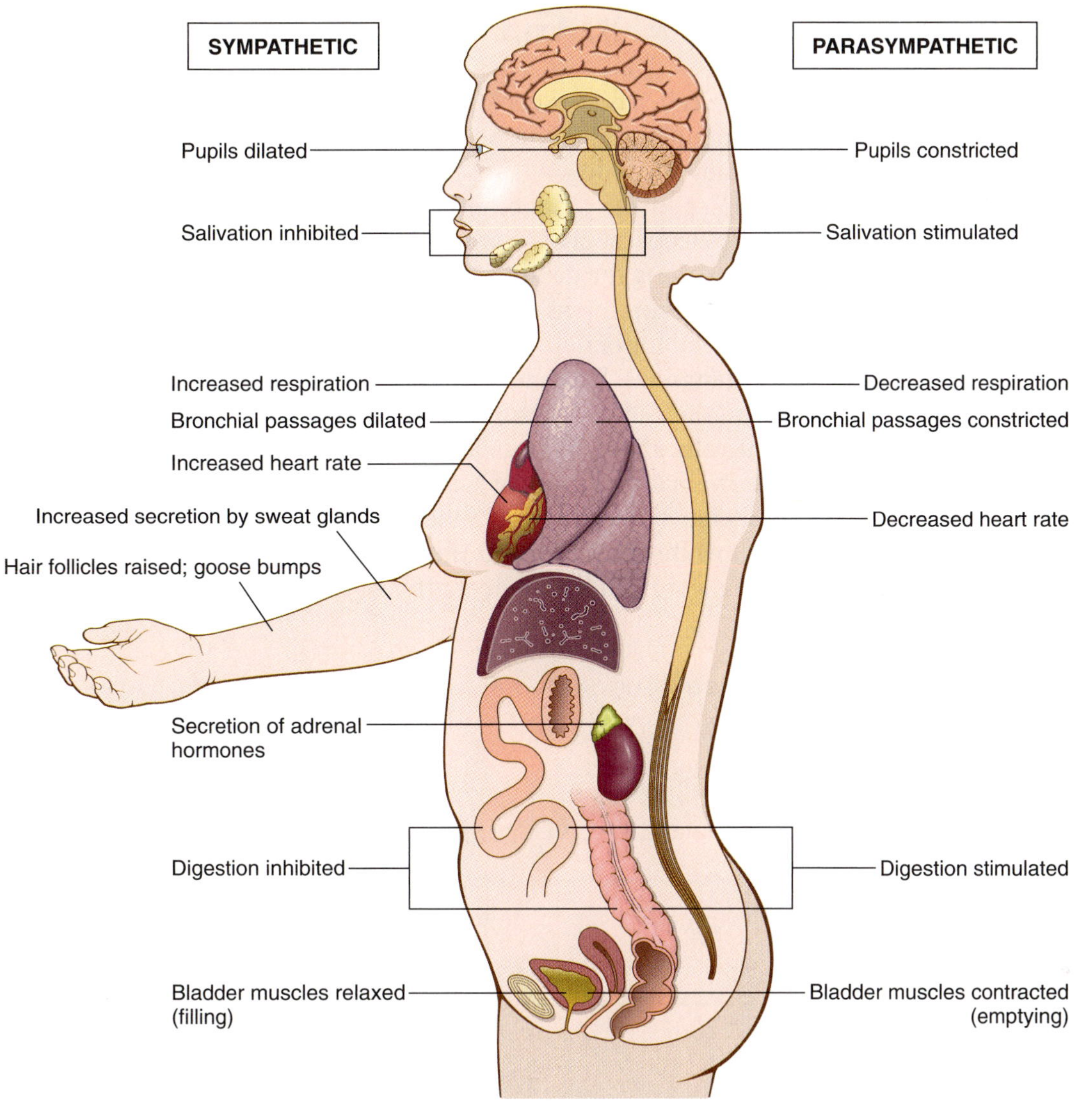

FIGURE 10-3 **Actions of parasympathetic and sympathetic nerves.**

Parasympathetic nerves slow down heart rate, lower blood pressure, and stimulate intestinal contractions to clear the rectum. Figure 10-3 shows the differences in actions between the sympathetic and parasympathetic nerves.

Figure 10-4 summarizes the divisions of the central and peripheral nervous systems.

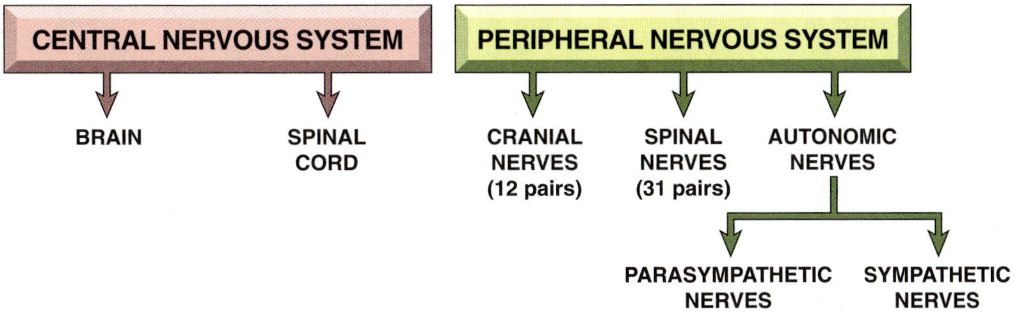

FIGURE 10-4 **Divisions of the central nervous system (CNS) and peripheral nervous system (PNS).** The autonomic nervous system is a part of the peripheral nervous system.

NEURONS, NERVES, AND GLIAL CELLS

A **neuron** is an individual nerve cell, a microscopic structure. Impulses pass along the parts of a nerve cell in a definite manner and direction. The parts of a neuron are pictured in Figure 10-5; label it as you study the following.

A **stimulus** begins an impulse in the branching fibers of the neuron, which are called **dendrites** [1]. A change in the electrical charge of the dendrite membranes is thus begun, and the nervous impulse moves along the dendrites like the movement of falling dominoes. The impulse, traveling in only one direction, next reaches the **cell body** [2], which contains the **cell nucleus** [3]. Small collections of nerve cell bodies outside the brain and spinal cord are called **ganglia** (*singular:* **ganglion**). Extending from the cell body is the **axon** [4], which carries the impulse away from the cell body. Axons can be covered with a fatty tissue called myelin. The purpose of this **myelin sheath** [5] is to insulate the axon and speed transmission of the electrical impulse. Demyelination is loss of the myelin insulating the nerve fiber and is characteristic of multiple sclerosis, an acquired illness affecting the CNS.

The myelin sheath gives a white appearance to the nerve fiber—hence the term white matter, as in parts of the spinal cord and the white matter of the brain and most peripheral

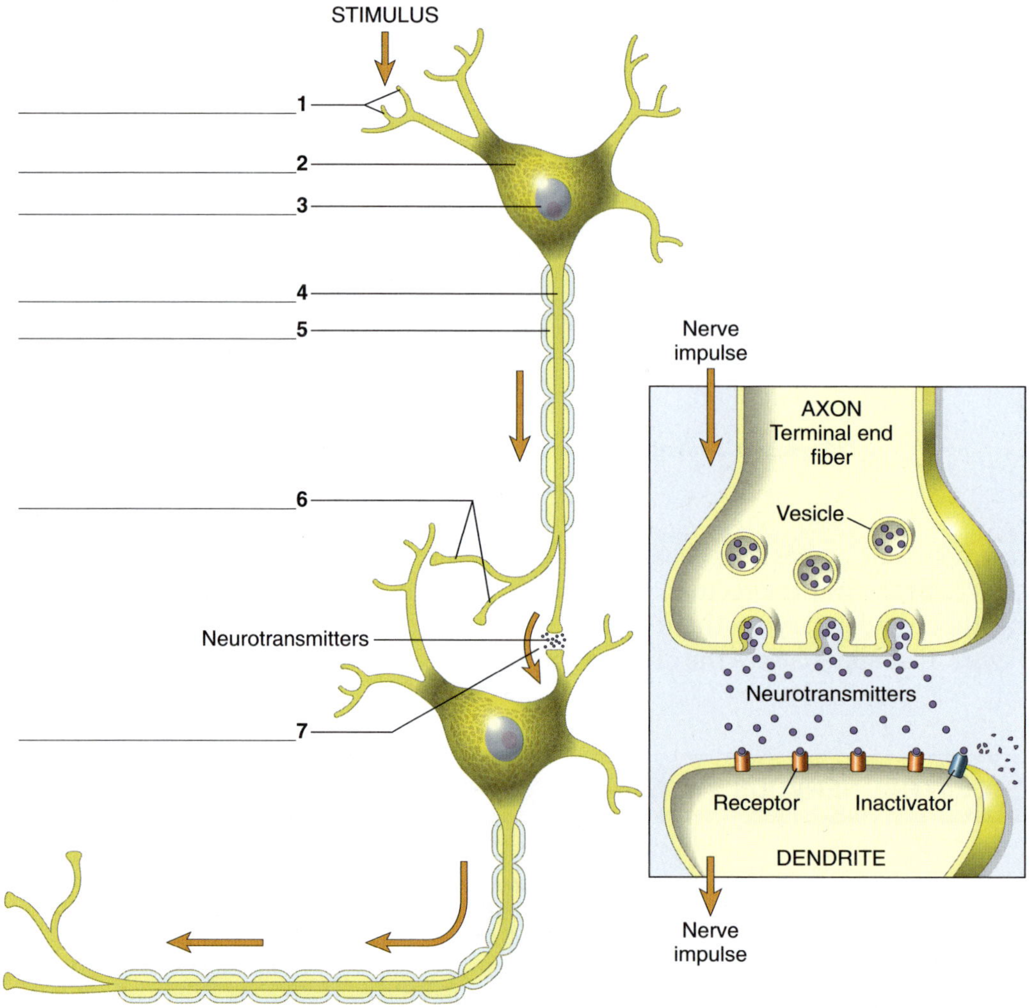

FIGURE 10-5 Parts of a neuron and the pathway of a nervous impulse. Neurons are the **parenchymal** (essential) **cells** of the nervous system. The *boxed drawing* shows what happens in a synapse: Vesicles store neurotransmitters in the terminal end fibers of axons. Receptors on the dendrites pick up the neurotransmitters. Inactivators end the activity of neurotransmitters when they have finished their job.

nerves. The gray matter of the brain and spinal cord is composed of the cell bodies of neurons that appear gray because they are not covered by a myelin sheath.

The nervous impulse passes through the axon to leave the cell via the **terminal end fibers** [6] of the neuron. The space where the nervous impulse jumps from one neuron to another is called the **synapse** [7]. The transfer of the impulse across the synapse depends on the release of a chemical substance, called a **neurotransmitter,** by the neuron that brings the impulse to the synapse. See the boxed diagram in Figure 10-5. Tiny sacs (vesicles) containing the neurotransmitter are located at the ends of neurons, and they release the neurotransmitter into the synapse. **Acetylcholine, norepinephrine, epinephrine (adrenaline), dopamine, serotonin,** and **endorphins** are examples of neurotransmitters.

Whereas a neuron is a microscopic structure within the nervous system, a **nerve** is macroscopic, able to be seen with the naked eye. A nerve consists of a bundle of dendrites and axons that travel together like strands of rope. Peripheral nerves that carry impulses *to* the brain and spinal cord from stimulus receptors like the skin, eye, ear, and nose are **afferent** or **sensory nerves;** those that carry impulses *from* the CNS to organs that produce responses, such as muscles and glands, are **efferent** or **motor nerves.**

Neurons and nerves are the **parenchyma** of the nervous system. Parenchyma is the essential distinguishing tissue of an organ. In the brain and spinal cord, neurons, which conduct electrical impulses, are the parenchymal tissue. **Stroma** of an organ is the connective and supportive tissue of an organ. The stromal tissue of the nervous system consists of the **glial (neuroglial) cells,** which make up its supportive framework and help it ward off infection. Glial cells do not transmit impulses. They are far more numerous than neurons and can reproduce.

There are four types of supporting or glial cells (see Figure 10-6). **Astrocytes (astroglial cells)** are star-like in appearance (astr/o means star) and transport water and salts between capillaries and neurons. **Microglial cells** are small cells with many branching processes (dendrites). As phagocytes, they protect neurons in response to inflammation. **Oligodendroglial cells (oligodendrocytes)** have few (olig/o means few or scanty) dendrites. These cells form the myelin sheath in the CNS. By contrast, **ependymal cells** (Greek *ependyma* means upper garment) line membranes within the brain and spinal cord where CSF is produced and circulates.

Glial cells, particularly the astrocytes, are associated with blood vessels and regulate the passage of potentially harmful substances from the blood into the nerve cells of the brain. This protective barrier between the blood and brain cells is called the **blood-brain barrier (BBB).** This barrier consists of special lining (endothelial) cells, which along with astrocytes separate capillaries from nerve cells. Delivery of chemotherapeutic drugs to treat brain tumors is thus difficult, because the BBB blocks drug access to brain tissues. Figure 10-6 illustrates glial cells.

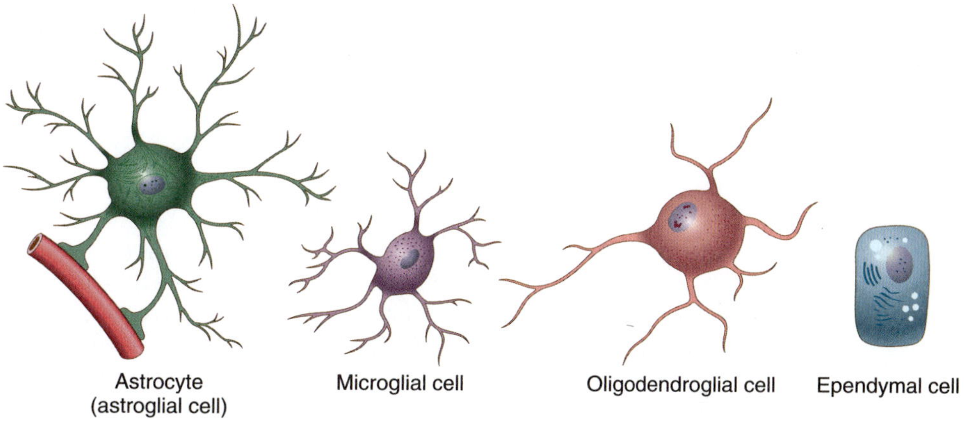

FIGURE 10-6 Glial cells (neuroglial cells). These are the supportive, protective, and connective tissue cells of the CNS. Glial cells are **stromal** (framework) **tissue**, whereas neurons carry nervous impulses.

THE BRAIN

The brain controls body activities. In the human adult, it weighs about 3 pounds and has many different parts, all of which control different aspects of body functions.

The largest part of the brain is the "thinking" area, or **cerebrum.** On the surface of the cerebrum, nerve cells lie in sheets, which make up the **cerebral cortex.** These sheets, arranged in folds called **gyri,** are separated from each other by grooves known as **sulci.** The brain is divided in half, a right side and a left side, which are called **cerebral hemispheres.** Each hemisphere is subdivided into four major lobes named for the cranial (skull) bones that overlie them. Figure 10-7 shows these lobes—frontal, parietal, occipital, and temporal—as well as gyri and sulci.

The cerebrum has many functions. Thought, judgment, memory, association, and discrimination take place within it. In addition, sensory impulses are received through afferent cranial nerves, and when registered in the cortex, they are the basis for perception. Cranial nerves carry motor impulses from the cerebrum to muscles and glands, and these produce movement and activity. Figure 10-7 shows the location of some of the centers in the cerebral cortex that control speech, vision, smell, movement, hearing, and thought processes.

In the middle of the cerebrum are spaces, or canals, called **ventricles** (pictured in Figure 10-8). They contain a watery fluid that flows throughout the brain and around the spinal cord. This fluid is **cerebrospinal fluid (CSF),** and it protects the brain and spinal cord from shock by acting like a cushion. CSF usually is clear and colorless and contains lymphocytes, sugar, and proteins. Spinal fluid can be withdrawn for diagnosis or relief of pressure on the brain; this is called a **lumbar puncture (LP).** For this procedure, a hollow needle is inserted

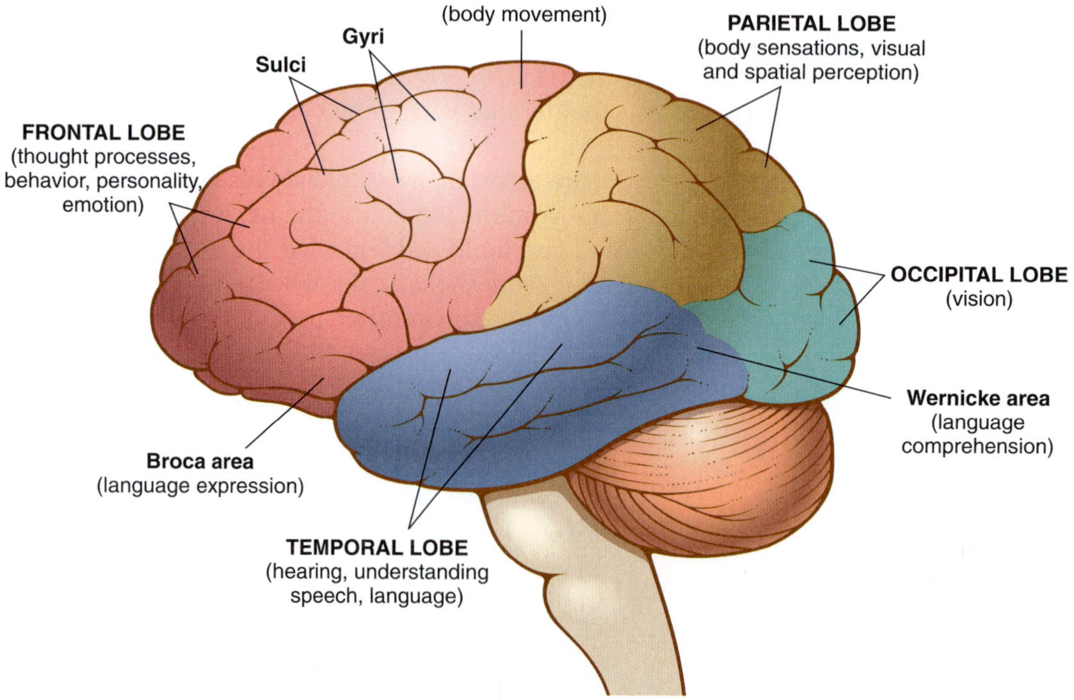

FIGURE 10-7 **Left cerebral hemisphere** (lateral view). **Gyri** (convolutions) and **sulci** (fissures) are indicated. Notice the lobes of the cerebrum and the functional centers that control speech, vision, movement, hearing, thinking, and other processes. Neurologists believe that the two hemispheres have different abilities. The **left brain** is more concerned with language, mathematical functioning, reasoning, and analytical thinking. The **right brain** is more active in spatial relationships, art, music, emotions, and intuition.

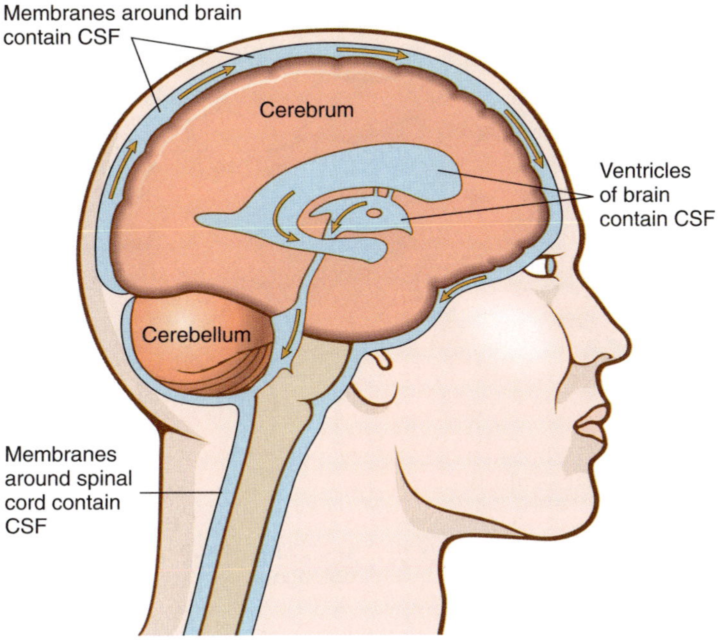

FIGURE 10-8 Circulation of cerebrospinal fluid (CSF) in the brain (ventricles) and around the spinal cord. CSF is formed within the ventricles and circulates between the membranes around the brain and within the spinal cord. CSF empties into the bloodstream through the membranes surrounding the brain and spinal cord.

10

into the lumbar region of the spinal column below the region where the nervous tissue of the spinal cord ends, and CSF is withdrawn.

Two other important parts of the brain are the **thalamus** and the **hypothalamus** (Figure 10-9). The thalamus acts like a triage center. It decides what is important and what is not, selectively processing and relaying sensory information to the cerebral cortex. The thalamus also plays a major role in maintaining levels of awareness and consciousness. The hypothalamus (below the thalamus) contains neurons that control body temperature, sleep, appetite, sexual desire, and emotions such as fear and pleasure. The hypothalamus also regulates the release of hormones from the pituitary gland at the base of the brain and integrates the activities of the sympathetic and parasympathetic nervous systems.

The following structures within the brain lie in the back and below the cerebrum and connect the cerebrum with the spinal cord: cerebellum, pons, and medulla oblongata. The pons and medulla are part of the **brainstem.**

The **cerebellum** functions to coordinate voluntary movements and to maintain balance and posture.

The **pons** is a part of the brainstem that literally means bridge. It contains nerve fiber tracts that connect the cerebellum and cerebrum with the rest of the brain. Nerves to the eyes and face lie here.

The **medulla oblongata,** also in the brainstem, connects the spinal cord with the rest of the brain. Nerve tracts cross from right to left and left to right in the medulla oblongata. For example, nerve cells that control movement of the left side of the body are found in the right half of the cerebrum. These cells send out axons that cross over (decussate) to the opposite side of the brain in the medulla oblongata and then travel down the spinal cord.

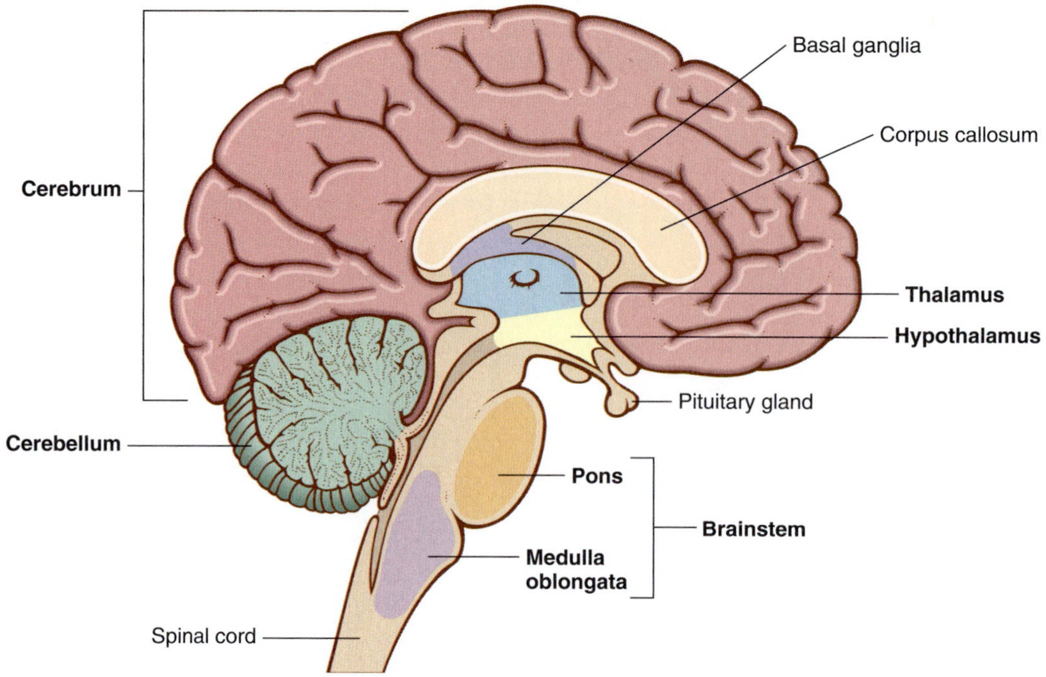

FIGURE 10-9 Parts of the brain: cerebrum, thalamus, hypothalamus, cerebellum, pons, and medulla oblongata. Note the location of the pituitary gland below the hypothalamus. The **basal ganglia** (a group of cells) regulate intentional movements of the body. The **corpus callosum** lies in the center of the brain and connects the two hemispheres (halves).

10

In addition, the medulla oblongata contains three important vital centers that regulate internal activities of the body:

1. **Respiratory center**—controls muscles of respiration in response to chemicals or other stimuli
2. **Cardiac center**—slows the heart rate when the heart is beating too rapidly
3. **Vasomotor center**—affects (constricts or dilates) the muscles in the walls of blood vessels, thus influencing blood pressure

Figure 10-9 shows the locations of the thalamus, hypothalamus, cerebellum, pons, and medulla oblongata. Table 10-1 reviews the functions of these parts of the brain.

TABLE 10-1 FUNCTIONS OF THE PARTS OF THE BRAIN

Structure	Function(s)
Cerebrum	Thinking, personality, sensations, movements, memory
Thalamus	Relay station ("triage center") for sensory impulses; control of awareness and consciousness
Hypothalamus	Body temperature, sleep, appetite, emotions, control of the pituitary gland
Cerebellum	Coordination of voluntary movements and balance
Pons	Connection of nerves (to the eyes and face)
Medulla oblongata	Nerve fibers cross over, left to right and right to left; contains centers to regulate heart, blood vessels, and respiratory system

THE SPINAL CORD AND MENINGES

SPINAL CORD

The **spinal cord** is a column of nervous tissue extending from the medulla oblongata to the second lumbar vertebra within the vertebral column. Below the end of the spinal cord is the **cauda equina** (Latin for "horse's tail"), a fan of nerve fibers (see Figure 10-1, page 345). The spinal cord carries all the nerves to and from the limbs and lower part of the body, and it is the pathway for impulses going to and from the brain. A cross-sectional view of the spinal cord (Figure 10-10) reveals an inner region of **gray matter** (containing cell bodies and dendrites) and an outer region of **white matter** (containing the nerve fiber tracts with myelin sheaths) conducting impulses to and from the brain.

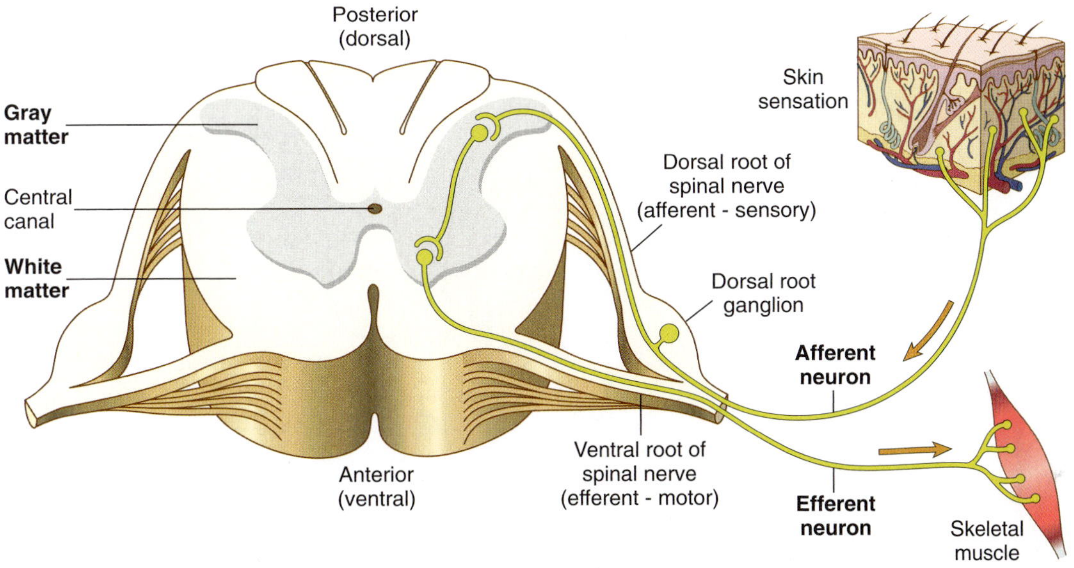

FIGURE 10-10 **The spinal cord, showing gray and white matter** (transverse view). **Afferent neurons** bring impulses from a sensory receptor (such as the skin) into the spinal cord. **Efferent neurons** carry impulses from the spinal cord to effector organs (such as skeletal muscle). The central canal is the space through which CSF travels.

MENINGES

The **meninges** are three layers of connective tissue membranes that surround the brain and spinal cord. Label Figure 10-11 as you study the following description of the meninges.

The outermost membrane of the meninges is the **dura mater** [1]. This thick, tough membrane contains channels (dural sinuses) that contain blood. The **subdural space** [2] is below the dural membrane. The second layer surrounding the brain and spinal cord is the **arachnoid membrane** [3]. The arachnoid (spider-like) membrane is loosely attached to the other meninges by web-like fibers, so there is a space for fluid between the fibers and the third membrane. This is the **subarachnoid space** [4], containing CSF. The third layer of the meninges, closest to the brain and spinal cord, is the **pia mater** [5]. It contains delicate (Latin *pia*) connective tissue with a rich supply of blood vessels. Most physicians refer to the pia and arachnoid membranes together as the pia-arachnoid.

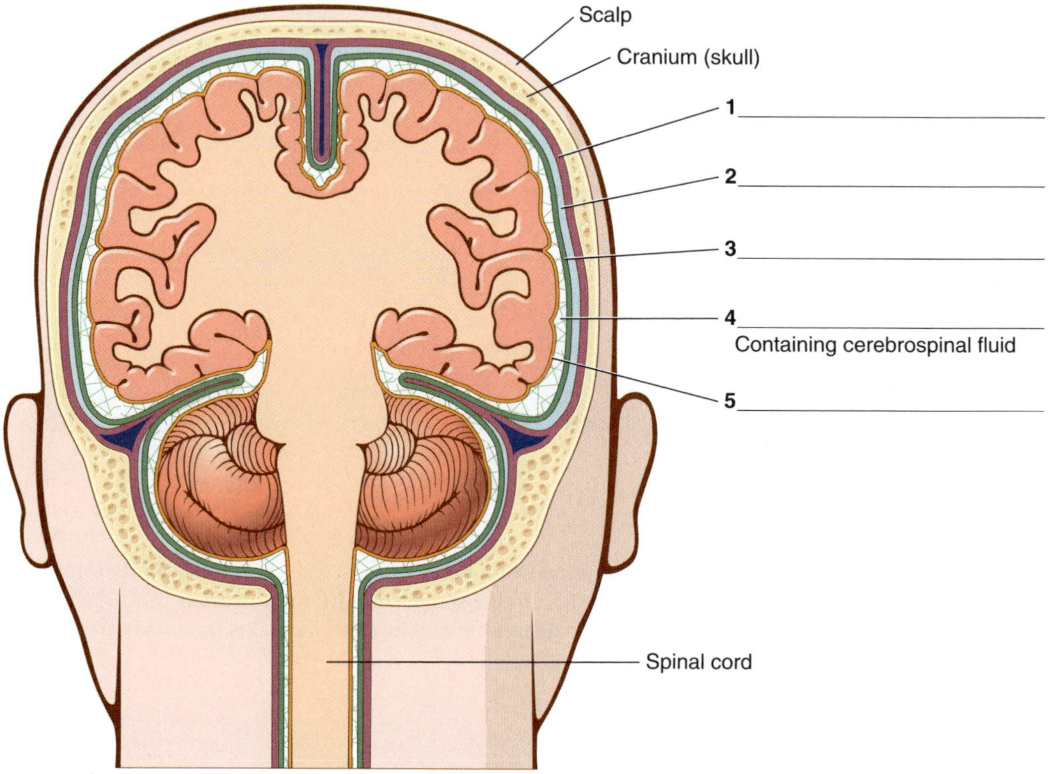

FIGURE 10-11 **The meninges,** posterior view.

VOCABULARY

This list reviews the new terms introduced in the text. Short definitions reinforce your understanding of the terms. Refer to the Pronunciation of Terms section for help with unfamiliar or more difficult words.

acetylcholine	Neurotransmitter chemical released at the ends of nerve cells.
afferent nerve	Carries messages *toward* the brain and spinal cord (sensory nerve). Afferent comes from *af-* (a form of *ad-*, meaning toward) and *-ferent* (meaning carrying).
arachnoid membrane	Middle layer of the three membranes (meninges) that surround the brain and spinal cord. The Greek *arachne* means spider.
astrocyte	Type of glial (neuroglial) cell that transports water and salts from capillaries.
autonomic nervous system	Nerves that control involuntary body functions of muscles, glands, and internal organs.
axon	Microscopic fiber that carries the nervous impulse along a nerve cell.
blood-brain barrier	Protective separation between the blood and brain cells. This makes it difficult for substances (such as anticancer drugs) to penetrate capillary walls and enter the brain.
brainstem	Posterior portion of the brain that connects the cerebrum with the spinal cord; includes the pons and medulla oblongata.
cauda equina	Collection of spinal nerves below the end of the spinal cord.
cell body	Part of a nerve cell that contains the nucleus.
central nervous system (CNS)	The brain and the spinal cord.
cerebellum	Posterior part of the brain that coordinates muscle movements and maintains balance.
cerebral cortex	Outer region of the cerebrum, containing sheets of nerve cells; gray matter of the brain.
cerebrospinal fluid (CSF)	Circulates throughout the brain and spinal cord.
cerebrum	Largest part of the brain; responsible for voluntary muscular activity, vision, speech, taste, hearing, thought, and memory.
cranial nerves	Twelve pairs of nerves that carry messages to and from the brain with regard to the head and neck (except the vagus nerve).
dendrite	Microscopic branching fiber of a nerve cell that is the first part to receive the nervous impulse.
dura mater	Thick, outermost layer of the meninges surrounding and protecting the brain and spinal cord. Latin for "hard mother."
efferent nerve	Carries messages *away from* the brain and spinal cord; motor nerve. Efferent comes from *ef-* (meaning away from) and *-ferent* (meaning to carry).
ependymal cell	Glial cell that lines membranes within the brain and spinal cord and helps form cerebrospinal fluid.

ganglion (*plural*: **ganglia**)	Collection of nerve cell bodies in the peripheral nervous system.
glial cell (neuroglial cell)	Supportive and connective nerve cell that does not carry nervous impulses. Examples are astrocytes, microglial cells, ependymal cells, and oligodendrocytes. Glial cells can reproduce themselves, as opposed to neurons.
gyrus (*plural*: **gyri**)	Sheet of nerve cells that produces a rounded ridge on the surface of the cerebral cortex; convolution.
hypothalamus	Portion of the brain beneath the thalamus; controls sleep, appetite, body temperature, and secretions from the pituitary gland.
medulla oblongata	Part of the brain just above the spinal cord; controls breathing, heartbeat, and the size of blood vessels; nerve fibers cross over here.
meninges	Three protective membranes that surround the brain and spinal cord.
microglial cell	Phagocytic glial cell that removes waste products from the central nervous system.
motor nerve	Carries messages away from the brain and spinal cord to muscles and organs; efferent nerve.
myelin sheath	Covering of white fatty tissue that surrounds and insulates the axon of a nerve cell. Myelin speeds impulse conduction along axons.
nerve	Macroscopic cord-like collection of fibers (axons and dendrites) that carry electrical impulses.
neuron	Nerve cell that carries impulses throughout the body; parenchyma of the nervous system.
neurotransmitter	Chemical messenger released at the end of a nerve cell. It stimulates or inhibits another cell, which can be a nerve cell, muscle cell, or gland cell. Examples of neurotransmitters are acetylcholine, norepinephrine, dopamine, and serotonin.
oligodendroglial cell	Glial cell that forms the myelin sheath covering axons. Also called oligodendrocyte.
parasympathetic nerves	Involuntary, autonomic nerves that regulate normal body functions such as heart rate, breathing, and muscles of the gastrointestinal tract.
parenchyma	Essential, distinguishing tissue of any organ or system. The parenchyma of the nervous system includes the neurons and nerves that carry nervous impulses. Parenchymal cells of the liver are hepatocytes, and parenchymal tissue of the kidney includes the nephrons, where urine is formed. Note the pronunciation: păr-ĔN-kĭ-mă.
peripheral nervous system	Nerves outside the brain and spinal cord: cranial, spinal, and autonomic nerves.
pia mater	Thin, delicate inner membrane of the meninges.
plexus (*plural*: **plexuses**)	Large, interlacing network of nerves. Examples are lumbosacral, cervical, and brachial (brachi/o means arm) plexuses. The term originated from the Indo-European *plek*, meaning to weave together.
pons	Part of the brain anterior to the cerebellum and between the medulla and the rest of the midbrain (Latin *pons* means bridge). It is a bridge connecting various parts of the brain.

receptor	Organ that receives a nervous stimulus and passes it on to afferent nerves. The skin, ears, eyes, and taste buds are receptors.
sciatic nerve	Nerve extending from the base of the spine down the thigh, lower leg, and foot. **Sciatica** is pain or inflammation along the course of the nerve.
sensory nerve	Carries messages toward the brain and spinal cord from a receptor; afferent nerve.
spinal nerves	Thirty-one pairs of nerves arising from the spinal cord.
stimulus (*plural*: **stimuli**)	Agent of change (light, sound, touch) in the internal or external environment that evokes a response.
stroma	Connective and supporting tissue of an organ. Glial cells are the stromal tissue of the brain.
sulcus (*plural*: **sulci**)	Depression or groove in the surface of the cerebral cortex; fissure.
sympathetic nerves	Autonomic nerves that influence bodily functions involuntarily in times of stress.
synapse	Space through which a nervous impulse travels between nerve cells or between nerve and muscle or glandular cells. From the Greek *synapsis*, a point of contact.
thalamus	Main relay center of the brain. It conducts impulses between the spinal cord and the cerebrum; incoming sensory messages are relayed through the thalamus to appropriate centers in the cerebrum. Latin *thalamus* means room. The Romans, who named this structure, thought this part of the brain was hollow, like a little room.
vagus nerve	Tenth cranial nerve (cranial nerve X); its branches reach to the larynx, trachea, bronchi, lungs, aorta, esophagus, and stomach. Latin *vagus* means wandering. Unlike the other cranial nerves, the vagus leaves the head and "wanders" into the abdominal and thoracic cavities.
ventricles of the brain	Canals in the brain that contain cerebrospinal fluid. Ventricles are also found in the heart. They are the two lower chambers of the heart.

TERMINOLOGY

This section is divided into terms that describe organs and structures of the nervous system and those that relate to neurologic signs and symptoms. Write the meanings of the medical terms in the spaces provided.

ORGANS AND STRUCTURES

COMBINING FORM	MEANING	TERMINOLOGY	MEANING
cerebell/o	cerebellum	cerebellar	______________________
cerebr/o	cerebrum	cerebrospinal fluid	______________________
		cerebral cortex *Cortical means pertaining to the cortex or outer area of an organ.*	______________________

COMBINING FORM	MEANING	TERMINOLOGY	MEANING
dur/o	dura mater	subdural hematoma *Remember: Hematomas are not tumors of blood, but are collections of blood.*	______________________
		epidural hematoma *Figure 10-12 shows subdural, epidural, and intracerebral hematomas.*	______________________
encephal/o	brain	encephalitis	______________________
		encephalopathy	______________________
		anencephaly *This is a congenital brain malformation; it is not compatible with life and may be detected with amniocentesis or ultrasonography of the fetus.*	______________________
gli/o	glial cells	glioblastoma *This is a highly malignant tumor (-blast means immature). Gliomas are tumors of glial (neuroglial) cells.*	______________________
lept/o	thin, slender	leptomeningeal *The pia and arachnoid membranes are known as the leptomeninges because of their thin, delicate structure.*	______________________
mening/o, meningi/o	membranes, meninges	meningeal	______________________
		meningioma *Slowly growing, benign tumor.*	______________________
		myelomeningocele *Neural tube defect caused by failure of the neural tube to close during embryonic development. This abnormality occurs in infants born with spina bifida. See page 363.*	______________________

10

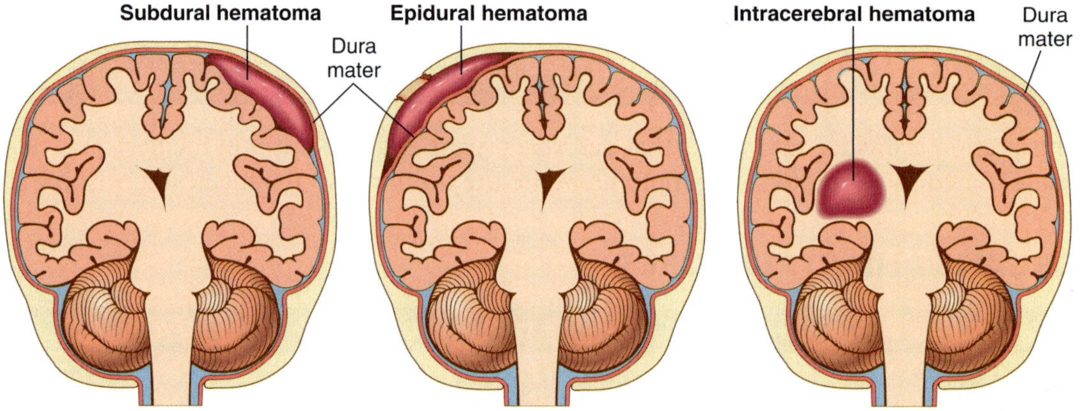

FIGURE 10-12 Hematomas. A **subdural hematoma** results from the tearing of veins between the dura and arachnoid membranes. It often is the result of blunt trauma, such as from blows to the head in boxers or in elderly patients who have fallen out of bed. An **epidural hematoma** occurs between the skull and the dura as the result of a ruptured meningeal artery, usually after a fracture of the skull. An **intracerebral hematoma** is caused by bleeding directly into brain tissue, such as can occur in the case of uncontrolled hypertension (high blood pressure).

COMBINING FORM	MEANING	TERMINOLOGY	MEANING
my/o	muscle	myoneural	______________
myel/o	spinal cord (means bone marrow in other contexts)	myelopathy	______________
		poliomyelitis *Polio- means gray matter. This viral disease affects the gray matter of the spinal cord, leading to paralysis of muscles that rely on the damaged neurons. Effective vaccines developed in the 20th century have made "polio" relatively uncommon.*	______________
neur/o	nerve	neuropathy	______________
		polyneuritis	______________
pont/o	pons	cerebellopontine *The suffix -ine means pertaining to.*	______________
radicul/o	nerve root (of spinal nerves)	radiculopathy ***Sciatica** is a radiculopathy affecting the sciatic nerve root in the back. A herniated disk is a common cause leading to pain, weakness, or numbness down the leg. See the **"In Person"** story on page 377.*	______________
		radiculitis *This condition often results in pain and loss of function.*	______________
thalam/o	thalamus	thalamic	______________
thec/o	sheath (refers to the meninges)	intrathecal injection *Chemicals, such as chemotherapeutic drugs, can be delivered into the subarachnoid space.*	______________
vag/o	vagus nerve (10th cranial nerve)	vagal *This cranial nerve has branches to the head and neck, as well as to the chest.*	______________

SIGNS AND SYMPTOMS

COMBINING FORM OR SUFFIX	MEANING	TERMINOLOGY	MEANING
alges/o, -algesia	excessive sensitivity to pain	analgesia	______________
		hypalgesia *Diminished sensation to pain. (Notice that the o in hypo- is dropped.) Hyperalgesia is increased sensitivity to pain.*	______________

myel/o and my/o

Don't confuse these combining forms. **Myel/o** means spinal cord or bone marrow, while **my/o** means muscle. Another pair to watch out for is **pyel/o** (renal pelvis of the kidney) and **py/o** (pus).

Neuropathies

Neuropathies are diseases of peripheral nerves. They can affect motor, sensory, and autonomic functions. **Polyneuropathies** affect many nerves, while **mononeuropathies** affect individual nerves.

COMBINING FORM OR SUFFIX	MEANING	TERMINOLOGY	MEANING
-algia	pain (see page 376 for information on pain medications)	neuralgia ***Trigeminal neuralgia*** *involves flashes of pain radiating along the course of the trigeminal nerve (fifth cranial nerve).*	
		cephalgia *Headaches may result from vasodilation (widening) of blood vessels in tissues surrounding the brain or from tension in neck and scalp muscles.*	
caus/o	burning	causalgia *Intense burning pain following injury to a sensory nerve.*	
comat/o	deep sleep (coma)	comatose *A* ***coma*** *is a state of unconsciousness from which the patient cannot be aroused. Semicomatose refers to a stupor (unresponsiveness) from which a patient can be aroused. In an irreversible coma (brain death), there is complete unresponsitivity to stimuli, no spontaneous breathing or movement, and a flat electroencephalogram (EEG) tracing.*	
esthesi/o, -esthesia	feeling, nervous sensation	anesthesia *Lack of normal sensation (e.g., absence of sense of touch or pain). Two common types of regional anesthesia are spinal and epidural (caudal) blocks (Figure 10-13).* ***Anesthetics*** *are agents that reduce or eliminate sensation. General and local anesthetics are listed in Table 21-2, page 887.*	
		hyperesthesia *A light touch with a pin may provoke increased sensation. Diminished sensitivity to pain is called hypesthesia.*	
		paresthesia *Par- (from para-) means abnormal. Paresthesias include tingling, burning, and "pins and needles" sensations.*	
kines/o, kinesi/o -kinesia, -kinesis, -kinetic	movement	bradykinesia	
		hyperkinesis *Amphetamines (CNS stimulants) are used to treat hyperkinesia in children, but the mechanism of their action is not understood.*	
		dyskinesia *Condition marked by involuntary, spasmodic movements.* ***Tardive*** *(occurring late)* ***dyskinesia*** *may develop in people who receive certain antipsychotic drugs for extended periods.*	
		akinetic	
-lepsy	seizure	epilepsy *See page 365.*	
		narcolepsy *Sudden, uncontrollable compulsion to sleep (narc/o = stupor, sleep). Amphetamines and stimulant drugs are prescribed to prevent attacks.*	

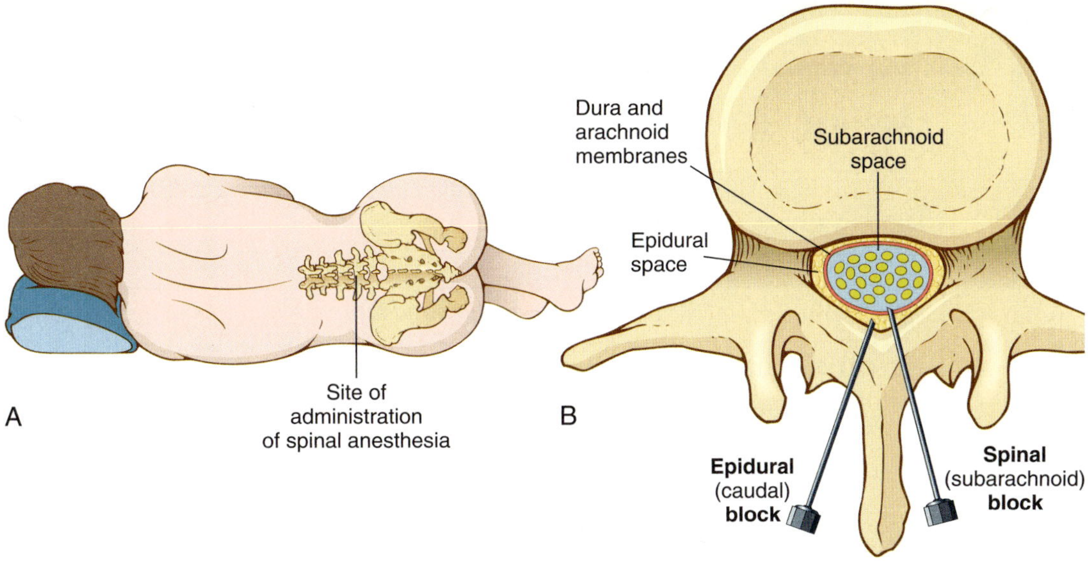

FIGURE 10-13 **A, Positioning of a patient for spinal anesthesia. B,** Cross-sectional view of the spinal cord showing injection sites for **epidural** and **spinal blocks (anesthesia).** Epidural (caudal) anesthesia is achieved by injecting an agent into the epidural space and is commonly used in obstetrics. Spinal anesthesia is achieved by injecting a local anesthetic into the subarachnoid space. Patients may experience loss of sensation and paralysis of feet, legs, and abdomen.

COMBINING FORM OR SUFFIX	MEANING	TERMINOLOGY	MEANING
lex/o	word, phrase	dyslexia	____ *This is a developmental reading disorder occurring when the brain does not properly recognize, process, and interpret language.*
-paresis	weakness	hemiparesis	____ *Affects either right or left side (half) of the body.* ***Paresis*** *also is used by itself to mean partial paralysis or weakness of muscles.*
-phasia	speech	aphasia	____ *Difficulty with speech.* ***Motor*** *(also called Broca or expressive)* ***aphasia*** *is present when the patient knows what he or she wants to say but cannot pronounce it. The patient with* ***sensory aphasia*** *has difficulty understanding language and may pronounce (articulate) words easily but use them inappropriately.*
-plegia	paralysis (loss or impairment of the ability to move parts of the body)	hemiplegia	____ *Affects the right or left half of the body and results from a stroke or other brain injury. The hemiplegia is contralateral to the brain lesion because motor nerve fibers from the right half of the brain cross to the left side of the body (in the medulla oblongata).*
		paraplegia	____ *Originally, the term paraplegia meant a stroke (paralysis) on one side (para-). Now, however, the term means paralysis of both legs and the lower part of the body caused by injury or disease of the spinal cord or cauda equina.*
		quadriplegia	____ *Quadri- means four. All four extremities are affected. Injury is at the cervical level of the spinal cord.*

10

COMBINING FORM OR SUFFIX	MEANING	TERMINOLOGY	MEANING
-praxia	action	apraxia ____________ *Movements and behavior are not purposeful. A patient with motor apraxia cannot use an object or perform a task. Motor weakness is not the cause.*	
-sthenia	strength	neurasthenia ____________ *Nervous exhaustion and fatigue, often following depression.*	
syncop/o	to cut off, cut short	syncopal ____________ ***Syncope** (SĬN-kō-pē) means fainting; sudden and temporary loss of consciousness caused by inadequate flow of blood to the brain. The term comes from a Greek word meaning cutting into pieces—thus, a fainting spell meant one's strength was "cut off." Remember: Syncopal means pertaining to fainting and is an adjective. A patient can experience a syncopal episode.*	
tax/o	order, coordination	ataxia ____________ *Condition of decreased coordination. Persistent unsteadiness on the feet can be caused by a disorder involving the cerebellum.*	

PATHOLOGY

10

The bones of the skull, the vertebral column, and the meninges, containing CSF, provide a hard box with an interior cushion around the brain and spinal cord. In addition, glial cells surrounding neurons form a blood-brain barrier that prevents many potentially harmful substances in the bloodstream from gaining access to neurons. However, these protective factors are counterbalanced by the extreme sensitivity of nerve cells to oxygen deficiency (brain cells die in a few minutes when deprived of oxygen).

Neurologic disorders may be classified in the following categories:

- Congenital
- Degenerative, movement, and seizure
- Infectious (meningitis and encephalitis)
- Neoplastic (tumors)
- Traumatic
- Vascular (stroke)

CONGENITAL DISORDERS

hydrocephalus

Abnormal accumulation of fluid (CSF) in the brain.

If circulation of CSF in the brain or spinal cord is impaired, fluid accumulates under pressure in the ventricles of the brain. To relieve pressure on the brain, a catheter (shunt) can be placed from the ventricle of the brain into the peritoneal space (ventriculoperitoneal shunt) or right atrium of the heart so that the CSF is continuously drained from the brain.

Hydrocephalus also can occur in adults as a result of tumors and infections.

spina bifida

Congenital defects in the lumbar spinal column caused by imperfect union of vertebral parts (neural tube defect).

In **spina bifida occulta,** the vertebral defect is covered over with skin and evident only on x-ray or other imaging examination. **Spina bifida cystica** is a more severe form, with cyst-like protrusions. In **meningocele,** the meninges protrude to the outside of the body, and in **myelomeningocele** (or meningomyelocele), both the spinal cord and meninges protrude (Figure 10-14A and B).

The etiology of neural tube defects is unknown. Defects originate in the early weeks of pregnancy as the spinal cord and vertebrae develop. Prenatal diagnosis is helped by imaging methods and testing maternal blood samples for alpha-fetoprotein.

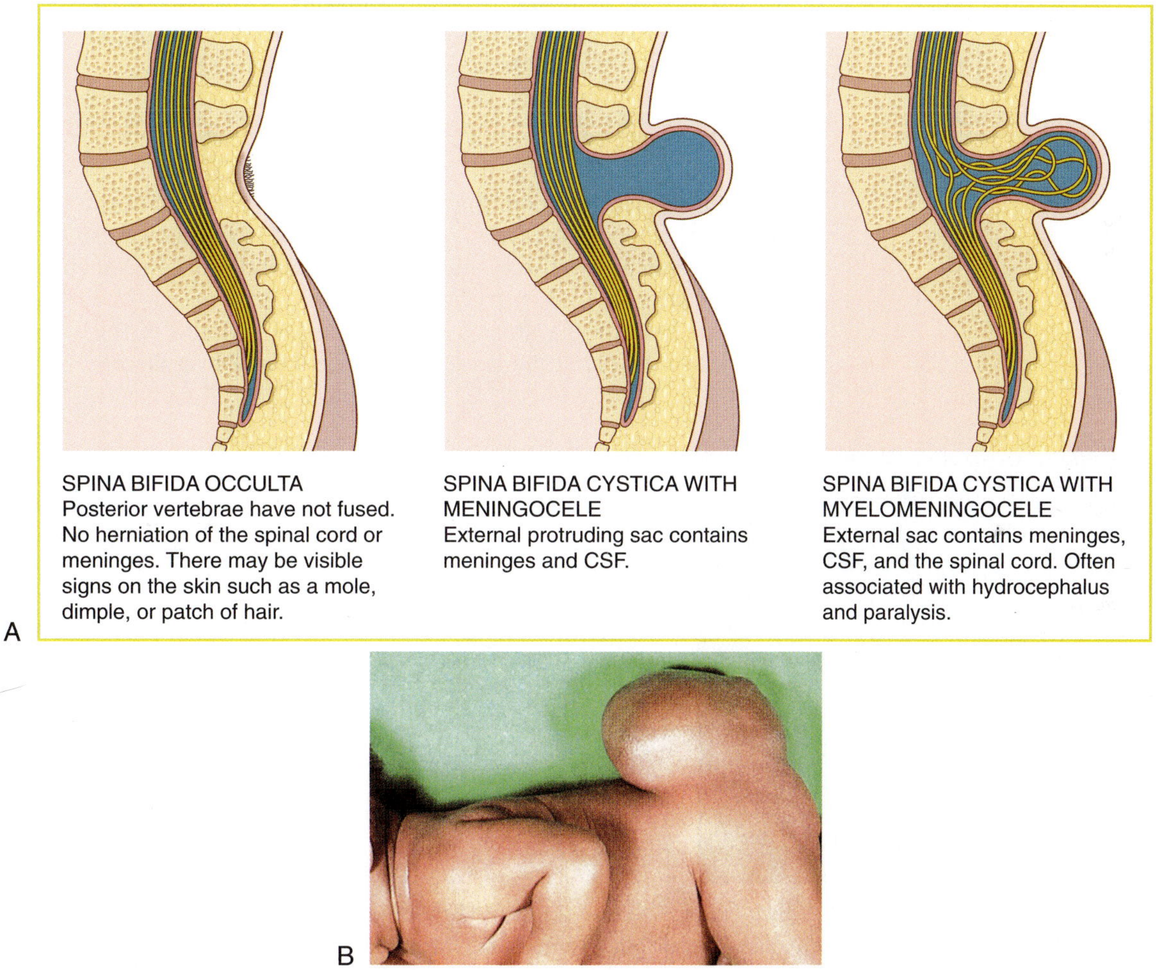

FIGURE 10-14 **A, Spina bifida** (neural tube defects). **B, Spina bifida cystica** with **myelomeningocele.**

DEGENERATIVE, MOVEMENT, AND SEIZURE DISORDERS

Alzheimer disease (AD)

Brain disorder marked by gradual and progressive mental deterioration (dementia), personality changes, and impairment of daily functioning.

Characteristics of AD include confusion, memory failure, disorientation, restlessness, and speech disturbances. Anxiety, depression, and emotional disturbances can occur as well. The disease sometimes begins in middle life with slight defects in memory and behavior, but can worsen after the age of 70. On autopsy there is atrophy of the cerebral cortex and widening of the cerebral sulci, especially in the frontal and temporal regions (Figure 10-15A and B). Microscopic examination shows **senile plaques** resulting from degeneration of neurons and **neurofibrillary tangles** (bundles of fibrils in the cytoplasm of a neuron) in the cerebral cortex. Deposits of **amyloid** (a protein) occur in neurofibrillary tangles, senile plaques, and blood vessels. The cause of AD remains unknown, although genetic factors may play a role. A mutation on chromosome 14 has been linked to familial cases. There is as yet no effective treatment.

amyotrophic lateral sclerosis (ALS)

Degenerative disorder of motor neurons in the spinal cord and brainstem.

ALS manifests in adulthood. Signs and symptoms are weakness and atrophy of muscles in the hands, forearms, and legs; difficulty in swallowing and talking and dyspnea develop as the throat and respiratory muscles become affected. Etiology (cause) and cure for ALS both are unknown.

A famous baseball player, Lou Gehrig, became a victim of this disease in the mid-1900s, so the condition became known as **Lou Gehrig disease.**

10

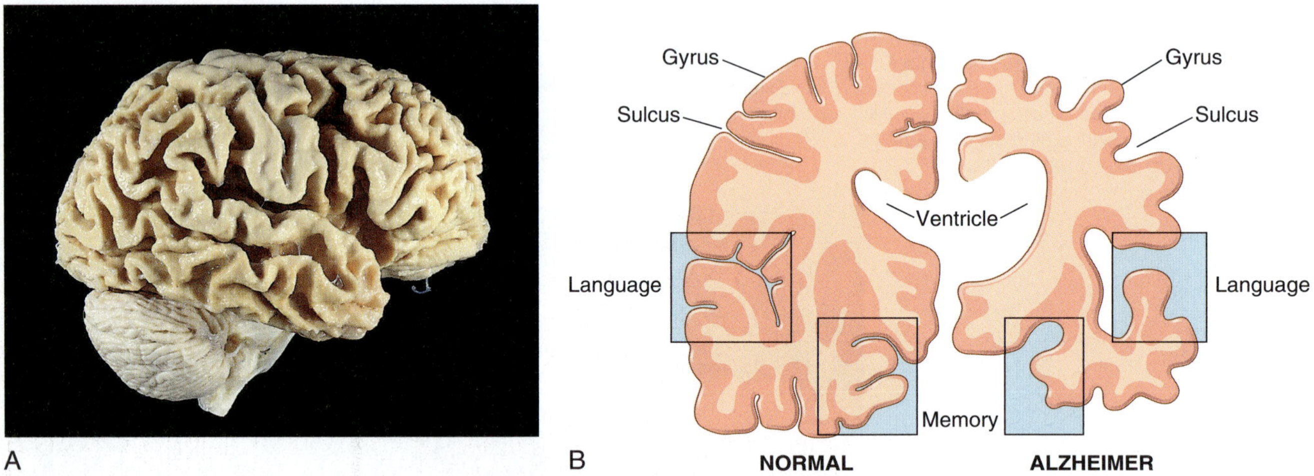

FIGURE 10-15 **A, Alzheimer disease.** Generalized loss of brain parenchyma (neuronal tissue) results in narrowing of the cerebral gyri and widening of the sulci. **B,** Cross-sectional comparison of a normal brain and a brain from a person with Alzheimer disease.

epilepsy

Chronic brain disorder characterized by recurrent seizure activity.

Seizures are abnormal, sudden discharges of electrical activity within the brain. Seizures are often symptoms of underlying brain pathologic conditions, such as brain tumors, meningitis, vascular disease, or scar tissue from a head injury. **Tonic-clonic seizures (grand mal** or **ictal events)** are characterized by a sudden loss of consciousness, falling down, and then tonic contractions (stiffening of muscles) followed by clonic contractions (twitching and jerking movements of the limbs). These convulsions often are preceded by an **aura,** which is a peculiar sensation experienced by the affected person before onset of a seizure. Dizziness, numbness, and visual or olfactory (sense of smell) disturbances are examples of an aura. **Absence seizures** are a form of seizure consisting of momentary clouding of consciousness and loss of awareness of the person's surroundings. These include **petit mal seizures** in children. Drug therapy (anticonvulsants) is used for control of epileptic seizures. After seizures, there may be neurologic symptoms such as weakness called **postictal events.**

In **temporal lobe epilepsy,** seizures begin in the temporal lobe (on each side of the brain near the ears) of the brain. The most common type of seizure is a **complex partial seizure.** Complex means impaired consciousness and partial indicates not generalized. Commonly these patients have seizures that cause them to pause in whatever they are doing, become confused, and have memory problems.

The term epilepsy comes from the Greek *epilepsis*, meaning a laying hold of. The Greeks thought a victim of a seizure was laid hold of by some mysterious force. The word ictal originates from the Latin *ictus*, meaning a blow or a stroke.

Huntington disease (Huntington chorea)

Hereditary disorder marked by degenerative changes in the cerebrum leading to abrupt involuntary movements and mental deterioration.

This condition typically begins in adulthood and results in personality changes, along with choreic (meaning dance-like) movements (uncontrollable, irregular, jerking movements of the arms and legs and facial grimacing).

The genetic defect in patients with Huntington disease is located on chromosome 4. Patients can be tested for the gene; however, no cure exists, and management is symptomatic.

multiple sclerosis (MS)

Destruction of the myelin sheath on neurons in the CNS and its replacement by plaques of sclerotic (hard) tissue.

One of the leading causes of neurologic disability in persons 20 to 40 years of age, MS is a chronic disease often marked by long periods of stability (remission) and worsening (relapse). **Demyelination** (loss of myelin insulation) prevents the conduction of nerve impulses through the axon and causes paresthesias, muscle weakness, unsteady **gait** (manner of walking), and paralysis. There may be visual (blurred and double vision) and speech disturbances as well. Areas of scarred myelin (plaques) can be seen on MRI scans of the brain (Figure 10-16B). Etiology is unknown but probably involves an autoimmune disease of lymphocytes reacting against myelin. Drugs that are commonly used to treat MS are corticosteroids (to reduce inflammation), interferons (to slow the rate of MS symptoms), and glatiramer (to block the immune system's attack on myelin).

Epilepsy and Seizures

Epilepsy is a brain disorder in which at least two or more seizures appear spontaneously and recurrently. Having a single seizure does not mean that the affected person has epilepsy.

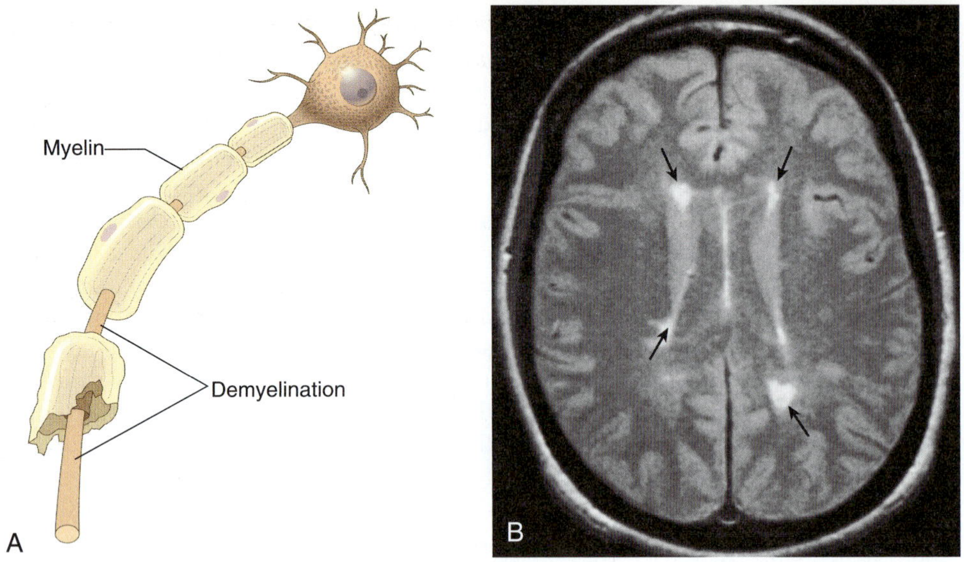

FIGURE 10-16 Multiple sclerosis. A, Demyelination of a nerve cell. **B,** This MRI scan shows multiple abnormal white areas that correspond to MS plaques *(arrows)*. The plaques are scar tissue that forms when myelin sheaths are destroyed.

myasthenia gravis (MG)

Autoimmune neuromuscular disorder characterized by weakness of voluntary muscles.

MG is a chronic autoimmune disorder. Antibodies block the ability of acetylcholine (neurotransmitter) to transmit the nervous impulse from nerve to muscle cell. Onset of symptoms usually is gradual. Brainstem signs are prominent and include ptosis of the upper eyelid, double vision (diplopia), and facial weakness. Respiratory paralysis is the main clinical concern. Therapy to reverse symptoms includes anticholinesterase drugs, which inhibit the enzyme that breaks down acetylcholine. Immunosuppressive therapy is used, including intravenous immunoglobin as well as medications such as corticosteroids (prednisone) and methotrexate. **Thymectomy** is also a method of treatment and is beneficial to many patients.

palsy

Paralysis (partial or complete loss of motor function).

Cerebral palsy is partial paralysis and lack of muscular coordination caused by loss of oxygen (hypoxia) or blood flow to the cerebrum during pregnancy or in the perinatal period. **Bell palsy** (or Bell's palsy) (Figure 10-17) is paralysis on one side of the face. The likely cause is a viral infection, and therapy is directed against the virus (antiviral drugs) and nerve swelling.

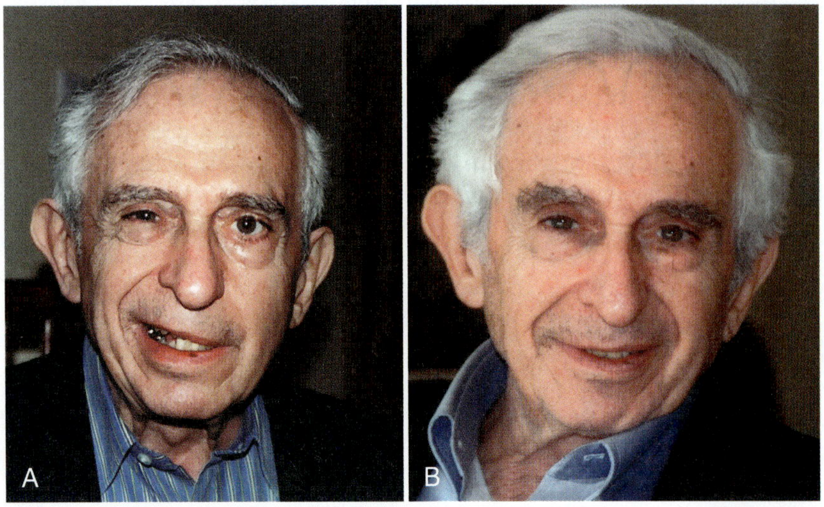

FIGURE 10-17 A, Bell palsy. Notice the paralysis on the left side of this man's face: The eyelid does not close properly, the forehead is not wrinkled as would be expected, and there is clear paralysis of the lower face. **B,** The palsy spontaneously resolved after 6 months.

Parkinson disease (parkinsonism)

Degeneration of neurons in the basal ganglia, occurring in later life and leading to tremors, weakness of muscles, and slowness of movement.

This slowly progressive condition is caused by a deficiency of **dopamine,** a neurotransmitter made by cells in the basal ganglia (see Figure 10-9). Motor disturbances include stooped posture, shuffling gait, and muscle stiffness (rigidity). Other signs are a typical "pill-rolling" tremor of hands and a characteristic mask-like lack of facial expression. See Figure 10-18.

Therapy with drugs such as levodopa plus carbidopa (Sinemet) to increase dopamine levels in the brain is **palliative** (relieving symptoms but not curative). Implantation of fetal brain tissue containing dopamine-producing cells is an experimental treatment but has produced uncertain results.

Tourette syndrome

Involuntary, spasmodic, twitching movements; uncontrollable vocal sounds; and inappropriate words.

These involuntary movements, usually beginning with twitching of the eyelid and muscles of the face with verbal outbursts, are called **tics.** Although the cause of Tourette syndrome is not known, it is associated with either an excess of dopamine or a hypersensitivity to dopamine. Psychological problems do not cause Tourette syndrome, but physicians have had some success in treating it with the anti-psychotic drug haloperidol (Haldol), antidepressants, and mood stabilizers.

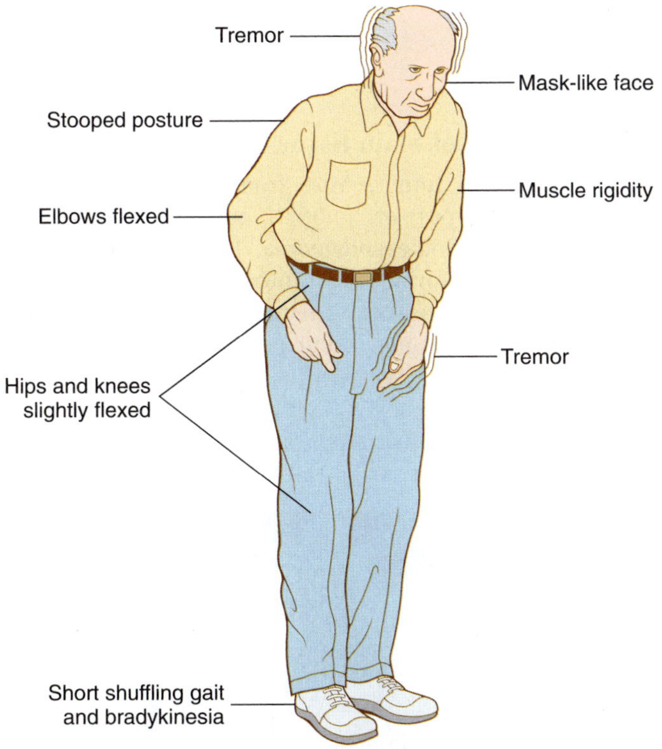

FIGURE 10-18 **Primary symptoms of Parkinson disease** are tremors in hands, arms, legs, jaw, and face; rigidity or stiffness of limbs and trunk; bradykinesia (shuffling gait), stooped posture, and masklike facies.

INFECTIOUS DISORDERS

herpes zoster (shingles)

Viral infection affecting peripheral nerves.

Blisters and pain spread along peripheral nerves (see Figure 10-19A) and are caused by inflammation due to a herpesvirus **(herpes zoster),** the same virus that causes chickenpox (varicella). Reactivation of the chickenpox virus (herpes varicella-zoster), which remains in the body after the person had chickenpox, occurs. Painful blisters follow the underlying route of cranial or spinal nerves around the trunk of the body; zoster means girdle. Zostavax is a vaccine to prevent shingles. It does not treat shingles and is recommended for people 60 years of age and older.

meningitis

Inflammation of the meninges; leptomeningitis.

This condition can be caused by bacteria (pyogenic meningitis) or viruses (aseptic or viral meningitis). Signs and symptoms are fever and signs of meningeal irritation, such as headache, photophobia (sensitivity to light), and a stiff neck. Lumbar punctures are performed to examine CSF. Physicians use antibiotics to treat the more serious pyogenic form, and antivirals for the viral form.

human immunodeficiency virus (HIV) encephalopathy

Brain disease and dementia occurring with AIDS.

Many patients with AIDS develop neurologic dysfunction. In addition to encephalitis and dementia (loss of mental functioning), some patients develop brain tumors and other infections.

NEOPLASTIC DISORDERS

brain tumor

Abnormal growth of brain tissue and meninges.

Most primary brain tumors arise from glial cells **(gliomas)** or the meninges **(meningiomas).** Types of gliomas include **astrocytoma** (Figure 10-19B), **oligodendroglioma,** and **ependymoma.** The most malignant form of astrocytoma is **glioblastoma multiforme** (-blast means immature) (see Figure 10-19B). Tumors can cause swelling **(cerebral edema)** and hydrocephalus. If CSF pressure is increased, swelling also may occur near the optic nerve (at the back of the eye). Other symptoms include severe headache and new seizures. Gliomas are removed surgically, and radiotherapy is used for tumors that are not completely resected. Steroids are given to reduce swelling after surgery.

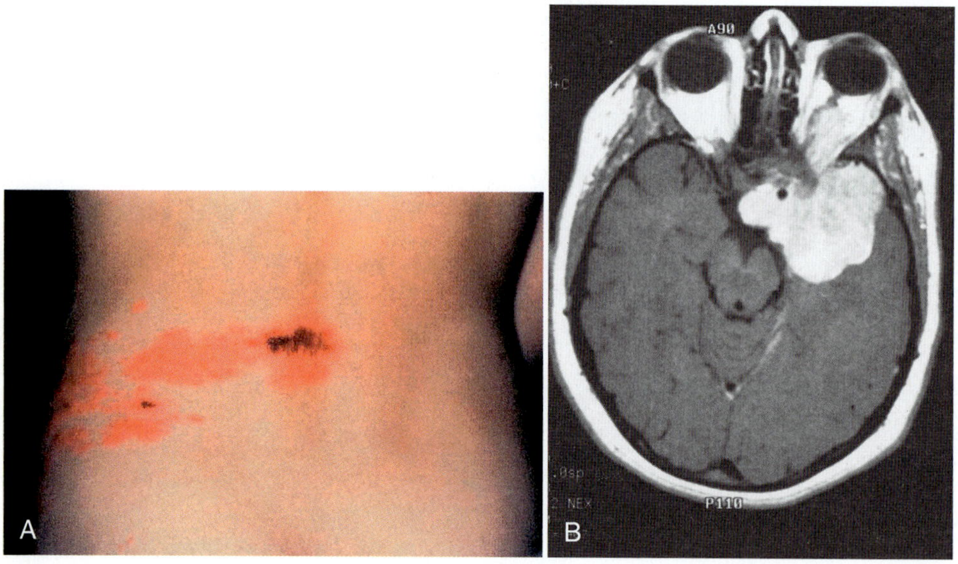

FIGURE 10-19 **A, Shingles. B, Glioblastoma** as seen on MRI.

Meningiomas usually are benign and surrounded by a capsule, but they may cause compression and distortion of the brain.

Tumors in the brain also may be single or multiple metastatic growths. Most arise from the lung, breast, skin (melanoma), kidney, and gastrointestinal tract and spread to the brain.

TRAUMATIC DISORDERS

cerebral concussion

Type of traumatic brain injury caused by a blow to the head.

There is usually no evidence of structural damage to brain tissue and loss of consciousness may not occur. Rest is very important after a concussion because it allows the brain to heal. Doctors recommend avoiding demanding mental and physical activities.

cerebral contusion

Bruising of brain tissue as a result of direct trauma to the head.

A cerebral contusion usually is associated with a fracture of the skull, as well as with with edema and an increase in intracranial pressure. Subdural and epidural hematomas occur (see Figure 10-12), leading to permanent brain injury with altered memory or speech or development of epilepsy.

VASCULAR DISORDERS

cerebrovascular accident (CVA)

Disruption in the normal blood supply to the brain; stroke.

This condition, also known as a **cerebral infarction,** is the result of impaired oxygen supply to the brain. There are three types of strokes (Figure 10-20):

1. **Thrombotic**—blood clot **(thrombus)** in the arteries leading to the brain, resulting in occlusion (blocking) of the vessel. Atherosclerosis leads to this common type of stroke as blood vessels become blocked over time. Before total occlusion occurs, a patient may experience symptoms that point to the gradual occlusion of blood vessels. These short episodes of neurologic dysfunction are known as **transient ischemic attacks (TIAs).**

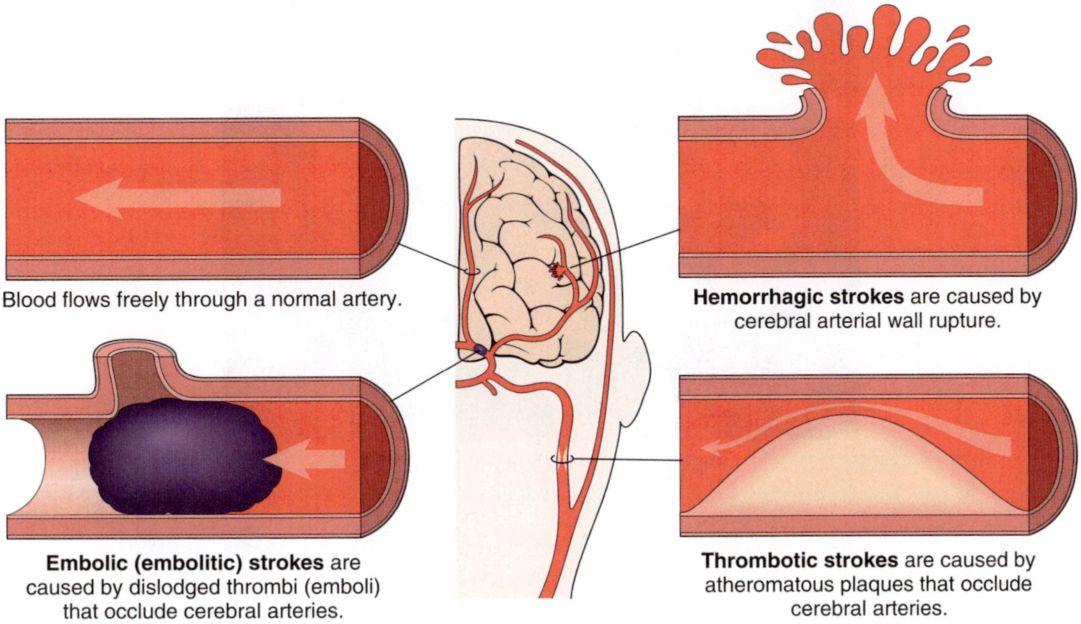

FIGURE 10-20 Three types of strokes: embolic, hemorrhagic, and thrombotic.

2. **Embolic**—an **embolus** (a dislodged thrombus) travels to cerebral arteries and occludes a small vessel. This type of stroke occurs very suddenly.
3. **Hemorrhagic**—a blood vessel, such as the cerebral artery, breaks and bleeding occurs. This type of stroke can be fatal and results from advancing age, atherosclerosis, or high blood pressure, all of which result in degeneration of cerebral blood vessels. With small hemorrhages, the body reabsorbs the blood and the patient makes good recovery with only slight disability. In a younger patient, cerebral hemorrhage usually is caused by mechanical injury associated with skull fracture or rupture of an arterial **aneurysm** (weakened area in the vessel wall that balloons and may eventually burst). See Figure 10-21.

The major risk factors for stroke are hypertension, diabetes, smoking, and heart disease. Other risk factors include obesity, substance abuse (cocaine), and elevated cholesterol levels.

Thrombotic strokes are treated with antiplatelet or anticoagulant (clot-dissolving) therapy. **Tissue plasminogen activator (tPA)** may be started shortly after the onset of a stroke. Surgical intervention with carotid endarterectomy (removal of the atherosclerotic plaque along with the inner lining of the affected carotid artery) is also possible.

migraine

Severe, recurring, unilateral, vascular headache.

Prodromal symptoms are known as an **aura** (peculiar sensations that precede the onset of illness). Symptoms of aura are temporary visual and sensory disturbances, including flashes of light and zigzag lines. Sensitivity to sound (phonophobia) and light (photophobia) are associated with the migraine itself. Migraine pain is believed to be related to dilation of the blood vessels. Treatment to prevent a migraine attack includes medications such as sumatriptan succinate (Imitrex) that target serotonin receptors on blood vessels and nerves. Drugs of this type reduce inflammation and restrict dilation of blood vessels.

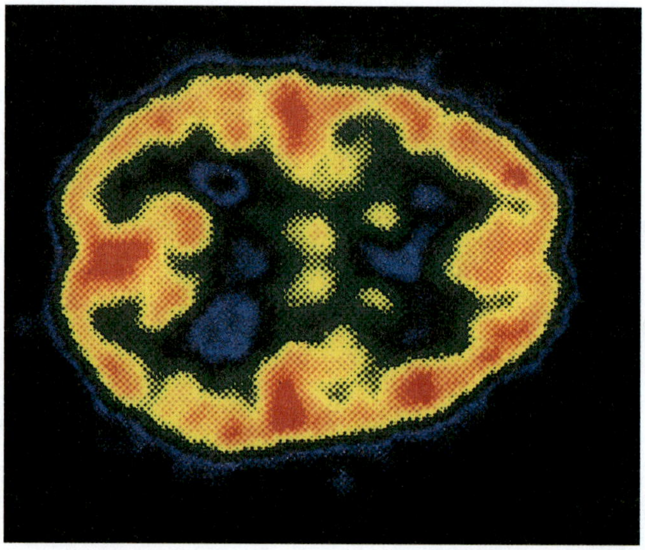

FIGURE 10-21 Cerebral aneurysm.

STUDY SECTION

The following list reviews the new terms used in the Pathology section. Practice spelling each term and know its meaning.

absence seizure Form of seizure consisting of momentary clouding of consciousness and loss of awareness of surroundings.

aneurysm Enlarged, weakened area in an arterial wall, which may rupture, leading to hemorrhage and CVA (stroke).

astrocytoma Malignant tumor of astrocytes (glial brain cells).

aura Peculiar symptom or sensation occurring before the onset (prodromal) of an attack of migraine or an epileptic seizure.

dementia Mental decline and deterioration.

demyelination Destruction of myelin on axons of neurons (as in multiple sclerosis).

dopamine CNS neurotransmitter, deficient in patient with Parkinson disease.

embolus Clot of material that travels through the bloodstream and suddenly blocks a vessel.

gait Manner of walking.

ictal event Pertaining to a sudden, acute onset, as with the convulsions of an epileptic seizure.

occlusion Blockage.

palliative Relieving symptoms but not curing them.

thymectomy Removal of the thymus gland (a lymphocyte-producing gland in the chest); used as treatment for myasthenia gravis.

TIA Transient ischemic attack.

tic Involuntary movement of a small group of muscles, as of the face; characteristic of Tourette syndrome.

tonic-clonic seizure Major (grand mal) convulsive seizure marked by sudden loss of consciousness, stiffening of muscles, and twitching and jerking movements.

10

LABORATORY TESTS AND CLINICAL PROCEDURES

LABORATORY TESTS

cerebrospinal fluid analysis **Samples of CSF are examined.**

CFS analysis measures protein, glucose, red (RBC) and white (WBC) blood cells as well as other chemical contents of the CSF. CSF analysis can also detect tumor cells (via cytology), bacteria, and viruses. These studies are used to diagnose infection, tumors, or multiple sclerosis.

CLINICAL PROCEDURES

X-Ray Tests

cerebral angiography **X-ray imaging of the arterial blood vessels in the brain after injection of contrast material.**

Contrast is injected into the femoral artery (in the thigh), and x-ray motion pictures are taken. These images diagnose vascular disease (aneurysm, occlusion, hemorrhage) in the brain.

computed tomography (CT) of the brain — **Computerized x-ray technique that generates multiple images of the brain and spinal cord.**

Contrast material may be injected intravenously to highlight abnormalities. The contrast leaks through the **blood-brain barrier** from blood vessels into the brain tissue and shows tumors, aneurysms, bleeding, brain injury, skull fractures, and blood clots. Operations are performed using the CT scan as a road map. CT scans are also particularly useful for visualizing blood and bone.

Magnetic Resonance Techniques

magnetic resonance imaging (MRI) — **Magnetic field and pulses of radiowave energy create images of the brain and spinal cord.**

MRI is better than CT at evaluation of brain parenchyma. It is excellent for viewing brain damage related to infection, inflammation or tumors. It also is used to look for causes of headaches, to help diagnose a stroke, and detect bleeding problems and head injury. Contrast material may be used to enhance images. **Magnetic resonance angiography (MRA)** produces images of blood vessels using magnetic resonance techniques.

Radionuclide Studies

positron emission tomography (PET) scan — **Radioactive glucose is injected and then detected in the brain to image the metabolic activity of cells.**

PET scans provide valuable information about the function of brain tissue in patients, to detect malignancy and to evaluate brain abnormalities in Alzheimer disease, stroke, schizophrenia, and epilepsy (Figure 10-22). Combined **PET-CT scanners** provide images that pinpoint the location of abnormal metabolic activity within the brain.

Ultrasound Examination

Doppler ultrasound studies — **Sound waves detect blood flow in the carotid and intracranial arteries.**

The carotid artery carries blood to the brain. These studies detect occlusion in blood vessels.

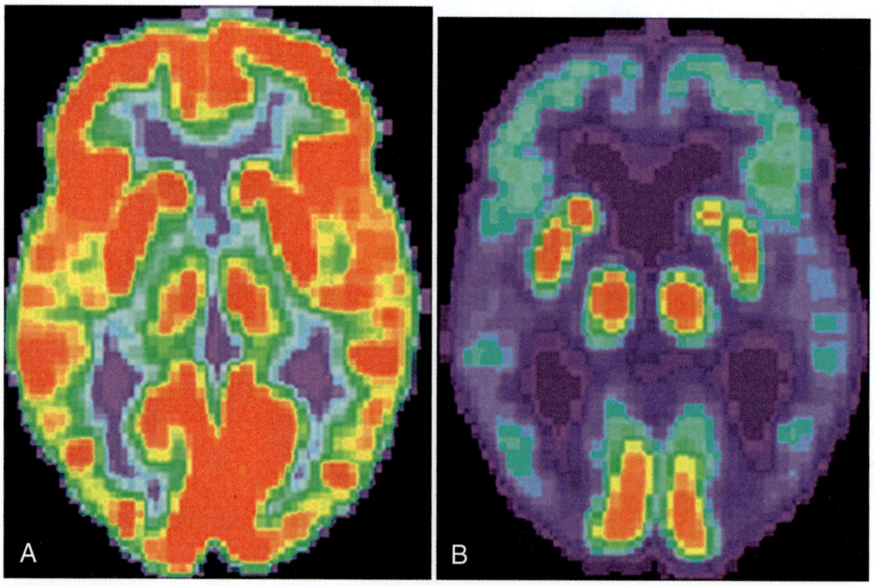

FIGURE 10-22 **PET scans. A, Normal brain. B, Brain affected by Alzheimer disease.** Red and yellow areas indicate high neural activity. Blue and purple indicate low neural activity.

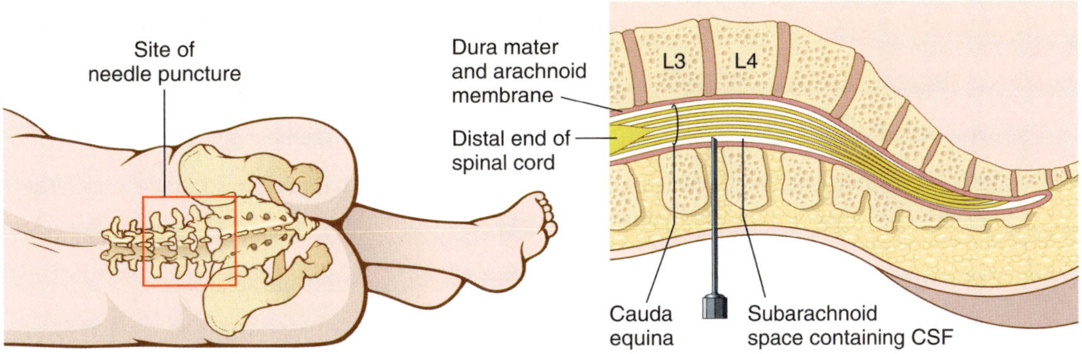

FIGURE 10-23 Lumbar puncture. The patient lies laterally, with the knees drawn up to the abdomen and the chin brought down to the chest. This position increases the spaces between the vertebrae. The lumbar puncture needle is inserted between the third and fourth (or the fourth and fifth) lumbar vertebrae and then is advanced to enter the subarachnoid space.

Other Procedures

electroencephalography (EEG)

Recording of the electrical activity of the brain.

EEG demonstrates seizure activity resulting from brain tumors, other diseases, and injury to the brain. It can also help define diffuse cortical dysfunction (encephalopathies).

lumbar puncture (LP)

CSF is withdrawn from between two lumbar vertebrae for analysis (Figure 10-23).

A device to measure the pressure of CSF may be attached to the end of the needle after it has been inserted. Injection of intrathecal medicines may be administered as well. Some patients experience headache after LP. An informal name for this procedure is "spinal tap."

stereotactic radiosurgery

Use of a specialized instrument to locate and treat targets in the brain.

The stereotactic instrument is fixed onto the skull and guides the insertion of a needle by three-dimensional measurement. A **Gamma Knife** (high-energy radiation beam) is used to treat deep and often inaccessible intracranial brain tumors and abnormal blood vessel masses **(arteriovenous malformations)** without surgical incision. **Proton stereotactic radiosurgery (PSRS)** delivers a uniform dose of proton radiation to a target and spares surrounding normal tissue (Figure 10-24 A and B).

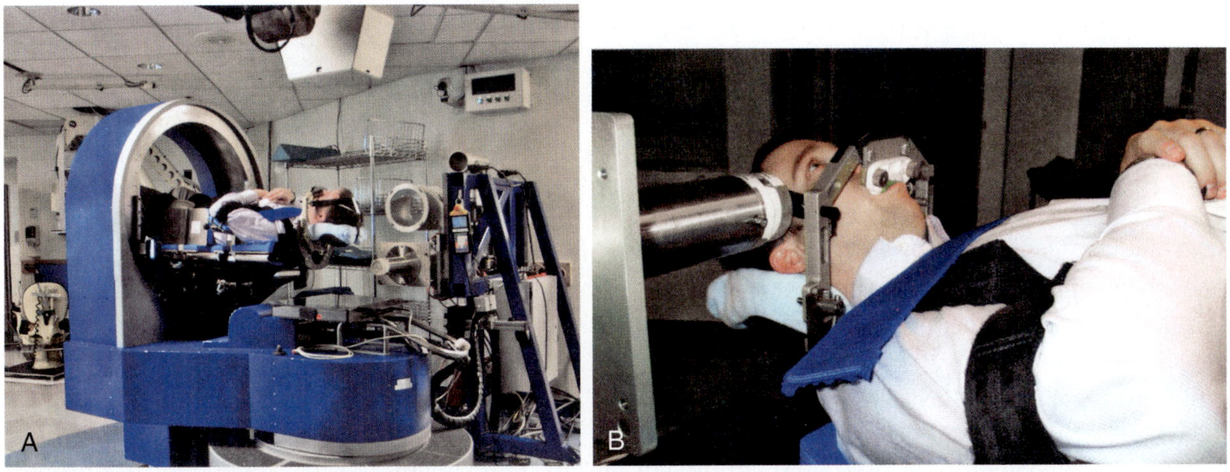

FIGURE 10-24 A, Patient in position on **stereotactic proton unit, ready to take an alignment x-ray. B, Stereotactic frame** holds the head in place for treatment with proton beam radiosurgery. *(Courtesy Department of Radiation Therapy, Massachusetts General Hospital, Boston.)*

10

ABBREVIATIONS

AD	Alzheimer disease
AFP	alpha-fetoprotein; elevated levels in amniotic fluid and maternal blood are associated with congenital malformations of the nervous system, such as anencephaly and spina bifida
ALS	amyotrophic lateral sclerosis—Lou Gehrig disease
AVM	arteriovenous malformation; congenital tangle of arteries and veins in the cerebrum
BBB	blood-brain barrier
CNS	central nervous system
CSF	cerebrospinal fluid
CT	computed tomography
CVA	cerebrovascular accident
EEG	electroencephalography
GABA	gamma-aminobutyric acid (neurotransmitter)
ICP	intracranial pressure (normal pressure is 5 to 15 mm Hg)
LP	lumbar puncture
MAC	monitored anesthetic care
MG	myasthenia gravis
MRA	magnetic resonance angiography
MRI	magnetic resonance imaging
MS	multiple sclerosis
½P	hemiparesis
PCA	patient-controlled analgesia
PET	positron emission tomography
PNS	peripheral nervous system
PSRS	proton stereotactic radiosurgery
Sz	seizure
TBI	traumatic brain injury
TENS	transcutaneous electrical nerve stimulation; technique using a battery-powered device to relieve acute and chronic pain
TIA	transient ischemic attack; temporary interference with the blood supply to the brain
TLE	temporal lobe epilepsy
tPA	tissue plasminogen activator; a clot-dissolving drug used as therapy for stroke

PRACTICAL APPLICATIONS

Answers to the following case report and case study are on page 387.

CASE REPORT: CEREBRAL INFARCTION

This patient was admitted on January 14 with a history of progressive right hemiparesis for the previous 1 to 2 months; fluctuating numbness of the right arm, thorax, and buttocks; jerking of the right leg; periods of speech arrest; diminished comprehension in reading; and recent development of a hemiplegic gait. He is suspected of having a left parietal tumor [the parietal lobes of the cerebrum are on either side under the roof of the skull].

Examinations done before hospitalization included skull films, EEG, and CSF analysis, which were all normal. After admission, an MRI was abnormal in the left parietal region, as was the EEG.

An MRA study to assess cerebral blood vessels was attempted, but the patient became progressively more restless and agitated after sedation, so the procedure was stopped. During the recovery phase from the sedation, the patient was alternately somnolent [sleepy] and violent, but it was later apparent that he had developed almost a complete aphasia and right hemiplegia.

In the next few days, he became more alert, although he remained dysarthric [from the Greek *arthroun*, to utter distinctly] and hemiplegic.

MRI and MRA with the patient under general anesthesia on January 19 showed complete occlusion of the left internal carotid artery with cross-filling of the left anterior and middle cerebral arteries from the right internal carotid circulation.

Final diagnosis: Left CVA caused by left internal carotid artery occlusion.

[Figure 10-25 shows the common carotid arteries and their branches within the head and brain.]

Questions about the Case Report

1. The patient was admitted with a history of
   a. Right-sided paralysis caused by a previous stroke
   b. Paralysis on the left side of his body
   c. Increasing paresis on the right side of his body
2. The patient also has experienced periods of
   a. Aphasia and dyslexia
   b. Dysplastic gait
   c. Apraxia and aphasia
3. After his admission, where did the MRI show an abnormality?
   a. Right posterior region of the brain
   b. Left and right sides of the brain
   c. Left side of the brain
4. What test determined the final diagnosis?
   a. EEG for both sides of the brain
   b. CSF analysis and cerebral angiography
   c. MRI and MRA
5. What was the final diagnosis?
   a. A stroke; ischemic tissue in the left cerebrum caused by blockage of an artery
   b. Cross-filling of blood vessels from the left to the right side of the brain
   c. Cerebral palsy on the left side of the brain with cross-filling of two cerebral arteries

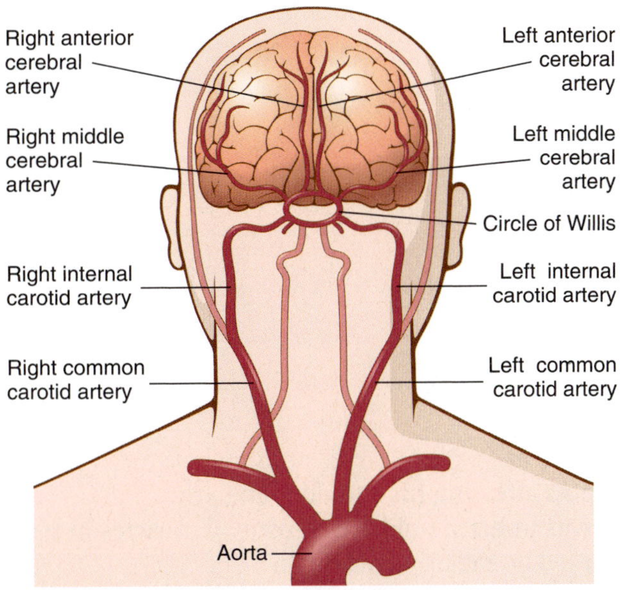

FIGURE 10-25 Common carotid arteries and their branches.

PAIN MEDICATIONS

Pain is a major symptom in many medical conditions. Both the area of injury and how the brain deals with it affect the sensations of pain. Medications to relieve pain (analgesics) act in different ways:

- Nonsteroidal anti-inflammatory drugs (NSAIDS) relieve pain by stopping inflammation. Examples are nonprescription drugs, such as ibuprofen (Advil, Motrin, Excedrin), aspirin (Anacin, Ascriptin, Bufferin), and naproxen (Aleve). Other NSAIDS that require a prescription are Toradol (ketorolac) and Feldine (pivoxicain).
- Acetaminophen (Tylenol) relieves fever and mild pain but is not an anti-inflammatory drug. It is not clear how acetaminophen works.
- Narcotics relieve pain by affecting receptors in the brain to control the perception of pain. Examples are morphine, codeine, oxycodone, and hydrocodone, Combinations of narcotics and acetaminophen are Vicodin (acetaminophen with hydrocodone) and Percocet (acetaminophen with oxycodone).

NEUROPATHIC PAIN AND CASE STUDY

Neuropathic pain is a unique type of pain that accompanies illnesses and trauma. Patients describe this pain as:

- radiating or spreading
- an electric shock–like sensation
- hot or burning
- shooting, piercing, darting, or stabbing (lancinating)
- abnormal skin sensations (paresthesias): numbness, tingling, “pins and needles”
- pain to light touch
- extreme sensitivity to ordinary, innocuous stimuli
- often independent of movement

Case Study

10

A 68-year-old man awoke one morning with severe pain in his right shoulder. On turning his head or lifting his shoulder, he experienced extreme discomfort and lancinating pain. The pain was a sharp, burning pain that moved across his shoulder and down into his right arm. Finding a comfortable position lying down was difficult. A cervical MRI study showed no bone abnormalities, whereas a neurologic examination provided evidence of damage to multiple peripheral nerves. He developed weakness of his shoulder muscles and was unable to lift his right arm. Final diagnosis was brachial plexus neuritis [also known as Parsonage-Turner syndrome]. The cause of the condition is unknown, but it may be related to a flu vaccination he received 2 weeks previously. Treatment consisted of pain medication and physical therapy to rehabilitate weakened muscles in his arm and shoulder.

Questions about the Case Study

1. The cervical MRI study showed
   a. Damage to the vertebrae in the neck
   b. Nerve entrapment in the upper spine
   c. Damage to multiple peripheral nerves
   d. Normal vertebrae in the neck
2. Lancinating pain is
   a. Pain to light touch
   b. Characterized by paresthesia
   c. Stabbing, piercing, shooting
   d. Characterized by numbness and tingling
3. The patient’s diagnosis is best described as
   a. Inflammation of cervical nerve roots affecting his shoulder and arm
   b. Inflammation of a network of nerves in his shoulder that control muscles in his arm
   c. First stages of a heart attack, marked by radiating arm pain
   d. Autoimmune disorder affecting voluntary muscles in his shoulder and arm

IN PERSON

This is a first person account of a woman in her mid-forties living with sciatica.

Five years ago, I wouldn't have believed that reaching into a laundry basket could change my my life. But in January 2009, it did.

I had gotten my first-ever backache a few days earlier, after a long car trip. A Google search instructed me to apply ice for the first 48 hours and then heat, if the pain persisted. My husband took over the kids' school day routine while I recuperated. That third morning, I could hear my younger son rifling around for his favorite sweatshirt; I knew it was at the foot of my bed waiting to be sorted. In the instant it took to reach into the laundry basket for that sweatshirt, my back went from dull ache to a crippling pain that radiated all the way down my left leg, to the tip of my left foot.

An MRI confirmed the diagnosis: spinal disc herniation, protruding onto the sciatic nerve root, causing the leg pain. Surgery being presented as a last resort, I embarked on a crash course of physical therapy, NSAIDs, oral steroids, muscle relaxants, epidural steroid injections, and lots and lots of patience. I saw gradual improvement for about three months, to the point that I was able to resume a modified daily routine.

Then, the improvement stopped. Conventional treatment had run its course. I was at the "last resort" stage. So I "cried uncle" and requested a surgical consult. The surgeon ordered a follow-up MRI, which showed good news: there had been much improvement to the herniation. To my surprise, the MRI also revealed that the sciatic nerve was now free and clear of impingement. If the nerve was back to normal, why was I still in such pain? Because, it turns out, the nerve was injured by its ordeal. Not uncommon, I was reassured. This development took the surgical option off the table. After all, the goal of the surgery would have been to relieve the affected nerve from compression by the protruding disc. In my case, even the relieved nerve was causing problems, and that meant not surgery, but more patience. The wait began: to see whether the the nerve would repair itself—I was told that could take years—or worse, whether I was facing permanent nerve damage.

Three years later the verdict seems clear: my sciatic nerve sustained what appears to be permanent damage. To this day, I have not regained full use of my left leg. Along with chronic, dull pain, there are also paresthesias—simultaneous burning and numbness along the path of the sciatic nerve accompanied by constant, involuntary muscle spasms. I've lost my Achilles jerk reflex, and so unresponsive is my left foot that I can't feel it hit the ground when I'm walking.

In those critical first months, I thought my options were either resolving the herniation with surgery or resolving it without surgery. It never once occurred to me that, four years later, the injury would remain unresolved.

There's always a new treatment, or specialist, or drug that shows promise or really worked for a friend of a friend. Until recently, it felt like I was giving up hope if I didn't pursue each lead. Now I'm focusing more on adapting to my new circumstances than on finding a "cure." I don't want my whole life to revolve around sciatica. I found a medication which reduces the chronic pain to more of an annoyance than a crisis (with occasional flare-ups).

I missed my old life and wanted it back. At the risk of sounding like a late night pharmaceutical ad, I'm not giving up; I'm going on.

AUTHOR'S NOTE: Everyone's experience with sciatica is unique. I recently experienced the condition myself, resulting from a L4-L5 disk herniation. After 7 months of pain radiating down right leg, I had microdiskectomy surgery, which fortunately alleviated my pain and sciatica.

EXERCISES

Remember to check your answers carefully with the Answers to Exercises, page 385.

A Match the following neurologic structures with their meanings as given below.

astrocyte	dendrite	neuron
axon	meninges	oligodendroglial cell
cauda equina	myelin sheath	plexus
cerebral cortex		

1. microscopic fiber leading from the cell body that carries the nervous impulse along a nerve cell ____________________
2. large, interlacing network of nerves ____________________
3. three protective membranes surrounding the brain and spinal cord ____________________
4. microscopic branching fiber of a nerve cell that is the first part to receive the nervous impulse ____________________
5. outer region of the largest part of the brain; composed of gray matter ____________________
6. glial cell that transports water and salts between capillaries and nerve cells ____________________
7. glial cell that produces myelin ____________________
8. a nerve cell that transmits a nerve impulse ____________________
9. collection of spinal nerves below the end of the spinal cord at the level of the second lumbar vertebra ____________________
10. fatty tissue that surrounds the axon of a nerve cell ____________________

B Give the meanings of the following terms.

1. dura mater ____________________
2. central nervous system ____________________
3. peripheral nervous system ____________________
4. arachnoid membrane ____________________
5. hypothalamus ____________________
6. synapse ____________________
7. sympathetic nerves ____________________
8. medulla oblongata ____________________
9. pons ____________________
10. cerebellum ____________________

11. thalamus ______________________

12. ventricles of the brain ______________________

13. brainstem ______________________

14. cerebrum ______________________

15. ganglion ______________________

C **Match the following terms with the meanings or associated terms below.**

glial cells	neurotransmitter	sensory nerves
gyri	parenchymal cell	subarachnoid space
motor nerves	pia mater	sulci

1. innermost meningeal membrane ______________________
2. carry messages away from (efferent) the brain and spinal cord to muscles and glands

   ____
3. carry messages toward (afferent) the brain and spinal cord from receptors ______________________
4. grooves in the cerebral cortex ______________________
5. contains cerebrospinal fluid ______________________
6. elevations in the cerebral cortex ______________________
7. chemical that is released at the end of a nerve cell and stimulates or inhibits another cell

   (example: acetylcholine) ______________________
8. essential cell of the nervous system; a neuron ______________________
9. connective and supportive (stromal) tissue ______________________

10

D **Circle the correct term for the given definition.**

1. disease of the brain **(encephalopathy, myelopathy)**
2. part of the brain that controls muscular coordination and balance **(cerebrum, cerebellum)**
3. collection of blood above the dura mater **(subdural hematoma, epidural hematoma)**
4. inflammation of the pia and arachnoid membranes **(leptomeningitis, causalgia)**
5. condition of absence of a brain **(hypalgesia, anencephaly)**
6. inflammation of the gray matter of the spinal cord **(poliomyelitis, polyneuritis)**
7. pertaining to the membranes around the brain and spinal cord **(cerebellopontine, meningeal)**
8. disease of nerve roots (of spinal nerves) **(neuropathy, radiculopathy)**
9. hernia of the spinal cord and meninges **(myelomeningocele, meningioma)**
10. pertaining to the tenth cranial nerve **(thalamic, vagal)**

E Give the meanings of the following terms.

1. cerebral cortex ______________________________
2. intrathecal ______________________________
3. polyneuritis ______________________________
4. thalamic ______________________________
5. myelopathy ______________________________
6. meningioma ______________________________
7. glioma ______________________________
8. subdural hematoma ______________________________

F Match the following neurologic symptoms with the meanings below.

aphasia	dyslexia	narcolepsy
ataxia	hemiparesis	neurasthenia
bradykinesia	hyperesthesia	paraplegia
causalgia	motor apraxia	syncope

1. reading disorder ______________________________
2. condition of decreased coordination ______________________________
3. condition of slow movement ______________________________
4. condition of increased sensation ______________________________
5. seizure of sleep; uncontrollable compulsion to sleep ______________________________
6. difficulty with speech ______________________________
7. inability to perform a task ______________________________
8. weakness in the right or left half of the body ______________________________
9. severe burning pain due to nerve injury ______________________________
10. paralysis in the lower part of the body ______________________________
11. fainting ______________________________
12. nervous exhaustion (lack of strength) and fatigue ______________________________

G Give the meanings of the following terms.

1. analgesia ______________________________
2. motor aphasia ______________________________
3. paresis ______________________________
4. quadriplegia ______________________________
5. asthenia ______________________________

10

6. comatose ______________________________
7. paresthesia ______________________________
8. hyperkinesis ______________________________
9. anesthesia ______________________________
10. causalgia ______________________________
11. akinetic ______________________________
12. hypalgesia ______________________________
13. dyskinesia ______________________________
14. migraine ______________________________

H Match the following terms with their descriptions below. The terms in boldface are clues!

Alzheimer disease	Huntington disease	myasthenia gravis
amyotrophic lateral sclerosis	hydrocephalus	Parkinson disease
Bell palsy	multiple sclerosis	myelomeningocele
epilepsy		

1. Destruction of myelin sheath (demyelination) and its replacement by **hard** plaques ______________________________
2. Sudden, transient disturbances of brain function cause **seizures** ______________________________
3. The **spinal** column is imperfectly joined (a **split** in a vertebra occurs), and part of the meninges and spinal cord can herniate out of the spinal cavity ______________________________
4. **Atrophy** of muscles and paralysis caused by damage to motor neurons in the spinal cord and brainstem ______________________________
5. Patient displays bizarre, abrupt, involuntary, **dance**-like movements, as well as decline in mental functions ______________________________
6. Cerebrospinal **fluid** accumulates in the **head** (in the ventricles of the brain) ______________________________
7. **Loss of muscle strength** due to the inability of a neurotransmitter (acetylcholine) to transmit impulses from nerve cells to muscle cells ______________________________
8. Degeneration of nerves in the basal ganglia occurring in later life, leading to tremors, shuffling gait, and muscle stiffness; **dopamine** (neurotransmitter) is deficient in the brain ______________________________
9. Deterioration of mental capacity **(dementia)**; autopsy shows cerebral cortex atrophy, widening of cerebral sulci, and microscopic neurofibrillary tangles ______________________________
10. Unilateral facial **paralysis** ______________________________

I **Give the meanings of the following terms for abnormal conditions.**

1. astrocytoma ______
2. pyogenic meningitis ______
3. Tourette syndrome ______
4. cerebral contusion ______
5. cerebrovascular accident ______
6. cerebral concussion ______
7. herpes zoster ______
8. cerebral embolus ______
9. cerebral thrombosis ______
10. cerebral hemorrhage ______
11. cerebral aneurysm ______
12. HIV encephalopathy ______

J **Match the term in Column I with the letter of its associated term or meaning in Column II.**

COLUMN I

1. ataxia ______
2. aura ______
3. transient ischemic attack ______
4. tonic-clonic seizure ______
5. herpes zoster ______
6. palliative ______
7. dopamine ______
8. occlusion ______
9. absence seizure ______
10. glioblastoma multiforme ______

COLUMN II

A. relieving, but not curing
B. virus that causes chickenpox and shingles
C. uncoordinated gait
D. neurotransmitter
E. peculiar sensation experienced by patient before onset of seizure
F. malignant brain tumor of immature glial cells
G. major epileptic seizure; ictal event
H. blood flow to the brain stops for a brief period of time
I. minor epileptic seizure
J. blockage

K **Describe what happens in the following two procedures.**

1. MRI of the brain ______
2. stereotactic radiosurgery with Gamma Knife ______

______

L **Match the following easily confused terms with their meanings below.**

analgesia	ataxia	neurasthenia
anesthesia	dyskinesia	paresis
aphasia	dyslexia	paresthesia
apraxia	hyperkinesia	

1. lack of nerve strength ____________________
2. inability to speak ____________________
3. inability to perform purposeful actions ____________________
4. condition of insensitivity to pain ____________________
5. condition of loss of sensation ____________________
6. sensations of tingling, numbness, or "pins and needles" ____________________
7. lack of coordination ____________________
8. excessive movement ____________________
9. abnormal, involuntary, spasmodic movements ____________________
10. developmental reading disorder ____________________
11. partial paralysis ____________________

M **Give the meanings of the following abbreviations and then select the letter of the best association for each.**

COLUMN I

1. EEG ____________ ______
2. PET ____________ ______
3. AFP ____________ ______
4. MS ____________ ______
5. MRI ____________ ______
6. LP ____________ ______
7. CVA ____________ ______
8. AD ____________ ______
9. TIA ____________ ______
10. CSF ____________ ______

COLUMN II

A. Gradually progressive dementia
B. Stroke; embolus, hemorrhage, or thrombosis are etiologic factors
C. Intrathecal medications can be administered through this procedure.
D. This fluid is analyzed for abnormal blood cells, chemicals, and protein.
E. Procedure to diagnose abnormal electrical activity in the brain
F. Neurologic symptoms and/or signs due to temporary interference of blood supply to the brain
G. High levels in amniotic fluid and maternal blood are associated with spina bifida.
H. Diagnostic procedure that allows excellent visualization of soft tissue in the brain
I. Radioactive materials, such as glucose, are taken up by the brain, and images recorded.
J. Destruction of the myelin sheath in the CNS occurs with plaques of hard scar tissue.

N **Circle the terms that complete the meanings of the sentences.**

1. Maria had such severe headaches that she could find relief only with strong analgesics. Her condition of **(spina bifida, migraine, epilepsy)** was debilitating.
2. Paul was in a coma after his high-speed car accident. His physicians were concerned that he had suffered a **(palsy, myelomeningocele, contusion and subdural hematoma)** as a result of the accident.
3. Dick went to the emergency department complaining of dizziness, nausea, and headache. The physician, suspecting increased ICP, prescribed corticosteroids, and Dick's symptoms disappeared. They returned, however, when the steroids were discontinued. A/an **(MRI study of the brain, electroencephalogram, CSF analysis)** revealed a large brain lesion. It was removed surgically and determined to be a/an **(embolus, glioblastoma multiforme, migraine)**.
4. Dorothy felt weakness in her hand and numbness in her arm, and noticed blurred vision, all signs of **(herpes zoster, meningitis, TIA)**. Her physician requested **(myelography, MRA, lumbar puncture)** to assess any damage to cerebral blood vessels and possible stroke.
5. When Bill noticed ptosis and muscle weakness in his face, he reported these symptoms to his doctor. The doctor diagnosed his condition as **(Tourette syndrome, Huntington disease, myasthenia gravis)** and prescribed **(dopamine, anticonvulsants, anticholinesterase drugs)**, which relieved his symptoms.
6. To rule out bacterial **(epilepsy, encephalomalacia, meningitis)**, Dr. Phillips, a pediatrician, requested that a/an **(EEG, PET scan, LP)** be performed on the febrile (feverish) child.
7. Eight-year-old Barry reversed his letters and had difficulty learning to read and write words. His family physician diagnosed his problem as **(aphasia, dyslexia, ataxia)**.
8. After his head hit the steering wheel during a recent automobile accident, Clark noticed **(hemiparesis, paraplegia, hyperesthesia)** on the left side of his body. A head CT scan revealed **(narcolepsy, neurasthenia, subdural hematoma)**.
9. For her 35th birthday, Elizabeth's husband threw her a surprise party. She was so startled by the crowd that she experienced a weakness of muscles and loss of consciousness. Friends placed her on her back in a horizontal position with her head low to improve blood flow to her brain. She soon recovered from her **(myoneural, syncopal, hyperkinetic)** episode.
10. Near his 65th birthday, Edward began having difficulty remembering recent events. Over the next 5 years, he developed **(dyslexia, dementia, seizures)** and was diagnosed with **(multiple sclerosis, myasthenia gravis, Alzheimer disease)**.
11. Elderly Mrs. Smith had been taking an antipsychotic drug for 5 years when she began exhibiting lip smacking and darting movements of her tongue. Her doctor described her condition as **(radiculitis, tardive dyskinesia, hemiparesis)** and discontinued her drug. The condition, acquired after use of the drug, would be considered **(iatrogenic, congenital, ictal)**.

O **Complete the spelling of the following terms based on their meanings.**

1. part of the brain that controls sleep, appetite, temperature, and secretions of the pituitary gland: hypo______________________________
2. pertaining to fainting: syn______________________________
3. abnormal tingling sensations: par______________________________
4. slight paralysis: par______________________________
5. inflammation of a spinal nerve root: ______________________________itis
6. inability to speak correctly: a______________________________
7. movements and behavior that are not purposeful: a______________________________
8. lack of muscular coordination: a______________________________
9. developmental reading disorder: dys______________________________
10. excessive movement: hyper______________________________
11. paralysis in one half (right or left) of the body: ______________________________plegia
12. paralysis in the lower half of the body: ______________________________plegia
13. paralysis in all four limbs: ______________________________plegia
14. nervous exhaustion and fatigue: neur______________________________

ANSWERS TO EXERCISES

A

1. axon
2. plexus
3. meninges
4. dendrite
5. cerebral cortex
6. astrocyte
7. oligodendroglial cell
8. neuron
9. cauda equina
10. myelin sheath

B

1. outermost meningeal layer surrounding the brain and spinal cord
2. brain and the spinal cord
3. nerves outside the brain and spinal cord; cranial, spinal, and autonomic nerves
4. middle meningeal membrane surrounding the brain and spinal cord
5. part of the brain below the thalamus; controls sleep, appetite, body temperature, and secretions from the pituitary gland
6. space through which a nervous impulse is transmitted from a nerve cell to another nerve cell or to a muscle or gland cell
7. autonomic nerves that influence body functions involuntarily in times of stress
8. part of the brain just above the spinal cord that controls breathing, heartbeat, and the size of blood vessels
9. part of the brain anterior to the cerebellum and between the medulla and the upper parts of the brain; connects these parts of the brain
10. posterior part of the brain that coordinates voluntary muscle movements
11. part of the brain below the cerebrum; relay center that conducts impulses between the spinal cord and the cerebrum
12. canals in the interior of the brain that are filled with CSF
13. lower portion of the brain that connects the cerebrum with the spinal cord (includes the pons and the medulla)
14. largest part of the brain; controls voluntary muscle movement, vision, speech, hearing, thought, memory
15. collection of nerve cell bodies outside the brain and spinal cord

C

1. pia mater
2. motor nerves
3. sensory nerves
4. sulci
5. subarachnoid space
6. gyri
7. neurotransmitter
8. parenchymal cell
9. glial cells

D

1. encephalopathy
2. cerebellum
3. epidural hematoma
4. leptomeningitis
5. anencephaly
6. poliomyelitis
7. meningeal
8. radiculopathy
9. myelomeningocele
10. vagal

E

1. outer region of the cerebrum (contains gray matter)
2. pertaining to within a sheath through the meninges and into the subarachnoid space
3. inflammation of many nerves
4. pertaining to the thalamus
5. disease of the spinal cord
6. tumor of the meninges
7. tumor of neuroglial cells (a brain tumor)
8. mass of blood below the dura mater (outermost meningeal membrane)

F

1. dyslexia
2. ataxia
3. bradykinesia
4. hyperesthesia
5. narcolepsy
6. aphasia
7. motor apraxia
8. hemiparesis
9. causalgia
10. paraplegia
11. syncope
12. neurasthenia

G

1. lack of sensitivity to pain
2. difficulty in speaking (patient cannot articulate words but can understand speech and knows what she or he wants to say)
3. weakness and partial loss of movement
4. paralysis in all four extremities (damage is to the cervical part of the spinal cord)
5. no strength (weakness)
6. pertaining to coma (loss of consciousness from which the patient cannot be aroused)
7. condition of abnormal sensations (prickling, tingling, burning)
8. excessive movement
9. condition of no sensation or nervous feeling
10. severe burning pain from injury to peripheral nerves
11. pertaining to without movement
12. diminished sensation to pain
13. impairment of the ability to perform voluntary movements
14. recurrent vascular headache with severe pain of unilateral onset and photophobia (sensitivity to light)

H

1. multiple sclerosis
2. epilepsy
3. myelomeningocele
4. amyotrophic lateral sclerosis
5. Huntington disease
6. hydrocephalus
7. myasthenia gravis
8. Parkinson disease
9. Alzheimer disease
10. Bell palsy

I

1. tumor of neuroglial brain cells (astrocytes)
2. inflammation of the meninges (bacterial infection with pus formation)
3. involuntary spasmodic, twitching movements (tics), uncontrollable vocal sounds, and inappropriate word
4. bruising of brain tissue as a result of direct trauma to the head
5. disruption of the normal blood supply to the brain; stroke or cerebral infarction
6. traumatic brain injury caused by a blow to the head
7. neurologic condition caused by infection with herpes zoster virus; blisters form along the course of peripheral nerves
8. blockage of a blood vessel in the cerebrum caused by material from another part of the body that suddenly occludes the vessel
9. blockage of a blood vessel in the cerebrum caused by the formation of a clot within the vessel
10. collection of blood in the brain (can cause a stroke)
11. widening of a blood vessel (artery) in the cerebrum; the aneurysm can burst and lead to a CVA
12. brain disease (dementia and encephalitis) caused by infection with AIDS virus

J

1. C
2. E
3. H
4. G
5. B
6. A
7. D
8. J
9. I
10. F

K

1. use of magnetic waves to create an image (in frontal, transverse, or sagittal plane) of the brain
2. an instrument (stereotactic) is fixed onto the skull and locates a target by three-dimensional measurement; gamma radiation or proton beams are used to treat deep brain lesions

L

1. neurasthenia
2. aphasia
3. apraxia
4. analgesia
5. anesthesia
6. paresthesia
7. ataxia
8. hyperkinesia
9. dyskinesia
10. dyslexia
11. paresis

M

1. electroencephalography: E
2. positron emission tomography: I
3. alpha-fetoprotein: G
4. multiple sclerosis: J
5. magnetic resonance imaging: H
6. lumbar puncture: C
7. cerebrovascular accident: B
8. Alzheimer disease: A
9. transient ischemic attack: F
10. cerebrospinal fluid: D

N

1. migraine
2. contusion and subdural hematoma
3. MRI of the brain; glioblastoma multiforme
4. TIA; MRA
5. myasthenia gravis; anticholinesterase drugs
6. meningitis; LP
7. dyslexia
8. hemiparesis; subdural hematoma
9. syncopal
10. dementia; Alzheimer disease
11. tardive dyskinesia; iatrogenic

O

1. hypothalamus
2. syncopal
3. paresthesias
4. paresis
5. radiculitis
6. aphasia
7. apraxia
8. ataxia
9. dyslexia
10. hyperkinesis
11. hemiplegia
12. paraplegia
13. quadriplegia
14. neurasthenia

Answers to Practical Applications

Case Report: Cerebral Infarction

1. c
2. a
3. c
4. c
5. a

Neuropathic Pain and Case Study

1. d
2. c
3. b

PRONUNCIATION OF TERMS

To test your understanding of the terminology in this chapter, write the meaning of each term in the space provided. In addition, you may wish to cover the terms and write them by looking at your definitions. Make sure your spelling is correct. The page number after each term indicates where it is defined or used in the book, so you can easily check your responses. You will find complete definitions for all of these terms and their audio pronunciations on the Evolve website.

Pronunciation Guide

ā as in āpe	ă as in ăpple
ē as in ēven	ĕ as in ĕvery
ī as in īce	ĭ as in ĭnterest
ō as in ōpen	ŏ as in pŏt
ū as in ūnit	ŭ as in ŭnder

Vocabulary and Combining Forms and Terminology

TERM	PRONUNCIATION	MEANING
acetylcholine (355)	ăs-ē-tĭl-KŌ-lēn	
afferent nerve (355)	ĂF-fĕr-ĕnt nĕrv	
akinetic (360)	ā-kĭ-NĔT-ĭk	
analgesia (359)	ăn-ăl-JĒ-zē-ă	
anencephaly (359)	ăn-ĕn-SĔF-ă-lē	
anesthesia (360)	ăn-ĕs-THĒ-zē-ă	
aphasia (361)	ă-FĀ-zē-ă	
apraxia (362)	Ā-PRĂK-sē-ă	
arachnoid membrane (355)	ă-RĂK-noyd MĔM-brān	
astrocyte (355)	ĂS-trō-sīt	
ataxia (362)	ă-TĂK-sē-ă	
autonomic nervous system (355)	ăw-tō-NŌM-ĭk NĔR-vŭs SĬS-tĕm	
axon (355)	ĂK-sŏn	
blood-brain barrier (355)	blŭd-brĀn BĂ-rē-ĕr	
bradykinesia (360)	brĀ-dē-kĭ-NĒ-zē-ă	
brainstem (355)	BRĀN-stĕm	
cauda equina (355)	KĂW-dă ĕ-KWĪ-nă	
causalgia (360)	kăw-ZĂL-jă	
cell body (355)	sĕl BŎD-ē	
central nervous system (355)	SĔN-trăl NĔR-vŭs SĬS-tĕm	
cephalgia (360)	sĕ-FĂL-jă	
cerebellar (357)	sĕr-ĕ-BĔL-ăr	

TERM	PRONUNCIATION	MEANING
cerebellopontine (359)	sĕr-ĕ-bĕl-ō-PŎN-tēn	
cerebellum (355)	sĕr-ĕ-BĔL-ŭm	
cerebral cortex (355)	sĕ-RĒ-brăl (*or* SĔR-ĕ-brăl) KŎR-tĕks	
cerebrospinal fluid (355)	sĕ-rē-brō-SPĪ-năl FLOO-ĭd	
cerebrum (355)	sĕ-RĒ-brŭm	
coma (360)	KŌ-mă	
comatose (360)	KŌ-mă-tōs	
cranial nerves (355)	KRĀ-nē-ăl nĕrvz	
dendrite (355)	DĔN-drīt	
dura mater (355)	DŪR-ă MĂ-tĕr	
dyslexia (361)	dĭs-LĔK-sē-ă	
dyskinesia (360)	dĭs-kĭ-NĒ-zē-ă	
efferent nerve (355)	ĔF-fĕr-ĕnt nĕrvz	
encephalitis (358)	ĕn-sĕf-ă-LĪ-tĭs	
encephalopathy (358)	ĕn-sĕf-ă-LŎP-ă-thē	
ependymal cell (355)	ĕp-ĔN-dĭ-măl sĕl	
epidural hematoma (358)	ĕp-ĕ-DŪ-răl hē-mă-TŌ-mă	
ganglion (356)	GĂNG-lē-ŏn	
glial cell (356)	GLĒ-ăl sĕl	
glioblastoma (358)	glē-ō-blă-STŌ-mă	
gyrus; gyri (356)	JĪ-rŭs; JĪ-rē	
hemiparesis (361)	hĕm-ē-pă-RĒ-sĭs	
hemiplegia (361)	hĕm-ē-PLĒ-jă	
hypalgesia (359)	hīp-ăl-GĒ-zē-ă	
hyperesthesia (360)	hī-pĕr-ĕs-THĒ-zē-ă	
hyperkinesis (360)	hī-pĕr-kĭ-NĒ-sĭs	
hypothalamus (356)	hī-pō-THĂL-ă-mŭs	
intrathecal injection (359)	ĭn-tră-THĒ-kăl ĭn-JĔK-shun	
leptomeningeal (358)	lĕp-tō-mĕn-ĭn-JĒ-ăl	
medulla oblongata (356)	mĕ-DŪL-ă (*or* mĕ-DŬL-ă) ŏb-lŏn-GĂ-tă	

10

TERM	PRONUNCIATION	MEANING
meningeal (358)	mĕ-NĬN-jē-ăl *or* mĕ-nĭn-JĒ-ăl	
meninges (356)	mĕ-NĬN-jēz	
meningioma (358)	mĕ-nĭn-jē-Ō-mă	
microglial cell (356)	mī-krō-GLĒ-ăl sĕl	
motor nerve (356)	MŌ-tĕr nĕrv	
myelin sheath (356)	MĪ-ĕ-lĭn shēth	
myelomeningocele (358)	mī-ĕ-lō-mĕ-NĬN-gō-sēl	
myelopathy (359)	mī-ĕ-LŎP-ă-thē	
myoneural (359)	mī-ō-NŪR-ăl	
narcolepsy (360)	NĂR-kō-lĕp-sē	
nerve (356)	nĕrv	
neuralgia (360)	nūr-ĂL-jă	
neurasthenia (362)	nūr-ăs-THĒ-nē-ă	
neuroglial cells (349)	nūr-ō-GLĒ-ăl cells	
neuron (356)	NŪR-ŏn	
neuropathy (359)	nūr-ŎP-ă-thē	
neurotransmitter (356)	nūr-ō-trănz-MĬT-ĕr	
oligodendroglial cell (356)	ŏl-ĭ-gō-dĕn-drō-GLĒ-ăl sĕl	
paraplegia (361)	păr-ă-PLĒ-jă	
parasympathetic nerves (356)	păr-ă-sĭm-pă-THĔT-ĭk nĕrvz	
parenchyma (356)	păr-ĔN-kĭ-mă	
paresis (361)	pă-RĒ-sĭs	
paresthesia (360)	păr-ĕs-THĒ-zē-ă	
peripheral nervous system (356)	pĕ-RĬF-ĕr-ăl NĔR-vŭs SĬS-tĕm system	
pia mater (356)	PĒ-ă MĂ-tĕr	
plexus (356)	PLĔK-sŭs	
poliomyelitis (359)	pō-lē-ō-mī-ĕ-LĪ-tĭs	
polyneuritis (359)	pŏl-ē-nŭ-RĪ-tĭs	
pons (356)	pŏnz	
quadriplegia (361)	kwŏd-rĭ-PLĒ-jă	

TERM	PRONUNCIATION	MEANING
radiculitis (359)	ră-dĭk-ū-LĪ-tĭs	
radiculopathy (359)	ră-dĭk-ū-LŎP-ă-thē	
receptor (357)	rē-SĔP-tŏr	
sciatic nerve (357)	sī-ĂT-ĭk nĕrv	
sciatica (357)	sī-ĂT-ĭ-kă	
sensory nerve (357)	SĔN-sō-rē nĕrv	
spinal nerves (357)	SPĪ-năl nĕrvz	
stimulus (357)	STĬM-ū-lŭs	
stroma (357)	STRŌ-mă	
subdural hematoma (358)	sŭb-DŪ-răl hē-mă-TŌ-mă	
sulcus; sulci (357)	SŬL-kŭs; SŬL-sī	
sympathetic nerves (357)	sĭm-pă-THĔT-ĭk nĕrvz	
synapse (357)	SĬN-ăps	
syncopal (362)	SĬN-kō-păl	
syncope (362)	SĬN-kō-pē	
thalamic (359)	THĂL-ă-mĭk *or* thă-LĂM-ĭk	
thalamus (357)	THĂL-ă-mŭs	
trigeminal neuralgia (360)	trī-GĔM-ĭn-ăl nūr-ĂL-jă	
vagal (359)	VĀ-găl	
vagus nerve (357)	VĀ-gŭs nĕrv	
ventricles of the brain (357)	VĔN-trĭ-klz of the brĀn	

Pathology, Laboratory Tests, and Clinical Procedures

TERM	PRONUNCIATION	MEANING
absence seizure (371)	ĂB-sĕns SĒ-zhŭr	
Alzheimer disease (364)	ĂLZ-hī-mĕr dĭ-ZĒZ	
amyotrophic lateral sclerosis (364)	ā-mī-ō-TRŌ-fĭk LĂ-tĕr-ăl sklĕ-RŌ-sĭs	
aneurysm (371)	ĂN-ūr-ĭ-zĭm	
astrocytoma (371)	ăs-trō-sī-TŌ-mă	
aura (371)	āW-ră	

10

TERM	PRONUNCIATION	MEANING
Bell palsy (366)	bĕl PĂL-zē	
brain tumor (368)	BRĀN TŪ-mĕr	
cerebral angiography (371)	sĕ-RĒ-brăl ăn-jē-ŎG-ră-fē	
cerebral concussion (369)	sĕ-RĒ-brăl kŏn-KŬS-shŭn	
cerebral contusion (369)	sĕ-RĒ-brăl kŏn-TOO-shŭn	
cerebral hemorrhage (370)	sĕ-RĒ-brăl HĔM-ōr-ĭj	
cerebral palsy (366)	sĕ-RĒ-brăl (*or* SĔR-ĕ-brăl) PĂL-zē	
cerebrospinal fluid analysis (371)	sĕ-rē-brō-SPĪ-năl FLOO-ĭd ă-NĂL-ĭ-sĭs	
cerebrovascular accident (369)	sĕ-rē-brō-VĂS-kū-lăr ĂK-sĭ-dĕnt	
computed tomography (372)	kŏm-PŪ-tĕd tō-MŎG-ră-fē	
dementia (371)	dĕ-MĔN-shē-ă	
demyelination (371)	dē-mī-ĕ-lĭ-NĀ-shun	
dopamine (371)	DŌ-pă-mēn	
Doppler ultrasound studies (372)	DŎP-lĕr ŬL-tră-sound STŬ-dēz	
electroencephalography (373)	ĕ-lĕk-trō-ĕn-sĕf-ă-LŎG-ră-fē	
embolus (371)	ĔM-bō-lŭs	
epilepsy (365)	ĔP-ĭ-lĕp-sē	
gait (371)	GĀT	
glioblastoma (368)	glē-ō-blăs-TŌ-mă	
herpes zoster (368)	HĔR-pēz ZŎS-tĕr	
HIV encephalopathy (368)	HIV ĕn-sĕf-ă-LŎP-ă-thē	
Huntington disease (365)	HŬN-ting-tŏn dĭ-ZĒZ	
hydrocephalus (362)	hī-drō-SĔF-ă-lŭs	
ictal event (371)	ĬK-tăl ē-VĔNT	
lumbar puncture (373)	LŬM-băr PŬNK-shŭr	
magnetic resonance imaging (372)	măg-NĔT-ĭk RĔ-zō-nănce ĬM-ă-jĭng	
meningitis (368)	mĕn-ĭn-JĪ-tĭs	
meningocele (363)	mĕ-NĬN-gō-sĕl	

TERM	PRONUNCIATION	MEANING
migraine (370)	MĪ-grān	________________
multiple sclerosis (365)	MŬL-tĭ-pl sklĕ-RŌ-sĭs	________________
myasthenia gravis (366)	mī-ăs-THĒ-nē-ă GRĂ-vĭs	________________
occlusion (371)	ō-KLŪ-zhŭn	________________
palliative (371)	PĂ-lē-ă-tĭv	________________
palsy (366)	PAWL-zē	________________
Parkinson disease (367)	PĂR-kĭn-sŭn dĭ-ZĒZ	________________
positron emission tomography (372)	PŎS-ĭ-trŏn ē-MĬ-shŭn tō-MŎG-ră-fē	________________
shingles (368)	SHĬNG-ŭlz	________________
spina bifida (363)	SPĪ-nă BĬF-ĭ-dă	________________
stereotactic radiosurgery (373)	stĕ-rē-ō-TĂK-tĭk rā-dē-ō-SŬR-gĕr-ē	________________
thrombus (369)	THRŎM-bŭs	________________
tic (371)	TĬK	________________
tonic-clonic seizure (371)	TŎN-ĭk-KLŎ-nĭk SĒ-zhŭr	________________
Tourette syndrome (367)	tŭ-RĔT SĬN-drōm	________________
transient ischemic attack (369)	TRĂN-zē-ĕnt ĭs-KĒ-mĭk ă-TĂK	________________

REVIEW SHEET

Write the meanings of the word parts in the spaces provided. Check your answers with the information in the chapter or in the Glossary (Medical Word Parts—English) at the end of the book.

Combining Forms

COMBINING FORM	MEANING	COMBINING FORM	MEANING
alges/o	______	lex/o	______
angi/o	______	mening/o, meningi/o	______
caus/o	______	my/o	______
cephal/o	______	myel/o	______
cerebell/o	______	narc/o	______
cerebr/o	______	neur/o	______
comat/o	______	olig/o	______
crani/o	______	pont/o	______
cry/o	______	radicul/o	______
dur/o	______	spin/o	______
encephal/o	______	syncop/o	______
esthesi/o	______	tax/o	______
gli/o	______	thalam/o	______
hydr/o	______	thec/o	______
kines/o, kinesi/o	______	troph/o	______
lept/o	______	vag/o	______

Prefixes

PREFIX	MEANING	PREFIX	MEANING
a-, an-	______	micro-	______
dys-	______	para-	______
epi-	______	polio-	______
hemi-	______	poly-	______
hyper-	______	quadri-	______
hypo-	______	sub-	______
intra-	______		

10

Suffixes

SUFFIX	MEANING	SUFFIX	MEANING
-algesia	________________	-ose	________________
-algia	________________	-paresis	________________
-blast	________________	-pathy	________________
-cele	________________	-phagia	________________
-esthesia	________________	-phasia	________________
-gram	________________	-plegia	________________
-graphy	________________	-praxia	________________
-ine	________________	-ptosis	________________
-itis	________________	-sclerosis	________________
-kinesia, -kinesis	________________	-sthenia	________________
-kinetic	________________	-tomy	________________
-lepsy	________________	-trophy	________________
-oma	________________		

Match the neurologic pathology in Column I with associated terms and descriptions in Column II.

COLUMN I		COLUMN II
1. Alzheimer's	_____	A. destruction of myelin sheath on neurons in CNS
2. ALS	_____	B. stroke; disruption in normal blood supply to the brain
3. epilepsy	_____	C. shingles; viral infection affecting peripheral nerves
4. MS	_____	D. progressive dementia; memory failure; senile plaques and neurofibrillary tangles
5. Parkinson's	_____	E. brain tumor; malignant astrocytoma
6. herpes zoster	_____	F. degeneration of neurons in basal ganglia; tremors, bradykinesia, and shuffling gait
7. glioblastoma multiforme	_____	G. recurrent seizure disorder; tonic-clonic and absence types
8. CVA	_____	H. degeneration of motor neurons in spinal cord and brain stem; weakness and muscle atrophy

evolve *Please visit the Evolve website for additional exercises, games, and images related to this chapter.*

CHAPTER 11

Cardiovascular System

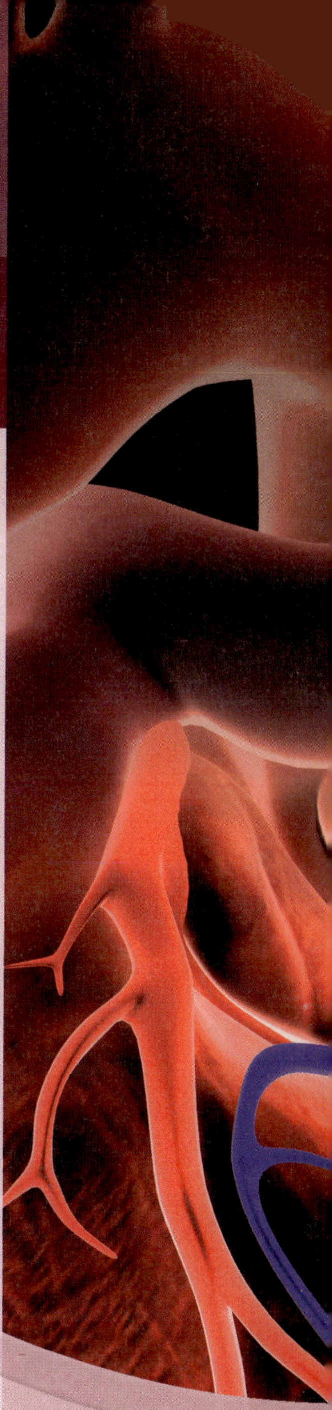

This chapter is divided into the following sections:

CHAPTER GOALS

- Name the parts of the heart and associated blood vessels and their functions in the circulation of blood.
- Trace the pathway of blood through the heart.
- Identify and describe major pathologic conditions affecting the heart and blood vessels.
- Define combining forms that relate to the cardiovascular system.
- Describe important laboratory tests and clinical procedures pertaining to the cardiovascular system, and recognize relevant abbreviations.
- Apply your new knowledge to understand medical terms in their proper context, such as in medical reports and records.

INTRODUCTION

Body cells are dependent on a constant supply of nutrients and oxygen. When the supplies are delivered and then chemically combined, they release the energy necessary to do the work of each cell. How does the body ensure that oxygen and food will be delivered to all of its cells? The cardiovascular system, consisting of the heart (a powerful muscular pump) and blood vessels (fuel line and transportation network), performs this important work. This chapter explores terminology related to the heart and blood vessels.

BLOOD VESSELS AND THE CIRCULATION OF BLOOD

BLOOD VESSELS

There are three types of blood vessels in the body: **arteries, veins,** and **capillaries.**

Arteries are large blood vessels that carry blood away from the heart. Their walls are lined with connective tissue, muscle tissue, and elastic fibers, with an innermost layer of epithelial cells called **endothelium.** Endothelial cells, found in all blood vessels, secrete factors that affect the size of blood vessels, reduce blood clotting, and promote the growth of blood vessels. Because arteries carry blood away from the heart, they must be strong enough to withstand the high pressure of the pumping action of the heart. Their elastic walls allow them to expand as the heartbeat forces blood into the arterial system throughout the body.

Smaller branches of arteries are **arterioles.** Arterioles are thinner than arteries and carry the blood to the tiniest of blood vessels, the capillaries.

Capillaries have walls that are only one endothelial cell in thickness. These delicate, microscopic vessels carry nutrient-rich, oxygenated blood from the arteries and arterioles to the body cells. Their thin walls allow passage of oxygen and nutrients out of the bloodstream and into cells. There, the nutrients are burned in the presence of oxygen (catabolism) to release energy. At the same time, waste products such as carbon dioxide and water pass out of cells and into the thin-walled capillaries. Waste-filled blood then flows back to the heart in small **venules,** which combine to form larger vessels called veins.

Veins have thinner walls compared with arteries. They conduct blood (that has given up most of its oxygen) toward the heart from the tissues. Veins have little elastic tissue and less connective tissue than that typical of arteries, and blood pressure in veins is extremely low compared with pressure in arteries. In order to keep blood moving back toward the heart, veins have **valves** that prevent the backflow of blood and keep the blood moving in one direction. Muscular action also helps the movement of blood in veins. Figure 11-1 illustrates the differences in blood vessels. Figure 11-2 reviews their characteristics and relationship to one another.

Blood Vessels and Blood

What color is blood? Blood is bright red in arteries (contains oxygen) and dark red (maroon) in veins (contains carbon dioxide). From the outside of the body, blood in veins ***appears*** blue because the color reflects off the skin.

How much blood is in the body? The average adult has about 5 quarts (4.7 liters) of blood in his or her body.

What is the length of all the blood vessels? The total length of all the blood vessels in the body is 60,000 miles!

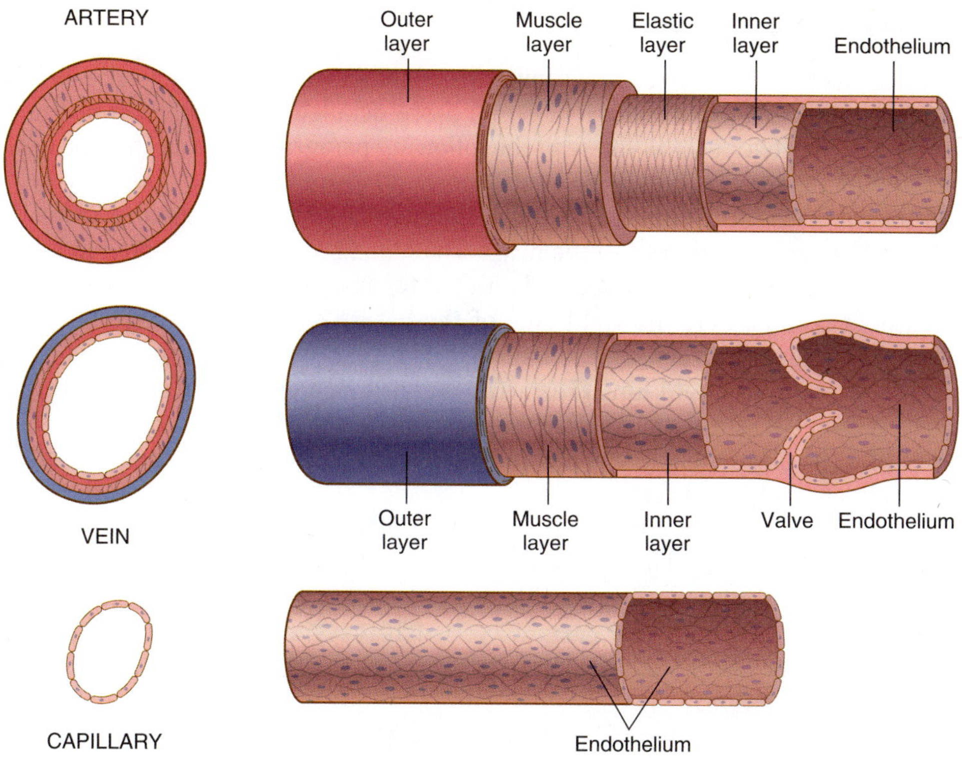

FIGURE 11-1 **Blood vessels.** Observe the differences in thickness of walls among an artery, a vein, and a capillary. All three vessels are lined with endothelium. Endothelial cells actively secrete substances that prevent clotting and regulate the tone of blood vessels. Examples of endothelial secretions are endothelium-derived relaxing factor (EDRF) and endothelin (a vasoconstrictor).

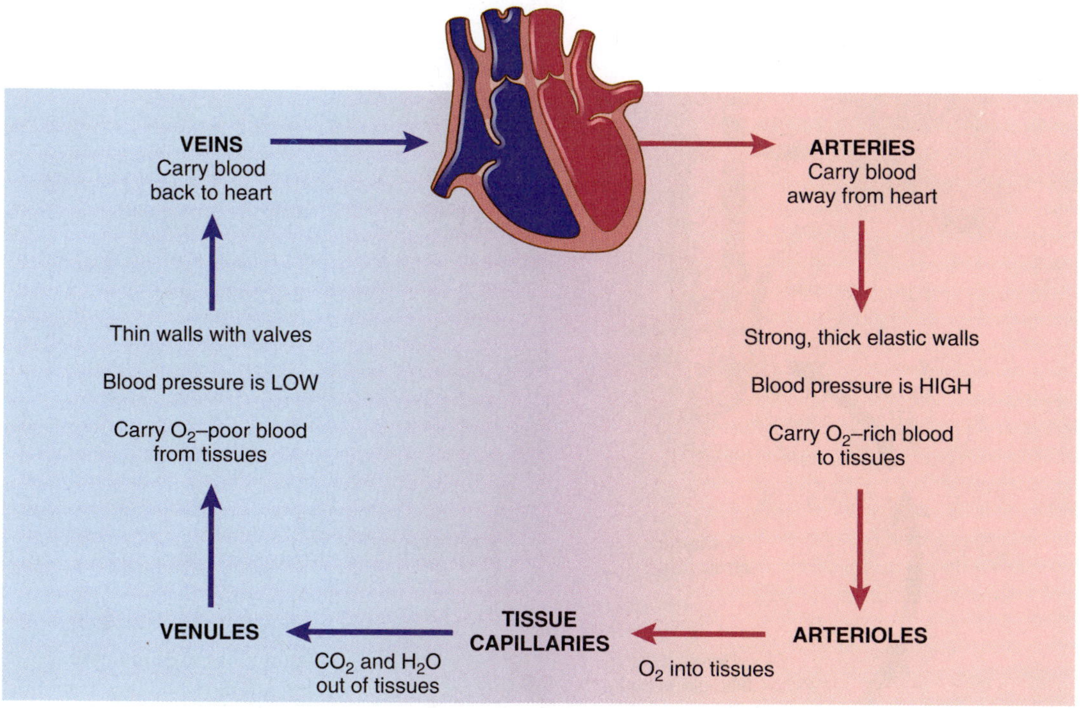

FIGURE 11-2 **Relationship and characteristics of blood vessels.**

CIRCULATION OF BLOOD

Arteries, arterioles, veins, venules, and capillaries, together with the heart, form a circulatory system for the flow of blood. Figure 11-3 is a more detailed representation of the entire circulatory system. Refer to it as you read the following paragraphs. (Note that the numbers in the following paragraphs correspond with those in Figure 11-3.)

Blood that is deficient in oxygen flows through two large veins, the **venae cavae** [1], on its way from the tissue capillaries to the heart. The blood became oxygen-poor at the tissue capillaries when oxygen left the blood and entered the body cells.

Oxygen-poor blood enters the **right side of the heart** [2] and travels through that side and into the **pulmonary artery** [3], a vessel that divides in two: one branch leading to the left lung, the other to the right lung. The arteries continue dividing and subdividing within the lungs, forming smaller and smaller vessels (arterioles) and finally reaching the **lung capillaries** [4]. The pulmonary artery is unusual in that it is the only artery in the body that carries blood deficient in oxygen.

While passing through the lung (pulmonary) capillaries, blood absorbs the oxygen that entered the body during inhalation. The newly oxygenated blood next returns immediately to the heart through **pulmonary veins** [5]. The pulmonary veins are unusual in that they are the only veins in the body that carry oxygen-rich **(oxygenated)** blood. The circulation of blood through the vessels from the heart to the lungs and then back to the heart again is the **pulmonary circulation.**

Oxygen-rich blood enters the **left side of the heart** [6] from the pulmonary veins. The muscles in the left side of the heart pump the blood out of the heart through the largest

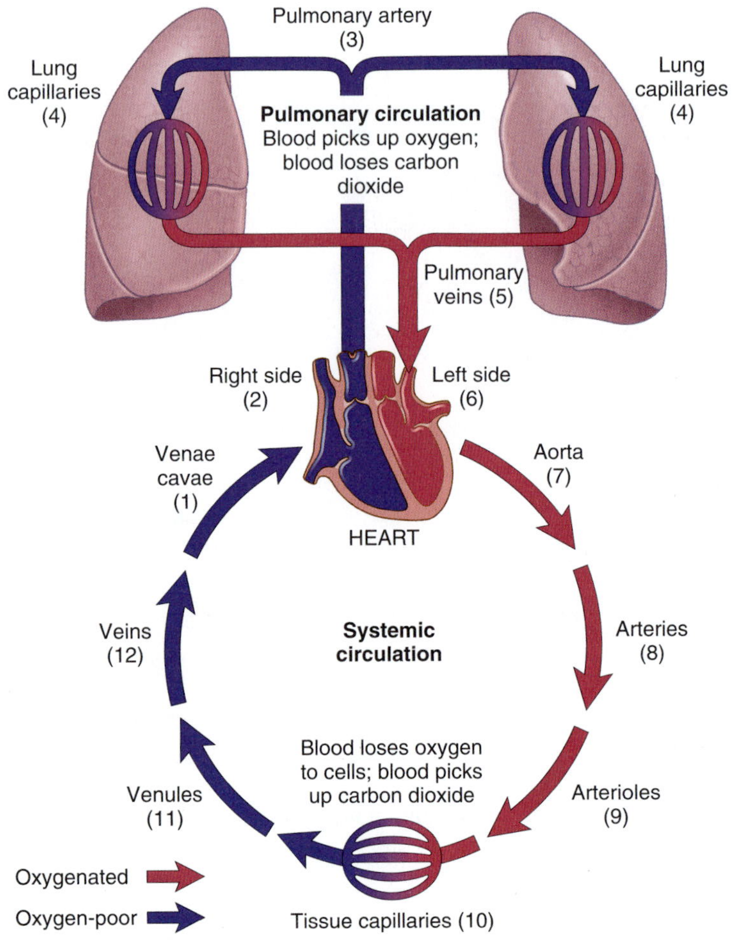

FIGURE 11-3 Schematic diagram of the **pulmonary circulation** (blood flow from the heart to lung capillaries and back to the heart) and **systemic circulation** (blood flow from the heart to tissue capillaries and back to the heart).

single artery in the body, the **aorta** [7]. The aorta moves up at first (ascending aorta) but then arches over dorsally and runs downward (descending aorta) just in front of the vertebral column. The aorta divides into numerous branches called **arteries** [8] that carry the oxygenated blood to all parts of the body. The names of some of these arterial branches will be familiar to you: brachial (brachi/o means arm), axillary, splenic, gastric, and renal arteries. The **carotid** arteries supply blood to the head and neck.

The relatively large arterial vessels branch further to form smaller **arterioles** [9]. The arterioles, still containing oxygenated blood, branch into smaller **tissue capillaries** [10], which are near the body cells. Oxygen leaves the blood and passes through the thin capillary walls to enter the body cells. There, food is broken down, in the presence of oxygen, and energy is released.

This chemical process also releases **carbon dioxide (CO_2)** as a waste product. Carbon dioxide passes out from the cell into the tissue capillaries at the same time that oxygen enters. Thus the blood returning to the heart from tissue capillaries through **venules** [11] and **veins** [12] is filled with carbon dioxide but is depleted of oxygen.

As this oxygen-poor blood enters the heart from the venae cavae, the circuit is complete. The pathway of blood from the heart to the tissue capillaries and back to the heart is the **systemic circulation.**

Figure 11-4 shows the aorta, selected arteries, and pulse points. The **pulse** is the beat of the heart as felt through the walls of arteries.

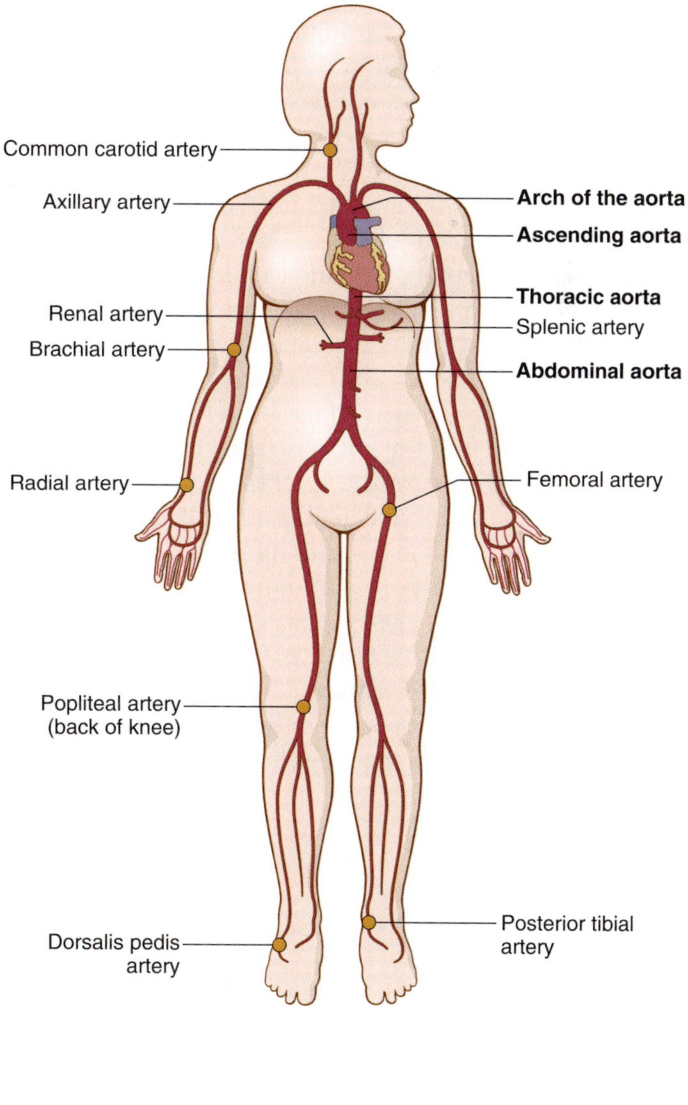

FIGURE 11-4 The aorta and arteries. *Solid gold dots* indicate pulse points in arteries. These are areas in which the **pulse** expansion and contraction of a superficial artery can be felt.

11

ANATOMY OF THE HEART

The human heart weighs less than a pound, is roughly the size of an adult fist, and lies in the thoracic cavity, just behind the breastbone in the mediastinum (between the lungs).

The heart is a pump consisting of four chambers: two upper chambers called **atria** (*singular:* **atrium**) and two lower chambers called **ventricles.** It is actually a double pump, bound into one organ and synchronized very carefully. Blood passes through each pump in a definite pattern. Pump station number one, on the right side of the heart, sends oxygen-deficient blood to the lungs, where the blood picks up oxygen and releases its carbon dioxide. The newly oxygenated blood returns to the left side of the heart to pump station number two and does not mix with the oxygen-poor blood in pump station number one. Pump station number two then forces the oxygenated blood out to all parts of the body. At the body tissues, the blood loses its oxygen, and on returning to the heart, to pump station number one, blood poor in oxygen (rich in carbon dioxide) is sent out to the lungs to begin the cycle anew.

Label Figure 11-5 as you learn the names of the parts of the heart and the vessels that carry blood to and from it.

Oxygen-poor blood enters the heart through the two largest veins in the body, the **venae cavae.** The **superior vena cava** [1] drains blood from the upper portion of the body, and the **inferior vena cava** [2] carries blood from the lower part of the body.

The venae cavae bring oxygen-poor blood that has passed through all of the body to the **right atrium** [3], the thin-walled upper right chamber of the heart. The right atrium contracts to force blood through the **tricuspid valve** [4] (cusps are the flaps of the valves) into the **right ventricle** [5], the lower right chamber of the heart. The cusps of the tricuspid valve form a one-way passage designed to keep the blood flowing in only one direction. As the right ventricle contracts to pump oxygen-poor blood through the **pulmonary valve** [6] into the **pulmonary artery** [7], the tricuspid valve stays shut, thus preventing blood from pushing back into the right atrium. The pulmonary artery then branches to carry oxygen-deficient blood to each lung.

The blood that enters the lung capillaries from the pulmonary artery soon loses its large quantity of carbon dioxide into the lung tissue, and the carbon dioxide is expelled. At the same time, oxygen enters the capillaries of the lungs and is brought back to the heart via the **pulmonary veins** [8]. The newly oxygenated blood enters the **left atrium** [9] of the heart from the pulmonary veins. The walls of the left atrium contract to force blood through the **mitral valve** [10] into the **left ventricle** [11].

The left ventricle has the thickest walls of all four heart chambers (three times the thickness of the right ventricular wall). It must pump blood with great force so that the blood travels through arteries to all parts of the body. The left ventricle propels the blood through the **aortic valve** [12] into the **aorta** [13], which branches to carry blood all over the body. The aortic valve closes to prevent return of aortic blood to the left ventricle.

In Figure 11-6, notice that the four chambers of the heart are separated by partitions called **septa** (*singular:* **septum**). (Label Figure 11-6 as you read these paragraphs.) The **interatrial septum** [1] separates the two upper chambers (atria), and the **interventricular septum** [2], a muscular wall, lies between the two lower chambers (ventricles).

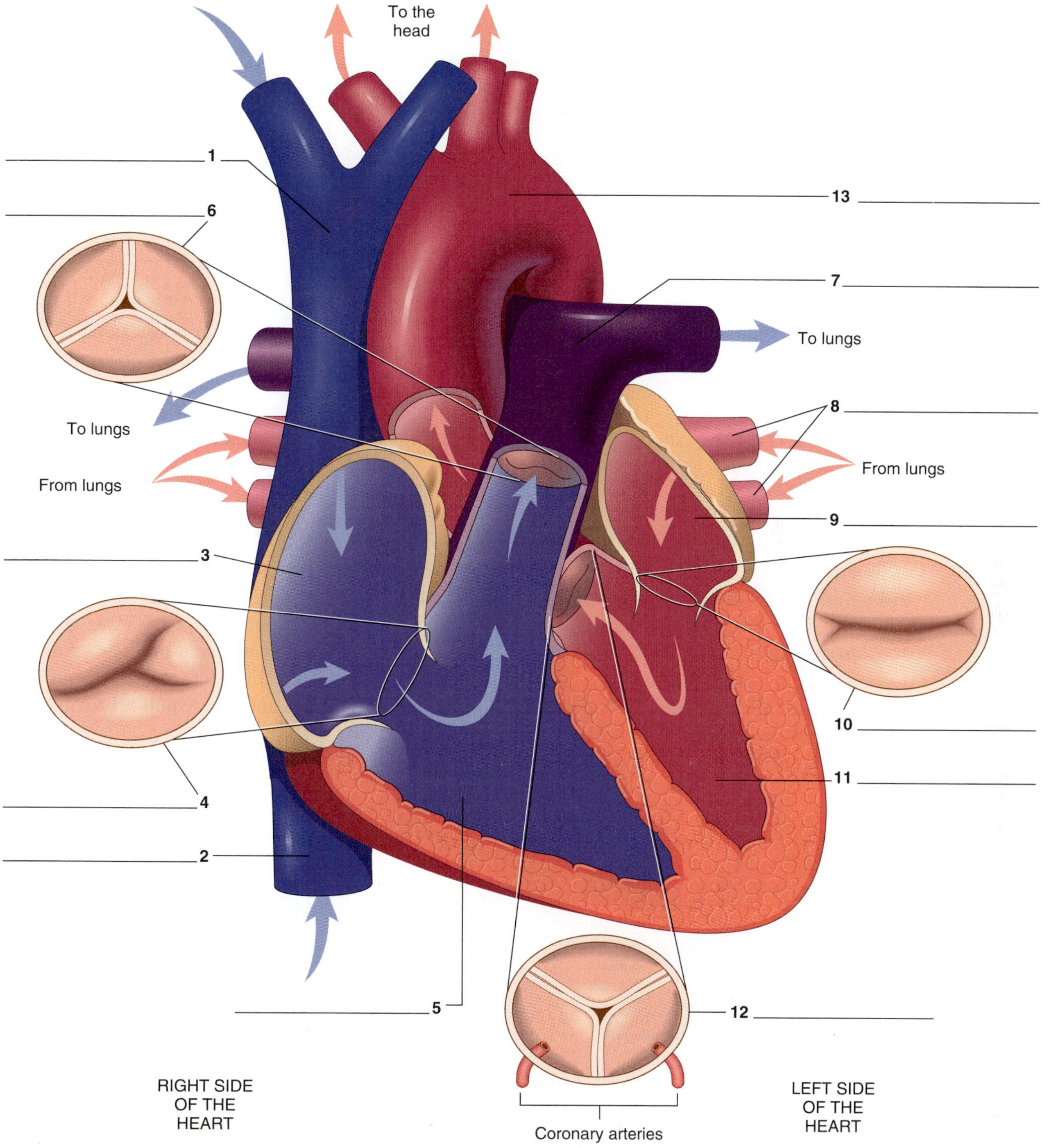

FIGURE 11-5 **Structure of the heart.** *Blue arrows* indicate oxygen-poor blood flow. *Red arrows* show oxygenated blood flow.

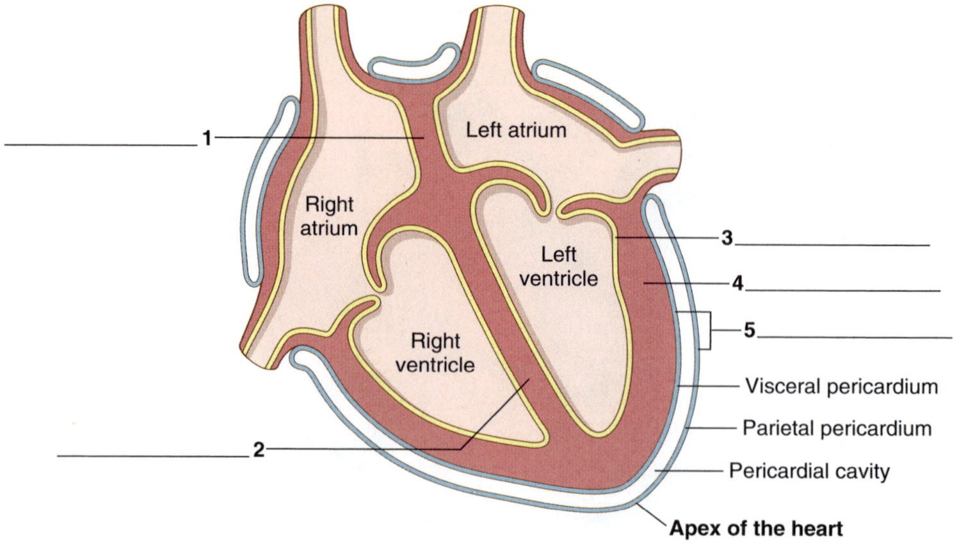

FIGURE 11-6 The walls of the heart and pericardium. Note that the **apex of the heart** is the conical (shaped like a cone) lower tip of the heart.

Figure 11-6 shows the three layers of the heart. The **endocardium** [3], a smooth layer of endothelial cells, lines the interior of the heart and heart valves. The **myocardium** [4], the middle, muscular layer of the heart wall, is its thickest layer. The **pericardium** [5], a fibrous and membranous sac, surrounds the heart. It is composed of two layers, the **visceral pericardium,** adhering to the heart, and the **parietal** (parietal means wall) **pericardium,** lining the outer fibrous coat. The **pericardial cavity** (between the visceral and the parietal pericardial layers) normally contains 10 to 15 mL of pericardial fluid, which lubricates the membranes as the heart beats.

Figure 11-7 reviews the pathway of blood through the heart.

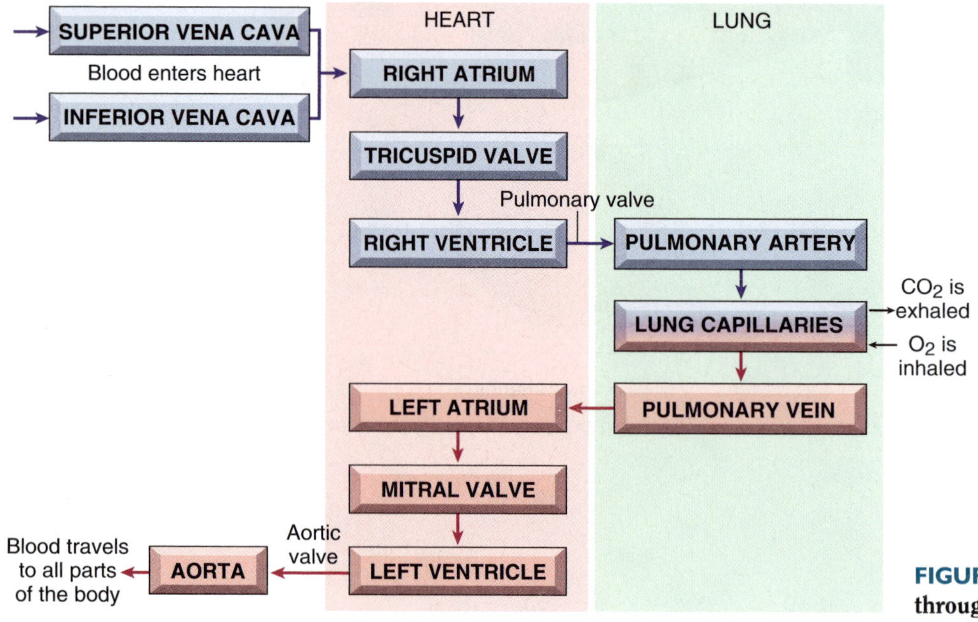

FIGURE 11-7 Pathway of blood through the heart.

PHYSIOLOGY OF THE HEART

HEARTBEAT AND HEART SOUNDS

There are two phases of the heartbeat: **diastole** (relaxation) and **systole** (contraction). Diastole occurs when the ventricle walls relax and blood flows into the heart from the venae cavae and the pulmonary veins. The tricuspid and mitral valves open in diastole, as blood passes from the right and left atria into the ventricles. The pulmonary and aortic valves close during diastole (Figure 11-8).

Systole occurs next, as the walls of the right and left ventricles contract to pump blood into the pulmonary artery and the aorta. Both the tricuspid and the mitral valves are closed during systole, thus preventing the flow of blood back into the atria (see Figure 11-8).

This diastole-systole cardiac cycle occurs between 70 and 80 times per minute (100,000 times a day). The heart pumps about 3 ounces of blood with each contraction. This means that about 5 quarts of blood are pumped by the heart in 1 minute (75 gallons an hour and about 2000 gallons a day).

Closure of the heart valves is associated with audible sounds, such as "lubb-dubb," which can be heard on listening to a normal heart with a stethoscope. The "lubb" is associated with closure of the tricuspid and mitral valves at the beginning of systole, and the "dubb" with the closure of the aortic and pulmonary valves at the end of systole. The "lubb" sound is called the first heart sound (S1) and the "dubb" is the second heart sound (S2) because the normal cycle of the heartbeat starts with the beginning of systole. Sometimes the flow of blood through the valves can produce an abnormal swishing sound known as a **murmur.**

CONDUCTION SYSTEM OF THE HEART

What keeps the heart at its perfect rhythm? Although the heart has nerves that affect its rate, they are not primarily responsible for its beat. The heart starts beating in the embryo before it is supplied with nerves, and continues to beat in experimental animals even when the nerve supply is cut.

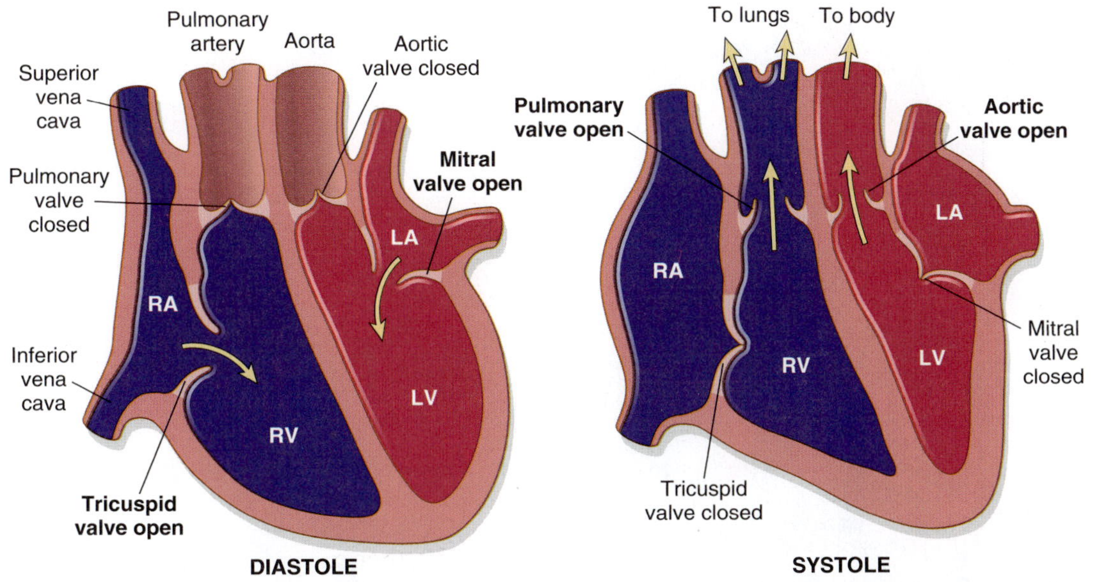

FIGURE 11-8 Phases of the heartbeat: diastole and systole. During diastole, the tricuspid and mitral valves are open as blood enters the ventricles. During systole, the pulmonary and aortic valves are open as blood is pumped to the pulmonary artery and aorta. LA, left atrium; LV, left ventricle; RA, right atrium; RV, right ventricle.

Label Figure 11-9 as you read the following. Primary responsibility for initiating the heartbeat rests with a small region of specialized muscle tissue in the posterior portion of the right atrium, where an electrical impulse originates. This is the **sinoatrial node (SA node)** or **pacemaker** [1] of the heart. The current of electricity generated by the pacemaker causes the walls of the atria to contract and force blood into the ventricles.

Almost like ripples in a pond of water when a stone is thrown, the wave of electricity passes from the pacemaker to another region of the myocardium. This region is within the interatrial septum and is the **atrioventricular node (AV node)** [2]. The AV node immediately sends the excitation wave to a bundle of specialized muscle fibers called the **atrioventricular bundle,** or **bundle of His** [3]. Within the interventricular septum, the bundle of His divides into the **left bundle branch** [4] and the **right bundle branch** [5], which form the conduction myofibers that extend through the ventricle walls and contract on stimulation. Thus systole occurs and blood is pumped away from the heart. A short rest period follows, and then the pacemaker begins the wave of excitation across the heart again.

The record used to detect these electrical changes in heart muscle as the heart beats is an **electrocardiogram** (**ECG** or **EKG**). The normal ECG tracing shows five waves, or **deflections,** that represent the electrical changes as a wave of excitation spreads through the heart. The deflections are called **P, QRS,** and **T** waves. Figure 11-10 illustrates P, QRS, and T waves on a normal ECG tracing.

Heart rhythm (originating in the SA node and traveling through the heart) is called **normal sinus rhythm (NSR).** Sympathetic nerves speed up the heart rate during conditions of emotional stress or vigorous exercise. Parasympathetic nerves slow the heart rate when there is no need for extra pumping.

BLOOD PRESSURE

Blood pressure is the force that the blood exerts on the arterial walls. This pressure is measured with a **sphygmomanometer** (Figure 11-11).

The sphygmomanometer consists of a rubber bag inside a cloth cuff that is wrapped around the upper arm, just above the elbow. The rubber bag is inflated with air using a hand

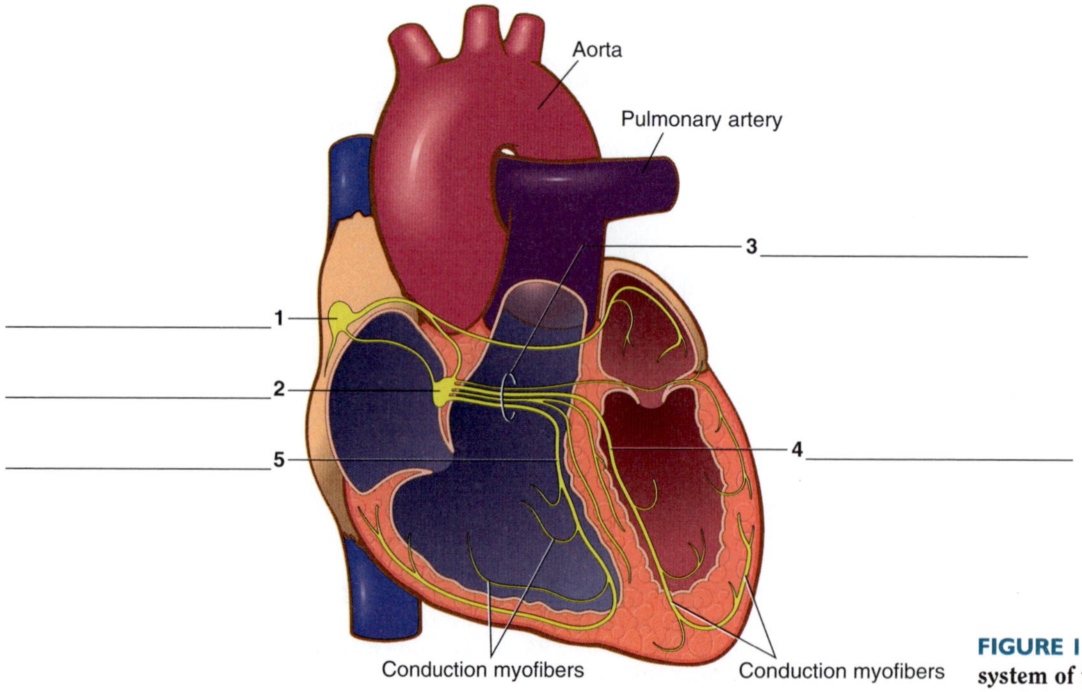

FIGURE 11-9 Conduction system of the heart.

11

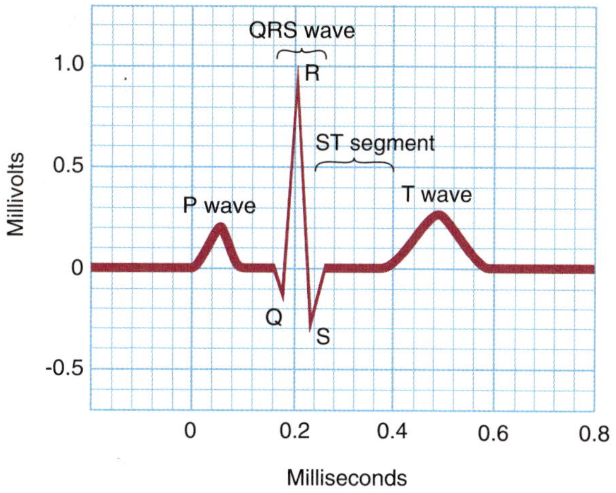

FIGURE 11-10 Electrocardiogram. P wave = spread of excitation wave over the atria just before contraction; **QRS wave** = spread of excitation wave over the ventricles as the ventricles contract; **T wave** = electrical recovery and relaxation of ventricles. A heart attack or myocardial infarction (MI) can be recognized by an elevation in the **ST segment** of the electrocardiographic tracing. Thus, one type of MI is an ST elevation MI **(STEMI)**.

bulb pump. As the bag is pumped up, the pressure within it increases and is measured on a recording device attached to the cuff.

The brachial artery in the upper arm is compressed by the air pressure in the bag. When there is sufficient air pressure in the bag to stop the flow of blood, the pulse in the lower arm (where the observer is listening with a stethoscope) drops.

Air is then allowed to escape from the bag and the pressure is lowered slowly, allowing the blood to begin to make its way through the gradually opening artery. At the point when the person listening with the stethoscope first hears the sounds of the pulse beats, the reading on the device attached to the cuff shows the higher, systolic blood pressure (pressure in the artery when the left ventricle is contracting to force the blood into the aorta and other arteries).

As air continues to escape, the sounds become progressively louder. Finally, when a change in sound from loud to soft occurs, the observer makes note of the pressure on the recording device. This is the diastolic blood pressure (pressure in the artery when the ventricles relax and the heart fills, receiving blood from the venae cavae and pulmonary veins).

Blood pressure is expressed as a fraction—for example, 120/80 mm Hg, in which the upper number (120) is the systolic pressure and the lower number (80) is the diastolic pressure. Hypertension, or high blood pressure, is defined as blood pressure greater than 140/90 mmHg. Both systolic and diastolic hypertension are associated with increased risk of heart attack and stroke.

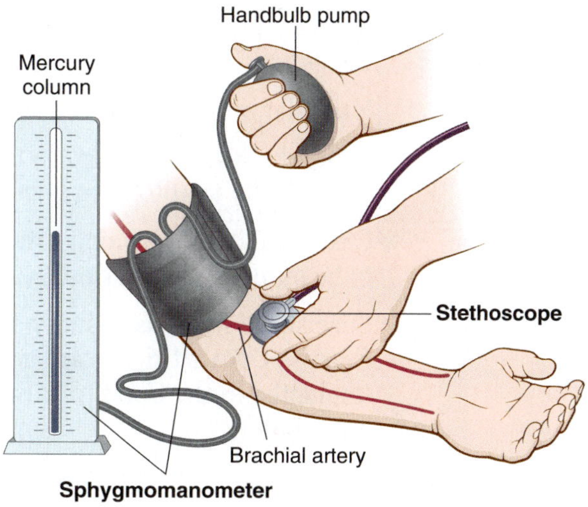

FIGURE 11-11 Measurement of blood pressure with a sphygmomanometer and stethoscope.

VOCABULARY

This list reviews new terms introduced in the text. Short definitions reinforce your understanding of the terms. See page 449 of this chapter for pronunciation of terms.

aorta	Largest artery in the body.
apex of the heart	Lower tip of the heart.
arteriole	Small artery.
artery	Largest type of blood vessel; carries blood away from the heart to all parts of the body. Notice that artery and away begin with an "a."
atrioventricular bundle (bundle of His)	Specialized muscle fibers connecting the atria with the ventricles and transmitting electrical impulses between them. His is pronounced "hiss."
atrioventricular node (AV node)	Specialized tissue in the wall between the atria. Electrical impulses pass from the pacemaker (SA node) through the AV node and the atrioventricular bundle or bundle of His toward the ventricles.
atrium (*plural*: **atria**)	One of two upper chambers of the heart.
capillary	Smallest blood vessel. Materials pass to and from the bloodstream through the thin capillary walls.
carbon dioxide (CO_2)	Gas (waste) released by body cells, transported via veins to the heart, and then to the lungs for exhalation.
coronary arteries	Blood vessels that branch from the aorta and carry oxygen-rich blood to the heart muscle.
deoxygenated blood	Blood that is oxygen-poor.
diastole	Relaxation phase of the heartbeat. (From Greek *diastole*, dilation.)
electrocardiogram	Record of the electricity flowing through the heart. The electricity is represented by waves or deflections called P, QRS, or T.
endocardium	Inner lining of the heart.
endothelium	Innermost lining of blood vessels.
mitral valve	Valve between the left atrium and the left ventricle; bicuspid valve.
murmur	Abnormal swishing sound caused by improper closure of the heart valves.
myocardium	Muscular, middle layer of the heart.
normal sinus rhythm	Heart rhythm originating in the sinoatrial node with a rate in patients at rest of 60 to 100 beats per minute.
oxygen	Gas that enters the blood through the lungs and travels to the heart to be pumped via arteries to all body cells.
pacemaker (sinoatrial node)	Specialized nervous tissue in the right atrium that begins the heartbeat. An artificial cardiac pacemaker is an electronic apparatus implanted in the chest to stimulate heart muscle that is weak and not functioning.
pericardium	Double-layered membrane surrounding the heart.

pulmonary artery	Artery carrying oxygen-poor blood from the heart to the lungs.
pulmonary circulation	Flow of blood from the heart to the lungs and back to the heart.
pulmonary valve	Valve positioned between the right ventricle and the pulmonary artery.
pulmonary vein	One of two pairs of vessels carrying oxygenated blood from the lungs to the left atrium of the heart.
pulse	Beat of the heart as felt through the walls of the arteries.
septum (*plural*: **septa**)	Partition or wall dividing a cavity; such as between the right and left atria (interatrial septum) and right and left ventricles (interventricular septum).
sinoatrial node (SA node)	Pacemaker of the heart.
sphygmomanometer	Instrument to measure blood pressure.
systemic circulation	Flow of blood from body tissue to the heart and then from the heart back to body tissues.
systole	Contraction phase of the heartbeat. (From Greek *systole,* contraction.)
tricuspid valve	Located between the right atrium and the right ventricle; it has three (tri-) leaflets, or cusps.
valve	Structure in veins or in the heart that temporarily closes an opening so that blood flows in only one direction.
vein	Thin-walled vessel that carries blood from body tissues and lungs back to the heart. Veins contain valves to prevent backflow of blood.
vena cava (*plural*: **venae cavae**)	Largest vein in the body. The superior and inferior venae cavae return blood to the right atrium of the heart.
ventricle	One of two lower chambers of the heart.
venule	Small vein.

TERMINOLOGY

Write the meaning of the medical term in the space provided.

COMBINING FORM	MEANING	TERMINOLOGY	MEANING
angi/o	vessel	angiogram	______________
		angioplasty	______________
aort/o	aorta	aortic stenosis	______________
arter/o, arteri/o	artery	arteriosclerosis	______________
		arterial anastomosis *From the Greek anastomoien, providing a mouth.*	______________
		arteriography	______________
		endarterectomy *See page 431.*	______________

COMBINING FORM	MEANING	TERMINOLOGY	MEANING
ather/o	yellowish plaque, fatty substance (Greek *athere* means porridge)	atheroma *The suffix -oma means mass or collection. Atheromas are collections of plaque that protrude into the **lumen** (opening) of an artery, weakening the muscle lining.*	______
		atherosclerosis *The major form of arteriosclerosis in which deposits of yellow plaque (atheromas) containing cholesterol and lipids are found within the lining of the artery (Figure 11-12).*	______
		atherectomy	______
atri/o	atrium, upper heart chamber	atrial	______
		atrioventricular	______
brachi/o	arm	brachial artery	______
cardi/o	heart	cardiomegaly	______
		cardiomyopathy *One type of cardiomyopathy is **hypertrophic cardiomyopathy**—abnormal thickening of heart muscle, usually in the left ventricle. The ventricle has to work harder to pump blood. The condition may be inherited or develop over time because of high blood pressure or aging. Often the cause is unknown (idiopathic).*	______
		bradycardia *Slower than 60 beats per minute. Normal pulse is about 60 to 80 beats per minute. Brady- means slow.*	______
		tachycardia *Faster than 100 beats per minute. Supraventricular tachycardia (SVT) involves rapid beats coming from the atria (above the ventricles) and causing palpitation (abnormal sensations in the chest). Tachy- means fast.*	______
		cardiogenic shock *Results from failure of the heart in its pumping action. **Shock** is circulatory failure associated with inadequate delivery of oxygen and nutrients to body tissues.*	______
cholesterol/o	cholesterol (a lipid substance)	hypercholesterolemia ***Statins** are drugs that work by blocking a key enzyme in the production of cholesterol by the liver.*	______
coron/o	heart	coronary arteries *These arteries come down over the top of the heart like a crown (corona); see Figure 11-22A, page 426.*	______

ather/o, arteri/o, arthr/o

These three combining forms are easily confused.

ather/o = yellowish plaque
arteri/o = artery
arthr/o = joint

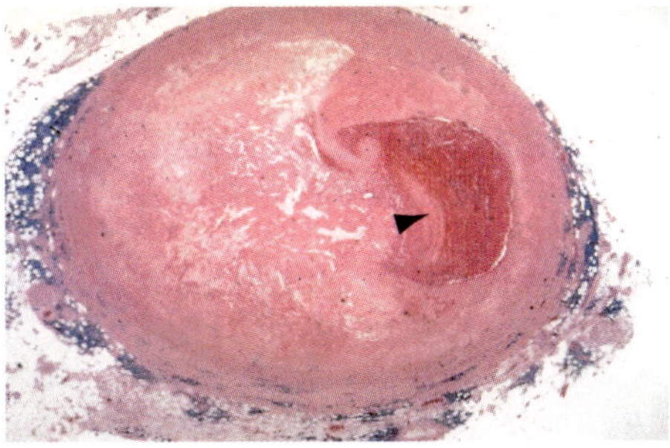

FIGURE 11-12 **Atherosclerosis.** *Arrow* points to accumulated plaque in lumen of an artery. *(Courtesy Sid Murphree, MD, Department of Pathology, University of Texas Southwestern Medical School, Dallas, Texas.)*

COMBINING FORM	MEANING	TERMINOLOGY	MEANING
cyan/o	blue	cyanosis ____ *This bluish discoloration of the skin indicates diminished oxygen content of the blood.*	
myx/o	mucus	myxoma ____ *A benign tumor derived from connective tissue, with cells embedded in soft mucoid stromal tissue. These rare tumors occur most frequently in the left atrium.*	
ox/o	oxygen	hypoxia ____ *Inadequate oxygen in tissues.* ***Anoxia*** *is an extreme form of hypoxia.*	
pericardi/o	pericardium	pericardiocentesis ____	
phleb/o	vein	phlebotomy ____ *A phlebotomist is trained in opening veins for phlebotomy.*	
		thrombophlebitis ____ *Often shortened to phlebitis. If the affected vein is deep within a muscle, the condition is* ***deep vein thrombosis (DVT).***	
rrhythm/o	rhythm	arrhythmia ____ ***Dysrhythmia*** *is also used to describe an abnormal heart rhythm. Notice that one "r" is dropped.*	
sphygm/o	pulse	sphygmomanometer ____ *A sphygmomanometer measures pressure.*	
steth/o	chest	stethoscope ____ *A misnomer because the examination is by ear, not by eye.* ***Auscultation*** *means listening to sounds within the body, typically using a stethoscope.*	
thromb/o	clot	thrombolysis ____	

COMBINING FORM	MEANING	TERMINOLOGY	MEANING
valvul/o, valv/o	valve	valvuloplasty *A balloon-tipped catheter dilates a cardiac valve.*	______________________
		mitral valvulitis *Commonly associated with rheumatic fever, an inflammatory disease caused by inadequate treatment of a streptococcal infection. An autoimmune reaction occurs, leading to inflammation and damage to heart valves. (See Figure 11-19, page 420.)*	______________________
		valvotomy	______________________
vas/o	vessel	vasoconstriction *Constriction means to tighten or narrow.*	______________________
		vasodilation	______________________
vascul/o	vessel	vascular	______________________
ven/o, ven/i	vein	venous *A venous cutdown is a small surgical incision to permit access to a collapsed vein. An intravenous infusion is delivery of fluids into a vein.*	______________________
		venipuncture *This procedure is performed for phlebotomy or to start an intravenous infusion.*	______________________
ventricul/o	ventricle, lower heart chamber	interventricular septum	______________________

PATHOLOGY: THE HEART AND BLOOD VESSELS

HEART

arrhythmias

Abnormal heart rhythms (dysrhythmias).

Arrhythmias are problems with the conduction or electrical system of the heart. More than 4 million Americans have recurrent cardiac arrhythmias.

Examples of cardiac arrhythmias are:

1. **bradycardia and heart block (atrioventricular block)**

Failure of proper conduction of impulses from the SA node through the AV node to the atrioventricular bundle (bundle of His).

Damage to the SA node may cause its impulses to be too weak to activate the AV node and impulses fail to reach the ventricles. The heart beats slowly and bradycardia results. If the failure occurs only occasionally, the heart misses a beat in a rhythm at regular intervals (partial heart block). If no impulses reach the AV node from the SA node, the ventricles contract slower than the atria and are not coordinated. This is complete heart block.

Right and left bundle branch block (RBBB and LBBB) are common types of heart block. They involve delay or failure of impulses traveling through the right and left bundle branches to the ventricles.

Implantation of an artificial **cardiac pacemaker** overcomes arrhythmias and keeps the heart beating at the proper rate. The pacemaker power source is a generator that contains a computer and lithium battery. It is implanted under the skin just below the collarbone, with leads (wires) to both chambers, usually on the right side of the heart. A newer type of pacemaker, called a **biventricular pacemaker**, treats delays and abnormalities in ventricular contractions (dysynergy) and also can relieve symptoms and improve quality of life in patients with congestive heart failure. It reduces exacerbations of heart failure that require hospital admission (Figure 11-13C).

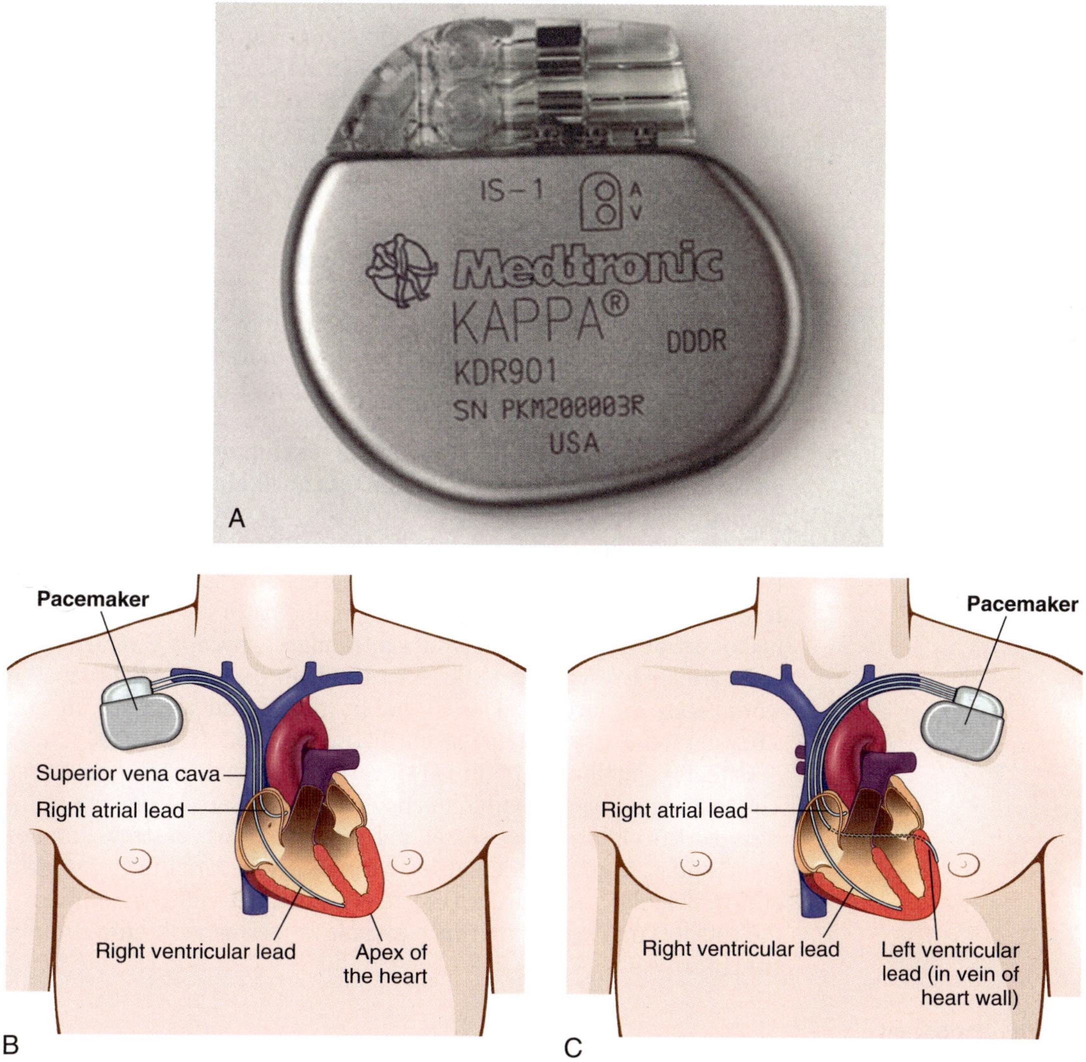

FIGURE 11-13 **A, A dual-chamber, rate-responsive pacemaker** *(actual size shown)* is designed to detect body movement and automatically increase or decrease paced heart rates based on levels of physical activity. **B, Cardiac pacemaker** with leads in the right atrium and right ventricle enable it to sense and pace in both heart chambers. **C, Biventricular pacemaker** with leads in the right atrium and the right and left ventricles to synchronize ventricular contractions.

How Does a Pacemaker Work?

The pacemaker leads (wires) detect the heart's own electrical activity and transmit that information to the generator (computer). The computer analyzes the heart's signals and decides when and where to pace. If the rate is slow, the generator emits a signal to stimulate contraction and increase the rate. Pacemakers with multiple leads can pace the atrium and ventricle in proper sequence. Rate-responsive pacemakers have sensors that detect body movement and breathing to then determine the best heart rate.

2. flutter

Rapid but regular contractions, usually of the atria.

Heart rhythm may reach up to 300 beats per minute. Atrial flutter is often symptomatic of heart disease and frequently requires treatment such as medication, electrical cardioversion, or catheter ablation (see below under fibrillation).

3. fibrillation

Very rapid, random, inefficient, and irregular contractions of the heart (350 beats or more per minute).

Atrial fibrillation (AF) is the most common type of cardiac arrhythmia, affecting 5% to 10% of 70- to 80-year-old people and greater than 15% of individuals in their 80s. Electrical impulses move randomly throughout the atria, causing the atria to quiver instead of contracting in a coordinated rhythm. Common symptoms are **palpitations** (uncomfortable sensations in the chest from missed heartbeats), fatigue, and shortness of breath. Patients with **paroxysmal AF** (irregular heartbeats occur periodically and episodically) and **permanent** or **persistent AF** (irregular heartbeats continue indefinitely) are at risk for stroke. This is because ineffective atrial contractions can lead to the formation of blood clots in the left atrial appendage (the area where clots form) that may travel to the brain. Also, sometimes AF can make the heart beat very fast for long periods of time, leading to weakening of the heart muscle.

In **ventricular fibrillation (VF),** electrical impulses move randomly throughout the ventricles. This life-threatening situation may result in sudden cardiac death or **cardiac arrest** (sudden stoppage of heart movement) unless help is provided immediately. If treatment is immediate, VF can be interrupted with **defibrillation** (application of an electrical shock). Defibrillation stops electrical activity in the heart for a brief moment so that normal rhythm takes over. Medications such as **digoxin, beta-blockers,** and **calcium channel blockers** convert fibrillation to normal sinus rhythm.

An **implantable cardioverter-defibrillator (ICD)** is a small electrical device that is implanted inside the chest (near the collarbone) to sense arrhythmias and terminate them with an electric shock. Candidates for ICDs are people who have had or are at high risk for having ventricular tachycardia, ventricular fibrillation, and cardiac arrest. **Automatic external defibrillators (AEDs)** may be found in workplaces, airports, and other public places and are used in an emergency situation to reverse ventricular fibrillation.

Catheter ablation is a minimally invasive treatment to treat cardiac arrhythmias. The technique, using radiofrequency energy delivered from the tip of a catheter inserted through a blood vessel and into the heart, destroys tissue that causes arrhythmias. Supraventricular tachycardia (SVT), atrial flutter, atrial fibrillation, and ventricular tachycardia (VT) may be treated with ablation when clinically indicated. This procedure may provide a permanent cure in many clinical situations.

Palpitation/Palpation

Don't confuse *palpitation* with *palpation*, which means to touch, feel, or examine with the hands and fingers.

congenital heart disease **Abnormalities in the heart at birth.**

The following conditions are congenital anomalies resulting from some failure in the development of the fetal heart.

1. **coarctation of the aorta (CoA)** **Narrowing (coarctation) of the aorta.**

   Figure 11-14A shows coarctation of the aorta. Surgical treatment consists of removal of the constricted region and end-to-end anastomosis of the aortic segments.

2. **patent ductus arteriosus (PDA)** **Passageway (ductus arteriosus) between the aorta and the pulmonary artery remains open (patent) after birth.**

   The ductus arteriosus normally closes after birth, but in this congenital condition it remains open (see Figure 11-14B), resulting in the flow of oxygenated blood from the aorta into the pulmonary artery. PDA occurs in premature infants, causing cyanosis, fatigue, and rapid breathing. Although the defect often closes on its own within months after birth, treatment may be necessary if patency continues. Treatments include use of a drug (indomethacin) to promote closure; surgery via catheterization (with coil embolization to "plug" the ductus); and ligation (tying off) via a small incision between the ribs.

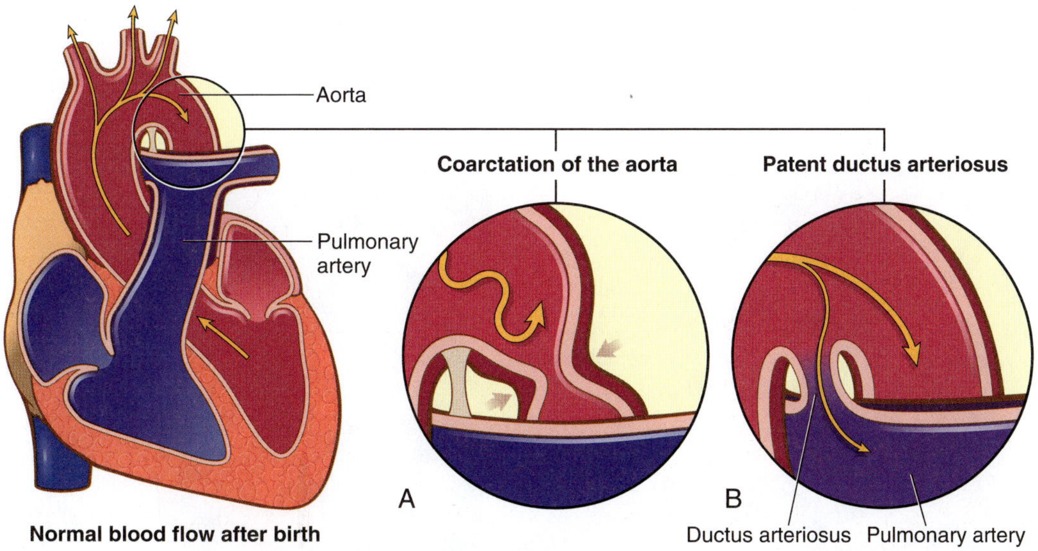

FIGURE 11-14 **A, Coarctation of the aorta.** Localized narrowing of the aorta reduces the supply of blood to the lower part of the body. **B, Patent ductus arteriosus.** The ductus arteriosus fails to close after birth, and blood from the aorta flows through it into the pulmonary artery.

3. septal defects

Small holes in the wall between the atria (atrial septal defects) or the ventricles (ventricular septal defects). Figure 11-15A shows a ventricular septal defect.

Although many septal defects close spontaneously, others require open heart surgery to close the hole between heart chambers. Septal defects are closed while maintaining a general circulation by means of a **heart-lung machine.** This machine, connected to the patient's circulatory system, relieves the heart and lungs of pumping and oxygenation functions during heart surgery.

Alternatively, septal defects may be repaired with a less invasive catheter technique using a device (Amplatzer device) in the defect to close it.

4. tetralogy of Fallot (fă-LŌ)

Congenital malformation involving four (tetra-) distinct heart defects.

The condition, named for Etienne Fallot, the French physician who described it in 1888, is illustrated in Figure 11-15B. The four defects are:

- **Pulmonary artery stenosis.** Pulmonary artery is narrow or obstructed.
- **Ventricular septal defect.** Large hole between two ventricles lets venous blood pass from the right to the left ventricle and out to the aorta without oxygenation.
- **Shift of the aorta to the right.** Aorta overrides the interventricular septum. Oxygen-poor blood passes from the right ventricle to the aorta.
- **Hypertrophy of the right ventricle.** Myocardium works harder to pump blood through a narrowed pulmonary artery.

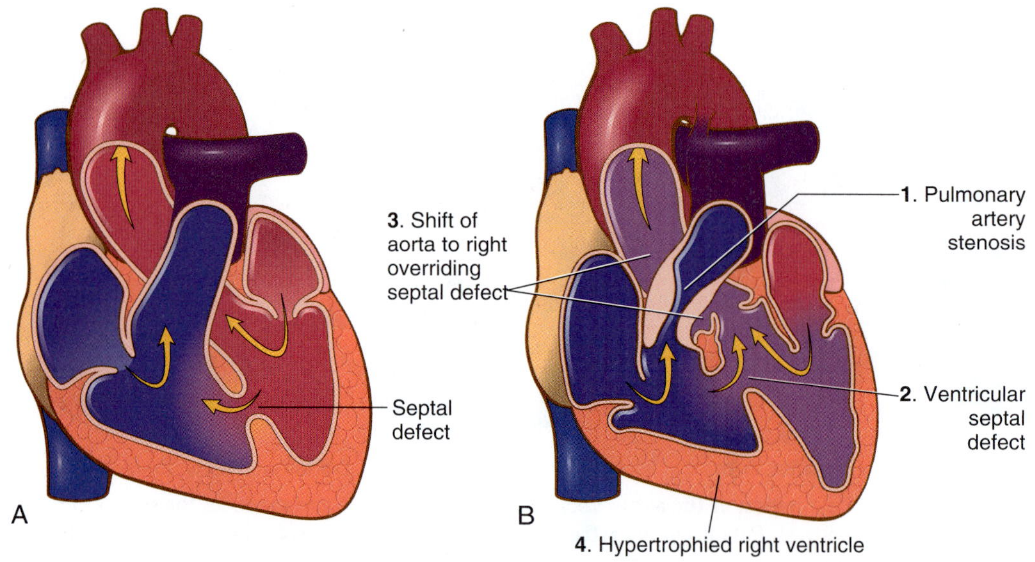

FIGURE 11-15 **A, Ventricular septal defect.** A hole in the ventricular septum causes blood to flow from the left ventricle to the right and into the lings via the pulmonary artery. **B, Tetralogy of Fallot** showing the four defects. The flow of blood is indicated by the *arrows*.

An infant with this condition is described as a "blue baby" because of the extreme degree of **cyanosis** present at birth. Surgery for tetralogy of Fallot includes a patch closure of the ventricular septal defect and removing obstruction to the outflow at the pulmonary artery.

Other congenital conditions such as **transposition of the great arteries (TGA)** (pulmonary artery arises from the left ventricle and the aorta from the right ventricle) cause cyanosis and hypoxia as well. Surgical correction of TGA involves an arterial switch procedure (pulmonary artery and aorta are reconnected in their proper positions).

congestive heart failure (CHF)

Heart is unable to pump its required amount of blood.

There are two types of congestive heart failure: systolic and diastolic. In **systolic CHF,** left ventricular dysfunction results in a low ejection fraction (the amount of blood that leaves the left ventricle). Less blood is pumped from the heart. In **diastolic CHF,** the heart can contract normally but is "stiff" or less compliant when relaxed or filling with blood. Fluid backs up in the lungs and other parts of the body. The most common cause of diastolic CHF is hypertension.

Symptoms of CHF include shortness of breath, exercise intolerance, and fluid retention. **Pulmonary edema** (fluid accumulation in the lungs) and swelling or edema in the legs, feet, and ankles are common. Treatment includes lowering dietary intake of sodium and the use of diuretics to promote fluid loss.

Angiotensin-converting enzyme (ACE) inhibitors (type I), beta-blockers, spironolactone (increases excretion of water and sodium by the kidney), and **digoxin** are also used.

If drug therapy and lifestyle changes fail to control congestive heart failure, heart transplantation may be the only treatment option. While waiting for a transplant, patients may need a device to assist the heart's pumping. A **left ventricular assist device (LVAD)** is a booster pump implanted in the abdomen, with a cannula (tube) inserted into the left ventricle. It pumps blood out of the heart to all parts of the body. LVAD may be used either as a "bridge to transplant" or as a "destination" therapy when heart transplantation is not possible. Because of the severe shortage of donor hearts, research efforts are directed at developing total artificial hearts.

coronary artery disease (CAD)

Disease of the arteries surrounding the heart.

The coronary arteries are a pair of blood vessels that arise from the aorta and supply oxygenated blood to the heart. After blood leaves the heart via the aorta, a portion is at once led back over the surface of the heart through the coronary arteries.

CAD usually is the result of **atherosclerosis.** This is the deposition of fatty compounds on the inner lining of the coronary arteries (any other artery can be similarly affected). The ordinarily smooth lining of the artery becomes roughened as the atherosclerotic plaque collects in the artery.

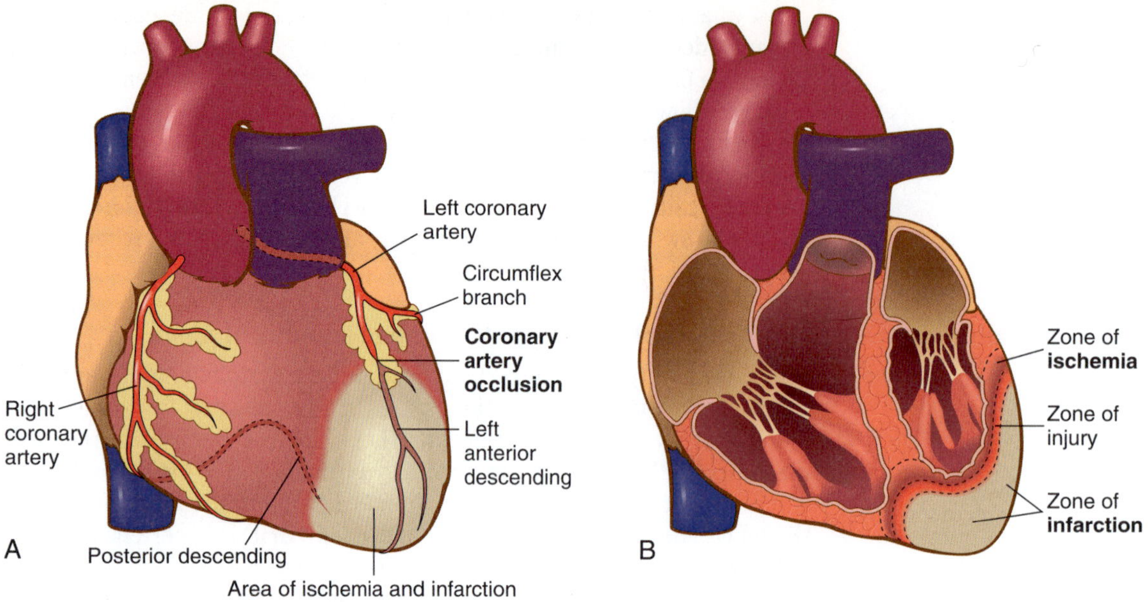

FIGURE 11-16 **A, Ischemia and infarction** produced by **coronary artery occlusion. B,** Internal view of the heart showing an area damaged by **myocardial infarction.**

The plaque first causes plugging of the coronary artery. Next, the roughened lining of the artery may rupture or cause abnormal clotting of blood, leading to **thrombotic occlusion** (blocking of the coronary artery by a clot). Blood flow is decreased **(ischemia)** or stopped entirely, leading to death **(necrosis)** of a part of the myocardium. This sequence of events constitutes a **myocardial infarction,** or heart attack, and the area of dead myocardial tissue is known as an infarct. The infarcted area is eventually replaced by scar tissue. Figure 11-16 shows coronary arteries branching from the aorta and illustrates coronary artery occlusion leading to ischemia and infarction of heart muscle. Figure 11-17 is a photograph of myocardium after an acute myocardial infarction.

Acute coronary syndromes (ACSs) are conditions caused by myocardial ischemia. These conditions are **unstable angina** (chest pain at rest or chest pain of increasing frequency) and **myocardial infarction** (Figure 11-18).

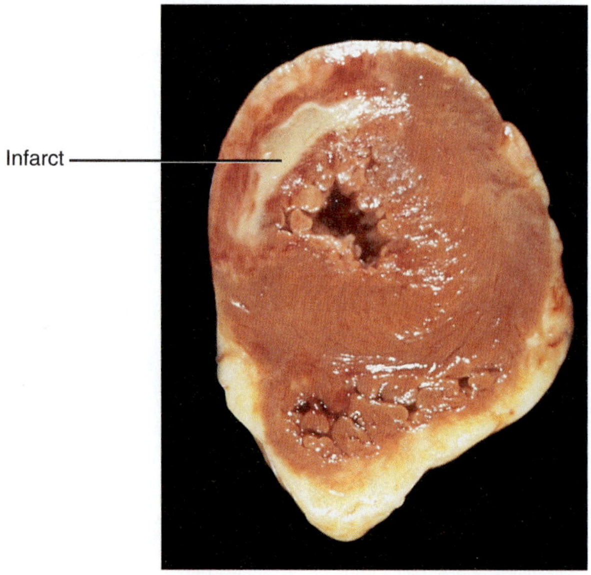

FIGURE 11-17 **Acute myocardial infarction (MI),** 5 to 7 days old. The infarct is visible as a well-demarcated, pale yellow lesion in the posterolateral region of the left ventricle. The border of the infarct is surrounded by a dark red zone of acute inflammation.

Patients with ACSs benefit from early angiography (x-ray imaging of coronary arteries) and PCI (percutaneous coronary intervention with a balloon catheter and stents) or CABG (coronary artery bypass grafting) to improve blood flow to the heart muscle (revascularization). Drugs used to treat ACSs are anticoagulants and antiplatelet agents such as aspirin and clopidogrel (Plavix), prasugrel (Effient) and ticagrelor (Brilinta).

For acute attacks of angina, **nitroglycerin** is given sublingually (under the tongue). This drug, one of several called **nitrates,** is a vasodilator that increases coronary blood flow and lowers blood pressure. Nitrates also produce venodilation to reduce venous return and decrease myocardial oxygen consumption, both of which help decrease the work of the heart.

Physicians advise patients to avoid risk factors such as smoking, obesity, and lack of exercise, and they prescribe effective drugs to prevent CAD and ACSs. These drugs include **aspirin** (to prevent clumping of platelets), **beta-blockers** (to reduce the force and speed of the heartbeat and to lower blood pressure), **ACE inhibitors** (to reduce high blood pressure and the risk of future heart attack even if the patient is not hypertensive), **calcium channel blockers** (to relax muscles in blood vessels), and **statins** (to lower cholesterol levels).

Cardiac surgeons perform an open heart operation called **coronary artery bypass grafting (CABG)** to treat CAD by replacing clogged vessels. Interventional cardiologists perform **percutaneous coronary intervention (PCI),** in which catheterization with balloons and stents opens clogged coronary arteries.

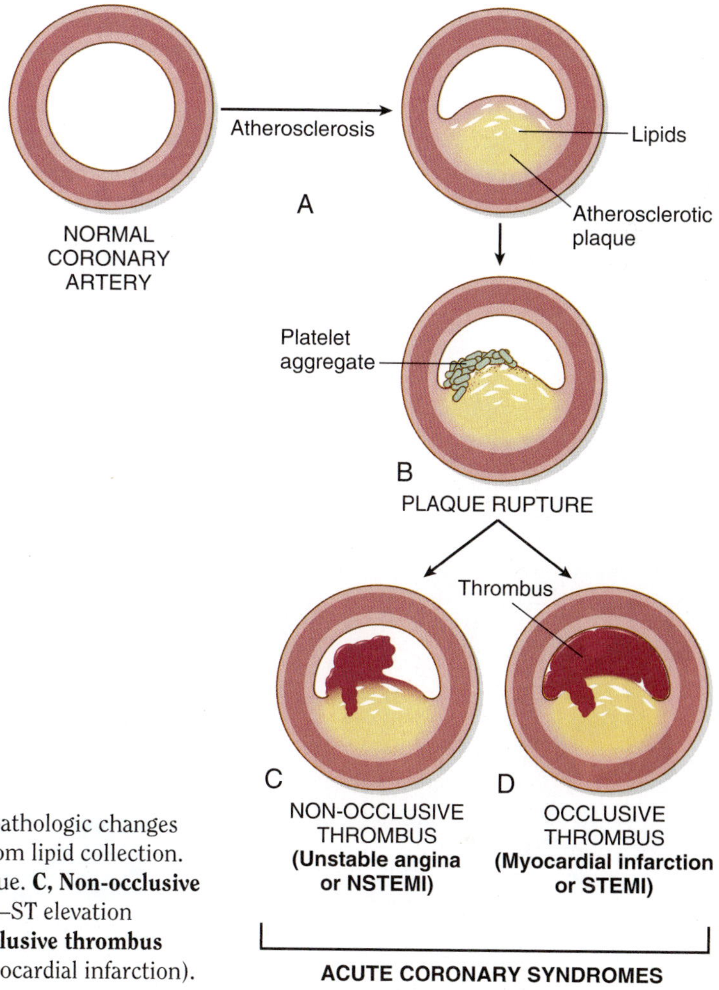

FIGURE 11-18 **Acute coronary syndromes:** sequence of pathologic changes leading to cardiac event. **A, Atherosclerotic plaque** forms from lipid collection. **B, Plaque rupture,** causing platelet aggregation on the plaque. **C, Non-occlusive thrombus** forms, causing **unstable angina** or **NSTEMI** (non–ST elevation myocardial infarction). **D,** Alternatively, formation of an **occlusive thrombus** leads to a **myocardial infarction** or **STEMI** (ST elevation myocardial infarction).

endocarditis

Inflammation of the inner lining of the heart.

Damage to the heart valves from infection **(bacterial endocarditis)** produces lesions called **vegetations** (resembling cauliflower) that break off into the bloodstream as **emboli** (material that travels through the blood). The emboli can lodge in other vessels, leading to a transient ischemic attack (TIA), or stroke, or in small vessels of the skin, where multiple pinpoint hemorrhages known as **petechiae** (from the Italian *petechio*, a flea bite) form. Antibiotics can cure bacterial endocarditis.

hypertensive heart disease

High blood pressure affecting the heart.

This condition results from narrowing of arterioles, which leads to increased pressure in arteries. The heart is affected (left ventricular hypertrophy) because it pumps more vigorously to overcome the increased resistance in the arteries.

mitral valve prolapse (MVP)

Improper closure of the mitral valve.

This condition occurs because the mitral valve enlarges and prolapses into the left atrium during systole. The physician hears a midsystolic click on **auscultation** (listening with a stethoscope). Most people with MVP live normal lives, but prolapsed valves can on rare occasion become infected.

murmur

Extra heart sound, heard between normal beats.

Murmurs are heard with the aid of a stethoscope and usually are caused by a valvular defect or disease that disrupts the smooth flow of blood in the heart. They also are heard in cases of interseptal defects, in which blood flows abnormally between chambers through holes in the septa. Functional murmurs are not caused by valve or septal defects and do not seriously endanger a person's health.

A **bruit** (BRŪ-ē) is an abnormal sound or murmur heard on auscultation. A **thrill,** which is a vibration felt on palpation of the chest, often accompanies a murmur.

pericarditis

Inflammation of the membrane (pericardium) surrounding the heart.

In most instances, pericarditis results from disease elsewhere in the body (such as pulmonary infection). Bacteria and viruses cause the condition, or the etiology may be idiopathic. Malaise, fever, and chest pain occur, and auscultation with a stethoscope often reveals a **pericardial friction rub** (heard as a scraping or grating sound). Compression of the heart caused by collection of fluid in the pericardial cavity is **cardiac tamponade** (tăm-pō-NŎD). Treatment includes anti-inflammatory drugs and other agents to manage pain. If the pericarditis is infective, antibiotics or antifungals are prescribed, depending on the microorganisms detected in specimens obtained by pericardiocentesis.

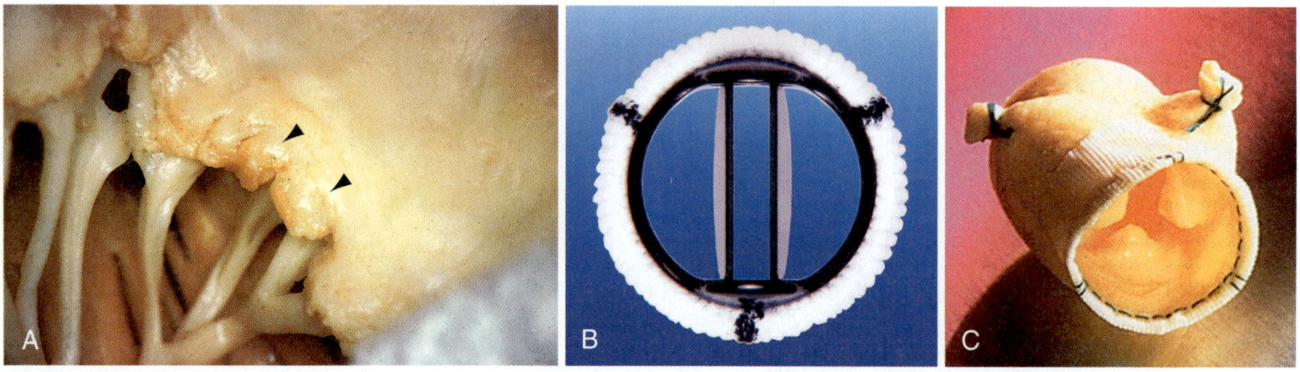

FIGURE 11-19 **A,** Acute rheumatic **mitral valvulitis** with chronic rheumatic heart disease. Small vegetations are visible along the line of closure of the mitral valve leaflet *(arrows)*. Previous episodes of rheumatic valvulitis have caused fibrous thickening and fusion of the chordae tendineae of the valves. **B, Artificial heart valve. C, Porcine xenograft** valve. A xenograft valve (Greek *xen/o* means stranger) is tissue that is transferred from an animal of one species (pig) to one of another species (human).

rheumatic heart disease

Heart disease caused by rheumatic fever.

Rheumatic fever is a childhood disease that follows a streptococcal infection. The heart valves can be damaged by inflammation and scarred (with **vegetations**), so that they do not open and close normally (Figure 11-19A). **Mitral stenosis**, atrial fibrillation, and congestive heart failure, caused by weakening of the myocardium, also can result from rheumatic heart disease. Treatment consists of reduced activity, drugs to control arrhythmia, surgery to repair a damaged valve, and anticoagulant therapy to prevent emboli from forming. Artificial and porcine (pig) valve implants can replace deteriorated heart valves (Figure 11-19B and C).

BLOOD VESSELS

aneurysm

Local widening (dilation) of an arterial wall.

An aneurysm (Greek *aneurysma*, widening) usually is caused by atherosclerosis and hypertension or a congenital weakness in the vessel wall. Aneurysms are common in the aorta but may occur in peripheral vessels as well. The danger of an aneurysm is rupture and hemorrhage. Treatment depends on the vessel involved, the site, and the health of the patient. In aneurysms of small vessels in the brain **(berry aneurysms)**, treatment is occlusion of the vessel with small clips. For larger arteries, such as the aorta, the aneurysm is resected and a synthetic graft is sewn within the affected vessel. Figure 11-20A shows an abdominal aortic aneurysm (called "AAA"), and Figure 11-20B illustrates a synthetic graft in place. Stent grafts also may be placed less invasively as an alternative to surgery in some patients.

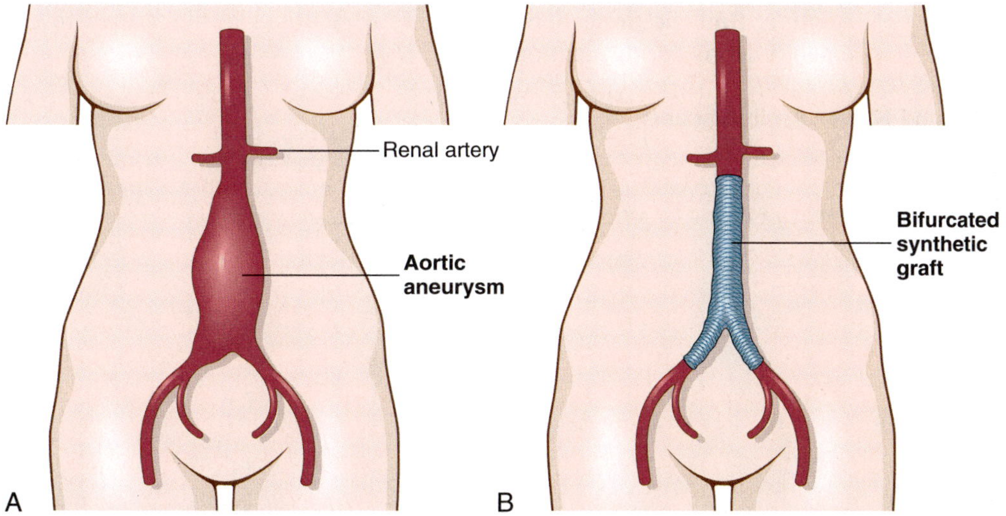

FIGURE 11-20 **A, Abdominal aortic aneurysm (AAA).** A **dissecting aortic aneurysm** is a splitting or dissection of the wall of the aorta by blood entering a tear or hemorrhage within the walls of the vessel. **B, Bifurcated synthetic graft** in place. Stent graft procedures for AAA are **EVAR** (endovascular aneurysm repair) and **TEVAR** (thoracic endovascular aneurysm repair).

Aortic Aneurysms and Marfan Syndrome

Aortic aneurysms are often associated with Marfan syndrome, a genetic disorder marked by long, thin fingers, great arm span, ocular lens dislocation, and loose joints. Abraham Lincoln is thought to have had Marfan syndrome, and the syndrome has also been diagnosed in basketball and volleyball players who have died suddenly as a result of ruptured aortic aneurysms.

deep vein thrombosis (DVT)

Blood clot (thrombus) forms in a large vein, usually in a lower limb.

This condition may result in a **pulmonary embolism** (clot travels to the lung) if not treated effectively. Anticoagulants (blood-thinning drugs) such as heparin and warfarin (Coumadin) are used to prevent DVTs and pulmonary emboli (PEs).

hypertension (HTN)

High blood pressure.

Most high blood pressure is **essential hypertension,** with no identifiable cause. In adults, a blood pressure of 140/90 mm Hg or greater is considered high. Diuretics, ACE inhibitors, calcium channel blockers, and beta-blockers, are used to treat essential hypertension. Losing weight, limiting sodium (salt) intake, stopping smoking, and reducing fat in the diet also can reduce blood pressure.

In **secondary hypertension,** the increase in pressure is caused by another associated lesion, such as glomerulonephritis, pyelonephritis, or disease of the adrenal glands.

peripheral arterial disease (PAD)

Blockage of arteries carrying blood to the legs, arms, kidneys and other organs.

Any artery can be affected, such as the **carotid** (neck), **femoral** (thigh), or **popliteal** (back of the knee). A sign of PAD in the lower extremities is **intermittent claudication** (absence of pain or discomfort in a leg at rest, but pain, tension, and weakness after walking has begun). Treatment is exercise, avoidance of nicotine (which causes vessel constriction), and control of risk factors such as hypertension, hyperlipidemia, and diabetes. Surgical treatment includes endarterectomy and bypass grafting (from the normal proximal vessel around the diseased area to a normal vessel distally).

Percutaneous treatments include balloon angioplasty, atherectomy, and stenting. **Embolic protection devices** are parachute-like filters used to capture embolic debris during stenting.

Warfarin (Coumadin) and Newer Anticoagulants

While the oral anticoagulant, warfarin, is used to prevent or treat thrombo-embolic diseases, treatment with warfarin requires careful monitoring, and is complicated by drug-drug or drug-food interactions. Newer anticoagulants that address these limitations have been approved recently by the FDA for anticoagulation in atrial fibrillation and will likely be expanded to DVT and PE.

Raynaud (rā-NŌ) **disease**

Recurrent episodes of pallor and cyanosis primarily in fingers and toes.

Of uncertain cause, this disorder is marked by intense constriction and vasospasm of arterioles often of young, otherwise healthy women. Episodes can be triggered by cold temperatures, emotional stress, or cigarette smoking. Protecting the body from cold and use of vasodilators are effective treatments.

Raynaud phenomenon is a similar condition of arterial insufficiency but is secondary to arterial narrowing from other conditions, such as atherosclerosis, systemic lupus erythematosus, or scleroderma.

varicose veins

Abnormally swollen and twisted veins, usually occurring in the legs.

This condition is caused by damaged valves that fail to prevent the backflow of blood (Figure 11-21A to C). The blood then collects in the veins, which distend to many times their normal size. Because of the slow flow of blood in the varicose veins and frequent injury to the vein, thrombosis may occur as well. **Hemorrhoids** (piles) are varicose veins near the anus.

Physicians now treat varicose veins with sclerotherapy (injections with sclerosing solution) or laser and pulsed-light treatments to seal off veins. Surgical interventions such as vein stripping and ligation are used less frequently.

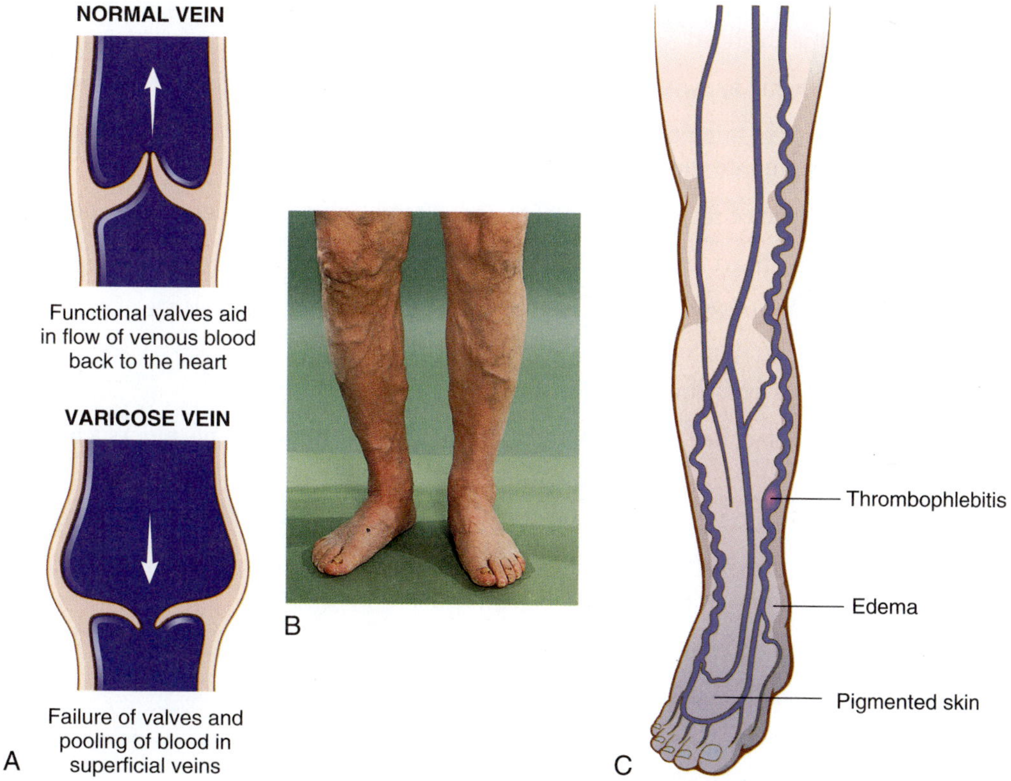

FIGURE 11-21 **A, Valve function in normal vein and varicose vein. B, Varicose veins. C,** The slow flow in veins increases susceptibility to **thrombophlebitis** (clot formation), **edema,** and **pigmented skin** (blood pools in the lower parts of the leg and fluid leaks from distended small capillaries). If a thrombus becomes loosened from its place in the vein, it can travel to the lungs (pulmonary embolism) and block a blood vessel there.

STUDY SECTION

Practice spelling each term and know its meaning.

acute coronary syndromes (ACSs)	Unstable angina and myocardial infarction (heart attack), which are consequences of plaque rupture in coronary arteries.
angina (pectoris)	Chest pain resulting from myocardial ischemia. Stable angina occurs predictably with exertion; unstable angina is chest pain that occurs more often and with less exertion.
angiotensin-converting enzyme (ACE) inhibitor	Antihypertensive drug that blocks the conversion of angiotensin I to angiotensin II, causing blood vessels to dilate. It prevents heart attacks, CHF, stroke, and death. See Table 21-6 on page 893 for names of ACE inhibitors and other cardiovascular drugs.
auscultation	Listening for sounds in blood vessels or other body structures, typically using a stethoscope.
beta-blocker	Drug used to treat angina, hypertension, and arrhythmias. It blocks the action of epinephrine (adrenaline) at receptor sites on cells, slowing the heartbeat and reducing the workload on the heart.
biventricular pacemaker	Device enabling ventricles to beat together (in synchrony) so that more blood is pumped out of the heart.
bruit	Abnormal blowing or swishing sound heard during auscultation of an artery or organ.
calcium channel blocker	Drug used to treat angina and hypertension. It dilates blood vessels by blocking the influx of calcium into muscle cells lining vessels.
cardiac arrest	Sudden, unexpected stoppage of heart action, often leading to sudden cardiac death.
cardiac tamponade	Pressure on the heart caused by fluid in the pericardial space.
claudication	Pain, tension, and weakness in a leg after walking has begun, but absence of pain at rest.
digoxin	Drug that treats arrhythmias and strengthens the heartbeat.
embolus (*plural:* **emboli**)	Clot or other substance that travels to a distant location and suddenly blocks a blood vessel.
infarction	Area of dead tissue.
nitrates	Drugs used in the treatment of angina. They dilate blood vessels, increasing blood flow and oxygen to myocardial tissue.
nitroglycerin	Nitrate drug used in the treatment of angina.
occlusion	Closure of a blood vessel due to blockage.
palpitations	Uncomfortable sensations in the chest related to cardiac arrhythmias, such as premature ventricular contractions (PVCs).
patent	Open.
pericardial friction rub	Scraping or grating noise heard on auscultation of the heart; suggestive of pericarditis.
petechiae	Small, pinpoint hemorrhages.
statins	Drugs used to lower cholesterol in the bloodstream.
thrill	Vibration felt over an area of turmoil in blood flow (as a blocked artery).
vegetations	Clumps of platelets, clotting proteins, microorganisms, and red blood cells on diseased heart valves.

LABORATORY TESTS AND CLINICAL PROCEDURES

LABORATORY TESTS

BNP test

Measurement of BNP (brain natriuretic peptide) in blood.

BNP is elevated in patients with heart failure, and it is useful in the diagnosis of CHF in patients with dyspnea who come to the emergency department. Its presence also identifies patients at risk for complications when presenting with acute coronary syndromes (e.g., myocardial infarction and unstable angina). It is secreted when the heart becomes overloaded, and it acts as a diuretic to help heart function return to normal.

The reference to brain in this substance originates from its initial identification from the brain of a pig.

cardiac biomarkers

Chemicals are measured in the blood as evidence of a heart attack.

Damaged heart muscle releases chemicals into the bloodstream. The substances tested for are **troponin-I (cTnI)** and **troponin-T (cTnT).** Troponin is a heart muscle protein released into circulation after myocardial injury.

lipid tests (lipid profile)

Measurement of cholesterol and triglycerides (fats) in a blood sample.

High levels of lipids are associated with atherosclerosis. The general guideline for total cholesterol in the blood is less than 200 mg/dL. **Saturated fats** (of animal origin, such as milk, butter, and meats) increase cholesterol in the blood, whereas **polyunsaturated fats** (of vegetable origin, such as corn and safflower oil) decrease blood cholesterol.

Treatment of hyperlipidemia includes proper diet (low-fat, high-fiber intake) and exercise. Niacin (a vitamin) also helps reduce lipids. Drug therapy includes **statins,** which reduce the risk of heart attack, stroke, and cardiovascular death. Statins lower cholesterol by reducing its production in the liver. Examples are simvastatin (Zocor), atorvastatin (Lipitor), and pravastatin (Pravachol).

lipoprotein electrophoresis

Lipoproteins (combinations of fat and protein) are physically separated and measured in a blood sample.

Examples of lipoproteins are **low-density lipoprotein (LDL)** and **high-density lipoprotein (HDL).** High levels of LDL are associated with atherosclerosis. The National Guideline for LDL is less than 130 mg/dL in normal persons and less than 70 mg/dL in patients with CAD, PAD, and diabetes mellitus. High levels of HDL protect adults from atherosclerosis. Factors that increase HDL are estrogen, exercise, and alcohol in moderation.

CLINICAL PROCEDURES: DIAGNOSTIC

X-Ray and Electron Beam Tests

angiography

X-ray imaging of blood vessels after injection of contrast material.

Arteriography is x-ray imaging of arteries after injection of contrast via a catheter into the aorta or an artery.

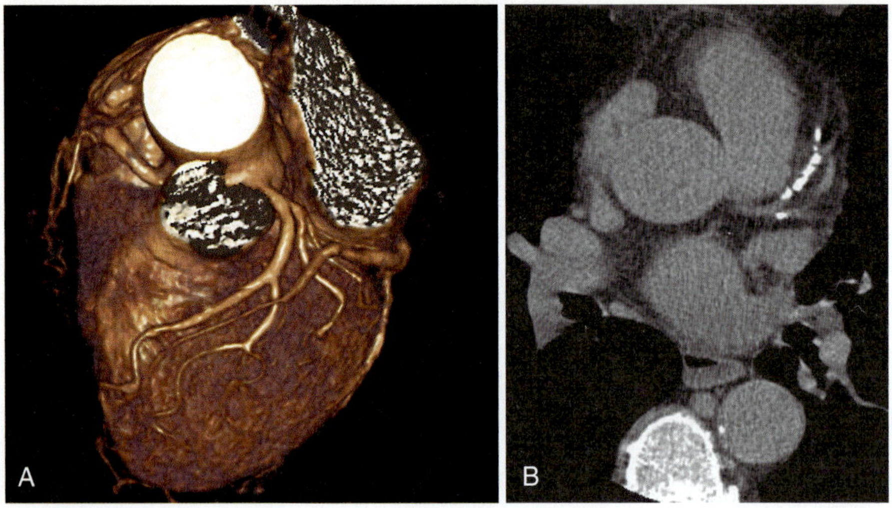

FIGURE 11-22 **A, Computed tomography angiography (CTA) showing coronary arteries.** High radiation is a drawback to the use of CTA. **B, Electron beam computed tomography** showing significant calcification *(white areas)* in the coronary arteries, indicating advanced coronary artery disease. ***(A,** Courtesy Massachusetts General Hospital, Boston.)*

computed tomography angiography (CTA)

Three-dimensional x-ray images of the heart and coronary arteries using computed tomography (64-slice CT scanner).

This newer technique takes hundreds of images of the heart per second. Cross-sectional images are assembled by computer into a three-dimensional picture. It is less invasive than angiography (contrast material is injected into a small peripheral vein with a small needle) and provides excellent views of the coronary arteries for diagnosis of coronary artery disease (Figure 11-22A).

digital subtraction angiography (DSA)

Video equipment and a computer produce x-ray images of blood vessels.

After taking an initial x-ray picture and storing it in a computer, physicians inject contrast material and take a second image of that area. The computer compares the two images and subtracts digital data for the first from the second, leaving an image of vessels with contrast.

electron beam computed tomography (EBCT *or* EBT)

Electron beams and CT identify calcium deposits in and around coronary arteries to diagnose early CAD.

A **coronary artery calcium score** is derived to indicate future risk of heart attack and stroke (see Figure 11-22B).

Ultrasound Examination

Doppler ultrasound studies

Sound waves measure blood flow within blood vessels.

An instrument focuses sound waves on blood vessels, and echoes bounce off red blood cells. The examiner can hear various alterations in blood flow caused by vessel obstruction. **Duplex ultrasound** combines Doppler and conventional ultrasound to allow physicians to image the structure of blood vessels and measure the speed of blood flow. Carotid artery occlusion, aneurysms, varicose veins, and other vessel disorders can be diagnosed with duplex ultrasound.

Coronary Artery Calcium Score

0-99	low risk
100-399	intermediate risk
>400	high risk

A calcium score >400 is associated with a nearly 25% chance of a heart attack or stroke occurring within 10 years.

echocardiography (ECHO)

Echoes generated by high-frequency sound waves produce images of the heart (Figure 11-23A).

ECHOs show the structure and movement of the heart. In **transesophageal echocardiography (TEE),** a transducer placed in the esophagus provides ultrasound and Doppler information (Figure 11-23B). This technique detects cardiac masses, prosthetic valve function, aneurysms, and pericardial fluid.

Nuclear Cardiology

positron emission tomography (PET) scan

Images show blood flow and myocardial function following uptake of radioactive glucose.

PET scanning can detect CAD, myocardial function, and differences between ischemic heart disease and cardiomyopathy.

technetium Tc 99m sestamibi scan

Technetium Tc 99m sestamibi injected intravenously is taken up in cardiac tissue, where it is detected by scanning.

This scan is used in persons who have had an MI, to assess the amount of damaged heart muscle. It also is used with an exercise tolerance test **(ETT-MIBI).** Sestamibi is a radioactive tracer compound used to define areas of poor blood flow in heart muscle.

thallium 201 scan

Concentration of radioactive thallium is measured to give information about blood supply to the heart muscle.

Thallium studies show the viability of heart muscle. Infarcted or scarred myocardium shows up as "cold spots."

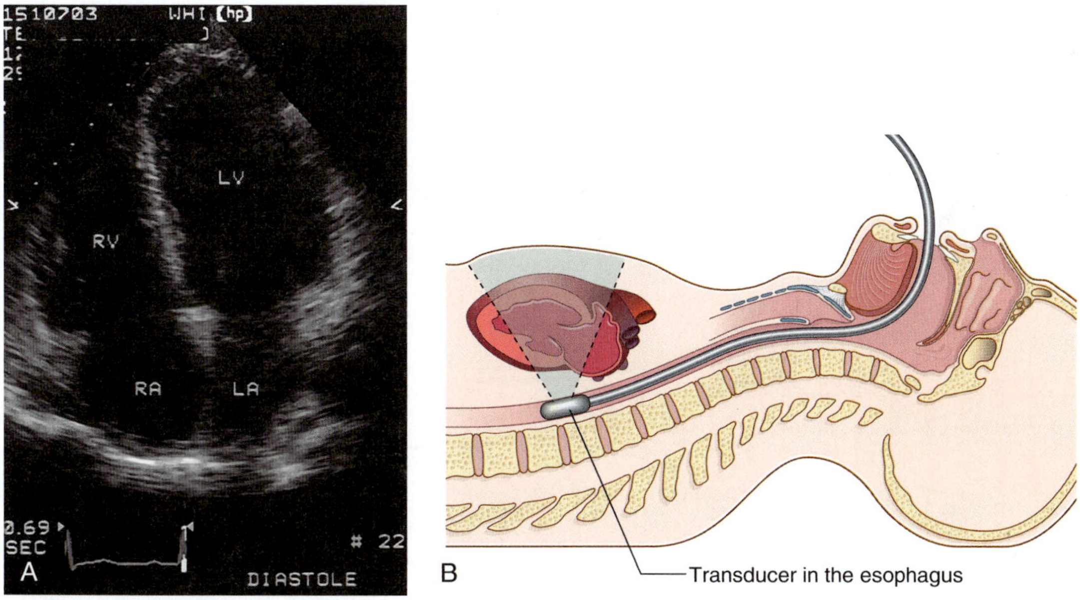

FIGURE 11-23 **A, Echocardiogram.** Notice that in this view, the ventricles are above the atria. **B, Transesophageal echocardiography.**

Magnetic Resonance Imaging (MRI)

cardiac MRI

Images of the heart are produced using radiowave energy in a magnetic field.

These images in multiple planes give information about left and right ventricular function, wall thickness, and fibrosis, aneurysms, cardiac output, and patency of peripheral and coronary arteries. The magnetic waves emitted during MRI could interfere with implanted pacemakers because of their metal content and heat generation, so it is currently contraindicated for a patient with a pacemaker to undergo cardiac MRI. However, new MRI-safe pacemakers have been approved. **Magnetic resonance angiography (MRA)** is a type of MRI that gives highly detailed images of blood vessels. Physicians use MRA to view arteries and blockage inside arteries. **Gadolinium** is the most common contrast agent used for MRI procedures.

Other Diagnostic Procedures

cardiac catheterization

Thin, flexible tube is guided into the heart via a vein or an artery.

This procedure detects pressures and patterns of blood flow in the heart. Contrast may be injected and x-ray images taken of the heart and blood vessels (Figure 11-24). This procedure may be used in diagnosis and treatment of heart conditions (see under percutaneous coronary intervention [PCI] on page 431).

electrocardiography (ECG)

Recording of electricity flowing through the heart.

Continuous monitoring of a patient's heart rhythm in hospitals is performed via **telemetry** (electronic transmission of data—tele/o means distant). Sinus rhythm begins in the SA node, and the normal rate is between 60 to 100 beats per minute. Figure 11-25 shows ECG strips for normal sinus rhythm and several types of dysrhythmias (abnormal rhythms).

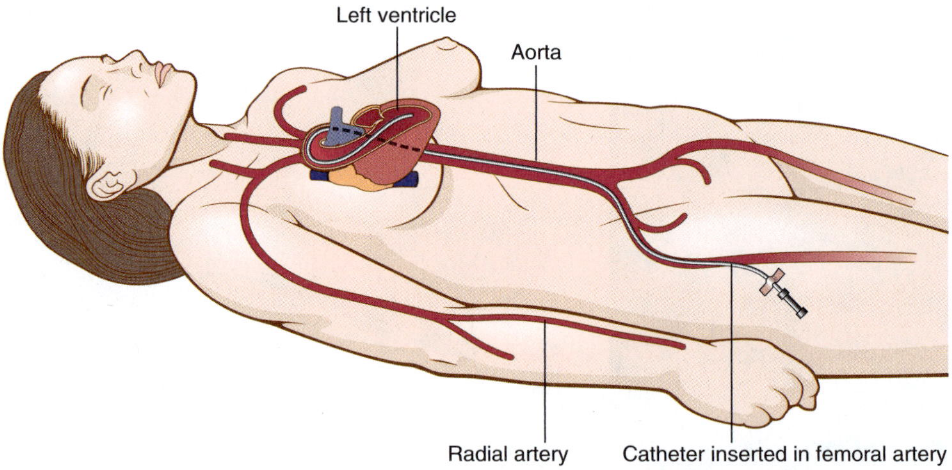

FIGURE 11-24 Left-sided cardiac catheterization. The catheter is passed retrograde (backward) from the femoral artery into the aorta and then into the left ventricle. Catheterization also is performed using the radial artery by an increasing number of interventional cardiologists. For right-sided cardiac catheterization, the cardiologist inserts a catheter through the femoral vein and advances it to the right atrium and right ventricle and into the pulmonary artery.

Holter monitoring — **An ECG device is worn during a 24-hour period to detect cardiac arrhythmias.**

Rhythm changes are correlated with symptoms recorded in a diary.

stress test — **Exercise tolerance test (ETT) determines the heart's response to physical exertion (stress).**

A common protocol uses 3-minute stages at set speeds and elevations of a treadmill. Continual monitoring of vital signs and ECG rhythms is important in the diagnosis of CAD and left ventricular function.

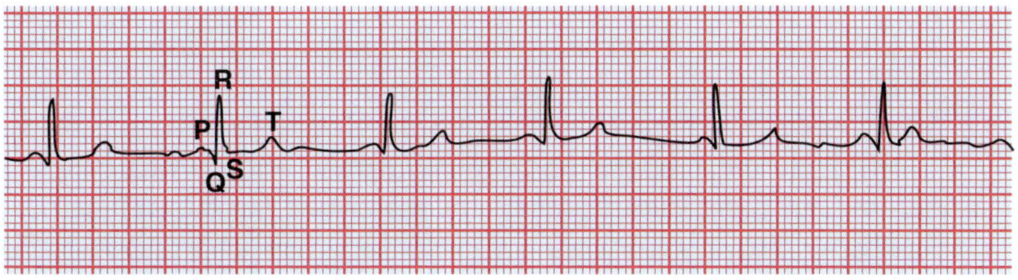

A

Normal sinus rhythm. Notice the regularity of the P, QRS, and T waves.

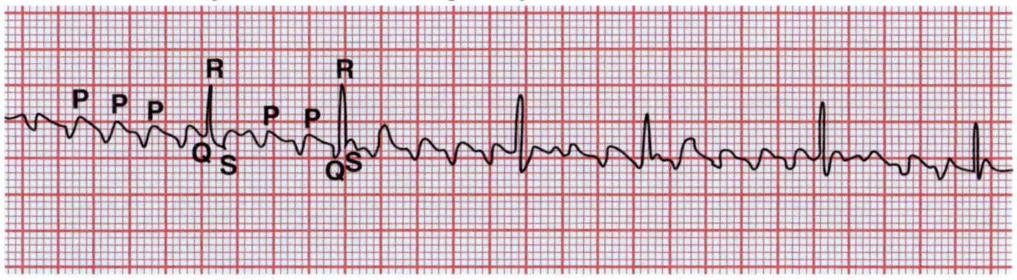

B

Atrial flutter. Notice the rapid atrial rate (P wave) compared with the slower. ventricular rate (QRS)

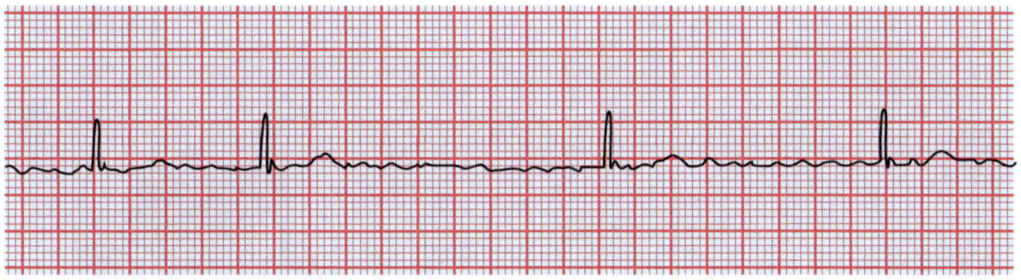

C

Atrial fibrillation. P waves are replaced by irregular and rapid fluctuations. There are no effective atrial contractions.

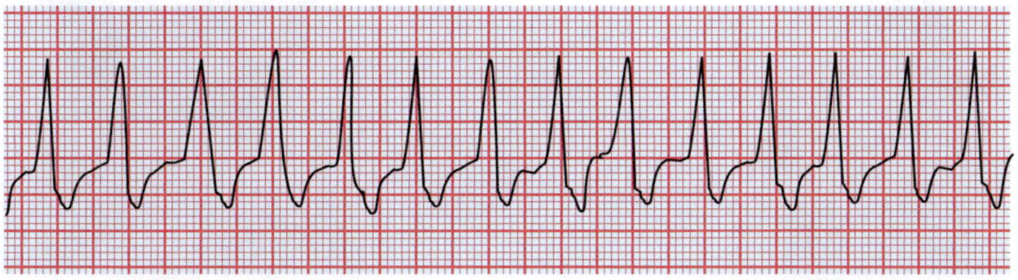

D

Ventricular tachycardia. Ventricular rate may be as high as 250 beats per minute. The rhythm is regular, but the atria are not contributing to ventricular filling and blood output is poor.

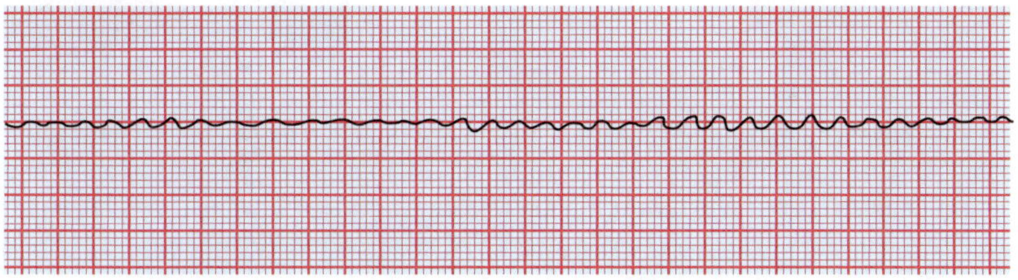

E

Ventricular fibrillation. Notice the abnormal, irregular waves. Ventricles in fibrillation cannot pump blood effectively. Circulation stops and sudden cardiac death follows if fibrillation is not reversed.

FIGURE 11-25 **ECG rhythm strips showing normal sinus rhythm and dysrhythmias (arrhythmias).**

CLINICAL PROCEDURES: TREATMENT

catheter ablation

Brief delivery of radiofrequency energy to destroy areas of heart tissue that may be causing arrhythmias

A catheter is guided through a vein in the leg to the vena cava and into the heart. The abnormal electrical pathway is located and ablated (destroyed) via energy emitted from the catheter. See Figure 11-26A.

coronary artery bypass grafting (CABG)

Arteries and veins are anastomosed to coronary arteries to detour around blockages.

Internal mammary (breast) and radial (arm) arteries and saphenous (leg) vein grafts are used to keep the myocardium supplied with oxygenated blood (Figure 11-26B). Cardiac surgeons perform minimally invasive CABG surgery using smaller incisions instead of the traditional sternotomy to open the chest. Vein and artery grafts are removed endoscopically through small incisions as well.

Although most operations are performed with a heart-lung machine ("on-pump"), an increasing number are performed "off-pump" with a beating heart. See the ***In Person*** story, on page 436, of a man who underwent coronary artery bypass graft surgery.

defibrillation

Brief discharges of electricity are applied across the chest to stop dysrhythmias (ventricular fibrillation).

For patients at high risk for sudden cardiac death from ventricular dysrhythmias, an **implantable cardioverter-defibrillator (ICD)** or **automatic implantable cardioverter-defibrillator (AICD)** is placed in the upper chest.

Cardioversion is another technique using lower energy to treat atrial fibrillation, atrial flutter, and supraventricular tachycardia.

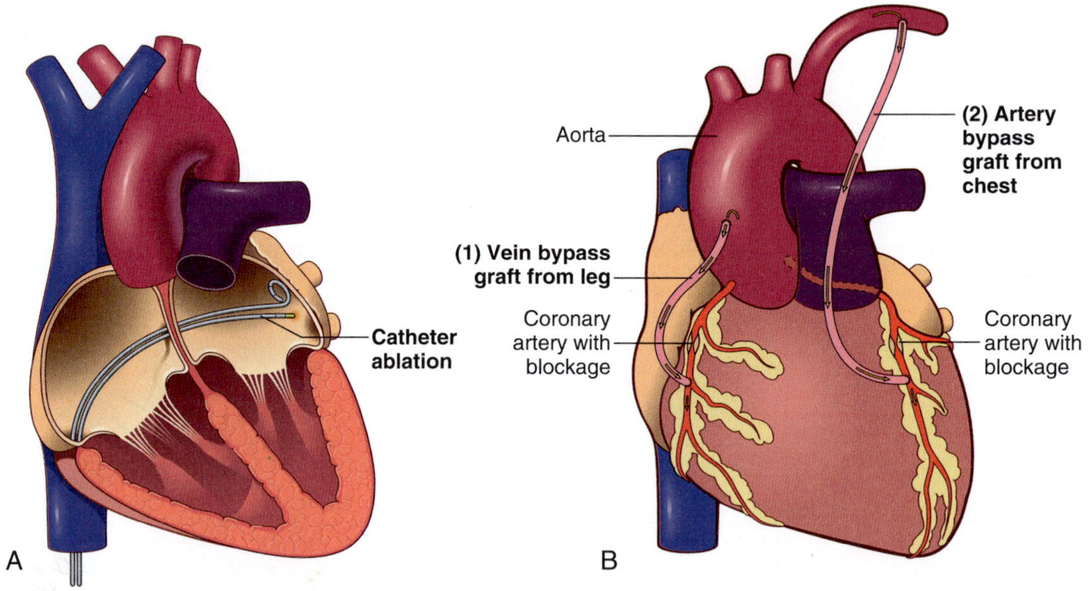

FIGURE 11-26 **A, Catheter ablation.** SVT, atrial flutter, AF, and VT may be treated with ablation when clinically indicated. **B, Coronary artery bypass grafting (CABG)** surgery with anastomosis of vein and arterial grafts. **(1)** A section of a vein is removed from the leg and anastomosed (upside down because of its directional valves) to a coronary artery, to bypass an area of arteriosclerotic blockage. **(2)** An internal mammary artery is grafted to a coronary artery to bypass a blockage.

endarterectomy

Surgical removal of plaque from the inner layer of an artery.

Fatty deposits (atheromas) and thromboses are removed to open clogged arteries. **Carotid endarterectomy** is a procedure to remove plaque buildup in the carotid artery to reduce risk of stroke.

extracorporeal circulation

Heart-lung machine diverts blood from the heart and lungs while the heart is repaired.

Blood leaves the body, enters the heart-lung machine, where it is oxygenated, and then returns to a blood vessel (artery) to circulate through the bloodstream. The machine uses the technique of **extracorporeal membrane oxygenation (ECMO).**

heart transplantation

A donor heart is transferred to a recipient.

While waiting for a transplant, a patient may need a **left ventricular assist device (LVAD),** which is a booster pump implanted in the abdomen with a cannula (flexible tube) to the left ventricle.

percutaneous coronary intervention (PCI)

Balloon-tipped catheter is inserted into a coronary artery to open the artery; stents are put in place.

An interventional cardiologist places the catheter in the femoral or radial artery and then threads it up the aorta into the coronary artery. **Stents** (expandable slotted tubes that serve as permanent scaffolding devices) create wide lumens and make restenosis less likely. Newer **drug-eluting stents (DESs)** are coated with polymers that elute (release) antiproliferative drugs to prevent scar tissue formation leading to restenosis (Figure 11-27). Stents are also placed in carotid, renal, and other peripheral arteries.

PCI techniques include percutaneous transluminal coronary angioplasty (PTCA), stent placement, laser angioplasty (a small laser on the tip of a catheter vaporizes plaque), and atherectomy.

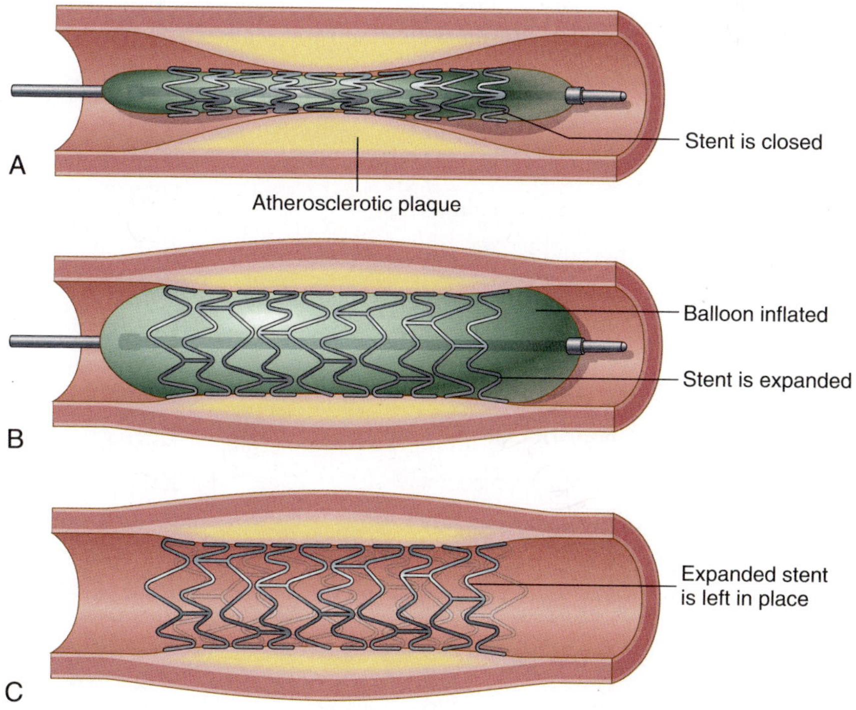

FIGURE 11-27 Placement of an intracoronary artery drug-eluting stent. A, The stent is positioned at the site of the lesion. **B,** The balloon is inflated, expanding the stent and compressing the plaque. **C,** When the balloon is withdrawn, the stent supports the artery and releases a drug to reduce the risk of restenosis. Stents are stainless-steel scaffolding devices that help hold open arteries, such as the coronary, renal, and carotid arteries.

thrombolytic therapy — **Drugs to dissolve clots are injected into the bloodstream of patients with coronary thrombosis.**

Tissue plasminogen activator **(tPA)** and **streptokinase** restore blood flow to the heart and limit irreversible damage to heart muscle. The drugs are given within 12 hours after the onset of a heart attack. Thrombolytic agents reduce the mortality rate in patients with myocardial infarction by 25%.

transcatheter aortic valve replacement (TAVR) — **Placement of a balloon-expandable aortic heart valve into the body via a catheter.**

The catheter is guided into the heart through the femoral artery, and a stent valve device is inserted via the catheter. This is a new minimally invasive catheter-based technology used to treat aortic stenosis.

ABBREVIATIONS

AAA	abdominal aortic aneurysm
ACE inhibitor	angiotensin-converting enzyme inhibitor
ACLS	advanced cardiac life support; CPR plus drugs and defibrillation
ACS	acute coronary syndrome
ADP	adenosine diphosphate; ADP blockers are used to prevent cardiovascular-related death, heart attack, and strokes and after all stent procedures
AED	automatic external defibrillator
AF, a-fib	atrial fibrillation
AICD	automatic implantable cardioverter-defibrillator
AMI	acute myocardial infarction
ARVD	arrhythmogenic right ventricular dysplasia
AS	aortic stenosis
ASD	atrial septal defect
AV, A-V	atrioventricular
AVR	aortic valve replacement
BBB	bundle branch block
BNP	brain natriuretic peptide; elevated in congestive heart failure
BP	blood pressure
CABG	coronary artery bypass grafting
CAD	coronary artery disease
CCU	coronary care unit
Cath	catheterization
CHF	congestive heart failure
CK	creatine kinase; released into the bloodstream after injury to heart or skeletal muscles
CoA	coarctation of the aorta
CPR	cardiopulmonary resuscitation
CRT	cardiac resynchronization therapy; biventricular pacing
CTNI *or* **cTnI; CTNT** *or* **cTnT**	cardiac troponin-I and cardiac troponin-T; troponin is a protein released into the bloodstream after myocardial injury
DES	drug-eluting stent
DSA	digital subtraction angiography
DVT	deep vein thrombosis
ECMO	extracorporeal membrane oxygenation
ECG; *also seen as* **EKG**	electrocardiography
ECHO	echocardiography
EF	ejection fraction; measure of the amount of blood that pumps out of the heart with each beat
EPS	electrophysiology study; electrode catheters are inserted into veins and threaded into the heart and electrical conduction is measured (tachycardias are provoked and analyzed)

ETT	exercise tolerance test
ETT-MIBI	exercise tolerance test combined with a radioactive tracer (sestamibi) scan
EVAR	endovascular aneurysm repair
HDL	high-density lipoprotein; high blood levels are associated with lower incidence of coronary artery disease
HTN	hypertension (high blood pressure)
IABP	intra-aortic balloon pump; used to support patients in cardiogenic shock
ICD	implantable cardioverter-defibrillator
LAD	left anterior descending (coronary artery)
LDL	low-density lipoprotein
LMWH	low-molecular-weight heparin
LV	left ventricle
LVAD	left ventricular assist device
LVH	left ventricular hypertrophy
MI	myocardial infarction
MUGA	multiple-gated acquisition scan; a radioactive test of heart function
MVP	mitral valve prolapse
NSR	normal sinus rhythm
NSTEMI	non–ST elevation myocardial infarction
PAC	premature atrial contraction
PAD	peripheral arterial disease
PCI	percutaneous coronary intervention
PDA	patent ductus arteriosus; posterior descending artery
PE	pulmonary embolus
PVC	premature ventricular contraction
SA, S-A node	sinoatrial node
SCD	sudden cardiac death
SOB	shortness of breath
SPECT	single photon emission computed tomography; used for myocardial imaging with sestamibi scans
STEMI	ST elevation myocardial infarction
SVT	supraventricular tachycardia; rapid heartbeats arising from the atria and causing palpitations, SOB, and dizziness
TAVR	transcatheter aortic valve replacement
TEE	transesophageal echocardiography
TEVAR	thoracic endovascular aneurysm repair
TGA	transposition of the great arteries
tPA	tissue-type plasminogen activator; a drug used to prevent thrombosis
UA	unstable angina; chest pain at rest or of increasing frequency
VF	ventricular fibrillation
VSD	ventricular septal defect
VT	ventricular tachycardia
WPW	Wolff-Parkinson-White syndrome; an abnormal ECG pattern often associated with paroxysmal tachycardia

PRACTICAL APPLICATIONS

Answers to Practical Applications are found on page 449.

OPERATING ROOM SCHEDULE: GENERAL HOSPITAL

Match the operative treatment in Column I with the appropriate surgical indication (diagnosis) in Column II.

COLUMN I		COLUMN II
1. coronary artery bypass grafting	_____	A. Congestive heart failure
2. left carotid endarterectomy	_____	B. Cardiac tamponade (fluid in the space surrounding the heart)
3. sclerosing injections and laser treatment	_____	C. Atherosclerotic occlusion of a main artery leading to the head
4. LV aneurysmectomy	_____	D. Congenital hole in the wall of the upper chamber of the heart
5. atrial septal defect repair	_____	E. Disabling angina and extensive coronary atherosclerosis despite medical therapy
6. left ventricular assist device	_____	F. Peripheral vascular disease
7. pericardiocentesis	_____	G. Heart block
8. aortic valve replacement	_____	H. Varicose veins
9. pacemaker implantation	_____	I. Protrusion of the wall of a lower heart chamber
10. femoral-popliteal bypass grafting	_____	J. Aortic stenosis

CLINICAL CASES: WHAT'S YOUR DIAGNOSIS?

Case 1: A 24-year-old woman with a history of palpitations [heartbeat is unusually strong, rapid, or irregular, so that patient is aware of it] and vague chest pains enters the hospital. With the patient supine, you hear a midsystolic click that is followed by a grade 3/6 [moderately loud—6/6 is loud and 1/6 is quiet] honking murmur.

1. Your diagnosis is
   a. Tetralogy of Fallot
   b. Mitral valve prolapse
   c. Raynaud disease
   d. Congestive heart failure

Case 2: Mr. Smith was admitted to the telemetry unit for cardiac monitoring after an episode of chest pain. His cardiac enzymes (CK, troponin-T, and troponin-I) were slightly elevated, and the ECG showed elevation in the ST segment. An angiogram reveals plaque blocking the LAD. PCI with DES is recommended.

1. What did the ECG reveal?
   a. NSTEMI and unstable angina
   b. Aortic aneurysm
   c. CHF
   d. STEMI

2. Your diagnosis for this patient is
   a. Heart attack
   b. Rheumatic heart disease
   c. Unstable angina
   d. Patent ductus arteriosus

3. What treatment is recommended?
   a. Coronary artery bypass grafting
   b. Catheterization with drug-eluting stent placement
   c. Defibrillation and cardioversion
   d. Thrombolytic drugs

Case 3: A 42-year-old female runner recovering from an upper respiratory infection comes to the ED complaining of chest pain that is sharp and constant, worse when she is lying down and decreased with sitting up and leaning forward. Serum CK and troponin I levels rule out an acute MI. The ED physician auscultates a pericardial friction rub.

1. What's your diagnosis for this patient?
   a. Myocardial ischemia
   b. Unstable angina and NSTEMI
   c. Endocarditis
   d. Pericarditis

2. The danger of this condition is the risk for progression to
   a. Cardiac tamponade
   b. Aneurysm
   c. Pulmonary embolism
   d. Claudication

IN PERSON

This is a first-person account of coronary artery bypass surgery.

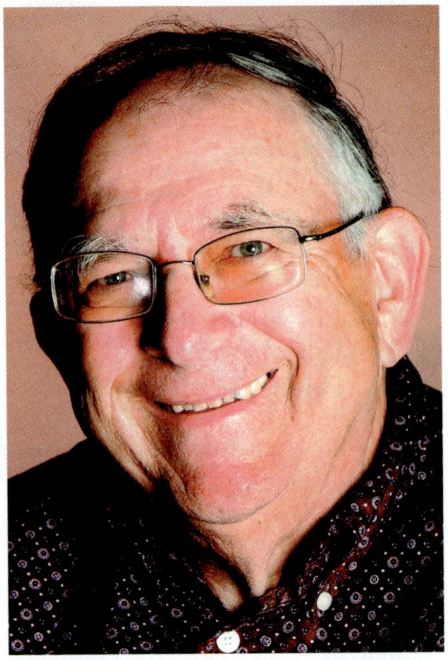

Possible heart attack? You have to be kidding. I had none of the supposed symptoms—shortness of breath or chest pain. Instead, I had bouts of atrial fibrillation off and on for several months. I got tired easily, and I could feel my blood pressure drop. After lying down for about an hour, I was fine, but in November 2010 I decided to get it checked out.

My cardiologist decided to do a stress test. He put me on a treadmill, which seemed like an eternity, and then did some ultrasound on me. I work out every day on a treadmill and a recumbent bike, so the test on the treadmill wasn't that difficult, although I loved the words "just a couple of seconds to go."

The cardiologist at Johns Hopkins told me after the stress test that it appeared that I had a slight blockage of an artery. No problem, I thought.

Angioplasty was recommended. During angioplasty, a catheter was inserted up my right arm and, although I was lightly sedated, I still felt it, particularly when the doctor hit a problem and had to make a slight correction. I was certain that they would put in a stent and I'd be home by the weekend. "No," said my doctor. "You have three blockages and will need bypass surgery." I thought he must be talking about someone else. That can't be me!

The blockages did not require immediate surgery. After all, I was pain free and asymptomatic. Still, I asked for an early date for surgery and it was set for January, 11, 2011. That was 1/11/11. How odd.

The triple coronary artery bypass opened me like a beached tuna, and made me an official member of the "zipper club." The atrial fibrillation was fixed with radio-frequency ablation.

After surgery I had to lie on my back, which meant minimal sleep for a week. Lasix (a diuretic) was my biggest problem, along with a dozen pills I had to take far too often. According to my surgeon, who visited me a day later, things went well, and I was up and walking the hallways of Hopkins with the help of a nurse and a walker.

I went home in a week. The toughest part of the ordeal, oddly enough, was trying to get to the bathroom in time and the bumpy ride home. Those bumps made me hold that pillow as close as I could. Ouch.

After I returned home, two nurses came for home care, and they were fabulous. I lost about 20 pounds prior to the surgery and another 17 pounds afterwards. I went from 210 pounds to around 173 pounds.

Nowadays, I eat no red meat, nothing with butter, and as little fat and salt as possible. In order words, I eat fish primarily. I work out every day (between 30 and 60 minutes), and I have regular checkups with my cardiologist.

I was lucky that the atrial fibrillation alerted my physicians to a deeper problem that may have resulted in a heart attack or even death. Secondly, I was fortunate to have some true professionals on hand to get me through the darkest days of my life. Many people who had bypass surgery told me I would have more energy after surgery due to my new plumbing. That hasn't occurred yet, but I still have hope, and will continue to work toward that goal.

Stan Ber was born in Maine, is a graduate of Bowdoin College, and has been a sports editor and columnist for two newspapers in Howard County, Maryland for the past 41 years. He was inducted into the County's Sports Hall of Fame in 2009.

EXERCISES

Remember to check your answers carefully with the Answers to Exercises, page 446.

A Match the following structures with their descriptions below.

aorta	inferior vena cava	superior vena cava
arteriole	mitral valve	tricuspid valve
atrium	pulmonary artery	ventricle
capillary	pulmonary vein	venule

1. valve that lies between the right atrium and the right ventricle ________________
2. smallest blood vessel ________________
3. carries oxygenated blood from the lungs to the heart ________________
4. largest artery in the body ________________
5. brings oxygen-poor blood into the heart from the upper parts of the body ________________
6. upper chamber of the heart ________________
7. carries oxygen-poor blood to the lungs from the heart ________________
8. small artery ________________
9. valve that lies between the left atrium and the left ventricle ________________
10. brings blood from the lower half of the body to the heart ________________
11. small vein ________________
12. lower chamber of the heart ________________

B Trace the path of blood through the heart. Begin as the blood enters the right atrium from the venae cavae (and include the valves within the heart).

1. *right atrium*	7. ________________
2. ________________	8. ________________
3. ________________	9. ________________
4. ________________	10. ________________
5. ________________	11. ________________
6. *capillaries of the lung*	12. *aorta*

C Complete the following sentences.

1. The pacemaker of the heart is the ______________________________.
2. The sac-like membrane surrounding the heart is the ______________________________.
3. The wall of the heart between the right and the left atria is the ______________________________.
4. The relaxation phase of the heartbeat is called ______________________________.
5. Specialized conductive tissue in the wall between the ventricles is the ______________________________.
6. The inner lining of the heart is the ______________________________.
7. The contractive phase of the heartbeat is called ______________________________.
8. A gas released as a metabolic product of catabolism is ______________________________.
9. Specialized conductive tissue at the base of the wall between the two upper heart chambers is the ______________________________.
10. The inner lining of the pericardium, adhering to the outside of the heart, is the ______________________________.
11. An abnormal heart sound due to improper closure of heart valves is a ______________________________.
12. The beat of the heart as felt through the walls of arteries is called the ______________________________.

D Complete the following terms using the given definitions.

1. hardening of arteries: arterio______________________
2. disease condition of heart muscle: cardio______________________
3. enlargement of the heart: cardio______________________
4. inflammation of a vein: phleb______________________
5. condition of rapid heartbeat: ______________________cardia
6. condition of slow heartbeat: ______________________cardia
7. high levels of cholesterol in the blood: hyper______________________
8. surgical repair of a valve: valvulo______________________
9. condition of deficient oxygen: hyp______________________
10. pertaining to an upper heart chamber: ______________________al
11. narrowing of the mitral valve: mitral ______________________
12. breakdown of a clot: thrombo______________________

E **Give the meanings of the following terms.**

1. cyanosis ____________________
2. phlebotomy ____________________
3. arterial anastomosis ____________________
4. cardiogenic shock ____________________
5. atheroma ____________________
6. arrhythmia ____________________
7. sphygmomanometer ____________________
8. stethoscope ____________________
9. mitral valvulitis ____________________
10. atherosclerosis ____________________
11. vasoconstriction ____________________
12. vasodilation ____________________

F **Match the following pathologic conditions of the heart with their meanings below.**

atrial septal defect	endocarditis	mitral valve prolapse
coarctation of the aorta	fibrillation	patent ductus arteriosus
congestive heart failure	flutter	pericarditis
coronary artery disease	hypertensive heart disease	tetralogy of Fallot

1. inflammation of the inner lining of the heart ____________________
2. rapid but regular atrial or ventricular contractions ____________________
3. small hole between the upper heart chambers; congenital anomaly ____________________
4. improper closure of the valve between the left atrium and ventricle during systole ____________________
5. blockage of the arteries surrounding the heart leading to ischemia ____________________
6. high blood pressure affecting the heart ____________________
7. rapid, random, ineffectual, and irregular contractions of the heart ____________________
8. inflammation of the sac surrounding the heart ____________________
9. inability of the heart to pump its required amount of blood ____________________
10. congenital malformation involving four separate heart defects ____________________
11. congenital narrowing of the large artery leading from the heart ____________________
12. a duct between the aorta and the pulmonary artery, which normally closes soon after birth, remains open ____________________

II

G Give the meanings of the following terms.

1. heart block ______
2. cardiac arrest ______
3. palpitations ______
4. artificial cardiac pacemaker ______
5. thrombotic occlusion ______
6. angina ______
7. myocardial infarction ______
8. necrosis ______
9. infarction ______
10. ischemia ______
11. nitroglycerin ______
12. digoxin ______
13. bruit ______
14. thrill ______
15. acute coronary syndromes ______
16. pericardial friction rub ______
17. deep vein thrombosis ______
18. biventricular pacemaker ______

H Match the following terms with their descriptions.

aneurysm	essential hypertension	Raynaud disease
auscultation	murmur	rheumatic heart disease
claudication	peripheral arterial disease	secondary hypertension
emboli	petechiae	vegetations

1. lesions that form on heart valves after damage by infection ______________
2. clots that travel to and suddenly block a blood vessel ______________
3. small, pinpoint hemorrhages ______________
4. an extra heart sound, heard between normal beats and caused by a valvular defect or condition that disrupts the smooth flow of blood through the heart ______________
5. listening with a stethoscope ______________
6. heart disease caused by rheumatic fever ______________
7. high blood pressure in arteries when the etiology is idiopathic ______________
8. high blood pressure related to kidney disease ______________
9. episodes of ischemia with pallor and numbness in fingers and toes caused by a temporary constriction of arterioles in the skin ______________
10. local widening of an artery ______________
11. pain, tension, and weakness in a limb after walking has begun ______________
12. blockage of arteries in the lower extremities; etiology is atherosclerosis ______________

I Give short answers for the following.

1. Types of drugs used to treat acute coronary syndromes include ______________ ______________.
2. When damaged valves in veins fail to prevent the backflow of blood, a condition (swollen, twisted vein) that results is ______________.
3. Swollen, twisted veins in the rectal region are called ______________.
4. Name the four defects in tetralogy of Fallot from their descriptions:
   a. narrowing of the artery leading to the lungs from the heart ______________
   b. gap in the wall between the ventricles ______________
   c. the large vessel leading from the left ventricle moves over the interventricular septum ______________
   d. excessive development of the wall of the right lower heart chamber ______________ ______________

J Select from the list of cardiac tests and procedures to complete the definitions below.

angiography (arteriography)	defibrillation	lipid tests (profile)
cardiac biomarkers	echocardiography	lipoprotein electrophoresis
cardiac MRI	electrocardiography	stress test
coronary artery bypass grafting	endarterectomy	thallium 201 scan

1. surgical removal of plaque from the inner lining of an artery ______________________
2. application of brief electrical discharges across the chest to stop ventricular fibrillation and pulseless ventricular tachycardia ______________________
3. measurement of levels of fatty substances (cholesterol and triglycerides) in the bloodstream ______________________
4. measurement of the heart's response to physical exertion (patient monitored while jogging on a treadmill) ______________________
5. measurement of troponin-T and troponin-I after myocardial infarction ______________________
6. injection of contrast into vessels and x-ray imaging ______________________
7. recording of the electricity in the heart ______________________
8. intravenous injection of a radioactive substance and measurement of its accumulation in heart muscle ______________________
9. use of echoes from high-frequency sound waves to produce images of the heart ______________________
10. separation of HDL and LDL from a blood sample ______________________
11. anastomosis of vessel grafts to existing coronary arteries to maintain blood supply to the myocardium ______________________
12. beaming of magnetic waves at the heart to produce images of its structure ______________________

K Give the meanings for the following terms.

1. digital subtraction angiography ____________________
2. heart transplantation ____________________
3. ETT-MIBI ____________________
4. Doppler ultrasound ____________________
5. Holter monitoring ____________________
6. thrombolytic therapy ____________________
7. extracorporeal circulation ____________________
8. cardiac catheterization ____________________
9. percutaneous coronary intervention ____________________
10. drug-eluting stent ____________________
11. electron beam computed tomography ____________________
12. CT angiography ____________________

L Identify the following cardiac dysrhythmias from their abbreviations.

1. AF ____________________
2. VT ____________________
3. VF ____________________
4. PVC ____________________
5. PAC ____________________

M Identify the following abnormal cardiac conditions from their abbreviations.

1. CHF ____________________
2. VSD ____________________
3. MI ____________________
4. PDA ____________________
5. MVP ____________________
6. AS ____________________
7. CAD ____________________
8. ASD ____________________

N Match the following abbreviations for cardiac tests and procedures with their explanations below.

BNP	ECMO	LDL
CRT	ETT	LVAD
cTnI or cTnT	ETT-MIBI	RFA
ECHO	ICD	TEE

1. cardiac serum enzyme test for myocardial infarction ____________________
2. booster pump implanted in the abdomen with a cannula leading to the heart as a "bridge to transplant" ____________________
3. ultrasound imaging of the heart using transducer within the esophagus ____________________
4. device implanted in the chest that senses and corrects arrhythmias by shocking the heart ____________________
5. catheter delivery of a high-frequency current to damage a small portion of the heart muscle and reverse an abnormal heart rhythm ____________________
6. procedure to determine the heart's response to physical exertion (stress) ____________________
7. cardiac imaging using high-frequency sound waves pulsed through the chest wall and bounced off heart structures ____________________
8. radioactive test of heart function with stress test ____________________
9. technique using heart-lung machine to divert blood from the heart and lungs while the heart is being repaired ____________________
10. biventricular pacing to correct serious abnormal ventricular rhythms ____________________
11. lipoprotein sample is measured ____________________
12. brain chemical measured to identify patients at risk for complications after MI and with CHF ____________________

O Spell the term correctly from its definition.

1. pertaining to the heart: ____________________ary
2. not a normal heart rhythm: arr____________________
3. abnormal condition of blueness: ____________________osis
4. relaxation phase of the heartbeat: ____________________tole
5. chest pain: ____________________ pectoris
6. inflammation of a vein: ____________________itis
7. widening of a vessel: vaso____________________
8. enlargement of the heart: cardio____________________
9. hardening of arteries with fatty plaque: ____________________sclerosis
10. swollen veins in the rectal region: ____________________oids

P **Match the following terms with their meanings below.**

aneurysmorrhaphy	catheter ablation	pericardiocentesis
atherectomy	embolectomy	STEMI
BNP test	endarterectomy	thrombolytic therapy
CABG	PCI	valvotomy

1. incision of a heart valve ____________________
2. removal of a clot that has traveled into a blood vessel and suddenly caused occlusion ____________________
3. coronary artery bypass grafting (to relieve ischemia) ____________________
4. surgical puncture to remove fluid from the pericardial space ____________________
5. insertion of a balloon-tipped catheter and stents into a coronary artery ____________________
6. removal of the inner lining of an artery to make it wider ____________________
7. suture (repair) of a ballooned-out portion of an artery ____________________
8. removal of plaque from an artery ____________________
9. type of acute coronary syndrome ____________________
10. use of streptokinase and tPA to dissolve clots ____________________
11. brief delivery of radiofrequency energy destroys areas of heart tissue to treat arrhythmias ____________________
12. measures a peptide elevated in patients with heart failure ____________________

Q **Select the boldface term that best completes each sentence.**

1. Bill was having pain in his chest that radiated up his neck and down his arm. He called his family physician, who thought Bill should report to the local hospital's emergency department (ED) immediately. The first test performed in the ED was a/an **(stress test, ECG, CABG)**.
2. Dr. Kelly explained to the family that their observation of the bluish color of baby Charles's skin helped her make the diagnosis of a/an **(thrombotic, aneurysmal, septal)** defect in the baby's heart, which needed immediate attention.
3. Mr. Duggan had a fever of unknown origin. When the doctors completed an echocardiogram and saw vegetations on his mitral valve, they suspected **(bacterial endocarditis, hypertensive heart disease, angina)**.
4. Claudia's hands turned red, almost purple, whenever she went out into the cold or became stressed. Her physician thought it might be wise to evaluate her for **(varicose veins, Raynaud disease, intermittent claudication)**.
5. Daisy's heart felt like it was skipping beats every time she drank coffee. Her physician suggested that she wear a/an **(Holter monitor, LVAD, CABG)** for 24 hours to assess the nature of the arrhythmia.

6. Paola's father and grandfather died of heart attacks. Her physician tells her that she has inherited a tendency to accumulate fats in her bloodstream. Blood tests reveal high levels of **(enzymes, lipids, nitroglycerin)**. Discussing her family history with her **(gynecologist, hematologist, cardiologist)**, she understands that she has familial **(hypocholesterolemia, hypercholesterolemia, cardiomyopathy)**.

7. While exercising, Bernard experienced a pain (cramp) in his calf muscle. The pain disappeared when he was resting. After performing **(Holter monitoring, Doppler ultrasound, echocardiography)** on his leg to assess blood flow, Dr. Shaw found **(stenosis, fibrillation, endocarditis)**, indicating poor circulation. She recommended a daily exercise program, low-fat diet, careful foot care, and antiplatelet drug therapy to treat Bernard's intermittent **(palpitations, hypertension, claudication)**.

8. Carol noticed that her 6-week-old son Louis had a slightly bluish or **(jaundiced, cyanotic, diastolic)** coloration to his skin. She consulted a pediatric **(dermatologist, hematologist, cardiologist)**, who performed **(echocardiography, PET scan, endarterectomy)** and diagnosed Louis's condition as **(endocarditis, congestive heart disease, tetralogy of Fallot)**.

9. Seventy-eight-year-old John Smith has had coronary artery disease and high blood pressure for the past 10 years. His history included an acute heart attack, or **(MI, PDA, CABG)**. He often was tired and complained of **(dyspnea, nausea, migraine headaches)** and swelling in his ankles. His physician diagnosed his condition as **(aortic aneurysm, congestive heart failure, congenital heart disease)** and recommended restricted salt intake, diuretics, and an **(ACE inhibitor, antibiotic, analgesic)**.

10. Sarah had a routine checkup that included **(auscultation, vasoconstriction, vasodilation)** of her chest with a **(catheter, stent, stethoscope)** to listen to her heart. Her physician noticed a midsystolic murmur characteristic of **(DVT, MVP, LDL)**. An echocardiogram confirmed the diagnosis.

ANSWERS TO EXERCISES

A

1. tricuspid valve
2. capillary
3. pulmonary vein
4. aorta
5. superior vena cava
6. atrium
7. pulmonary artery
8. arteriole
9. mitral valve
10. inferior vena cava
11. venule
12. ventricle

B

1. right atrium
2. tricuspid valve
3. right ventricle
4. pulmonary valve
5. pulmonary artery
6. capillaries of the lung
7. pulmonary veins
8. left atrium
9. mitral valve
10. left ventricle
11. aortic valve
12. aorta

C

1. sinoatrial (SA) node
2. pericardium
3. interatrial septum
4. diastole
5. atrioventricular bundle or bundle of His
6. endocardium
7. systole
8. carbon dioxide (CO_2)
9. atrioventricular (AV) node
10. visceral pericardium (the outer lining is the parietal pericardium)
11. murmur
12. pulse

D

1. arteriosclerosis
2. cardiomyopathy
3. cardiomegaly
4. phlebitis
5. tachycardia
6. bradycardia
7. hypercholesterolemia
8. valvuloplasty
9. hypoxia
10. atrial
11. mitral stenosis
12. thrombolysis

E

1. bluish discoloration of the skin owing to deficient oxygen in the blood
2. incision of a vein
3. new connection between arteries
4. circulatory failure due to poor heart function
5. mass of yellowish plaque (fatty substance)
6. abnormal heart rhythm
7. instrument to measure blood pressure
8. instrument to listen to sounds within the chest
9. inflammation of the mitral valve
10. hardening of arteries with a yellowish, fatty substance (plaque)
11. narrowing of a vessel
12. widening of a vessel

F

1. endocarditis
2. flutter
3. atrial septal defect
4. mitral valve prolapse
5. coronary artery disease
6. hypertensive heart disease
7. fibrillation
8. pericarditis
9. congestive heart failure
10. tetralogy of Fallot
11. coarctation of the aorta
12. patent ductus arteriosus

G

1. failure of proper conduction of impulses through the AV node to the atrioventricular bundle (bundle of His)
2. sudden unexpected stoppage of heart action
3. uncomfortable sensations in the chest associated with arrhythmias
4. battery-operated device that is placed in the chest and wired to send electrical current to the heart to establish a normal sinus rhythm
5. blockage of a vessel by a clot
6. chest pain resulting from insufficient oxygen being supplied to the heart muscle (ischemia)
7. area of necrosis (tissue death in the heart muscle; heart attack)
8. abnormal condition of death (dead tissue)
9. damage or death of tissue due to deprivation of oxygen
10. blood is held back from an area of the body
11. nitrate drug used in the treatment of angina
12. drug that treats arrhythmias and strengthens the heartbeat
13. abnormal sound (murmur) heard on auscultation
14. vibration felt on palpation of the chest
15. consequences of plaque rupture in coronary arteries; MI and unstable angina
16. scraping or grating noise on auscultation of heart; indicates pericarditis
17. clot formation in a large vein, usually in lower limb
18. device enabling ventricles to beat in synchrony; cardiac resynchronization therapy

H

1. vegetations
2. emboli
3. petechiae
4. murmur
5. auscultation
6. rheumatic heart disease
7. essential hypertension
8. secondary hypertension
9. Raynaud disease
10. aneurysm
11. claudication
12. peripheral arterial disease

I

1. beta-blockers, ACE inhibitors, statins, aspirin, calcium channel blockers
2. varicose veins
3. hemorrhoids
4. a. pulmonary artery stenosis
   b. ventricular septal defect
   c. shift of the aorta to the right
   d. hypertrophy of the right ventricle

J

1. endarterectomy
2. defibrillation
3. lipid tests (profile)
4. stress test
5. cardiac biomarkers
6. angiography (arteriography)
7. electrocardiography
8. thallium 201 scan
9. echocardiography
10. lipoprotein electrophoresis
11. coronary artery bypass grafting
12. cardiac MRI

K

1. Video equipment and a computer produce x-ray pictures of blood vessels by taking two pictures (without and with contrast) and subtracting the first image (without contrast) from the second.
2. A donor heart is transferred to a recipient.
3. Exercise tolerance test combined with a radioactive tracer scan.
4. An instrument that focuses sound waves on a blood vessel to measure blood flow.
5. A compact version of an electrocardiograph is worn during a 24-hour period to detect cardiac arrhythmias.
6. Treatment with drugs (streptokinase and tPA) to dissolve clots after a heart attack.
7. A heart-lung machine is used to divert blood from the heart and lungs during surgery. The machine oxygenates the blood and sends it back into the bloodstream.
8. A catheter (tube) is inserted into an artery or vein and threaded into the heart chambers. Contrast can be injected to take x-ray pictures, patterns of blood flow can be detected, and blood pressures can be measured.
9. A balloon-tipped catheter is inserted into a coronary artery to open the artery; stents are put in place.
10. Stents are expandable slotted tubes that are placed in arteries during PCI. They release polymers that prevent plaque from reforming.
11. Electron beams and CT identify calcium deposits in and around coronary arteries to diagnose CAD.
12. X-ray images of the heart and coronary arteries obtained using CT technology.

L

1. atrial fibrillation
2. ventricular tachycardia
3. ventricular fibrillation
4. premature ventricular contraction
5. premature atrial contraction

M

1. congestive heart failure
2. ventricular septal defect
3. myocardial infarction
4. patent ductus arteriosus
5. mitral valve prolapse
6. aortic stenosis
7. coronary artery disease
8. atrial septal defect

N

1. cTnI or cTnT: cardiac troponin-I and troponin-T
2. LVAD: left ventricular assist device
3. TEE: transesophageal echocardiography
4. ICD: implantable cardioverter-defibrillator
5. RFA: radiofrequency catheter ablation
6. ETT: exercise tolerance test
7. ECHO: echocardiography
8. ETT-MIBI: exercise tolerance test with sesta<u>mibi</u> scan
9. ECMO: extracorporeal membrane oxygenation
10. CRT: cardiac resynchronization therapy
11. LDL: low-density lipoprotein; high levels indicate risk for CAD
12. BNP: brain natriuretic peptide

O

1. coronary
2. arrhythmia
3. cyanosis
4. diastole
5. angina pectoris
6. phlebitis
7. vasodilation
8. cardiomegaly
9. atherosclerosis
10. hemorrhoids

P

1. valvotomy
2. embolectomy
3. CABG
4. pericardiocentesis
5. PCI
6. endarterectomy
7. aneurysmorrhaphy
8. atherectomy
9. STEMI (ST segment elevation myocardial infarction)
10. thrombolytic therapy
11. catheter ablation
12. BNP test

Q

1. ECG
2. septal
3. bacterial endocarditis
4. Raynaud disease
5. Holter monitor
6. lipids; cardiologist; hypercholesterolemia
7. Doppler ultrasound; stenosis; claudication
8. cyanotic; cardiologist; echocardiography; tetralogy of Fallot
9. MI; dyspnea; congestive heart failure; ACE inhibitor
10. auscultation; stethoscope; MVP

Answers to Practical Applications

Operating Room Schedule

1. E	5. D	8. J
2. C	6. A	9. G
3. H	7. B	10. F
4. I		

Clinical Cases: What's Your Diagnosis?

Case 1	*Case 2*	*Case 3*
1. b	1. d	1. d
	2. a	2. a
	3. b	

PRONUNCIATION OF TERMS

To test your understanding of the terminology in this chapter, write the meaning of each term in the space provided. In addition, you may wish to cover the terms and write them by looking at your definitions. Make sure your spelling is correct. The page number after each term indicates where it is defined or used in the book, so you can easily check your responses. You will find complete definitions for all of these terms and their audio pronunciations on the Evolve website.

Pronunciation Guide

ā as in āpe	ă as in ăpple
ē as in ēven	ĕ as in ĕvery
ī as in īce	ĭ as in ĭnterest
ō as in ōpen	ŏ as in pŏt
ū as in ūnit	ŭ as in ŭnder

Vocabulary and Terminology

TERM	PRONUNCIATION	MEANING
angiogram (409)	ĂN-jē-ō-grăm	______________
angioplasty (409)	ĂN-jē-ō-plăs-tē	______________
anoxia (411)	ă-NŎK-sē-ă	______________
aorta (408)	ā-ŌR-tă	______________
aortic stenosis (409)	ā-ŌR-tĭk stĕ-NŌ-sĭs	______________
apex of the heart (408)	Ā-pĕks of the hărt	______________
arrhythmia (411)	ā-RĬTH-mē-ă	______________
arterial anastomosis (409)	ăr-TĒ-rē-ăl ă-năs-tō-MŌ-sĭs	______________
arteriography (409)	ăr-tē-rē-ŎG-ră-fē	______________
arteriole (408)	ăr-TĒ-rē-ōl	______________
arteriosclerosis (409)	ăr-tē-rē-ō-sklĕ-RŌ-sĭs	______________
artery (408)	ĂR-tĕ-rē	______________
atherectomy (410)	ă-thĕ-RĔK-tō-mē	______________
atheroma (410)	ăth-ĕr-Ō-mă	______________
atherosclerosis (410)	ăth-ĕr-ō-sklĕ-RŌ-sĭs	______________

TERM	PRONUNCIATION	MEANING
atrial (410)	Ā-trē-ăl	
atrioventricular bundle (408)	ā-trē-ō-vĕn-TRĬK-ū-lăr BŬN-dl	
atrioventricular node (408)	ā-trē-ō-vĕn-TRĬK-ū-lăr nōd	
atrium; atria (408)	Ā-trē-ŭm; Ā-trē-ă	
brachial artery (410)	BRĀ-kē-ăl ĂR-tĕ-rē	
bradycardia (410)	brād-ē-KĂR-dē-ă	
bundle of His (408)	BŬN-dl of Hĭss	
capillary (408)	KĂP-ĭ-lăr-ē	
carbon dioxide (408)	KĂR-bŏn dī-ŎK-sīd	
cardiogenic shock (410)	kăr-dē-ō-JĔN-ĭk shŏk	
cardiomegaly (410)	kăr-dē-ō-MĔG-ă-lē	
cardiomyopathy (410)	kăr-dē-ō-mī-ŎP-ă-thē	
coronary arteries (408)	KŎR-ō-năr-ē ĂR-tĕ-rēz	
cyanosis (411)	sī-ă-NŌ-sĭs	
deoxygenated blood (408)	dē-ŎK-sĭ-jĕ-NĀ-tĕd blŭd	
diastole (408)	dī-ĂS-tō-lē	
electrocardiogram (408)	ĕ-lĕk-trō-KĂR-dē-ō-grăm	
endocardium (408)	ĕn-dō-KĂR-dē-ŭm	
endothelium (408)	ĕn-dō-THĒ-lē-um	
hypercholesterolemia (410)	hī-pĕr-kō-lĕs-tĕr-ŏl-Ē-mē-ă	
hypoxia (411)	hī-PŎK-sē-ă	
interventricular septum (412)	ĭn-tĕr-vĕn-TRĬK-ū-lăr SĔP-tŭm	
mitral valve (408)	MĪ-trăl vălv	
mitral valvulitis (412)	MĪ-trăl văl-vū-LĪ-tĭs	
myocardium (408)	mī-ō-KĂR-dē-ŭm	
myxoma (411)	mĭk-SŌ-mă	
normal sinus rhythm (408)	NŎR-măl SĪ-nus RĬ-thĕm	
oxygen (408)	ŎK-sĭ-jĕn	
pacemaker (408)	PĀS-mā-kĕr	
pericardiocentesis (411)	pĕr-ĭ-kăr-dē-ō-sĕn-TĒ-sĭs	
pericardium (408)	pĕr-ĭ-KĂR-dē-ŭm	

TERM	PRONUNCIATION	MEANING
phlebotomy (411)	flĕ-BŎT-ō-mē	
pulmonary artery (408)	PŬL-mō-nĕr-ē ĂR-tĕr-ē	
pulmonary circulation (408)	PŬL-mō-nĕr-ē sĕr-kū-LĀ-shŭn	
pulmonary valve (409)	PŬL-mō-nĕr-ē vălv	
pulmonary vein (409)	PŬL-mō-nĕr-ē vān	
pulse (409)	pŭls	
septum; septa (409)	SĔP-tŭm; SĔP-tă	
sinoatrial node (409)	sī-nō-Ā-trē-ăl nōd	
sphygmomanometer (409)	sfĭg-mō-mă-NŎM-ĕ-tĕr	
stethoscope (411)	STĔTH-ō-skōp	
systemic circulation (409)	sĭs-TĔM-ĭk sĕr-kū-LĀ-shŭn	
systole (409)	SĬS-tō-lē	
tachycardia (410)	tăk-ē-KĂR-dē-ă	
thrombolysis (411)	thrŏm-BŎL-ĭ-sĭs	
thrombophlebitis (411)	thrŏm-bō-flĕ-BĪ-tĭs	
tricuspid valve (409)	trī-KŬS-pĭd vălv	
valve (409)	vălv	
valvotomy (412)	văl-VŎT-ō-mē	
valvuloplasty (412)	văl-vū-lō-PLĂS-tē	
vascular (412)	VĂS-kū-lăr	
vasoconstriction (412)	văz-ō-kŏn-STRĬK-shŭn	
vasodilation (412)	văz-ō-dī-LĀ-shŭn	
vein (409)	vān	
vena cava; venae cavae (409)	VĒ-nă KĀ-vă; VĒ-nē KĀ-vē	
venipuncture (412)	vĕ-nĭ-PŬNK-chŭr	
venous (412)	VĒ-nŭs	
ventricle (409)	VĔN-trĭ-kl	
venule (409)	VĔN-ūl	

Pathology, Laboratory Tests, and Clinical Procedures

TERM	PRONUNCIATION	MEANING
ACE inhibitor (424)	ĀCE ĭn-HĬB-ĭ-tŏr	
acute coronary syndromes (424)	ă-KŪT kŏr-ō-NĂR-ē SĬN-drōmz	
aneurysm (421)	ĂN-ū-rĭzm	
angina (424)	ăn-JĪ-nă *or* ĂN-jĭ-nă	
angiography (425)	ăn-jē-ŎG-ră-fē	
atrioventricular block (412)	ā-trē-ō-vĕn-TRĬK-ū-lăr blŏk	
atrial fibrillation (414)	Ā-trē-ăl fĭb-rĭ-LĀ-shŭn	
auscultation (424)	ăw-skŭl-TĀ-shŭn	
beta-blocker (424)	BĀ-tă-BLŎK-ĕr	
biventricular pacemaker (424)	bī-vĕn-TRĬK-ū-lăr PĀS-mā-kĕr	
BNP test (425)	BNP tĕst	
bruit (424)	BRŪ-ē	
calcium channel blocker (424)	KĂL-sē-ŭm CHĂ-nĕl BLŎK-ĕr	
cardiac arrest (424)	KĂR-dē-ăk ā-RĔST	
cardiac catheterization (428)	KĂR-dē-ăk kăth-ĕ-tĕr-ĭ-ZĀ-shŭn	
cardiac MRI (428)	KĂR-dē-ăk MRI	
cardiac biomarkers (425)	KĂR-dē-ăk BĪ-ō-mar-kerz	
cardiac tamponade (424)	KĂR-dē-ăk tăm-pō-NŎD	
cardioversion (430)	kăr-dē-ō-VĔR-zhŭn	
catheter ablation (430)	KĂTH-ĕ-tĕr ăb-LĀ-shŭn	
claudication (424)	klăw-dĕ-KĀ-shŭn	
coarctation of the aorta (415)	kō-ărk-TĀ-shŭn of the ā-ŎR-tă	
computed tomography angiography (426)	kŏm-PŪ-tĕd tō-MŎG-ră-fē ăn-jē-ŎG-ră-fē	
congenital heart disease (415)	kŏn-GĔN-ĭ-tăl hărt dĭ-ZĒZ	
congestive heart failure (417)	kŏn-GĔS-tĭv hărt FĀL-ŭr	
coronary artery disease (417)	kŏr-ō-NĂR-ē ĂR-tĕ-rē dĭ-ZĒZ	
coronary artery bypass grafting (430)	kŏr-ō-NĂR-ē ĂR-tĕ-rē BĪ-păs GRĂF-tĭng	
deep vein thrombosis (422)	dēp vān thrŏm-BŌ-sĭs	
defibrillation (430)	dē-fĭb-rĭ-LĀ-shun	

TERM	PRONUNCIATION	MEANING
digoxin (424)	dĭ-JŎK-sĭn	
digital subtraction angiography (426)	DĬJ-ĭ-tăl sŭb-TRĂK-shŭn ăn-jē-ŎG-ră-fē	
Doppler ultrasound (426)	DŎP-lĕr ŬL-tră-sŏnd	
dysrhythmia (412)	dĭs-RĬTH-mē-ă	
echocardiography (427)	ĕk-ō-kăr-dē-ŌG-ră-fē	
electrocardiography (428)	ē-lĕk-trō-kăr-dē-ŎG-ră-fē	
electron beam computed tomography (426)	ē-LĔK-trŏn bēm kŏm-PŪ-tĕd tō-MŎG-ră-fē	
embolus; emboli (424)	ĔM-bō-lŭs; ĔM-bō-lī	
endarterectomy (431)	ĕnd-ăr-tĕr-ĔK-tō-mē	
endocarditis (420)	ĕn-dō-kăr-DĪ-tĭs	
extracorporeal circulation (431)	ĕks-tră-kŏr-PŎR-ē-ăl sĕr-kū-LĀ-shŭn	
fibrillation (414)	fĭb-rĭ-LĀ-shŭn	
flutter (414)	FLŬ-tĕr	
heart block (412)	hărt blŏk	
heart transplantation (431)	hărt trănz-plăn-TĀ-shŭn	
hemorrhoids (423)	HĔM-ō-roydz	
Holter monitoring (429)	HŌL-tĕr MŎN-ĭ-tĕ-rĭng	
hypertension (422)	hī-pĕr-TĔN-shŭn	
hypertensive heart disease (420)	hī-pĕr-TĔN-sĭv hărt dĭ-ZĒZ	
implantable cardioverter-defibrillator (414)	ĭm-PLĂNT-ă-bŭl kăr-dē-ō-VĔR-tĕr dē-FĬB-rĭ-lā-tŏr	
infarction (424)	ĭn-FĂRK-shŭn	
ischemia (423)	ĭs-KĒ-mē-ă	
left ventricular assist device (417)	lĕft vĕn-TRĬ-kū-lăr ă-SĬST dē-VĪS	
lipid tests (425)	LĬ-pĭd tĕsts	
lipoprotein electrophoresis (425)	lī-pō-PRŌ-tēn ē-lĕk-trō-fŏr-Ē-sĭs	
mitral stenosis (421)	MĪ-trăl stĕ-NŌ-sĭs	
mitral valve prolapse (420)	MĪ-trăl vălv PRŌ-laps	
murmur (420)	MŬR-mĕr	

TERM	PRONUNCIATION	MEANING
myocardial infarction (418)	mī-ō-KĂR-dē-ăl ĭn-FĂRK-shŭn	
nitrates (424)	nī-TRĀTZ	
nitroglycerin (424)	nī-trō-GLĬS-ĕr-ĭn	
occlusion (424)	ŏ-KLŪ-jŭn	
palpitations (424)	păl-pĭ-TĀ-shŭnz	
patent (424)	PĀ-tĕnt	
patent ductus arteriosus (415)	PĀ-tĕnt DŬK-tŭs ăr-tēr-ē-Ō-sŭs	
percutaneous coronary intervention (431)	pĕr-kū-TĀ-nē-ŭs KŎR-ō-năr-ē ĭn-tĕr-VĔN-shŭn	
pericardial friction rub (424)	pĕr-ĭ-KĂR-dē-ăl FRĬK-shŭn rŭb	
pericarditis (420)	pĕr-ĭ-kăr-DĪ-tĭs	
peripheral arterial disease (422)	pĕ-RĬ-fĕr-ăl ăr-TĒ-rē-ăl dĭ-ZĒZ	
petechiae (424)	pĕ-TĒ-kē-ē	
positron emission tomography (427)	pŏs-ĭ-tron ē-MĬSH-un tō-MŎG-ră-fē	
Raynaud disease (423)	rā-NŌ dĭ-ZĒZ	
rheumatic heart disease (421)	roo-MĂT-ik hărt dĭ-ZĒZ	
septal defects (416)	SĔP-tăl DĒ-fĕkts	
statins (424)	STĂ-tĭnz	
stress test (429)	STRĔS tĕst	
telemetry (428)	tĕl-ĔM-ĕ-trē	
tetralogy of Fallot (416)	tĕ-TRĂL-ō-jē of fă-LŌ	
technetium Tc99m sestamibi scan (427)	tĕk-NĒ-shē-ŭm Tc99m sĕs-tă-MĬ-bē skăn	
thallium 201 scan (427)	THĂL-ē-um 201 skăn	
thrill (424)	thrĭl	
thrombolytic therapy (432)	thrŏm-bō-LĬ-tĭk THĔ-ră-pē	
thrombotic occlusion (418)	thrŏm-BŎT-ĭk ŏ-KLŪ-zhĕn	
transcatheter aortic valve replacement (432)	trănz-KĂTH-ĕ-tĕr ā-ŎR-tĭk valve rē-PLĀS-mĕnt	
varicose veins (423)	VĂR-ĭ-kōs vānz	
vegetations (424)	vĕj-ĕ-TĀ-shŭnz	

REVIEW SHEET

Write the meanings of each word part in the space provided. Check your answers with the information in the chapter or in the Glossary (Medical Word Parts—English) at the end of the book.

Combining Forms

COMBINING FORM	MEANING	COMBINING FORM	MEANING
aneurysm/o	______	ox/o	______
angi/o	______	pericardi/o	______
aort/o	______	phleb/o	______
arter/o, arteri/o	______	pulmon/o	______
ather/o	______	rrhythm/o	______
atri/o	______	sphygm/o	______
axill/o	______	steth/o	______
brachi/o	______	thromb/o	______
cardi/o	______	valv/o	______
cholesterol/o	______	valvul/o	______
coron/o	______	vas/o	______
cyan/o	______	vascul/o	______
isch/o	______	ven/o, ven/i	______
my/o	______	ventricul/o	______
myx/o	______		

Suffixes

SUFFIX	MEANING	SUFFIX	MEANING
-constriction	______	-oma	______
-dilation	______	-osis	______
-emia	______	-plasty	______
-graphy	______	-sclerosis	______
-lysis	______	-stenosis	______
-megaly	______	-tomy	______
-meter	______		

Prefixes

PREFIX	MEANING	PREFIX	MEANING
a-, an-	________________	hypo-	________________
brady-	________________	inter-	________________
de-	________________	peri-	________________
dys-	________________	tachy-	________________
endo-	________________	tetra-	________________
hyper-	________________	tri-	________________

Use the following terms to complete the chart below.

aorta	lung capillaries	right atrium
inferior vena cava	mitral valve	right ventricle
left atrium	pulmonary artery	superior vena cava
left ventricle	pulmonary vein	tricuspid valve

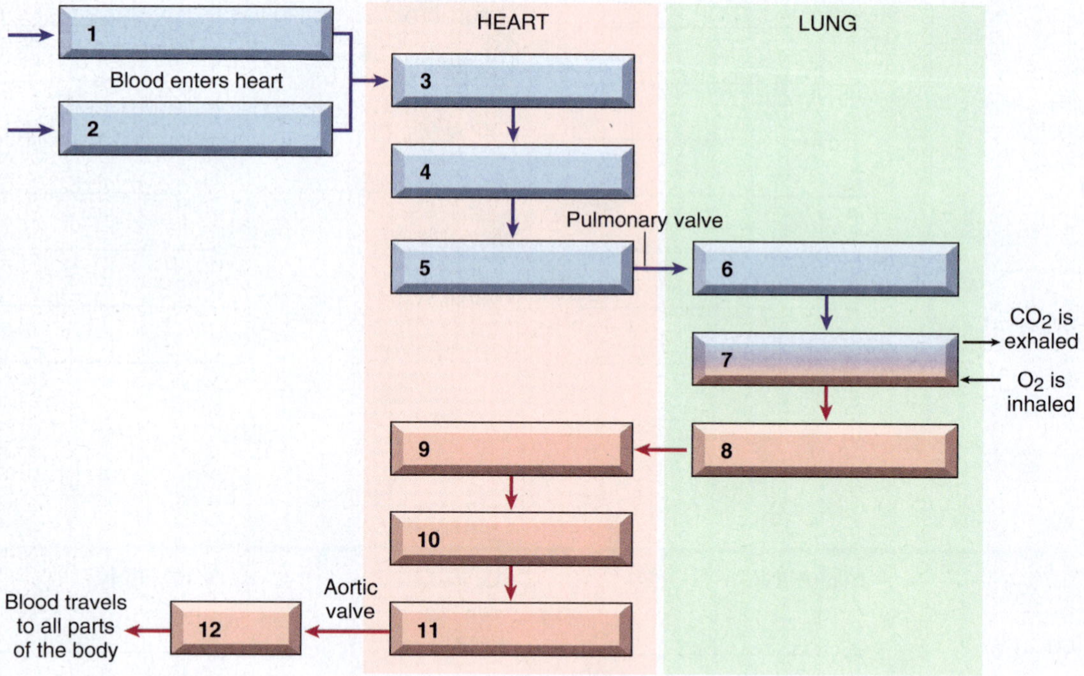

evolve *Please visit the Evolve website for additional exercises, games, and images related to this chapter.*

CHAPTER 12

Respiratory System

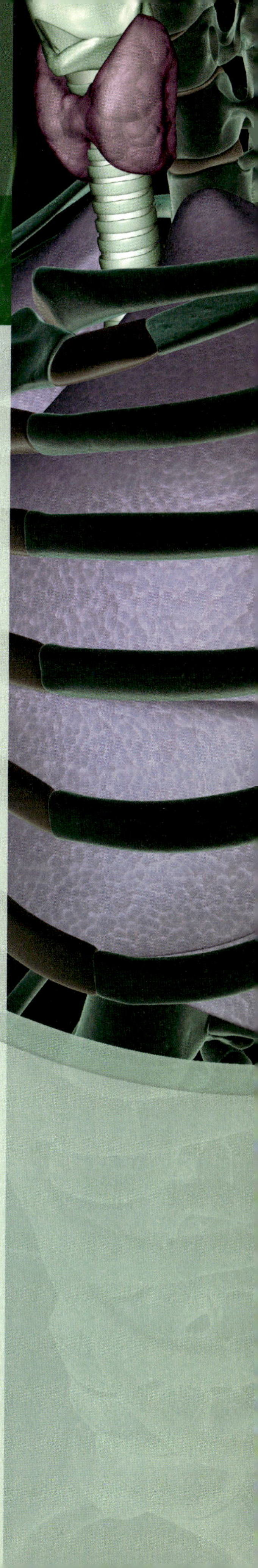

This chapter is divided into the following sections:

CHAPTER GOALS

- Name the organs of the respiratory system and their location and function.
- Identify pathologic conditions that affect the respiratory system.
- Learn medical terms that pertain to respiration.
- Describe important clinical procedures related to the respiratory system, and recognize relevant abbreviations.
- Apply your new knowledge to understanding medical terms in their proper contexts, such as medical reports and records.

INTRODUCTION

We usually think of **respiration** as the mechanical process of breathing, the exchange of air between the lungs and the external environment. This exchange of air at the lungs is called **external respiration.** In external respiration, oxygen is inhaled (inhaled air contains about 21% oxygen) into the air spaces (sacs) of the lungs and immediately passes into tiny blood vessels (capillaries) surrounding the air spaces. Simultaneously, carbon dioxide, a gas produced when oxygen and food combine in cells, passes from the capillary blood vessels into the air spaces of the lungs to be exhaled.

Whereas external respiration occurs between the outside environment and the capillary blood of the lungs, another form of respiration occurs simultaneously between the individual body cells and the tiny capillary blood vessels that surround them. This is **internal (cellular) respiration,** which involves an exchange of gases at the level of the cells within all organs of the body. Here, oxygen passes out of the capillaries into tissue cells. At the same time, carbon dioxide passes from tissue cells into the capillaries to travel to the lungs for exhalation.

ANATOMY AND PHYSIOLOGY OF RESPIRATION

Label Figure 12-1 as you read the following paragraphs.

Air enters the body via the **nose** [1] through two openings called nostrils or **nares.** Air then passes through the **nasal cavity** [2], lined with a mucous membrane and fine hairs **(cilia)** to help filter out foreign bodies, as well as to warm and moisten the air. **Paranasal sinuses** [3] are hollow, air-containing spaces within the skull that communicate with the nasal cavity. They, too, have a mucous membrane lining. Besides producing mucus, a lubricating fluid, the sinuses lighten the bones of the skull and help produce sound.

After passing through the nasal cavity, the air next reaches the **pharynx (throat).** There are three divisions of the pharynx. The first is the **nasopharynx** [4]. It contains the **pharyngeal tonsils,** or **adenoids** [5], which are collections of lymphatic tissue. They are more prominent in children and, if enlarged, can obstruct air passageways. Below the nasopharynx and closer to the mouth is the second division of the pharynx, the **oropharynx** [6]. The **palatine tonsils** [7], two rounded masses of lymphatic tissue, are in the oropharynx. The third division of the pharynx, the **laryngopharynx** [8], serves as a common passageway for food from the mouth and air from the nose. It divides into the **larynx (voice box)** [9] and the **esophagus** [10].

The esophagus leads into the stomach and carries food to be digested. The larynx contains the vocal cords and is surrounded by pieces of cartilage for support. The thyroid cartilage is the largest and in men is commonly referred to as the Adam's apple. As expelled air passes the vocal cords, they vibrate to produce sounds. The tension of the vocal cords determines the high or low pitch of the voice.

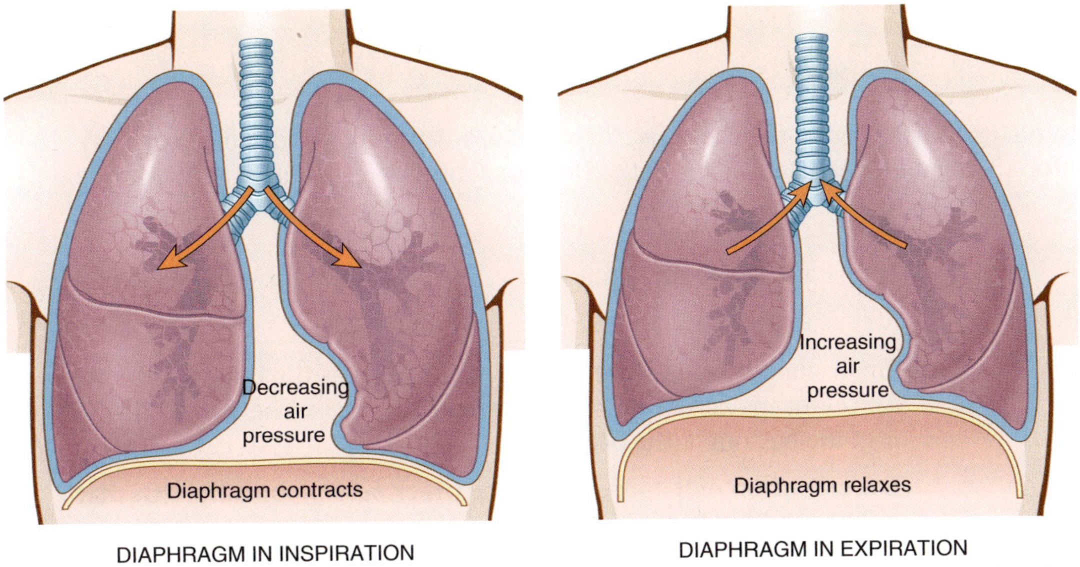

FIGURE 12-3 **Position of the diaphragm during inspiration (inhalation) and expiration (exhalation).**

increasing air pressure in the chest. Air then is expelled out of the lungs to equalize the pressure; this is **exhalation (expiration).**

Figure 12-3 shows the position of the diaphragm in inspiration and in expiration.

Figure 12-4 is a flow diagram of the pathway of air from the nose, where air enters the body, to the capillaries of the lungs, where oxygen enters the bloodstream.

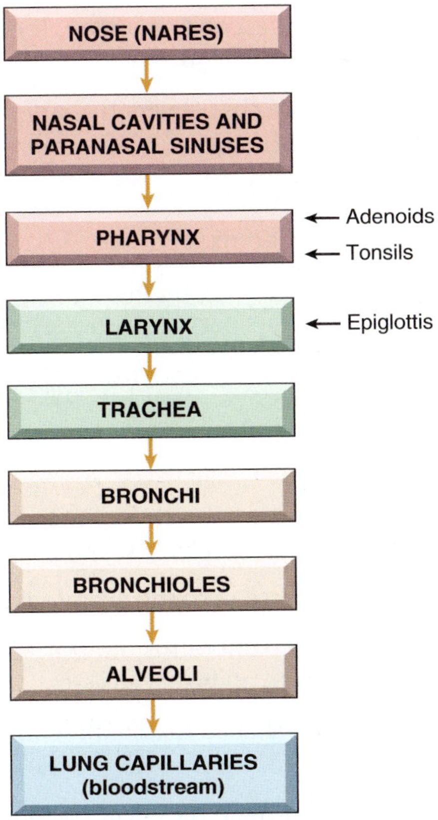

FIGURE 12-4 **Pathway of air from the nose to the capillaries of the lungs.**

12

VOCABULARY

This list reviews terminology introduced in the previous section. Short definitions and additional information will reinforce your understanding. Refer to the Pronunciation of Terms on page 494 for help with difficult or unfamiliar words.

adenoids	Lymphatic tissue in the nasopharynx; pharyngeal tonsils.
alveolus (*plural*: **alveoli**)	Air sac in the lung.
apex of the lung	Tip or uppermost portion of the lung. An apex is the tip of a structure. **Apical** means pertaining to or located at the apex. The apex of the heart is at the bottom of the heart.
base of the lung	Lower portion of the lung; from the Greek *basis*, foundation. **Basilar** means located at or in the base.
bronchioles	Smallest branches of the bronchi. Terminal bronchioles lead to alveolar ducts.
bronchus (*plural*: **bronchi**)	Branch of the trachea (windpipe) that is a passageway into the lung; bronchial tube.
carbon dioxide (CO_2)	Gas produced by body cells when oxygen and carbon atoms from food combine; exhaled through the lungs.
cilia	Thin hairs attached to the mucous membrane epithelium lining the respiratory tract. They clear bacteria and foreign substances from the lung. Cigarette smoke impairs the function of cilia.
diaphragm	Muscle separating the chest and abdomen. It contracts to pull air into the lungs and relaxes to push air out.
epiglottis	Lid-like piece of cartilage that covers the larynx, preventing food from entering the larynx and trachea during swallowing.
expiration	Breathing out (exhalation).
glottis	Slit-like opening to the larynx.
hilum of the lung	Midline region where the bronchi, blood vessels, and nerves enter and exit the lungs. **Hilar** means pertaining to (at) the hilum.
inspiration	Breathing in (inhalation).
larynx	Voice box; containing the vocal cords.
lobe	Division of a lung.
mediastinum	Region between the lungs in the chest cavity. It contains the trachea, heart, lymph nodes, aorta, esophagus, and bronchial tubes.
nares	Openings through the nose carrying air into the nasal cavities.
oxygen (O_2)	Gas that makes up 21 percent of the air. It passes into the bloodstream at the lungs and travels to all body cells.
palatine tonsil	One of a pair of almond-shaped masses of lymphatic tissue in the oropharynx (palatine means pertaining to the roof of the mouth).
paranasal sinus	One of the air cavities in the bones near the nose.
parietal pleura	Outer layer of pleura lying closer to the ribs and chest wall.

pharynx	Throat; including the nasopharynx, oropharynx, and laryngopharynx.
pleura	Double-layered membrane surrounding each lung.
pleural cavity	Space between the folds of the pleura.
pulmonary parenchyma	Essential parts of the lung, responsible for respiration; bronchioles and alveoli.
respiration	Process of moving air into and out of the lungs; breathing
trachea	Windpipe.
visceral pleura	Inner layer of pleura lying closer to the lung tissue.

TERMINOLOGY

Write the meanings of the medical terms in the spaces provided.

COMBINING FORMS

COMBINING FORM	MEANING	TERMINOLOGY	MEANING
adenoid/o	adenoids	adenoidectomy	________________
		adenoid hypertrophy	________________
alveol/o	alveolus, air sac	alveolar	________________
bronch/o bronchi/o	bronchial tube, bronchus	bronchospasm *This tightening of the bronchus is a chief characteristic of asthma and bronchitis.*	________________
		bronchiectasis *Caused by weakening of the bronchial wall from infection.*	________________
		bronchodilator *This drug causes dilation, or enlargement, of the opening of a bronchus to improve ventilation to the lungs. An example is albuterol, delivered via an inhaler.*	________________
		bronchopleural *A **bronchopleural fistula** is an abnormal connection between the bronchial tube and the pleural cavity (space). Occurring as a result of lung disease or surgical complication, this can cause an air leak into the pleural space.*	________________
bronchiol/o	bronchiole, small bronchus	bronchiolitis *This is an acute viral infection occurring in infants younger than 18 months of age.*	________________
capn/o	carbon dioxide	hypercapnia	________________
coni/o	dust	pneumoconiosis *See page 472.*	________________

12

COMBINING FORM	MEANING	TERMINOLOGY	MEANING
cyan/o	blue	cyanosis ______ *Caused by deficient oxygen in the blood.*	
epiglott/o	epiglottis	epiglottitis ______ *Characterized by fever, sore throat, and an erythematous, swollen epiglottis.*	
laryng/o	larynx, voice box	laryngeal ______	
		laryngospasm ______ *Spasm of laryngeal muscles that closes the larynx.*	
		laryngitis ______	
lob/o	lobe of the lung	lobectomy ______ *Figure 12-5 shows four different types of pulmonary resections.*	

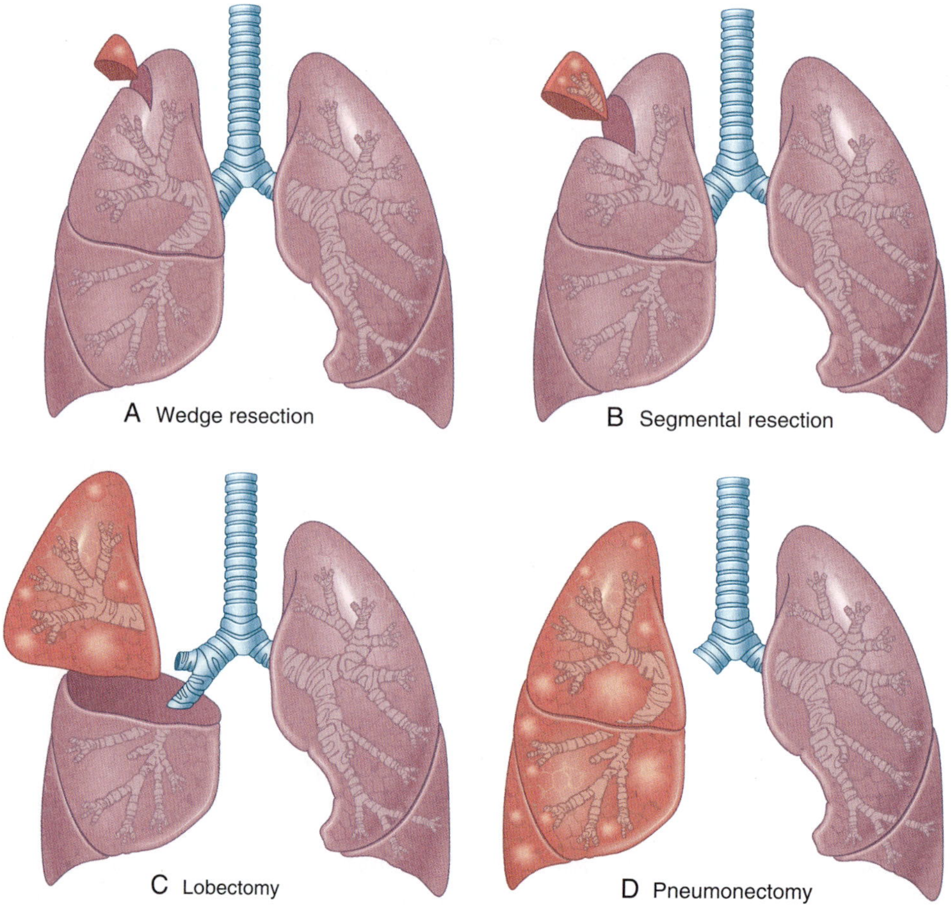

FIGURE 12-5 **Pulmonary resections. A, Wedge resection** is the removal of a small, localized area of diseased tissue near the surface of the lung. Pulmonary function and structure are relatively unchanged after healing. **B, Segmental resection** is the removal of a bronchiole and its alveoli (one or more lung segments). The remaining lung tissue expands to fill the previously occupied space. **C, Lobectomy** is the removal of an entire lobe of the lung. After lobectomy, the remaining lung increases in size to fill the space in the thoracic cavity. **D, Pneumonectomy** is the removal of an entire lung. Techniques such as removal of ribs and elevation of the diaphragm are used to reduce the size of the empty thoracic space.

COMBINING FORM	MEANING	TERMINOLOGY	MEANING
mediastin/o	mediastinum	mediastinoscopy *An endoscope is inserted through an incision in the chest.*	________________
nas/o	nose	paranasal sinuses *Para- means near in this term.*	________________
		nasogastric intubation	________________
orth/o	straight, upright	orthopnea *An abnormal condition in which breathing (-pnea) is easier in the upright position. A major cause of orthopnea is congestive heart failure (the lungs fill with fluid when the patient is lying flat). Physicians assess the degree of orthopnea by the number of pillows a patient requires to sleep comfortably (e.g., two-pillow orthopnea).*	________________
ox/o	oxygen	hypoxia *Tissues have a decreased amount of oxygen, and cyanosis can result.*	________________
pector/o	chest	expectoration *Clearing of secretions from the airway by coughing or spitting. This sputum can contain mucus, blood, cellular debris, pus, and microorganisms.*	________________
pharyng/o	pharynx, throat	pharyngeal	________________
phon/o	voice	dysphonia *Hoarseness or other voice impairment.*	________________
phren/o	diaphragm	phrenic nerve *The motor nerve to the diaphragm.*	________________
pleur/o	pleura	pleurodynia *The suffix -dynia means pain. The intercostal muscles or pleura are inflamed, causing pain during breathing.*	________________
		pleural effusion *An **effusion** is the escape of fluid from blood vessels or lymphatics into a cavity or into tissue spaces.*	________________

COMBINING FORM	MEANING	TERMINOLOGY	MEANING
pneum/o, pneumon/o	air, lung	pneumothorax *The suffix -thorax means chest. Because of a hole in the lung, air accumulates in the pleural cavity, between the layers of the pleura (Figure 12-6).*	
		pneumonectomy	
pulmon/o	lung	pulmonary	
rhin/o	nose	rhinoplasty	
		rhinorrhea *Commonly known as "runny nose."*	
sinus/o	sinus, cavity	sinusitis	
spir/o	breathing	spirometer	
		expiration *Note that the s is omitted (when it's preceded by an x).*	
		respiration ***Cheyne-Stokes respirations** are marked by rhythmic changes in the depth of breathing (rapid breathing and then absence of breathing). The pattern occurs every 45 seconds to 3 minutes. The cause may be heart failure or brain damage, both of which affect the respiratory center in the brain.*	

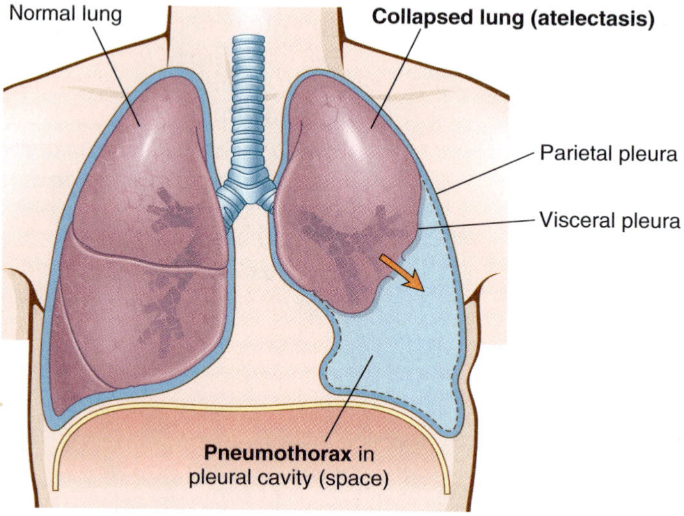

FIGURE 12-6 Pneumothorax. Air gathers in the pleural cavity, causing the lung to collapse. When this happens, the lung cannot fill up with air, breathing becomes more difficult, and the body gets less oxygen. Onset of pneumothorax is marked by sudden, sharp chest pain with difficulty breathing.

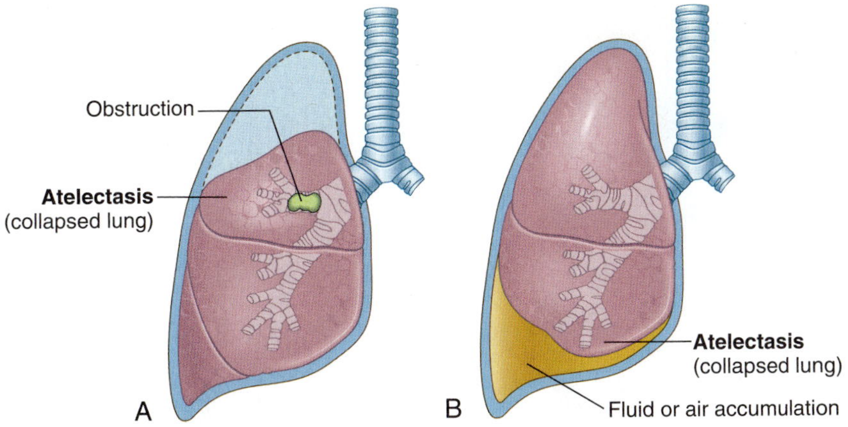

FIGURE 12-7 **Two forms of atelectasis. A,** An obstruction prevents air from reaching distal airways, and alveoli collapse. The most frequent cause is blockage of a bronchus by a mucous or mucopurulent (pus-containing) plug, as might occur postoperatively. **B,** Accumulations of fluid, blood, or air within the pleural cavity collapse the lung. This can occur with congestive heart failure (poor circulation leads to fluid buildup in the pleural cavity), pneumonia, trauma, or a pneumothorax.

COMBINING FORM	MEANING	TERMINOLOGY	MEANING
tel/o	complete	atelectasis *Collapsed lung; incomplete expansion (-ectasis) of a lung (Figure 12-7). Atelectasis may occur after surgery when a patient experiences pain and does not take deep breaths, preventing full expansion of the lungs.*	
thorac/o	chest	thoracotomy	
		thoracic	
tonsill/o	tonsils	tonsillectomy *The oropharyngeal (palatine) tonsils are removed.*	
trache/o	trachea, windpipe	tracheotomy	
		tracheal stenosis *Injury to the trachea from trauma, a burn, or serious infection can cause scarring and contraction that obstructs the flow of air. For example, having an endotracheal tube in place for a prolonged period may lead to tracheal injury or the formation of scar tissue.*	

SUFFIXES

SUFFIX	MEANING	TERMINOLOGY	MEANING
-ema	condition	empyema *Em- at the beginning of this term means in. Empyema (pyothorax) is a collection of pus in the pleural cavity.*	
-osmia	smell	anosmia	

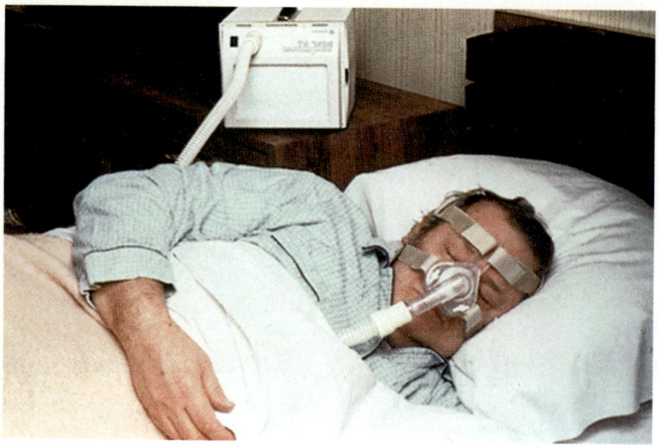

FIGURE 12-8 This man is sleeping with a **nasal CPAP (continuous positive airway pressure)** mask in place. The pressure supplied by air coming from the compressor opens the oropharynx and nasopharynx.

SUFFIX	MEANING	TERMINOLOGY	MEANING
-pnea	breathing	apnea ***Sleep apnea** is sudden cessation of breathing during sleep. It can result in hypoxia, leading to cognitive impairment, hypertension, and arrhythmias.* ***Obstructive sleep apnea (OSA)*** *involves narrowing or occlusion in the upper airway.* ***Continuous positive airway pressure (CPAP)*** *is gentle ventilatory support used to keep the airways open (Figure 12-8).*	
		dyspnea *Dys- means abnormal here and is associated with shortness of breath (SOB).* ***Paroxysmal*** *(sudden)* ***nocturnal*** *(at night)* ***dyspnea*** *may be experienced by patients with congestive heart failure when they recline in bed. Patients often describe the sensation as "air hunger."*	
		hyperpnea *An increase in the depth of breathing, occurring normally with exercise and abnormally with any condition in which the supply of oxygen is inadequate.*	
		tachypnea *Tachy- means fast. Excessively rapid and shallow breathing; hyperventilation.*	
-ptysis	spitting	hemoptysis *Blood is coughed up from the bronchial tubes and lungs; occurs with bronchitis or pneumonia, but also with tuberculosis, cancer, bronchiectasis, and pulmonary embolism.*	
-sphyxia	pulse	asphyxia *This condition, literally meaning lack of pulse, is severe hypoxia leading to hypoxemia, hypercapnia, loss of consciousness, and death.*	
-thorax	pleural cavity, chest	hemothorax	
		pyothorax *Empyema of the chest.*	

PATHOLOGY

DIAGNOSTIC TERMS

auscultation

Listening to sounds within the body.

This procedure, performed with a stethoscope, is used chiefly for listening to the passage of air into and out of the lungs and listening to heart sounds. It is helpful to diagnose conditions of the lungs, pleura, heart, and abdomen, as well as to determine the condition of the fetus during pregnancy.

percussion

Tapping on a surface to determine the difference in the density of the underlying structure.

Tapping over a solid organ produces a dull sound without resonance. Percussion over an air-filled structure, such as the lung, produces a resonant, hollow note. When the lungs or the pleural space are filled with fluid and become more dense, as in pneumonia, resonance is replaced by dullness.

pleural rub

Scratchy sound produced by pleural surfaces rubbing against each other.

Pleural rub (also called a **friction rub**) occurs when the pleura are roughened and thickened by inflammation, infection, scarring, or neoplastic cells. It is heard on auscultation and can be felt by placing the fingers on the chest wall.

rales (crackles)

Fine crackling sounds heard on auscultation (during inhalation) when there is fluid in the alveoli.

These popping or clicking sounds can be heard in patients with pneumonia, bronchiectasis, or acute bronchitis. The French word *rale* means rattle.

rhonchi (*singular:* **rhonchus**)

Loud rumbling sounds heard on auscultation of bronchi obstructed by sputum.

These coarse rumbling sounds resemble snoring and are usually caused by secretions in larger bronchial tubes.

sputum

Material expelled from the bronchi, lungs, or upper respiratory tract by spitting.

Purulent (containing pus) sputum often is green or brown. It results from infection and may be seen with asthma. Blood-tinged sputum is suggestive of tuberculosis or malignancy. For a **sputum culture**, the specimen is maintained in a nutrient medium to promote growth of a pathogen. **Culture and sensitivity (C&S)** studies identify the sputum pathogen and determine which antibiotic will be effective in destroying or reducing its growth.

stridor

Strained, high-pitched sound heard on inspiration caused by obstruction in the pharynx or larynx.

Common causes of stridor include throat abscess, airway injury, croup, allergic reaction, or epiglottitis and laryngitis.

wheezes

Continuous high-pitched whistling sounds produced during breathing.

Wheezes are heard when air is forced through narrowed or obstructed airways. Patients with asthma commonly experience wheezing as bronchi narrow and tighten.

UPPER RESPIRATORY DISORDERS

croup

Acute viral infection of infants and children with obstruction of the larynx, accompanied by barking cough and stridor.

The most common causative agents are influenza viruses or **respiratory syncytial virus (RSV).**

diphtheria

Acute infection of the throat and upper respiratory tract caused by the diphtheria bacterium *(Corynebacterium).*

Inflammation occurs, and a leathery, opaque membrane (Greek *diphthera*, leather membrane) forms in the pharynx and trachea.

Immunity to diphtheria (by production of antibodies) is induced by the administration of weakened toxins (antigens) beginning between the sixth and eighth weeks of life. These injections usually are given as combination vaccines with pertussis and tetanus toxins and so are called **DPT** injections.

epistaxis

Nosebleed.

Epistaxis is a Greek word meaning a dropping. It commonly results from irritation of nasal mucous membranes, trauma, vitamin K deficiency, clotting abnormalities, blood-thinning medications (such as aspirin and warfarin), or hypertension.

pertussis

Whooping cough; highly contagious bacterial infection of the pharynx, larynx, and trachea caused by *Bordetella pertussis*.

Pertussis is characterized by **paroxysmal** (violent, sudden) spasms of coughing that ends in a loud "whooping" inspiration.

BRONCHIAL DISORDERS

asthma

Chronic bronchial inflammatory disorder with airway obstruction due to bronchial edema and constriction and increased mucus production.

Associated signs and symptoms of asthma are dyspnea, wheezing, and cough. Etiology can involve allergy or infection. Triggers for asthmatic attacks include exercise, strong odors, cold air, stress, allergens (e.g., tobacco smoke, pet dander, dust, molds, pollens, foods), and medications (aspirin, beta-blockers).

Asthma treatments are:

- Fast-acting agents for acute symptoms; example is an albuterol inhaler **(bronchodilator).**
- Long-acting agents for long term control; examples are glucocorticoids (inhaled), oral steroids (anti-inflammatory drugs), and leukotriene blockers such as Singulair.

Other conditions, such as gastroesophageal reflux disease (GERD), sinusitis, and allergic rhinitis can exacerbate asthma.

bronchiectasis

Chronic dilation of a bronchus secondary to infection.

This condition is caused by chronic infection with loss of elasticity of the bronchi. Secretions puddle and do not drain normally. Signs and symptoms are cough, fever, and expectoration of foul-smelling, **purulent** (pus-containing) sputum. Treatment is **palliative** (noncurative) and includes antibiotics, mucolytics, bronchodilators, respiratory therapy, and surgical resection if other therapies are not effective.

chronic bronchitis

Inflammation of bronchi persisting over a long time; type of chronic obstructive pulmonary disease (COPD).

Infection and cigarette smoking are etiologic factors. Signs and symptoms include excessive secretion of often infected mucus, a productive cough, and obstruction of respiratory passages. Chronic bronchitis and emphysema (lung disease in which air exchange at the alveoli is severely impaired) are types of **chronic obstructive pulmonary disease (COPD).**

cystic fibrosis (CF)

Inherited disorder of exocrine glands resulting in thick mucinous secretions in the respiratory tract that do not drain normally.

This is a genetic disorder caused by a mutation in a gene. It can be diagnosed by newborn screening blood test, sweat test, and genetic testing. CF affects the epithelium (lining cells) of the respiratory tract, leading to chronic airway obstruction, infection, bronchiectasis, and sometimes respiratory failure. It also involves exocrine glands, such as the pancreas (insufficient secretion of digestive enzymes leads to poor growth) and sweat glands (salty tasting skin). There is no known cure, but therapy includes antibiotics, aerosolized medications, chest physiotherapy, and replacement of pancreatic enzymes. Lung transplantation becomes necessary for some patients. It can restore lung function and prolong life.

LUNG DISORDERS

atelectasis

Collapsed lung; incomplete expansion of alveoli, (Figure 12-7 page 467).

In atelectasis, the bronchioles and alveoli (pulmonary parenchyma) resemble a collapsed balloon.

emphysema

Hyperinflation of air sacs with destruction of alveolar walls (Figure 12-9A and B).

Loss of elasticity and the breakdown of alveolar walls result in expiratory flow limitation. There is a strong association between cigarette smoking and emphysema. As a result of the destruction of lung parenchyma, including blood vessels, pulmonary artery pressure rises and the right side of the heart must work harder to pump blood. This leads to right ventricular hypertrophy and right heart failure **(cor pulmonale).**

Emphysema and chronic bronchitis are both forms of **COPD.**

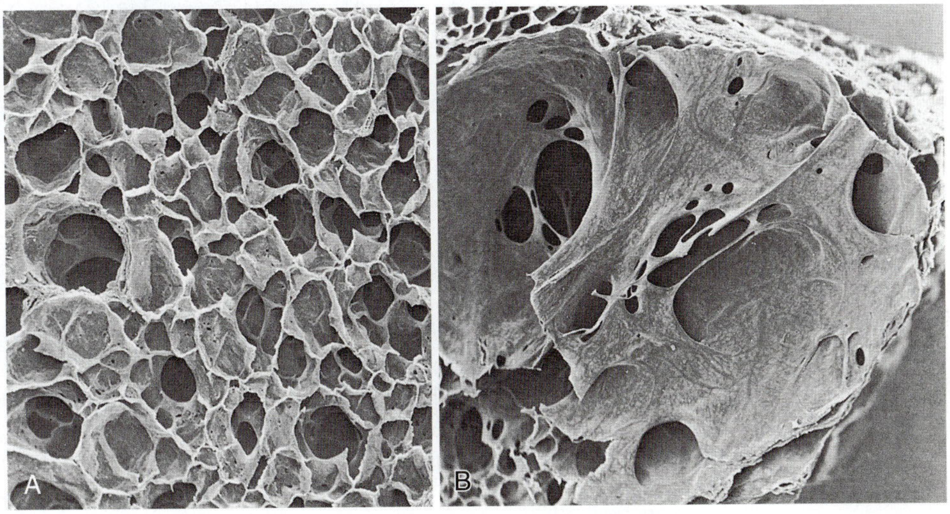

FIGURE 12-9 A, Normal lung tissue. B, Emphysema. Notice the overinflation of air sacs and destruction of alveolar walls.

Atelectasis: Common causes

- Bronchial obstruction—by secretions or tumor
- Complications following surgery—poor breathing ability
- Chest wounds—air (pneumothorax), fluid (pleural effusion), or blood (hemothorax) accumulate in the pleural cavity

lung cancer

Malignant tumor arising from the lungs and bronchi (Figure 12-10).

This group of cancers, often associated with cigarette smoking, is the most frequent fatal malignancy. Lung cancers are divided into two general categories: **non–small cell lung cancer (NSCLC)** and **small cell lung cancer (SCLC).**

NSCLC accounts for 90% of lung cancers and comprises three main types: adenocarcinoma (derived from mucus-secreting cells), squamous cell carcinoma (derived from the lining cells of the upper airway), and large cell lung cancer. When lung cancer is diagnosed, physicians assess the *stage* of the tumor (determined by its size, lymph node involvement, and any distant areas of spread) to prepare a protocol for treatment.

For localized tumors, surgery may be curative. Staging of NSCLC by assessing mediastinal lymph nodes is critical. If nodes are negative, the patient is a good candidate for surgery. If nodes are positive, multimodality treatment (chemotherapy and irradiation), with or without surgery, is an option. Doctors treat metastatic disease (to liver, brain, and bones) with palliative chemotherapy and/or radiation therapy.

In some patients, often nonsmokers, NSCLC may be caused by a mutation (change) in epithelial lung tissue. An example is a mutation in the epidermal growth factor receptor (EGFR), which is sensitive to treatment with EGFR inhibitors (Iressa and Tarceva). This is an example of targeted drug therapy for cancer.

SCLC derives from small, round ("oat" cells) cells found in pulmonary epithelium. It grows rapidly early and quickly spreads outside the lung. Treatment with radiation therapy and chemotherapy may lead to remissions.

pneumoconiosis

Abnormal condition caused by dust in the lungs, with chronic inflammation, infection, and bronchitis (Figure 12-11A).

Various forms are named according to the type of dust particle inhaled: **anthracosis**—coal (anthrac/o) dust (black lung disease); **asbestosis**—asbestos (asbest/o) particles (in shipbuilding and construction trades); **silicosis**—silica (silic/o = rocks) or glass (grinder's disease).

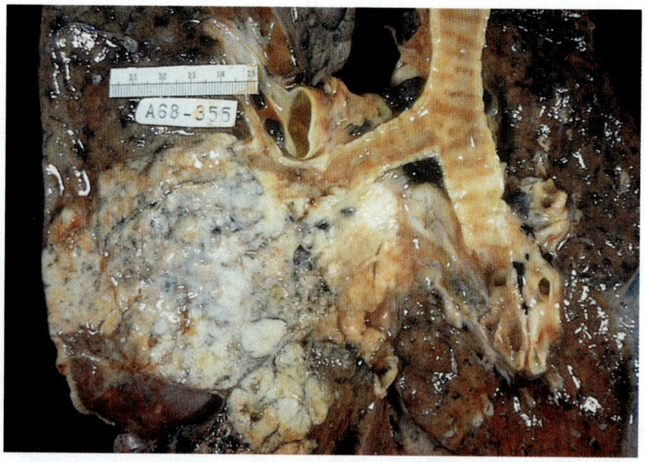

FIGURE 12-10 **Lung cancer.** The gray-white tumor tissue is infiltrating the substance of the lung. This tumor was identified as a squamous cell carcinoma. Squamous cell carcinomas arise in major bronchi and spread to local hilar lymph nodes.

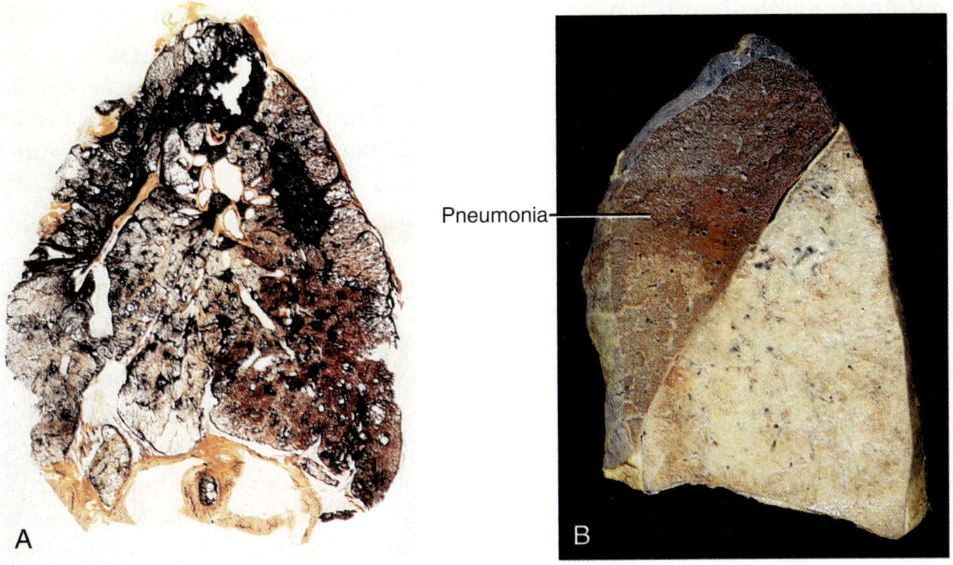

FIGURE 12-11 **A, Anthracosis** or black lung disease. Notice the dark black deposits of coal dust throughout the lung. **B, Lobar pneumonia** (at autopsy). Notice that the condition affects a lobe of the lung. The patient's signs and symptoms included fever, chills, cough, dark sputum, rapid shallow breathing, and hypoxia. If diagnosis is made early, antibiotic therapy is successful.

pneumonia

Acute inflammation and infection of alveoli, which fill with pus or products of the inflammatory reaction.

Etiologic agents are pneumococci, staphylococci, and other bacteria, fungi, or viruses. Infection damages alveolar membranes so that an **exudate** (fluid, blood cells, and debris) consolidates the alveoli (sacs become "glued" together, making air exchange less effective). An **infiltrate** is a fluid-filled area within the lungs as seen on a chest x-ray or CT scan. **Lobar pneumonia** (see Figure 12-11B) involves an entire lobe of a lung. **Bronchopneumonia** is a limited form of infection that produces patchy consolidation (abscesses) in the lung parenchyma. Treatment includes appropriate antibiotics and, if necessary, oxygen and mechanical ventilation in severe cases. See the ***In Person*** account on page 484 of a woman with recurring pneumonia.

Community-acquired pneumonia results from a contagious respiratory infection, caused by a variety of viruses and bacteria (especially *Mycoplasma* bacteria). It usually is treated at home with oral antibiotics.

Hospital-acquired pneumonia or **nosocomial pneumonia** is acquired during hospitalization (Greek *nosokomeion* means hospital). For example, patients may contract pneumonia while on mechanical ventilation or as a hospital-acquired infection.

Aspiration pneumonia is caused by material, such as food or vomitus, lodging in bronchi or lungs. It is a danger in the elderly, Alzheimer disease patients, stroke victims, and people with esophageal reflux and feeding tubes.

X-ray images of a normal chest and one with pneumonia are on page 476.

pulmonary abscess

Large collection of pus (bacterial infection) in the lungs.

pulmonary edema

Fluid in the air sacs and bronchioles.

This condition most often is caused by the inability of the heart to pump blood (congestive heart failure). Blood backs up in the pulmonary blood vessels, and fluid seeps out into the alveoli and bronchioles. Acute pulmonary edema requires immediate medical attention, including drugs (diuretics), oxygen in high concentrations, and keeping the patient in a sitting position (to decrease venous return to the heart).

12

pulmonary embolism (PE)

Clot or other material lodges in vessels of the lung (Figure 12-12A and B).

The clot (embolus) travels from distant veins, usually in the legs. Occlusion can produce an area of dead (necrotic) tissue; this is a **pulmonary infarction.** PE often causes acute pleuritic chest pain (pain on inspiration) and may be associated with blood in the sputum, fever, and respiratory insufficiency. CT angiography is the primary diagnostic tool for pulmonary emboli.

pulmonary fibrosis

Formation of scar tissue in the connective tissue of the lungs.

This condition may be the result of chronic inflammation or irritation caused by tuberculosis, pneumonia, or pneumoconiosis.

sarcoidosis

Chronic inflammatory disease in which small nodules (granulomas) develop in lungs, lymph nodes, and other organs.

The cause of sarcoidosis is unknown. Bilateral hilar lymphadenopathy or lung involvement is visible on chest x-ray in most cases. Many patients are asymptomatic and retain adequate pulmonary function. Sarcoidosis may affect the brain, heart, liver, and other organs. Other patients have more active disease and impaired pulmonary function. Corticosteroid drugs are used to prevent progression of the illness.

tuberculosis (TB)

Infectious disease caused by *Mycobacterium tuberculosis*; lungs usually are involved, but any organ in the body may be affected.

Rod-shaped bacteria called **bacilli** invade the lungs, producing small tubercles (from Latin *tuber*, a swelling) of infection. Early TB usually is asymptomatic and detected on routine chest x-ray studies. Signs and symptoms of advanced disease are cough, weight loss, night sweats, hemoptysis, and pleuritic pain. Antituberculosis chemotherapy (isoniazid, rifampin) is effective in most cases. Immunocompromised patients are particularly susceptible to antibiotic-resistant TB. It is important and often necessary to treat TB with several drugs at the same time to prevent drug resistance.

The PPD skin test (see page 480) is given to most hospital and medical employees because TB is highly contagious. A positive PPD test, in the absence of infection, requires treatment with isoniazid.

12

PLEURAL DISORDERS

mesothelioma

Rare malignant tumor arising in the pleura.

Mesotheliomas are derived from mesothelium, which forms the lining of the pleural surface. These tumors are caused by asbestos exposure.

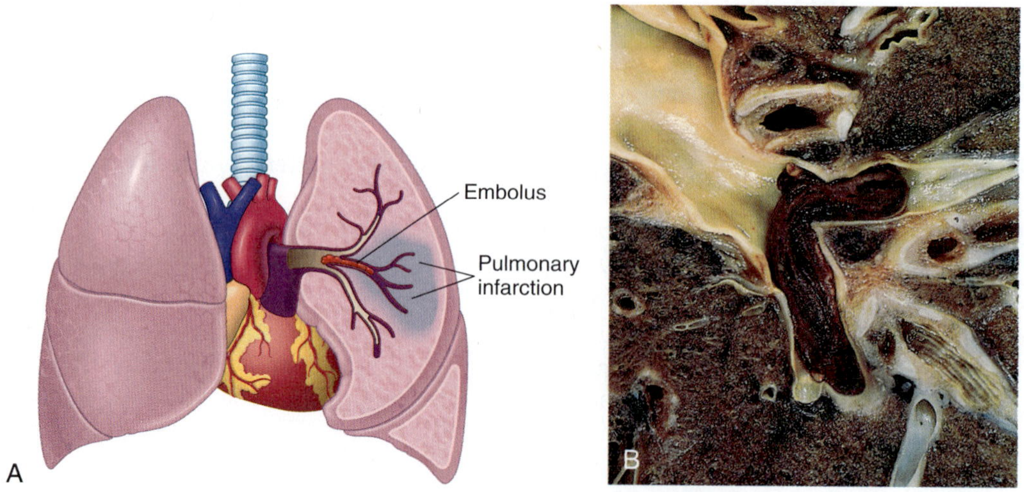

FIGURE 12-12 Pulmonary embolism (A and B).

pleural effusion

Abnormal accumulation of fluid in the pleural space (cavity).

Two types of pleural effusions are **exudates** (fluid from tumors and infections) and **transudates** (fluid from congestive heart failure, pulmonary embolism, or cirrhosis).

pleurisy (pleuritis)

Inflammation of the pleura.

This condition causes pleurodynia and dyspnea and, in chronic cases, pleural effusion.

pneumothorax

Collection of air in the pleural space.

Pneumothorax may occur in the course of a pulmonary disease (emphysema, carcinoma, tuberculosis, or lung abscess) when a break in the lung surface releases air into the pleural space. This allows communication between an alveolus or bronchus and the pleural cavity. It may also follow trauma and perforation of the chest wall or prolonged high-flow oxygen delivered by a respirator in an intensive care unit (ICU).

Pleurodesis (-desis means to bind) is the artificial production of adhesions between the parietal and visceral pleura for treatment of persistent pneumothorax and severe pleural effusion. This is accomplished by using talc powder or drugs, such as antibiotics, that cause irritation and scarring of the pleura.

STUDY SECTION

Practice spelling each term and know its meaning.

anthracosis	Coal dust accumulates in the lungs.
asbestosis	Asbestos particles accumulate in the lungs.
bacilli (*singular*: **bacillus**)	Rod-shaped bacteria (cause of tuberculosis).
chronic obstructive pulmonary disease (COPD)	Chronic condition of persistent obstruction of air flow through bronchial tubes and lungs. COPD is caused by smoking, air pollution, chronic infection, and, in a minority of cases, asthma. Patients with predominant **chronic bronchitis** COPD are referred to as "blue bloaters" (cyanotic, stocky build), whereas those with predominant **emphysema** are called "pink puffers" (short of breath, but with near-normal blood oxygen levels, and no change in skin color).
cor pulmonale	Failure of the right side of the heart to pump a sufficient amount of blood to the lungs because of underlying lung disease.
exudates	Fluid, cells, and other substances (pus) that filter from cells or capillaries ooze into lesions or areas of inflammation.
hydrothorax	Collection of fluid in the pleural cavity.
infiltrate	Collection of fluid or other material within the lung, as seen on a chest film, CT scan, or other radiologic image.
palliative	Relieving symptoms, but not curing the disease.
paroxysmal	Pertaining to a sudden occurrence, such as a spasm or seizure; oxysm/o means sudden.
pulmonary infarction	Area of necrosis (death of lung tissue).
purulent	Containing pus.
silicosis	Disease due to silica or glass dust in the lungs; occurs in mining occupations.

CLINICAL PROCEDURES

X-RAY TESTS

chest x-ray (CXR)

Radiographic image of the thoracic cavity (chest film).

Chest x-rays are taken in the frontal (coronal) plane as posteroanterior (PA) or anteroposterior (AP) views and in the sagittal plane as lateral views. Figure 12-13A and B shows a normal chest film and an x-ray film of the chest with pneumonia.

computed tomography (CT) scan of the chest

Computer-generated series of x-ray images show thoracic structures in cross section and other planes.

This test is for diagnosis of lesions difficult to assess by conventional x-ray studies, such as those in the lungs, mediastinum, and pleura.

CT pulmonary angiography (CTPA) is the combination of CT scanning and angiography. It is useful to examine the pulmonary circulation in the diagnosis of a pulmonary embolism.

MAGNETIC IMAGING

magnetic resonance imaging (MRI) of the chest

Magnetic waves create detailed images of the chest in frontal, lateral (sagittal), and cross-sectional (axial) planes.

This test is helpful in defining mediastinal tumors (such as those of Hodgkin disease) difficult to assess by CT scan.

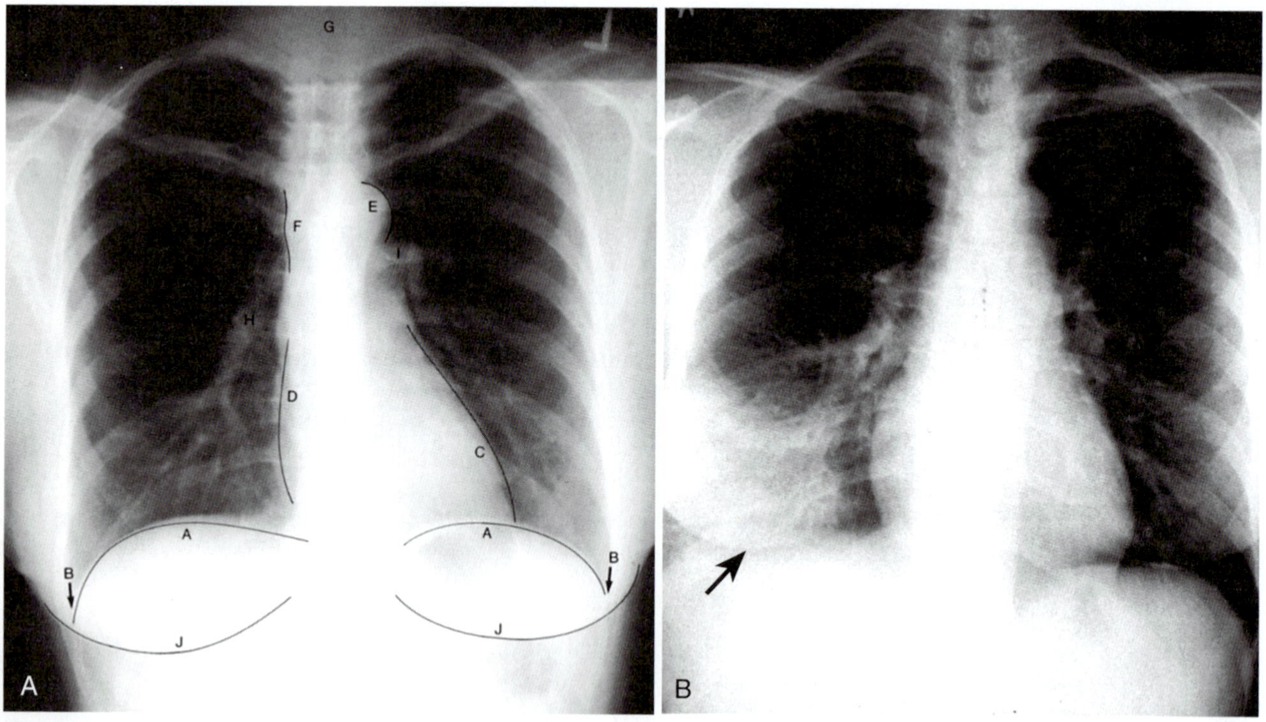

FIGURE 12-13 **A,** A **normal chest x-ray** appearance. The image is taken from the posteroanterior (PA) view (picture was taken back to front). The *backward L* in the upper corner is placed on the film to indicate the left side of the patient's chest. A, Diaphragm; B, costophrenic angle; C, left ventricle; D, right atrium; E, aortic arch; F, superior vena cava; G, trachea; H, right bronchus; I, left bronchus; J, breast shadows. Air-filled lung spaces appear black. **B, Pneumonia** of the right lung shown on an x-ray image of the chest.

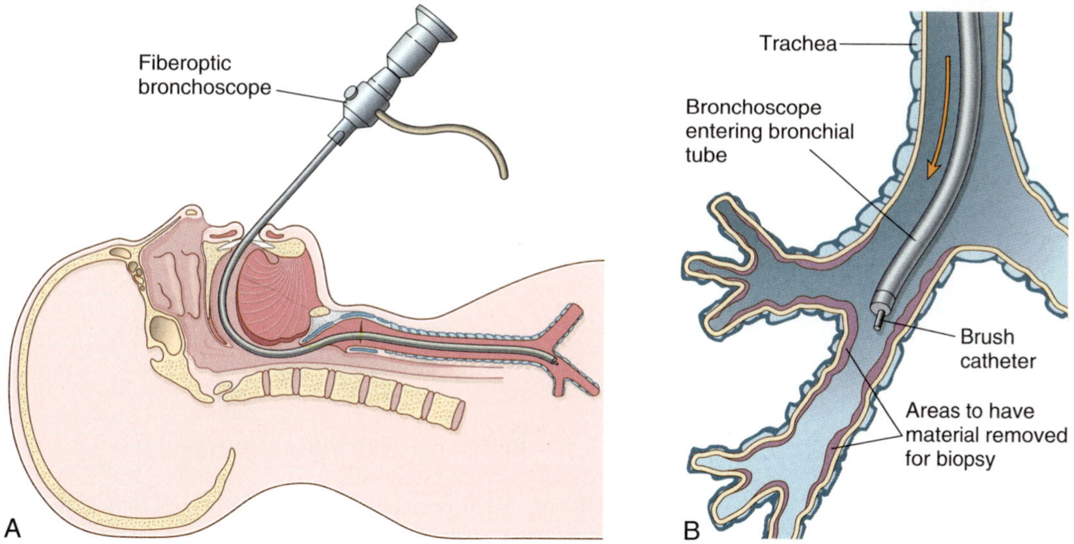

FIGURE 12-14 **A, Fiberoptic bronchoscopy.** A bronchoscope is passed through the nose, throat, larynx, and trachea into a bronchus. **B,** A **bronchoscope,** with brush catheter, in place in a bronchial tube.

NUCLEAR MEDICINE TESTS

positron emission tomography (PET) scan of the lung

Radioactive glucose is injected and images reveal metabolic activity in the lungs.

This scanning technique can identify malignant tumors, which have higher metabolic activity. It is also used to assess small nodules seen on a CT scan.

ventilation-perfusion (V/Q) scan

Detection device records radioactivity in the lung after injection of a radioisotope or inhalation of small amount of radioactive gas (xenon).

This test can identify areas of the lung not receiving adequate air flow (ventilation) or blood flow (perfusion). Q is the symbol for blood volume or rate of blood flow.

12

OTHER PROCEDURES

bronchoscopy

Fiberoptic endoscope examination of the bronchial tubes.

A physician places the bronchoscope through the throat, larynx, and trachea into the bronchi for diagnosis, biopsy, or collection of secretions. In **bronchoalveolar lavage (bronchial washing),** fluid is injected and withdrawn. In **bronchial brushing,** a brush is inserted through the bronchoscope and is used to scrape off tissue (Figure 12-14).

Endobronchial ultrasound (EBUS) is performed during bronchoscopy to diagnose and stage lung cancer. An EBUS-guided forceps biopsy allows for sampling of small (<3 cm) peripheral lesions endoscopically.

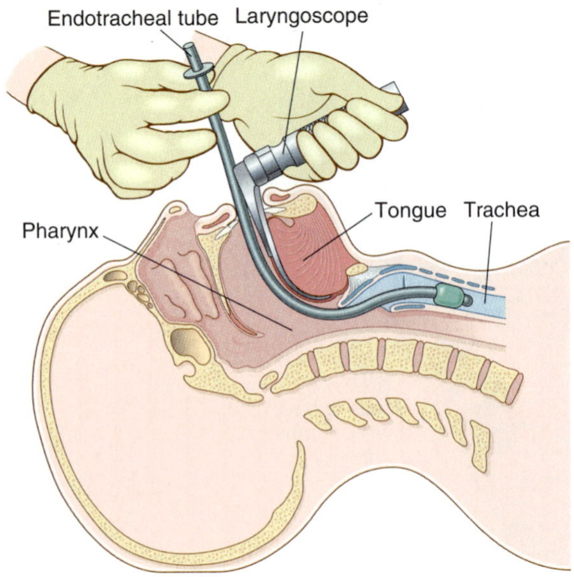

FIGURE 12-15 Endotracheal intubation. The patient is in a supine position; the head is hyperextended, the lower portion of the neck is flexed, and the mouth is opened. A **laryngoscope** is used to hold the airway open, to expose the vocal cords, and as a guide for placing the tube into the trachea.

endotracheal intubation

Placement of a tube through the mouth into the pharynx, larynx, and trachea to establish an airway (Figure 12-15).

This procedure also allows the patient to be placed on a mechanical **ventilator** (an apparatus that moves air into and out of the lungs).

laryngoscopy

Visual examination of the voice box.

A lighted, flexible endoscope is passed through the mouth or nose into the larynx.

12

lung biopsy

Removal of lung tissue followed by microscopic examination.

Specimens may be obtained by bronchoscopy, thoracotomy (open-lung biopsy), or by needle biopsy through the chest wall.

mediastinoscopy

Endoscopic visual examination of the mediastinum.

An incision is made above the breastbone (suprasternal) for inspection and biopsy of lymph nodes in the underlying space (mediastinum).

pulmonary function tests (PFTs)

Tests that measure the ventilation mechanics of the lungs: airway function, lung volume, and the capacity of the lungs to exchange oxygen and carbon dioxide efficiently. See Figure 12-16.

PFTs are used for many reasons: (1) to evaluate patients with shortness of breath (SOB); (2) to monitor lung function in patients with known respiratory disease; (3) to evaluate disability; and (4) to assess lung function before surgery. A **spirometer** measures the volume and rate of air passing into and out of the lung.

PFTs determine if lung disease is obstructive, restrictive, or both. In **obstructive lung disease,** airways are narrowed, which results in resistance to air flow during breathing. A hallmark PFT abnormality in obstructive disease is decreased expiratory flow rate or **FEV_1** (forced expiratory volume in the first second of expiration). Examples of obstructive lung diseases are asthma, COPD, bronchiectasis, cystic fibrosis, and bronchiolitis.

In **restrictive lung disease,** expansion of the lung is limited by disease that affects the chest wall, pleura, or lung tissue itself. A hallmark PFT abnormality in restrictive disease is decreased **total lung capacity (TLC).** Examples of lung conditions that stiffen and scar the lung are pulmonary fibrosis, radiation damage to the lung, and pneumoconiosis. Other causes of restrictive lung disease are neuromuscular conditions that affect the lung, such as myasthenia gravis, muscular dystrophy, and diaphragmatic weakness and paralysis.

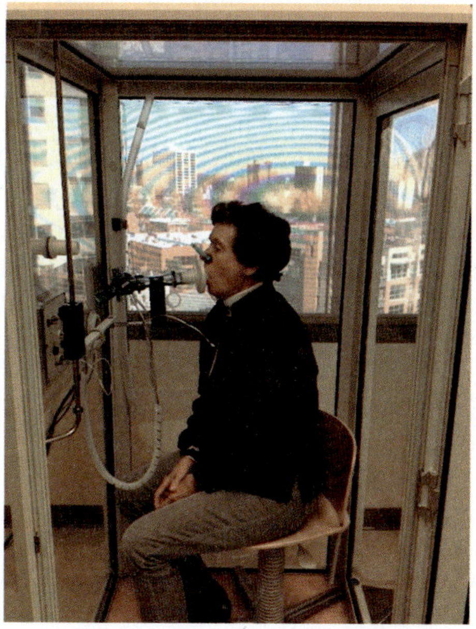

FIGURE 12-16 An individual undergoing a **pulmonary function test**.

The ability of gas to diffuse across the alveolar-capillary membrane is assessed by determining the diffusion capacity of the lung for carbon monoxide **(DL_{CO})**. A patient breathes in a small amount of carbon monoxide (CO), and the length of time it takes the gas to enter the bloodstream is measured.

thoracentesis

Surgical puncture to remove fluid from the pleural space.

This procedure is used to obtain pleural fluid for diagnosis or to therapeutically drain a pleural effusion (Figure 12-17).

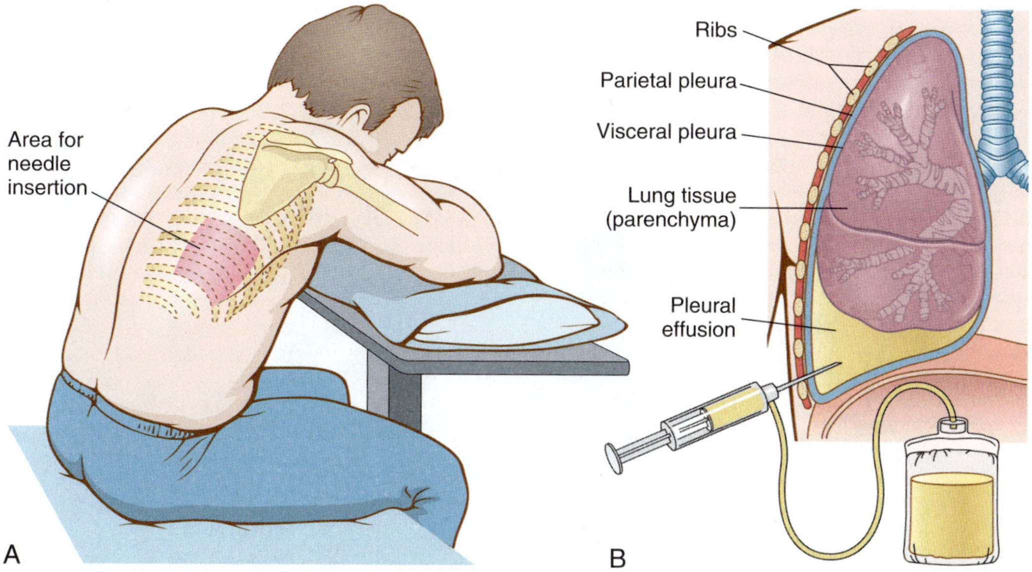

FIGURE 12-17 **Thoracentesis. A,** The patient is sitting in the correct position for the procedure; it allows the chest wall to be pulled outward in an expanded position. **B,** The needle is inserted close to the base of the effusion so that gravity can help with drainage, but it is kept as far away from the diaphragm as possible.

thoracotomy

Large surgical incision of the chest.

The incision is large, cutting into bone, muscle, and cartilage. It is necessary for lung biopsies and resections (lobectomy and pneumonectomy).

thoracoscopy (thorascopy)

Visual examination of the chest via small incisions and use of an endoscope.

Video-assisted thoracic surgery (VATS) allows the surgeon to view the chest from a video monitor. The thorascope (thoracoscope) is equipped with a camera that magnifies the image on the monitor. Thoracoscopy can diagnose and treat conditions of the lung, pleura, and mediastinum.

tracheostomy

Surgical creation of an opening into the trachea through the neck.

A tube is inserted to create an airway. The tracheostomy tube may be permanent as well as an emergency device (Figure 12-18). A **tracheotomy** is the incision necessary to create a tracheostomy.

tuberculin test

Determines past or present tuberculous infection based on a positive skin reaction.

Examples are the **Heaf test** and the **tine test,** using purified protein derivative **(PPD)** applied with multiple punctures of the skin, and the **Mantoux test,** using PPD given by intradermal injection.

tube thoracostomy

A flexible, plastic chest tube is passed into the pleural space through an opening in the chest.

This procedure is used to continuously remove air (pneumothorax), fluid (pleural effusion), or pus (empyema). See Figure 12-19.

12

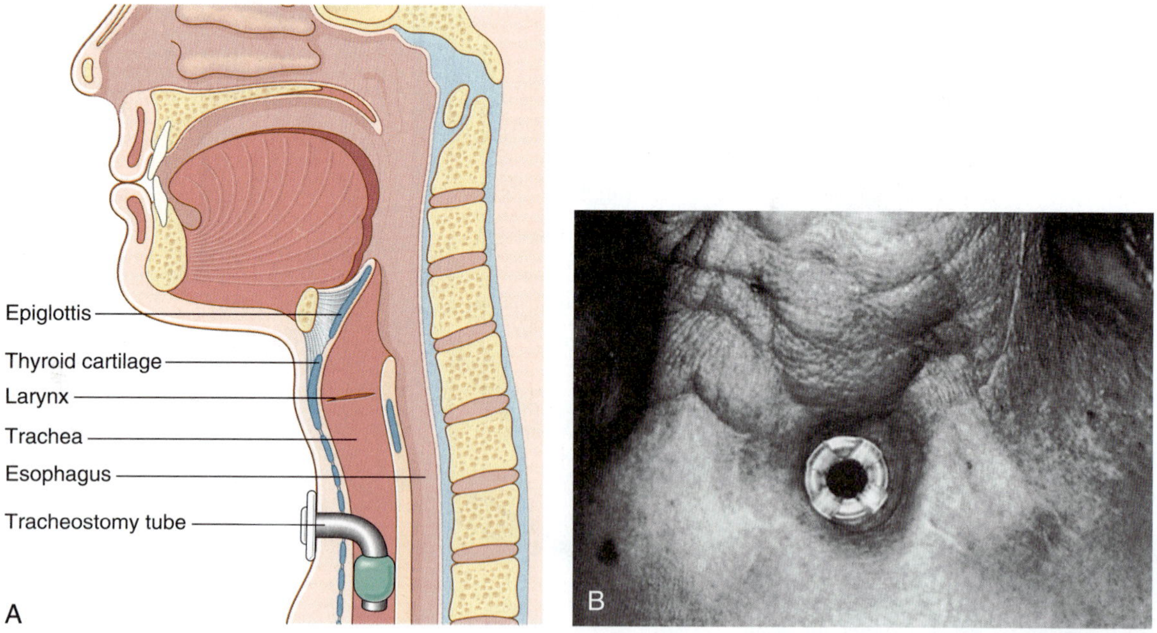

FIGURE 12-18 **A, Tracheostomy tube** in place. **B, Healed tracheostomy** after laryngectomy.

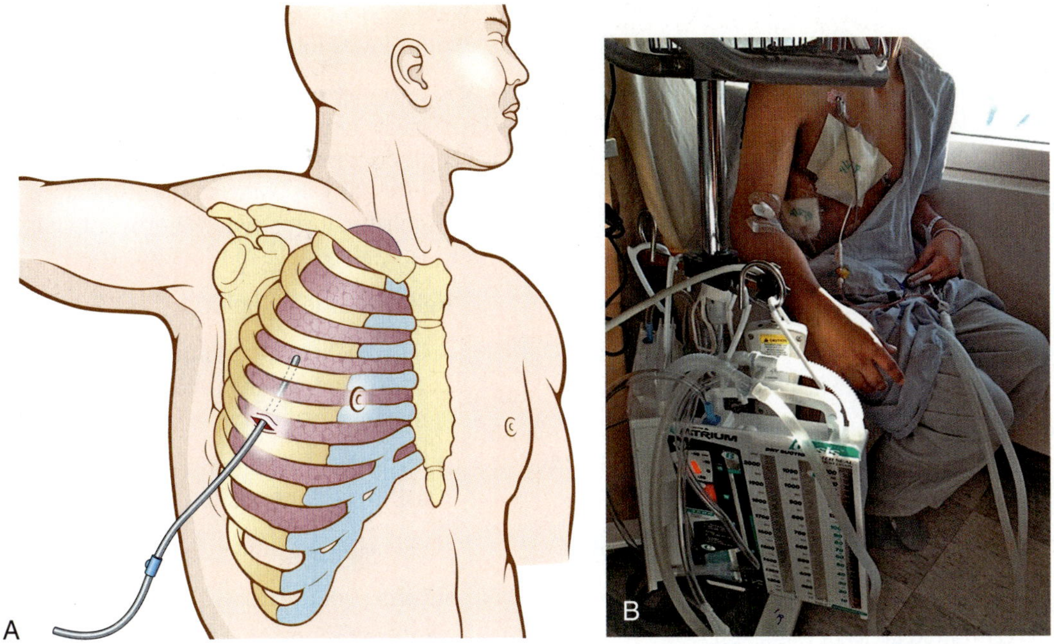

FIGURE 12-19 **A, Tube thoracostomy. B,** A patient with two **thoracostomy tubes** draining a pleural effusion in two different areas of the chest.

ABBREVIATIONS

ABGs	arterial blood gases
AFB	acid-fast bacillus—the type of organism that causes tuberculosis
ARDS	acute respiratory distress syndrome—severe, sudden lung injury caused by acute illness
BAL	bronchoalveolar lavage
Bronch	bronchoscopy
CF	cystic fibrosis
CO_2	carbon dioxide
COPD	chronic obstructive pulmonary disease—airway obstruction associated with emphysema and chronic bronchitis
CPAP	continuous positive airway pressure
CPR	cardiopulmonary resuscitation—three basic steps (CAB): C, *c*irculation restored by external cardiac compression; A, *a*irway opened by tilting the head; B, *b*reathing restored by mouth-to-mouth breathing
C&S	culture and sensitivity testing (of sputum)
CTPA	computed tomography pulmonary angiography
CXR	chest x-ray [film]
DL_{CO}	diffusion capacity of the lung for carbon monoxide
DOE	dyspnea on exertion
DPT	diphtheria, pertussis, tetanus—toxoids for vaccination of infants, to provide immunity to these diseases
FEV_1	forced expiratory volume in 1 second
FVC	forced vital capacity—amount of gas that can be forcibly and rapidly exhaled after a full inspiration
ICU	intensive care unit
LLL	left lower lobe (of lung)
LUL	left upper lobe (of lung)
MDI	metered-dose inhaler—used to deliver aerosolized medications to patients
NSCLC	non–small cell lung cancer
O_2	oxygen

OSA	obstructive sleep apnea
$Paco_2$	carbon dioxide partial pressure—measure of the amount of carbon dioxide in arterial blood
Pao_2	oxygen partial pressure—a measure of the amount of oxygen in arterial blood
PCP	*Pneumocystis* pneumonia—a type of pneumonia seen in patients with AIDS or other immunosuppression
PE	pulmonary embolism
PEP	positive expiratory pressure—mechanical ventilator strategy in which the patient takes a deep breath and then exhales through a device that resists air flow (helps refill underventilated areas of the lung)
PEEP	positive end-expiratory pressure—common mechanical ventilator setting in which airway pressure is maintained above atmospheric pressure
PFTs	pulmonary function tests
PND	paroxysmal nocturnal dyspnea
PPD	purified protein derivative—substance used in a tuberculosis test
RDS	respiratory distress syndrome—in the newborn infant, condition marked by dyspnea and cyanosis and related to absence of surfactant, a substance that permits normal expansion of lungs; also called hyaline membrane disease
RLL	right lower lobe (of lung)
RSV	respiratory syncytial virus—common cause of bronchiolitis, bronchopneumonia, and the common cold, especially in children (in tissue culture, forms syncytia or giant cells, so that cytoplasm flows together)
RUL	right upper lobe (of lung)
RV	residual volume—amount of air remaining in lungs at the end of maximal expiration
SABA	short-acting beta agonist (for relief of asthma symptoms)
SCLC	small cell lung cancer
SOB	shortness of breath
TB	tuberculosis
TLC	total lung capacity—volume of gas in the lungs at the end of maximal inspiration; equals VC plus RV
URI	upper respiratory infection
V_T	tidal volume—amount of air inhaled and exhaled during a normal ventilation
VATS	video-assisted thoracic surgery (thoracoscopy)
VC	vital capacity—equals inspiratory reserve volume plus expiratory reserve volume plus tidal volume
V/Q scan	ventilation-perfusion scan—radioactive test of lung ventilation and blood perfusion throughout the lung capillaries (lung scan)

PRACTICAL APPLICATIONS

Reproduced here are actual medical reports using terms that you have studied in this and previous chapters. Explanations of more difficult terms are added in brackets. Answers to the questions for the autopsy report are on page 493.

CASE REPORT

A 22-year-old known heroin abuser was admitted to an emergency department comatose with shallow respirations. Routine laboratory studies and chest x-ray studies were done after the patient was aroused. He was then transferred to the ICU. He complained of left-sided chest pain. Examination of the chest x-ray showed three fractured ribs on the right and a large right pleural effusion. Further questioning of a friend revealed that he had fallen and struck the corner of a table after injecting heroin.

The diagnosis was traumatic hemothorax secondary to rib fractures, and a chest tube was inserted into the right pleural space. No blood could be obtained despite maneuvering of the tube. Another chest x-ray showed that the tube was correctly placed in the right pleural space, but the fractured ribs and pleural effusion were on the left. The radiologist then realized that he had reversed the first film. A second tube was inserted into the left pleural space, and 1500 mL [6 to 7 cups] of blood was evacuated.

AUTOPSY REPORT

Adenocarcinoma, bronchogenic, left lung, with extensive mediastinal, pleural, and pericardial involvement. Metastasis to tracheobronchial lymph nodes, liver, lumbar vertebrae. Pulmonary emboli, multiple, recent, with recent infarct of left lower lobe. The tumor apparently originated at the left main bronchus and extends peripherally. Parenchyma (alveoli) is particularly atelectatic with a centrally located area of hemorrhage in the lower lobe.

Questions about the Autopsy Report

1. What was the patient's primary disease?
   a. Blood clots in the lung
   b. Mediastinal, pleural, and pericardial inflammation
   c. Lung cancer
2. Which was *not* an area of metastasis?
   a. Backbones
   b. Bone marrow
   c. Hepatocytes
3. What event probably was the cause of death?
   a. Infarction of lung tissue caused by pulmonary emboli
   b. COPD
   c. Myocardial infarction
4. What best describes the pulmonary parenchyma in the lower left lobe?
   a. Alveoli are filled with tumor.
   b. Alveoli are collapsed, with central area of bleeding.
   c. Alveoli are filled with pus and blood.

X-RAY AND BRONCHOSCOPY REPORTS

1. *CXR*: Complete opacification of left hemithorax with deviation of mediastinal structures of right side. Massive pleural effusion.
2. *Chest tomograms*: Mass most compatible with LUL bronchogenic carcinoma. Possible left paratracheal adenopathy or direct involvement of mediastinum.
3. *Bronchoscopy*: Larynx, trachea, **carina** [area of bifurcation or forking of the trachea], and left lung all within normal limits. On the right side there was irregularity and roughening of the bronchial mucosa on the lateral aspect of the bronchial wall. This irregularity extended into the RUL, and the apical and posterior segments [divisions of lobes of the lung] each contained inflamed irregular mucosa. Conclusion: Suspicious for infiltrating tumor, but may be nonspecific inflammation. Bronchial washings, brushings, and bxs [biopsies] taken. Bronchial biopsy diagnosis: squamous cell carcinoma. Washings and brushings showed no malignant cells.

12

IN PERSON

This is a first-person account of a woman with recurring pneumonia.

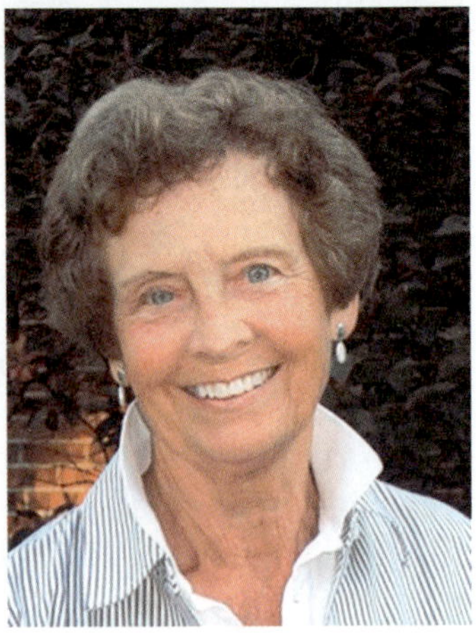

While growing up in West Virginia in the 1940s and 50s, I was frighteningly aware of the prevalence of lung diseases. With coal mining at its peak, large numbers of miners suffered and died from black lung disease. Tuberculosis was not uncommon and neither was pneumonia. Little did I imagine, then or in 1999, when I first contracted the disease, that recurring pneumonia would become my most troublesome medical issue.

As bitterly cold temperatures persisted during the winter of 1999, I was not particularly concerned about a lingering cold and cough. But when I developed a low-grade fever and decreased energy, a chest x-ray confirmed that I had pneumonia in my left lung (lower lobe). My doctor prescribed a one-week course of antibiotics and reassured me that the diagnosis was not unusual. I quickly improved and a follow-up x-ray showed that the pneumonia had cleared. My doctor then suggested that I receive the pneumonia vaccine, which produces antibodies against many types of pneumococcal bacteria. End of story. Or so I thought.

In October of 2001, at age 60, I began training to run the Boston Marathon. A few days after a long training run in January of 2002, cough and cold symptoms, a low-grade fever, and rather marked fatigue set in. The thought of pneumonia did not cross my mind initially. But, when symptoms didn't improve, a visit to my doctor and chest x-ray confirmed my second diagnosis of pneumonia, again in my left lower lobe. I felt some relief when my physician, a pulmonologist and a serious runner himself, assured me that cold weather training had not caused the pneumonia. I recovered quickly, after a two-week course of antibiotics, and resumed training, completing the marathon in April. A follow-up chest CT performed in May showed no abnormal result, and a bronchoscopy in June ruled out any malignancy that might have led to pneumonia. Relieved, I assumed I was finished with pneumonia.

However, pneumonia wasn't finished with me. The next bout came three years later, in the right upper lobe. After antibiotic treatment, I managed to be pneumonia-free for the next six years. But in late July of 2011, I experienced a cold and cough in hot weather, which was quite unusual for me. Surely this can't be pneumonia. After all, it has been 6 years! I began to wonder when tightness in my upper chest and extreme fatigue followed the cold and cough symptoms. Sure enough, I had pneumonia once again. With this latest diagnosis, my doctor became more focused on identifying the possible underlying cause(s) of my recurring pneumonia.

The disease hit again just six months later, in December of 2011. After appearing to resolve following two weeks of antibiotics, the pneumonia returned less than a month later. Now, to see if there was an issue with my immune system, my doctor ordered immunoglobulin (antibody) testing. The results were normal. No clues here. Another pneumonia episode occurred in May of 2012, this time accompanied by a 104-degree fever. This one took a little longer to resolve, again with antibiotics. By this time my levels of bewilderment and anxiety were going up a notch with each episode.

With the referral of my doctor, I sought out a pulmonologist, one who specializes in the treatment of pneumonia, to undergo additional studies that might yield useful information. Over a two-day period, pulmonary function tests were conducted, and computers tracked the results. I was given albuterol, a substance that aids in breathing and is often administered to people who have asthma. But the albuterol did not increase my breathing efficiency significantly. Other tests ruled out various other abnormalities.

With all the information, gathered and evaluated by experts, what happens next? At this point, the doctors conclude that my pneumonia is probably idiopathic. They suggest that I have a follow-up CT scan and additional testing when pneumonia episodes actually occur. They also caution me about exposure around children and hospitalized patients. I asked my lung specialist if he thought this pneumonia puzzle would ever be resolved. His reply was, "Something is going on that we will eventually understand. We just haven't figured it out yet." Unsettling and stress producing as this has been, I know I am fortunate to be dealing with an illness that has, so far, responded to medication. Still, every time I get cold signs and symptoms, I worry. And I never take good health for granted.

Brenda Melson's professional career was in teaching, counseling, and college advising.

EXERCISES

Remember to check your answers carefully with the Answers to Exercises, page 492.

A Match the following anatomic structures with their descriptions below.

adenoids	epiglottis	paranasal sinuses
alveoli	hilum	parietal pleura
bronchi	larynx	pharynx
bronchioles	mediastinum	trachea
cilia	palatine tonsils	visceral pleura

1. outer fold of pleura lying closer to the ribs ______
2. collections of lymph tissue in the nasopharynx ______
3. windpipe ______
4. lid-like piece of cartilage that covers the voice box ______
5. branches of the windpipe that lead into the lungs ______
6. region between the lungs in the chest cavity ______
7. air-containing cavities in the bones around the nose ______
8. thin hairs attached to the mucous membrane lining the respiratory tract ______
9. inner fold of pleura closer to lung tissue ______
10. throat ______
11. air sacs of the lung ______
12. voice box ______
13. smallest branches of bronchi ______
14. collections of lymph tissue in the oropharynx ______
15. midline region of the lungs where bronchi, blood vessels, and nerves enter and exit the lungs ______

B Complete the following sentences.

1. The apical part of the lung is the ______.
2. The gas that passes into the bloodstream at the lungs is ______.
3. Breathing in air is called ______.
4. Divisions of the lungs are known as ______.

5. The gas produced by cells and exhaled through the lungs is ________________.
6. The space between the visceral and the parietal pleura is the ________________.
7. Breathing out air is called ________________.
8. The essential tissues of the lung that perform its main function are pulmonary ________________.
9. The exchange of gases in the lung is ________________ respiration.
10. The exchange of gases at the tissue cells is ________________ respiration.

C Give meanings for the following terms relating to respiratory disorders and structures.

1. bronchiectasis ________________
2. pleuritis ________________
3. pneumothorax ________________
4. anosmia ________________
5. laryngectomy ________________
6. nasopharyngitis ________________
7. phrenic ________________
8. alveolar ________________
9. glottis ________________
10. tracheal stenosis ________________

12

D Complete the medical terms for the following respiratory symptoms.

1. excessive carbon dioxide in the blood: hyper________________
2. breathing is easiest or possible only in an upright position: ________________pnea
3. difficult breathing: ________________pnea
4. condition of blueness of skin: ________________osis
5. spitting up blood: hemo________________
6. deficiency of oxygen: hyp________________
7. condition of pus in the pleural cavity: pyo________________ *or* em________________
8. hoarseness; voice impairment: dys________________
9. blood in the pleural cavity: hemo________________
10. nosebleed: epi________________

E Give the meanings of the following medical terms.

1. rales (crackles) ____________________
2. auscultation ____________________
3. sputum ____________________
4. percussion ____________________
5. rhonchi ____________________
6. pleural rub ____________________
7. purulent ____________________
8. paroxysmal nocturnal dyspnea ____________________
9. hydrothorax ____________________
10. pulmonary infarction ____________________
11. stridor ____________________
12. wheeze ____________________

F Match the following terms with the descriptions below.

asbestosis	croup	infiltrate
asthma	cystic fibrosis	lung cancer
atelectasis	diphtheria	pertussis
chronic bronchitis	emphysema	sarcoidosis

1. acute infectious disease of the throat caused by *Corynebacterium* ____________________
2. acute respiratory syndrome in children and infants that is marked by obstruction of the larynx and stridor ____________________
3. hyperinflation of air sacs with destruction of alveolar walls ____________________
4. inflammation of tubes that lead from the trachea, over a long period of time ____________________
5. chronic inflammatory disorder characterized by airway obstruction ____________________
6. lung or a portion of a lung is collapsed ____________________
7. malignant neoplasm originating in a lung or bronchus ____________________
8. whooping cough ____________________
9. a collection of fluid or other material within the lung as seen on chest film, CT scan, or other radiologic study ____________________
10. inherited disease of exocrine glands; mucous secretions lead to airway obstruction ____________________
11. type of pneumoconiosis; dust particles are inhaled ____________________
12. inflammatory disease in which small nodules form in lungs and lymph nodes ____________________

G **Use the following terms and abbreviations to complete the sentences below.**

CPAP	fibrosis	PaO_2
DL_{CO}	obstructive lung disease	palliative
exudate	OSA	restrictive lung disease
FEV_1	$PaCO_2$	rhonchi

1. Sarah had a pulmonary function test in which she inhaled as much air as she could and the air that she expelled in the first second was measured. The result of this PFT is a/an ____________________
2. Dr. Smith heard loud ____________________ when he auscultated Kate's chest. Her bronchial tubes were obstructed with thick mucous secretions.
3. Karl was asked to breathe in a small amount of carbon monoxide and then blood samples were taken to detect the gas in his bloodstream. This PFT assesses how well gases can diffuse across the alveolar membrane, and the result of the test is called ____________________.
4. Formation of scar tissue in the connective tissue of the lungs is pulmonary ____________________.
5. A purulent ____________________ consists of white blood cells, microorganisms (dead and alive), and other debris.
6. Myasthenia gravis and muscular dystrophy are examples of neuromuscular conditions that produce ____________________.
7. Chronic bronchitis and asthma are examples of ____________________.
8. Patients with a small pharyngeal airway that closes during sleep may experience ____________________.
9. With nasal ____________________, positive pressure (air coming from a compressor) opens the oropharynx and nasopharynx, preventing obstructive sleep apnea.
10. Doctors realized that they could not cure Jean's adenocarcinoma of the lung. They used ____________________ measures to relieve her uncomfortable symptoms.
11. During an apneic period, a patient experiences severe hypoxemia (decreased ____________________) and hypercapnia (increased ____________________).

12

H **Give the meanings of the following medical terms.**

1. pulmonary abscess ____________________
2. pulmonary edema ____________________
3. pneumoconiosis ____________________
4. pneumonia ____________________
5. pulmonary embolism ____________________

6. tuberculosis ______________________________
7. pleural effusion ______________________________
8. pleurisy ______________________________
9. anthracosis ______________________________
10. mesothelioma ______________________________
11. adenoid hypertrophy ______________________________
12. pleurodynia ______________________________
13. expectoration ______________________________
14. tachypnea ______________________________

I Match the clinical procedure or abbreviation with its description.

bronchoalveolar lavage	laryngoscopy	tracheostomy
bronchoscopy	mediastinoscopy	tube thoracostomy
CT pulmonary angiography	pulmonary function tests	tuberculin tests
endotracheal intubation	thoracentesis	V/Q scan

1. placement of a tube through the mouth into the trachea to establish an airway

   ____
2. injection or inhalation of radioactive material and recording images of its distribution in the lungs ______________________
3. tine and Mantoux tests ______________________
4. puncture of the chest wall to obtain fluid from the pleural cavity ______________________
5. tests that measure the ventilation mechanics of the lung ______________________
6. creation of an opening into the trachea through the neck to establish an airway

   ____
7. visual examination of the bronchi ______________________
8. injection of fluid into the bronchi, followed by withdrawal of the fluid for examination

   ____
9. insertion of an endoscope into the larynx to view the voice box ______________________
10. combination of computer-generated x-ray images and recording (with contrast) of blood flow in the lung ______________________
11. visual examination of the area between the lungs ______________________
12. continuous drainage of the pleural spaces from a chest tube placed through a small skin incision

    ____

J **Give the meanings of the following abbreviations and then select the letter of the sentence that is the best association for each.**

COLUMN I

1. DOE ______________________ _____
2. PND ______________________ _____
3. VATS ______________________ _____
4. CPR ______________________ _____
5. NSCLC ______________________ _____
6. ARDS ______________________ _____
7. COPD ______________________ _____
8. PFTs ______________________ _____
9. PPD ______________________ _____
10. DPT ______________________ _____

COLUMN II

A. Patients with congestive heart failure and pulmonary edema experience this symptom when they recline in bed.
B. Chronic bronchitis and emphysema are examples.
C. Substance used in the test for tuberculosis.
D. Adenocarcinoma and squamous cell carcinoma are types.
E. Visual examination of the chest via endoscope and a video monitor.
F. Injection in an infant to provide immunity.
G. A spirometer is used for these respiratory tests.
H. This symptom means that a patient has difficulty breathing and becomes short of breath when exercising.
I. Three basic steps: A, airway opened by tilting the head; B, breathing restored by mouth-to-mouth breathing; C, circulation restored by external cardiac compression.
J. A group of symptoms resulting in acute respiratory failure.

12

K **Match the respiratory system procedures with their meanings.**

laryngectomy	rhinoplasty	thoracotomy
lobectomy	thoracentesis	tonsillectomy
pneumonectomy	thoracoscopy (thorascopy)	

1. removal of lymph tissue in the oropharynx ______________________
2. surgical puncture of the chest to remove fluid from the pleural space ______________________
3. surgical repair of the nose ______________________
4. incision of the chest ______________________
5. removal of the voice box ______________________
6. removal of a region of a lung ______________________
7. endoscopic examination of the chest ______________________
8. pulmonary resection ______________________

L **Circle the boldface term that best completes the meaning of each sentence.**

1. Ruth was having difficulty taking a deep breath, and her chest x-ray showed accumulation of fluid in her pleural spaces. Dr. Smith ordered **(PPD, tracheotomy, thoracentesis)** to relieve the pressure on her lungs.

2. Dr. Wong used her stethoscope to perform **(percussion, auscultation, thoracentesis)** on the patient's chest.

3. Before making a decision to perform surgery on Mrs. Hope, an 80-year-old woman with lung cancer, her physicians ordered **(COPD, bronchoscopy, PFTs)** to determine the functioning of her lungs.

4. Sylvia produced yellow-colored sputum and had a high fever. Her physician told her that she probably had **(pneumonia, pulmonary embolism, pneumothorax)** and needed antibiotics.

5. The night before her thoracotomy for lung biopsy, Mrs. White was told by her anesthesiologist that he would place a/an **(thoracostomy tube, mediastinoscope, endotracheal tube)** down her throat to keep her airway open during surgery.

6. Early in her pregnancy, Sonya had a routine **(PET scan, CXR, MRI)** that revealed a/an **(epiglottic, alveolar, mediastinal)** mass in the area between her lungs. After delivery of her child, the mass was removed, and biopsy revealed a malignant thymoma (tumor of the thymus gland).

7. Five-year-old Seth was allergic to cats and experienced wheezing, coughing, and difficult breathing at night when he was trying to sleep. After careful evaluation by a **(cardiologist, pulmonologist, neurologist)**, his parents were told that Seth had **(pleurisy, sarcoidosis, asthma)** involving inflammation of his **(nasal passages, pharynx, bronchial tubes)**.

8. Six-year-old Daisy had a habit of picking her nose. During the winter months, heat in her family's house caused drying of her nasal **(mucus, mucous, pleural)** membranes. She had frequent bouts of **(epistaxis, croup, stridor)**.

9. Seventy-five-year-old Beatrice had been a pack-a-day smoker all of her adult life. Over the previous 3 months she noticed a persistent cough, weight loss, blood in her sputum **(hemoptysis, hematemesis, asbestosis)**, and dyspnea. A chest CT scan revealed a mass. Biopsy confirmed the diagnosis of **(tuberculosis, pneumoconiosis, adenocarcinoma)**, which is a type of **(small cell, non–small cell, lymph node)** lung cancer.

10. Carrie's lungs were normal at birth, but thick bronchial secretions soon blocked her **(arterioles, venules, bronchioles)**, which became inflamed. She was losing weight, and tests revealed inadequate amounts of pancreatic enzymes necessary for digestion of fats and proteins. Her pediatrician diagnosed her hereditary condition as **(chronic bronchitis, asthma, cystic fibrosis)**.

ANSWERS TO EXERCISES

A

1. parietal pleura
2. adenoids
3. trachea
4. epiglottis
5. bronchi
6. mediastinum
7. paranasal sinuses
8. cilia
9. visceral pleura
10. pharynx
11. alveoli
12. larynx
13. bronchioles
14. palatine tonsils
15. hilum

B

1. uppermost part
2. oxygen
3. inspiration; inhalation
4. lobes
5. carbon dioxide
6. pleural cavity
7. expiration; exhalation
8. parenchyma
9. external
10. internal

C

1. chronic dilation of a bronchus
2. inflammation of pleura
3. air in the chest (pleural cavity)
4. lack of sense of smell
5. removal of the voice box
6. inflammation of the nose and throat
7. pertaining to the diaphragm
8. pertaining to an air sac
9. opening to the larynx
10. narrowing of the windpipe

D

1. hypercapnia
2. orthopnea
3. dyspnea
4. cyanosis
5. hemoptysis
6. hypoxia
7. pyothorax; empyema
8. dysphonia
9. hemothorax
10. epistaxis

E

1. fine crackling sounds heard during inhalation when there is fluid in the alveoli
2. listening to sounds within the body
3. material expelled from the respiratory tract by deep coughing and spitting
4. tapping on the surface to determine the underlying structure
5. loud rumbling sounds on auscultation of chest; bronchi obstructed by sputum
6. scratching sound produced by pleural surfaces rubbing against each other (caused by inflammation or tumor cells)
7. pus-filled
8. sudden attack of difficult breathing associated with lying down at night (caused by congestive heart failure and pulmonary edema as the lungs fill with fluid)
9. fluid in the pleural cavity
10. area of dead tissue in the lung
11. strained, high-pitched inspirational sound
12. continuous high-pitched whistling sound produced during breathing when air is forced through a narrow space; heard in asthma

F

1. diphtheria
2. croup
3. emphysema
4. chronic bronchitis
5. asthma
6. atelectasis
7. lung cancer
8. pertussis
9. infiltrate
10. cystic fibrosis
11. asbestosis
12. sarcoidosis

G

1. FEV_1 (forced expiratory volume in first second)
2. rhonchi
3. DL_{CO} (diffusion capacity of the lung for carbon monoxide)
4. fibrosis
5. exudate
6. restrictive lung disease
7. obstructive lung disease
8. OSA: obstructive sleep apnea
9. CPAP: continuous positive airway pressure
10. palliative
11. PaO_2, $PaCO_2$

12

H

1. collection of pus in the lungs
2. swelling, fluid collection in the air sacs and bronchioles
3. abnormal condition of dust in the lungs
4. acute inflammation and infection of alveoli; they become filled with fluid and blood cells
5. floating clot or other material blocking the blood vessels of the lung
6. an infectious disease caused by rod-shaped bacilli and producing tubercles (nodes) of infection
7. collection of fluid in the pleural cavity
8. inflammation of pleura
9. abnormal condition of coal dust in the lungs (black lung disease)
10. malignant tumor arising in the pleura; composed of mesothelium (epithelium that covers the surfaces of membranes such as pleura and peritoneum)
11. excessive growth of cells in the adenoids (lymph tissue in the nasopharynx)
12. pain of the pleura (irritation of pleural surfaces leads to intercostal pain)
13. coughing up of material from the chest
14. rapid breathing; hyperventilation

I

1. endotracheal intubation
2. V/Q scan
3. tuberculin tests
4. thoracentesis
5. pulmonary function tests
6. tracheostomy
7. bronchoscopy
8. bronchoalveolar lavage
9. laryngoscopy
10. CT pulmonary angiography
11. mediastinoscopy
12. tube thoracostomy

J

1. dyspnea on exertion: H
2. paroxysmal nocturnal dyspnea: A
3. video-assisted thoracic surgery: E
4. cardiopulmonary resuscitation: I
5. non–small cell lung cancer: D
6. acute (adult) respiratory distress syndrome: J
7. chronic obstructive pulmonary disease: B
8. pulmonary function tests: G
9. purified protein derivative: C
10. diphtheria, pertussis, and tetanus: F

K

1. tonsillectomy
2. thoracentesis
3. rhinoplasty
4. thoracotomy
5. laryngectomy
6. lobectomy
7. thoracoscopy (thorascopy)
8. pneumonectomy

L

1. thoracentesis
2. auscultation
3. PFTs
4. pneumonia
5. endotracheal tube
6. CXR; mediastinal
7. pulmonologist; asthma; bronchial tubes
8. mucous; epistaxis
9. hemoptysis; adenocarcinoma; non–small cell
10. bronchioles; cystic fibrosis

Answers to Practical Applications

Autopsy Report

1. c
2. b
3. a
4. b

12

PRONUNCIATION OF TERMS

To test your understanding of the terminology in this chapter, write the meaning of each term in the space provided. In addition, you may wish to cover the terms and write them by looking at your definitions. Make sure your spelling is correct. The page number after each term indicates where it is defined or used in the book, so you can easily check your responses. You will find complete definitions for all of these terms and their audio pronunciations on the Evolve website.

Pronunciation Guide

ā as in āpe	ă as in ăpple
ē as in ēven	ĕ as in ĕvery
ī as in īce	ĭ as in ĭnterest
ō as in ōpen	ŏ as in pŏt
ū as in ūnit	ŭ as in ŭnder

Vocabulary and Terminology

TERM	PRONUNCIATION	MEANING
adenoidectomy (463)	ăd-ĕ-noyd-ĔK-tō-mē	
adenoid hypertrophy (463)	ĂD-ĕ-noyd hī-PĔR-trō-fē	
adenoids (462)	ĂD-ĕ-noydz	
alveolar (463)	ăl-VĒ-ō-lăr	
alveolus; alveoli (462)	ăl-VĒ-ō-lŭs; ăl-VĒ-ō-lī	
anosmia (467)	ăn-ŎS-mē-ă	
apex of the lung (462)	Ā-pĕkz of the lŭng	
apical (462)	Ā-pĭ-kăl	
apnea (468)	ĂP-nē-ă	
asphyxia (468)	ăs-FĬK-sē-ă	
atelectasis (467)	ă-tĕ-LĔK-tă-sĭs	
base of the lung (462)	bās of the lŭng	
bronchiectasis (463)	brŏng-kē-ĔK-tă-sĭs	
bronchioles (462)	BRŎNG-kē-ōlz	
bronchiolitis (463)	brŏng-kē-ō-LĪ-tĭs	
bronchodilator (463)	brŏng-kō-DĪ-lā-tĕr	
bronchopleural (463)	brŏng-kō-PLOO-răl	
bronchospasm (463)	BRŎNG-kō-spăzm	
bronchus; bronchi (462)	BRŎNG-kŭs; BRŎNG-kī	
carbon dioxide (462)	KĂR-bŏn dī-ŎK-sīd	
cilia (462)	SĬL-ē-ă	
cyanosis (464)	sī-ă-NŌ-sĭs	
diaphragm (462)	DĪ-ă-frăm	

12

TERM	PRONUNCIATION	MEANING
dysphonia (465)	dĭs-FŌ-nē-ă	______
dyspnea (468)	DĬSP-nē-ă	______
empyema (467)	ĕm-pī-Ē-mă	______
epiglottis (462)	ĕp-ĭ-GLŎT-ĭs	______
epiglottitis (464)	ĕp-ĭ-glŏ-TĪ-tĭs	______
expectoration (465)	ĕk-spĕk-tō-RĀ-shŭn	______
expiration (462)	ĕks-pĭr-RĀ-shŭn	______
glottis (462)	GLŎ-tĭs	______
hemoptysis (468)	hē-MŎP-tĭ-sĭs	______
hemothorax (468)	hē-mō-THŌ-răks	______
hilum of the lung (462)	HĪ-lŭm of the lŭng	______
hilar (462)	HĪ-lăr	______
hypercapnia (463)	hī-pĕr-KĂP-nē-ă	______
hyperpnea (468)	hī-PĔRP-nē-ă	______
hypoxia (465)	hī-PŎK-sē-ă	______
inspiration (462)	ĭn-spĭ-RĀ-shŭn	______
laryngeal (464)	lă-RĬN-jē-ăl *or* lăr-ĭn-JĒ-ăl	______
laryngospasm (464)	lă-RĬNG-gō-spăzm	______
laryngitis (464)	lă-rĭn-JĪ-tĭs	______
larynx (462)	LĂR-ĭnks	______
lobectomy (464)	lō-BĔK-tō-mē	______
mediastinoscopy (465)	mē-dē-ă-stī-NŎS-kō-pē	______
mediastinum (462)	mē-dē-ă-STĪ-nŭm	______
nares (462)	NĀ-rēz	______
nasogastric intubation (465)	nā-zō-GĂS-trĭk ĭn-too-BĀ-shŭn	______
orthopnea (465)	ŏr-THŎP-nē-ă	______
oxygen (462)	ŎKS-ĭ-jĕn	______
palatine tonsil (462)	PĂL-ĭ-tīn TŎN-sĭl	______
paranasal sinus (462)	pă-ră-NĀ-zăl SĪ-nŭs	______
parietal pleura (462)	pă-RĪ-ĕ-tăl PLOO-ră	______
pharyngeal (465)	fă-RĬN-jē-ăl *or* făr-ĭn-JĒ-ăl	______

12

TERM	PRONUNCIATION	MEANING
pharynx (463)	FĂR-ĭnkz	____
phrenic nerve (465)	FRĔN-ĭk nĕrv	____
pleura (463)	PLOOR-ă	____
pleural cavity (463)	PLOOR-ăl KĂ-vĭ-tē	____
pleurodynia (465)	ploor-ō-DĬN-ē-ă	____
pneumonectomy (466)	nū-mō-NĔK-tō-mē	____
pneumothorax (466)	nū-mō-THŌ-răks	____
pulmonary (466)	PŬL-mō-nār-ē	____
pulmonary parenchyma (463)	pŭl-mō-NĀR-ē pă-RĔN-kĭ-mă	____
pyothorax (468)	pī-ō-THŌ-răks	____
respiration (463)	rĕs-pĭ-RĀ-shĕn	____
rhinoplasty (466)	RĪ-nō-plăs-tē	____
rhinorrhea (466)	rī-nō-RĒ-ăh	____
sinusitis (466)	sī-nū-SĪ-tĭs	____
spirometer (466)	spī-RŎM-ĕ-tĕr	____
tachypnea (468)	tăk-ĬP-nē-ă	____
thoracic (467)	thōr-RĂ-sĭk	____
thoracotomy (467)	thōr-ră-KŎT-ō-mē	____
tonsillectomy (467)	tŏn-sĭ-LĔK-tō-mē	____
trachea (463)	TRĀ-kē-ă	____
tracheal stenosis (467)	TRĀ-kē-ăl stĕ-NŌ-sĭs	____
tracheotomy (467)	trā-kē-ŎT-ō-mē	____
visceral pleura (463)	VĬS-ĕr-ăl PLOOR-ă	____

Pathologic Conditions, Laboratory Tests, and Clinical Procedures

TERM	PRONUNCIATION	MEANING
anthracosis (475)	ăn-thră-KŌ-sĭs	____
asbestosis (475)	ăs-bĕs-TŌ-sĭs	____
asthma (470)	ĂZ-mă	____
atelectasis (471)	ă-tĕ-LĔK-tă-sĭs	____
auscultation (469)	ăw-skŭl-TĀ-shŭn	____

12

TERM	PRONUNCIATION	MEANING
bacilli (475)	bă-SĬL-ī	
bronchoalveolar lavage (477)	BRŎNG-kō-ăl-vē-Ō-lar lă-VĂJ	
bronchiectasis (470)	brŏng-kē-ĔK-tă-sĭs	
bronchoscopy (477)	brŏng-KŎS-kō-pē	
chronic bronchitis (470)	KRŎ-nĭk brŏng-KĪ-tĭs	
chronic obstructive pulmonary disease (475)	KRŎ-nĭk ŏb-STRŬK-tĭv PŬL-mō-nă-rē dĭ-ZĒZ	
computed tomography (476)	kŏm-PŪ-tĭd tō-MŎG-ră-fē	
cor pulmonale (475)	kŏr pŭl-mō-NĂ-lē	
croup (470)	kroop	
cystic fibrosis (471)	SĬS-tĭk fī-BRŌ-sĭs	
diphtheria (470)	dĭf-THĔR-ē-ă	
emphysema (471)	ĕm-fĭ-ZĒ-mă	
endotracheal intubation (478)	ĕn-dō-TRĀ-kē-ăl ĭn-tū-BĀ-shŭn	
epistaxis (470)	ĕp-ĭ-STĂK-sĭs	
exudate (475)	ĔK-sū-dāt	
hydrothorax (475)	hī-drō-THŎR-ăks	
infiltrate (475)	ĬN-fĭl-trāt	
laryngoscopy (478)	lăr-ĭng-GŎS-kō-pē	
lung biopsy (478)	lŭng BĪ-ŏp-sē	
lung cancer (472)	lŭng KĂN-sĕr	
magnetic resonance imaging of the chest (497)	măg-NĔ-tĭk RĔ-zō-năns ĬM-ă-gĭng of the chĕst	
mediastinoscopy (478)	mē-dē-ă-stī-NŎS-kō-pē	
mesothelioma (474)	mĕz-ō-thē-lē-Ō-mă	
obstructive lung disease (478)	ŏb-STRŬK-tĭv lŭng dĭ-ZĒZ	
palliative (475)	PĂL-ē-ă-tĭv	
paroxysmal (475)	păr-ŏk-SĬZ-măl	
percussion (469)	pĕr-KŬSH-ŭn	
pertussis (470)	pĕr-TŬS-ĭs	
pleural effusion (475)	PLOOR-ăl ĕ-FŪ-zhŭn	
pleural rub (469)	PLOOR-ăl rŭb	

12

TERM	PRONUNCIATION	MEANING
pleurisy (475)	PLOOR-ĭ-sē	
pneumoconiosis (472)	nū-mō-kō-nē-Ō-sĭs	
pneumonia (473)	nū-MŌ-nē-ă	
pneumothorax (475)	nū-mō-THŎR-ăks	
positron emission tomography (477)	PŎS-ĭ-trŏn ē-MĬ-shŭn tō-MŎG-ră-fē	
pulmonary abscess (473)	PŬL-mō-nă-rē ĂB-sĕs	
pulmonary edema (473)	PŬL-mō-nă-rē ĕ-DĒ-mă	
pulmonary embolism (474)	PŬL-mō-nă-rē ĔM-bō-lĭzm	
pulmonary fibrosis (474)	PŬL-mō-nă-rē fī-BRŌ-sĭs	
pulmonary function tests (478)	PŬL-mō-nă-rē FŬNK-shŭn tĕsts	
pulmonary infarction (475)	PŬL-mō-nă-rē ĭn-FĂRK-shŭn	
purulent (475)	PŪ-rū-lĕnt	
rales (469)	răhlz	
restrictive lung disease (478)	rē-STRĬK-tĭv lŭng dĭ-ZĒZ	
rhonchi (469)	RŎNG-kī	
sarcoidosis (474)	săr-koy-DŌ-sĭs	
silicosis (475)	sĭ-lĭ-KŌ-sĭs	
sputum (469)	SPŪ-tŭm	
sputum culture (469)	SPŪ-tŭm KŬL-chŭr	
stridor (469)	STRĪ-dŏr	
thoracentesis (479)	thō-ră-sĕn-TĒ-sĭs	
thoracotomy (480)	thō-ră-KŎ-tō-mē	
thoracoscopy (thorascopy) (480)	thō-ră-KŎS-kō-pē (thō-RĂS-kō-pē)	
tracheostomy (480)	trā-kē-ŎS-tō-mē	
tuberculin test (480)	too-BĔR-kū-lĭn tĕst	
tuberculosis (474)	too-bĕr-kū-LŌ-sĭs	
tube thoracostomy (480)	toob thŏr-ă-KŎS-tō-mē	
ventilation-perfusion scan (477)	vĕn-tĭ-LĀ-shŭn pĕr-FŪ-zhŭn scăn	
wheezes (469)	WĒZ-ĕz	

12

REVIEW SHEET

Write the meanings of the word parts in the spaces provided. Check your answers with the information in the chapter or in the Glossary (Medical Word Parts—English) at the end of the book.

Combining Forms

COMBINING FORM	MEANING	COMBINING FORM	MEANING
adenoid/o	______	pector/o	______
alveol/o	______	pharyng/o	______
bronch/o	______	phon/o	______
bronchi/o	______	phren/o	______
bronchiol/o	______	pleur/o	______
capn/o	______	pneum/o	______
coni/o	______	pneumon/o	______
cyan/o	______	pulmon/o	______
epiglott/o	______	py/o	______
hydr/o	______	rhin/o	______
laryng/o	______	sinus/o	______
lob/o	______	spir/o	______
mediastin/o	______	tel/o	______
nas/o	______	thorac/o	______
or/o	______	tonsill/o	______
orth/o	______	trache/o	______
ox/o	______		

Suffixes

SUFFIX	MEANING	SUFFIX	MEANING
-algia	______	-plasty	______
-capnia	______	-pnea	______
-centesis	______	-ptysis	______
-dynia	______	-rrhea	______
-ectasis	______	-scopy	______
-ectomy	______	-sphyxia	______
-ema	______	-stenosis	______
-lysis	______	-stomy	______
-osmia	______	-thorax	______
-oxia	______	-tomy	______
-phonia	______	-trophy	______

12

Prefixes

PREFIX	MEANING	PREFIX	MEANING
a-, an-	____________	hyper-	____________
brady-	____________	hypo-	____________
dys-	____________	para-	____________
em-	____________	per-	____________
eu-	____________	re-	____________
ex-	____________	tachy-	____________

Label the following lung abnormalities: atelectasis, pleural effusion, pneumothorax, and pulmonary edema.

A

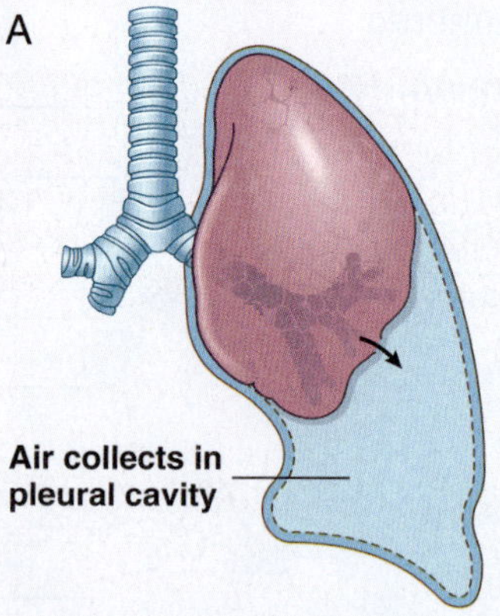

____

B

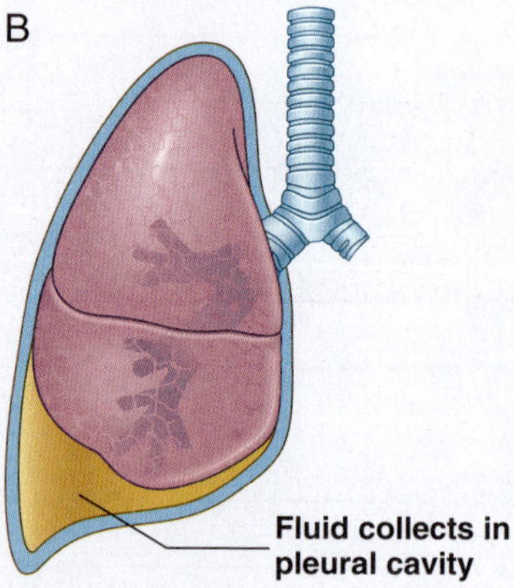

____

C

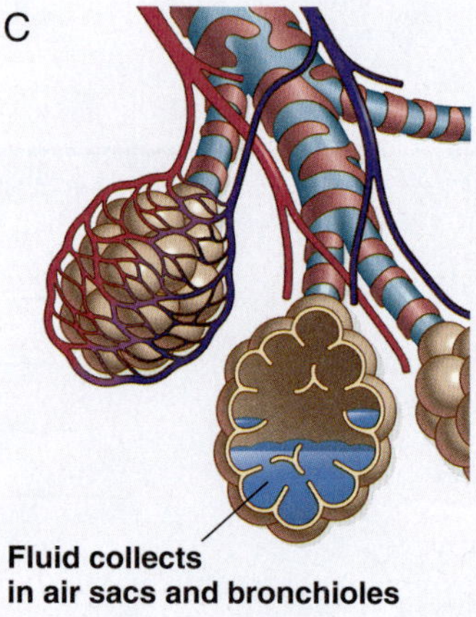

____

D

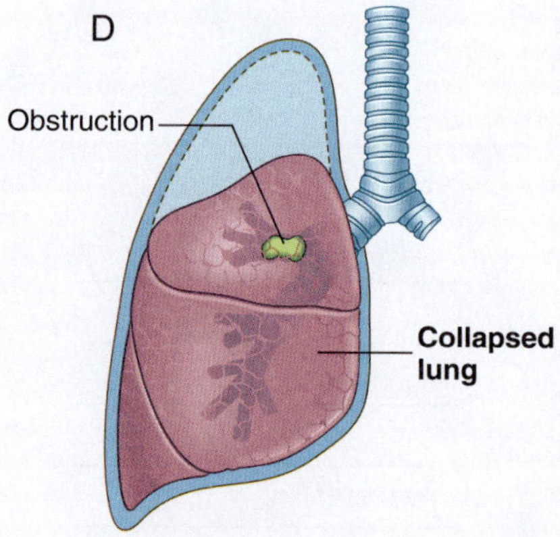

____

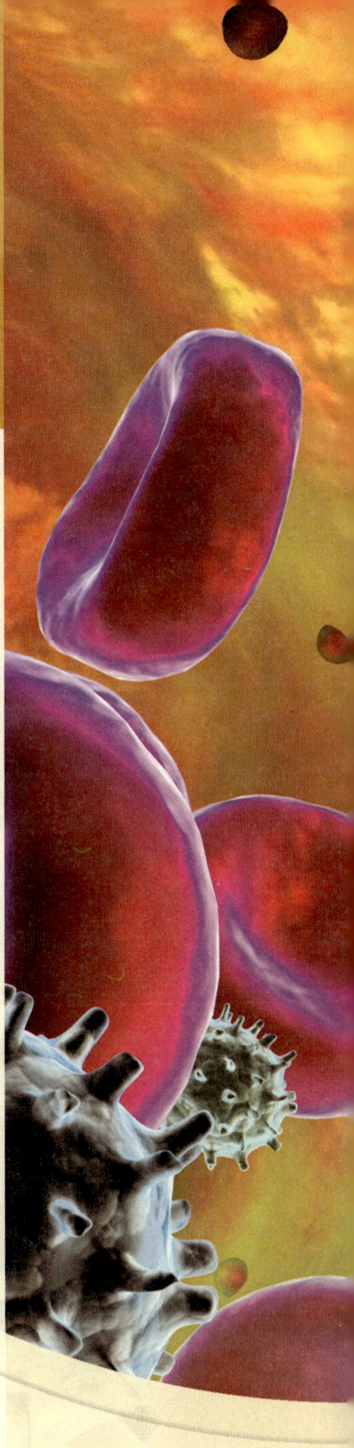

CHAPTER 13

Blood System

This chapter is divided into the following sections:

CHAPTER GOALS

- Identify terms relating to the composition, formation, and function of blood.
- Differentiate among the four major blood types.
- Identify terms related to blood clotting.
- Build words and recognize combining forms used in blood system terminology.
- Identify various pathologic conditions affecting blood.
- Describe various laboratory tests and clinical procedures used with hematologic disorders, and recognize relevant abbreviations.
- Apply your new knowledge to understanding medical terms in their proper contexts, such as medical reports and records.

INTRODUCTION

The primary function of blood is to maintain a constant environment for the other living tissues of the body. Blood transports nutrients, gases, and wastes to and from the cells of the body. Nutrients from food, digested in the stomach and small intestine, pass into the bloodstream through the lining cells of the small intestine. Blood then carries these nutrients to all body cells. Oxygen enters the body through the air sacs of the lungs. Red blood cells then transport the oxygen to cells throughout the body. Blood also helps remove the waste products released by cells. It carries gaseous waste (such as carbon dioxide) to the lungs to be exhaled. It carries chemical waste, such as urea, to the kidneys to be excreted in the urine.

Blood transports chemical messengers called hormones from their sites of secretion in glands, such as the thyroid or pituitary, to distant sites where they regulate growth, reproduction, and energy production. These hormones are discussed later in the endocrine chapter.

Finally, blood contains proteins, white blood cells and antibodies that fight infection, and platelets (thrombocytes) and other proteins that help the blood to clot.

COMPOSITION AND FORMATION OF BLOOD

Blood is composed of **cells,** or formed elements, suspended in a clear, straw-colored liquid called **plasma.** The cells normally constitute 45% of the blood volume and include **erythrocytes** (red blood cells), **leukocytes** (white blood cells), and **platelets** or **thrombocytes** (clotting cells). The remaining 55% of blood is plasma, a solution of water, proteins, sugar, salts, hormones, lipids, and vitamins.

CELLS

Beginning at birth, all blood cells originate in the marrow cavity of bones. Both the red blood cells that carry oxygen and the white blood cells that fight infection arise from the same blood-forming or **hematopoietic stem cells.** Under the influence of proteins in the blood and bone marrow, stem cells change their size and shape to become specialized, or **differentiated.** In this process, the cells change in size from large (immature cells) to small (mature forms), and the cell nucleus shrinks (in red cells, the nucleus actually disappears). Figure 13-1 illustrates these changes in the formation of blood cells. Use Figure 13-1 as a **reference** as you learn the names of mature blood cells and their earlier forms.

ERYTHROCYTES

As a red blood cell matures (from erythroblast to erythrocyte), it loses its nucleus and assumes the shape of a biconcave disk. This shape (a depressed or hollow surface on each side of the cell, resembling a cough drop with a thin central portion) allows for a large surface area so that absorption and release of gases (oxygen and carbon dioxide) can take place (Figure 13-2A and B). Red cells contain the unique protein **hemoglobin,** composed of **heme** (iron-containing pigment) and **globin** (protein). Hemoglobin enables the erythrocyte to carry oxygen. The combination of oxygen and hemoglobin (oxyhemoglobin) produces the bright red color of blood.

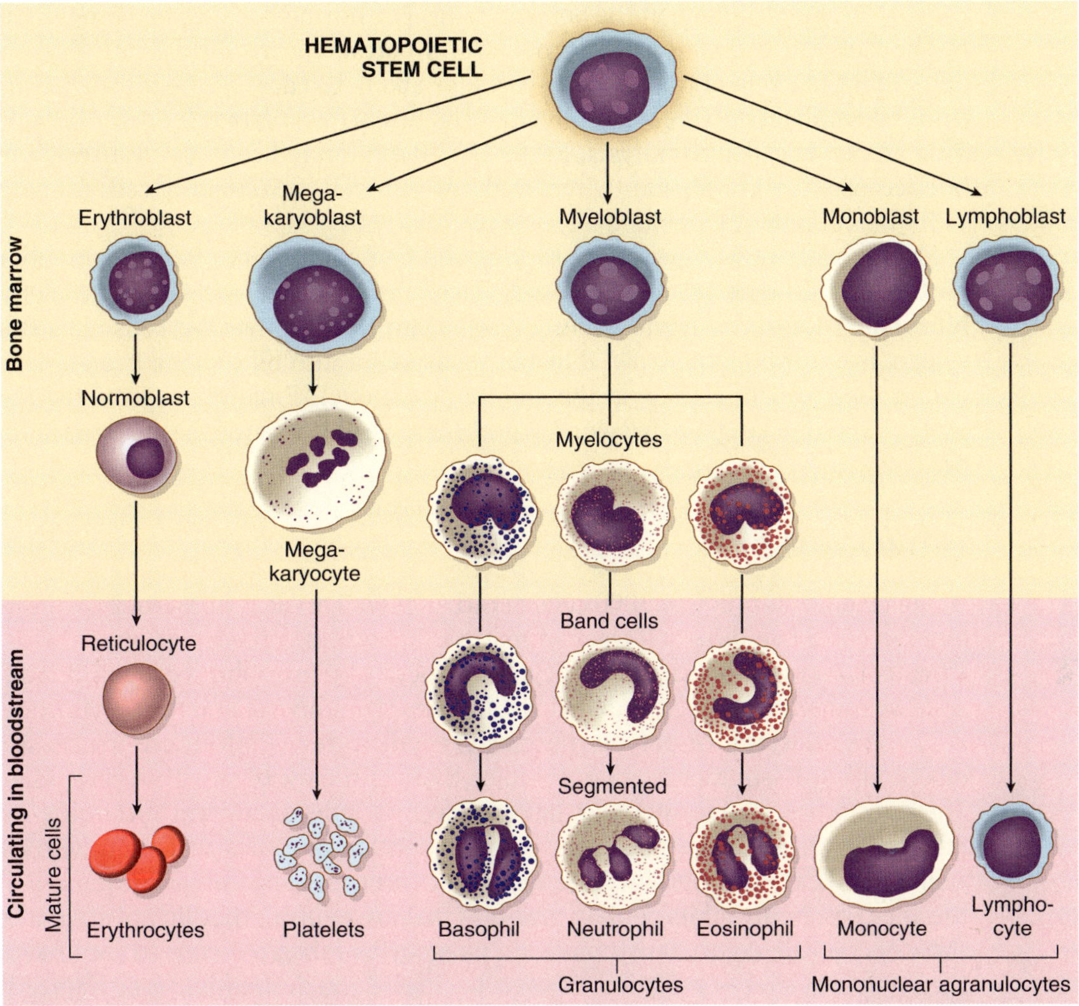

FIGURE 13-1 Stages in blood cell development (hematopoiesis). All blood cells originate from **hematopoietic stem cells. Progenitor cells** are derived from hematopoietic stem cells. **Myeloid progenitor cells** give rise to **erythroblasts, megakaryoblasts,** and **myeloblasts. Lymphoid progenitor cells** give rise to **monoblasts** and **lymphoblasts.** Notice that the suffix **-blast** indicates immature forms of all cells. **Band cells** are identical to **segmented granulocytes** except that the nucleus is U-shaped and its lobes are connected by a band rather than by a thin thread as in segmented forms.

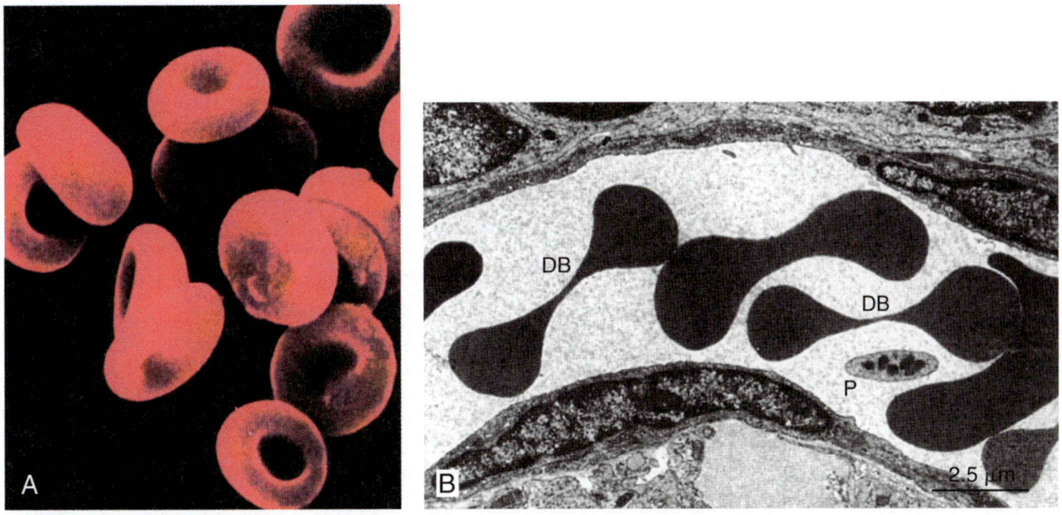

FIGURE 13-2 A, Normal erythrocytes (red blood cells). **B,** Electron micrograph showing **erythrocytes within a capillary.** Note the classic biconcave or "dumbbell" shape (DB) seen when the erythrocyte is cut through its thin central zone. A platelet (P) is seen as well.

13

Erythrocytes originate in the bone marrow. The hormone called **erythropoietin** (secreted by the kidneys) stimulates their production (**-poiesis** means formation). Erythrocytes live and fulfill their role of transporting gases for about 120 days in the bloodstream. After this time, **macrophages** (in the spleen, liver, and bone marrow) destroy the worn-out erythrocytes. This process is called **hemolysis.** From 2 to 10 million red cells are destroyed each second, but because they are constantly replaced, the number of circulating cells remains constant (4 to 6 million per μL of blood).

Macrophages break down erythrocytes and hemoglobin into heme and globin (protein) portions. The heme releases iron and decomposes into a yellow-orange pigment called **bilirubin.** The iron in hemoglobin is used again to form new red cells or is stored in the spleen, liver, or bone marrow. Bilirubin is excreted into bile by the liver, and from bile it enters the small intestine via the common bile duct. Finally it is excreted in the stool, where its color changes to brown. Figure 13-3 reviews the sequence of events in hemoglobin breakdown.

LEUKOCYTES

White blood cells (7000 to 9000 cells per μL of blood) are less numerous than erythrocytes, but there are five different types of mature leukocytes, shown in Figure 13-4. These are three polymorphonuclear granulocytic leukocytes (neutrophil, eosinophil, and basophil) and two mononuclear agranulocytic leukocytes (lymphocyte and monocyte).

The **granulocytes,** or **polymorphonuclear leukocytes (PMNs),** are the most numerous (about 60%). **Basophils** contain granules that stain dark blue with a basic (alkaline) dye. These granules contain heparin (an anticlotting substance) and histamine (a chemical released in allergic responses). **Eosinophils** contain granules that stain with eosin, a red acidic dye. These granules increase in allergic responses and engulf substances that trigger the allergies. **Neutrophils** contain granules that are neutral; they do not stain intensely and show only a pale color. Neutrophils are **phagocytes** (**phag/o** means to eat or swallow) that accumulate at sites of infection, where they ingest and destroy bacteria. Figure 13-5 shows phagocytosis by a neutrophil.

Specific proteins called **colony-stimulating factors** (CSFs) promote the growth of granulocytes in bone marrow. **G-CSF** (granulocyte CSF) and **GM-CSF** (granulocyte-macrophage CSF) are given to restore granulocyte production in cancer patients. **Erythropoietin,** like CSFs, can be produced by recombinant DNA techniques. It stimulates red blood cell production (erythropoiesis).

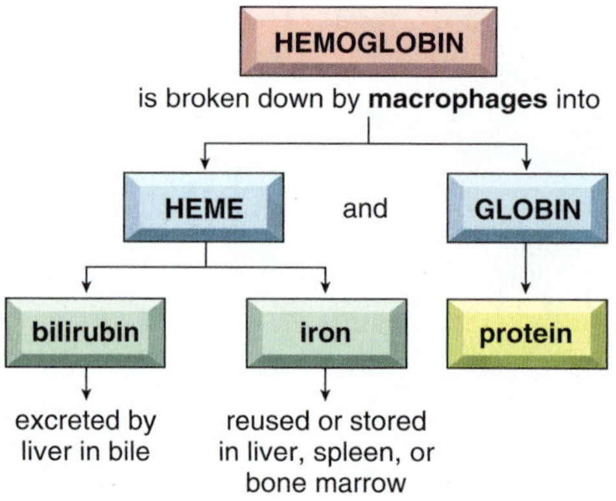

FIGURE 13-3 **The breakdown of hemoglobin.**

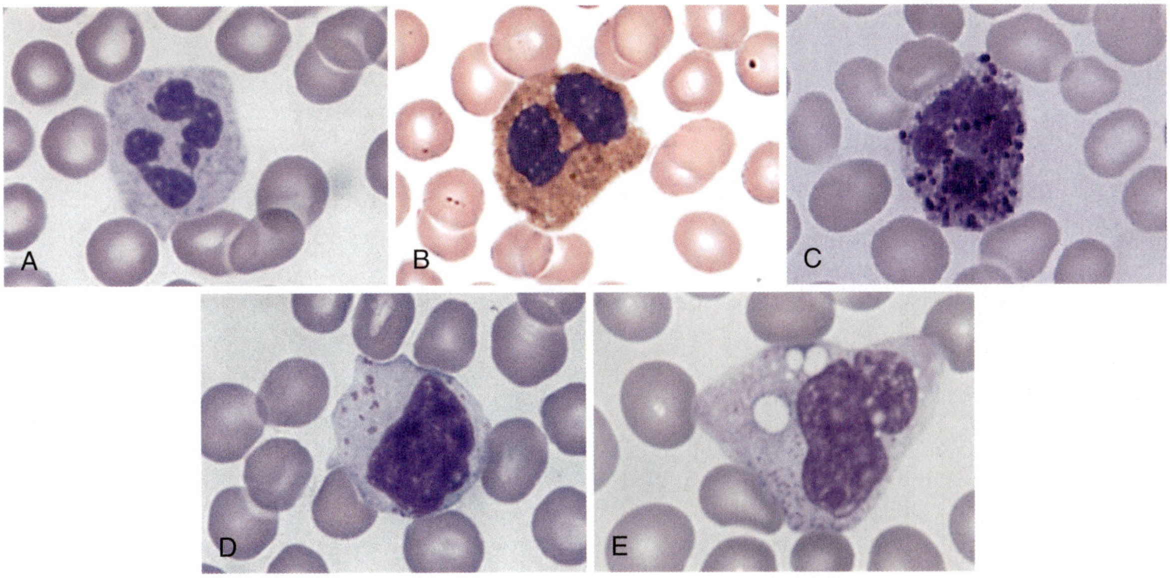

FIGURE 13-4 **Leukocytes. A, Neutrophil. B, Eosinophil. C, Basophil. D, Lymphocyte. E, Monocyte.**

Although all granulocytes are **polymorphonuclear** (they have multilobed nuclei), the term **polymorphonuclear granulocytes ("polys")** often describe the **neutrophil,** which is the most numerous of the granulocytes.

Mononuclear (containing one large nucleus) leukocytes do not have large numbers of granules in their cytoplasm, but they may have a few granules. These are **lymphocytes** and **monocytes** (see Figure 13-1). Lymphocytes are made in bone marrow and lymph nodes and circulate both in the bloodstream and in the parallel circulating system, the lymphatic system.

Lymphocytes play an important role in the **immune response** that protects the body against infection. They can directly attack foreign matter and, in addition, make **antibodies** that neutralize and can lead to the destruction of foreign **antigens** (bacteria and viruses). **Monocytes** are phagocytic cells that also fight disease. As **macrophages**, they move from the bloodstream into tissues and dispose of dead and dying cells and other tissue debris by phagocytosis.

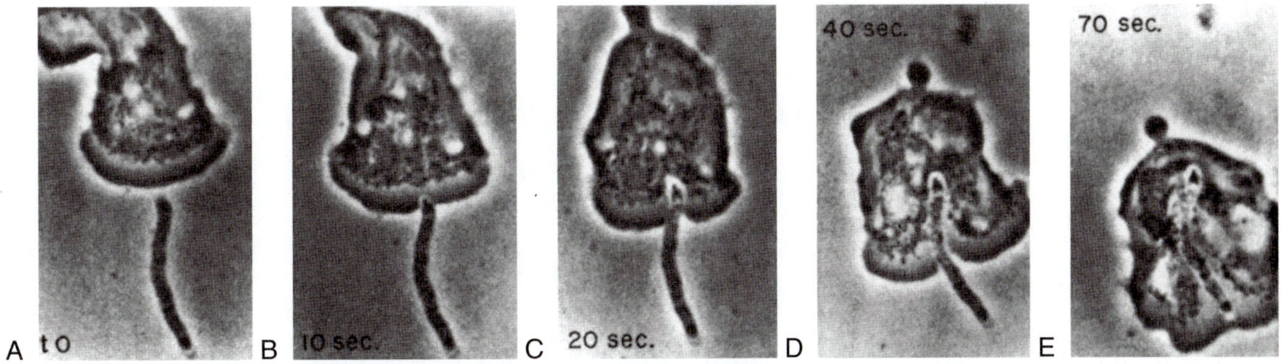

FIGURE 13-5 **Phagocytosis** (ingestion) of a bacterium by a neutrophil.

TABLE 13-1 LEUKOCYTES

Leukocyte	Normal Percentage in Blood	Function
Granulocytes		
Basophil	0-1	Responds to allergens; releases histamine and heparin
Eosinophil	1-4	Responds to parasitic infections and is a phagocyte in allergic reactions
Neutrophil	50-70	Major role in fighting bacterial infection; phagocyte
Mononuclear Cells		
Lymphocyte	20-40	Controls the immune response; makes antibodies to antigens
Monocyte	3-8	Phagocytic cell that becomes a macrophage and digests bacteria and tissue debris

Table 13-1 reviews the different types of leukocytes, their numbers in the blood, and their functions.

PLATELETS (THROMBOCYTES)

Platelets, actually blood cell fragments, are formed in bone marrow from giant cells with multilobed nuclei called **megakaryocytes** (Figure 13-6A and B). Tiny fragments of a megakaryocyte break off to form platelets. The main function of platelets is to help blood to clot. Specific terms related to blood clotting are discussed later in this chapter.

13

PLASMA

Plasma, the liquid part of the blood, consists of water, dissolved proteins, sugar, wastes, salts, hormones, and other substances. The four major plasma proteins are **albumin, globulins, fibrinogen,** and **prothrombin** (the last two are clotting proteins).

Albumin maintains the proper proportion (and concentration) of water in the blood. Because albumin cannot pass easily through capillary walls, it remains in the blood and

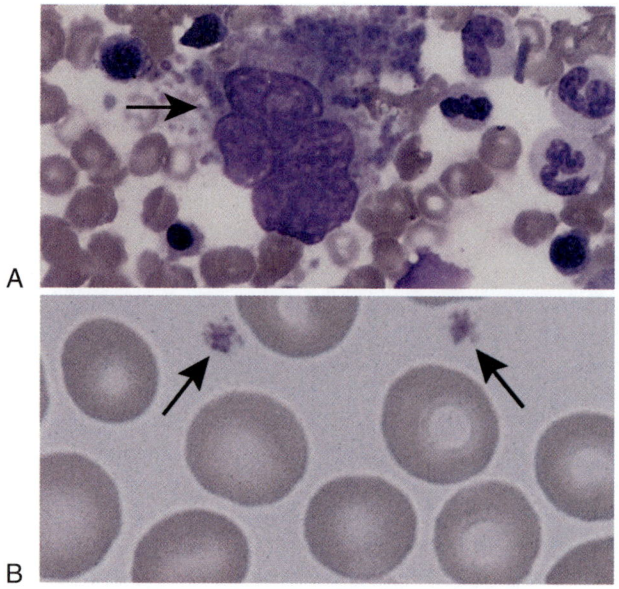

FIGURE 13-6 **A, Megakaryocyte B, Platelets.**

carries smaller molecules bound to its surface. It attracts water from the tissues back into the bloodstream and thus opposes the water's tendency to leave the blood and leak out into tissue spaces. **Edema** (swelling) results when too much fluid from blood "leaks" out into tissues. This happens in a mild form when a person ingests too much salt (water is retained in the blood and seeps out into tissues) and in a severe form when a person is burned in a fire. In this situation, albumin escapes from capillaries as a result of the burn injury. Then water cannot be held in the blood; it escapes through the skin, and blood volume drops.

Globulins are another component of blood and one of the plasma proteins. There are alpha, beta, and gamma globulins. The gamma globulins are **immunoglobulins,** which are antibodies that bind to and sometimes destroy antigens (foreign substances). Examples of immunoglobulin antibodies are **IgG** (found in high concentration in plasma) and **IgA** (found in breast milk, saliva, tears, and respiratory mucus). Other immunoglobulins are **IgM, IgD,** and **IgE.** Immunoglobulins are separated from other plasma proteins by **electrophoresis.** In this process, an electrical current passes through a solution of plasma. The different proteins in plasma separate as they migrate at different speeds to the source of the electricity.

Plasmapheresis (**-apheresis** means to remove) is the process of separating plasma from cells and then removing the plasma from the patient. In plasmapheresis, the entire blood sample is spun in a centrifuge machine, and the plasma, being lighter in weight than the cells, moves to the top of the sample.

Figure 13-7 reviews the composition of blood.

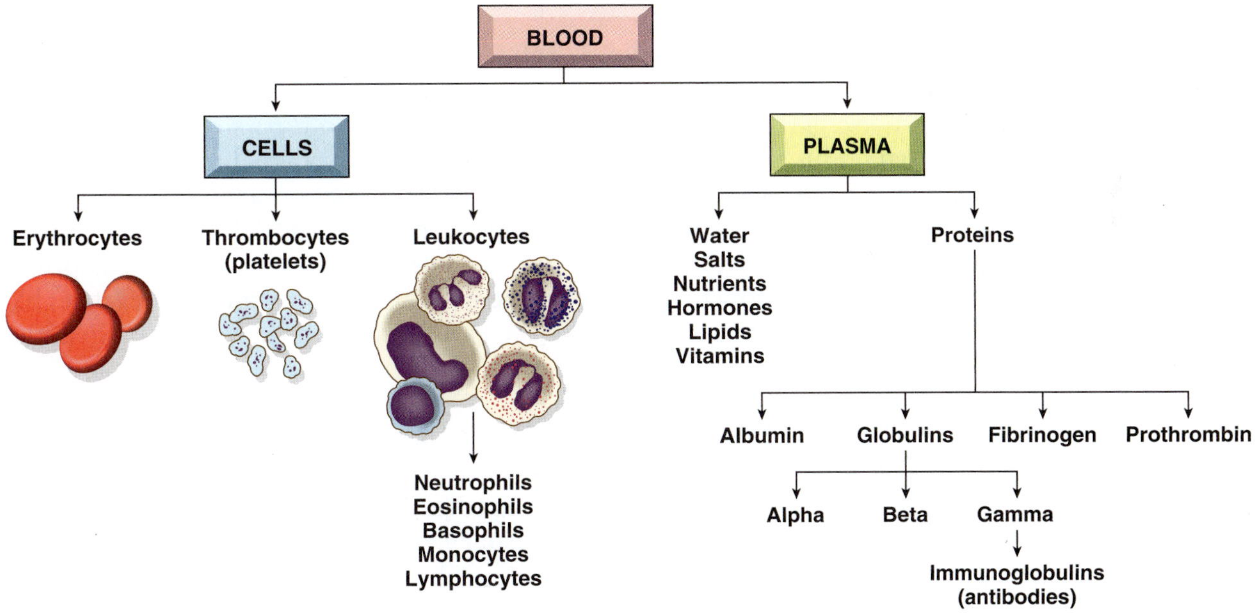

FIGURE 13-7 The composition of blood.

TABLE 13-2	BLOOD TYPES		
Type	**Percentage in Population**	**Red Cell Antigens**	**Serum Antibodies**
A	41	A	Yes (anti-B)
B	10	B	Yes (anti-A)
AB	4	A and B	No (anti-A or anti-B)
O	45	No A and B	Yes (anti-A and anti-B)

Blood Types

Transfusions of whole blood (cells and plasma) are used to replace blood lost after injury, during surgery, or in severe shock. A patient who is severely anemic and needs only red blood cells will receive a transfusion of **packed red cells** (whole blood with most of the plasma removed). Human blood falls into four main types: A, B, AB, and O. These types are based on the antigens on red blood cells and antibodies found in each person's serum (Table 13-2).

There are harmful effects of transfusing blood from a donor of one blood type into a recipient who has blood of another blood type. Therefore, before blood is transfused, both the blood donor and the blood recipient are tested, to make sure that the transfused blood will be compatible with the recipient's blood type. During transfusion, if blood is not compatible, then **hemolysis** (breakdown of red blood cells) occurs. This may be followed by excessive clotting in blood vessels **(disseminated intravascular coagulation,** or **DIC),** which is a life-threatening condition.

Besides A and B antigens, many other antigens are located on the surface of red blood cells. One of these is called the **Rh factor** (named because it was first found in the blood of a rhesus monkey). The term Rh positive (Rh+) refers to a person who is born with the Rh antigen on his or her red blood cells. An Rh negative (Rh–) person does not have the Rh antigen. See Chapter 4, page 118 for more information about the Rh factor. In clinical practice, blood types are named to indicate both Rh and ABO antigen status. If a woman has an A+ (A positive) blood type, for example, this means that she was born with both A antigen and Rh antigen on her red blood cells. If a man has a B– (B negative) blood type, this means he was born with the B antigen on his red blood cells but not Rh antigen.

Blood Clotting

Blood clotting, or **coagulation,** is a complicated process involving many different substances and chemical reactions. The final result (usually taking less than 15 minutes) is the formation of a **fibrin clot** from the plasma protein **fibrinogen.** The suffix -gen means giving rise to. Platelets are important in beginning the process following injury to tissues or blood vessels. The platelets become sticky and collect, or aggregate, at the site of injury. Then, in combination with tissue and clotting factors, plus calcium, prothrombin, and thrombin, fibrinogen is converted to fibrin to form a clot (Figure 13-8). One of the important clotting factors is factor VIII. It is missing in some people who are born with hemophilia. Other hemophiliacs are missing factor IX.

Why Is Type O the Universal Donor?

Type O blood does not contain A or B red cell antigens and therefore will not react with antibodies in any recipient's bloodstream. Anti-A and anti-B antibodies present in type O blood become diluted in the recipient's bloodstream and do not cause an adverse reaction.

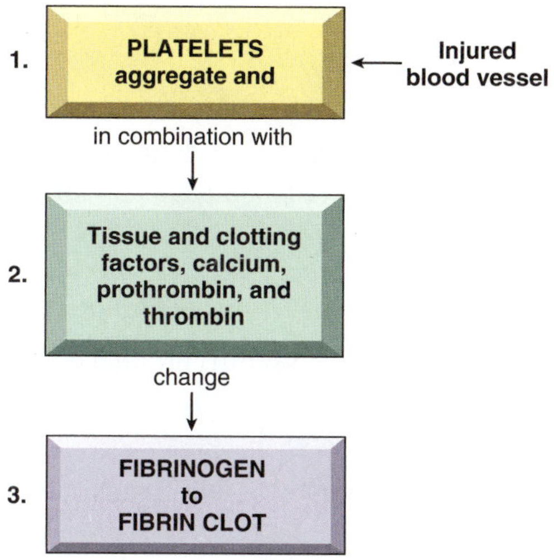

FIGURE 13-8 The sequence of events in blood clotting.

The fibrin threads form the clot by trapping red blood cells (Figure 13-9 shows a red blood cell trapped by fibrin threads). Then the clot retracts into a tight ball, leaving behind a clear fluid called **serum.** Normally, clots (thrombi) do not form in blood vessels unless the vessel is damaged or the flow of blood is impeded. **Anticoagulant substances** in the blood inhibit blood clotting, so clots do not form. **Heparin,** produced by tissue cells (especially in the liver), is an example of an anticoagulant. Other drugs such as **warfarin (Coumadin)** are given to patients with thromboembolic diseases to prevent the formation of clots.

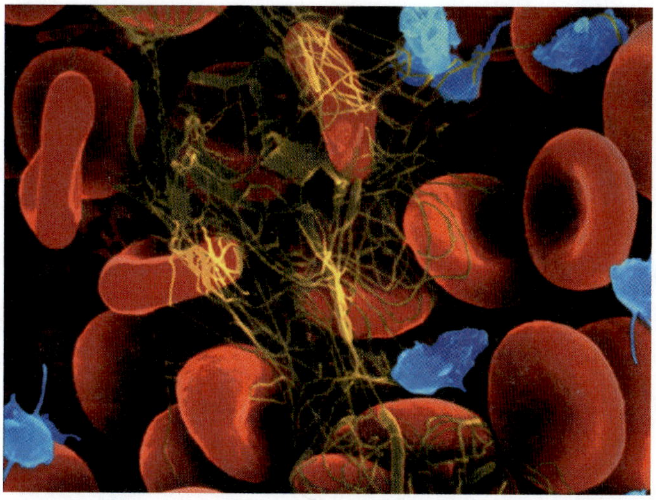

FIGURE 13-9 A red blood cell enmeshed in threads of fibrin.

13

VOCABULARY

This list reviews many of the new terms introduced in the text. Short definitions reinforce your understanding of the terms. Refer to the Pronunciation of Terms on page 538 for help with difficult or unfamiliar words.

albumin	Protein in blood; maintains the proper amount of water in the blood.
antibody (Ab)	Specific protein (immunoglobulin) produced by lymphocytes in response to bacteria, viruses, or other antigens. An antibody is specific to an antigen and inactivates it.
antigen	Substance (usually foreign) that stimulates the production of an antibody.
basophil	White blood cell containing granules that stain blue; associated with release of histamine and heparin.
bilirubin	Orange-yellow pigment in bile; formed by the breakdown of hemoglobin when red blood cells are destroyed.
coagulation	Blood clotting.
colony-stimulating factor (CSF)	Protein that stimulates growth of white blood cells (granulocytes).
differentiation	Change in structure and function of a cell as it matures; specialization.
electrophoresis	Method of separating serum proteins by electrical charge.
eosinophil	White blood cell containing granules that stain red; associated with allergic reactions.
erythroblast	Immature red blood cell.
erythrocyte	Red blood cell. There are about 5 million per microliter (μL) or cubic millimeter (mm^3) of blood.
erythropoietin (EPO)	Hormone secreted by the kidneys; stimulates red blood cell formation.
fibrin	Protein that forms the basis of a blood clot.
fibrinogen	Plasma protein that is converted to fibrin in the clotting process.
globulin	Plasma protein; alpha, beta, and gamma (immune) globulins are examples.
granulocyte	White blood cell with numerous dark-staining granules: eosinophil, neutrophil, and basophil.
hematopoietic stem cell	Cell in the bone marrow that gives rise to all types of blood cells.
hemoglobin	Blood protein containing iron; carries oxygen in red blood cells.
hemolysis	Destruction or breakdown of blood (red blood cells).
heparin	Anticoagulant found in blood and tissue cells.
immune reaction	Response of the immune system to foreign invasion.
immunoglobulin	Protein (globulin) with antibody activity; examples are IgG, IgM, IgA, IgE, IgD. Immun/o means protection.

leukocyte	White blood cell.
lymphocyte	Mononuclear leukocyte that produces antibodies.
macrophage	Monocyte that migrates from the blood to tissue spaces. As a phagocyte, it engulfs foreign material and debris. In the liver, spleen, and bone marrow, macrophages destroy worn out red blood cells.
megakaryocyte	Large platelet precursor cell found in the bone marrow.
monocyte	Leukocyte with one large nucleus. It is a cell that engulfs foreign material and debris. Monocytes become macrophages as they leave the blood and enter body tissues.
mononuclear	Pertaining to a cell (leukocyte) with a single round nucleus; lymphocytes and monocytes are mononuclear leukocytes.
myeloblast	Immature bone marrow that gives rise to granulocytes.
neutrophil	Granulocytic leukocyte formed in bone marrow. It is a phagocytic tissue-fighting cell. Also called a **polymorphonuclear leukocyte.**
plasma	Liquid portion of blood; contains water, proteins, salts, nutrients, lipids, hormones, and vitamins.
plasmapheresis	Removal of plasma from withdrawn blood by centrifuge. Collected cells are retransfused back into the donor. Fresh-frozen plasma or salt solution is used to replace withdrawn plasma.
platelet	Small blood fragment that collects at sites of injury to begin the clotting process.
polymorphonuclear	Pertaining to a white blood cell with a multi-lobed; neutrophil.
prothrombin	Plasma protein; converted to thrombin in the clotting process.
reticulocyte	Immature erythrocyte. A network of strands (reticulin) is seen after staining the cell with special dyes.
Rh factor	Antigen on red blood cells of Rh-positive (Rh^+) individuals. The factor was first identified in the blood of a rhesus monkey.
serum	Plasma minus clotting proteins and cells. Clear, yellowish fluid that separates from blood when it is allowed to clot. It is formed from plasma, but does not contain protein-coagulation factors.
stem cell	Unspecialized cell that gives rise to mature, specialized forms. A **hematopoietic stem cell** is the progenitor for all different types of blood cells.
thrombin	Enzyme that converts fibrinogen to fibrin during coagulation.
thrombocyte	Platelet.

TERMINOLOGY

Write the meanings of the medical terms in the spaces provided.

COMBINING FORMS

COMBINING FORM	MEANING	TERMINOLOGY	MEANING
bas/o	base (*alkaline*, the opposite of acid)	basophil *The suffix -phil means attraction to.*	____________
chrom/o	color	hypochromic *Hypochromic anemia is marked by a decreased concentration of hemoglobin in red blood cells.*	____________
coagul/o	clotting	anticoagulant	____________
		coagulopathy	____________
cyt/o	cell	cytology	____________
eosin/o	red, dawn, rosy	eosinophil	____________
erythr/o	red	erythroblast *-blast means immature.*	____________
granul/o	granules	granulocyte	____________
hem/o	blood	hemolysis *Destruction or breakdown of red blood cells. See hemolytic anemia, page 516.*	____________
hemat/o	blood	hematocrit *The suffix -crit means to separate. The hematocrit gives the percentage of red blood cells in a volume of blood. See page 521.*	____________
hemoglobin/o	hemoglobin	hemoglobinopathy	____________
is/o	same, equal	anisocytosis *An abnormality of red blood cells; they are of unequal (anis/o) size; -cytosis means an increase in the number of cells.*	____________
kary/o	nucleus	megakaryocyte	____________
leuk/o	white	leukopenia	____________
mon/o	one, single	monocyte *The cell has a single, rather than a multilobed, nucleus.*	____________
morph/o	shape, form	morphology	____________

COMBINING FORM	MEANING	TERMINOLOGY	MEANING
myel/o	bone marrow	myeloblast *The suffix -blast indicates an immature cell.*	
		myelodysplasia *This is a preleukemic condition.*	
neutr/o	neutral (neither base nor acid)	neutropenia *This term refers to neutrophils.*	
nucle/o	nucleus	polymorphonuclear	
phag/o	eat, swallow	phagocyte	
poikil/o	varied, irregular	poikilocytosis *Irregularity in the shape of red blood cells. Poikilocytosis occurs in certain types of anemia.*	
sider/o	iron	sideropenia	
spher/o	globe, round	spherocytosis *In this condition, the erythrocyte has a round shape, making the cell fragile and easily able to be destroyed.*	
thromb/o	clot	thrombocytopenia	

SUFFIXES

SUFFIX	MEANING	TERMINOLOGY	MEANING
-apheresis	removal, a carrying away	plasmapheresis *A centrifuge spins blood to remove plasma from the other parts of blood.*	
		leukapheresis	
		plateletpheresis *Note that the a of apheresis is dropped in this term. Platelets are removed from the donor's blood (and used in a patient), and the remainder of the blood is reinfused into the donor.*	
-blast	immature cell, embryonic	monoblast	

Don't confuse -apheresis with -phoresis

The suffix **-apheresis** (see page 522) refers to the removal of blood from a donor with a portion separated and retained and the remainder reinfused into the donor. The suffix **-phoresis** indicates transmission (as in **electrophoresis,** the transmission of electricity to separate substances).

SUFFIX	MEANING	TERMINOLOGY	MEANING
-cytosis	abnormal condition of cells (increase in cells)	macrocytosis *Macrocytes are erythrocytes that are larger (macro-) than normal.*	
		microcytosis *These are erythrocytes that are smaller (micro-) than normal. Table 13-3 reviews terms related to abnormalities of red blood cell morphology.*	
-emia	blood condition	leukemia *See page 518.*	
-gen	giving rise to; producing	fibrinogen *Fibrin is a protein that forms the basis of a blood clot.*	
-globin	protein	hemoglobin	
-globulin		immunoglobulin	
-lytic	pertaining to destruction	thrombolytic therapy *Used to dissolve clots.*	
-oid	derived or originating from	myeloid	
-osis	abnormal condition	thrombosis	
-penia	deficiency	granulocytopenia	
		pancytopenia	
-phage	eat, swallow	macrophage *A large phagocyte that destroys worn-out red blood cells and foreign material.*	
-philia	attraction for (an increase in cell numbers)	eosinophilia	
		neutrophilia	
-phoresis	carrying, transmission	electrophoresis	
-poiesis	formation	hematopoiesis	
		erythropoiesis ***Erythropoietin** is produced by the kidneys to stimulate erythrocyte formation.*	
		myelopoiesis	
-stasis	stop, control	hemostasis	

13

TABLE 13-3 ABNORMALITIES OF RED BLOOD CELL MORPHOLOGY

Abnormality	Description
Anisocytosis	Cells are **unequal** in size
Hypo**chromia**	Cells have reduced **color** (less hemoglobin)
Macrocytosis	Cells are **large**
Microcytosis	Cells are **small**
Poikilocytosis	Cells are **irregularly shaped**
Spherocytosis	Cells are **rounded**

PATHOLOGY

Any abnormal or pathologic condition of the blood generally is referred to as a blood **dyscrasia** (disease). The blood dyscrasias discussed in this section are organized in the following manner: diseases of red blood cells, disorders of blood clotting, diseases of white blood cells, and disease of the bone marrow.

DISEASES OF RED BLOOD CELLS

anemia

Deficiency in erythrocytes or hemoglobin.

The most common type of anemia is **iron deficiency anemia;** it is caused by a lack of iron, which is required for hemoglobin production (Figure 13-10).

Other types of anemia include:

1. aplastic anemia

Failure of blood cell production in the bone marrow.

The cause of most cases of aplastic anemia is unknown (idiopathic), but some have been linked to benzene exposure and to antibiotics such as chloramphenicol. **Pancytopenia** occurs when stem cells fail to produce leukocytes, platelets, and erythrocytes. Blood transfusions prolong life, allowing the marrow time to resume its normal functioning, and antibiotics control infections. Bone marrow transplantation and regimens of drugs that inhibit the immune system are successful treatments in cases in which spontaneous recovery is unlikely.

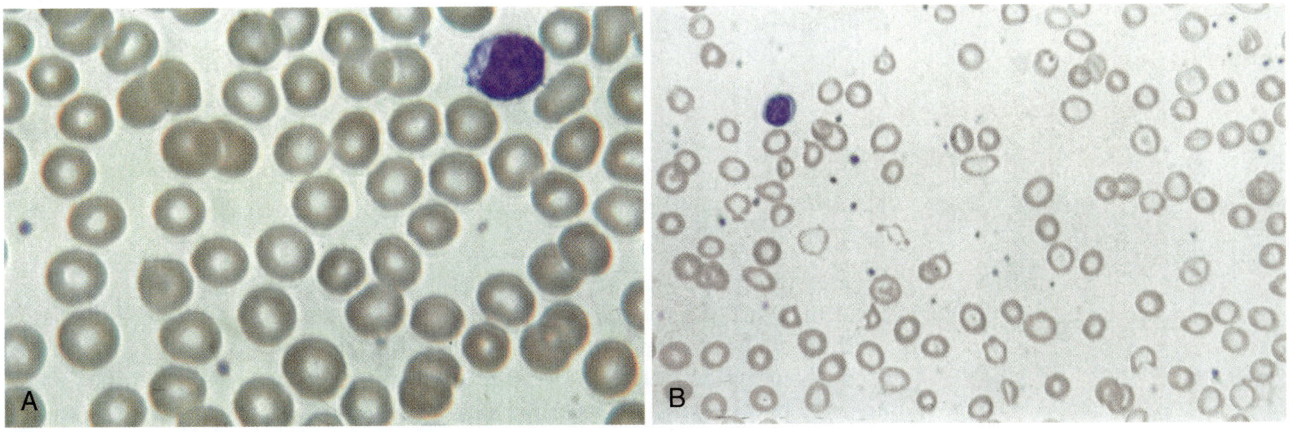

FIGURE 13-10 **Normal red blood cells and iron deficiency anemia. A, Normal red cells.** Erythrocytes are fairly uniform in size and shape. The red cells are normal in hemoglobin content (normochromic) and size (normocytic). **B, Iron deficiency anemia.** Many erythrocytes are small (**microcytic**) and have increased central pallor (**hypochromic**). Red cells in this slide show variation in size (**anisocytosis**) and shape (**poikilocytosis**).

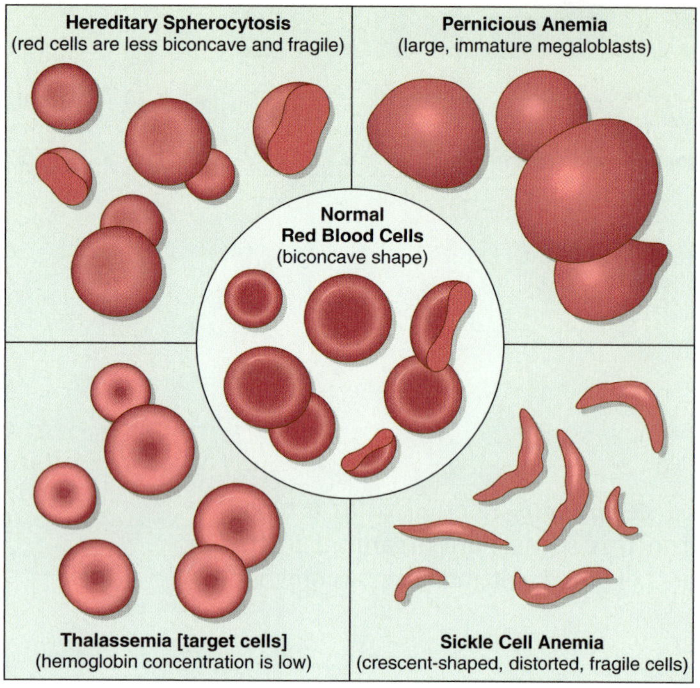

FIGURE 13-11 Normal red blood cells and the abnormal cells in several types of anemia.

2. hemolytic anemia

Reduction in red cells due to excessive destruction.

One example of hemolytic anemia is **congenital spherocytic anemia (hereditary spherocytosis).** Instead of their normal biconcave shape, erythrocytes become spheroidal. This rounded shape makes them fragile and easily destroyed (hemolysis). Shortened red cell survival results in increased reticulocytes in blood as the bone marrow compensates for hemolysis of mature erythrocytes. Because the spleen destroys red cells, removal of the spleen usually improves this anemia. Figure 13-11 shows the altered shape of erythrocytes in hereditary spherocytosis.

3. pernicious anemia

Lack of mature erythrocytes caused by inability to absorb vitamin B_{12} into the bloodstream.

Vitamin B_{12} is necessary for the proper development and maturation of erythrocytes. Although vitamin B_{12} is a common constituent of food (liver, kidney, sardines, egg yolks, oysters), it cannot be absorbed into the bloodstream without the aid of a special substance called **intrinsic factor** that is normally found in gastric juice. People with pernicious anemia lack this factor in their gastric juice, and the result is unsuccessful maturation of red blood cells, with an excess of large, immature, and poorly functioning cells in the bone marrow and large, often oval red cells (macrocytes) in the circulation. Treatment is administration (via injection) of vitamin B_{12} for life. Figure 13-11 illustrates cells in pernicious anemia. Pernicious means ruinous or hurtful.

4. sickle cell anemia

Hereditary disorder of abnormal hemoglobin producing sickle-shaped erythrocytes and hemolysis.

The crescent, or sickle, shape of the erythrocyte (see Figure 13-11) is caused by an abnormal type of hemoglobin (hemoglobin S) in the red cell. The distorted, fragile erythrocytes cannot pass through small blood vessels normally. This leads to thrombosis and infarction (local tissue death from ischemia). Signs and symptoms are arthralgias, acute attacks of abdominal pain, and ulcerations of the extremities. The genetic defect (presence of the hemoglobin S gene) is particularly prevalent in black persons of African or African American ancestry and appears with different degrees of severity. Individuals with the sickle cell trait inherit just one gene for the disorder and usually do not have symptoms.

5. thalassemia

Inherited defect in ability to produce hemoglobin, leading to hypochromia.

This condition, usually occurring in persons of Mediterranean background, manifests in varying forms and degrees of severity and usually leads to hypochromic anemia with diminished hemoglobin content in red cells (see Figure 13-11). *Thalassa* is a Greek word meaning sea.

hemochromatosis

Excess iron deposits throughout the body.

Hepatomegaly, cirrhosis, skin pigmentation, diabetes, and cardiac failure may occur.

polycythemia vera

General increase in red blood cells (erythremia).

Blood consistency is viscous (thick) because of greatly increased numbers of erythrocytes. The bone marrow is hyperplastic, and leukocytosis and thrombocytosis commonly accompany the increase in red blood cells. Treatment consists of reduction of red cell volume to normal levels by phlebotomy (removal of blood from a vein) and by suppressing blood cell production with myelotoxic drugs. Notice that that suffix here is -hemia, instead of -emia.

DISORDERS OF BLOOD CLOTTING

hemophilia

Excessive bleeding caused by hereditary lack of blood clotting factors (factor VIII or IX) necessary for blood clotting.

Although the platelet count of a hemophiliac patient is normal, deficiency in clotting factors (factor VIII or IX) results in a prolonged coagulation time. Patients with clotting factor deficiencies often bleed into weight-bearing joints, especially ankles and knees. See Figure 13-12. Treatment consists of administration of the deficient factor.

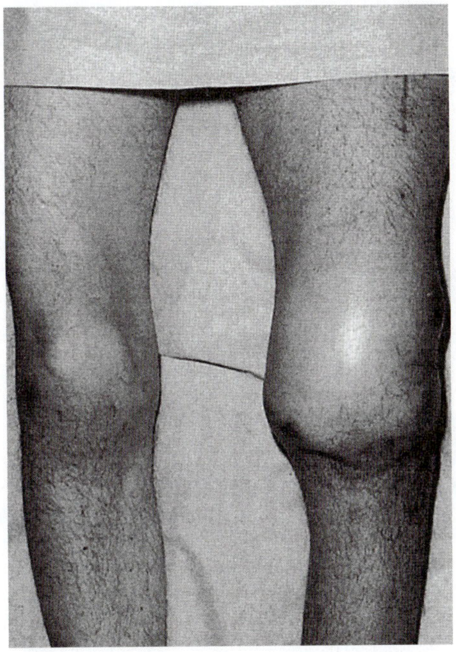

FIGURE 13-12 Lower limbs of a male with **hemophilia** showing the effect of recurrent hemorrhage into the knees. *(Courtesy Dr. G. Dolan, University Hospital, Nottingham, UK.)*

purpura

Multiple pinpoint hemorrhages and accumulation of blood under the skin.

Hemorrhages into the skin and mucous membranes produce red-purple discoloration of the skin. **Petechiae** are tiny purple or red flat spots appearing on the skin as a result of hemorrhages. **Ecchymoses** are larger blue or purplish patches on the skin (bruises) (Figure 13-13). Purpura can be caused by having too few platelets (thrombocytopenia). The cause may be immunologic, meaning the body produces an antiplatelet factor that harms its own platelets. **Autoimmune thrombocytopenic purpura** is a condition in which a patient makes an antibody that destroys platelets. Bleeding time is prolonged; splenectomy (the spleen is the site of platelet destruction) and drug therapy with corticosteroids are common treatments.

DISEASES OF WHITE BLOOD CELLS

leukemia

Increase in cancerous white blood cells (leukocytes).

Acute leukemias have common clinical characteristics: abrupt onset of symptoms, fatigue, fever, bleeding, bone pain, lymphadenopathy, splenomegaly, and hepatomegaly. If the disease has spread to the spinal canal, signs such as headache and vomiting may occur. In addition, because normal blood cells are crowded out, patients have little defense against infection.

Four types of leukemia are:

1. **Acute myelogenous (myelocytic) leukemia (AML).** Immature granulocytes (myeloblasts) predominate. Platelets and erythrocytes are diminished because of infiltration and replacement of the bone marrow by large numbers of myeloblasts (Figure 13-14A).

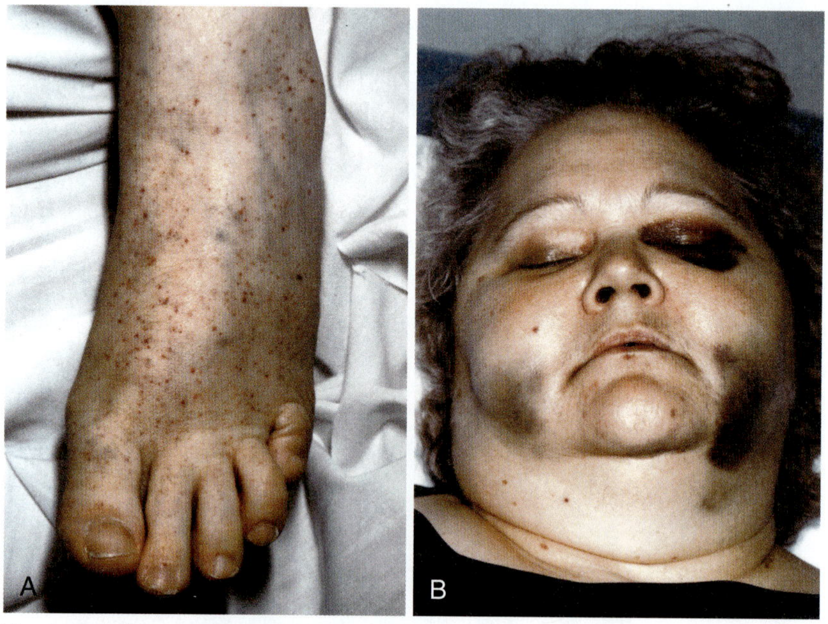

FIGURE 13-13 **A, Petechiae** result from bleeding from capillaries or small arterioles. **B, Ecchymoses** are larger and more extensive than petechiae.

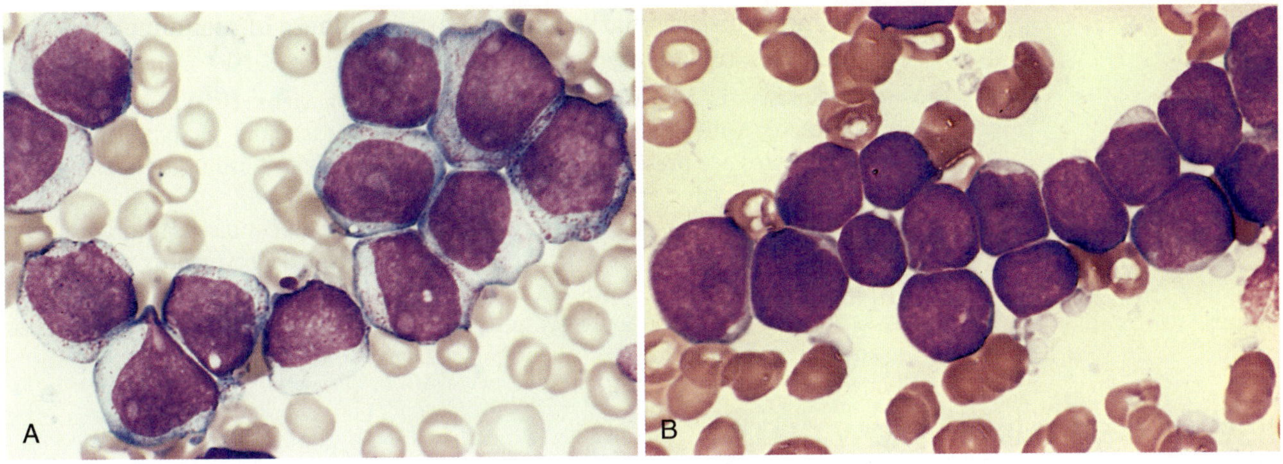

FIGURE 13-14 **Acute leukemia. A, Acute myeloblastic leukemia** (AML). Myeloblasts (immature granulocytes) predominate. There are large cells with small granules in their cytoplasm. AML affects primarily adults. A majority of patients achieve remission with intensive chemotherapy, but relapse is common. Hematopoietic stem cell transplantation may be a curative therapy. **B, Acute lymphoblastic leukemia** (ALL). Lymphoblasts (immature lymphocytes) predominate. ALL is a disease of children and young adults. Most children are cured with chemotherapy. *(Courtesy Dr. Robert W. McKenna, Department of Pathology, University of Texas Southwestern Medical School, Dallas.)*

2. **Acute lymphocytic leukemia (ALL).** Immature lymphocytes (lymphoblasts) predominate. This form is seen most often in children and adolescents; onset is sudden (see Figure 13-14B).
3. **Chronic myelogenous (myelocytic) leukemia (CML).** Both mature and immature granulocytes are present in large numbers in the marrow and blood. This is a slowly progressive illness with which patients (often adults older than 55) may live for many years without encountering life-threatening problems. New therapies (such as the drug Gleevec) target abnormal proteins responsible for malignancy and produce long-term control.
4. **Chronic lymphocytic leukemia (CLL).** Abnormal numbers of relatively mature lymphocytes predominate in the marrow, lymph nodes, and spleen. This most common form of leukemia usually occurs in the elderly and follows a slowly progressive course. It often does not require immediate treatment.

All forms of leukemia are treated with chemotherapy, using drugs that prevent cell division and selectively injure rapidly dividing cells. Effective treatment can lead to a **remission** (disappearance of signs and symptoms of disease). **Relapse** occurs when disease symptoms and signs reappear, necessitating further treatment.

Transplantation of normal bone marrow from donors of similar tissue type is successful in restoring normal bone marrow function in some patients with acute leukemia. This procedure is performed after high-dose chemotherapy, which is administered to eliminate the leukemic cells.

granulocytosis

Abnormal increase in granulocytes in the blood.

An increase in neutrophils in the blood may occur in response to infection or inflammation of any type. **Eosinophilia** is an increase in eosinophilic granulocytes, seen in certain allergic conditions, such as asthma, or in parasitic infections (tapeworm, pinworm). **Basophilia** is an increase in basophilic granulocytes seen in certain types of leukemia.

mononucleosis

Infectious disease marked by increased numbers of mononuclear leukocytes and enlarged cervical lymph nodes.

This disease is transmitted by the **Epstein-Barr virus (EBV).** Lymphadenitis is present, with fever, fatigue, asthenia (weakness), and pharyngitis. Atypical lymphocytes are present in the blood, liver, and spleen (leading to hepatomegaly and splenomegaly).

Mononucleosis usually is transmitted by direct oral contact (salivary exchange during kissing) and affects primarily young adults. No treatment is necessary for EBV infections. Antibiotics are not effective for self-limited viral illnesses. Rest during the period of acute symptoms and slow return to normal activities are advised.

DISEASE OF BONE MARROW CELLS

multiple myeloma

Malignant neoplasm of bone marrow.

The malignant cells (lymphocytes that produce antibodies) destroy bone tissue and cause overproduction of immunoglobulins, including **Bence Jones protein**, an immunoglobulin fragment found in urine. The condition leads to osteolytic lesions, hypercalcemia, anemia, renal damage, and increased susceptibility to infection. Treatment is with analgesics, radiotherapy, various doses of chemotherapy, and special orthopedic supports. Drugs such as thalidomide and Velcade (bortezomib) are **palliative** (relieving symptoms) and stop disease progression, which improves the outlook for this disease. **Autologous bone marrow transplantation (ABMT),** in which the patient serves as his or her own donor for stem cells, may lead to prolonged remission.

LABORATORY TESTS AND CLINICAL PROCEDURES

LABORATORY TESTS

antiglobulin test (Coombs test)

Test for the presence of antibodies that coat and damage erythrocytes.

This test determines the presence of antibodies in infants of Rh-negative women or in patients with autoimmune hemolytic anemia.

bleeding time

Time required for blood to stop flowing from a tiny puncture wound.

Normal time is 8 minutes or less. Either the Simplate or the Ivy method is used. Platelet disorders and the use of aspirin prolong bleeding time.

coagulation time

Time required for venous blood to clot in a test tube.

Normal time is less than 15 minutes.

complete blood count (CBC)

Determination of numbers of blood cells, hemoglobin concentration, hematocrit, and red cell values—MCH, MCV, MCHC (see Abbreviations).

erythrocyte sedimentation rate (ESR)

Speed at which erythrocytes settle out of plasma.

Venous blood is collected into an anticoagulant, and the blood is placed in a tube in a vertical position. The distance that the erythrocytes sink in a given period of time is the sedimentation rate. The rate increases with infections, joint inflammation, and tumor, which increase the fibrinogen content of the blood. Also called sed rate for short.

hematocrit (Hct)

Percentage of erythrocytes in a volume of blood.

A sample of blood is spun in a centrifuge so that the erythrocytes fall to the bottom of the sample.

hemoglobin test (H, Hg, Hgb, HGB)

Total amount of hemoglobin in a sample of peripheral blood.

platelet count

Number of platelets per cubic millimeter (mm^3) or microliter (μL) of blood.

Platelets normally average between 150,000 and 350,000 per mm^3 (cu mm) or μL.

prothrombin time (PT)

Test of the ability of blood to clot.

Prothrombin is one of the clotting factors (factor II) made by the liver. This test is used to monitor (follow) patients taking anticoagulant drugs. Another blood clotting test, **partial thromboplastin time (PTT)**, measures other clotting factors. Both PT and PTT are often done at the same time to check for bleeding problems.

red blood cell count (RBC)

Number of erythrocytes per cubic millimeter (mm^3) or microliter (μL) of blood.

The normal number is 4 to 6 million per mm^3 (or μL).

red blood cell morphology

Microscopic examination of a stained blood smear to determine the shape of individual red cells.

Abnormal morphology includes anisocytosis, poikilocytosis, and sickle cells.

white blood cell count (WBC)

Number of leukocytes per cubic millimeter (mm^3) or microliter (μL) of blood.

Automated counting devices record numbers within seconds. Normal number of leukocytes averages between 5000 and 10,000 per mm^3 (or μL).

white blood cell differential [count]

Percentages of different types of leukocytes in the blood.

Some instruments can produce an automated differential count, but otherwise the cells are stained and counted under a microscope by a technician. Percentages of neutrophils, eosinophils, basophils, monocytes, lymphocytes, and immature cells (bands) are determined. See page 526 for the normal differential values.

The term **shift to the left** describes an increase in immature neutrophils in the blood.

Shift to the Left

The phrase "**shift to the left**" derives from the early practice of reporting percentages of each WBC type across the top of a page, starting with blasts (immature cells) on the left and more mature cells on the right. An increase in immature neutrophils (as seen with severe infection) would be noted on the left-hand column of a form. Thus a "shift to the left" indicates an infection and the body's effort to fight it by making more neutrophils.

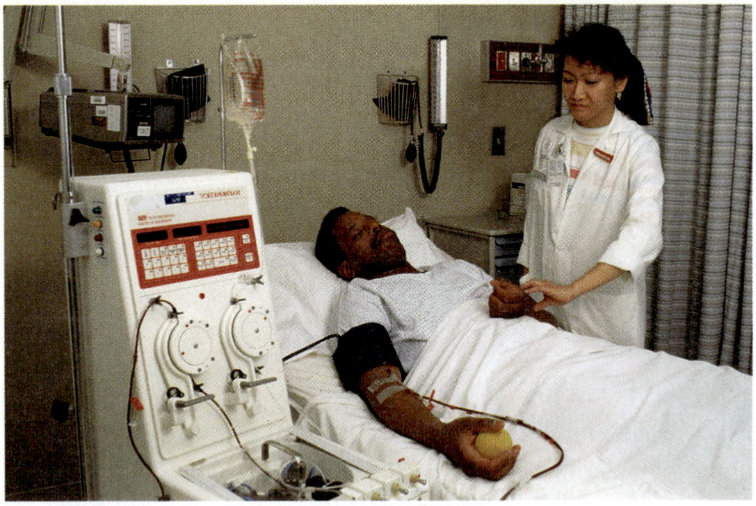

FIGURE 13-15 **Leukapheresis.** This machine is an automated blood cell separator that removes large numbers of white blood cells and returns red cells, platelets, and plasma to the patient.

CLINICAL PROCEDURES

apheresis

Separation of blood into component parts and removal of a select portion from the blood.

This procedure can remove toxic substances or autoantibodies from the blood and can collect blood cells. Leukapheresis, plateletpheresis, and plasmapheresis are examples (Figure 13-15). If plasma is removed from the patient and fresh plasma is given, the procedure is termed **plasma exchange.**

13

blood transfusion

Whole blood or cells are taken from a donor and infused into a patient.

Appropriate testing to ensure a match of red blood cell type (A, B, AB, or O) is essential. Tests also are performed to detect the presence of hepatitis and the acquired immunodeficiency syndrome (AIDS) virus (HIV). **Autologous transfusion** is the collection and later reinfusion of a patient's own blood or blood components. **Packed cells** are a preparation of red blood cells separated from liquid plasma and administered in severe anemia to restore levels of hemoglobin and red cells without overdiluting the blood with excess fluid.

bone marrow biopsy

Microscopic examination of a core of bone marrow removed with a needle.

This procedure is helpful in the diagnosis of blood disorders such as anemia, pancytopenias, and leukemia. Bone marrow also may be removed by brief suction produced by a syringe, which is termed a **bone marrow aspiration.** See Figure 13-16.

hematopoietic stem cell transplantation

Peripheral stem cells from a compatible donor are administered to a recipient.

Patients with malignancies, such as AML, ALL, CLL, CML, lymphoma and multiple myeloma, are candidates for this treatment. First the donor is treated with a drug that mobilizes stem cells into the blood. Then stem cells are removed from the donor, a process like leukapheresis in Figure 13-15. Meanwhile, the patient (recipient) undergoes a conditioning process in which radiation and chemotherapy drugs are administered to kill malignant marrow cells and inactivate the patient's immune system so that subsequently infused stem cells will not be rejected. A cell suspension containing the donor's stem cells, which will repopulate the bone marrow, is then given through a vein to the recipient. In **autologous stem cell transplantation,** the patient's own stem cells are collected, stored, and reinfused after potent chemotherapy. See the ***In Person*** story, page 528.

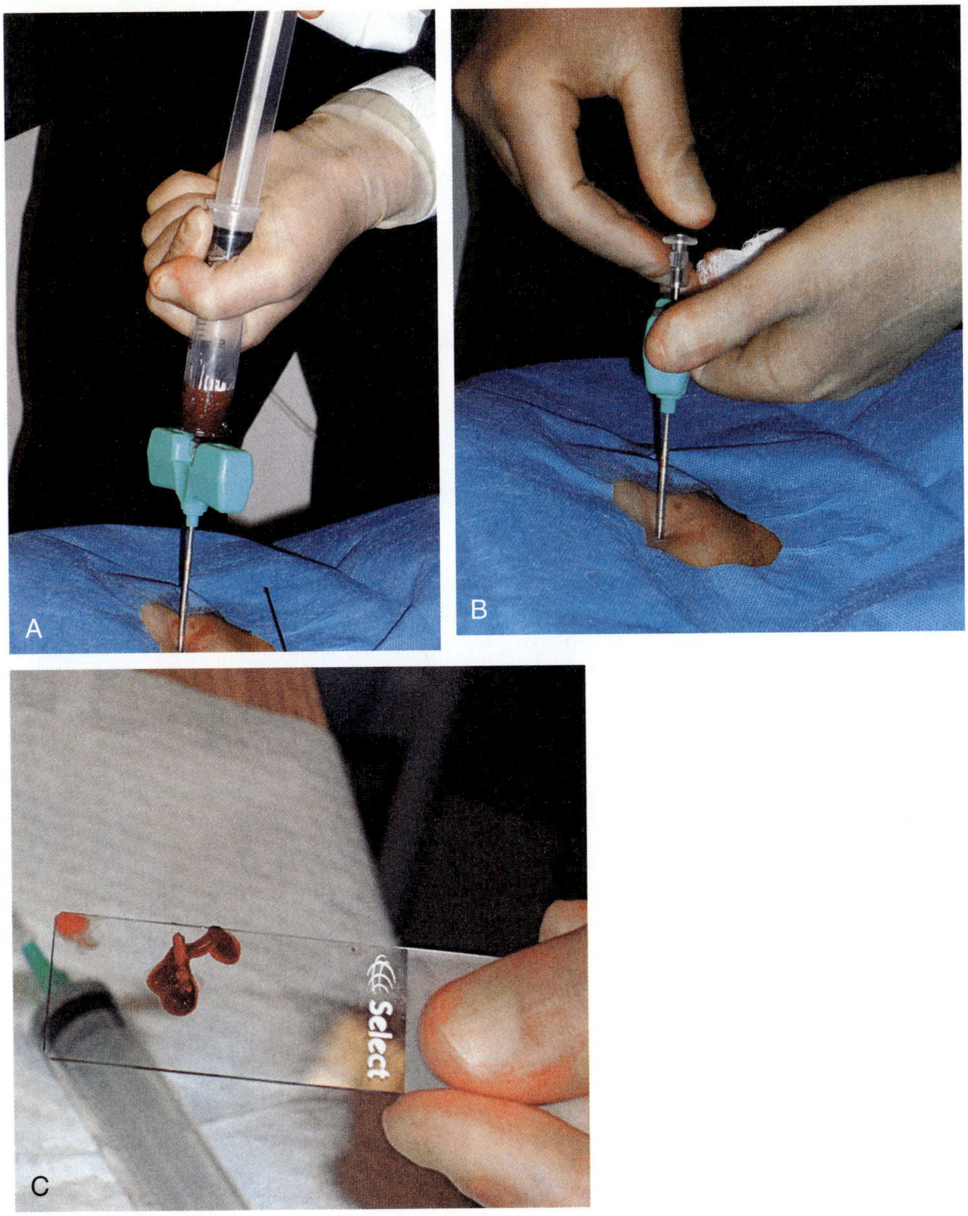

FIGURE 13-16 **Bone marrow aspiration and biopsy. A,** Placement of a bone marrow needle into the iliac crest (upper portion of hipbone) and aspiration of liquid bone marrow. **B,** Trephine needle is then inserted and anchored in the bone. **C,** A solid piece of bone marrow (biopsy sample) is then extracted through the needle.

Bone marrow transplantation follows the same procedure, except that bone marrow cells are used rather than peripheral stem cells (Figure 13-17). Problems encountered subsequently may include serious infection, **graft-versus-host disease (GVHD),** and relapse of the original disease despite the treatment.

In GVHD, the immunocompetent cells in the donor's tissue recognize the recipient's tissues as foreign and attack them. Because the recipient patient is totally immunosuppressed, his or her immune system cannot defend against the attack. Intensive prophylaxis (prevention) with **immunosuppressive drugs** is standard for patients undergoing **allogeneic transplants** (see Figure 13-17). These drugs include **cyclosporine** and **methotrexate**.

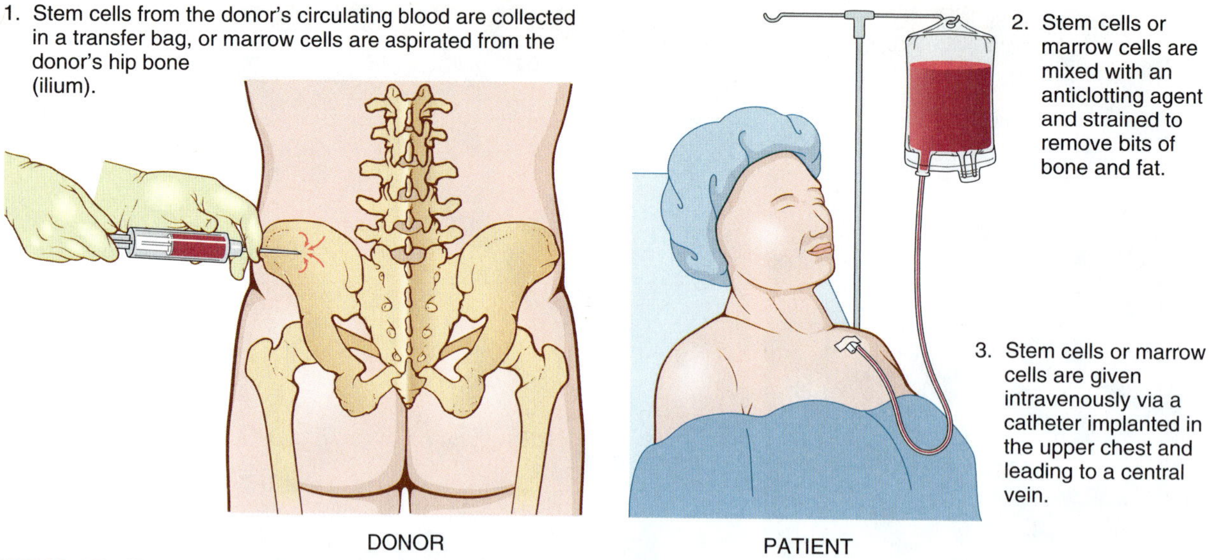

FIGURE 13-17 Hematopoietic stem cell and bone marrow transplantation. These procedures constitute **allogeneic** (all/o means other, different) **transplantation,** in which a relative or unrelated person having a close or identical HLA (human leukocyte antigen) type is the donor. It carries a high rate of morbidity (disease) and mortality (death) because of complications of incompatibility such as GVHD (graft-versus-host disease). In an **autologous transplantation,** stem cells or bone marrow cells are removed from the patient during a remission phase and given back to the patient after intensive chemotherapy (drug treatment).

ABBREVIATIONS

Ab	antibody
ABMT	autologous bone marrow transplantation—patient serves as his or her own donor for stem cells
ABO	four main blood types—A, B, AB, and O
ALL	acute lymphocytic leukemia
AML	acute myelogenous leukemia
ANC	absolute neutrophil count—total WBC times a measure of the number of bands and segs present in the blood; an ANC less than 1500 cells/uL is neutropenia
ASCT	autologous stem cell transplantation
bands	immature white blood cells (granulocytes)
baso	basophils
BMT	bone marrow transplantation
CBC	complete blood count
CLL	chronic lymphocytic leukemia
CML	chronic myelogenous leukemia
DIC	disseminated intravascular coagulation—bleeding disorder marked by reduction in blood clotting factors due to their use and depletion for intravascular clotting
diff	differential count (white blood cells)
EBV	Epstein-Barr virus; cause of mononucleosis
eos	eosinophils
EPO	erythropoietin
ESR	erythrocyte sedimentation rate
Fe	iron
G-CSF	granulocyte colony-stimulating factor—promotes neutrophil production
GM-CSF	granulocyte-macrophage colony-stimulating factor—promotes myeloid progenitor cells with differentiation to granulocytes
g/dL	gram per deciliter (1 deciliter = one tenth of a liter; 1 liter = 1.057 quarts)

GVHD	graft-versus-host disease—immune reaction of donor's cells to recipient's tissue
HCL	hairy cell leukemia—abnormal lymphocytes accumulate in bone marrow, leading to anemia, thrombocytopenia, neutropenia, and infection
Hct	hematocrit
Hgb, HGB	hemoglobin
H and H	hemoglobin and hematocrit
HLA	human leukocyte antigen
IgA, IgD, IgE, IgG, IgM	immunoglobulins
lymphs	lymphocytes
MCH	mean corpuscular hemoglobin—average amount of hemoglobin per cell
MCHC	mean corpuscular hemoglobin concentration—average concentration of hemoglobin in a single red cell; when MCHC is low, the cell is hypochromic
MCV	mean corpuscular volume—average volume or size of a single red blood cell; when MCV is high, the cells are macrocytic, and when low, the cells are microcytic
MDS	myelodysplastic syndrome—preleukemic condition (anemia, cytopenias, and possible transformation to AML)
mm^3	cubic millimeter—one millionth of a liter; 1 liter = 1.057 quarts
mono	monocyte
polys, PMNs, PMNLs	polymorphonuclear leukocytes; neutrophils, eosinophils, basophils
PT, pro time	prothrombin time
PTT	partial thromboplastin time
RBC	red blood cell; red blood cell count
sed rate	erythrocyte sedimentation rate
segs	segmented, mature white blood cells (neutrophils)
SMAC	Sequential Multiple Analyzer Computer—an automated chemistry system that determines substances in serum
μL	microliter—one millionth of a liter; 1 liter = 1.057 quarts
WBC	white blood cell; white blood cell count
WNL	within normal limits

PRACTICAL APPLICATIONS

The cases presented here are based on data from actual medical records. Use the table of normal values to help you decide on a probable diagnosis in each case. Answers to the questions are on page 538.

Normal Laboratory Values

WBC 4,500–11,000/mm³ or µL		**RBC**	M:	4.5-6.0 million per mm³ or µL
Differential:			F:	4.0-5.5 million per mm³ or µL
Segs (polys)	54-62%	**Hct**	M:	40-50%
Lymphs	20-40%		F:	37-47%
Eos	1-3%	**Hgb**	M:	14-16 g/dL
Baso	0-1%		F:	12-14 g/dL
Mono	3-7%	**Platelets** 150,000-350,000/mm³ or µL		

FIVE SHORT CLINICAL CASES

1. A 65-year-old woman visits her physician complaining of shortness of breath and swollen ankles. Lab tests reveal that her hematocrit is 18.0 and her hemoglobin 5.8. Her blood smear shows macrocytes and her blood level of vitamin B_{12} is very low. What is a likely diagnosis?
   a. Aplastic anemia
   b. Hemochromatosis
   c. Pernicious anemia

2. A 22-year-old college student visits the clinic with a fever, complaining of a sore throat. Blood tests show a WBC of 28,000 per mm³ with 95% myeloblasts (polys are 5%). Platelet count is 15,000 per mm³, hemoglobin is 10 g/dL, and the hematocrit is 22.5. What is your diagnosis?
   a. Chronic lymphocytic leukemia
   b. Acute myelogenous leukemia
   c. Thalassemia

3. A 35-year-old woman goes to her physician complaining of spots on her legs and bleeding gums. On examination, she has tiny purple spots covering her legs and evidence of dried blood in her mouth. Her CBC shows hemoglobin 14 g/dL, hematocrit 42%, WBC 5000/mm³ with normal differential, and platelet count 4000/mm³ (with megakaryocytes in bone marrow). What is your diagnosis?
   a. Sickle cell anemia
   b. Hemolytic anemia
   c. Autoimmune thrombocytopenic purpura

4. A 55-year-old man is admitted to the hospital after a motorcycle crash. He sustained right hemopneumothorax (blood and air in the chest cavity) requiring placement of a chest tube. His admission hemoglobin wa 11.4 g/dL and his hematocrit was 33.7%. On the 3rd day of hospitalization, his hemoglobin dropped to 7.5 g/dL and hematocrit fell to 22.4%. What do you think his physician should order?
   a. Bone marrow aspirate and biopsy
   b. Transfusion of packed red blood cells
   c. Leukapheresis

5. A 45-year-old woman has recently been traveling internationally and comes to the ED complaining of diarrhea, vomiting, and severe abdominal pain lasting for the previous two weeks. Her total WBC was elevated. Stool cultures reveal a parasitic infection. Which element of the differential do you expect to be elevated?
   a. Eosinophils
   b. Monocytes
   c. Segs (polys)

CASE REPORT

Four-year-old Sally has been running a low-grade fever for several weeks, with recurrent sore throat, earache, and cough. Her mother takes her to the family physician, who diagnoses her condition as otitis. Sally continues to be fatigued and anorexic. Her mother then notices bruising on her legs and arms. The family physician finally orders blood tests and an antibiotic drug. Peripheral blood tests reveal Hgb 7.4, platelet count 40,000, and WBC count 85,000 with 90% lymphoblasts. A bone marrow biopsy is ordered.

1. What's the likely diagnosis for this patient?
   a. AML
   b. CLL
   c. ALL
   d. CML
2. The probable cause of Sally's ecchymoses is
   a. Neutropenia
   b. Thrombocytopenia
   c. Anorexia
   d. Otitis
3. The likely explanation for Sally's fatigue is
   a. Anemia
   b. Sore throat and cough
   c. Thrombocytopenia
   d. Neutropenia
4. Treatment for Sally's condition is likely to be
   a. Prolonged antibiotic therapy
   b. IV feeding
   c. Surgery to repair the bone marrow
   d. Chemotherapy

IN PERSON

This is a first-person account of a woman undergoing an autologous stem cell transplant.

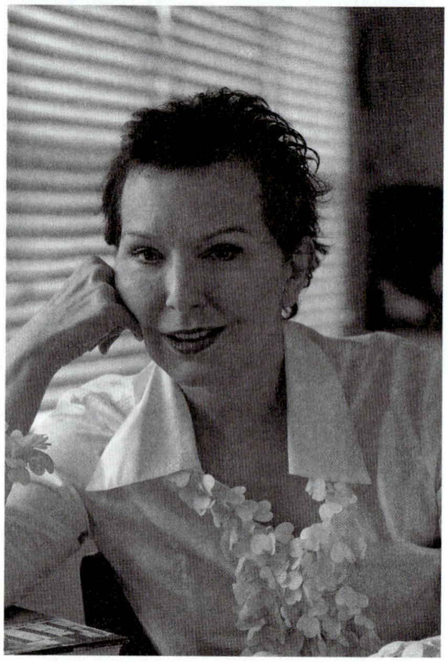

I was scheduled for a stem cell transplant to cure my recurrent primary central nervous system lymphoma, or PCNSL, a rare type of brain cancer. Until around fifteen years ago, stem cell transplants depended upon bone marrow from which to harvest the cells. Since then, scientists have discovered that there are actually more cells available in peripheral (circulating) blood than in marrow. Two medicines, Mozobil and Neupogen, aimed at stimulating enough stem cells to be collected from that peripheral source. Now, to prepare for my transplant, my daughter took me to Memorial Sloan-Kettering four consecutive nights for a Mozobil shot. Eight hours later, I had to return, after giving myself a Neupogen injection. In a peripheral autologous blood stem cell transplant, stem cells are collected from the circulating blood by apheresis, in which blood is withdrawn through a sterile needle, and passed through a machine that harvests stem cells into a container, while the remaining blood components are then transferred back into the patient's bloodstream. The fraction containing the blood stem cells is then frozen until needed for transplantation. Because patients get their own cells back, no chance exists for immune mismatch or graft-versus-host problems.

"Your blood has circulated through your body once—it takes an hour," the nurse explained that first day. "It will go around twice more, to sweep up all the stem cells it can, then you'll be done till tomorrow morning." That first day, I produced half of the total stem cells I would need for my treatment, emboldening me to make plans to return home after the next session. Instead, my collection slowed down and I squeezed out only another quarter of the necessary supply. I made enough stem cells the third day to reach the magic number, and was able to go home and wait for the hospital to call and say they'd scheduled me into their transplant schedule. A representative phoned two days later, laying out the next five weeks for me: I'd be admitted in eleven days to the transplant division, where I would remain, they hoped, for no more than a month. My (presumably clean) stem cells were safely stored in a freezer while I was to undergo intensive chemotherapy meant to destroy any lurking cancer cells in my brain (and of course, benign others in the medicine's take-no-prisoners path).

I was glad when the date arrived, and my husband Dennis moved me into my next month's home on the eighth floor of MSK, where we cheerfully commented on my having freedom to read as much as I wanted. I loved solitude, and I had so many books, loaded conveniently on my Kindle, that I planned to devour. What I had failed to understand is the nature of an autologous stem cell transplant, at least for primary CNS lymphoma. I was to be blasted, rendered helpless, with a trio of chemo agents able to pass through the blood-brain barrier, but not ordinarily available for treatment-as-a-threesome due to their combined viciousness: busulfan, thiotepa (mustard gas related), and cyclophosphamide (also a nitrogen mustard alkylating agent). I could risk receiving these killers because my uncontaminated stem cells were stored in the freezer. They would eventually replace my currently circulating blood that was being saturated with chemotherapy agents.

After nine days, my white blood count showed I was as low as I could go: I was at ground zero, "my second birthday." The blood we'd collected with the help of Mozobil and company was slowly thawed, for a few hours, and soon I was given a transfusion of my previously frozen blood, swarming with stem cells. Before long, I felt so sick I thought I was dying. Wearing diapers that had to be changed every twenty minutes, having rectal samples taken from my chafed, sometimes bloody "toilet skin" (as the nurse called it), being forced to sit up every minute, even at night, so that I could put the suction tube down my throat to keep from drowning in the rope-like mucositis, which ulcerated the membranes lining my digestive system. I could go on and on.

But as I'd been promised, nearly five weeks post-admission for the life-giving stem cell transplant, I was deemed ready to go home. For a month, however, our house operated like a medical office. That first week, I kept down half a shake a day. When I returned to Memorial for my first checkup, I had to stay an extra five hours for a hydration infusion. Four days later, my red blood count was low and I needed a transfusion—perfectly typical, Craig said cheerfully. By the second week, I'd started eating Cheerios with milk throughout the day, and my weight at least stabilized. I no longer looked like a skeleton.

At 100 days post-transplant, we could make love again. I worried that Dennis would find my scrawniness a turnoff, but he quickly forgot my new boy's body and enthusiastically helped me recapture my faith in our oneness. After all, we'd been through the battle and needed now to smell the perennial flowers. Turns out they're as colorful as ever.

Laura Claridge Oppenheimer is a writer with Farrar, Straus and Giroux, currently working on a biography of publisher Blanche Knopf.

EXERCISES

Remember to check your answers carefully with the Answers to Exercises, page 537.

A Match the following cells with their definitions as given below.

basophil
eosinophil
erythrocyte
hematopoietic stem cell
lymphocyte
monocyte
neutrophil
platelet

1. mononuclear white blood cell (agranulocyte) formed in lymph tissue; it is a phagocyte and the precursor of a macrophage ____________________
2. thrombocyte or cell fragment that helps blood clot ____________________
3. cell in the bone marrow that gives rise to different types of blood cells ____________________
4. mononuclear leukocyte formed in lymph tissue; produces antibodies ____________________
5. leukocyte with dense, reddish granules having an affinity for red acidic dye; associated with allergic reactions ____________________
6. red blood cell ____________________
7. leukocyte (polymorphonuclear granulocyte) formed in the bone marrow; granules do not stain intensely and have a pale color ____________________
8. leukocyte (granulocyte) with dark-staining blue granules; releases histamine and heparin ____________________

B Give the meanings of the following terms.

1. coagulation ____________________
2. granulocyte ____________________
3. mononuclear ____________________
4. polymorphonuclear ____________________
5. globulin ____________________
6. erythroblast ____________________
7. megakaryocyte ____________________
8. macrophage ____________________
9. hemoglobin ____________________
10. plasma ____________________
11. myeloblast ____________________

C Match the following terms with their definitions below.

albumin	colony-stimulating factor	globulin
antibody	differentiation	heparin
antigen	erythropoietin	plasma
bilirubin	fibrinogen	serum

1. liquid portion of blood ____________________
2. orange-yellow pigment produced from hemoglobin when red blood cells are destroyed

   ____
3. plasma protein converted to fibrin in clotting process ____________________
4. proteins in plasma; separated into alpha, beta, and gamma types ____________________
5. hormone secreted by the kidneys to stimulate bone marrow to produce red blood cells

   ____
6. substance (usually foreign) that stimulates production of an antibody ____________________
7. protein in blood that maintains the proper amount of water in the blood ____________________
8. specific protein produced by lymphocytes in response to antigens in the blood ____________________
9. anticoagulant found in blood and tissue cells ____________________
10. plasma minus clotting proteins and cells ____________________
11. change in structure and function of a cell as it matures ____________________
12. protein that stimulates growth of white blood cells ____________________

D Give short answers for the following.

1. Name four types of plasma proteins. ____________________

   ____
2. What is the Rh factor? ____________________
3. What is hemolysis? ____________________
4. A person with type A blood has ________ antigens and ________ antibodies in his or her blood.
5. A person with type B blood has ________ antigens and ________ antibodies in his or her blood.
6. A person with type O blood has ________ antigens and ________ antibodies in his or her blood.
7. A person with type AB blood has ________ antigens and ________ antibodies in his or her blood.
8. Can you transfuse blood from a type A donor into a type B recipient? ________ Why or why not?

   ____
9. Can you transfuse blood from a type AB donor into a type O recipient? Why or why not?

   ____
10. What is electrophoresis? ____________________

13

11. What is an immunoglobulin? ______________________________

12. What is differentiation? ______________________________

13. What is plasmapheresis? ______________________________

14. Why is type O the universal donor? ______________________________

E **Match the following terms related to clotting with their meanings as given below.**

coagulation	heparin	thrombin
fibrin	prothrombin	warfarin (Coumadin)
fibrinogen	serum	

1. anticoagulant substance found in liver cells, blood, and tissues ______________
2. protein thread that forms the basis of a blood clot ______________
3. plasma protein that is converted to thrombin in the clotting process ______________
4. plasma minus clotting proteins and cells ______________
5. drug given to patients to prevent formation of clots ______________
6. plasma protein that is converted to fibrin in the clotting process ______________
7. process of clotting ______________
8. enzyme that helps convert fibrinogen to fibrin ______________

13

F **Divide the following terms into component parts and give the meanings of the complete terms.**

1. anticoagulant ______________________________
2. hemoglobinopathy ______________________________
3. cytology ______________________________
4. leukopenia ______________________________
5. morphology ______________________________
6. megakaryocyte ______________________________
7. sideropenia ______________________________
8. phagocyte ______________________________
9. myelopoiesis ______________________________
10. plateletpheresis ______________________________
11. monoblast ______________________________
12. myelodysplasia ______________________________
13. hemostasis ______________________________
14. thrombolytic (therapy) ______________________________
15. hematopoiesis ______________________________

G Match the following terms with their meanings.

coagulopathy	leukapheresis	thrombocytopenia
eosinophilia	myeloid	thrombosis
hematocrit	neutropenia	

1. derived in bone marrow ______________________
2. deficiency of a type of white blood cell ______________________
3. percentage of red blood cells in a volume of blood ______________________
4. increase in a type of white blood cell (seen in allergies) ______________________
5. abnormal condition of clot formation ______________________
6. separation of white blood cells from a blood sample ______________________
7. disease of clotting process ______________________
8. deficiency of platelets ______________________

H Match the following terms concerning red blood cells with their meanings as given below.

anemia	hemoglobin	microcytosis
anisocytosis	hemolysis	poikilocytosis
erythropoiesis	hypochromic	polycythemia vera
hematocrit	macrocytosis	spherocytosis

1. any irregularity in the shape of red blood cells ______________________
2. oxygen-containing protein in red blood cells ______________________
3. formation of red blood cells ______________________
4. deficiency in numbers of red blood cells ______________________
5. destruction of red blood cells ______________________
6. pertaining to reduction of hemoglobin in red blood cells ______________________
7. variation in size of red blood cells ______________________
8. abnormal numbers of round, rather than normally biconcave-shaped, red blood cells

   ____
9. increase in number of small red blood cells ______________________
10. general increase in numbers of red blood cells; erythremia ______________________
11. increase in numbers of large red blood cells ______________________
12. separation of blood so that the percentage of red blood cells in relation to the volume of a blood sample is measured ______________________

I **Describe the problem in each of the following forms of anemia.**

1. iron deficiency anemia ______________________
2. pernicious anemia ______________________
3. sickle cell anemia ______________________
4. aplastic anemia ______________________
5. thalassemia ______________________

J **Give the meanings of the following terms for blood dyscrasias.**

1. purpura ______________________
2. granulocytosis ______________________
3. hemophilia ______________________
4. hemochromatosis ______________________
5. multiple myeloma ______________________
6. mononucleosis ______________________

K **Match the term in Column I with its meaning in Column II. Write the letter of the meaning in the space provided.**

COLUMN I

1. relapse ______
2. remission ______
3. palliative ______
4. Bence Jones protein ______
5. ecchymoses ______
6. pancytopenia ______
7. apheresis ______
8. eosinophilia ______
9. petechiae ______
10. packed cells ______

COLUMN II

A. Deficiency of all blood cells
B. Immunoglobulin fragment found in the urine of patients with multiple myeloma
C. Increase in numbers of granulocytes; seen in allergic conditions
D. Large blue or purplish patches on skin (bruises)
E. Symptoms of the disease return
F. Tiny purple or flat red spots on skin occurring as a result of small hemorrhages
G. Symptoms of the disease disappear
H. Separation of blood into its parts
I. Preparation of erythrocytes separated from plasma
J. Relieving but not curing

L Match the following laboratory test or clinical procedure with its description.

antiglobulin (Coombs) test
autologous transfusion
bleeding time
bone marrow biopsy
coagulation time
erythrocyte sedimentation rate
hematocrit
hematopoietic stem cell transplantation
platelet count
red blood cell count
red blood cell morphology
white blood cell differential

1. microscopic examination of a stained blood smear to determine the shape of individual red blood cells _______________
2. percentage of red blood cells in a volume of blood _______________
3. determines the number of clotting cells per mm^3 or μL of blood _______________
4. time required for venous blood to clot in a test tube _______________
5. speed at which erythrocytes settle out of plasma _______________
6. percentages of different types of leukocytes in the blood _______________
7. test for the presence of antibodies that coat and damage erythrocytes _______________
8. peripheral stem cells from a compatible donor are infused into a recipient's vein to repopulate the bone marrow _______________
9. time required for blood to stop flowing from a small puncture wound _______________
10. microscopic examination of a core of bone marrow removed with a needle _______________
11. number of erythrocytes per mm^3 or μL of blood _______________
12. blood is collected from and later reinfused into the same patient _______________

M Circle the boldface terms that best complete the meanings of the sentences.

1. Gary, a 1-year-old African American child, was failing to gain weight normally. He seemed pale and without energy. His blood tests showed a decreased hemoglobin (5.0 g/dL) and decreased hematocrit (16.5%). After a blood smear revealed abnormally shaped red cells, the physician told Gary's parents that their son had **(iron deficiency anemia, hemophilia, sickle cell anemia)**.
2. While in the hospital, Mr. Klein was told he had an elevated **(red blood cell, white blood cell, platelet)** count with a "shift to the left." This was information that confirmed his diagnosis of a systemic infection.
3. While Mr. Chen was taking warfarin (Coumadin), a blood thinner, his physician made sure to check his **(prothrombin time, hematocrit, sed rate)**.
4. Sixty-one-year-old Barbara's laboratory tests showed abnormal proteins in her plasma and Bence Jones protein in her urine. She had osteopenia and a fracture in one of her ribs. Her oncologist diagnosed her condition as **(mononucleosis, thrombocytopenic purpura, multiple myeloma)**. He prescribed analgesics and drugs such as thalidomide and bortezomib (Velcade).
5. Bobby was diagnosed at a very early age with a bleeding disorder called **(hemophilia, thalassemia, eosinophilia)**. He needed factor VIII regularly, especially after even the slightest traumatic injury.

6. Juan was a 9-year-old boy who suddenly noticed many black and blue marks all over his legs. He had a fever and was tired all the time. The physician did a blood test that revealed pancytopenia. A bone marrow biopsy confirmed the diagnosis of **(acute lymphocytic leukemia, polycythemia vera, aplastic anemia)**.

7. Alice and her friends had been staying up late for weeks, cramming for exams. She developed a sore throat and swollen lymph nodes in her neck and felt fatigued all the time. Dr. Smith did a blood test, and the results showed lymphocytosis and antibodies to EBV in the bloodstream. His diagnosis was **(leukapheresis, lymphocytopenia, mononucleosis)**.

8. Susan was experiencing heavy menstrual periods **(menorrhea, menorrhagia, hemoptysis)**. Because of the bleeding, she frequently felt tired and weak and probably was sideropenic. Her physician performed blood tests that revealed her problem as **(thrombocytopenia, pernicious anemia, iron deficiency anemia)**.

9. Dr. Harris examined a highly allergic patient and sent a blood sample to a specialist, a **(pulmonary, cardiovascular, hematologic)** pathologist. The specialist stained the blood smear and found an abundance of leukocytes with dense, reddish granules. She made the diagnosis of **(basophilia, eosinophilia, neutrophilia)**.

10. George's blood cell counts had been falling in recent weeks. His scheduled laparotomy was canceled because blood tests revealed **(pancytopenia, plasmapheresis, myelopoiesis)**. Bone marrow biopsy determined that the cause was **(hyperplasia, hypoplasia, differentiation)** of all cellular elements.

13

N **Give the meanings of the following abbreviations in Column I and then select the best association for each from sentences in Column II.**

COLUMN I

1. Hgb ______________________ _____
2. GVHD ______________________ _____
3. ALL ______________________ _____
4. PT ______________________ _____
5. CML ______________________ _____
6. EPO ______________________ _____
7. IgA, IgE, IgD ______________________ _____
8. CLL ______________________ _____
9. Hct ______________________ _____
10. AML ______________________ _____

COLUMN II

A. Blood protein that transports oxygen to tissues.
B. Malignant condition of white blood cells; immature granulocytes (myeloblasts) predominate.
C. Malignant condition of white blood cells; immature lymphocytes predominate.
D. Test used to follow patients who are taking certain anticoagulants.
E. Percentage of red cells in blood volume.
F. Malignant condition of white blood cells in which both mature and immature granulocytes are present; a slowly progressive illness.
G. Immune reaction of donor's cells/tissue to recipient's cells/tissue; a possible outcome of hematopoietic stem cell or bone marrow transplantation.
H. Proteins containing antibodies.
I. Malignant condition of white blood cells in which relatively mature lymphocytes predominate in lymph nodes, spleen, and bone marrow; usually seen in elderly patients.
J. Hormone that stimulates the growth of red blood cells.

ANSWERS TO EXERCISES

A

1. monocyte
2. platelet
3. hematopoietic stem cell
4. lymphocyte
5. eosinophil
6. erythrocyte
7. neutrophil
8. basophil

B

1. blood clotting
2. white blood cell with numerous, dark-staining granules (neutrophil, basophil, and eosinophil)
3. pertaining to a leukocyte with a single round nucleus; monocytes and lymphocytes are mononuclear leukocytes
4. pertaining to a white blood cell with a multi-lobed nucleus; neutrophil
5. plasma protein; alpha, beta, and gamma (immune) globulins are examples
6. immature red blood cell
7. large platelet precursor (forerunner) cell found in bone marrow
8. monocyte that migrates from blood to tissue spaces; phagocyte that engulfs foreign material and ingests red blood cells
9. blood protein containing iron; carries oxygen in erythrocytes
10. liquid portion of blood
11. immature bone marrow cell that gives rise to granulocytes

C

1. plasma
2. bilirubin
3. fibrinogen
4. globulin
5. erythropoietin
6. antigen
7. albumin
8. antibody
9. heparin
10. serum
11. differentiation
12. colony-stimulating factor

D

1. albumin, globulins, fibrinogen, and prothrombin
2. an antigen normally found on red blood cells of Rh+ individuals
3. destruction or breakdown of red blood cells
4. A; anti-B
5. B; anti-A
6. no A or B; anti-A and anti-B
7. A and B; no anti-A and no anti-B
8. no; A antigens will react with the anti-A antibodies in the type B recipient's bloodstream
9. no; A and B antigens will react with the anti-A and anti-B antibodies in the type O recipient's bloodstream
10. a method of separating serum proteins by electrical charge
11. protein with antibody activity; IgG, IgH, IgE
12. change in structure and function of a cell as it matures; specialization
13. removal by centrifuge of plasma from withdrawn blood
14. type O blood does not contain A or B antigens and therefore will not react with antibodies in any recipient's blood

E

1. heparin
2. fibrin
3. prothrombin
4. serum
5. warfarin (Coumadin)
6. fibrinogen
7. coagulation
8. thrombin

F

1. anti/coagul/ant—a substance that prevents clotting
2. hemoglobin/o/pathy—disease (abnormality) of hemoglobin
3. cyt/o/logy—study of cells
4. leuk/o/penia—deficiency of white (blood) cells
5. morph/o/logy—study of the shape or form (of cells)
6. mega/kary/o/cyte—cell with a large (mega-) nucleus (kary); platelet precursor
7. sider/o/penia—deficiency of iron
8. phag/o/cyte—cell that eats or swallows other cells
9. myel/o/poiesis—formation of bone marrow
10. platelet/pheresis—separation of platelets from the rest of the blood
11. mon/o/blast—immature monocyte
12. myel/o/dys/plasia—abnormal (ineffective) production of myeloid cells in bone marrow. Myeloid progenitor cells give rise to erythrocytes, granulocytes, and platelets
13. hem/o/stasis—controlling or stopping the flow of blood
14. thromb/o/lytic (therapy)—pertaining to treatment using drugs to destroy clots
15. hemat/o/poiesis—formation of blood cells

G

1. myeloid
2. neutropenia
3. hematocrit
4. eosinophilia
5. thrombosis
6. leukapheresis
7. coagulopathy
8. thrombocytopenia

H

1. poikilocytosis
2. hemoglobin
3. erythropoiesis
4. anemia
5. hemolysis
6. hypochromic
7. anisocytosis
8. spherocytosis
9. microcytosis
10. polycythemia vera
11. macrocytosis
12. hematocrit

I

1. lack of iron leading to insufficient hemoglobin production
2. lack of mature erythrocytes caused by inability to absorb vitamin B_{12} into the bloodstream (intrinsic factor is missing in gastric juice, so B_{12} is not absorbed)
3. hereditary disorder of abnormal hemoglobin producing sickle-shaped erythrocytes and hemolysis
4. failure of blood cell production in bone marrow
5. inherited defect in ability to produce hemoglobin, leading to hypochromia

J

1. multiple pinpoint hemorrhages and accumulation of blood under the skin (cause is deficiency of platelets)
2. abnormal increase in granulocytes in the blood (eosinophilia and basophilia)
3. excessive bleeding caused by hereditary lack of blood clotting factors
4. excessive iron deposits throughout the body
5. malignant neoplasm of bone marrow
6. infectious disease marked by increased numbers of mononuclear leukocytes and enlarged cervical lymph nodes

K

1. E
2. G
3. J
4. B
5. D
6. A
7. H
8. C
9. F
10. I

L

1. red blood cell morphology
2. hematocrit
3. platelet count
4. coagulation time
5. erythrocyte sedimentation rate
6. white blood cell differential
7. antiglobulin (Coombs) test
8. hematopoietic stem cell transplantation
9. bleeding time
10. bone marrow biopsy
11. red blood cell count
12. autologous transfusion

M

1. sickle cell anemia
2. white blood cell
3. prothrombin time
4. multiple myeloma
5. hemophilia
6. aplastic anemia
7. mononucleosis
8. menorrhagia; iron deficiency anemia
9. hematologic; eosinophilia
10. pancytopenia; hypoplasia

N

1. hemoglobin: A
2. graft-versus-host disease: G
3. acute lymphocytic leukemia: C
4. prothrombin time: D
5. chronic myelogenous (myelocytic) leukemia: F
6. erythropoietin: J
7. immunoglobulins: H
8. chronic lymphocytic leukemia: I
9. hematocrit: E
10. acute myelogenous (myelocytic) leukemia: B

Answers to Practical Applications

Five Short Clinical Cases

1. c
2. b
3. c
4. b
5. a

Case Report

1. c
2. b
3. a
4. d

PRONUNCIATION OF TERMS

To test your understanding of the terminology in this chapter, write the meaning of each term in the space provided. In addition, you may wish to cover the terms and write them by looking at your definitions. Make sure your spelling is correct. The page number after each term indicates where it is defined or used in the book, so you can easily check your responses. You will find complete definitions for all of these terms and their audio pronunciations on the Evolve website.

Pronunciation Guide

ā as in āpe	ă as in ăpple
ē as in ēven	ĕ as in ĕvery
ī as in īce	ĭ as in ĭnterest
ō as in ōpen	ŏ as in pŏt
ū as in ūnit	ŭ as in ŭnder

Vocabulary and Terminology

TERM	PRONUNCIATION	MEANING
albumin (510)	ăl-BŪ-mĭn	______
anisocytosis (512)	ăn-ī-sō-sī-TŌ-sĭs	______
antibody (510)	ĂN-tĭ-bŏd-ē	______
anticoagulant (512)	ăn-tĭ-cō-ĂG-ū-lănt	______
antigen (510)	ĂN-tĭ-jĕn	______
basophil (510)	BĀ-sō-fĭl	______
bilirubin (510)	bĭl-ĭ-ROO-bĭn	______
coagulation (510)	kō-ăg-ū-LĀ-shŭn	______
coagulopathy (512)	kō-ăg-ū-LŎP-ă-thē	______
colony-stimulating factor (510)	KŎL-ō-nē STĬM-ū-lā-tĭng FĂK-tŏr	______
cytology (512)	sī-TŎL-ō-jē	______
differentiation (510)	dĭf-ĕr-ĕn-shē-Ā-shŭn	______
electrophoresis (510)	ē-lĕk-trō-fō-RĒ-sis	______
eosinophil (510)	ē-ō-SĬN-ō-fĭl	______
eosinophilia (514)	ē-ō-sĭn-ō-FĬL-ē-ă	______
erythroblast (510)	ĕ-RĬTH-rō-blăst	______
erythrocyte (510)	ĕ-RĬTH-rō-sīt	______
erythropoiesis (514)	ĕ-rĭth-rō-poy-Ē-sĭs	______
erythropoietin (510)	ĕ-rĭth-rō-POY-ĕ-tĭn	______
fibrin (510)	FĪ-brĭn	______
fibrinogen (510)	fī-BRĬN-ō-jĕn	______
globulin (510)	GLŎB-ū-lĭn	______
granulocyte (512)	GRĂN-ū-lō-sīt	______
granulocytopenia (514)	grăn-ū-lō-sī-tō-PĒ-nē-ă	______
hematopoiesis (514)	hē-mă-tō-poy-Ē-sĭs	______

13

TERM	PRONUNCIATION	MEANING
hematopoietic stem cell (510)	hē-mă-tō-pō-EH-tĭk stĕm sĕl	________
hemoglobin (510)	HĒ-mō-glō-bĭn	________
hemoglobinopathy (512)	hē-mō-glō-bĭn-ŎP-ă-thē	________
hemolysis (510)	hē-MŎL-ĭ-sĭs	________
hemostasis (514)	hē-mō-STĀ-sĭs	________
heparin (510)	HĔP-ă-rĭn	________
hypochromic (512)	hī-pō-KRŌ-mĭk	________
immune reaction (510)	ĭm-MŪN rē-ĂK-shŭn	________
immunoglobulin (510)	ĭm-ū-nō-GLŎB-ū-lĭn	________
leukapheresis (513)	loo-kă-fĕ-RĒ-sĭs	________
leukocyte (511)	LOO-kō-sīt	________
leukopenia (512)	loo-kō-PĒ-nē-ă	________
lymphocyte (511)	LĬM-fō-sīt	________
macrocytosis (514)	măk-rō-sī-TŌ-sĭs	________
macrophage (511)	MĂK-rō-făj	________
megakaryocyte (511)	mĕg-ă-KĀR-ē-ō-sīt	________
microcytosis (514)	mī-krō-sī-TŌ-sĭs	________
monoblast (513)	MŎN-ō-blăst	________
monocyte (511)	MŎN-ō-sīt	________
mononuclear (511)	mŏn-ō-NŪ-klē-ăr	________
morphology (512)	mŏr-FŎL-ō-jē	________
myeloblast (511)	MĪ-ĕ-lō-blăst	________
myelodysplasia (513)	mī-ĕ-lō-dĭs-PLĀ-zhē-ă	________
myeloid (514)	MĪ-ĕ-loyd	________
myelopoiesis (514)	mī-ĕ-lō-poy-Ē-sĭs	________
neutropenia (513)	noo-trō-PĒ-nē-ă	________
neutrophil (511)	NOO-trō-fĭl	________
neutrophilia (514)	noo-trō-FĬL-ē-ă	________
pancytopenia (514)	păn-sī-tō-PĒ-nē-ă	________
phagocyte (513)	FĂG-ō-sīt	________
plasma (511)	PLĂZ-mă	________
plasmapheresis (511)	plăz-mă-fĕ-RĒ-sĭs	________
platelet (511)	PLĀT-lĕt	________
plateletpheresis (513)	plāt-lĕt-fĕ-RĒ-sĭs	________

13

TERM	PRONUNCIATION	MEANING
poikilocytosis (513)	poy-kĭ-lō-sī-TŌ-sĭs	________
polymorphonuclear (511)	pŏl-ē-mŏr-fō-NŪ-klē-ăr	________
prothrombin (511)	prō-THRŎM-bĭn	________
reticulocyte (511)	rĕ-TĬK-ū-lō-sīt	________
Rh factor (511)	R-h FĂK-tŏr	________
serum (511)	SĔ-rŭm	________
sideropenia (513)	sĭd-ĕr-ō-PĒ-nē-ă	________
spherocytosis (515)	sfĕr-ō-sī-TŌ-sĭs	________
stem cell (511)	STĔM sĕl	________
thrombin (511)	THRŎM-bĭn	________
thrombocyte (511)	THRŎM-bō-sīt	________
thrombocytopenia (513)	thrŏm-bō-sī-tō-PĒ-nē-ă	________
thrombolytic therapy (514)	thrŏm-bō-LĬ-tĭk THĔR-ă-pē	________
thrombosis (514)	thrŏm-BŌ-sĭs	________

Pathology, Laboratory Tests, and Clinical Procedures

TERM	PRONUNCIATION	MEANING
acute lymphocytic leukemia (519)	ă-KŪT lĭm-fō-SĬ-tĭk loo-KĒ-mē-ă	________
acute myelogenous leukemia (518)	ă-KŪT mī-ĕ-LŎJ-ĕ-nŭs loo-KĒ-mē-ă	________
anemia (515)	ă-NĒ-mē-ă	________
antiglobulin test (520)	ăn-tē-GLŎB-ū-lĭn tĕst	________
apheresis (522)	ă-fĕ-RĒ-sĭs	________
aplastic anemia (515)	ā-PLĂS-tĭk ă-NĒ-mē-ă	________
autologous transfusion (522)	ăw-TŎL-ō-gŭs trăns-FŪ-zhŭn	________
bleeding time (520)	BLĒ-dĭng tīm	________
blood transfusion (522)	blŭd trăns-FŪ-zhŭn	________
bone marrow biopsy (522)	bōn MĂ-rō BĪ-ŏp-sē	________
chronic lymphocytic leukemia (519)	KRŎ-nĭk lĭm-fō-SĬ-tĭk loo-KĒ-mē-ă	________
chronic myelogenous leukemia (519)	KRŎ-nĭk mī-ĕ-LŎJ-ĕ-nŭs loo-KĒ-mē-ă	________
coagulation time (520)	kō-ăg-ū-LĀ-shŭn tīm	________
complete blood count (520)	kŏm-PLĒT blŭd kount	________

13

TERM	PRONUNCIATION	MEANING
dyscrasia (515)	dĭs-KRĀ-zē-ă	
ecchymoses (518)	ĕk-kĭ-MŌ-sēs	
erythrocyte sedimentation rate (520)	ĕ-RĬTH-rō-sīt sĕd-ĭ-mĕn-TĀ-shŭn rāt	
granulocytosis (519)	grăn-ū-lō-sī-TŌ-sis	
hematocrit (521)	hē-MĂT-ō-krĭt	
hematopoietic stem cell transplant (522)	hē-mă-tō-poy-Ĕ-tĭk stĕm sĕl TRĂNS-plănt	
hemochromatosis (517)	hē-mō-krō-mă-TŌ-sĭs	
hemoglobin test (521)	HĒ-mō-glō-bĭn tĕst	
hemolytic anemia (516)	hē-mō-LĬ-tĭk ă-NĒ-mē-ă	
hemophilia (517)	hē-mō-FĬL-ē-ă	
intrinsic factor (516)	ĭn-TRĬN-sĭk FĂK-tŏr	
leukemia (518)	loo-KĒ-mē-ă	
mononucleosis (520)	mŏ-nō-nū-klē-Ō-sĭs	
multiple myeloma (520)	MŬL-tĭ-pl mī-ĕ-LŌ-mă	
palliative (520)	PĂL-ē-ă-tĭv	
pernicious anemia (516)	pĕr-NĬSH-ŭs ă-NĒ-mē-ă	
petechiae (518)	pĕ-TĒ-kē-ā	
platelet count (521)	PLĀT-lĕt kount	
polycythemia vera (517)	pŏl-ē-sī-THĒ-mē-ă VĔR-ă	
prothrombin time (521)	prō-THRŎM-bĭn tīm	
purpura (518)	PŬR-pū-ră	
red blood cell count (521)	rĕd blŭd sĕl kount	
red blood cell morphology (521)	rĕd blŭd sĕl mŏr-FŎL-ō-jē	
relapse (519)	RĒ-lăps	
remission (519)	rē-MĬSH-ŭn	
sickle cell anemia (516)	SĬK-l sĕl ă-NĒ-mē-ă	
thalassemia (517)	thăl-ă-SĒ-mē-ă	
white blood cell count (521)	wīt blŭd sĕl kount	
white blood cell differential (521)	wīt blŭd sĕl dĭ-fĕr-ĔN-shŭl	

REVIEW SHEET

Write the meanings of the word parts in the spaces provided. Check your answers with the information in the chapter or in the Glossary (Medical Word Parts—English) at the end of the book.

Combining Forms

COMBINING FORM	MEANING	COMBINING FORM	MEANING
bas/o	________	leuk/o	________
chrom/o	________	kary/o	________
coagul/o	________	mon/o	________
cyt/o	________	morph/o	________
eosin/o	________	myel/o	________
erythr/o	________	neutr/o	________
fibrin/o	________	nucle/o	________
granul/o	________	phag/o	________
hem/o	________	poikil/o	________
hemat/o	________	sider/o	________
hemoglobin/o	________	spher/o	________
is/o	________	thromb/o	________

Suffixes

SUFFIX	MEANING	SUFFIX	MEANING
-apheresis	________	-osis	________
-blast	________	-penia	________
-cytosis	________	-phage	________
-emia	________	-philia	________
-gen	________	-phoresis	________
-globin	________	-plasia	________
-globulin	________	-poiesis	________
-lytic	________	-stasis	________
-oid	________		

Prefixes

PREFIX	MEANING	PREFIX	MEANING
a-, an-	______	micro-	______
anti-	______	mono-	______
hypo-	______	pan-	______
macro-	______	poly-	______
mega-	______		

Components of blood: Study Figure 13-7, page 507 and fill in the blank boxes.

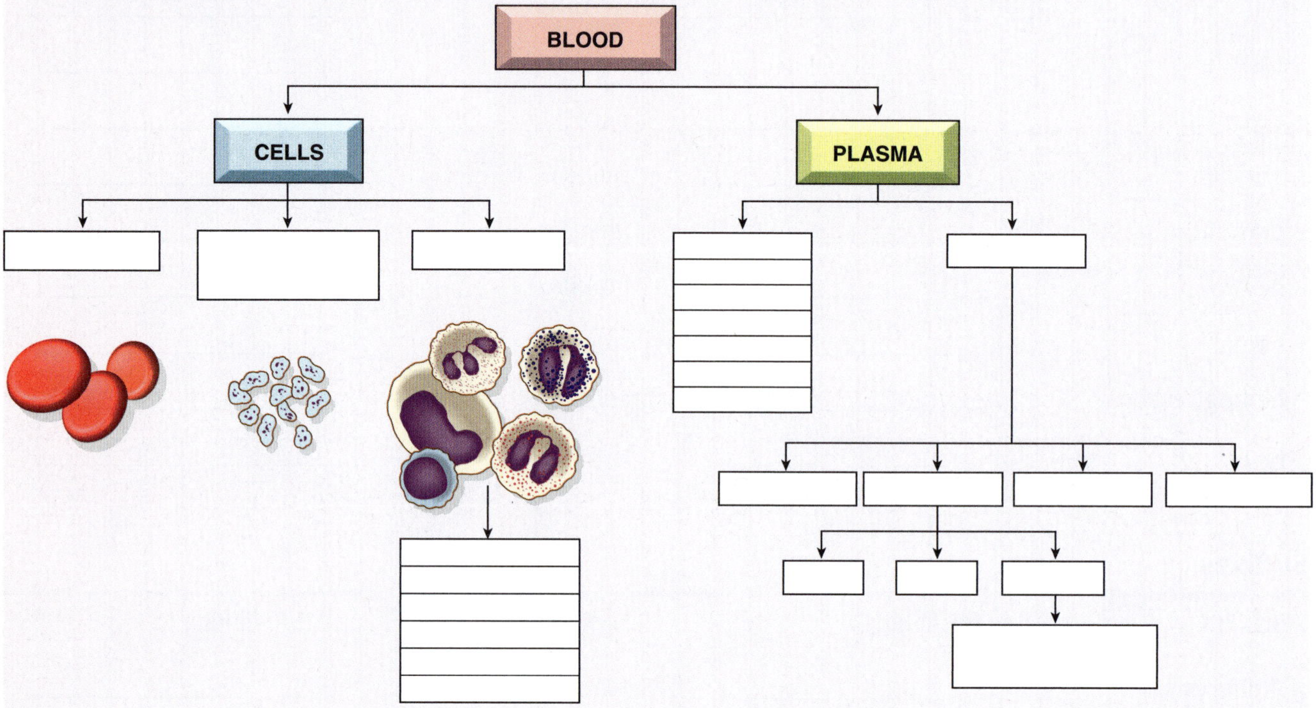

13

Please refer to the Evolve website for additional exercises, games, and images related to this chapter.

CHAPTER 14

Lymphatic and Immune Systems

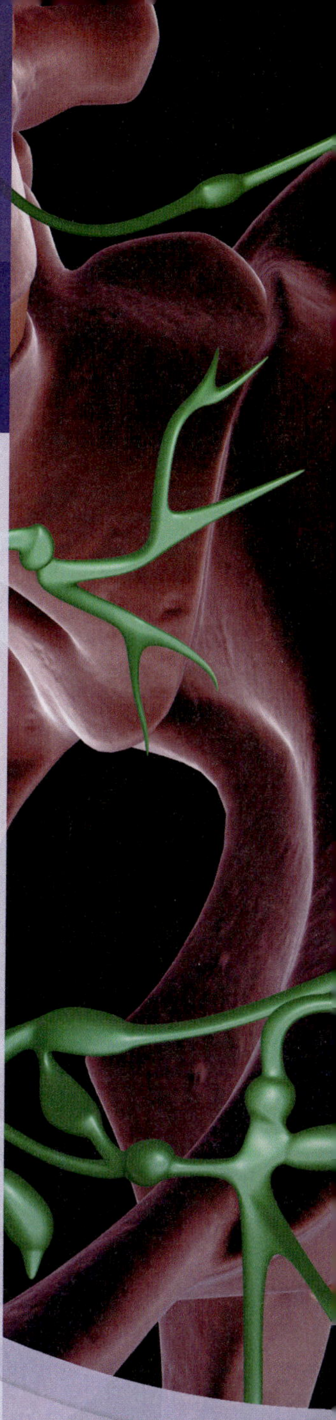

This chapter is divided into the following sections:

CHAPTER GOALS

- Identify the structures of the lymphatic and immune systems and understand how the systems work.
- Learn basic terminology, combining forms, and other word parts related to these systems.
- Recognize terms describing pathologic conditions.
- Identify laboratory tests, clinical procedures, and abbreviations.
- Apply your new knowledge to understanding medical terms in their proper contexts, such as medical reports and records.

INTRODUCTION

The lymphatic system and the immune system are considered together in this chapter because aspects of their functions in the body are very closely related.

Lymph is a clear, watery fluid that surrounds body cells and flows in a system of thin-walled lymph vessels (the lymphatic system) that extends throughout the body.

Lymph differs from blood, but it has a close relationship to the blood system. Lymph fluid does not contain erythrocytes or platelets, but it is rich in two types of white blood cells (leukocytes): **lymphocytes** and **monocytes**. The liquid part of lymph is similar to blood plasma in that it contains water, salts, sugar, and wastes of metabolism such as urea and creatinine, but it differs in that it contains less protein. Lymph actually originates from the blood. It is the same fluid that filters out of tiny blood capillaries into the spaces between cells. This fluid that surrounds body cells is called **interstitial fluid**. Interstitial fluid passes continuously into specialized thin-walled vessels called **lymph capillaries**, which are found coursing through tissue spaces (Figure 14-1). The fluid in the lymph capillaries, now called **lymph** instead of interstitial fluid, passes through larger lymphatic vessels and through clusters of lymph tissues **(lymph nodes)**, finally reaching large lymphatic vessels in the upper chest. Lymph enters these large lymphatic vessels, which then empty into the bloodstream. Figure 14-2 illustrates schematically the relationship between the blood and the lymphatic systems. Table 14-1 reviews the differences between lymph and blood.

The lymphatic system has several functions. First, it is a drainage system to transport needed proteins and fluid that have leaked out of the blood capillaries (and into the interstitial fluid) back to the bloodstream via the veins. Second, the lymphatic vessels in the intestines absorb lipids (fats) from the small intestine and transport them to the bloodstream.

14

A third function of the lymphatic system relates to the **immune system:** the defense of the body against foreign organisms such as bacteria and viruses. Lymphocytes and monocytes, originating in bone marrow, lymph nodes, and organs such as the spleen and thymus gland, protect the body by producing antibodies and by mounting a cellular attack on foreign cells and organisms.

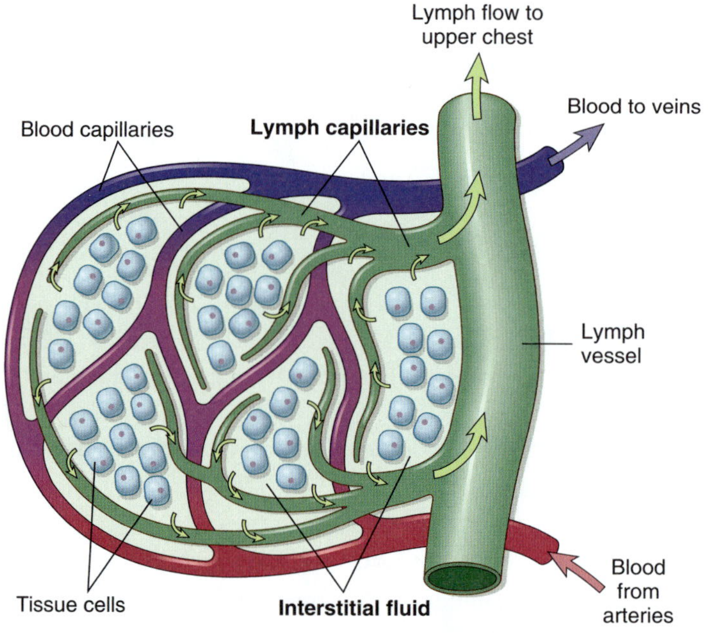

FIGURE 14-1 **Interstitial fluid and lymph capillaries.**

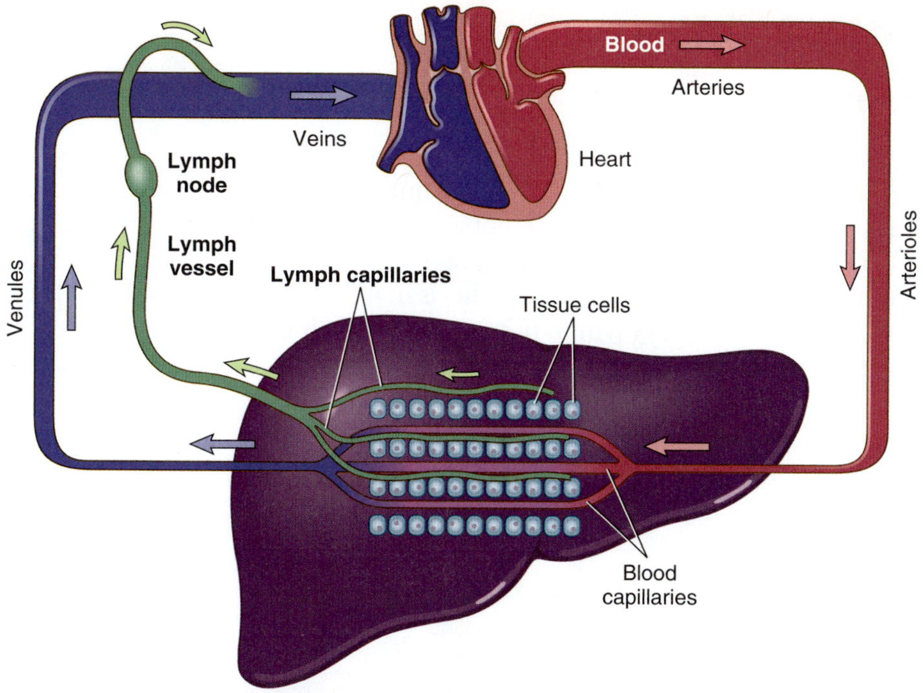

FIGURE 14-2 Relationship between the circulatory systems of blood and lymph.

TABLE 14-1 LYMPH AND BLOOD

Lymph (colorless)	Blood (red)
NO PUMP Fluid moved along by muscle movement and valves	**PUMP** Heart pumps blood through blood vessels
WHITE BLOOD CELLS Lymphocytes Monocytes	**ALL BLOOD CELLS** Erythrocytes (give blood its red color) Leukocytes Platelets
INTERSTITIAL FLUID Water Less protein and other plasma components Lipids (fats) from small intestine	**PLASMA** Water Proteins Salts, nutrients, lipids, and wastes

14

LYMPHATIC SYSTEM

ANATOMY

Label Figure 14-3A as you read the following paragraphs.

Lymph capillaries [1] begin at the spaces around cells throughout the body. Like blood capillaries, they are thin-walled tubes. Lymph capillaries carry lymph from the tissue spaces to larger **lymph vessels** [2]. Lymph vessels have thicker walls than those of lymph capillaries and, like veins, contain valves so that lymph flows in only one direction, toward the thoracic cavity. Collections of stationary lymph tissue, called **lymph nodes** [3], are located along the path of the lymph vessels.

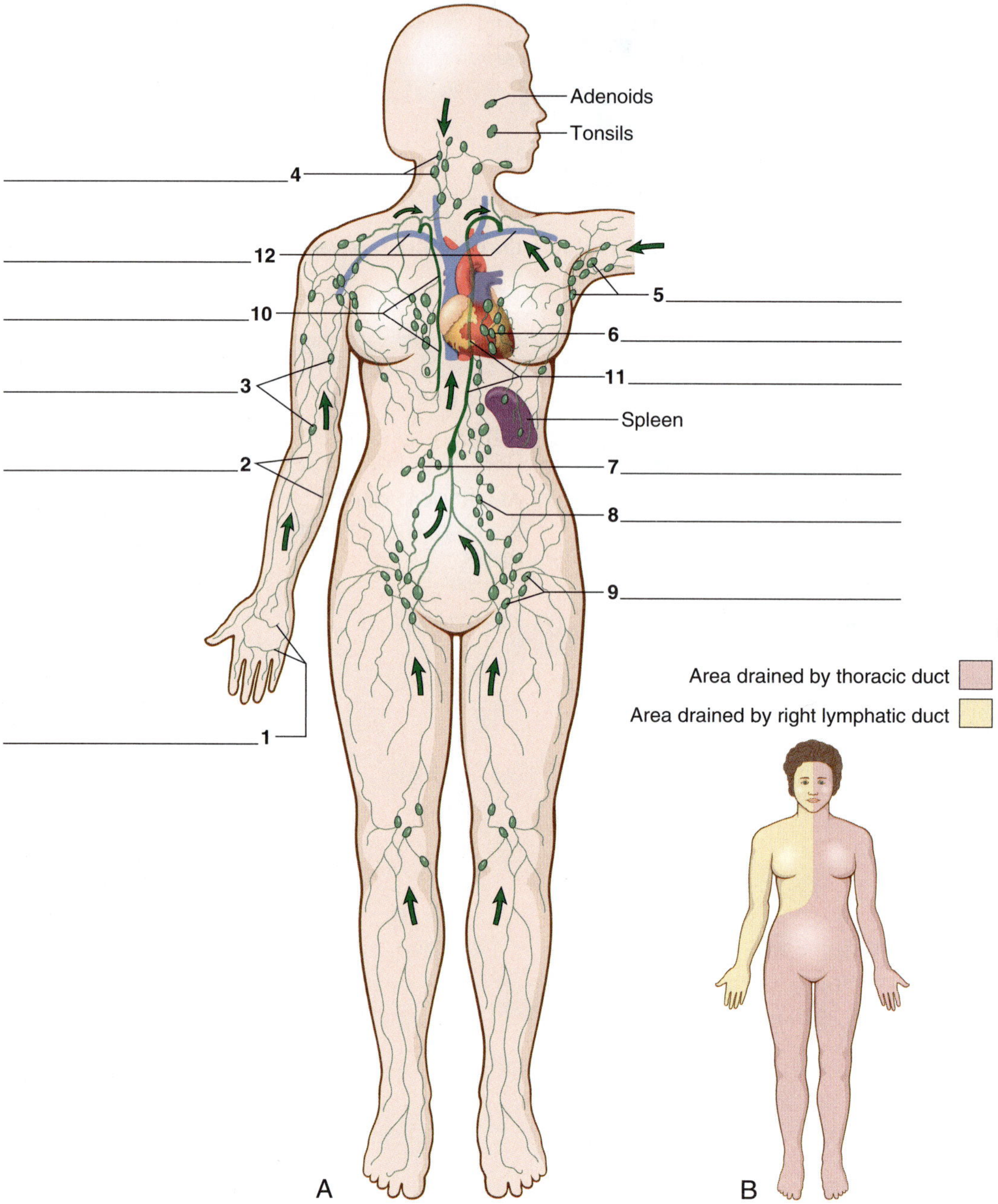

FIGURE 14-3 **Lymphatic system. A,** Label the figure according to the descriptions in the text. **B,** Note the different regions of the body drained by the right lymphatic duct and the thoracic duct.

Major sites of lymph node concentration are shown in Figure 14-3A. These are the **cervical** (neck) [4], **axillary** (armpit) [5], **mediastinal** (chest) [6], **mesenteric** (intestinal) [7], **paraaortic** (lumbar) [8], and **inguinal** (groin) [9] regions. Remember that **tonsils** are masses of lymph tissue in the throat near the back of the mouth (oropharynx), and **adenoids** are enlarged lymph tissue in the part of the throat near the nasal passages (nasopharynx).

Lymph vessels all lead toward the thoracic cavity and empty into two large ducts in the upper chest. These are the **right lymphatic duct** [10] and the **thoracic duct** [11]. The thoracic duct drains the lower body and the left side of the head, whereas the right lymphatic duct drains the right side of the head and the chest (a much smaller area) (see Figure 14-3B). Both ducts carry the lymph into **large veins** [12] in the neck, where the lymph then enters the bloodstream.

Lymph nodes not only produce lymphocytes but also filter lymph and trap substances from infectious, inflammatory, and cancerous lesions. Special cells called **macrophages**, located in lymph nodes (as well as in the spleen, liver, and lungs), swallow (phagocytose) foreign substances. When bacteria are present in lymph nodes that drain a particular area of the body, the nodes become swollen with collections of cells and their engulfed debris and become tender. Lymph nodes also fight disease when specialized lymphocytes called **B lymphocytes (B cells)**, which are present in the nodes, produce antibodies. Other lymphocytes present in nodes are **T lymphocytes (T cells)**. They attack bacteria and foreign cells by accurately recognizing a cell as foreign and destroying it. (See Figure 14-4.) B cells mature in bone marrow, while T cells originate in the thymus gland.

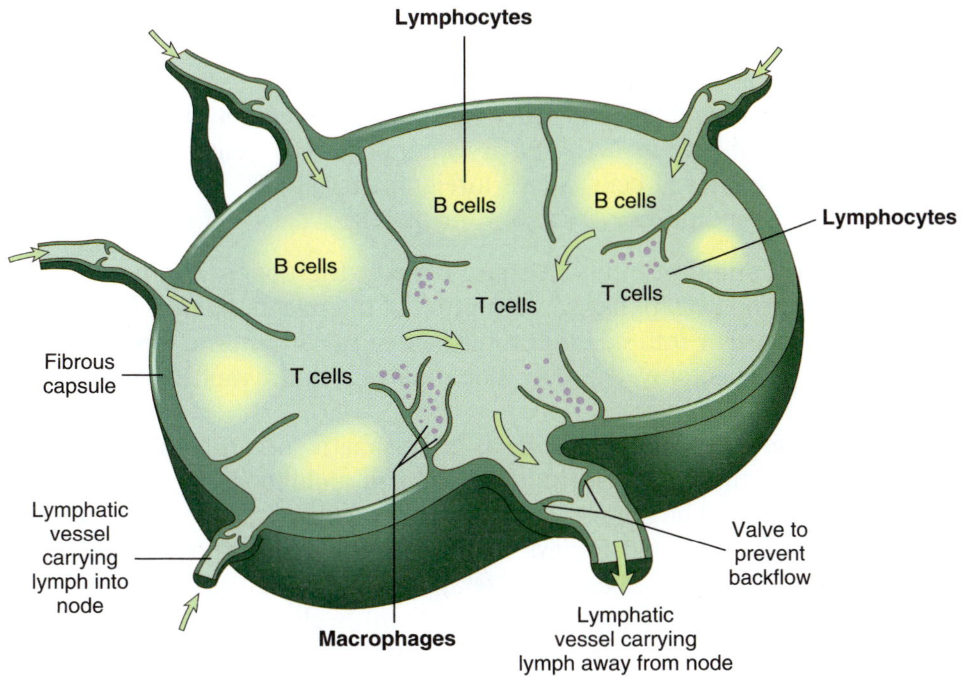

FIGURE 14-4 **Lymph node** containing **lymphocytes** (**B cells** and **T cells**) and **macrophages.**

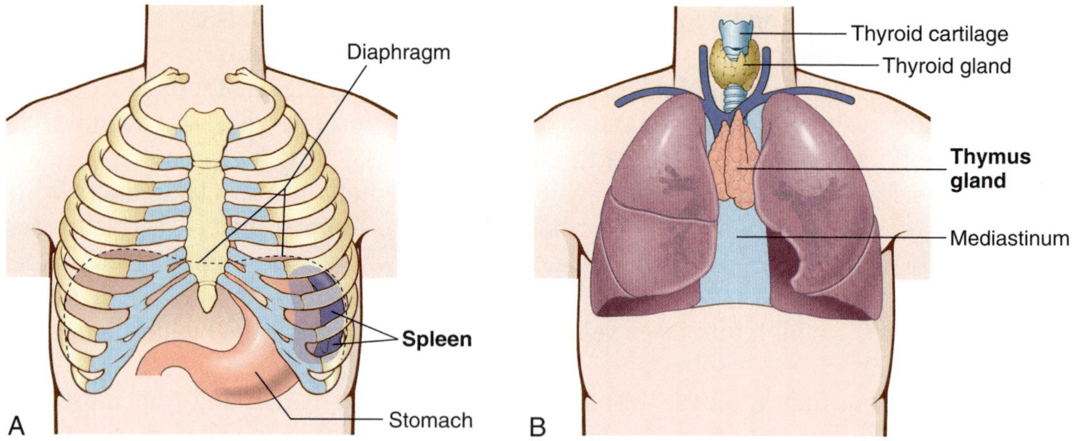

FIGURE 14-5 **A, Spleen** and adjacent structures. **B, Thymus gland** in its location in the mediastinum between the lungs.

SPLEEN AND THYMUS GLAND

The spleen and the thymus gland are specialized organs that are also a part of the lymphatic system.

The **spleen** (Figure 14-5A) is located in the left upper quadrant of the abdomen, next to the stomach. Although the spleen is not essential to life, it has several important functions:

1. **Destruction of old erythrocytes by macrophages.** In the slow-moving circulation of the spleen, red cell breakdown (hemolysis) liberates hemoglobin, which is converted to bilirubin in the liver and then is excreted into the bile.
2. **Filtration of microorganisms and other foreign material from the blood.**
3. **Activation of lymphocytes.** Activated B lymphocytes (B cells) produce antibodies. Activated T lymphocytes (T cells) attack foreign materials.
4. **Storage of blood**, especially erythrocytes and platelets.

The spleen is susceptible to injury. A sharp blow to the upper abdomen (as from the impact of a car's steering wheel) may cause rupture of the spleen. Massive hemorrhage can occur when the spleen is ruptured, and immediate surgical removal (splenectomy) may be necessary. After splenectomy, the liver, bone marrow, and lymph nodes take over the functions of the spleen.

The **thymus gland** (see Figure 14-5B) is a lymphatic organ located in the upper mediastinum between the lungs. During fetal life and childhood it is quite large, but it becomes smaller with age. The thymus gland is composed of nests of lymphoid cells resting on a platform of connective tissue. It plays an important role in the body's ability to protect itself from disease (immunity), especially in fetal life and during the early years of growth. It is known that a thymectomy (removal of the thymus gland) performed in an animal during the first weeks of life impairs the ability of the animal to make antibodies and to produce immune cells that fight against foreign antigens such as bacteria and viruses. Thus, the thymus gland is important in development of an effective immune system in childhood.

Early in development, in the thymus, lymphocytes learn to recognize and accept the body's own antigens as "self" or friendly. This acceptance of "self" antigens is called **tolerance**. When the tolerance process fails, immune cells react against normal cells, resulting in various pathologic conditions (autoimmune disease). See page 556, under **autoimmune disease** (aut/o = self).

14

IMMUNE SYSTEM

The immune system is specialized to defend the body against **antigens** (such as toxins, bacterial proteins, or foreign blood cells). This system includes **leukocytes** such as **neutrophils**, **monocytes**, and **macrophages**, which are phagocytes found in blood and tissues throughout the body. In addition, **lymphoid organs**, such as the lymph nodes, spleen, thymus gland, tonsils, and adenoids, produce **lymphocytes** and **antibodies**.

NATURAL AND ADAPTIVE IMMUNITY

Immunity is the body's ability to resist foreign organisms and toxins that damage tissues and organs. **Natural immunity** is **resistance present at birth**. It is not dependent on prior exposure to an antigen (infectious agent). An example of natural immunity is after a bacterial infection, white blood cells respond immediately to the intruding antigens. **Neutrophils** travel to the infected area and ingest bacteria. Other white blood cells, such as **monocytes**, **macrophages**, and **lymphocytes (NK** or **natural killer cells),** also participate in the body's natural immunity against infection.

In addition to natural immunity, a healthy person can develop **adaptive immunity**. This is the body's ability to **recognize** and **remember** specific antigens in an immune response. **Lymphocytes (T and B cells)** are part of adaptive immunity. **T cells recognize** and **remember** specific antigens and produce stronger attacks each time the antigen is encountered. **B cells** secrete **antibodies** against antigens. Think of what happens when you have a cold or the flu. You are exposed to a viral antigen. Your B cells secrete antibodies, which not only destroy the virus but remain in the blood so that when the virus reappears, at a later time, you have adaptive immunity to it! Another example of adaptive immunity is **vaccination**. You are given an injection of a killed virus (for example, poliovirus) that doesn't make you ill, but stimulates your B cells to secrete antibodies against that virus so that if you are exposed to it at a later time, you will have adaptive immunity.

There are instances when more immediate adaptive immunity is necessary. Poisons (toxins) that rapidly cause major damage (for example, snake venom) can be counteracted by giving ready-made antibodies, called **antitoxins**, produced in another organism. Injections of ready-made antibodies, such as **immunoglobulins**, can boost your adaptive immunity before you travel to a foreign country. Infants are given adaptive immunity when they receive **maternal antibodies** through the placenta or breast milk. Figure 14-6 reviews the general differences between natural and adaptive immunity.

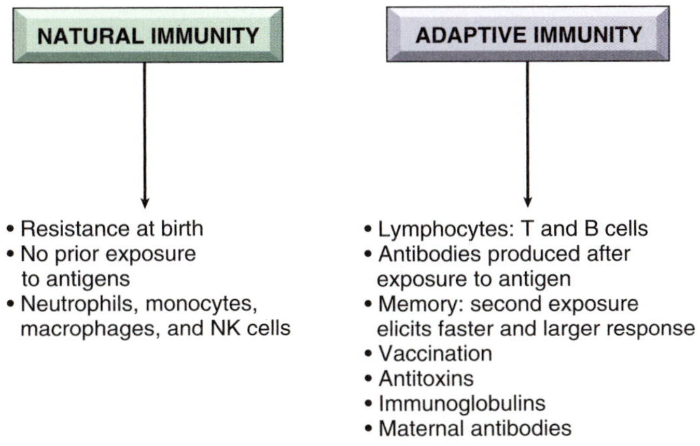

FIGURE 14-6 **Types of immunity.**

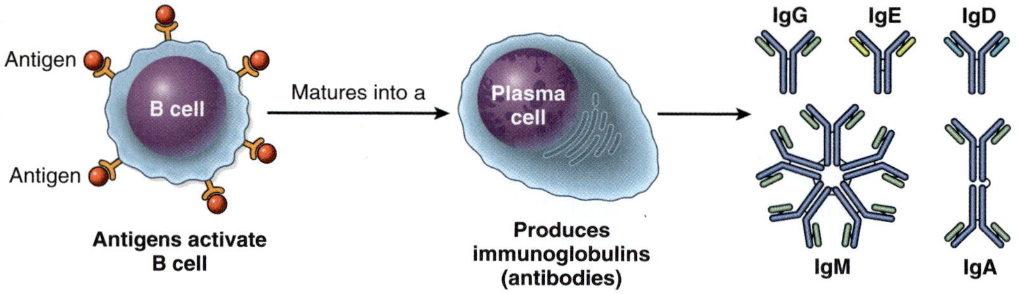

FIGURE 14-7 **Humoral immunity: B cell, plasma cell,** and **immunoglobulins.**

Adaptive immunity has two components: **humoral immunity** and **cell-mediated immunity**. Humoral immunity involves **B cells (B lymphocytes)**, while cell-mediated immunity involves **T cells (T lymphocytes)**. In **humoral immunity, B cells** produce **antibodies** after exposure to specific antigens (viruses and bacteria). This is what happens: The B cell matures into another cell called a **plasma cell**. It is the plasma cell that produces antibodies called **immunoglobulins**, which block the effects of antigens. Examples of immunoglobulins (**Ig = immunoglobulin**) are **IgM, IgA, IgG, IgE**, and **IgD**. One maternal immunoglobulin, **IgG**, crosses the placenta to provide immunity for newborns. Another, **IgE**, is important in allergic reactions and in fighting parasitic infections. Figure 14-7 reviews the relationship of a B cell, plasma cell, and immunoglobulins in humoral immunity.

Cell-mediated immunity does not involve antibodies. Rather, it involves several types of **T cells** with different functions. For example, **cytotoxic T cells (CD8+ T cells)** attach to antigens and directly kill them. Cytotoxic cells also secrete **cytokines (interferons and interleukins)**, which aid other cells in antigen destruction. **Helper T cells (CD4+ T cells)** assist B cells in making antibodies and they stimulate T cells to attack antigens. **Suppressor T cells** (also called **regulatory T cells** or **Tregs**) inhibit both B and T cells and prevent them from attacking the body's own good cells. Figure 14-8 reviews the types of T cells in cell-mediated immunity.

The adaptive immune system is helped by a number of other proteins and cells found in circulating blood. One of these is the **complement system**, a group of proteins that helps antibodies kill their target. Another warrior is the **dendritic cell,** which initiates adaptive immunity by presenting antigens to T and B cells, showing them precisely what they need to counteract. A number of cell types can present antigens to T cells, but dendritic cells are especially efficient at this task. Figure 14-9 reviews the roles of B cells, T cells, complement, and dendritic cells.

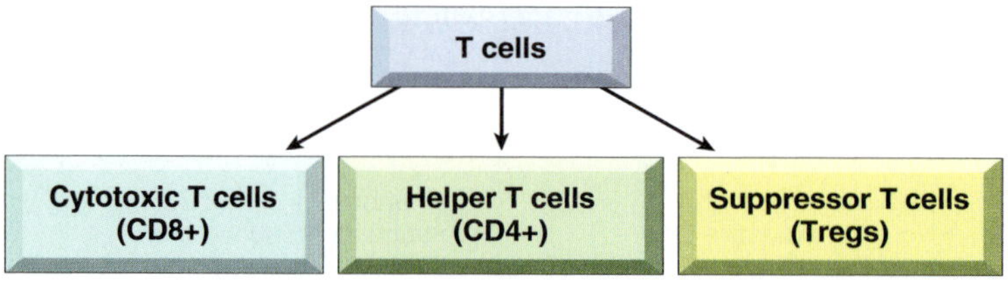

FIGURE 14-8 **Cell-mediated immunity:** Types of **T cells.**

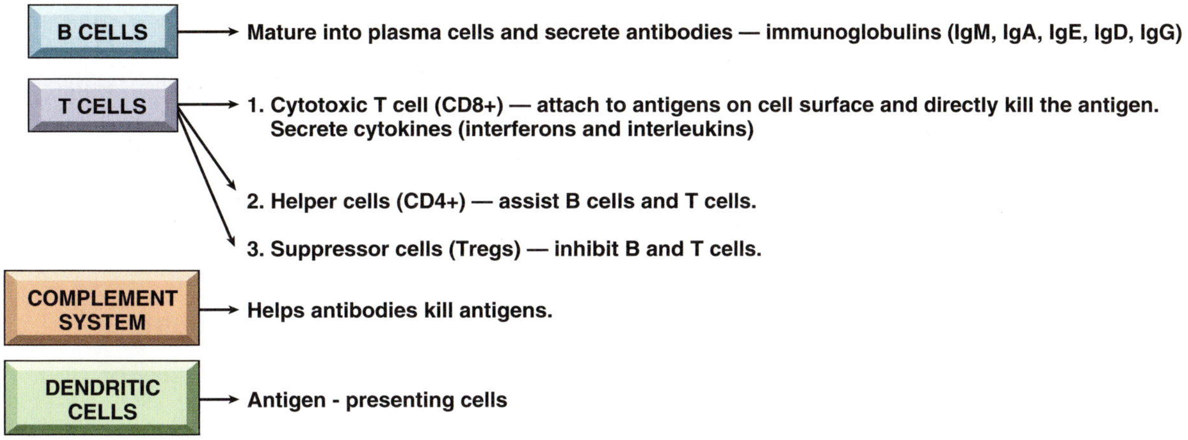

FIGURE 14-9 Functions of B cells, T cells, complement, and dendritic cells.

IMMUNOTHERAPY

Immunotherapy is the use of antibodies, B cells (producing antibodies), and T cells to treat disease such as cancer. Types of immunotherapy are:

Monoclonal antibodies (MoAb)—These are antibodies created in a laboratory by special reproductive (cloning) techniques. They are designed to attack specific cancer cells. An example of monoclonal antibody therapy is the drug rituximab (Rituxan), made to kill malignant lymphoma cells. The antibody may be linked to various toxins or radioactive particles and delivered to tumor cells, to enhance the killing effect.

Vaccines—These preparations contain antigens (proteins) from a patient's tumor cells. When they are injected, they stimulate the patient's own T cells to recognize and kill the cancerous cells. Vaccines may be injected or given as a nasal spray.

Transfer of immune cells—In bone marrow transplantation, T lymphocytes from a donor can replace a patient's immune system with new cells that recognize tumor cells as foreign and kill them.

Monoclonal antibodies and transfer of immune cells are passive immunotherapy (immune agents are given to the patient), while vaccination is active immunotherapy (the patient's own immune system is stimulated to do the work).

VOCABULARY

This list reviews many of the new terms introduced in the text. Short definitions reinforce your understanding of the terms. Refer to the Pronunciation of Terms on page 573 for help with unfamiliar or difficult words.

adaptive immunity	The ability to recognize and remember specific antigens and mount an attack on them. Humoral (B cells) and cell-mediated immunity (T cells) are examples.
adenoids	Mass of lymphatic tissue in the nasopharynx.
antibody	Protein produced by B cells to destroy antigens.
antigen	Substance that the body recognizes as foreign; evokes an immune response. Most antigens are proteins or protein fragments found on the surface of bacteria, viruses, or organ transplant tissue cells.

axillary nodes	Lymph nodes in the armpit (underarm).
B cell (B lymphocyte)	Lymphocyte that matures into a plasma cell to secrete antibodies. The B refers to the bursa of Fabricius, an organ in birds in which B cell differentiation and growth were first noted to occur.
cell-mediated immunity	T cells (cytotoxic, helper and suppressor) that respond to antigens and destroy them; a type of adaptive immunity.
cervical nodes	Lymph nodes in the neck region.
complement system	Proteins in the blood that help antibodies kill their target.
cytokines	Proteins secreted by cytotoxic T cells to aid in antigen destruction. Examples are interferons and interleukins.
cytotoxic T cell	Lymphocyte that directly kills antigens; called **CD8-positive T cell.**
dendritic cell	Antigen-presenting cell. Shows T and B cells what to attack.
helper T cell	Lymphocyte that aids B cells and stimulates T cells. Also called **CD4-positive T cell.**
humoral immunity	B cells produce antibodies after exposure to specific antigens; type of adaptive immunity.
immunity	Body's ability to resist foreign organisms and toxins that damage tissues and organs. This includes natural immunity and adaptive immunity. The word immunity comes from Latin *immunis,* meaning exempt or protected from.
immunoglobulins	Antibodies such as IgA, IgE, IgG, IgM, and IgD; secreted by plasma cells (mature B cells) in response to the presence of an antigen.
immunotherapy	Use of immune cells, antibodies, or vaccines to treat or prevent disease.
inguinal nodes	Lymph nodes in the groin region.
interferons	Proteins (cytokines) secreted by T cells and other cells to aid and regulate the immune response.
interleukins	Proteins (cytokines) that stimulate the growth of B and T lymphocytes.
interstitial fluid	Fluid in the spaces between cells. This fluid becomes lymph when it enters lymph capillaries.
lymph	Thin, watery fluid found within lymphatic vessels and collected from tissues throughout the body. Latin *lympha* means clear spring water.
lymph capillaries	Tiniest lymphatic vessels.
lymphoid organs	Lymph nodes, spleen, and thymus gland.
lymph node	Collection of stationary solid lymphatic tissue along lymph vessels; contains cells (lymphocytes and macrophages) that fight infection.
lymph vessel	Carrier of lymph throughout the body; lymphatic vessels empty lymph into veins in the upper part of the chest.
macrophage	Large phagocyte found in lymph nodes and other tissues of the body. Phag/o means to eat or swallow.
mediastinal nodes	Lymph nodes in the area between the lungs in the thoracic (chest) cavity.

mesenteric nodes	Lymph nodes in the mesentery (intestinal region).
monoclonal antibody	Antibody produced in a laboratory to attack antigens and to destroy cells; useful in immunotherapy.
natural immunity	Protection that an individual is born with to fight infection such as neutrophils, monocytes, macrophages, and NK cells. It is not antigen specific and does not elicit memory.
paraaortic nodes	Lymph nodes near the aorta in the lumbar (waist) area of the body.
plasma cell	Lymphocyte that secretes antibodies. It matures from B lymphocytes.
right lymphatic duct	Lymphatic vessel in the chest that drains lymph from the upper right part of the body. It empties lymph into a large vein in the neck.
spleen	Organ in the left upper quadrant of the abdomen that destroys worn-out red blood cells, activates lymphocytes, and stores blood.
suppressor T cell	Lymphocyte that inhibits the activity of B and T cells. Also called a **Treg (regulatory T cell)**.
T cell (T lymphocyte)	Lymphocyte that acts directly on antigens to destroy them or produce chemicals (cytokines) such as interferons and interleukins that are toxic to antigens.
tolerance	The ability of T lymphocytes to recognize and accept the body's own antigens as "self" or friendly. Once tolerance is established, the immune system will not react against the body.
thoracic duct	Large lymphatic vessel that drains lymph from the lower and left side of the body (head, neck, arm, and chest). It empties lymph into large veins in the neck.
thymus gland	Lymphoid organ in the mediastinum that conditions T cells to react to foreign cells and aids in the immune response.
tonsils	Masses of lymphatic tissue in the back of the oropharynx.
toxin	Poison; a protein produced by certain bacteria, animals, or plants.
vaccination	Exposure of an individual to a foreign protein (antigen) that provokes an immune response. The response will destroy any cell that possesses the antigen on its surface and will protect against infection. The term comes from the Latin *vacca,* cow—the first inoculations were given with organisms that caused the disease cowpox to produce immunity to smallpox.
vaccine	Weakened or killed microorganisms, toxins, or other proteins given to induce immunity to infection or disease.

14

TERMINOLOGY

Write the meanings of the medical terms in the spaces provided.

COMBINING FORMS

COMBINING FORM	MEANING	TERMINOLOGY	MEANING
immun/o	protection	autoimmune disease *Examples are rheumatoid arthritis and systemic lupus erythematosus. These are chronic, disabling diseases caused by the abnormal production of antibodies against normal body tissues. Signs and symptoms are inflammation of joints, skin rash, and fever. Glucocorticoid drugs (prednisone) and other immunosuppressants (azathioprine, methotrexate) are effective as treatment but make patients susceptible to infection.*	______
		immunoglobulin	______
		immunosuppression *This may occur because of exposure to drugs (corticosteroids) or as the result of disease (AIDS and cancer). Immunosuppressed patients are susceptible to infection with fungi,* Pneumocystis *bacteria, and other pathogens.*	______
lymph/o	lymph	lymphopoiesis	______
		lymphedema *Interstitial fluid collects within the spaces between cells as a result of obstruction of lymphatic vessels and nodes. Radiation therapy may destroy lymphatics and produce lymphedema, as in breast cancer treatment (Figure 14-10).*	______
		lymphocytopenia	______
		lymphocytosis	______
		lymphoid *The suffix -oid means resembling or derived from. Lymphoid organs include lymph nodes, spleen, and thymus gland.*	______

14

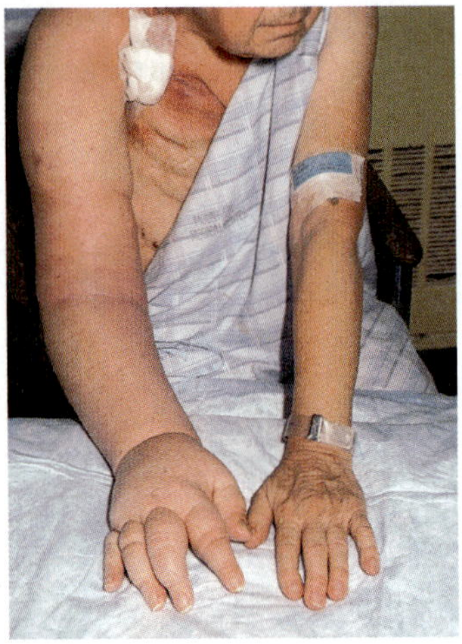

FIGURE 14-10 **Lymphedema** of right arm secondary to mastectomy, lymphadenectomy, and radiotherapy.

COMBINING FORM	MEANING	TERMINOLOGY	MEANING
lymphaden/o	lymph node (gland)	lymphadenopathy	______
		lymphadenitis	______
splen/o	spleen	splenomegaly	______
		Note that the combining form for spleen contains only one e.	
		splenectomy	______
		asplenia	______
		The condition may be congenital or result from surgical removal.	
		hypersplenism	______
		A syndrome marked by splenomegaly and often associated with blood cell destruction, anemia, leukopenia, and thrombocytopenia.	
thym/o	thymus gland	thymectomy	______
tox/o	poison	toxic	______

PREFIXES

PREFIX	MEANING	TERMINOLOGY	MEANING
ana-	again, anew	anaphylaxis	______
		The suffix -phylaxis means protection. This is an unusual hypersensitivity to previously encountered foreign proteins or other antigens. Vasodilation and a decrease in blood pressure can be life-threatening.	
inter-	between	interstitial fluid	______
		The suffix -stitial means pertaining to standing or positioned.	

14

PATHOLOGY

IMMUNODEFICIENCY

Some immunodeficiency disorders are present at birth. An example is **severe combined immunodeficiency disease (SCID).** Affected infants are born with a deficiency of B cells and T cells, resulting in a lack of immunity. The thymus is small, and children have little or no protection against infection.

acquired immunodeficiency syndrome (AIDS)

Group of clinical signs and symptoms associated with suppression of the immune system and marked by opportunistic infections, secondary neoplasms, and neurologic problems.

AIDS is caused by the **human immunodeficiency virus (HIV)**. HIV destroys **helper T cells** (also known as **CD4+ cells**, containing the CD4 protein antigen). This disrupts the immune response, allowing infections to occur. Infectious diseases associated with AIDS are called **opportunistic infections** because HIV lowers resistance and allows infection by bacteria and parasites that are easily otherwise contained by normal defenses. Table 14-2 lists many of these opportunistic infections; use the table as a reference.

TABLE 14-2 OPPORTUNISTIC INFECTIONS WITH AIDS

Infection	Description
candidiasis	Yeast-like fungus *(Candida)*, normally present in the mouth, skin, intestinal tract, and vagina, overgrows, causing infection of the mouth (thrush), respiratory tract, and skin.
cryptococcal infection (Crypto)	Yeast-like fungus *(Cryptococcus)* causes lung, brain, and blood infections. Pathogen is found in pigeon droppings and nesting places, air, water, and soil.
cryptosporidiosis	Parasitic infection of the gastrointestinal tract and brain and spinal cord. The pathogen, *Cryptosporidium*, is a one-celled organism commonly found in farm animals.
cytomegalovirus (CMV) infection	Virus causes enteritis and retinitis (inflammation of the retina at the back of the eye). Found in saliva, semen, cervical secretions, urine, feces, blood, and breast milk, but usually causes disease only when the immune system is compromised.
herpes simplex	Viral infection causes small blisters on the skin of the lips or nose or on the genitals. Herpes simplex virus also can cause encephalitis.
histoplasmosis (Histo)	Fungal infection caused by inhalation of dust contaminated with *Histoplasma capsulatum*; causes fever, chills, and lung infection. Pathogen is found in bird and bat droppings.
Mycobacterium avium-intracellulare (MAI) complex infection	Bacterial disease manifesting with fever, malaise, night sweats, anorexia, diarrhea, weight loss, and lung and blood infections.
***Pneumocystis* pneumonia (PCP)**	One-celled organism causes lung infection, with fever, cough, and chest pain. Pathogen is found in air, water, and soil and is carried by animals. Infection is treated with trimethoprim-sulfamethoxazole (Bactrim), a combination of antibiotics, or with pentamidine. Aerosolized pentamidine, which is inhaled, can prevent occurrence of PCP.
toxoplasmosis (Toxo)	Parasitic infection involving the central nervous system (CNS) and causing fever, chills, visual disturbances, confusion, hemiparesis (slight paralysis in half of the body), and seizures. Pathogen *(Toxoplasma)* is acquired by eating uncooked lamb or pork, unpasteurized dairy products, or raw eggs or vegetables.
tuberculosis (TB)	Bacterial disease (caused by *Mycobacterium tuberculosis*) involving the lungs, brain, and other organs. Signs and symptoms are fever, cough, loss of weight, anorexia, and blood in sputum.

Malignancies associated with AIDS are **Kaposi sarcoma** (a cancer arising from the lining cells of capillaries that produces dark purplish skin nodules) and **lymphoma** (cancer of lymph nodes). **Wasting syndrome**, marked by weight loss and decrease in muscular strength, appetite, and mental activity, also may occur with AIDS (Figure 14-11A and B).

Persons who were exposed to HIV and now have antibodies in their blood against this virus are **HIV-positive**. HIV is found in blood, semen, vaginal and cervical secretions, saliva, and other body fluids. Transmission of HIV may occur by three routes: sexual contact, blood inoculation (through sharing of contaminated needles, accidental needlesticks, or contact with contaminated blood or blood products), and passage of the virus from infected mothers to their newborns. Table 14-3 summarizes the common routes of transmission of HIV.

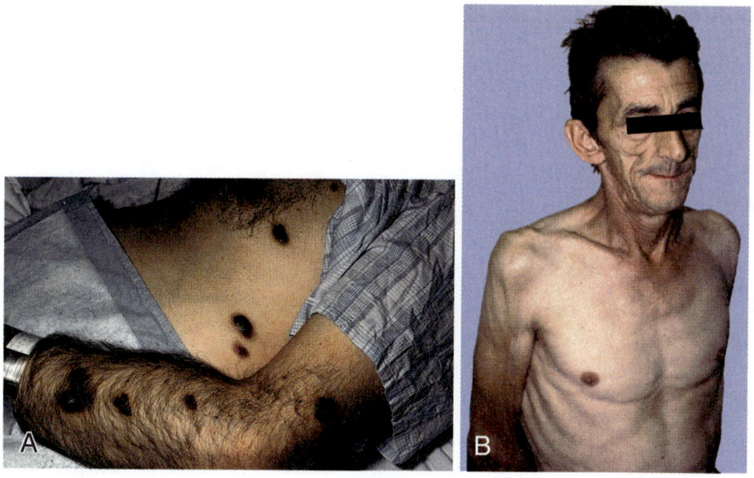

FIGURE 14-11 **A, Kaposi sarcoma. B, Wasting syndrome.**

HIV-infected patients may remain asymptomatic for as long as 10 years. Signs and symptoms associated with HIV infection are lymphadenopathy, neurologic disease, oral thrush (fungal infection), night sweats, fatigue, and evidence of opportunistic infections.

Some drugs that are used to treat AIDS are inhibitors of the viral enzyme called **reverse transcriptase (RT)**. After invading the helper T cell (carrying the CD4+ antigen), HIV releases reverse transcriptase to help it grow and multiply inside the cell. Examples of **reverse transcriptase inhibitors (RTIs)** are zidovudine and lamivudine (Epivir). A second class of anti-HIV drugs is the **protease inhibitors**. These drugs inhibit another viral enzyme called protease. HIV needs protease to reproduce. Use of combinations of protease inhibitors (nelfinavir, amprenavir) and RTIs is called **HAART (highly active antiretroviral therapy)**. This treatment has in many cases abolished evidence of viral infection in affected people.

TABLE 14-3 COMMON ROUTES OF TRANSMISSION OF AIDS VIRUS

Route	People Affected
Receptive oral and anal intercourse	Men and women
Receptive vaginal intercourse	Women
Sharing of needles and equipment (users of intravenous drugs)	Men and women
Contaminated blood (for transfusion) or blood products	Men and women (in hemophiliacs)
From mother, in utero or via breast feeding	Neonates

HYPERSENSITIVITY

allergy

Abnormal hypersensitivity acquired by exposure to an antigen.

Allergic (all/o = other) reactions occur when a sensitized person, who has previously been exposed to an agent **(allergen),** reacts violently to a subsequent exposure. This reaction varies in intensity from **allergic rhinitis** or hay fever (caused by pollen or animal dander) to **systemic anaphylaxis,** in which an extraordinary hypersensitivity reaction occurs throughout the body, leading to fall in blood pressure (hypotension), shock, respiratory distress, and edema (swelling) of the larynx. Anaphylaxis can be life-threatening, but the patient usually survives if the airways are kept open and treatment is given immediately (epinephrine and antihistamines).

Other allergies include **asthma** (pollens, dust, molds), **hives** (caused by food or drugs), and **atopic dermatitis** (rash from soaps, cosmetics, chemicals). Atopic means related to **atopy,** a hypersensitivity or allergic state arising from an inherited predisposition. A person who is atopic is prone to allergies (Figure 14-12).

MALIGNANCIES

lymphoma

Malignant tumor of lymph nodes and lymph tissue.

There are many types of lymphoma, varying according to the particular cell type and degree of differentiation. Some examples are:

Hodgkin disease—Malignant tumor of lymphoid tissue in the spleen and lymph nodes. This disease is characterized by **lymphadenopathy** (lymph nodes enlarge), splenomegaly, fever, weakness, and loss of weight and appetite. The diagnosis often is made by identifying a malignant cell **(Reed-Sternberg cell)** in the lymph nodes. If disease is localized, the treatment may be radiotherapy or chemotherapy. If the disease is more widespread, chemotherapy is given alone. There is a very high probability of cure with available treatments. Figure 14-13 illustrates staging of Hodgkin disease.

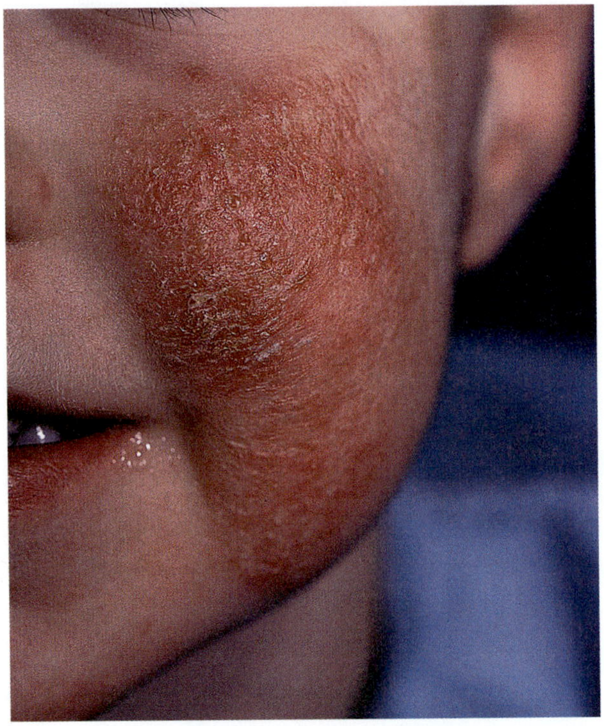

FIGURE 14-12 Atopic dermatitis.

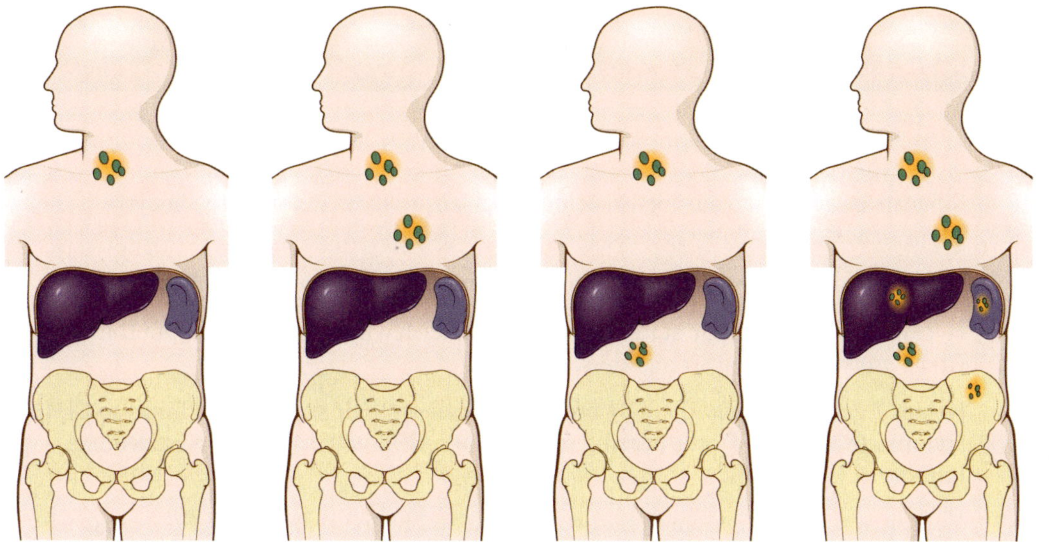

FIGURE 14-13 **Staging of Hodgkin disease** involves assessing the extent of spread of the disease. Lymph node biopsies, laparotomy with liver and lymph node biopsies, and splenectomy may be necessary for staging.

Non-Hodgkin lymphomas—These include **follicular lymphoma** (composed of collections of small lymphocytes in a follicle or nodule arrangement) and **large cell lymphoma** (composed of large lymphocytes that infiltrate nodes and tissues diffusely). Non-Hodgkin lymphomas are mostly B cell lymphomas and rarely T cell malignancies. Chemotherapy may cure or stop the progress of this disease.

multiple myeloma

Malignant tumor of bone marrow cells.

This is a tumor composed of **plasma cells** (antibody-producing B lymphocytes) associated with high levels of one of the specific immunoglobulins, usually IgG. **Waldenström macroglobulinemia** is another disorder of malignant B cells. This disease involves B cells that produce large quantities of IgM (a globulin of high molecular weight). Increased IgM concentration impairs the passage of blood through capillaries in the brain and eyes, causing a hyperviscosity syndrome (thickening of the blood).

thymoma

Malignant tumor of the thymus gland.

Often thymoma is associated with a neuromuscular disorder, myasthenia gravis. Many patients with thymoma have other associated autoimmune disorders such as systemic lupus erythematosus and rheumatoid arthritis.

Surgery is the principal method of treating thymoma; postoperative radiation therapy is used for patients with evidence of spread of the tumor.

STUDY SECTION

Practice spelling each term and know its meaning.

allergen	Substance capable of causing a specific hypersensitivity reaction in the body; a type of antigen.
anaphylaxis	Exaggerated or unusual hypersensitivity to foreign protein or other substance.
atopy	Hypersensitive or allergic state involving an inherited predisposition. From the Greek *atopia*, meaning strangeness.
CD4+ cells	Helper T cells that carry the CD4 protein antigen on their surface. HIV binds to CD4 and infects and kills T cells bearing this protein. AIDS patients have an inadequate number of CD4+ cells.
Hodgkin disease	Malignant tumor of lymphoid tissue in spleen and lymph nodes; Reed-Sternberg cell often is found on microscopic analysis.
human immunodeficiency virus (HIV)	Virus (retrovirus) that causes AIDS.
Kaposi sarcoma	Malignant lesion associated with AIDS; arises from the lining of capillaries and appears as red, purple, brown, or black skin nodules.
non-Hodgkin lymphomas	Group of malignant tumors involving lymphoid tissue. Examples are follicular lymphoma and large cell lymphoma.
opportunistic infections	Infectious diseases associated with AIDS; they occur because HIV infection lowers the body's resistance and allows infection by bacteria and parasites that normally are easily contained.
protease inhibitor	Drug that treats AIDS by blocking the production of protease, a proteolytic enzyme that helps create new viral pieces for HIV.
reverse transcriptase inhibitor (RTI)	Drug that treats AIDS by blocking reverse transcriptase, an enzyme needed to make copies of HIV.
wasting syndrome	Weight loss, decrease in muscular strength, appetite, and mental activity; associated with AIDS.

LABORATORY TESTS AND CLINICAL PROCEDURES

LABORATORY TESTS

CD4+ cell count

Measures the number of CD4+ T cells (helper T cells) in the bloodstream of patients with AIDS.

A normal count usually is between 500 and 1500 CD4+ cells per mm^3. If the CD4+ count falls below 250 to 200, it is recommended to start treatment with anti-HIV drugs.

ELISA

Screening test to detect anti-HIV antibodies in the bloodstream.

Antibodies to HIV begin to appear within 2 weeks of infection with HIV. If the result of this test is positive, it is confirmed with a **Western blot** test, which is more specific. ELISA is an abbreviation for enzyme-linked immunosorbent assay.

immunoelectrophoresis — **Test that separates immunoglobulins (IgM, IgG, IgE, IgA, IgD).**

This procedure detects the presence of abnormal levels of antibodies in patients with conditions such as multiple myeloma and Waldenström macroglobulinemia.

viral load test — **Measurement of the amount of AIDS virus (HIV) in the bloodstream.**

Two viral load tests are a PCR (polymerase chain reaction) assay and an NASBA (nucleic acid sequence–based amplification) test.

CLINICAL PROCEDURES

computed tomography (CT) scan — **X-ray imaging produces cross-sectional and other views of anatomic structures.**

These x-ray views show abnormalities of lymphoid organs, such as lymph nodes, spleen, and thymus gland.

ABBREVIATIONS

AIDS	acquired immunodeficiency syndrome
CD4+ cell	helper T cell
CD8+ cell	cytotoxic T cell
CMV	cytomegalovirus—causes opportunistic AIDS-related infection
Crypto	*Cryptococcus*—causes opportunistic AIDS-related infection
ELISA	enzyme-linked immunosorbent assay—test to detect anti-HIV antibodies
G-CSF	granulocyte colony-stimulating factor—cytokine that promotes neutrophil production
GM-CSF	granulocyte-macrophage colony-stimulating factor—cytokine secreted by macrophages to promote growth of myeloid progenitor cells and their differentiation to granulocytes
HAART	highly active antiretroviral therapy—use of combinations of drugs that are effective against AIDS
HD	Hodgkin disease
Histo	histoplasmosis—fungal infection seen in AIDS patients
HIV	human immunodeficiency virus—causes AIDS
HSV	herpes simplex virus
IgA, IgD, IgE, IgG, IgM	immunoglobulins
IL1 to IL15	interleukins
KS	Kaposi sarcoma
MAI	*Mycobacterium avium-intracellulare* (MAI) complex—group of pathogens that cause lung and systemic disease in immunocompromised patients
MoAb	monoclonal antibody
NHL	non-Hodgkin lymphoma
PCP	*Pneumocystis* pneumonia—opportunistic AIDS-related infection
PI	protease inhibitor
RTI	reverse transcriptase inhibitor—for example, zidovudine (Retrovir) or lamivudine (Epivir)
SCID	severe combined immunodeficiency disease
Treg	regulatory T cell (suppressor T cell)
Toxo	toxoplasmosis—parasitic infection associated with AIDS

PRACTICAL APPLICATIONS

Answers to the questions are on page 572.

MEDICAL TERMINOLOGY IN SENTENCES

1. In addition to the opportunistic infections and malignancies that typically characterize AIDS, pathology of the CNS occurs with some regularity. Specifically, CNS lymphomas, encephalitis, meningitis, progressive leukoencephalopathy, toxoplasmosis, and myelitis have been reported in patients with HIV infection. Dementia and delirium [clouding of consciousness] also have been reported as psychiatric complications.
2. Protease inhibitors interrupt HIV replication, blocking an enzyme called protease. When protease is blocked, HIV cannot infect new cells. Protease inhibitors can reduce HIV viral load in the blood and increase CD4+ T cell counts. Examples of protease inhibitors are indinavir (Crixivan) and nelfinavir (Viracept).
3. Lymph nodes that are nontender and rock-hard are suggestive of a diagnosis of metastatic carcinoma.
4. Infectious mononucleosis and Hodgkin disease are more common in young adults, whereas non-Hodgkin lymphoma and chronic lymphocytic leukemia are more common in middle-aged and elderly people.
5. Oral candidiasis (thrush) manifesting without a history of recent antibiotic therapy, chemotherapy, or immunosuppression may indicate the possibility of HIV infection or diabetes.

14

Questions about Medical Terminology In Sentences

1. What parts of the body commonly are affected by the AIDS virus?
   a. Kidney and urinary bladder
   b. Brain and spinal cord
   c. Pancreas and thyroid glands
2. Which CNS condition often is seen in AIDS patients?
   a. Inflammation of the brain and membranes around the brain
   b. Fluid collection in the brain
   c. Disk impinging on the spinal cord
3. Protease is a/an
   a. Antiviral enzyme
   b. Enzyme that helps HIV infect new cells
   c. Reverse transcriptase inhibitor
4. CD4+ T cell counts can be increased by
   a. High levels of HIV in the blood
   b. Protease inhibitors
   c. Lymphocyte-inhibiting agents
5. A diagnosis of metastatic carcinoma means
   a. The tumor has spread to a secondary location
   b. Lymph nodes are not usually affected
   c. The tumor is localized

6. Hodgkin disease
   a. Commonly affects elderly people
   b. Is a type of lymphoma affecting young adults
   c. Is an infectious disease

7. Which condition may indicate an AIDS virus infection?
   a. High blood sugar
   b. Oral leukoplakia
   c. Fungal infection of the mouth

SHORT CLINICAL CASES

Circle the correct answer for the diagnosis.

1. John was healthy until the age of 22 months, when he developed angioedema [swelling induced while eating a cookie containing peanut butter]. The symptoms disappeared in about an hour. A month later, while eating the same type of cookie, he started to vomit, became hoarse, had great difficulty in breathing, started to wheeze, and developed a swollen face. He was taken immediately to the ED of Children's Hospital, where he was given a subcutaneous injection of epinephrine [adrenaline]. Within minutes of the epinephrine injection, John's hoarseness decreased, the wheezing diminished, and his breathing was less labored. His parents were advised to avoid giving him foods containing peanuts in any form.

Diagnosis: **(multiple myeloma, acute systemic anaphylaxis, acquired immunodeficiency syndrome)**

2. Mark Scott is a 48-year-old band leader who has always been in good health. Six months ago he went to the ED at the local hospital complaining of fever and a swollen right hand from a cat scratch. He was admitted to the hospital for the hand infection. His blood lymphocyte count was very low, so a blood sample was sent to be tested for antibodies against HIV. Both ELISA and a Western blot revealed presence of anti-HIV antibodies. His CD4+ T-cell count was very low at 170 [normal is 500-1600]. Mr. Scott told his doctor that he had several homosexual encounters before his marriage. His physician prescribed trimethoprim-sulfamethoxazole for prophylaxis against *Pneumocystis* pneumonia, and Mark also was given HAART. After 5 weeks of therapy, his HIV viral load declined to undetectable levels and his CD4+ T cell count rose. He remains well and active and works full time.

Diagnosis: **(T cell lymphoma, severe combined immunodeficiency disease, acquired immunodeficiency syndrome)**

3. Mrs. Archer is a 55-year-old housewife who began to experience excessive fatigue. A blood sample revealed mild anemia and slightly lowered white blood cell count. Her sedimentation rate was elevated, and electrophoresis of serum proteins showed marked elevation of IgG. She returned for regular visits to her physician, and on each occasion serum IgG levels were gradually increasing. After she experienced sudden onset of upper back pain, a thoracic spine MRI study was performed and showed destruction of a portion of a vertebra. A bone marrow biopsy specimen showed a proliferation of plasma cells. She was given chemotherapy (vincristine, Adriamycin, and Decadron), but a year later she developed fever and chest pain. Chest x-ray revealed pneumonia, and antibiotics were given. Her outlook for survival is poor.

Diagnosis: **(Hodgkin disease, hemolytic anemia, multiple myeloma)**

IN PERSON

This is written by a medical oncologist who specializes in the treatment of lymphoma patients.

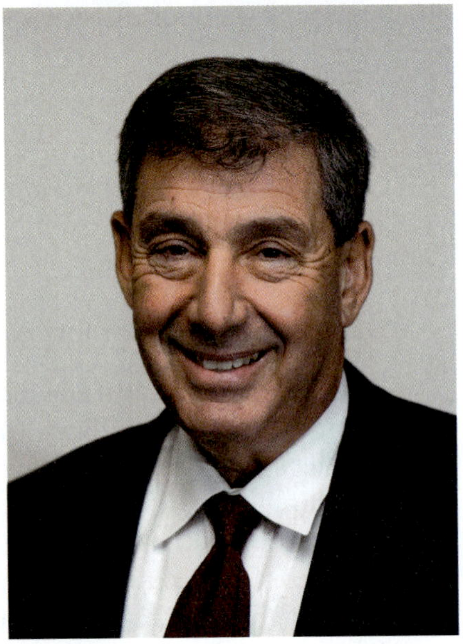

Of the many challenges of practicing medical oncology, the treatment of patients with lymphoma is among the most satisfying, and at times, most difficult. Lymphomas were the first common solid tumor to become curable with drugs alone. In 1969, investigators at the National Cancer Institute published their promising results with combination chemotherapy for Hodgkin disease. At that time, this was a tumor that was only treatable and curable with radiation therapy in a limited fraction of patients, when disease involved only a few lymph nodes. Very soon thereafter, chemotherapy proved curative for almost half of patients with a more aggressive disease (large B-cell lymphocytic lymphoma), a malignancy that affects 20,000 new subjects every year in the USA. In succeeding years, for patients not cured with conventional drugs, bone marrow transplant following ultra-high dose chemotherapy salvaged at least half of those patients who experienced a relapse of disease. New drugs, particularly monoclonal antibodies that attack proteins on the surface of tumors and initiate immune destruction of tumors, have added to that success. Thus, at present, by using chemotherapy, irradiation, and high-dose drug treatment, most lymphoma patients can be cured.

The experience of treating a lymphoma patient is not simple. It requires, first of all, making the correct diagnosis, which requires obtaining an adequate biopsy of the involved lymph nodes, bone marrow, or other disease sites. Secondly, the physician in charge of the case must establish the sites and extent of disease, and this requires sophisticated x-ray and even MR imaging of lungs, abdomen, bones, and even spinal canal. The choice of drug regimens and other treatment depend on making a correct assessment of these factors.

The doctor must explain all this to the patient so that he or she has a clear understanding of what lies ahead. This involves hospital outpatient visits for evaluation and treatment, including possible biopsy and repeat biopsy of sites of disease to establish whether the tumor has been effectively treated. I also spend considerable time with patients explaining the potential side effects of treatments, some of which can affect the lungs, heart, and immune system. In addition, patients need guidance following chemotherapy about susceptibility to serious infections when blood counts are low. Overall, the psychological stress and uncertainty of outcome plus the impact on work and family responsibilities make the need for support from friends and family crucial.

For most patients, all of these issues are successfully managed during treatment, and no experience is more gratifying for me, as an oncologist, than to achieve cure of a potentially lethal disease. All of this is accomplished at a price. For a few patients, the stresses of disease and its impact on family and work prove overwhelming. I call upon the intervention of social workers, nurses, and even psychiatrists to help my patients deal with the difficulty of disease and life-changing experiences. The added rigors of bone marrow transplantation increase the burden on patients who are not cured by conventional treatments. And, even more stressful and challenging are those patients, a minority to be sure, whose disease progresses despite all interventions, and who are destined not to survive. For these patients, experimental treatments at times are the best option, and again may reverse the downward course. Through it all, as a physician, I find that we must all work as a team to provide the best medical advice, psychological support, and hope for 60,000 new patients who develop lymphoma each year.

Dr. Bruce A. Chabner is a professor of medicine at Harvard Medical School and the Director of Clinical Research at the Massachusetts General Hospital Cancer Center.

EXERCISES

Remember to check your answers carefully with the Answers to Exercises, page 571.

A Match the following terms with the descriptions below.

adenoids	lymph node	thoracic duct
interstitial fluid	right lymphatic duct	thymus gland
lymph capillaries	spleen	

1. collection of stationary lymphatic tissue along lymph vessels ______________________
2. large lymphatic vessel that drains lymph from the lower and left side of the body ______________________
3. organ in the left upper quadrant of the abdomen that destroys worn-out erythrocytes, activates lymphocytes, and stores blood ______________________
4. mass of lymphatic tissue in the nasopharynx ______________________
5. lymphoid organ in the mediastinum that conditions T cells to react to foreign cells in the immune response ______________________
6. tiniest lymphatic vessels ______________________
7. large lymphatic vessel in the chest that drains lymph from the upper right part of the body ______________________
8. fluid in the spaces between cells ______________________

B Give the locations of the following lymph nodes.

1. inguinal nodes ______________________
2. axillary nodes ______________________
3. cervical nodes ______________________
4. mediastinal nodes ______________________
5. paraaortic nodes ______________________
6. mesenteric nodes ______________________

C Circle the correct answer in each sentence.

1. Cytotoxic T cells are **(CD8+ T cells, helper T cells, suppressor T cells)** and directly kill foreign cells.
2. Lymphocytes that directly act on antigens are **(B cells, T cells, macrophages)**.
3. CD4+ T cells are **(helper T cells, Tregs, B cells)** and are deficient in people with AIDS.
4. Lymphocytes that mature into plasma cells and secrete antibodies are **(B cells, T cells, macrophages)**.
5. The type of immunity in which B cells produce antibodies after exposure to antigens is **(natural immunity, cytotoxic immunity, humoral immunity)**.
6. The type of immunity that is the ability to recognize and remember specific antigens and mount an attack on them is **(adaptive immunity, natural immunity)**.

D Match the following cell names with their meanings as given below.

complement system	helper T cell	plasma cell
dendritic cell	macrophage	suppressor T cell

1. lymphocyte that matures from a B lymphocyte and secretes antibodies ____________________
2. large phagocyte found in lymph nodes and other tissues of the body ____________________
3. CD4+ T cell that aids B cells in recognizing antigens ____________________
4. Treg that inhibits the activity of B and T lymphocytes ____________________
5. proteins in the blood that help antibodies and T cells kill their target ____________________
6. antigen-presenting cell; shows B cells and T cells what to attack ____________________

14

E Match the terms in Column I with their descriptions in Column II. Write your answers in the spaces provided.

COLUMN I

1. immunoglobulins _____
2. toxins _____
3. helper T cells _____
4. suppressor T cells _____
5. cytotoxic T cells _____
6. plasma cells _____
7. interferons and interleukins _____

COLUMN II

A. Antibodies—IgA, IgE, IgG, IgM, IgD
B. Lymphocytes that aids B cells; CD4+ T cell
C. Poisons (antigens)
D. T lymphocytes that inhibit the activity of B and T cells
E. Cytokines secreted by cytotoxic T cells
F. Transformed B cells that secrete antibodies
G. T lymphocytes that directly kill foreign cells (CD8+ T cells)

F **Use the given definitions to build medical terms.**

1. removal of the spleen ________________
2. enlargement of the spleen ________________
3. formation of lymph ________________
4. malignant tumor of the thymus gland ________________
5. inflammation of lymph glands (nodes) ________________
6. deficiency of lymph cells ________________
7. pertaining to poison ________________
8. disease of lymph glands (nodes) ________________

G **Match the following terms with their meanings below.**

AIDS	Hodgkin disease	lymphoid organs
allergen	hypersplenism	thymectomy
anaphylaxis	lymphedema	

1. syndrome marked by enlargement of the spleen and associated with anemia, leukopenia, and thrombocytopenia ________________
2. extraordinary hypersensitivity to a foreign protein; marked by hypotension, shock, and respiratory distress ________________
3. antigen capable of causing allergy (hypersensitivity) ________________
4. disorder in which the immune system is suppressed by exposure to HIV ________________
5. removal of a mediastinal organ ________________
6. malignant tumor of lymphoid tissue in the lymph nodes and spleen; Reed-Sternberg cells are in lymph nodes ________________
7. spleen, thymus, and tonsils ________________
8. swelling of tissues due to interstitial fluid accumulation ________________

H **Match the following terms or abbreviations related to AIDS with their descriptions below.**

CD4+ T cells	Kaposi sarcoma	reverse transcriptase inhibitor
ELISA	opportunistic infections	viral load test
HAART	protease inhibitor	wasting syndrome
HIV		

1. malignant condition associated with AIDS (purplish skin nodules appear) ______________________
2. human immunodeficiency virus; the retrovirus that causes AIDS ______________________
3. white blood cells that are destroyed by the AIDS virus ______________________
4. group of infectious diseases associated with AIDS ______________________
5. measures the amount of HIV in blood ______________________
6. weight loss with decreased muscular strength, appetite, and mental activity ______________________
7. drug used to treat AIDS by blocking an enzyme needed to make copies of HIV ______________________
8. drug used to treat AIDS by blocking the production of an enzyme that creates new viral pieces for HIV ______________________
9. use of combinations of drugs to treat AIDS ______________________
10. test to detect anti-HIV antibodies ______________________

14

I **Complete the following terms according to the definitions provided. Pay close attention to the proper spelling of each term.**

1. chronic, disabling diseases caused by abnormal production of antibodies to normal tissue: auto______________________ diseases
2. a hypersensitivity or allergic state with an inherited predisposition: a______________________
3. a malignant tumor of lymph nodes; follicular and large cell are types of this disease: non______________________
4. fluid that lies between cells throughout the body: inter______________________ fluid
5. formation of lymphocytes or lymphoid tissue: lympho______________________
6. chronic swelling of a part of the body due to collection of fluid between tissues secondary to obstruction of lymph vessels and nodes: lymph______________________
7. an unusual or exaggerated allergic reaction to a foreign protein: ana______________________
8. introduction of altered antigens to produce an immune response and protection from disease: vac______________________
9. test that separates immunoglobulins: immuno______________________
10. antibody used in immunotherapy; produced in a laboratory to attack antigens and destroy cells: mono______________________ antibody

J **Circle the correct term(s) to complete each sentence.**

1. Mr. Blake had been HIV-positive for 5 years before he developed **(*Pneumocystis* pneumonia, thymoma, multiple myeloma)** and was diagnosed with **(Hodgkin disease, non-Hodgkin lymphoma, AIDS)**.
2. Mary developed rhinitis, rhinorrhea, and red eyes every spring when pollen was prevalent. She consulted her doctor about her severe **(hypersplenism, allergies, lymphadenitis)**.
3. Paul felt some marble-sized lumps in his left groin. His doctor told him that he had an infection in his foot and had developed secondary **(axillary, cervical, inguinal)** lymphadenopathy.
4. Mr. Jones was referred to a dermatologist and an oncologist when his primary physician noticed purple spots on his arms and legs. Because he had AIDS, his physician was concerned about the possibility of **(Kaposi sarcoma, splenomegaly, thrombocytopenic purpura)**.
5. Fifteen-year-old Peter was allergic to peanuts. His allergy was so severe that he carried epinephrine with him at all times to prevent **(adaptive immunity, anaphylaxis, immunosuppression)** in case he came in contact with peanut butter at school.
6. When she was in her mid-20s, Rona was diagnosed with a lymph node malignancy known as **(sarcoidosis, Kaposi sarcoma, Hodgkin disease)**. Because the disease was primarily in her chest, her **(inguinal, mediastinal, axillary)** lymph nodes were irradiated (radiation therapy), and she was cured. When she developed lung cancer in her mid-40s, her oncologist told her she had a/an **(iatrogenic, hereditary, metastatic)** radiation-induced secondary tumor.
7. Mary has suffered from hay fever, asthma, and chronic dermatitis ever since she was a young child. She has been particularly bothered by the severely pruritic (itching), erythematous (reddish) patches on her hands. Her dermatologist gave her topical steroids for her **(toxic, atopic, opportunistic)** dermatitis and told her to avoid soaps, cosmetics, and irritating chemicals.
8. Bernie noticed pain in his pelvis, spine, and ribs and was evaluated by his physician. Blood tests showed high levels of plasma cells and abnormal globulins. Increased numbers of plasma cells were revealed on **(chest x-ray, stem cell transplantation, bone marrow biopsy)**. Radiologic studies showed bone loss. The physician's diagnosis was multiple **(sclerosis, thymoma, myeloma)**.
9. AIDS is caused by **(herpes simplex virus, monoclonal antibodies, human immunodeficiency virus)**. Lymphocytes called **(CD4+ cells, suppressor cells, B cells)** are destroyed, leading to **(anaphylaxis, atopy, opportunistic infections)**.
10. Drugs used to treat AIDS are **(immunosuppressants, protease inhibitors, interferons)**. Other anti-AIDS drugs are **(reverse transcriptase inhibitors, monoclonal antibodies, immunoglobulins)**.

14

ANSWERS TO EXERCISES

A

1. lymph node
2. thoracic duct
3. spleen
4. adenoids
5. thymus gland
6. lymph capillaries
7. right lymphatic duct
8. interstitial fluid

B

1. groin region
2. armpit region
3. neck (of the body) region
4. space between the lungs in the chest
5 near the aorta in the lumbar area of the body
6. intestinal region

C

1. CD8+ T cells
2. T cells
3. helper T cells
4. B cells
5. humoral immunity
6. adaptive immunity

D

1. plasma cell
2. macrophage
3. helper T cell
4. suppressor T cell
5. complement system
6. dendritic cell

E

1. A
2. C
3. B
4. D
5. G
6. F
7. E

F

1. splenectomy
2. splenomegaly
3. lymphopoiesis
4. thymoma
5. lymphadenitis
6. lymphocytopenia
7. toxic
8. lymphadenopathy

G

1. hypersplenism
2. anaphylaxis
3. allergen
4. AIDS
5. thymectomy
6. Hodgkin disease
7. lymphoid organs
8. lymphedema

H

1. Kaposi sarcoma
2. HIV
3. CD4+ T cells
4. opportunistic infections
5. viral load test
6. wasting syndrome
7. reverse transcriptase inhibitor
8. protease inhibitor
9. HAART (highly active antiretroviral therapy)
10. ELISA (enzyme-linked immunosorbent assay)

I

1. autoimmune
2. atopy
3. non-Hodgkin lymphoma
4. interstitial
5. lymphopoiesis
6. lymphedema
7. anaphylaxis
8. vaccination
9. immunoelectrophoresis
10. monoclonal

J

1. *Pneumocystis* pneumonia; AIDS
2. allergies
3. inguinal
4. Kaposi sarcoma
5. anaphylaxis
6. Hodgkin disease; mediastinal; iatrogenic
7. atopic
8. bone marrow biopsy; myeloma
9. human immunodeficiency virus; CD4+ cells; opportunistic infections
10. protease inhibitors; reverse transcriptase inhibitors

Answers to Practical Applications

Medical Terminology Sentences

1. b
2. a
3. b
4. b
5. a
6. b
7. c

Short Clinical Cases

1. acute systemic anaphylaxis—Allergic reactions occur when already sensitized individuals are reexposed to the same allergen. The first exposure generates allergen-specific antibodies and/or T cells, and reexposure to the same allergen can produce a severe allergic reaction or anaphylaxis.
2. acquired immunodeficiency syndrome
3. multiple myeloma

PRONUNCIATION OF TERMS

To test your understanding of the terminology in this chapter, write the meaning of each term in the space provided. In addition, you may wish to cover the terms and write them by looking at your definitions. Make sure your spelling is correct. The page number after each term indicates where it is defined or used in the book, so you can easily check your responses. You will find complete definitions for all of these terms and their audio pronunciations on the Evolve website.

Pronunciation Guide

ā as in āpe	ă as in ăpple
ē as in ēven	ĕ as in ĕvery
ī as in īce	ĭ as in ĭnterest
ō as in ōpen	ŏ as in pŏt
ū as in ūnit	ŭ as in ŭnder

Vocabulary and Terminology

TERM	PRONUNCIATION	MEANING
adaptive immunity (553)	ă-DĀP-tĭv ĭ-MŪ-nĭ-tē	
adenoids (553)	ĂD-ĕ-noydz	
anaphylaxis (557)	ăn-ă-fă-LĂK-sĭs	
antibody (553)	ĂN-tĭ-bŏ-dē	
antigen (553)	ĂN-tĭ-jĕn	
asplenia (557)	ā-SPLĒN-ē-ă	
autoimmune disease (556)	aw-tō-ĭ-MŪN dĭ-ZĒZ	
axillary nodes (554)	ĂKS-ĭ-lăr-ē nōdz	
B cell (554)	B sĕl	
cell-mediated immunity (554)	sĕl mē-dē-Ā-tĕd ĭ-MŪN -ĭ-tē	
cervical nodes (554)	SĔR-vĭ-kl nōdz	
complement system (554)	CŎM-plĕ-mĕnt SĭS-tĕm	
cytokines (554)	SĪ-tō-kĭnz	
cytotoxic T cell (554)	sī-tō-TŎK-sĭk T sĕl	
dendritic cell (554)	dĕn-DRĬ-tĭk sĕl	
helper T cell (554)	HĔL-pĕr T sĕl	
humoral immunity (554)	HŪ-mĕr-ăl ĭm-MŪN-ĭ-tē	
hypersplenism (557)	hī-pĕr-SPLĔN-ĭzm	
immunity (554)	ĭm-MŪN-ĭ-tē	
immunoglobulins (554)	ĭm-ū-nō-GLŎB-ū-lĭnz	
immunosuppression (556)	ĭm-ū-nō-sŭ-PRĔ-shŭn	
immunotherapy (554)	ĭ-mū-nō-THĔR-ă-pē	

14

TERM	PRONUNCIATION	MEANING
inguinal node (554)	ĬNG-gwĭ-năl nōd	______
interferons (554)	ĭn-tĕr-FĒR-ŏnz	______
interleukins (554)	ĭn-tĕr-LOO-kĭnz	______
interstitial fluid (554)	ĭn-tĕr-STĬSH-ăl FLOO-ĭd	______
lymph (554)	lĭmf	______
lymphadenitis (557)	lĭm-făh-dĕ-NĪ-tĭs	______
lymphadenopathy (557)	lĭm-făd-ĕ-NŎP-ăh-thē	______
lymph capillaries (554)	lĭmf KĂP-ĭ-lă-rēz	______
lymphedema (556)	lĭmf-ĕ-DĒ-mă	______
lymph node (554)	lĭmf nōd	______
lymphocytes (546)	LĬM-fō-sītz	______
lymphocytosis (556)	lĭm-fō-sī-TŌ-sĭs	______
lymphocytopenia (556)	lĭm-fō-sī-tō-PĒ-nē-ă	______
lymphoid organs (554)	LĬM-foid ŎR-gănz	______
lymphopoiesis (556)	lĭm-fō-poy-Ē-sĭs	______
lymph vessel (554)	lĭmf VĔS-ĕl	______
macrophage (554)	MĂK-rō-fāj	______
mediastinal nodes (554)	mē-dē-ăs-TĪ-năl nōdz	______
mesenteric nodes (555)	mĕs-ĕn-TĔR-ĭk nōdz	______
monoclonal antibody (555)	mŏn-ō-KLŌ-năl ĂN-tĭ-bŏd-ē	______
natural immunity (555)	NĂ-tū-răl ĭm-MŪ-nĭ-tē	______
paraaortic nodes (555)	pă-ră-ā-ŎR-tĭk nōdz	______
plasma cell (555)	PLĂZ-mă sĕl	______
right lymphatic duct (555)	rīt lĭm-FĂ-tĭk dŭkt	______
spleen (555)	splēn	______
splenectomy (557)	splĕ-NĔK-tō-mē	______
splenomegaly (557)	splĕ-nō-MĔG-ă-lē	______
suppressor T cell (555)	sŭ-PRĔ-sŏr T sĕl	______
T cell (555)	T sĕl	______
thoracic duct (555)	thō-RĂ-sĭk dŭkt	______
thymectomy (557)	thī-MĔK-tō-mē	______
thymus gland (555)	THĪ-mŭs glănd	______
tolerance (555)	TŎL-ĕr-ăntz	______
tonsils (555)	TŎN-sĭlz	______

14

TERM	PRONUNCIATION	MEANING
toxic (557)	TŎK-sĭk	___
toxin (555)	TŎK-sĭn	___
vaccination (555)	văk-sĭ-NĀ-shŭn	___
vaccine (555)	văk-SĒN	___

Pathology and Laboratory Tests

TERM	PRONUNCIATION	MEANING
acquired immunodeficiency syndrome (557)	ă-KWĪRD ĭm-ū-nō-dĕ-FĬSH-ĕn-sē SĬN-drōm	___
allergen (562)	ĂL-ĕr-jĕn	___
allergy (560)	ĂL-ĕr-jē	___
atopy (562)	ĂT-ō-pē	___
CD4+ cell (562)	CD4 PŎS-ĭ-tĭv sĕl	___
ELISA (562)	ĕ-LĪ-ză	___
Hodgkin disease (562)	HŎJ-kĭn dĭ-ZĒZ	___
human immunodeficiency virus (562)	HŪ-măn ĭm-ū-nō-dĕ-FĬSH-ĕn-sē VĪ-rŭs	___
immunoelectrophoresis (563)	ĭm-ū-nō-ē-lĕk-trō-phŏr-Ē-sĭs	___
Kaposi sarcoma (562)	KĂ-pō-sē (*or* kă-PŌS-sē) săr-KŌ-mă	___
lymphoma (560)	lĭm-FŌ-mă	___
multiple myeloma (561)	MŬLT-ĭ-pl mī-ĕ-LŌ-mă	___
non-Hodgkin lymphoma (562)	nŏn-HŎJ-kĭn lĭm-FŌ-ma	___
opportunistic infections (562)	ŏp-pŏr-tū-NĬS-tĭk ĭn-FĔK-shŭnz	___
protease inhibitors (562)	PRŌ-tē-ās ĭn-HĬB-ĭ-tŏrz	___
reverse transcriptase inhibitors (562)	rē-VĔRS trăns-SCRĬPT-āz ĭn-HĬB-ĭ-tŏrz	___
severe combined immunodeficiency disease (557)	sĕ-VĒR kŏm-BĪND ĭm-ū-nō-dĕ-FĬSH-ĕn-sē dĭ-ZĒZ	___
thymoma (561)	thī-MŌ-mă	___
viral load test (563)	vī-răl lōd tĕst	___
wasting syndrome (562)	WĀST-ĭng SĬN-drōm	___
Western blot (562)	WĔS-tĕrn blŏt	___

14

REVIEW SHEET

Write the meaning of the word parts in the spaces provided. Check your answers with the information in the chapter or in the Glossary (Medical Word Parts—English) at the end of the book.

Combining Forms

COMBINING FORM	MEANING	COMBINING FORM	MEANING
axill/o	______	lymphaden/o	______
cervic/o	______	splen/o	______
immun/o	______	thym/o	______
inguin/o	______	tox/o	______
lymph/o	______		

Suffixes

SUFFIX	MEANING	SUFFIX	MEANING
-cytosis	______	-pathy	______
-edema	______	-penia	______
-globulin	______	-phylaxis	______
-megaly	______	-poiesis	______
-oid	______	-stitial	______
-oma	______	-suppression	______

Prefixes

PREFIX	MEANING	PREFIX	MEANING
ana-	______	inter-	______
auto-	______	retro-	______
hyper-	______		

evolve *Please refer to the Evolve website for additional exercises and images related to this chapter.*

CHAPTER 15

Musculoskeletal System

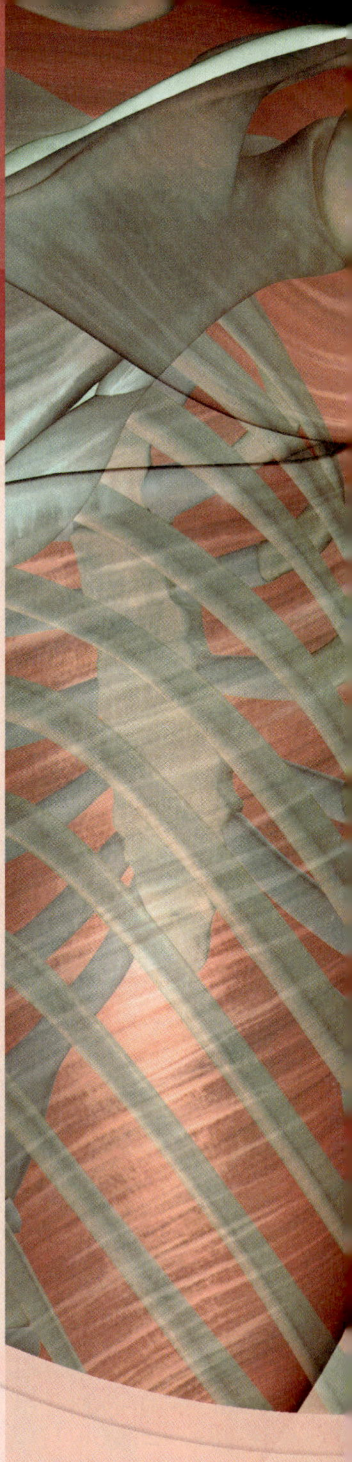

This chapter is divided into the following sections:

CHAPTER GOALS

- Define terms relating to the structure and function of bones, joints, and muscles.
- Describe the process of bone formation and growth.
- Locate and name the major bones of the body.
- Analyze the combining forms, prefixes, and suffixes used to describe bones, joints, and muscles.
- Explain various musculoskeletal disease conditions and terms related to bone fractures.
- Describe important laboratory tests and clinical procedures relating to the musculoskeletal system, and recognize relevant abbreviations.
- Apply your new knowledge to understanding medical terms in their proper contexts, such as medical reports and records.

INTRODUCTION

The musculoskeletal system includes the bones, muscles, and joints. All have important functions in the body.

Bones provide the framework on which the body is constructed and protect and support internal organs. Bones also assist the body in movement, because they serve as a point of attachment for muscles. The inner core of bones is composed of hematopoietic tissue (red bone marrow, which manufactures blood cells), whereas other parts of bone are storage areas for minerals necessary for growth, such as calcium and phosphorus.

Joints are the places at which bones come together. Several different types of joints are found within the body. The type of joint found in any specific location is determined by the need for greater or lesser flexibility of movement.

Muscles, whether attached to bones or to internal organs and blood vessels, are responsible for movement. Internal movement involves the contraction and relaxation of muscles found in viscera, and external movement is accomplished by the contraction and relaxation of muscles that are attached to the bones. **Tendons** are connective tissue that bind muscles to bones, while **ligaments** bind bones to other bones.

Orthopedists are physicians who treat (surgically and medically) bone, joint, and muscle conditions. Originally, orthopedics was a branch of medicine correcting deformities in children (**orth/o** means straight, **ped/o** means child). **Rheumatologists** are physicians (nonsurgical) who specialize primarily in joint problems, such as arthritis; in this context, **rheumat/o,** meaning watery flow, refers to joint fluid. **Physiatrists** are medical doctors whose focus is on rehabilitation after injury or illness to muscles, bones, and nerves.

15

Both a **medical doctor (MD)** and an **osteopathic physician (DO)** can specialize in orthopedics or rheumatology. MD and DO medical education programs are similar, and both kinds of physicians perform surgery as well as prescribe medication. An osteopath has added training in the musculoskeletal system, with an emphasis on body mechanics to promote good health. A **chiropractor** (**chir/o** means hand) is not a physician but has extensive and specialized training in using physical means to manipulate the spinal column, joints, and soft tissues. Chiropractic medicine considers that disease is related to pressure on nerves by spinal misalignment.

A **physical therapist** is a master's or doctoral degree–prepared health care professional who develops a treatment plan based on a physician's diagnosis. The goals of physical therapy (PT) are to restore function, improve mobility, and relieve pain.

BONES

FORMATION AND STRUCTURE

Formation

Bones are complete organs composed chiefly of connective tissue called **osseous** (bony) **tissue,** plus a rich supply of blood vessels and nerves. Osseous tissue consists of a combination of **osteocytes** (bone cells), dense connective tissue strands known as **collagen,** and intercellular **calcium salts.**

During fetal development, the bones of the fetus are composed of **cartilaginous tissue,** which resembles osseous tissue but is more flexible and less dense because of a lack of calcium salts in its intercellular spaces. As the embryo develops, the process of depositing calcium salts in the soft, cartilaginous tissue occurs and continues throughout the life of the individual after birth. The gradual replacement of cartilage and its intercellular substance by immature bone cells and calcium deposits is **ossification** (bone formation).

Osteoblasts are the immature osteocytes that produce the bony tissue that replaces cartilage during ossification. **Osteoclasts** (**-clast** is from the Greek word meaning to break) are large cells that function to reabsorb, or digest, bony tissue. Osteoclasts (also called **bone phagocytes**) digest bone tissue from the inner sides of bones thus enlarging the inner bone cavity so that the bone does not become overly thick and heavy. When a bone breaks, osteoblasts lay down the mineral bone matter (calcium salts) and osteoclasts remove excess bone debris (smooth out the bone).

Osteoblasts and osteoclasts work together in all bones throughout life, tearing down (osteoclasts) and rebuilding (osteoblasts) bony tissue. This allows bone to respond to mechanical stresses placed on it and thus enables it to be a living tissue, constantly rebuilding and renewing itself.

The formation of bone depends largely on a proper supply of **calcium** and **phosphorus** to the bone tissue. These minerals must be taken into the body along with a sufficient amount of vitamin D. Vitamin D helps calcium to pass through the lining of the small intestine and into the bloodstream. Once calcium and phosphorus are in the bones, osteoblastic activity produces an enzyme that forms calcium phosphate, a substance that gives bone its characteristic hard quality. It is the major calcium salt.

Not only are calcium and phosphorus part of the hard structure of bone tissue, but calcium also is stored elsewhere in bones, and small quantities are present in the blood. If the proper amount of calcium is lacking in the blood, nerve fibers are unable to transmit impulses effectively to muscles, the heart muscle becomes weak, and muscles attached to bones undergo spasms.

The necessary level of calcium in the blood is maintained by the parathyroid gland, which secretes a hormone that signals the release of calcium from bone storage. An excess of the hormone (caused by tumor or another pathologic process) will raise blood calcium at the expense of the bones, which become weakened by the loss of calcium.

Structure

There are 206 bones of various types in the body. **Long bones** are found in the thigh, lower leg, and upper and lower arm. These bones are very strong, are broad at the ends where they join with other bones, and have large surface areas for muscle attachment.

Short bones are found in the wrist and ankle and are small with irregular shapes. **Flat bones** are found covering soft body parts. These bones are the skull, shoulder blades, ribs, and pelvic bones. **Sesamoid bones** are small, rounded bones (resembling a sesame seed in shape). They are found near joints, and they increase the efficiency of muscles near a particular joint. The kneecap is the largest example of a sesamoid bone.

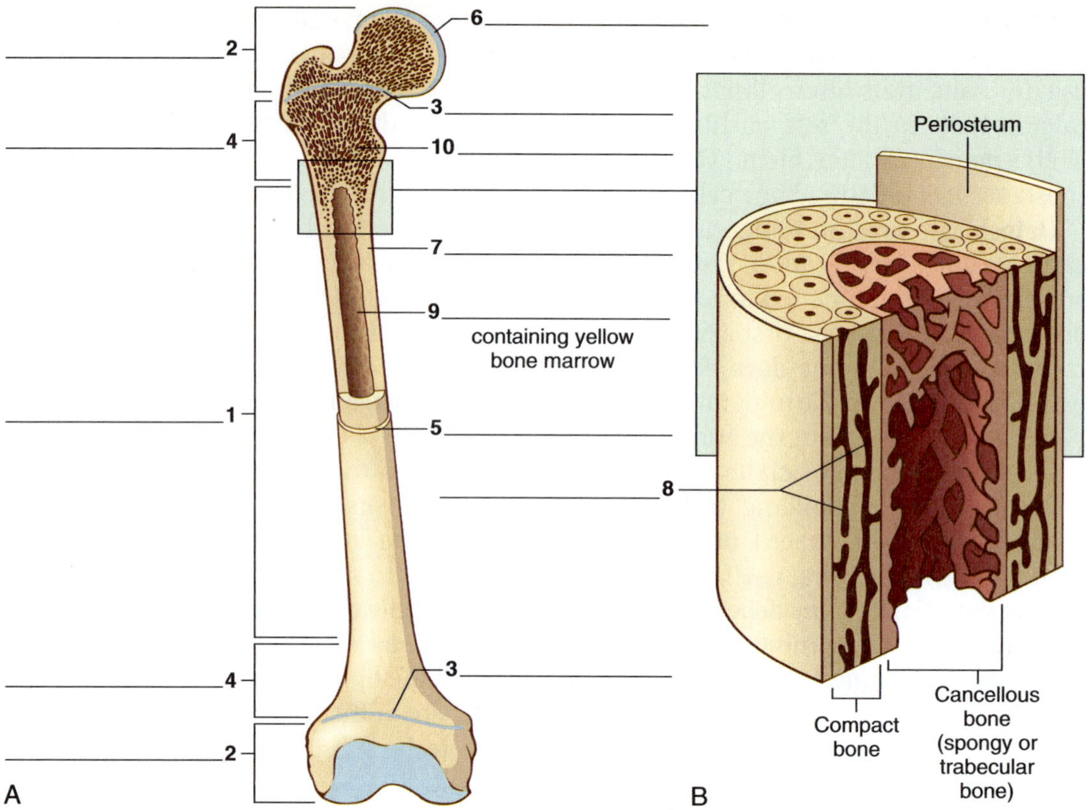

FIGURE 15-1 **A, Divisions of a long bone and interior bone structure. B, Composition of compact (cortical) bone.**

Figure 15-1A shows the anatomic divisions of a long bone such as the thigh bone or upper arm bone. Label the figure as you read the following.

The shaft, or middle region, of a long bone is called the **diaphysis** [1]. Each end of a long bone is called an **epiphysis** [2]. The **epiphyseal line** or **plate** [3] represents an area of cartilage tissue that is constantly being replaced by new bone tissue as the bone grows; it also is commonly known as the growth plate. Cartilage cells at the edges of the epiphyseal plate form new bone, which is responsible for lengthening bones during childhood and adolescence. The plate calcifies and disappears when the bone has achieved its full growth. The **metaphysis** [4] is the flared portion of the bone; it lies between the epiphysis and the diaphysis. It is adjacent to the epiphyseal plate.

The **periosteum** [5] is a strong, fibrous, vascular membrane that covers the surface of long bones, except at the ends of the epiphyses. It has an extensive nerve supply as well. Bones other than long bones are also covered by the periosteum.

The ends of long bones and the surface of any bone that meets another bone to form a joint are covered with **articular cartilage** [6]. When two bones come together to form a joint, the bones themselves do not touch precisely. The articular cartilage that caps the end of one bone comes into contact with that of the other bone. Articular cartilage is a very smooth, strong, and slick tissue. It cushions the joint and allows it to move smoothly and efficiently. Unlike the cartilage of the epiphyseal plate, which disappears when a bone achieves its full growth, articular cartilage is present throughout life.

Compact (cortical) bone [7] is a layer of hard, dense bone that lies under the periosteum in all bones and is located chiefly around the diaphysis of long bones. Within the compact bone is a system of small canals containing blood vessels that bring oxygen and nutrients to the bone and remove waste products such as carbon dioxide. Figure 15-1B shows these channels, called **haversian canals** [8], in the compact bone. Compact bone is tunneled out in the central shaft of the long bones by a **medullary cavity** [9] that contains **yellow bone marrow.** Yellow marrow is composed chiefly of fat cells.

Cancellous bone [10], sometimes called **spongy** or **trabecular bone,** is much more porous and less dense than compact bone. The mineral matter in it is laid down in a series of separated bony fibers that make up a spongy latticework. These interwoven fibers, called **trabeculae,** are found largely in the epiphyses and metaphyses of long bones and in the middle portion of most other bones of the body as well. Spaces in cancellous bone contain **red bone marrow.** The red marrow consists of immature and mature blood cells in various stages of development. **Hematopoiesis** is formation of all types of blood cells in the bone marrow.

In an adult, the ribs, pelvic bone, sternum (breastbone), and vertebrae, as well as the epiphyses of long bones, contain red bone marrow within cancellous tissue. Red marrow in the medullary cavity of long bones is plentiful in young children but decreases through the years and is replaced by yellow marrow.

PROCESSES AND DEPRESSIONS IN BONES

Bone processes are enlarged areas that extend out from bones to serve as attachments for muscles, tendons, and ligaments. Bone depressions are openings or hollow regions serving as connections between bones, or passageways for blood vessels and nerves. Table 15-1 lists various processes and depressions for your reference.

TABLE 15-1 PROCESSES AND DEPRESSIONS IN BONES

Process (Refer to Figure 15-2)	**Description**	
1. Bone head	Rounded end of a bone	
2. Condyle	Rounded knuckle-like process	
3. Epicondyle	Small rounded process above the condyle	
4. Trochanters	Large and small processes for tendon attachments	
5. Tuberosity (tubercle)	Small round elevation where tendons and muscles attach	
Depression	**Description**	**Example**
Fissure	Narrow groove or slit-like opening	Orbital (eye socket) fissure (Figure 15-5)
Foramen	Opening for blood vessels and nerves	Foramen magnum of the skull (Figure 15-4)
Fossa	Shallow cavity in or on a bone	Olecranon (elbow) fossa on humerus (Figure 15-2)
Sinus	Hollow cavity within bone	Sinuses of the skull (Figure 15-6)

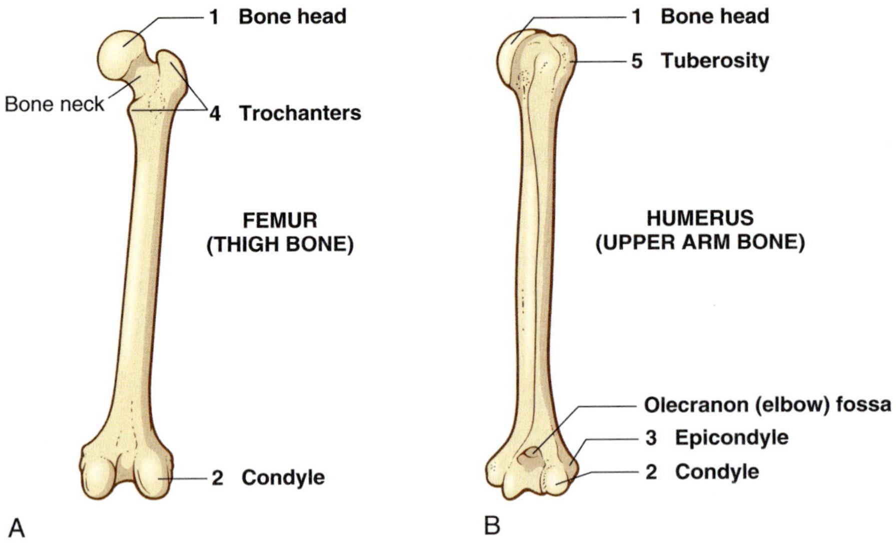

FIGURE 15-2 **Bone processes on the femur** (thigh bone) **(A)** and **humerus** (upper arm bone) **(B)**. The **bone neck** separates the bone head from the rest of the bone. A **fossa** is a shallow depression or cavity in a bone. The fossa on the humerus is a space for the olecranon process on the lower arm bone (ulna) when the elbow is extended.

CRANIAL BONES

The bones of the skull, or cranium, protect the brain and structures related to it, such as the sense organs. Muscles for controlling head movements and chewing motions are connected to the cranial bones. The cranial bones join each other at joints called **sutures.**

The cranial bones of a newborn child are not completely joined. There are gaps of unossified tissue in the skull at birth. These are called soft spots, or **fontanelles** ("little fountains"). The pulse of blood vessels can be felt (palpated) under the skin in those areas.

Figure 15-3 illustrates the bones of the cranium. Label them as you read the following descriptions:

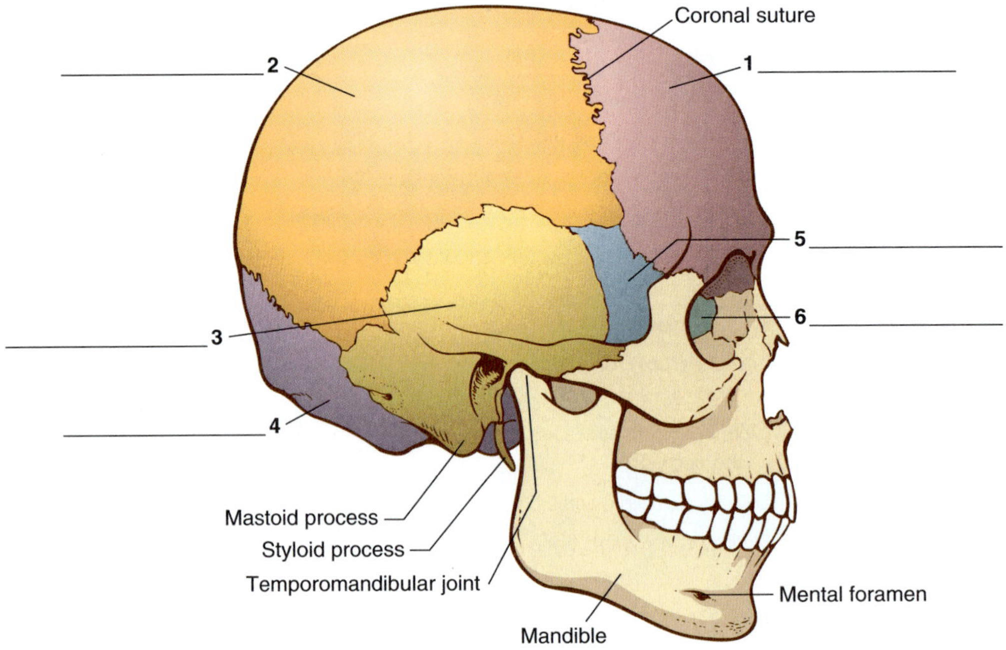

FIGURE 15-3 **Cranial bones,** lateral view. The **mental** (ment/o = chin) **foramen** is the opening in the mandible that allows blood vessels and nerves to enter and leave. The **coronal suture** is the connection across the skull between the two parietal bones and the frontal bone.

Frontal bone [1]—forms the forehead and the roof of the bony sockets that contain the eyes.

Parietal bone [2]—the two bones (one on each side of the skull) that form the roof and upper part of the sides of the cranium.

Temporal bone [3]—the two bones that form the lower sides and base of the cranium. Each bone encloses an ear and contains a fossa for joining with the mandible (lower jawbone). The **temporomandibular joint (TMJ)** is the area of connection between the temporal and mandibular bones. The **mastoid process** is a round (**mast/o** means breast) process of the temporal bone behind the ear. The **styloid process** (**styl/o** means pole or stake) projects downward from the temporal bone.

Occipital bone [4]—forms the back and base of the skull and joins the parietal and temporal bones, forming a suture. The inferior portion of the occipital bone has an opening called the **foramen magnum** through which the spinal cord passes (see Figure 15-4).

Sphenoid bone [5]—the bat-shaped bone that extends behind the eyes and forms part of the base of the skull. Because it joins with the frontal, occipital, and ethmoid bones, it serves as an anchor to hold those skull bones together (**sphen/o** means wedge). The **sella turcica** (meaning Turkish saddle) is a depression in the sphenoid bone in which the pituitary gland is located (see Figure 15-4).

Ethmoid bone [6]—the thin, delicate bone that supports the nasal cavity and forms part of the sockets of the eyes. It is composed primarily of spongy, cancellous bone, which contains numerous small holes (**ethm/o** means sieve).

Study Figure 15-4, which shows these cranial bones as viewed from above downward, toward the floor of the cranial cavity.

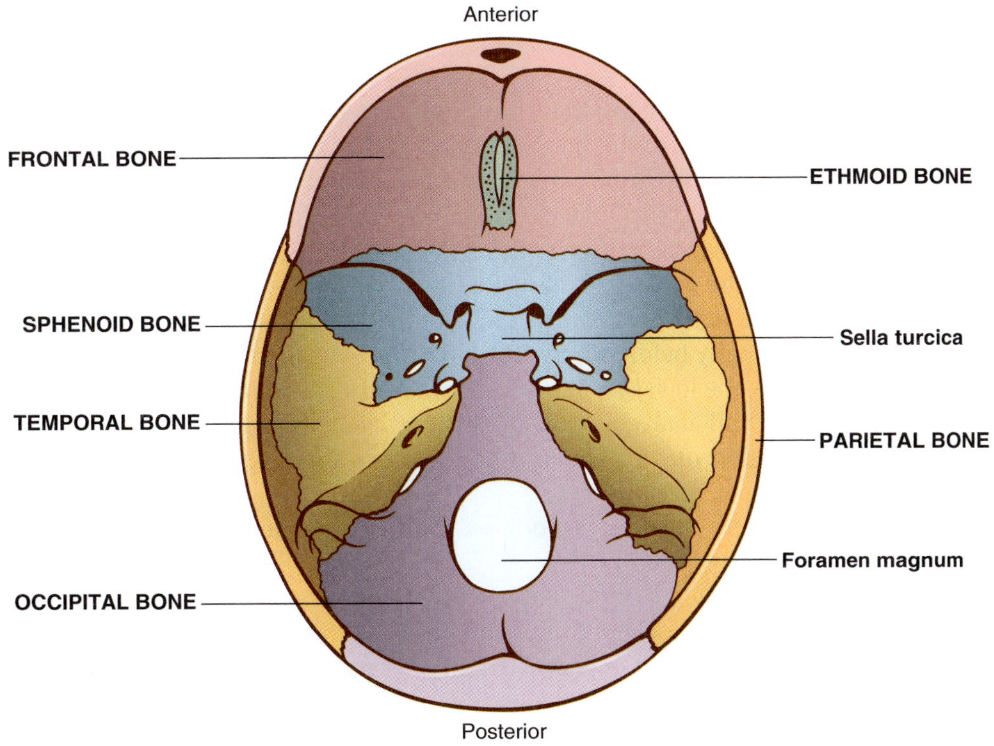

FIGURE 15-4 **Cranial bones,** viewed from above downward, to the floor of the cranial cavity.

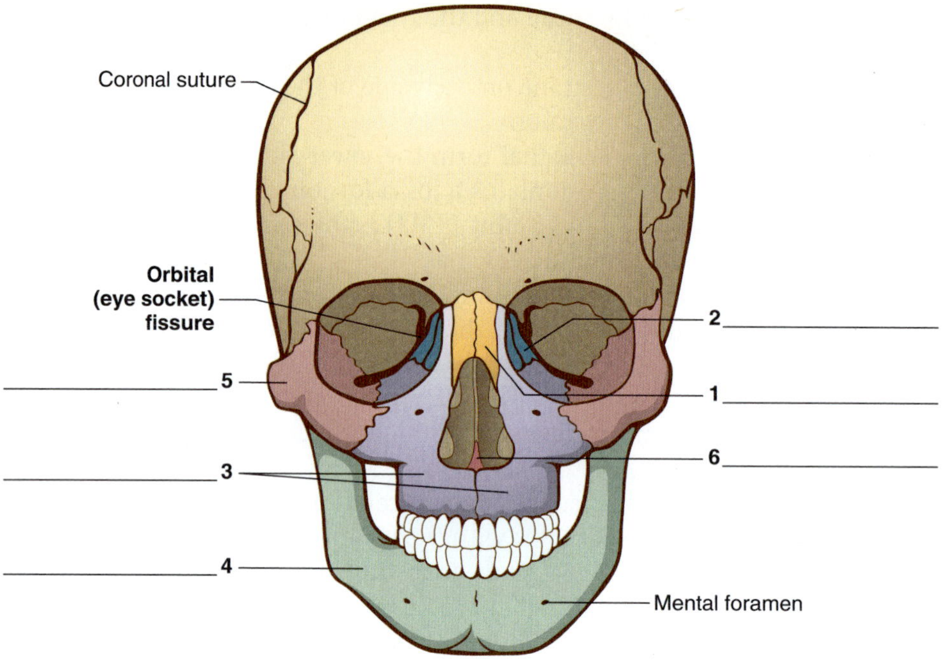

FIGURE 15-5 **Facial bones.**

15

FACIAL BONES

All of the facial bones except one are joined together by sutures, so they are immovable. The mandible (lower jawbone) is the only facial bone capable of movement. This ability is necessary for activities such as mastication (chewing) and speaking.

Figure 15-5 shows the facial bones; label it as you read the following descriptions of the facial bones:

Nasal bones [1]—the two slender bones that support the bridge of the nose (**nas/o** means nose). They join with the frontal bone superiorly and form part of the nasal septum.

Lacrimal bones [2]—the two small, thin bones located at the corner of each eye. The lacrimal (**lacrim/o** means tear) bones contain fossae for the lacrimal gland (tear gland) and canals for the passage of the lacrimal duct.

Maxillary bones [3]—the two large bones that compose the massive upper jawbones **(maxillae).** They are joined by a suture in the median plane. If the two bones do not come together normally before birth, the condition known as **cleft palate** results.

Mandibular bone [4]—the lower jawbone **(mandible).** Both the maxilla and the mandible contain the sockets called **alveoli** in which the teeth are embedded. The mandible joins the skull at the region of the temporal bone, forming the temporomandibular joint (TMJ) on either side of the skull.

Zygomatic bones [5]—the two bones, one on each side of the face, that form the high portion of the cheek.

Vomer [6]—the thin, single, flat bone that forms the lower portion of the nasal septum.

Sinuses, or air cavities, are located in specific places within the cranial and facial bones to lighten the skull and warm and moisten air as it passes through. Figure 15-6 shows the sinuses of the skull.

Table 15-2 reviews the cranial and facial bones with the location of each bone.

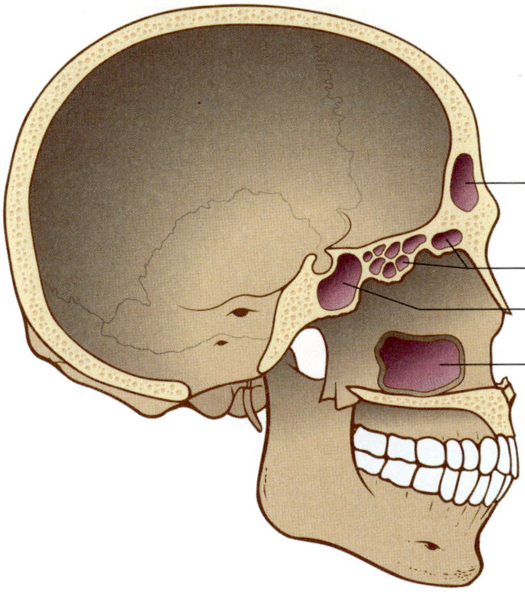

FIGURE 15-6 Sinuses of the skull.

TABLE 15-2 CRANIAL AND FACIAL BONES

CRANIAL BONES	LOCATION
Ethmoid bone	Supports nasal cavity and eye sockets
Frontal bone	Forehead; part of eye sockets
Occipital bone	Back and base of skull
Parietal bones	Top and sides of skull
Sphenoid bone	Base of skull and behind eyes (bat-shaped bone)
Temporal bones	Lower sides and back of skull
FACIAL BONES	**LOCATION**
Lacrimal bones	Corners of each eye
Mandible	Lower jawbone
Maxillae	Upper jawbones
Nasal bones	Bridge and septum of nose
Vomer	Nasal septum (thin, flat bone)
Zygomatic bones	Cheek bones

VERTEBRAL COLUMN AND STRUCTURE OF VERTEBRAE

The **vertebral (spinal) column** is composed of 26 bone segments, called vertebrae, that are arranged in five divisions from the base of the skull to the tailbone. The bones are separated by pads of cartilage called **intervertebral disks** (discs).

Figure 15-7A illustrates the general structure of a vertebra. Although the individual vertebrae in the separate regions of the spinal column are all slightly different in structure, they do have several parts in common.

A vertebra is composed of an inner, thick, round anterior portion called the **vertebral body** [1]. Between the body of one vertebra and the body of the vertebra lying beneath or above is an **intervertebral disk (disc).** This is a pad of cartilage that provides flexibility and absorbs shocks to the vertebral column (see Figure 15-7B). A spinal disk herniation occurs when a tear in a disk causes a portion of the disk to bulge out into the neural canal.

The posterior portion of a vertebra (vertebral arch) consists of a single **spinous process** [2], a **transverse process** [3] on each side of the spinous process, and a bar-like **lamina** [4] between each transverse process and the spinous process. The **neural canal** [5] is the space between the vertebral body and the vertebral arch through which the spinal cord passes. Figure 15-7B shows a lateral view of several vertebrae. Note the location of the spinal cord running through the neural canal.

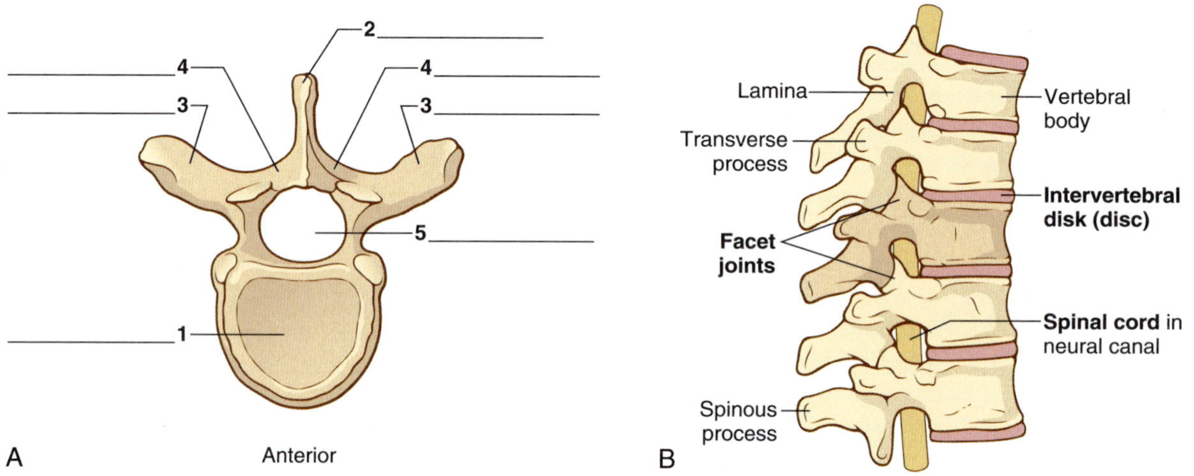

FIGURE 15-7 **A, General structure of a vertebra,** viewed from above. **B, Series of vertebrae,** lateral view, to show the position of the spinal cord behind the vertebral bodies and intervertebral disks. **Facet** (fă-SET) **joints** connect the vertebrae to each other. They are important in guiding and limiting the movement of the spinal column. When facet joints become inflamed and arthritic, they lead to narrowing of the neural canal and **spinal stenosis**.

Figure 15-8 illustrates the divisions of the vertebral column: cervical, thoracic, lumbar, sacrum, and coccyx.

The first seven bones of the vertebral column, forming the bony aspect of the neck, are the **cervical (C1 to C7) vertebrae.** These vertebrae do not articulate (join) with the ribs.

The second set of 12 vertebrae is known as the **thoracic (T1 to T12) vertebrae.** These vertebrae articulate with the 12 pairs of ribs.

The third set of five vertebral bones is the **lumbar (L1 to L5) vertebrae.** They are the strongest and largest of the backbones. Like the cervical vertebrae, these bones do not articulate with the ribs.

The **sacral vertebrae (sacrum)** are five separate bones that fuse in a young child. In an adult, the sacrum is a slightly curved, triangularly shaped bone.

The **coccyx** is the tailbone, and it, too, is a fused bone, having been formed from four small coccygeal bones.

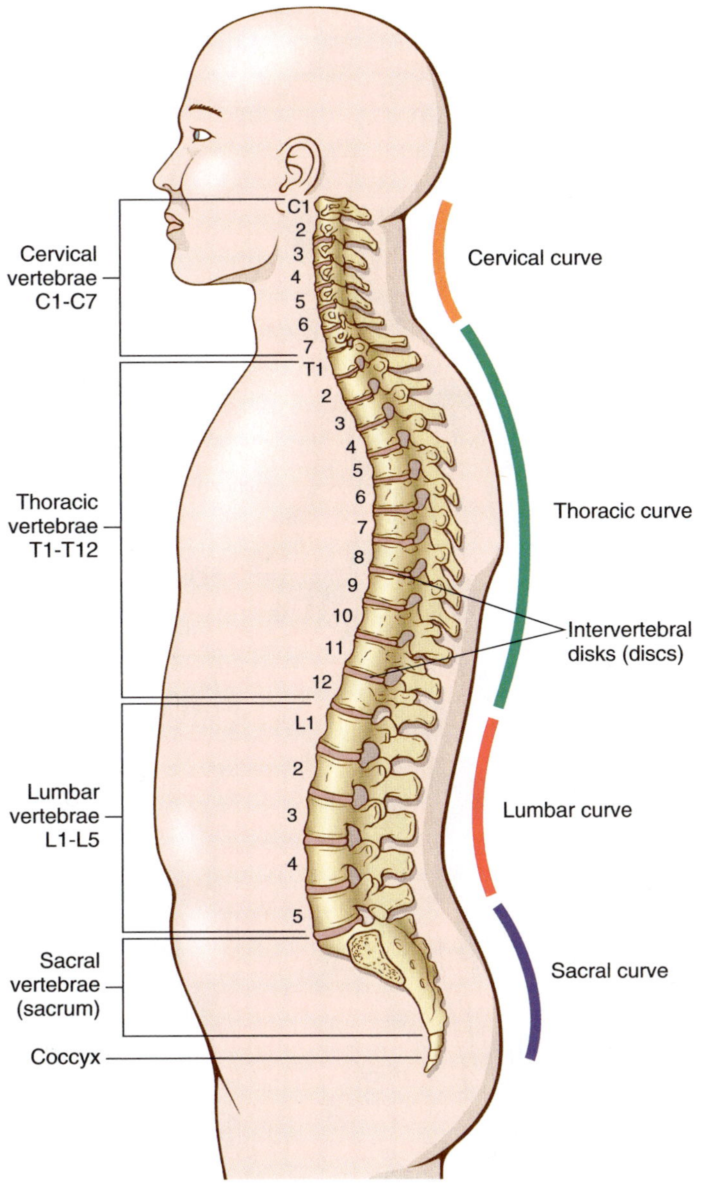

FIGURE 15-8 Vertebral column. Notice the four curves of the vertebral column. The sacral and thoracic curvatures are present at birth. The cervical curvature develops when the infant holds the head erect. The lumbar curvature develops as the infant begins to stand and walk.

BONES OF THE THORAX, PELVIS, AND EXTREMITIES

Label Figure 15-9 as you read the following descriptions of the bones of the thorax (chest cavity), pelvis (hip bone), and extremities (arms, hands, legs, and feet):

Bones of the Thorax

Clavicle [1]—collar bone; a slender bone, positioned ventrally, one on each side, connecting the breastbone (sternum) to each shoulder blade (scapula).

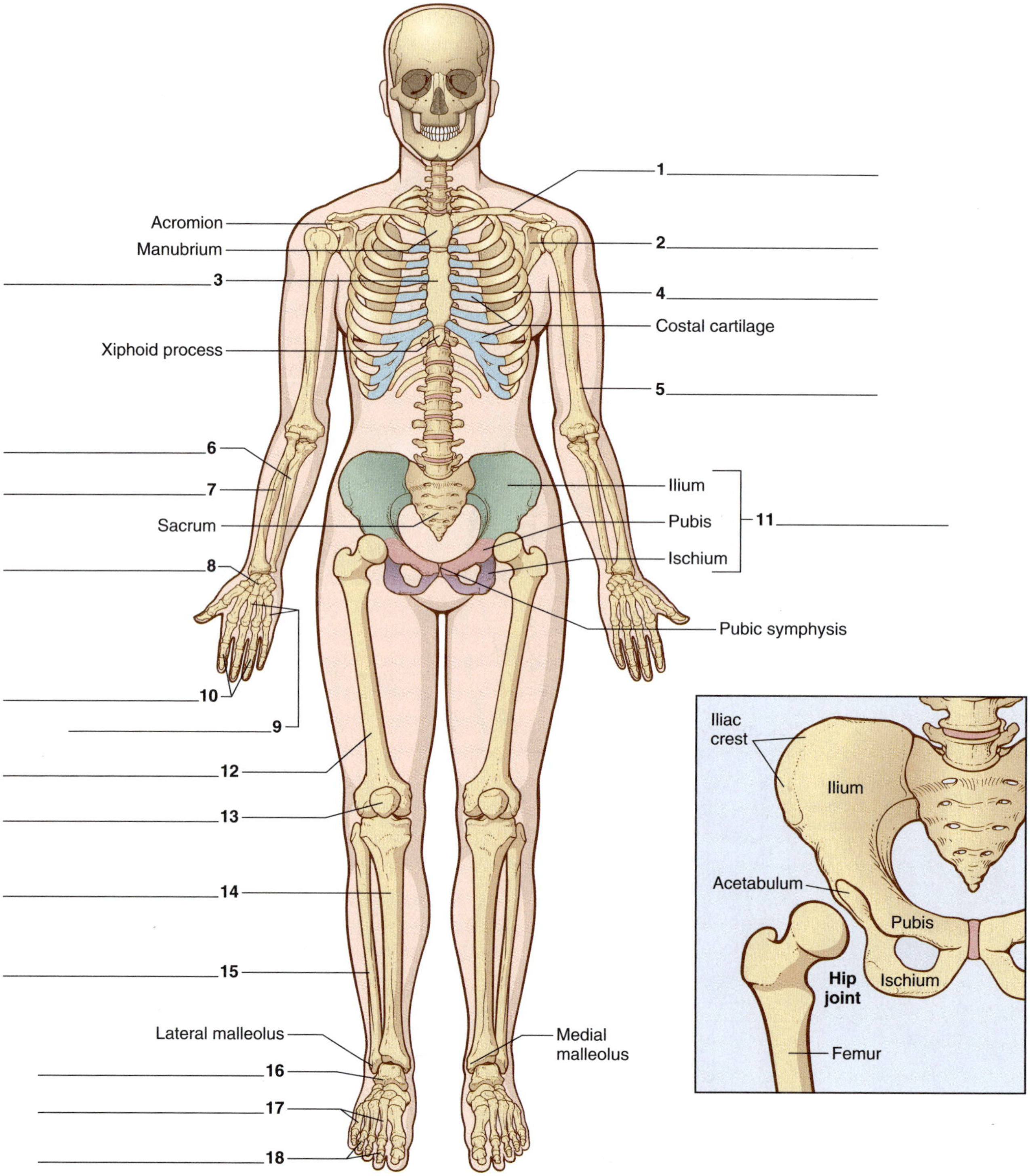

FIGURE 15-9 **Bones of the thorax, pelvis, and extremities.**

Scapula [2] (*plural*: **scapulae**)—shoulder blade; one of two flat, triangular bones on each dorsal side of the thorax. The extension of the scapula that joins with the clavicle to form a joint above the shoulder is called the **acromion** (**acr/o** means extremity, **om/o** means shoulder). The joint formed by these two bones is known as the acromioclavicular (AC) joint. Figure 15-10A shows a posterior view of the scapula.

Sternum [3]—breastbone; a flat bone extending ventrally down the midline of the chest. The upper part of the sternum articulates on the sides with the clavicle and ribs, and the lower, narrower portion is attached to the ribs, diaphragm, and abdominal muscles. The lowest portion of the sternum is the **xiphoid process** (**xiph/o** means sword). The uppermost portion is the **manubrium** (from a Latin term meaning handle).

Ribs [4]—There are 12 pairs of ribs. The first 7 pairs join the sternum anteriorly through cartilaginous attachments called **costal cartilages.** Ribs 1 to 7 are called **true ribs.** They join with the sternum anteriorly and with the vertebral column posteriorly. Ribs 8 to 10 are called **false ribs.** They join with the vertebral column posteriorly but join the 7th rib anteriorly instead of attaching to the sternum. Ribs 11 and 12 are the **floating ribs** because they are completely free at their anterior ends. Figure 15-10A shows a posterior view of the rib cage.

Bones of the Arm and Hand

These are described with the subject in the anatomic position—standing, with the arms held at the sides and the palms forward.

Humerus [5]—upper arm bone; the large head of the humerus is rounded and joins with the glenoid fossa of the scapula to form the shoulder or glenoid humeral joint (see Figure 15-10A). A cuff of cartilage, called a **labrum,** allows the humerus to move in the glenoid fossa (see Figure 15-10B).

Ulna [6]—medial lower arm (forearm) bone; the proximal bony process of the ulna at the elbow is called the **olecranon** (elbow bone). The olecranon is the bony point of the elbow when the elbow is bent.

Radius [7]—lateral lower arm (forearm) bone (in line with the thumb).

Carpals [8]—wrist bones; there are two rows of four bones in the wrist.

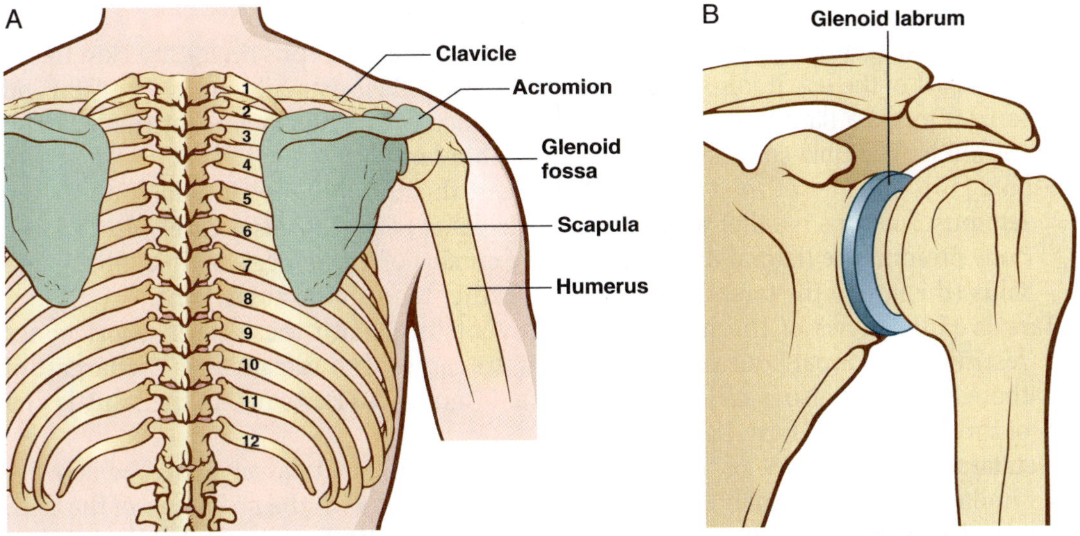

FIGURE 15-10 **A, Scapulae and rib cage,** posterior view. The **glenoid fossa** is the depression in the scapula into which the humerus fits. **B,** The **labrum** is a cuff of cartilage in the glenoid fossa that forms a cap for the end of the humerus to move in. A **labrum tear** can occur with a shoulder injury.

Metacarpals [9]—the five bones of the palm of the hand.

Phalanges [10] (*singular*: **phalanx**)—finger bones. Each finger (except the thumb) has three phalanges: a proximal, a middle, and a distal phalanx. The thumb has only two phalanges: a proximal and a distal phalanx.

Bones of the Pelvis

Pelvic girdle [11]—pelvis. This collection of bones supports the trunk of the body and articulates with the femur to form the hip joint. The adult pelvis is composed of three pairs of fused bones: the ilium, ischium, and pubis.

Ilium—uppermost and largest portion of the pelvis. Dorsally, the two parts of the ilium do not meet. Rather, they join the sacrum on either side to form the sacroiliac joints. The connection between the iliac bones and the sacrum is very firm, and very little motion occurs at these joints. The superior part of the ilium is the **iliac crest.** It is filled with red bone marrow and serves as an attachment for abdominal wall muscles.

Ischium—inferior or lower part of the pelvis. The ischium and the tendons and muscles attached to it are what you sit on.

Pubis—anterior part of the pelvis. The two pubic bones join by way of a cartilaginous disk. This area is called the **pubic symphysis.** Like the sacroiliac joints, this area is quite rigid.

Pelvic cavity—region within the ring of bone formed by the pelvic girdle. The rectum, sigmoid colon, bladder, and female reproductive organs lie within the pelvic cavity and are protected by the rigid architecture of the pelvic girdle. See Chapter 2, page 55, for comparison of the male pelvis and the female pelvis.

Bones of the Leg and Foot

15

Femur [12]—thigh bone; this is the longest bone in the body. At its proximal end it has a rounded head that fits into a depression, or socket, in the pelvis. This socket is called the **acetabulum.** The acetabulum was named because of its resemblance to a rounded cup the Romans used for vinegar *(acetum)*. The head of the femur and the acetabulum form a ball-and-socket joint otherwise known as the **hip joint.** See inset in Figure 15-9.

Patella [13]—kneecap; this is a small, flat bone that lies in front of the articulation between the femur and one of the lower leg bones called the tibia. It is a sesamoid bone surrounded by protective tendons and held in place by muscle attachments. Together with the femur and the tibia, it forms the knee joint.

Tibia [14]—larger of the two bones of the lower leg; the tibia runs under the skin in the front part of the leg. It joins with the femur and patella proximally, and at its distal end (ankle) forms a flare that is the bony prominence (medial **malleolus**) at the inside of the ankle. The tibia commonly is called the **shin bone.**

Fibula [15]—smaller of the two lower leg bones; this thin bone, well hidden under the leg muscles, runs parallel to the tibia. At its distal part, it forms a flare, which is the bony prominence (lateral **malleolus**) on the outside of the ankle. The tibia, fibula, and **talus** (the first of the tarsal bones) come together to form the **ankle joint.**

Tarsals [16]—bones of the hind part of the foot (hindfoot); these seven short bones resemble the carpal bones of the wrist but are larger. The **calcaneus** is the largest of these bones and also is called the **heel bone** (Figure 15-11). As noted, the **talus** is one of three bones that form the ankle joint.

Metatarsals [17]—bones of the midfoot; there are five metatarsal bones, which are similar to the metacarpals of the hand. Each articulates with the phalanges of the toes.

Phalanges of the toes [18]—bones of the forefoot; as in the digits of the hand, there are two phalanges in the big toe and three in each of the other toes.

Figure 15-11 illustrates the bones of the foot. Table 15-3 reviews bones and bone processes and their common names.

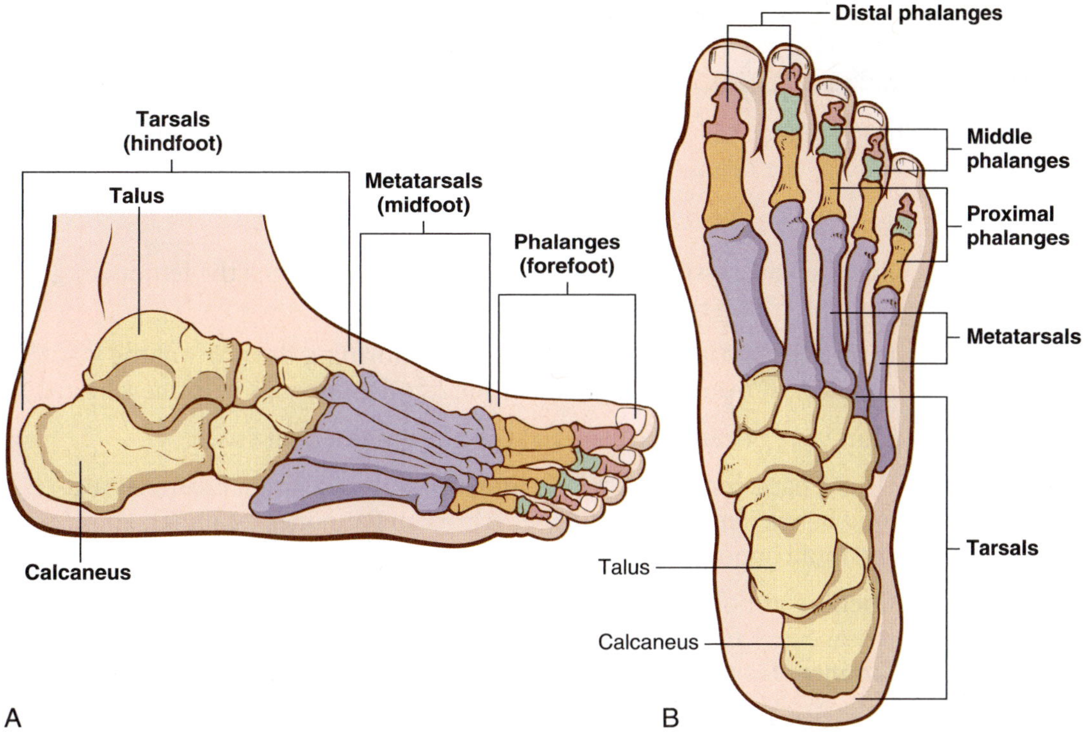

FIGURE 15-11 **A, Bones of the foot,** lateral view. **B, Bones of the foot,** as viewed from above.

TABLE 15-3 BONES OR PROCESSES AND THEIR COMMON NAMES

Bone or Process	Common Name	Bone or Process	Common Name
Acetabulum	Hip socket	Metacarpals	Hand bones
Calcaneus	Heel	Metatarsals	Midfoot bones
Carpals	Wrist bones	Olecranon	Elbow
Clavicle	Collar bone	Patella	Kneecap
Coccyx	Tailbone	Phalanges	Finger and toe bones
Cranium	Skull	Pubis	Anterior part of the pelvic bone
Femur	Thigh bone	Radius	Forearm bone—thumb side
Fibula	Smaller of the two lower leg bones	Scapula	Shoulder blade
Humerus	Upper arm bone	Sternum	Breastbone
Ilium	Upper part of pelvic bone	Tarsals	Hindfoot bones
Ischium	Inferior or lower part of the pelvic bone	Tibia	Shin bone—larger of the two lower leg bones
Malleolus	Ankle	Ulna	Forearm bone—little finger side
Mandible	Lower jawbone	Vertebra	Backbone/spine
Maxilla	Upper jawbone		

VOCABULARY—BONES

This list reviews many of the new terms related to bones introduced in the text. Short definitions reinforce your understanding of the terms. Refer to the Pronunciation of Terms on page 641 for help with unfamiliar or difficult terms.

acetabulum	Rounded depression, or socket, in the pelvis that joins the femur (thigh bone), forming the hip joint.
acromion	Outward extension of the shoulder blade forming the point of the shoulder. It overlies the shoulder joint and articulates with the clavicle.
articular cartilage	Thin layer of cartilage covering the bone in the joint space.
bone	Dense, hard connective tissue composing the skeleton. Examples are long bones (femur), short bones (carpals), flat bones (scapula), and sesamoid bones (patella).
bone depression	Opening or hollow region serving as a connection for bones, or passageways for blood vessels and nerves. Examples are **fissure**, **foramen**, **fossa**, and **sinus**.
bone process	Enlarged area that extends from bones as an attachment for muscles, tendons, and ligaments. Examples are **bone head**, **condyle**, **epicondyle**, **trochanter**, **tubercle**, and **tuberosity**.
calcium	One of the mineral constituents of bone. **Calcium phosphate** is the major calcium salt in bones.
cancellous bone	Spongy, porous, bone tissue in the inner part of a bone.
cartilage	Flexible, rubbery connective tissue. It is found in the immature skeleton, at the epiphyseal growth plate, and on joint surfaces.
collagen	Dense, connective tissue protein strands found in bone and other tissues.
compact bone	Hard, dense bone tissue, usually found around the outer portion of bones.
cranial bones	Skull bones: **ethmoid, frontal, occipital, parietal, sphenoid,** and **temporal.**
diaphysis	Shaft, or mid-portion, of a long bone.
disk (disc)	Flat, round, plate-like structure. An intervertebral disk is a fibrocartilaginous substance between two vertebrae.
epiphyseal plate	Cartilaginous area at the ends of long bones where lengthwise growth takes place in the immature skeleton.
epiphysis	Each end of a long bone; the area beyond the epiphyseal plate.
facial bones	Bones of the face: **lacrimal, mandibular, maxillary, nasal, vomer,** and **zygomatic.**
fontanelle	Soft spot (incomplete bone formation) between the skull bones of an infant.
foramen magnum	Opening of the occipital bone through which the spinal cord passes.

haversian canals	Minute spaces filled with blood vessels; found in compact bone.
ligament	Fibrous tissue connecting bones to other bones.
malleolus	Round process on both sides of the ankle joint. The lateral malleolus is part of the fibula, and the medial malleolus is part of the tibia.
manubrium	Upper portion of the sternum; articulates with the medial aspect of the clavicle.
mastoid process	Round projection on the temporal bone behind the ear.
medullary cavity	Central, hollowed-out area in the shaft of a long bone.
metaphysis	Flared portion of a long bone, between the diaphysis (shaft) and the epiphyseal plate (in this term, meta- means between).
olecranon	Large process on the proximal end of the ulna; the point of the flexed elbow.
orthopedist	Medical doctor who specializes in bone, joint, and muscle conditions.
osseous tissue	Bone tissue.
ossification	Process of bone formation.
osteoblast	Bone cell that helps form bony tissue.
osteoclast	Bone cell that absorbs and removes unwanted bony tissue.
periosteum	Membrane surrounding bones; rich in blood vessels and nerve tissue.
phosphorus	Mineral substance found in bones in combination with calcium.
physiatrist	Medical doctor specializing in rehabilitation (physic/o means function).
pubic symphysis	Area of confluence (coming together) of the two pubic bones in the pelvis. They are joined (sym- = together, -physis = to grow) by a fibrocartilaginous disk.
red bone marrow	Found in cancellous bone; site of hematopoiesis.
ribs	Twelve pairs of curved bones that form the chest wall. True ribs are the first 7 pairs; false ribs are pairs 8 to 10; floating ribs are pairs 11 and 12.
sella turcica	Depression in the sphenoid bone where the pituitary gland is located.
sinus	Hollow air cavity within a bone.
styloid process	Pole-like process extending downward from the temporal bone on each side of the skull.
suture	Immovable joint between bones, such as the skull (cranium).
temporomandibular joint	Connection on either side of the head between the temporal bone of the skull and mandibular bone of the jaw.
tendon	Fibrous connective tissue connecting muscles and bones.
trabeculae	Supporting bundles of bony fibers in cancellous (spongy) bone.
vertebra	Individual segment of the spine composed of the vertebral body, vertebral arch, spinous process, transverse process, and lamina, enclosing the neural canal.
xiphoid process	Lower, narrow portion of the sternum.
yellow bone marrow	Fatty tissue found in the medullary cavity of most adult long bones.

TERMINOLOGY—BONES

The following word parts pertaining to bones are divided into two groups: general terms and terms related to specific bones. Write the meanings of the medical terms in the spaces provided.

General Terms

COMBINING FORMS

COMBINING FORM	MEANING	TERMINOLOGY	MEANING
calc/o, calci/o	calcium	hypercalcemia	_______________
		decalcification *de- means less or lack of; -fication is the process of making.*	_______________
kyph/o	humpback, hunchback (posterior curvature in the thoracic region)	kyphosis *This term (from Greek meaning hill or mountain) indicates a hump on the back. The affected person's height is reduced, and kyphosis may lead to pressure on the spinal cord or peripheral nerves (Figure 15-12).*	_______________
lamin/o	lamina (part of the vertebral arch)	laminectomy *An operation often performed to relieve the symptoms of compression of the spinal cord or spinal nerve roots. It involves removal of the lamina and spinous process.*	_______________
lord/o	curve, swayback (anterior curvature in the lumbar region)	lordosis *The normal anterior curvature of the lumbar spine becomes exaggerated (see Figure 15-12). The word lordosis is derived from Greek, describing a person leaning backward in a lordly fashion.*	_______________

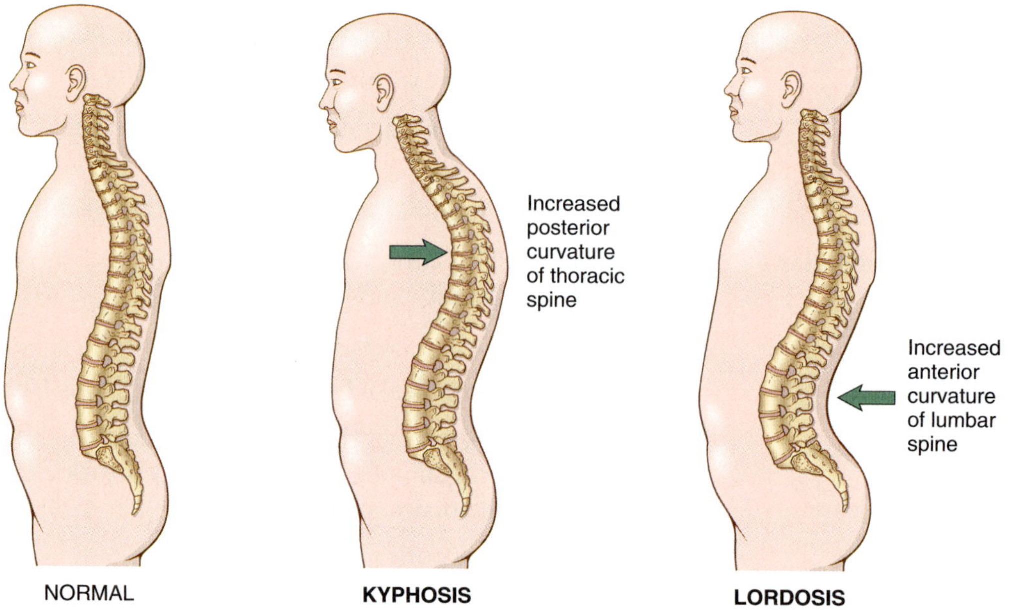

FIGURE 15-12 **Kyphosis** and **lordosis.**

COMBINING FORM	MEANING	TERMINOLOGY	MEANING
lumb/o	loins, lower back	lumbar	_______________
		lumbosacral	_______________
myel/o	bone marrow	myelopoiesis	_______________
orth/o	straight	orthopedics *Ped/o means child.*	_______________
oste/o	bone	osteitis ***Osteitis deformans** is better known as **Paget disease.** Bones become weak and painful, especially in the spine, skull, pelvis, and legs.*	_______________
		osteodystrophy	_______________
		osteogenesis ***Osteogenesis imperfecta** is a genetic disorder involving defective development of bones that are brittle and fragile; fractures occur with the slightest trauma.*	_______________
scoli/o	crooked, bent (lateral curvature)	scoliosis *The spinal column is bent abnormally to the side. Scoliosis is the most common spinal deformity in adolescent girls (Figure 15-13).*	_______________

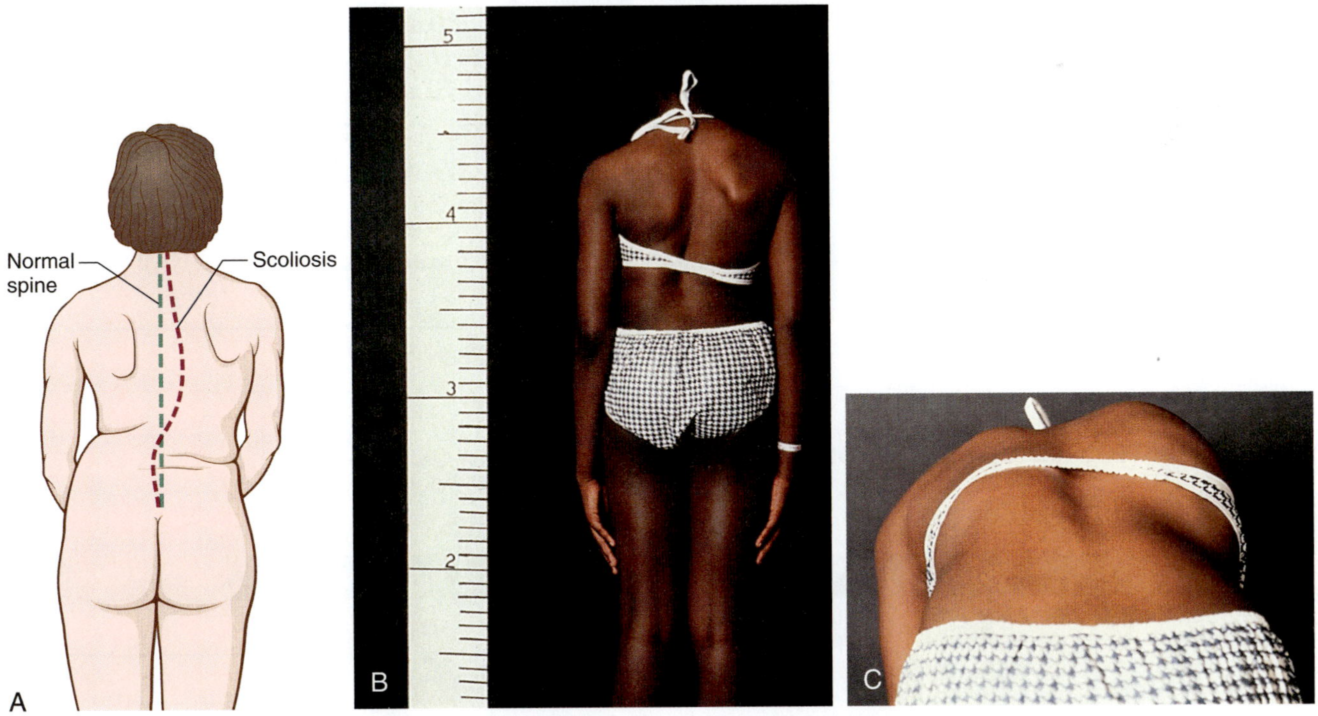

FIGURE 15-13 Moderate thoracic idiopathic adolescent scoliosis. A, Normal spine and **scoliosis. B,** Notice the **scapular asymmetry** in the upright position. This results from rotation of the spine and attached rib cage. **C,** Bending forward reveals a mild rib hump deformity.

COMBINING FORM	MEANING	TERMINOLOGY	MEANING
spondyl/o (used to make words about conditions of the structure)	vertebra	spondylosis	______ *Degeneration of the intervertebral disks in the cervical, thoracic, and lumbar regions. Signs and symptoms include pain and restriction of movement.*
vertebr/o (used to describe the structure itself)	vertebra	vertebroplasty	______ *Percutaneous vertebroplasty relieves pain caused by compression fractures of the vertebrae. Medical cement is used to fill in the cracks and strengthen bone.*

SUFFIXES

SUFFIX	MEANING	TERMINOLOGY	MEANING
-blast	embryonic or immature cell	osteoblast	______ *This cell synthesizes collagen and protein to form bone tissue.*
-clast	to break	osteoclast	______ *This cell breaks down bone to remove bone tissue.*
-listhesis	slipping	spondylolisthesis	______ *(Pronounced spŏn-dĭ-lō-lĭs-THĒ-sĭs.) The forward slipping (subluxation) of a vertebra over a lower vertebra.*
-malacia	softening	osteomalacia	______ *A condition in which vitamin D deficiency leads to decalcification of bones; known as rickets in children.*
-physis	to grow	epiphysis	______
		pubic symphysis	______
-porosis	pore, passage	osteoporosis	______ *Loss of bony tissue with decreased mass of bone. See page 600.*
-tome	instrument to cut	osteotome	______ *This surgical chisel is designed to cut bone.*

Terms Related to Specific Bones

COMBINING FORMS

COMBINING FORM	MEANING	TERMINOLOGY	MEANING
acetabul/o	acetabulum (hip socket)	acetabular	______
calcane/o	calcaneus (heel)	calcaneal	______ *The calcaneus is one of the tarsal (hindfoot) bones.*
carp/o	carpals (wrist bones)	carpal	______

COMBINING FORM	MEANING	TERMINOLOGY	MEANING
clavicul/o	clavicle (collar bone)	supraclavicular *Supra- means above.*	________
cost/o	ribs (true ribs, false ribs, and floating ribs)	subcostal	________
		chondrocostal *Cartilage that is attached to the ribs.*	________
crani/o	cranium (skull)	craniotomy	________
		craniotome	________
femor/o	femur (thigh bone)	femoral	________
fibul/o	fibula (smaller lower leg bone)	fibular *See perone/o.*	________
humer/o	humerus (upper arm bone)	humeral	________
ili/o	ilium (upper part of pelvic bone)	iliac	________
ischi/o	ischium (posterior part of pelvic bone)	ischial	________
malleol/o	malleolus (process on each side of the ankle)	malleolar *The medial malleolus is at the distal end of the tibia, and the lateral malleolus is at the distal end of the fibula.*	________
mandibul/o	mandible (lower jawbone)	mandibular	________
maxill/o	maxilla (upper jawbone)	maxillary	________
metacarp/o	metacarpals (hand bones)	metacarpectomy	________
metatars/o	metatarsals (foot bones)	metatarsalgia	________
olecran/o	olecranon (elbow)	olecranal	________
patell/o	patella (kneecap)	patellar	________
pelv/i	pelvis (hipbone)	pelvimetry	________

15

COMBINING FORM	MEANING	TERMINOLOGY	MEANING
perone/o	fibula	peroneal	________________
phalang/o	phalanges (finger and/or toe bones)	phalangeal	________________
pub/o	pubis (anterior part of the pelvic bone)	pubic	________________
radi/o	radius (forearm bone—thumb side)	radial	________________
scapul/o	scapula (shoulder blade)	scapular	________________
stern/o	sternum (breastbone)	sternal	________________
tars/o	tarsals (bones of the hindfoot)	tarsectomy	________________
tibi/o	tibia (shin bone)	tibial	________________
uln/o	ulna (forearm bone—little finger side)	ulnar	________________

PATHOLOGY—BONES

Ewing sarcoma

Rare malignant tumor arising in bone; most often occurring in children.

Pain and swelling are common, especially if the tumor involves the shaft (medullary cavity) of a long bone. This tumor usually occurs at an early age between 5 and 15 years, and combined treatment with surgery, radiotherapy, and chemotherapy represents the best chance for cure (60% to 70% of patients are cured if metastasis has not occurred).

exostosis

Bony growth (benign) arising from the surface of bone.

Osteochondromas (composed of cartilage and bone) are benign **exostoses** usually found on the metaphyses of long bones near the epiphyseal plates. Ex- means out; -ostosis is condition of bones.

A **bunion** is a swelling of the metatarsophalangeal joint near the base of the big toe and is accompanied by the buildup of soft tissue and underlying bone at the distal/medial aspect of the first metatarsal.

Peroneal/Peritoneal/Perineal

Peroneal means pertaining to the fibula (smaller of two lower leg bones). Don't confuse this term with ***peritoneal,*** meaning pertaining to the peritoneum (membrane surrounding the abdominal organs), and **perineal,** meaning pertaining to the area between the rectum and the vagina in females, and between the rectum and scrotal sac in males.

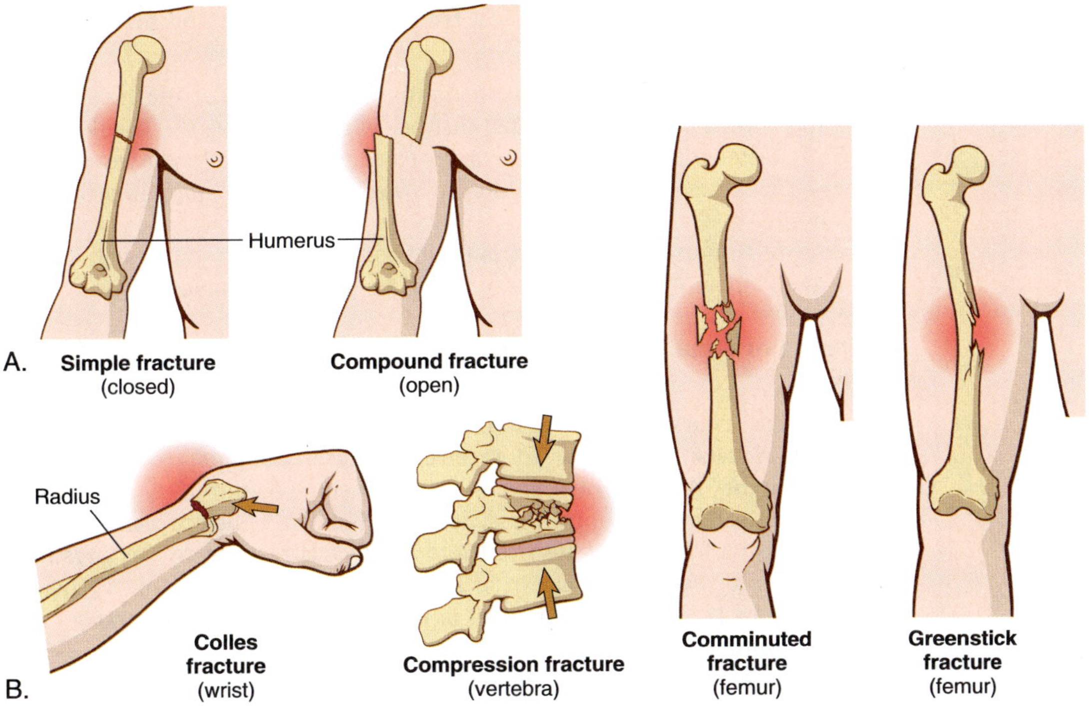

FIGURE 15-14 **A, Simple** and **compound** fractures. **B, Types of fractures.** A **pathologic fracture** is caused by disease of bones (tumor, infection, osteoporosis) that causes them to weaken.

fracture

Traumatic breaking of a bone.

In a **simple (closed) fracture,** the bone is broken but there is no open wound in the skin. In a **compound (open) fracture,** the bone is broken and a fragment of bone protrudes through an open wound in the skin. See Figure 15-14A. **Crepitus** is the crackling sound produced when ends of bones rub each other or rub against roughened cartilage. Table 15-4 lists different types of fractures and their descriptions. Figure 15-14B illustrates these fractures.

Treatment of fractures involves **reduction,** which is restoration of the bone to its normal position. A **closed reduction** is manipulative reduction without a surgical incision; in an **open reduction,** an incision is made for access to the fracture site. A **cast** (solid mold of the body part) is applied to fractures to immobilize the injured bone after a closed reduction. The abbreviation **ORIF** means open reduction/internal fixation. Often this involves insertion of metal plates, screws, rods, or pins to stabilize the bone.

TABLE 15-4 **TYPES OF FRACTURES** (see Figure 15-14B)

Type	Description
Colles	Near the wrist at distal end of the radius
Comminuted	Bone is splintered and crushed into several pieces
Compression	Bone collapses or is compressed; occurs in vertebrae
Greenstick	Bone is partially broken; breaks on one surface and bends on another; often occurring in forearm
Impacted	One fragment is driven firmly into the other; at the head of the femur or head of the humerus (not pictured)

osteogenic sarcoma (osteosarcoma)

Common malignant tumor arising from osteoblasts, found primarily in children and adolescents.

Osteoblasts multiply, forming large, bony tumors, especially at the ends of long bones (half of the lesions are located just below or just above the knee) (Figure 15-15). Metastasis (spread of tumor) takes place through the bloodstream, often affecting the lungs. Surgical resection followed by chemotherapy improves the survival rate.

Malignant tumors from other parts of the body (breast, prostate, lung, thyroid gland, and kidney) that metastasize to bones are **metastatic bone lesions.**

osteomalacia

Softening of bone, with inadequate amounts of mineral (calcium) in the bone.

Osteomalacia occurs primarily as a disease of infancy and childhood and is then known as **rickets.** Bones fail to receive adequate amounts of calcium and phosphorus; they become soft, bend easily, and become deformed.

In affected patients, vitamin D is deficient in the diet, which prevents calcium and phosphorus from being absorbed into the bloodstream from the intestines. Vitamin D is formed by the action of sunlight on certain compounds (such as cholesterol) in the skin; thus, rickets is more common in large, smoky cities during the winter months.

Treatment most often consists of administration of large daily doses of vitamin D and an increase in dietary intake of calcium and phosphorus.

osteomyelitis

Inflammation of the bone and bone marrow secondary to infection.

Bacteria enter the body through a wound and spread to the bone. Children are affected most often, and the infection usually occurs near the ends of long bones of the legs and arms. Adults can be affected too, usually as the result of an open fracture.

The lesion begins as an inflammation with pus collection. Pus tends to spread down the medullary cavity and outward to the periosteum. Antibiotic therapy corrects the condition if the infection is treated quickly. If treatment is delayed, an **abscess** can form. An abscess is a walled-off area of infection that can be difficult or impossible to penetrate with antibiotics. Surgical drainage of an abscess usually is necessary.

osteoporosis

Decrease in bone density (mass); thinning and weakening of bone.

Osteopenia is a condition in which bone mineral density is lower than normal. In some cases, it is a precursor to osteoporosis. In osteoporosis, the interior of bones is diminished in structure, as if the steel skeleton of a building had rusted and deteriorated (Figure 15-16). The condition commonly occurs in older women as a consequence of estrogen deficiency with menopause. Lack of estrogen promotes

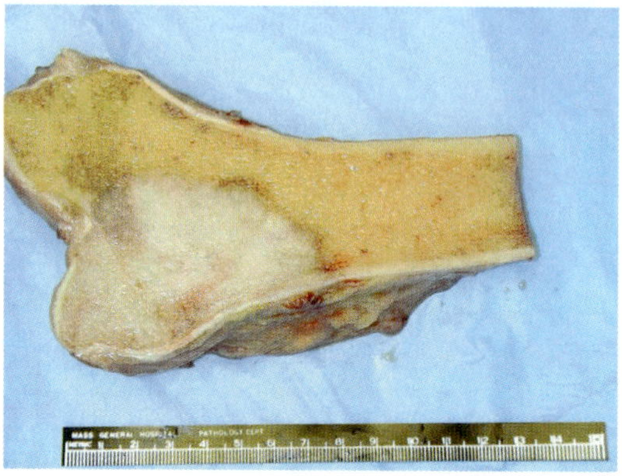

FIGURE 15-15 Osteosarcoma. The tumor has grown through the cortex of the bone and elevated the periosteum. *(Courtesy Dr. Francis Hornicek, Massachusetts General Hospital Department of Orthopedics, Boston.)*

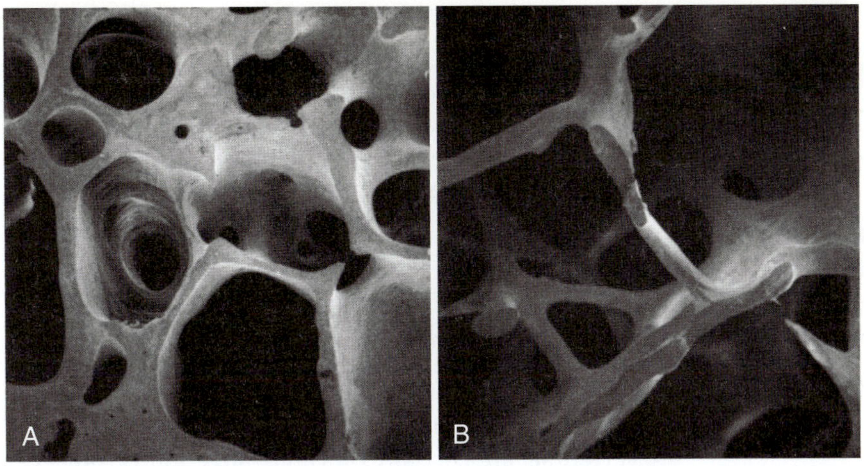

FIGURE 15-16 Scanning electron micrograph of normal bone (A) and **bone with osteoporosis (B).** Notice the thinning and wide separation of the trabeculae in the osteoporotic bone.

excessive bone resorption (osteoclast activity) and less bone deposition. Weakened bones are subject to fracture (as in the hip); loss of height and kyphosis occur as vertebrae collapse (Figure 15-17).

Osteoporosis can occur with atrophy caused by disuse, as in a limb that is in a cast, in the legs of a person with paraplegia, or in a bedridden patient. It also may occur in men as part of the aging process and in patients who have received corticosteroids (hormones made by the adrenal gland and used to treat inflammatory conditions).

Treatment and prevention of osteoporosis are critical to maintaining strong bones and avoiding fractures of the spine, hip, or wrist.

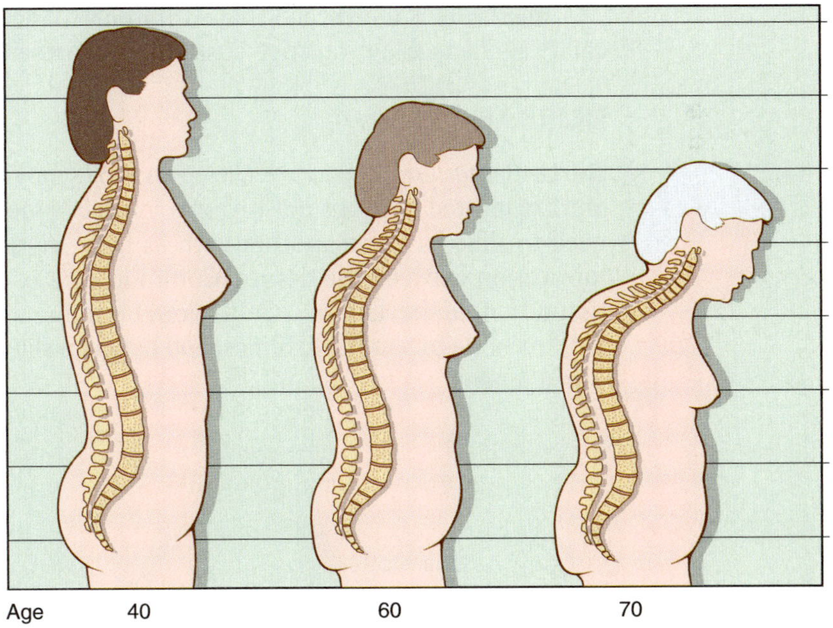

FIGURE 15-17 Kyphosis. Loss of bone mass due to osteoporosis produces posterior curvature of the spine in the thoracic region. A normal spine is shown at the age of 40 years, and osteoporotic changes are illustrated at the ages of 60 and 70 years. The changes in the spine can cause a loss of as much as 6 to 9 inches in height.

Preventing Osteoporosis

Prevention of osteoporosis includes the following:

- Balanced diet rich in calcium and vitamin D
- Weight-bearing and resistance exercise
- Reduction of smoking and alcohol intake
- Checking bone mineral density (BMD) with a DEXA test (see page 619)
- Medications when appropriate—such as bisphosphonates (Fosamax, Boniva) and selective estrogen receptor modulators (SERMs—Raloxifene, Evista) and hormone replacement therapy (HRT)

talipes

Congenital abnormality of the hindfoot (involving the talus).

Talipes (Latin *talus* = ankle, *pes* = foot) is a congenital anomaly. The most common form is **talipes equinovarus** (**equin/o** = horse), or **clubfoot.** The infant cannot stand with the sole of the foot flat on the ground. The defect can be corrected by applying orthopedic casts in the early months of infancy or, if that fails, by surgery.

JOINTS

TYPES OF JOINTS

A **joint (articulation)** is a coming together of two or more bones. Some joints are immovable, such as the **suture joints** between the skull bones. Other joints, such as those between the vertebrae, are partially movable. Most joints, however, allow considerable movement. These freely movable joints are called **synovial joints.** Examples of synovial joints are the ball-and-socket type (the hip and shoulder joints) and the hinge type (elbow, knee, and ankle joints). Label the structures in Figure 15-18 as you read the following description of a synovial joint.

The bones in a synovial joint are surrounded by a **joint capsule** [1] composed of fibrous tissue. **Ligaments** (thickened fibrous bands of connective tissue) anchor one bone to another and thereby add considerable strength to the joint capsule in critical areas. Bones at the joint are covered with a smooth, glistening white tissue called the **articular cartilage** [2]. The **synovial membrane** [3] lies under the joint capsule and lines the **synovial cavity** [4] between the bones. The synovial cavity is filled with a special lubricating fluid produced by the synovial membrane. This **synovial fluid** contains water and nutrients that nourish as well as lubricate the joints so that friction on the articular cartilage is minimal.

A **meniscus** is a crescent-shaped fibrocartilaginous structure that partly divides a joint cavity and acts as a protective cushion. It is present in the knee (see Figure 15-19).

BURSAE

Bursae (*singular*: **bursa**) are closed sacs of synovial fluid lined with a synovial membrane and are located near but not within a joint. Bursae are present wherever two types of tissue need to slide past one another with as little friction as possible. Bursae serve as layers of lubrication between the tissues. Common sites of bursae are between **tendons** (connective tissue that connects a muscle to bone) and bones, between **ligaments** (connective tissue binding bone to bone) and bones, and between skin and bones in areas where bony anatomy is prominent.

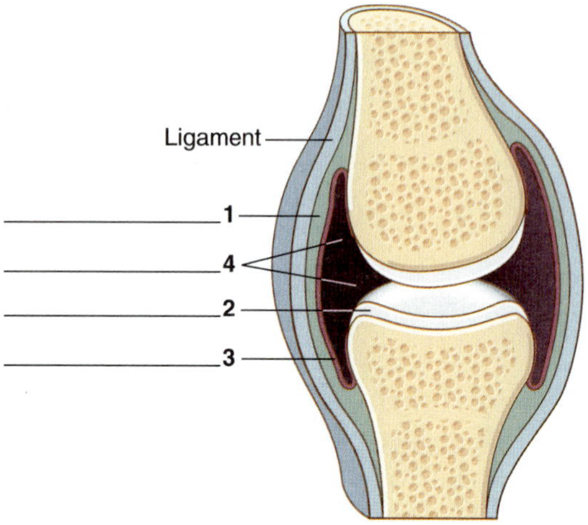

FIGURE 15-18 **Structure of a synovial joint.**

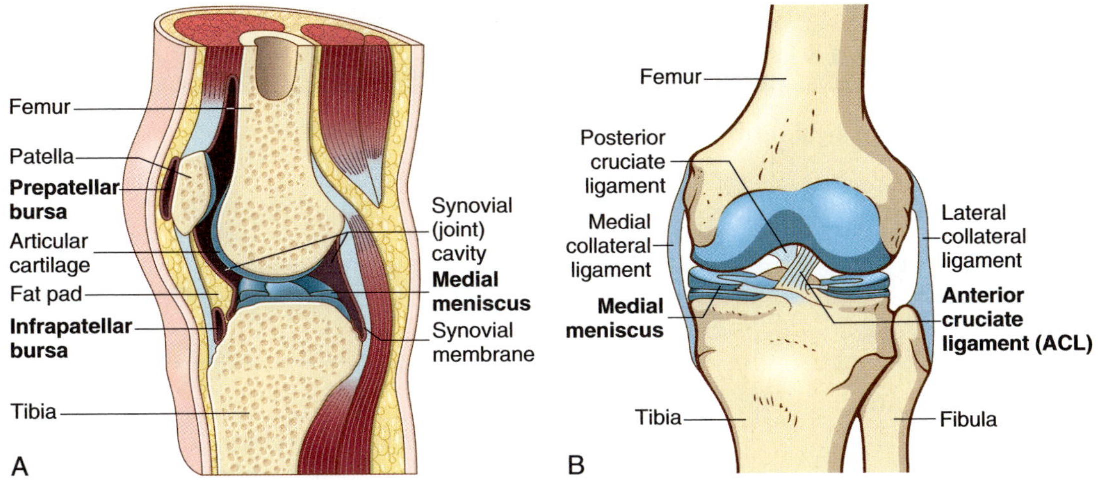

FIGURE 15-19 **A, Sagittal (lateral) section of the knee showing the medial meniscus** (plural menisci), and **bursae.** A "torn cartilage" in the knee is a damaged meniscus and is frequently repaired with arthroscopic surgery. **B, Frontal section of the knee.** Notice the **anterior cruciate ligament (ACL),** which may be damaged ("torn ligament") with knee injury. Reconstruction of the ACL can require extensive surgery, and months of physical therapy may be required before return of normal function. See case study, page 624.

Some common locations of bursae are at the elbow joint (olecranon bursa), knee joint (prepatellar bursa), and shoulder joint (subacromial bursa). Figure 15-19A shows a lateral view of the knee joint with bursae. Figure 15-19B is a frontal (anterior/posterior) view of the knee showing ligaments that provide stability for the joint.

VOCABULARY—JOINTS

This list reviews many new terms related to joints introduced in the text. Short definitions reinforce your understanding of the terms. Refer to the Pronunciation of Terms on page 645 for help with unfamiliar or difficult terms.

articular cartilage	Smooth, glistening white tissue that covers the surface of a joint.
articulation	Any type of joint.
bursa (*plural*: **bursae**)	Sac of fluid near a joint; promotes smooth sliding of one tissue against another.
ligament	Connective tissue binding bones to other bones; supports, strengthens, and stabilizes the joint.
meniscus	Crescent-shaped fibrocartilaginous structure found in the knee.
suture joint	Immovable joint, such as between the bones of the skull.
synovial cavity	Space between bones at a synovial joint; contains synovial fluid produced by the synovial membrane.
synovial fluid	Viscous (sticky) fluid within the synovial cavity. Synovial fluid is similar in viscosity to egg white; this accounts for the origin of the term (syn- = like, ov/o = egg).
synovial joint	A freely movable joint.
synovial membrane	Tissue lining the synovial cavity; it produces synovial fluid.
tendon	Connective tissue that binds muscles to bones.

TERMINOLOGY—JOINTS

Write the meanings of the medical terms in the spaces provided.

COMBINING FORMS

COMBINING FORM	MEANING	TERMINOLOGY	MEANING
ankyl/o	stiff	ankylosis	______________
arthr/o	joint	arthroplasty	______________
		Replacement arthroplasty is replacement of one or both bone ends by a prosthesis (artificial part) of metal or plastic. See page 618. Carpometacarpal arthroplasty is a treatment for arthritis in the thumb (at the basal joint).	
		arthrotomy	______________
		hemarthrosis	______________
		hydrarthrosis	______________
		Synovial fluid collects abnormally in the joint.	
		polyarthritis	______________
articul/o	joint	articular cartilage	______________
		Inflammation of articular cartilage is arthritis, whereas a "torn cartilage" is specifically a tear of a meniscus.	
burs/o	bursa	bursitis	______________
		Causes of this periarticular condition may be related to stress placed on the bursa or to diseases such as gout or rheumatoid arthritis. The bursa becomes inflamed and movement is limited and painful. Intrabursal injection of corticosteroids and also rest and splinting of the limb are helpful in treatment.	
chondr/o	cartilage	achondroplasia	______________
		This is an inherited condition in which the bones of the arms and legs fail to grow to normal size because of a defect in cartilage and bone formation. Dwarfism results, characterized by short limbs and a normal-sized head and trunk. See page 80.	
		chondroma	______________
		chondromalacia	______________
		***Chondromalacia patellae** is a softening and roughening of the articular cartilaginous surface of the kneecap, resulting in pain, a grating sensation, and mechanical "catching" behind the patella with joint movement.*	
ligament/o	ligament	ligamentous	______________

15

Ankylosis/Alkalosis

Ankylosis is a condition of joint stiffening or immobilization. Don't confuse this term with *alkalosis,* meaning increased alkalinity (pH) of blood and tissues.

COMBINING FORM	MEANING	TERMINOLOGY	MEANING
rheumat/o	watery flow	rheumatologist ______ *Various forms of arthritis are marked by collection of fluid in joint spaces.*	
synov/o	synovial membrane	synovitis ______	
ten/o	tendon	tenorrhaphy ______ tenosynovitis ______ *Synov/o here refers to the sheath (covering) around the tendon.*	
tendin/o	tendon	tendinitis ______ *Also spelled tendonitis.*	

SUFFIXES

SUFFIX	MEANING	TERMINOLOGY	MEANING
-desis	to bind, tie together	arthrodesis ______ *Bones are fused across the joint space by surgery (artificial ankylosis). This operation is performed when a joint is very painful, unstable, or chronically infected.*	
-stenosis	narrowing	spinal stenosis ______ *Narrowing of the neural (spinal) canal in the lumbar spine. Symptoms (pain, paresthesias, urinary retention, bowel incontinence) come from compression of the cauda equina (nerves that spread out from the lower end of the spinal cord like a horse's tail). See Figure 15-20.*	

15

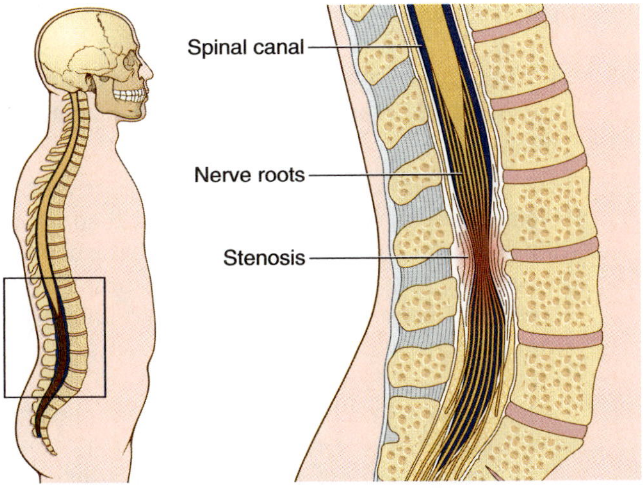

FIGURE 15-20 Spinal stenosis. Wear-and-tear effects of aging can lead to narrowing of the spinal (neural) canal.

PATHOLOGY—JOINTS

arthritis

Inflammation of any joint.

Some of the more common forms are:

1. **ankylosing spondylitis**

Chronic, progressive arthritis with stiffening of joints, primarily of the spine.

Bilateral sclerosis (hardening) of the sacroiliac joints is a diagnostic sign. Joint changes are similar to those seen in rheumatoid arthritis, and the condition can respond to corticosteroids and anti-inflammatory drugs.

2. **gouty arthritis (gout)**

Inflammation and painful swelling of joints caused by excessive uric acid in the body.

A congenital defect in the metabolism of uric acid causes too much of it to accumulate in blood **(hyperuricemia),** joints, and soft tissues near joints. The "pointy" uric acid crystals (salts) destroy the articular cartilage and damage the synovial membrane, often resulting in excruciating pain. The joint chiefly affected is the big toe; hence, the condition often is called **podagra** (pod/o = foot, -agra = excessive pain). Treatment consists of drugs to lower uric acid production (allopurinol) and to prevent inflammation (colchicine and indomethacin) and a special diet that avoids foods that are rich in uric acid, such as red meats, red wines, and fermented cheeses.

3. **osteoarthritis (OA)**

Progressive, degenerative joint disease with loss of articular cartilage and hypertrophy of bone (formation of osteophytes, or bone spurs) at articular surfaces.

This condition, also known as **degenerative joint disease,** can occur in any joint, but occurs mainly in the spine, hips, and knees of older people. It is marked by a narrowing of the joint space (due to loss of cartilage). Treatment consists of aspirin and nonsteroidal anti-inflammatory drugs (NSAIDs) to reduce inflammation and pain and physical therapy to loosen impaired joints. Figure 15-21 compares a normal joint and those with changes characteristic of osteoarthritis and rheumatoid arthritis.

End-stage osteoarthritis is the most common reason for joint replacement surgery (total joint arthroplasty).

4. **rheumatoid arthritis (RA)**

Chronic joint condition with inflammation and pain; caused by an autoimmune reaction against joint tissue, particularly the synovial membrane.

The small joints of the hands and feet are affected first, and larger joints later. Women are more commonly afflicted than men. Synovial membranes become inflamed and thickened, damaging the articular cartilage and preventing easy movement (see Figure 15-21). Sometimes fibrous tissue forms and calcifies, creating a **bony ankylosis** (pathologic union) at the joint and preventing any movement at all. Swollen, painful joints accompanied by **pyrexia** (fever) are symptoms.

Diagnosis is by a blood test that shows the presence of the rheumatoid factor (an antibody) and x-ray images revealing changes around the affected joints. Treatment consists of heat applications and drugs such as aspirin and other NSAIDs and corticosteroids to reduce inflammation and pain. Disease-modifying antirheumatic drugs (DMARDs) such as methotrexate and gold salts also are used.

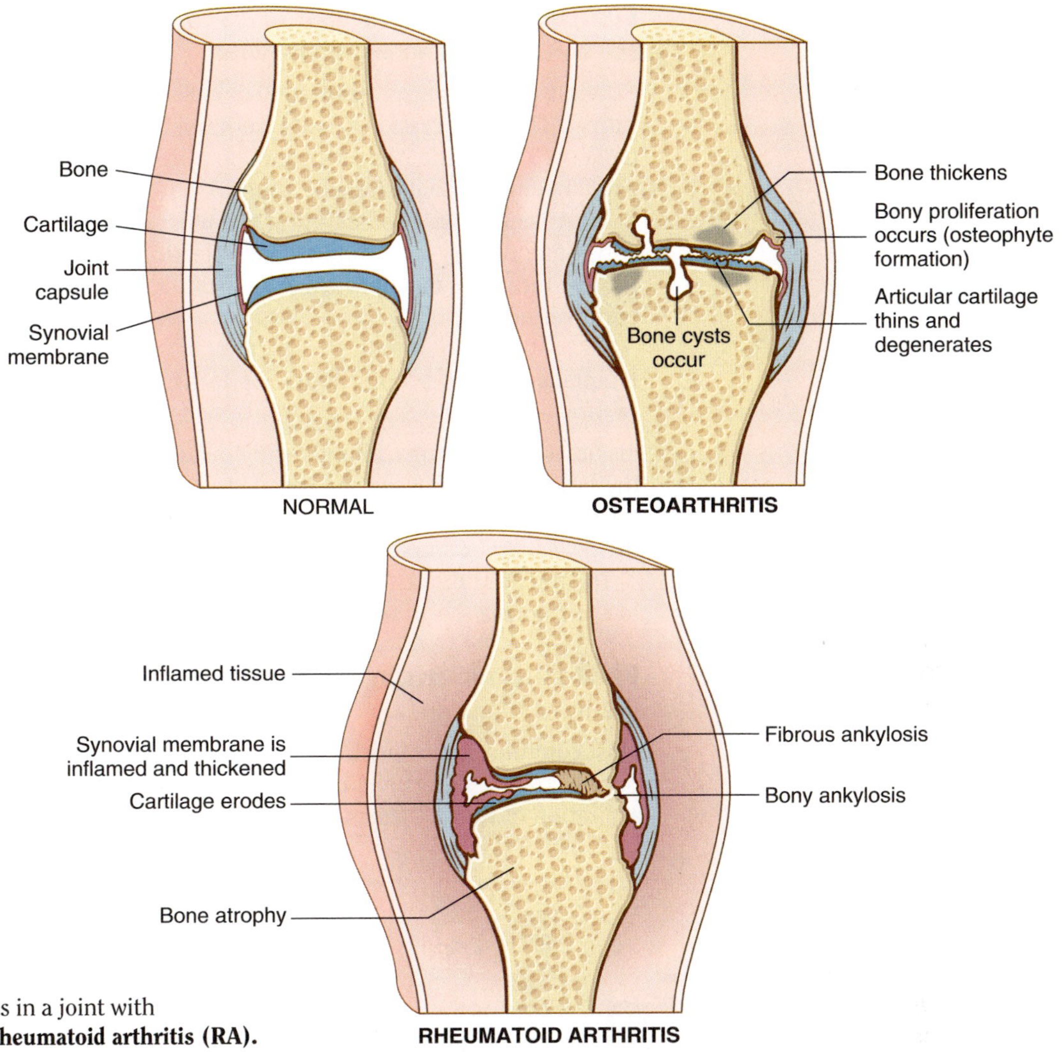

FIGURE 15-21 Changes in a joint with **osteoarthritis (OA)** and **rheumatoid arthritis (RA).**

bunion

Enlargement of bone or tissue around the joint at the base of the big toe (metatarsophalangeal joint).

Chronic irritation from ill-fitting shoes can cause a buildup of soft tissue and underlying bone. Bunionectomy (removal of a bony exostosis and associated soft tissue) is indicated if other measures (changing shoes and use of anti-inflammatory agents) fail. See Figure 15-22. Another name for a bunion is **hallux** (great toe) **valgus** (abnormal angulation of the toe).

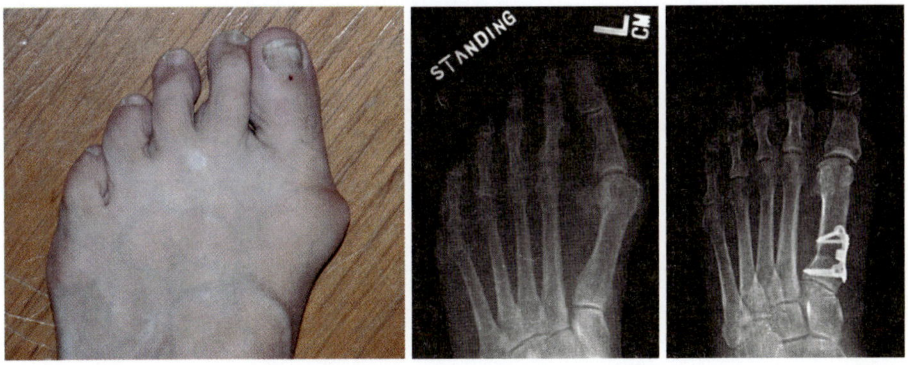

FIGURE 15-22 The photograph shows a **bunion** of the left foot. The first x-ray is before **bunionectomy,** and the second is after surgery to remove tissue and realign the bones. *(Courtesy Dr. Sidra Ezrahi and Dr. Richard de Asia, Massachusetts General Hospital, Boston.)*

15

carpal tunnel syndrome (CTS)

Compression of the median nerve as it passes between the ligament and the bones and tendons of the wrist.

CTS is caused by compression of the median nerve (see Figure 15-23) in the carpal tunnel. The compression results from swelling and/or inflammation of the flexor tendons. The thumb, the index and long (middle) fingers, and the radial half of the ring finger become dysesthetic (numb).

Treatment consists of splinting the wrist during sleep to immobilize it, use of anti-inflammatory medications, and injection of cortisone into the carpal tunnel. If these measures fail, surgical release of the transverse carpal ligament is usually curative.

dislocation

Displacement of a bone from its joint.

Dislocated bones do not articulate with each other. The most common cause of dislocations is trauma. **Shoulder dislocation** (disruption of articulation between the head of the humerus and the glenoid fossa of the scapula) and **hip dislocation** (disruption of articulation between the head of the femur and the acetabulum of the pelvis) are examples.

Treatment of dislocations involves **reduction,** which is restoration of the bones to their normal positions. A **subluxation** is a partial or incomplete dislocation.

ganglion cyst

Fluid-filled sac arising from joint capsules or tendons, typically in the hand.

Most common in the wrist, but can occur in the shoulder, knee, hip, or ankle. See Figure 15-24. Treatment ranges from immobilization and reduced activity to aspiration of fluid if necessary.

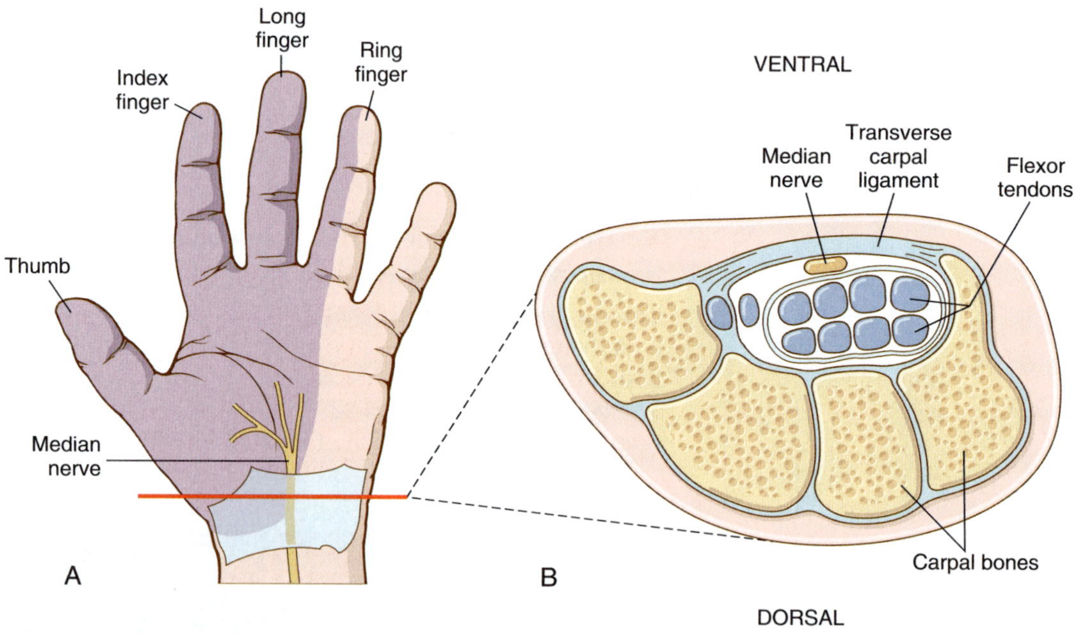

FIGURE 15-23 **Carpal tunnel syndrome (CTS). A,** The median nerve's sensory distribution in the thumb, first three fingers, and palm. **B,** Cross section of a left hand at the level indicated in **(A)**. Note the position of the median nerve between the carpal ligament and the tendons and carpal bones.

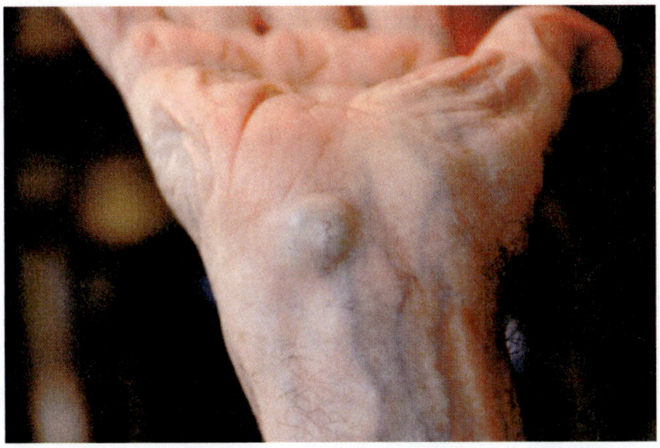

FIGURE 15-24 **Ganglion** cyst on the wrist. This is commonly known as a Bible cyst because a frequent treatment in the past was to strike the ganglion with a Bible to rupture it.

herniation of an intervertebral disk (disc)

Abnormal protrusion of an intervertebral disk into the spinal canal or spinal nerves.

This condition is commonly referred to as a **"slipped disk."** Pain is experienced as the inner portion of the disk (nucleus pulposus) presses on spinal nerves or on the spinal cord. See Figure 15-25A. Low back pain and **sciatica** (pain radiating down the leg) are symptoms when the disk protrudes in the lumbar spine. See Figure 15-25B. Neck pain and burning pain radiating down an arm are characteristic of a herniated disk in the cervical spine. Physical therapy, drugs for pain, and epidural cortisone injections may help initially. In patients with chronic or recurrent disk herniation, **microdiskectomy** (removal of a portion of the protruding disk) may be advised. See Figure 15-26A. In microendoscopic surgery, the disk is removed by inserting a tube through the skin and aspirating the disk through the tube.

15

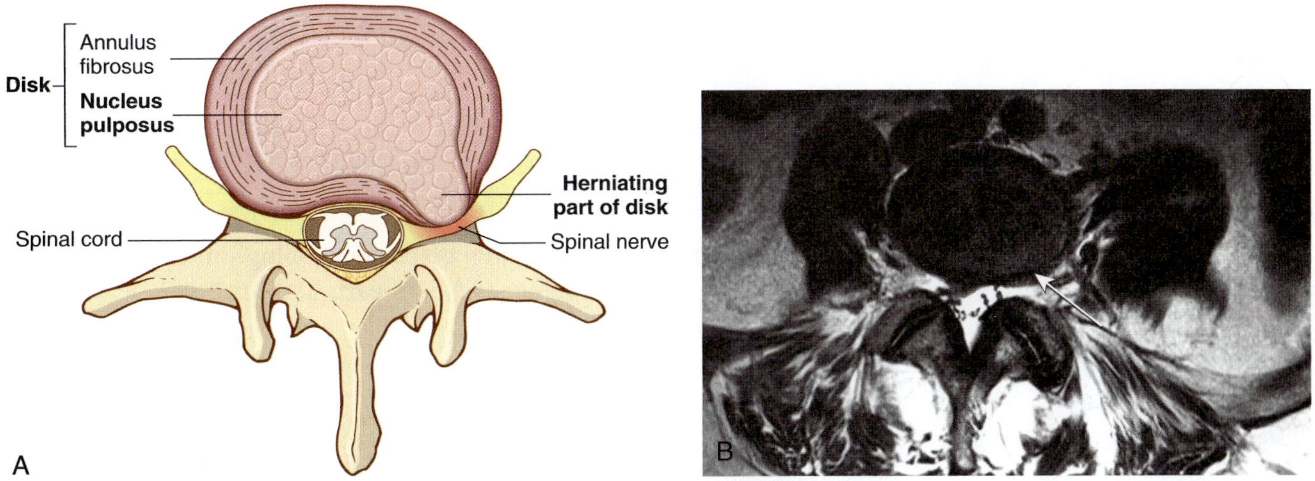

FIGURE 15-25 **A, Herniation of an intervertebral disk** (view from above the vertebra). The inner portion (nucleus pulposus) of the disk can be seen pressing on the spinal nerve. The condition is also known as **herniated nucleus pulposus (HNP). B, MRI showing a herniated disk impinging on the sciatic nerve root.**

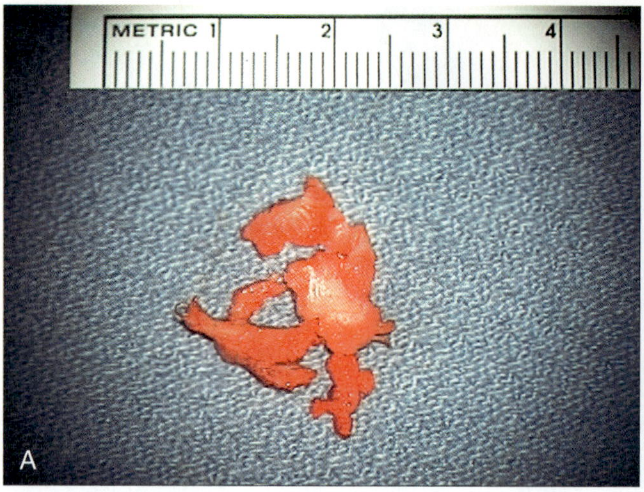

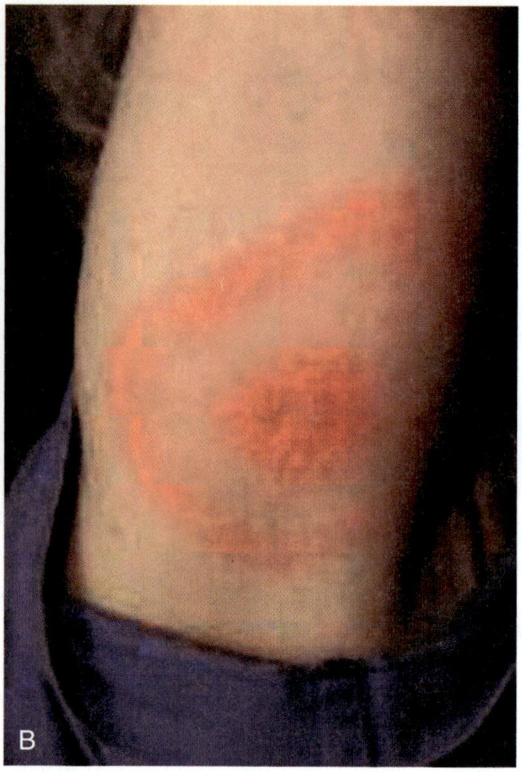

FIGURE 15-26 **A, After microdiskectomy, fragments of the herniated disk are removed and shown here.** *Courtesy of Jean-Valéry Coumans, Massachusetts General Hospital.* **B, "Bull's eye" rash in Lyme disease.**

15

Lyme disease (Lyme arthritis)

Disorder marked by arthritis, myalgia, and malaise; cause is a bacterium carried by a tick.

It was first reported in Old Lyme, Connecticut, and is now found throughout the eastern coastal region of the United States. It is often marked by a "bull's eye" rash at the site of the tick bite. See Figure 15-26B. The condition is treated with antibiotics. In some cases, Lyme disease can affect the nervous system. See In Person account on page 622.

sprain

Trauma to ligaments without rupture.

A **strain** is an injury involving the overstretching of muscle. Application of gentle compressive wraps is an immediate measure to relieve pain and minimize swelling caused by sprains and strains. Application of ice and elevation of the extremity are also helpful.

systemic lupus erythematosus (SLE)

Chronic inflammatory autoimmune disease involving joints, skin, kidneys, central nervous system (CNS), heart, and lungs.

This condition affects connective tissue (specifically a protein component called **collagen**) in tendons, ligaments, bones, and cartilage all over the body. Typically, there is a red, scaly rash over the nose and cheeks ("butterfly" rash) (Figure 15-27). Patients, usually women, experience joint pain in several joints (polyarthralgia), pyrexia (fever), kidney inflammation, and malaise. SLE is an autoimmune disease that is diagnosed by the presence of abnormal antibodies in the blood and characteristic white blood cells called LE cells. Treatment involves giving corticosteroids, hormones made by the adrenal gland that are used to treat inflammatory conditions.

The name **lupus,** meaning wolf, has been used since the 13th century, because people with lupus looked like their skin had been affected by wolf bites.

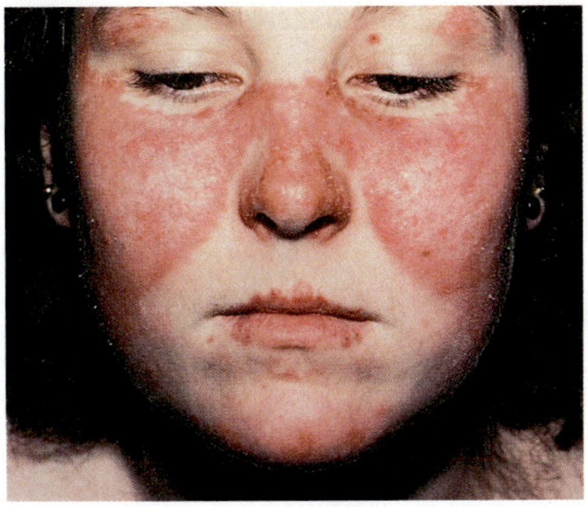

FIGURE 15-27 **Butterfly rash** that may accompany systemic lupus erythematosus.

Muscles

TYPES OF MUSCLES

There are three types of muscles in the body. Label Figure 15-28 as you read the following descriptions of the various types of muscles.

Striated muscle [1] makes up the **voluntary** or **skeletal muscles** that move all bones, as well as controlling facial expression and eye movements. Through the central and peripheral nervous systems, we have conscious control over these muscles. Striated muscle fibers (cells) have a pattern of dark and light bands, or fibrils, in their cytoplasm. Fibrous tissue that envelops and separates muscles is called **fascia,** which contains the muscle's blood, lymph, and nerve supply.

15

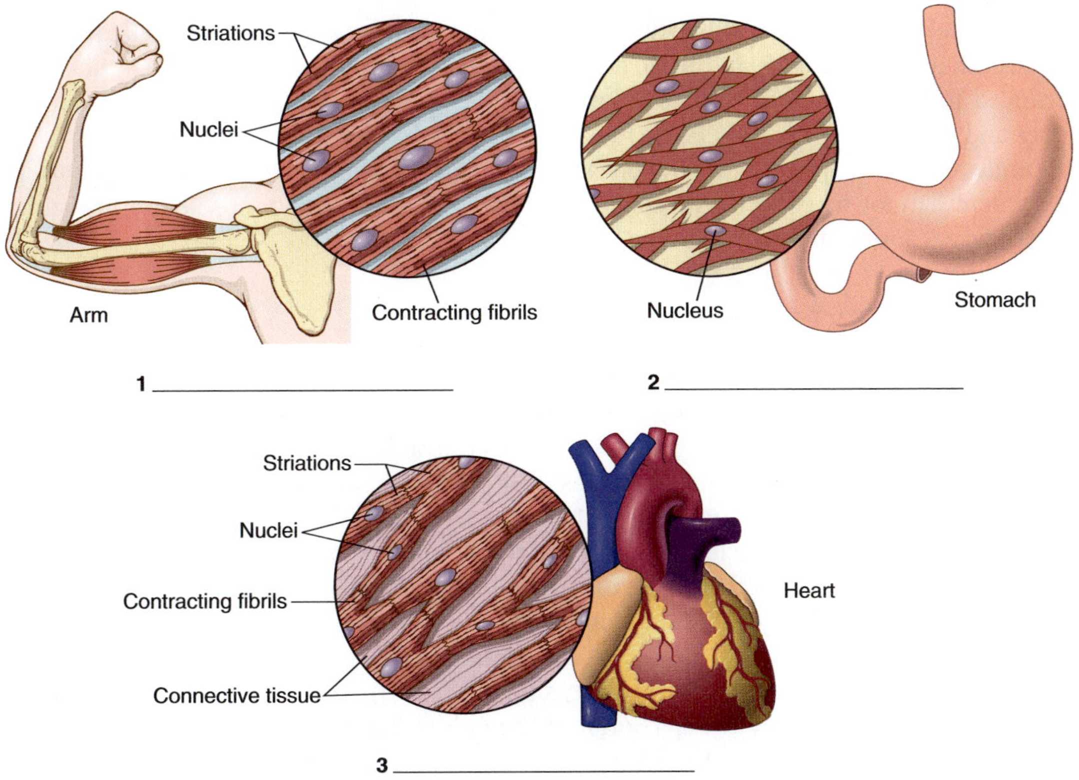

FIGURE 15-28 **Types of muscles.**

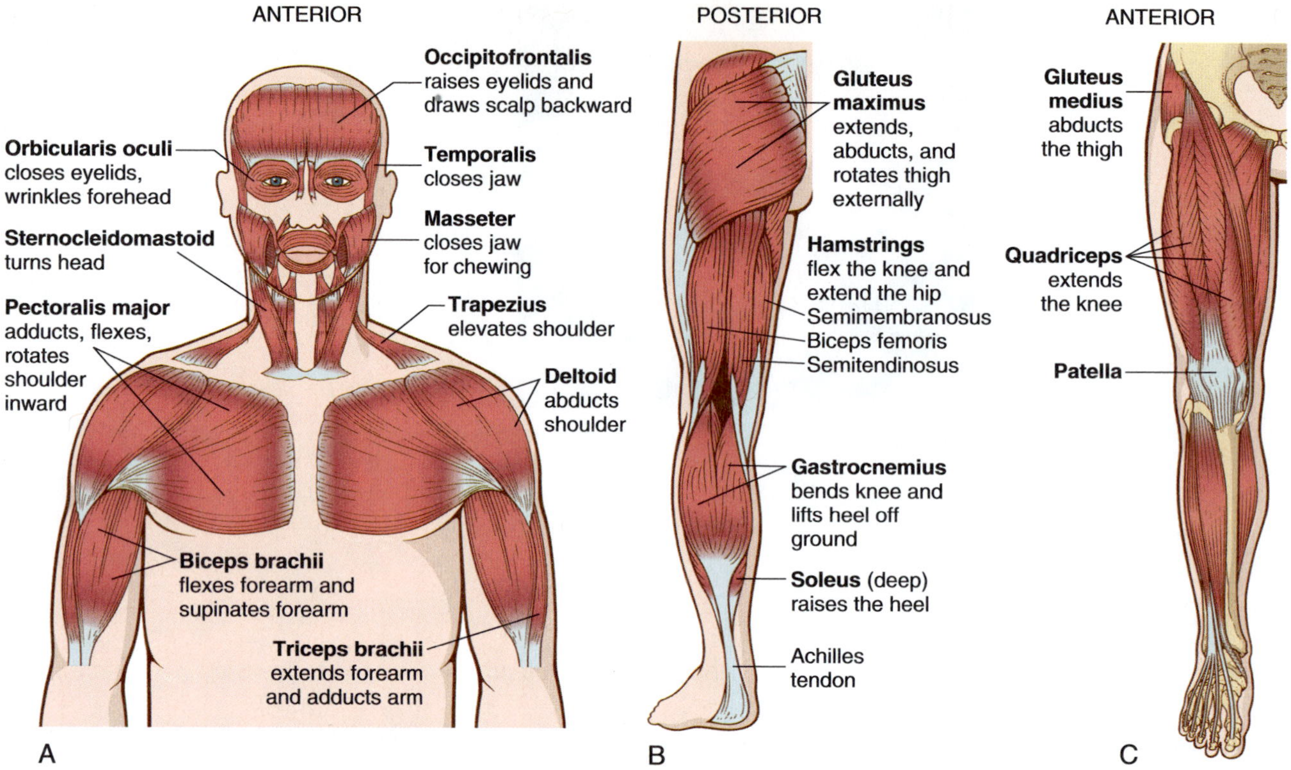

FIGURE 15-29 **(A) Selected muscles of the head, neck, torso, and arm and their functions. (B) Selected muscles of the posterior and anterior aspect of the leg and their functions.** The Evolve site contains additional anterior and posterior images of major muscles and their functions.

15

Smooth muscle [2] makes up the **involuntary** or **visceral muscles** that move internal organs such as the digestive tract, blood vessels, and secretory ducts leading from glands. These muscles are controlled by the autonomic nervous system. They are called smooth because they have no dark and light fibrils in their cytoplasm. Skeletal muscle fibers are arranged in bundles, whereas smooth muscle forms sheets of fibers as it wraps around tubes and vessels.

Cardiac muscle [3] is striated in appearance but is like smooth muscle in its action. Its movement cannot be consciously controlled. The fibers of cardiac muscle are branching fibers and are found in the heart.

ACTIONS OF SKELETAL MUSCLES

Skeletal (striated) muscles (more than 600 in the human body) are the muscles that move bones. Figure 15-29 shows some skeletal muscles of the head, neck, and torso and muscles of the posterior aspect of the leg. When a muscle contracts, one of the bones to which it is joined remains virtually stationary as a result of other muscles that hold it in place. The point of attachment of the muscle to the stationary bone is called the **origin (beginning)** of that muscle. When the muscle contracts, however, another bone to which it is attached does move. The point of junction of the muscle to the bone that moves is called the **insertion** of the muscle. Most often, the origin of a muscle lies proximal in the skeleton, whereas its insertion lies distal.

Figure 15-30 shows the biceps and triceps muscles in the upper arm. One origin of the biceps is at the scapula, and its insertion is at the radius. Tendons are the connective tissue bands that connect muscles to the bones.

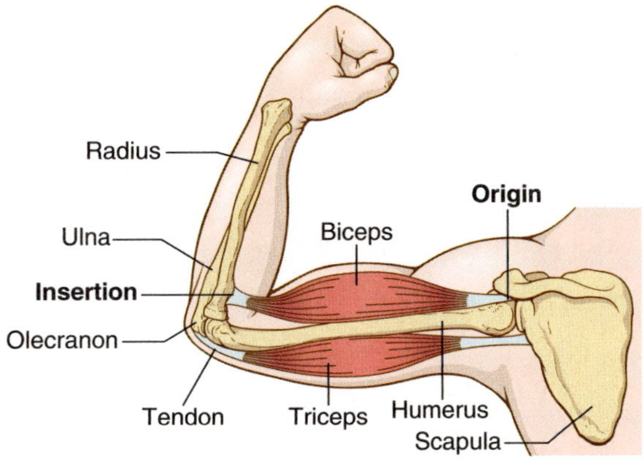

FIGURE 15-30 Origin and insertion of the biceps in the arm. Note also the origin of the triceps at the scapula and the insertion at the olecranon of the ulna.

Muscles can perform a variety of actions. Some of the terms used to describe those actions are listed here, with a short description of the specific type of movement performed (See Figure 15-31 on page 614).

ACTION	MEANING
flexion	Decreasing the angle between two bones; bending a limb.
extension	Increasing the angle between two bones; straightening out a limb.
abduction	Movement away from the midline of the body.
adduction	Movement toward the midline of the body.
rotation	Circular movement around an axis (central point). **Internal rotation** is toward the center of the body and **external rotation** is away from the center of the body.
dorsiflexion	Decreasing the angle of the ankle joint so that the foot bends backward (upward). This is the opposite movement of stepping on the gas pedal when driving a car.
plantar flexion	Motion that extends the foot downward toward the ground as when pointing the toes or stepping on the gas pedal. Plant/o means sole of the foot.
supination	As applied to the hand and forearm, the act of turning the palm up. As applied to the foot, it is outward roll of the foot during normal motion.
pronation	As applied to the hand and forearm, the act of turning the palm down. As applied to the foot, it is inward roll of the foot during normal motion.

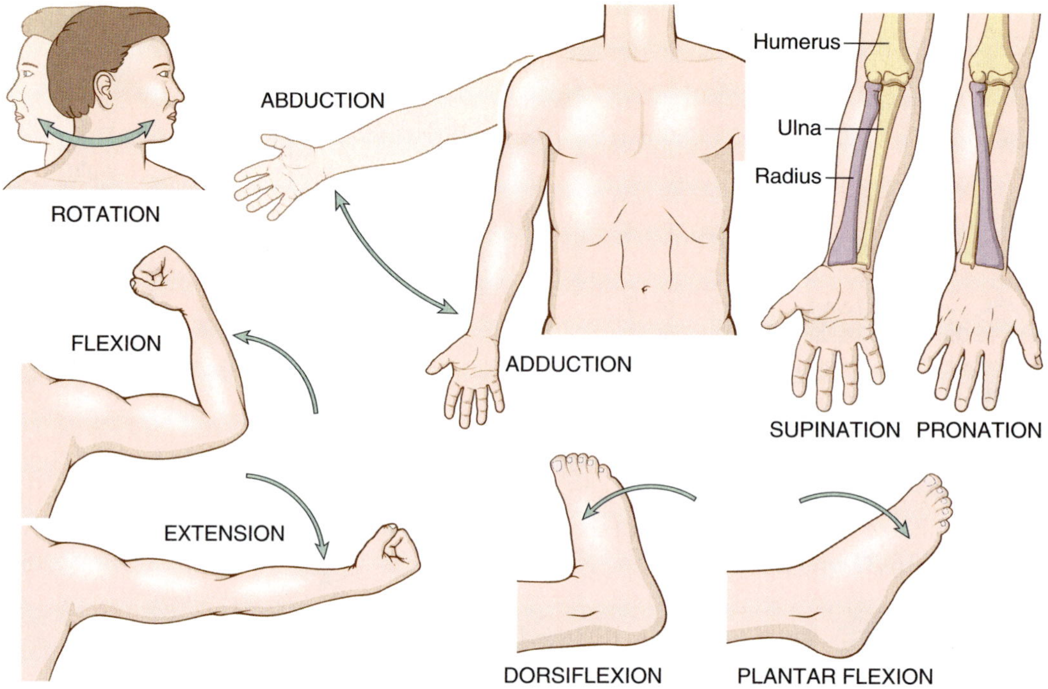

FIGURE 15-31 Types of muscular actions.

15

VOCABULARY—MUSCLES

This list reviews many of the new terms related to muscle introduced in the text. Short definitions reinforce your understanding of the terms. Refer to the Pronunciation of Terms on p. 645 for help with unfamiliar or difficult terms.

abduction	Movement away from the midline of the body.
adduction	Movement toward the midline of the body.
dorsiflexion	Backward (upward) bending of the foot.
extension	Straightening of a flexed limb.
fascia	Fibrous membrane separating and enveloping muscles.
flexion	Bending a limb; decreasing the angle between bones.
insertion of a muscle	Connection of the muscle to a bone that moves.
origin of a muscle	Connection of the muscle to a stationary bone.
plantar flexion	Bending the sole of the foot downward toward the ground.
pronation	Turning the palm downward.
rotation	Circular movement around a central point. **Internal rotation** is toward the center of the body. **External rotation** is away from the center of the body.
striated muscle	Muscle connected to bones; voluntary or skeletal muscle.
supination	Turning the palm upward.
visceral muscle	Muscle connected to internal organs; involuntary or smooth muscle.

TERMINOLOGY—MUSCLES

Write the meanings of the medical terms in the spaces provided.

COMBINING FORMS

COMBINING FORM	MEANING	TERMINOLOGY	MEANING
fasci/o	fascia (forms sheaths enveloping muscles)	fasciotomy *Fascia is cut to relieve tension or pressure on muscles. See Figure 15-32.*	_______________
fibr/o	fibrous connective tissue	fibromyalgia *Chronic pain and stiffness in muscles, joints, and fibrous tissue, especially of the back, shoulders, neck, hips, and knees. Fatigue is a common complaint. Cause is unknown, and treatment includes physical therapy, stress relief methods, and medications such as Cymbalta (duloxetine) and Lyrica (pregabalin).*	_______________
leiomy/o	smooth (visceral) muscle that lines the walls of internal organs	leiomyoma	_______________
		leiomyosarcoma	_______________

15

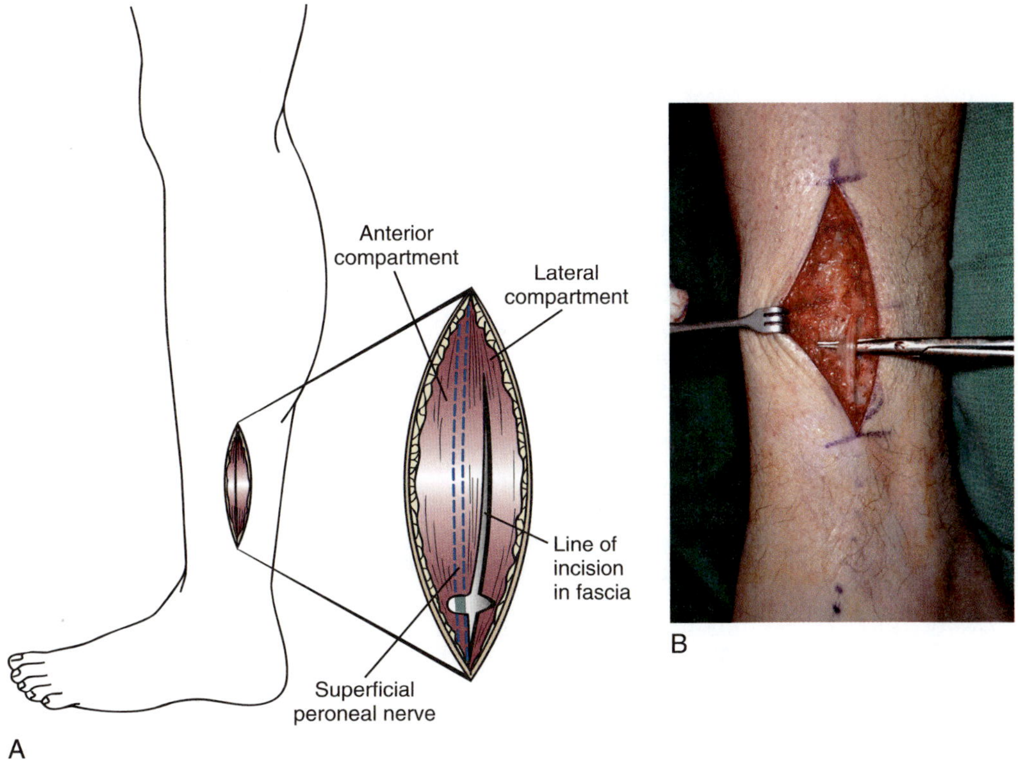

FIGURE 15-32 **A, Fasciotomy** as treatment for **compartment syndrome,** which is the compression of muscle, blood vessels, and nerves inside a closed space (compartment) of the body. It most often involves the lower leg. **B, Clinical photograph of fasciotomy and exposed superficial peroneal nerve.**

COMBINING FORM	MEANING	TERMINOLOGY	MEANING
my/o	muscle	myalgia	____________
		electromyography	____________
		myopathy	____________
myocardi/o	heart muscle	myocardial	____________
myos/o	muscle	myositis	____________
plant/o	sole of the foot	plantar flexion	____________
rhabdomy/o	skeletal (striated) muscle connected to bones	rhabdomyoma	____________
		rhabdomyosarcoma	____________
sarc/o	muscle and flesh	sarcopenia ____________ *Loss of muscle mass and strength associated with aging. Exercise and strength training can help preserve and enhance muscle mass at any age.*	

SUFFIXES

15

SUFFIX	MEANING	TERMINOLOGY	MEANING
-asthenia	lack of strength	myasthenia gravis ____________ *Muscles lose strength because of a failure in transmission of the nervous impulse from the nerve to the muscle cell.*	
-trophy	development, nourishment	atrophy ____________ *Decrease in size of an organ or tissue.*	
		hypertrophy ____________ *Increase in size of an organ or tissue.*	
		amyotrophic ____________ *In **amyotrophic lateral sclerosis** (Lou Gehrig disease), muscles deteriorate (paralysis occurs) as a result of degeneration of nerves in the spinal cord and lower region of the brain.*	

PREFIXES

PREFIX	MEANING	TERMINOLOGY	MEANING
ab-	away from	abduction ____________ *Duct/o means to lead.*	
ad-	toward	adduction	____________
dorsi-	back	dorsiflexion	____________

PREFIX	MEANING	TERMINOLOGY	MEANING
poly-	many, much	polymyalgia *__Polymyalgia rheumatica__ is a syndrome marked by aching and morning stiffness in the shoulder, hip, or neck for longer than 1 month.*	________________

PATHOLOGY—MUSCLES

muscular dystrophy

Group of inherited diseases characterized by progressive weakness and degeneration of muscle fibers without involvement of the nervous system.

Duchenne muscular dystrophy is the most common form. Muscles appear to enlarge **(pseudohypertrophy)** as fat replaces functional muscle cells that have degenerated and atrophied. Onset of muscle weakness occurs soon after birth, and diagnosis can be made by muscle biopsy and electromyography. The disease predominantly affects males; muscle weakness produces stumbling, falling, lordosis, winged (prominent) scapulae, and cardiac problems.

polymyositis

Chronic inflammatory myopathy.

This condition is marked by symmetrical muscle weakness and pain, often accompanied by a rash around the eyes and on the face and limbs. Evidence that polymyositis is an autoimmune disorder is growing stronger, and some patients recover completely with immunosuppressive therapy.

15

LABORATORY TESTS AND CLINICAL PROCEDURES

LABORATORY TESTS

antinuclear antibody test (ANA)

Detects an antibody present in serum of patients with systemic lupus erythematosus (SLE) and other autoimmune diseases.

erythrocyte sedimentation rate (ESR)

Measures time it takes for erythrocytes to settle to the bottom of a test tube.

Elevated ESR is associated with inflammatory disorders such as rheumatoid arthritis, tumors, and infections, and with chronic infections of bone and soft tissue.

rheumatoid factor test (RF)

Serum is tested for the presence of an antibody found in patients with rheumatoid arthritis.

serum calcium (Ca)

Measurement of calcium level in serum.

Hypercalcemia may be caused by disorders of the parathyroid gland and malignancy that affects bone metabolism. Hypocalcemia is seen in critically ill patients with burns, sepsis, and acute renal failure.

serum creatine kinase (CK)

Measurement of the enzyme creatine kinase in serum.

This enzyme normally is present in skeletal and cardiac muscle. Increased levels occur in muscular dystrophy, polymyositis, and with traumatic injuries.

uric acid test — **Measurement of uric acid in serum.**
High levels are associated with gouty arthritis.

CLINICAL PROCEDURES

arthrocentesis — **Surgical puncture to remove fluid from the joint space.**
Synovial fluid is removed for analysis.

arthrography — **Taking x-ray images after injection of contrast material into a joint.**

arthroplasty — **Surgical repair or replacement of a joint.**

Total hip arthroplasty or **total hip replacement (THR)** is replacement of the femoral head and acetabulum with prostheses that are fastened into the bone (Figure 15-33).

In a **total knee replacement (TKR)** a metal prosthesis covers the end of the femur, and a tibial component made of metal and plastic covers the tip end of the tibia. See page 625 for a clinical case showing TKR and page 626 for an ***In Person*** account of the procedure.

Other examples of arthroplasties are **resection arthroplasty** (small portion of a bone is removed to repair the joint; acromioclavicular joint is a common location), **interposition arthroplasty** (new tissue taken from another place is placed between damaged surface of elbow joint), and **revision arthroplasty** (an operation to replace a failing prosthetic joint).

15

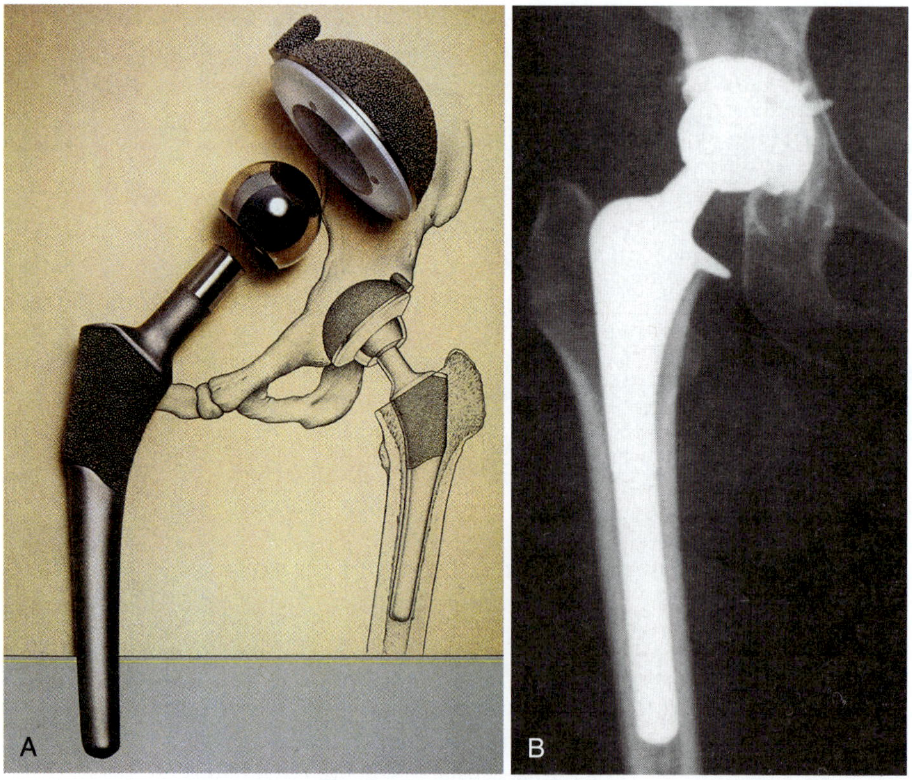

FIGURE 15-33 **A, Acetabular and femoral components of a total hip arthroplasty. B,** Radiograph showing a hip after a cementless Harris-Galante implant. The bone grows into the porous metal to stabilize it to the skeleton.

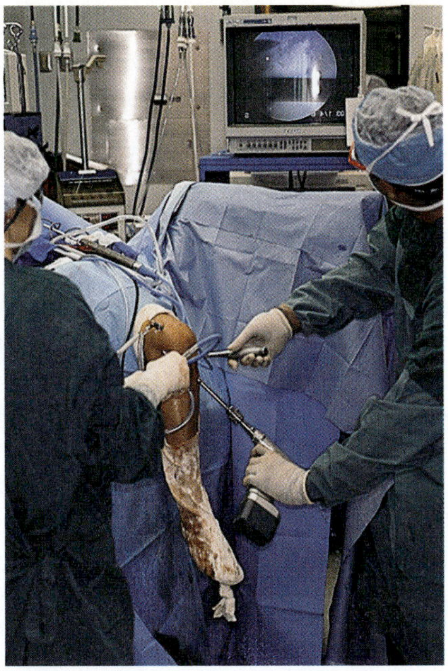

FIGURE 15-34 **Knee arthroscopy in progress.** Notice the monitor in the background. An arthroscope is used in the diagnosis and treatment of pathologic changes.

arthroscopy

Visual examination of a joint with an arthroscope and television camera.

An orthopedist passes small surgical instruments into a joint (knee, shoulder, ankle, wrist, hip) to evaluate and/or remove and repair damaged tissue (Figure 15-34).

bone density test (bone densitometry)

Low-energy x-ray absorption in bones of the spinal column, pelvis, and wrist is used to measure bone mass.

An x-ray detector measures how well x-rays penetrate through bones (Figure 15-35). Areas of decreased density indicate osteopenia and osteoporosis. Also called **dual-energy x-ray absorptiometry (DEXA** *or* **DXA).**

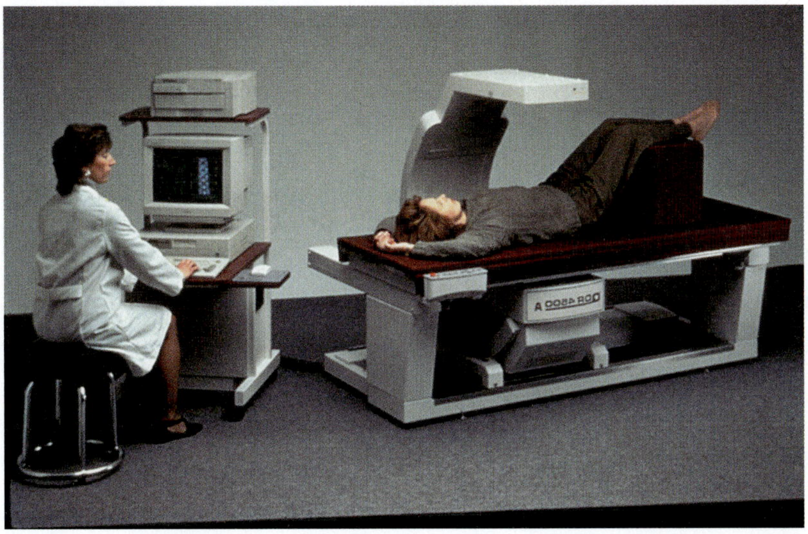

FIGURE 15-35 Patient undergoing **bone density test** or **dual energy x-ray absorptiometry** (**DEXA** or **DXA**).

bone scan — **Uptake of a radioactive substance is measured in bone.**

A nuclear medicine physician uses a special scanning device to detect areas of increased uptake (tumors, infection, inflammation, stress fractures) (Figure 15-36).

computed tomography (CT) — **X-ray beam and computer provide cross-sectional and other images.**

CT scans identify bone abnormalities, and musculo-skeletal trauma.

diskography — **X-ray examination of cervical or lumbar intervertebral disk after injection of contrast into nucleus pulposus (interior of the disk).**

electromyography (EMG) — **Recording the strength of muscle contraction as a result of electrical stimulation.**

magnetic resonance imaging (MRI) — **Magnetic field creates images of soft tissue.**

MRI shows soft tissue conditions in greater detail than that achieved with CT.

muscle biopsy — **Removal of muscle tissue for microscopic examination.**

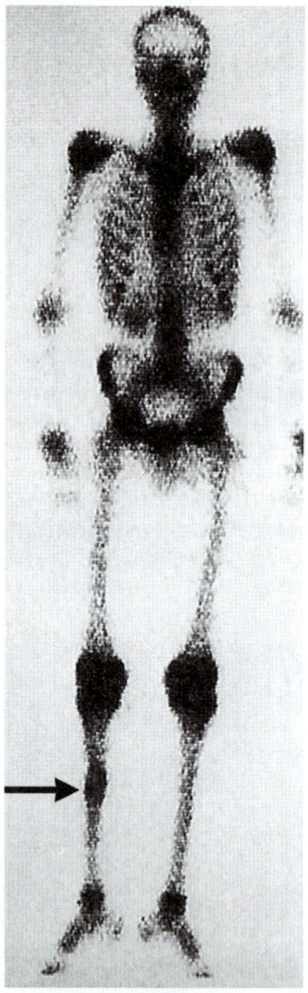

FIGURE 15-36 **A technetium-99m bone scan of a skeleton** showing an area of increased radioactive uptake on the right tibia *(arrow)* that indicates a bone tumor.

ABBREVIATIONS

AC	acromioclavicular (joint)
ACL	anterior cruciate ligament of the knee
ANA	antinuclear antibody—indicator of systemic lupus erythematosus
BKA	below-knee amputation
BMD	bone mineral density
C1 to C7	cervical vertebrae
Ca	calcium
CK	creatine kinase—enzyme elevated in muscle disease
CMC	carpometacarpal (joint)
CTS	carpal tunnel syndrome
DEXA *or* **DXA**	dual-energy x-ray absorptiometry—a test of bone mineral density
DMARD	disease-modifying antirheumatic drug
DO	doctor of osteopathy
DTRs	deep tendon reflexes
EMG	electromyography
ESR (sed rate)	erythrocyte sedimentation rate—indicates inflammation
HNP	herniated nucleus pulposus
IM	intramuscular
L1 to L5	lumbar vertebrae
NSAID	nonsteroidal anti-inflammatory drug—often prescribed to treat musculoskeletal disorders
OA	osteoarthritis
ORIF	open reduction (of fracture)/internal fixation
ortho	orthopedics (*or* orthopaedics)
OT	occupational therapy—helps patients with impaired musculoskeletal function perform activities of daily living and function in work-related situations
P	phosphorus
PT	physical therapy—helps patients regain use of muscles and joints after injury or surgery
RA	rheumatoid arthritis
RF	rheumatoid factor
ROM	range of motion
SLE	systemic lupus erythematosus
T1 to T12	thoracic vertebrae
TKR	total knee replacement/arthroplasty
THR	total hip replacement/arthroplasty
TMJ	temporomandibular joint

IN PERSON

This first-person account was written by a woman diagnosed with neurological Lyme disease.

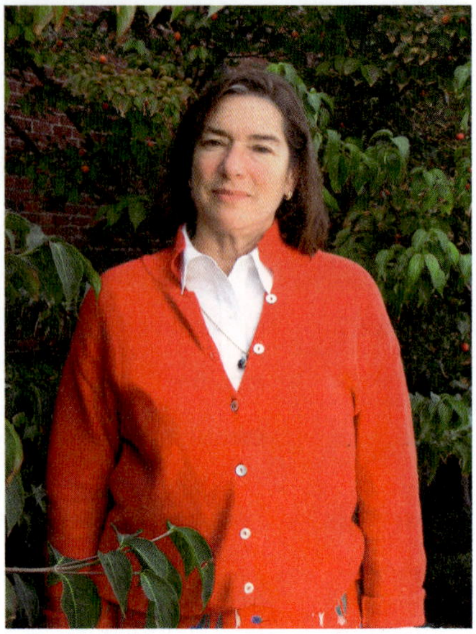

Weeding the garden and pruning the shrubs are chores I have willingly performed many, many times with no ill effects except an occasional backache, some scratches, and the misery of poison ivy. To avoid bending over I would often kneel or sit down in the garden. In late June 2009 I not only got quite dirty, but unknowingly connected with a deer tick and developed acute neurological Lyme disease. One day shortly after working in the garden, I developed a fever and noticed a rash all over my trunk. I figured I had a summer virus that would go away in a few days. I never suspected Lyme disease. There was no tick and no telltale "bulls-eye" pattern in the rash. Indeed, I did feel fine in just a few days—the respite lasted just one day, however. The next day, I had another rash and was feeling poorly. My husband Paul drove me to the doctor's office where a physician's assistant took some blood and gave me a prescription for doxycycline. I had taken just four doses when my condition worsened alarmingly. I lost my balance and could barely lift my head up while lying in bed. Mental processing was slow and I was having difficulty with word finding—more than the usual memory lapses of a healthy 67-year-old. When I called the doctor's office, I was told to stop taking the doxycycline as I could be having an allergic reaction. We went back to the doctor's office, where I was put into an ambulance and sent to the hospital.

15

Neurologists and infectious disease specialists examined me over the next five days and ordered tests, e.g., an MRI (to rule out stroke), EMGs (there was delayed nerve conduction in my legs), and a lumbar puncture (spinal tap). The doctors first suspected Guillain-Barré syndrome, a scary paralyzing autoimmune disease, but the blood work indicated that my condition was Lyme disease. I learned that in Lyme disease, the bite of an infected deer tick releases a spirochete (bacterium) into the bloodstream and can affect joints, the nervous system, and other organs.

My treatment was a course of intravenous antibiotics. A PICC (peripherally inserted central catheter) was implanted in my upper arm leading to the superior vena cava to gain access to my bloodstream. I was given a prescription for a powerful antibiotic called ceftriaxone (though I was not allergic to the first antibiotic, doxycycline, after all) and I was allowed to go home. I reclined in a hospital bed in the dining room and received excellent nursing care from my husband, a college professor, who, luckily, could be at home with me 24/7. Paul carefully infused 2000 mg of ceftriaxone daily and kept the PICC sterile. He also held on to me in the bathtub where I sat on a bathtub chair and helped me wash my hair. Now that was an experience!

Physical therapists, occupational therapists. and visiting nurses came to the house over the next three weeks. I had to practice writing my name and the numbers 1 to 10. I had to coordinate getting out of bed and standing up–without holding on to the bed. I learned to walk and balance on one foot by holding on to the kitchen counter. I went up stairs slowly holding on to the banister for dear life and went down stairs on my bottom like a crab. Eventually, I had a walker, then a cane, and Paul escorted me on short trips around the top of the driveway. During this time, I also made follow-up visits to doctors. I had strength in my legs and feet but was still wobbly mentally and physically. One day I was able to walk by myself in the neighborhood–this a triumph for a woman who was used to a 3½ mile daily walk and long bike rides. I also exercised in the shallow end of our swimming pool. But I could not drive until the neurological symptoms resolved. This was the only thing Paul and I fought about! The first time he took me for a "driving test," he flunked me. I was indignant, to say the least. In another few weeks my timing and coordination had improved and I was able to drive and begin to take long walks and bike rides once again. I also joined a health club to vary my exercise routine and have kept at it ever since. I no longer get down and dirty when I pull weeds in the garden.

Elizabeth F. Fideler, EdD is an independent researcher and author of Women Still at Work: Professionals Over Sixty and On the Job (Rowman & Littlefield, 2012). She has two children and five grandchildren.

PRACTICAL APPLICATIONS

This section contains an x-ray report, an orthopedic operating room schedule, a case report with findings presented in SOAP format, and a short clinical case. Explanations of more difficult or unfamiliar terms are given in brackets. Answers to the matching questions are found on page 640.

MEDICAL REPORT: RESULTS OF CHEST X-RAY EXAMINATION

PA [posteroanterior] and lateral chest: The heart is enlarged in its transverse diameter. The lungs are fully expanded and free of active disease.

Thoracic spine shows a scoliosis of the upper thoracic spine convex to the left. There is 50% wedge compression fracture of T6 and slight wedge compression fracture of T5. There is also anterior wedge compression fracture of T12.

Lumbar spine shows 90% compression fractures of L1 and L3 with 30% compression fractures of L2 and L5. All bones are markedly osteoporotic. There is calcification within the aortic arch. There are gallstones in the right upper quadrant. The findings in the spine are most compatible with osteoporotic compression fractures. During the procedure, the patient had a sickable [syncopal—this word was incorrectly transcribed!] episode and fell, striking her head. A skull series, done at no cost to the patient, shows no evidence of bony fracture. The pineal gland is calcified and has a midline location. The sella turcica is normal.

OPERATING ROOM SCHEDULE I

Match the operation in Column I with an accompanying diagnosis or indication for surgery from Column II.

COLUMN I

1. Excision, osteochondroma, R calcaneus _____
2. TMJ arthroscopy with probable arthrotomy _____
3. L4–5 laminectomy and diskectomy _____
4. Arthroscopy, left knee _____
5. Open reduction, malleolar fracture _____
6. R occipital craniotomy with tumor resection _____
7. Excision, distal end right clavicle, with prob. acromioplasty _____
8. Open reduction and internal fixation of the acetabulum _____

COLUMN II

A. Fracture of the ankle
B. ACL rupture
C. Neoplastic lesion in brain
D. Exostosis on heel bone
E. Pelvic fracture
F. Pain and malocclusion of jawbones
G. Lower back pain radiating down one leg
H. Pain in shoulder joint with bone spur (exostosis) evident on x-ray

15

CASE REPORT—SOAP FORMAT: ACL INJURY

[Note: **SOAP** stands for **S**ubjective, **O**bjective, **A**ssessment, and **P**lan.]
S: Patient reports that she fell and twisted her right knee while skiing last month. She notes that she felt a "pop" and experienced immediate pain and swelling of the knee. X-ray was negative for fracture, but an MRI revealed a torn ACL [anterior cruciate ligament]. Patient underwent an ACL reconstruction using a patellar tendon autograft 1 week ago. Pain is 3/10 at rest and 6/10 during weight-bearing. Her goals are to decrease pain, walk normally, and return to prior level of functioning, including skiing and soccer.
O: *Gait:* Ambulates with Bledsoe [hinged] brace and bilateral axillary crutches.

	Left	*Right*
Range of Motion:		
Extension	0°	0°
Flexion	140°	90°
Strength:		
Quadriceps	5/5	3+/5
Hamstrings	5/5	4–/5
Gluteus medius	5/5	4–/5
Gluteus maximus	5/5	4–/5
Gastroc/soleus	5/5	4–/5
Girth (mid-patella):	15″	16″

A: Patient is a 20-year-old female presenting with signs and symptoms consistent with status post-ACL reconstruction. Impairments include gait disturbance, decreased range of motion, decreased strength, edema, pain, and decreased functional activities.

P: Treatment will include manual therapy, therapeutic exercise modalities, patient education, and gait training.

SHORT CLINICAL CASE: OA OF THE KNEE

A 65-year-old woman has been suffering from right knee joint stiffness, aching pain, and limited movement that is worse when she rises in the morning or after inactivity. She has been taking acetaminophen (Tylenol) and other NSAIDs (Motrin or Advil) to cope with the pain.

An x-ray of her knees (see Figure 15-37A) shows deterioration of articular cartilage in the right knee with narrowing of the joint space. See left knee for comparison. Surgery is recommended for TKR and was performed (see Figure 15-37B and C). Follow-up x-ray (Figure 15-37D) shows the prosthesis in place. After a successful healing of the incision and removal of surgical clips, the patient had several months of PT and is walking normally without pain.

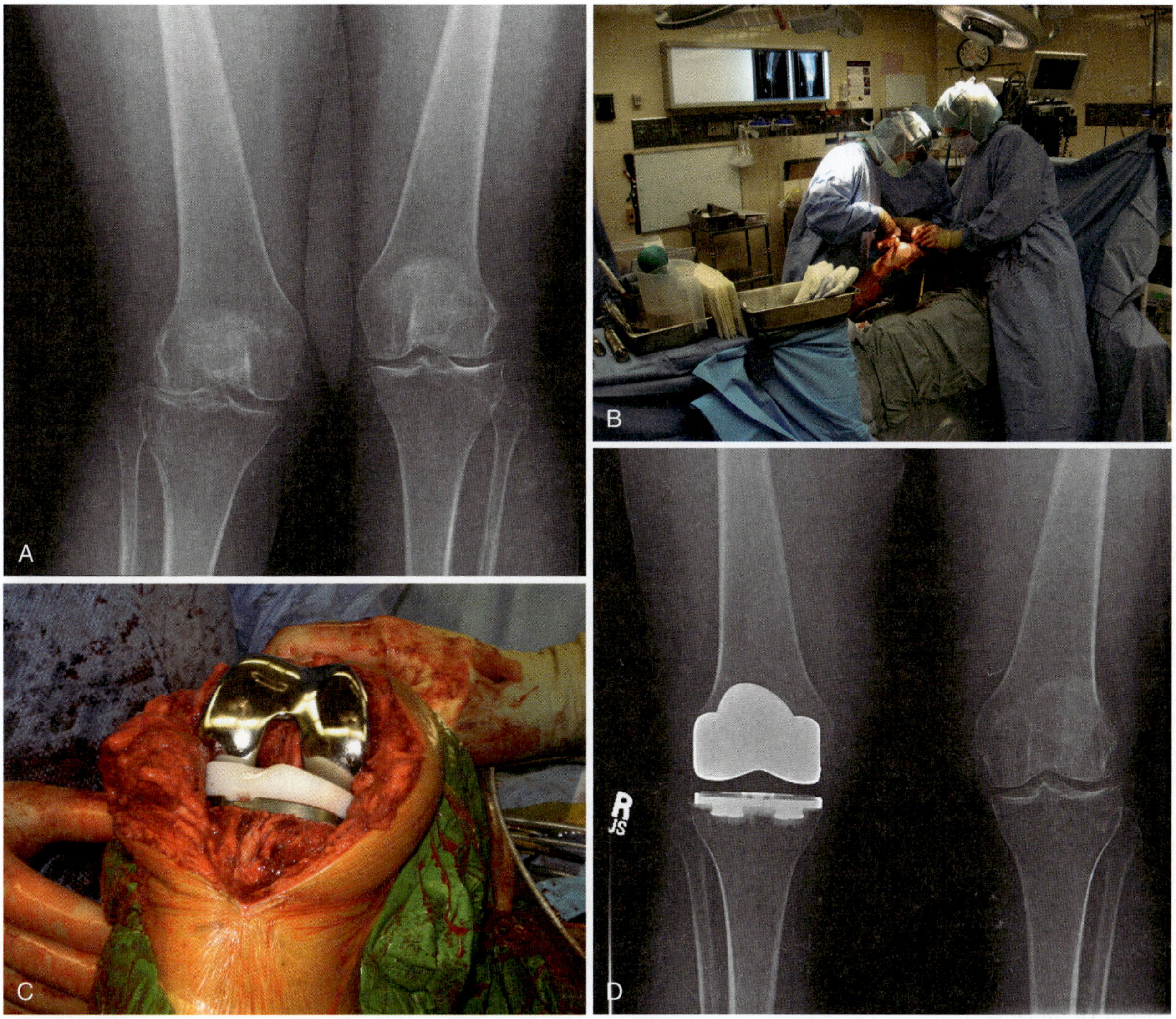

FIGURE 15-37 **A,** X-ray of knees showing **osteoarthritis** in right knee. **B,** Patient undergoing **total knee replacement (TKR).** **C,** **Prosthetic device** in place. **D,** X-ray of knees after TKR. *(Courtesy Dr. Sidra Ezrahi and Dr. Dennis Burke, Massachusetts General Hospital, Boston.)*

IN PERSON

The following is a first-person narrative describing the experience of a woman of a "certain age" (in her words) who had a knee replacement procedure.

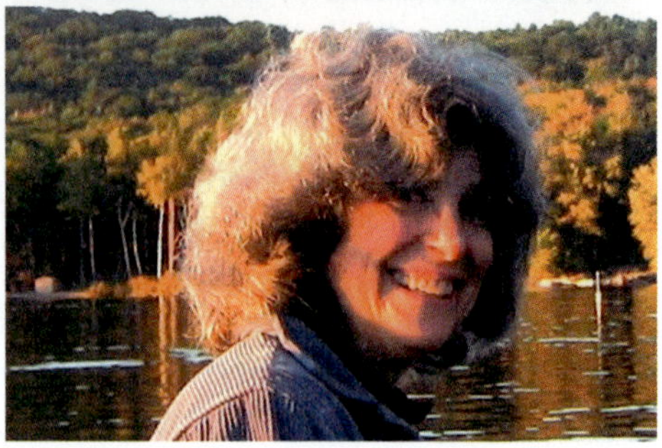

Writing about my TKR [total knee replacement] more than two years after the operation is a singular experience. The main advantage of the passage of time is that—unlike psychic trauma, which seems to make inroads in the very structure of our brains—the release of the body from physical pain leaves amnesia in its wake. If that were not the case, no woman would ever have a second child—and no biped a second knee replacement. I know, even if my body doesn't remember, that I endured much pain in the aftermath of the surgery and for many weeks thereafter. In fact, unlike most other physical ailments, joint replacement necessitates working through the pain in order to regain mobility. It's when you feel you simply cannot bend it any more that you "start" working. ... So the pain is actually functional, and rather relentless. And yet I know—and accept—that sometime in the not-too-distant future, my left knee will follow my right in seeking a replacement. And that is because the osteoarthritis that depleted the first is depleting the second, and all my glucosamine-chondroitin pills, my quad exercises, my frequent massages, and even my nightshade-free diet are at best only putting off by several months or a year the inevitable.

I had endured many years of diminishing mobility in my right leg, alleviated somewhat by occasional cortisone shots and two arthroscopic surgeries (while stitching the second arthroscopic wound, my Israeli orthopedist said, "Nothing more to be done with this one ... next stop: total knee replacement!') With all the research that I did in preparation for the Big Surgery, I became convinced—and still hold some version of this conviction—that TKR entails sawing the leg in two, like Houdini's blonde assistant in the box, and then screwing it back together with better screws. It didn't change that image much when my orthopedic surgeon at MGH [Massachusetts General Hospital], Dr. Dennis Burke, surely the best in his field in the universe, assured me that he is, in his spare time, a master carpenter. ...

Okay—as this narrative demonstrates, the truth is a bit more complex and less grotesque. Still the procedure is very radical and involves major trauma to all the supporting muscles, tendons, nerves, and blood vessels. Hence a long period of recuperation is involved. I took advantage of the extra day that was offered to me at MGH (bless Medicare!) for a total hospitalization of five days, during which I had to learn how to perform the most basic functions in new ways. I found, after many trials, that a walker is preferable to crutches. Both are hard on the hands but the walker is more stable, and the attachable basket is a boon.

For those of a "certain age" who are contemplating TKR, the question of where to do the rehab is crucial. If, as I did, you have the conditions to recover at home, that is preferable. The necessary conditions are, first, a partner or caregiver who is available 24/7 for the first few days and who doesn't decide to take a prolonged vacation after that ... The second relates to the physical conditions at home. Preferably the living area should all be on one level; although climbing stairs becomes one of the protocols of physical therapy, it takes a while to get to that point, and one is not very steady until that time. Easy access to bathrooms and to other living areas is crucial. The third necessary condition is the availability of the physical therapist. Living in the summer and fall months in rural New Hampshire, I was fortunate to qualify for the services of the local VNA [Visiting Nurse Association], and a marvelous physical therapist visited me three times a week for about six weeks. In between visits, I worked hard to win her approval and, although it seemed at first like tackling Everest to lift my leg even one inch off the floor, let alone walk, within about six weeks I could drive, even if I was getting around outside with crutches; within two months I had regained good mobility, and six months later I was as good as new, and ever so grateful. ...

Although I consider this procedure to be nothing short of miraculous, like any major elective surgery, one should not undertake it unless the pain of daily life outweighs its joys. ... when the doctors ask you about the pain, on a scale of 1 to 10, take them seriously. Don't undergo this surgery until it hovers around 8 or 9 ... And then—well, enjoy the results!

Sidra DeKoven Ezrahi is a professor of Comparative Literature at the Hebrew University and is a Guggenheim Fellow. She divides her time between Jerusalem, Israel and Wilmot, New Hampshire.

EXERCISES

Remember to check your answers carefully with the Answers to Exercises, page 638.

A Complete the following sentences.

1. Bones are composed of a type of connective tissue called ______________________ tissue.
2. Bone cells are called ______________________.
3. The bones of a fetus are composed mainly of ______________________.
4. Immature bone cells called ______________________ produce bony tissue.
5. Large bone cells called ______________________ digest bone tissue to shape the bone and smooth it out.
6. Mineral substances needed for bone development are ______________________ and ______________________.
7. Round, small bone covering the knee joint is a/an ______________________ bone.
8. Shaft of a long bone is the ______________________.
9. Ends of a long bone are the ______________________.
10. Cartilaginous area at the end of a long bone where growth takes place is the ______________________.
11. Red bone marrow is found in spongy or ______________________ bone.
12. Yellow bone marrow is composed of ______________________ tissue.
13. The strong membrane surrounding the surface of a bone is the ______________________.
14. Hard, dense bone tissue lying under the periosteum is ______________________.
15. A series of canals containing blood vessels lie within the outer dense tissue of bone and are called the______________________ canals.
16. A thin layer of cartilage covering the ends of bones at the joints is ______________________.
17. The ______________________ is a central, hollowed-out area in the shaft of long bones.
18. Two physicians who treat bones and bone diseases are a/an______________________ and a/an ______________________.
19. A practitioner who manipulates the patient's spinal column to relieve pressure on nerves is a/an ______________________.
20. Medical doctor who specializes in restoring patients to functional activity after injuries to bones, nerves, and muscles is a/an ______________________.

B **Match the following cranial and facial bones with their meanings as given below.**

ethmoid bone	maxilla	sphenoid bone
frontal bone	nasal bone	temporal bone
lacrimal bones	occipital bone	vomer
mandible	parietal bone	zygomatic bone

1. forms the roof and upper side parts of the skull ____________________
2. delicate bone, composed of spongy, cancellous tissue; supports the nasal cavity and orbits of the eye ____________________
3. forms the back and base of the skull ____________________
4. forms the forehead ____________________
5. bat-shaped bone extending behind the eyes to form the base of the skull ____________________
6. bone near the ear and connecting to the lower jaw ____________________
7. cheekbone ____________________
8. bone that supports the bridge of the nose ____________________
9. thin, flat bone forming the lower portion of the nasal septum ____________________
10. lower jawbone ____________________
11. upper jawbone ____________________
12. two paired bones, one located at the corner of each eye ____________________

15

C **Identify the following parts associated with a vertebra.** See Figure 15-7, page 586.

1. space through which the spinal cord passes ____________________
2. piece of cartilage between two vertebrae ____________________
3. posterior part of a vertebra ____________________
4. anterior part of a vertebra ____________________

D **Name the five divisions of the spinal column.**

1. ____________________
2. ____________________
3. ____________________
4. ____________________
5. ____________________

E **Give the medical names of the following bones.**

1. shoulder blade ______________________
2. upper arm bone ______________________
3. breastbone ______________________
4. thigh bone ______________________
5. finger bones ______________________
6. hand bones ______________________
7. forearm bone (little finger side) ______________________
8. forearm bone (thumb side) ______________________
9. collar bone ______________________
10. wrist bones ______________________
11. backbone ______________________
12. kneecap ______________________
13. shin bone (larger of two lower leg bones) ______________________
14. smaller of two lower leg bones ______________________
15. three parts of the pelvis ______________, ______________, and ______________
16. midfoot bones ______________________

F **Give the meanings of the following terms associated with bones.**

1. foramen magnum ______________________
2. calcaneus ______________________
3. acromion ______________________
4. xiphoid process ______________________
5. lamina ______________________
6. malleolus ______________________
7. acetabulum ______________________
8. pubic symphysis ______________________
9. olecranon ______________________
10. fontanelle ______________________
11. mastoid process ______________________
12. styloid process ______________________

G Give the meanings of the following terms.

1. osteogenesis ______
2. hypercalcemia ______
3. spondylosis ______
4. epiphyseal ______
5. decalcification ______
6. ossification ______
7. osteitis ______
8. costoclavicular ______

H Build medical terms for the following definitions.

1. pertaining to the shoulder blade ______
2. instrument to cut the skull ______
3. pertaining to the upper arm bone ______
4. pertaining to below the kneecap ______
5. softening of cartilage ______
6. pertaining to a toe bone ______
7. removal of hand bones ______
8. pertaining to the shin bone ______
9. pertaining to the heel bone ______
10. poor bone development ______
11. removal of the lamina of the vertebral arch ______
12. pertaining to the sacrum and ilium ______

I Give medical terms for the following.

1. formation of bone marrow ______________________
2. clubfoot ______________________
3. humpback ______________________
4. high levels of calcium in the blood ______________________
5. benign tumors arising from the bone surface ______________________
6. brittle bone disease ______________________
7. lateral curvature of the spine ______________________
8. anterior curvature of the spine ______________________
9. forward slipping (subluxation) of a vertebra over a lower vertebra ______________________
10. instrument to cut bone ______________________

J Give the meanings of the following terms.

1. osteoporosis ______________________
2. osteomyelitis ______________________
3. osteogenic sarcoma ______________________
4. crepitus ______________________
5. osteomalacia ______________________
6. abscess ______________________
7. osteopenia ______________________
8. Ewing sarcoma ______________________
9. metastatic bone lesion ______________________
10. compound fracture ______________________
11. simple fracture ______________________
12. open reduction ______________________

K Complete the following sentences.

1. Immovable joint, as in the skull bones, is called a ______________________.
2. Connective tissue that binds muscles to bones is a/an ______________________.
3. Another term for a joint is a/an ______________________.
4. Connective tissue that binds bones to other bones is a/an ______________________.
5. Fluid found in a joint is called ______________________.
6. The membrane that lines the joint cavity is the ______________________.
7. Sac of fluid near a joint is a/an ______________________.
8. Smooth cartilage that covers the surface of bones at joints is ______________________.
9. Surgical repair of a joint is called ______________________.
10. Inflammation surrounding a joint is known as ______________________.

L Complete the following terms based on the definitions provided.

1. inflammation of a tendon: ______________________itis
2. tumor (benign) of cartilage: ______________________oma
3. tumor (malignant) of cartilage: ______________________oma
4. incision of a joint: arthr______________________
5. softening of cartilage: chondro______________________
6. abnormal condition of blood in the joint: ______________________osis
7. inflammation of a sac of fluid near the joint: ______________________itis
8. doctor who specializes in treatment of joint disorders: ______________________logist
9. abnormal condition of a stiffened, immobile joint: ______________________osis
10. suture of a tendon: ten______________________

M Select from the following terms to name the abnormal conditions described below.

achondroplasia	dislocation	osteoarthritis
ankylosing spondylitis	ganglion cyst	rheumatoid arthritis
bunion	gouty arthritis	systemic lupus erythematosus
carpal tunnel syndrome	Lyme disease	tenosynovitis

1. an inherited condition in which the bones of the arms and the legs fail to grow normally because of a defect in cartilage and bone formation; type of dwarfism ____________________
2. degenerative joint disease; chronic inflammation of bones and joints ____________________
3. inflammation of joints caused by excessive uric acid in the body (hyperuricemia) ____________________
4. chronic joint disease; inflamed and painful joints owing to autoimmune reaction against normal joint tissue, and synovial membranes become swollen and thickened ____________________
5. tick-borne bacterium causes this condition marked by arthritis, myalgia, malaise, and neurologic and cardiac symptoms ____________________
6. abnormal swelling of a metatarsophalangeal joint ____________________
7. cystic mass arising from a tendon in the wrist ____________________
8. chronic, progressive arthritis with stiffening of joints, especially of the spine (vertebrae) ____________________
9. chronic inflammatory disease affecting not only the joints but also the skin (butterfly rash on the face), kidneys, heart, and lungs ____________________
10. inflammation of a tendon sheath ____________________
11. compression of the median nerve in the wrist as it passes through an area between a ligament tendons, bones, and connective tissue ____________________
12. displacement of a bone from its joint ____________________

N Give the meanings of the following terms.

1. subluxation ____________________
2. arthrodesis ____________________
3. pyrexia ____________________
4. podagra ____________________
5. sciatica ____________________

6. herniation of an intervertebral disk ________________
7. laminectomy ________________
8. sprain ________________
9. strain ________________
10. hyperuricemia ________________
11. fasciotomy ________________

O Circle the term that best fits the given definition.

1. fibrous membrane separating and enveloping muscles: **(fascia, flexion)**
2. movement away from the midline of the body: **(abduction, adduction)**
3. connection of the muscle to a stationary bone: **(insertion, origin)** of the muscle
4. connection of the muscle to a bone that moves: **(insertion, origin)** of the muscle
5. muscle that is connected to internal organs; involuntary muscle: **(skeletal, visceral)** muscle
6. muscle that is connected to bones; voluntary muscle: **(skeletal, visceral)** muscle
7. pain of many muscles: **(myositis, polymyalgia)**
8. pertaining to heart muscle: **(myocardial, myasthenia)**
9. process of recording electricity within muscles: **(muscle biopsy, electromyography)**
10. increase in development (size) of an organ or tissue: **(hypertrophy, atrophy)**

15

P Match the term for muscle action in Column I with its meaning in Column II. Write the letter of your answer in the space provided.

COLUMN I		COLUMN II
1. extension	_______	A. movement away from the midline
2. rotation	_______	B. turning the palm down
3. flexion	_______	C. turning the palm up
4. adduction	_______	D. straightening out a limb or joint
5. supination	_______	E. bending the sole of the foot downward
6. abduction	_______	F. circular movement around an axis
7. pronation	_______	G. bending a limb
8. dorsiflexion	_______	H. movement toward the midline
9. plantar flexion	_______	I. backward (upward) bending of the foot

Q Give the meanings of the following abnormal conditions affecting muscles.

1. leiomyosarcoma ______________________
2. rhabdomyoma ______________________
3. polymyositis ______________________
4. fibromyalgia ______________________
5. muscular dystrophy ______________________
6. myasthenia gravis ______________________
7. amyotrophic lateral sclerosis ______________________
8. sarcopenia ______________________

R Match the term in Column I with its meaning in Column II. Write the letter of your answer in the space provided.

COLUMN I

1. antinuclear antibody test ______
2. serum creatine kinase ______
3. uric acid test ______
4. rheumatoid factor test ______
5. bone scan ______
6. muscle biopsy ______
7. arthroscopy ______
8. acetylcholine ______
9. calcium ______
10. arthrography ______

COLUMN II

A. Radioactive substance is injected and traced in dense, hard connective tissue.
B. Chemical found in myoneural space.
C. Test for presence of an antibody found in the serum of patients with rheumatoid arthritis.
D. Substance necessary for proper bone development.
E. Visual examination of a joint.
F. Test tells if patient has gouty arthritis.
G. Test tells if patient has systemic lupus erythematosus.
H. Removal of soft connective tissue for microscopic examination.
I. Process of taking x-ray pictures of a joint.
J. Elevated blood levels of this enzyme are found in muscular disorders.

15

S Circle the term that best completes the meaning of the sentence.

1. Selma, a 40-year-old secretary, had been complaining of wrist pain with tingling sensations in her fingers for months. Dr. Ayres diagnosed her condition as **(osteomyelitis, rheumatoid arthritis, carpal tunnel syndrome)**.
2. Bill was a marathon runner who developed compartment syndrome in his left lower leg (calf). He had severe pain, and his orthopedist recommended **(tenorrhaphy, arthroplasty, fasciotomy)** to cut through the fibrous connective tissue and relieve pressure. A skin graft was needed later to close the wound.
3. Sally was experiencing chronic muscle pain and stiffness in her shoulder, back, knees, and hips. Most of all she was very tired all the time. Her doctor diagnosed her condition as **(myasthenia gravis, fibromyalgia, sarcopenia)** and prescribed medication for fatigue and pain plus physical therapy.

4. Paul had a skiing accident and tore ligaments in his knee. Dr. Miller recommended **(electromyography, hypertrophy, arthroscopic surgery)** to repair the ligaments.

5. For several months after her first pregnancy Elsie noticed a red rash on her face and cheeks. Her joints were giving her pain and she had a slight fever. Her ANA was elevated and her doctor suspected that she had **(SLE, polymyositis, muscular dystrophy)**.

6. David injured his left knee while playing basketball. He was scheduled for arthroscopic repair of his **(ACL, SLE, TMJ)**. However, because of his height and the length of the ligament, his **(rheumatologist, orthopedist, chiropractor)** decided to do "open" surgery.

7. James has significant lower back pain radiating down his left leg. This condition is called **(fibromyalgia, sciatica, talipes)**. MRI shows an intervertebral **(disk, bunion, exostosis)** impinging on spinal nerves at the **(L5–S1, C2–C3, T3–T5)** level. Bed rest produced no improvement. His orthopedist decided to perform a **(tenorrhaphy, microdiskectomy, bunionectomy)** to relieve pressure on his nerves.

8. Bruce spent 2 weeks hiking and vacationing on Nantucket Island. A week later he developed a "bull's-eye" rash on his chest (from a tick bite), fever, muscle pain, and a swollen, tender right ankle. His physician ordered a blood test that revealed **(antigens, antibodies)** to a spirochete bacterium. The physician told Bruce he had contracted **(ankylosing spondylitis, polymyositis, Lyme disease)**.

9. Scott likes to eat rich food. Lately he has noticed pain and tenderness in his right toe, called **(talipes, podagra, rickets)**, and also hard, lumpy deposits over his elbows. His doctor orders a serum uric acid test; the result is abnormally high, revealing **(hemarthrosis, hyperuricemia, hypercalcemia)**, consistent with a diagnosis of **(rheumatoid arthritis, gouty arthritis, osteoarthritis)**.

10. Sara, a 70-year-old widow, has persistent midback pain, and her **(CXR, ESR, EMG)** shows compression fractures of her **(scapula, femur, vertebrae)** and thinning of her bones. A bone density scan confirms the diagnosis of **(osteomyelitis, osteomalacia, osteoporosis)**, and her doctor prescribes calcium, vitamin D, and Fosamax.

T Give meanings for the abbreviations in Column I. Then select the letter in Column II of the best association for each.

COLUMN I

1. ROM ____________ ______
2. NSAID ____________ ______
3. TMJ ____________ ______
4. EMG ____________ ______
5. ACL ____________ ______
6. SLE ____________ ______
7. C1 to C5 ____________ ______
8. T1 to T12 ____________ ______
9. THR ____________ ______
10. ORIF ____________ ______

COLUMN II

A. Connection between the lower jawbone and a bone of the skull
B. Band of fibrous tissue connecting bones in the knee
C. Bones of the spinal column in the chest region
D. Test of strength of electrical transmission within muscle
E. This autoimmune disease affects joints, skin, and other body tissues
F. Measurement in degrees of a circle assesses the extent a joint can be flexed or extended
G. Bones of the spinal column in the neck region
H. Drug used to treat joint diseases
I. Procedure to repair compound fracture
J. Arthroplasty

U **Match the images in Figure 15-38 with the descriptions below, and give a medical term for the abnormal condition.**

1. Children who are born with a condition of muscle deterioration and wasting have winged scapulae ____________________
2. Children are born with this deformity of the talus ____________________
3. This deformity is often the result of a chronic, inflammatory, autoimmune disorder that affects joints, leading to bony ankylosis and inflamed, thickened synovial membranes ____________________
4. Bleeding disorders can lead to this accumulation of blood in and around a joint ____________________
5. Inflammation of a bursa causes this abnormality ____________________
6. Fluid-filled cyst arising from joint capsules or tendons ____________________

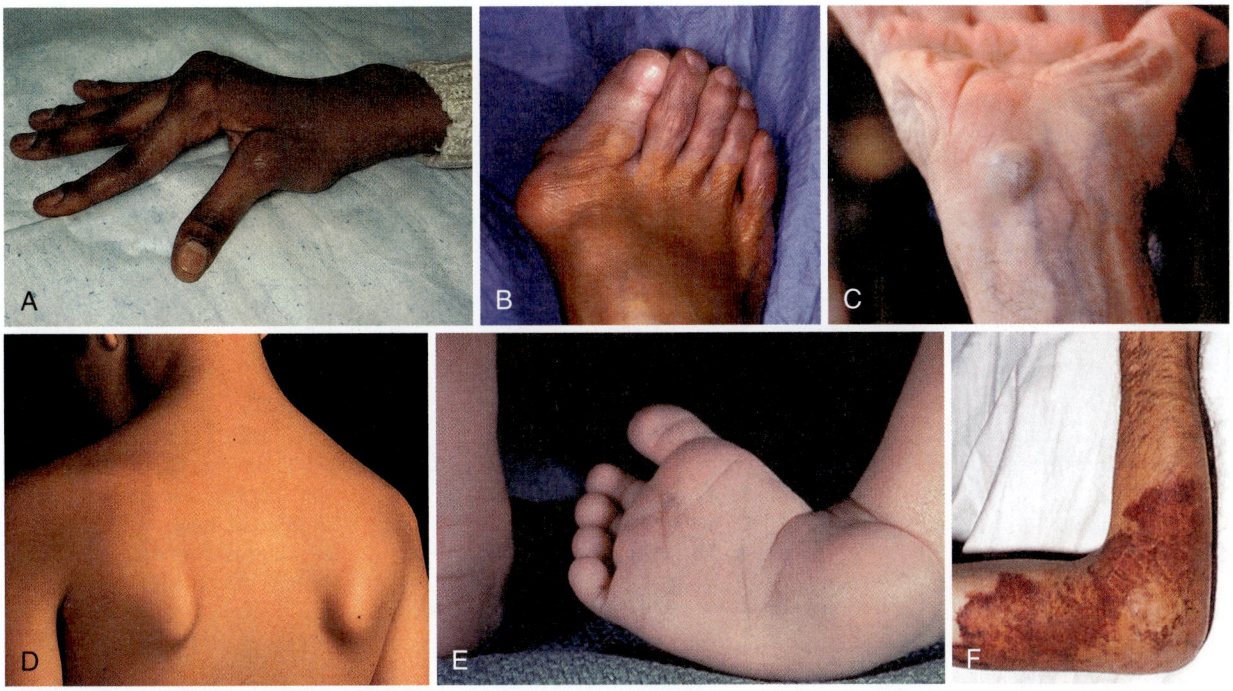

FIGURE 15-38 ***A,*** *From Swartz MH: Textbook of Physical Diagnosis, History and Examination, 5th ed., Philadelphia, Saunders, 2006;* ***B*** *and* ***E,*** *from Canale ST, Beaty JH: Campbell's Operative Orthopaedics, 11th ed., St. Louis, Mosby, 2008;* ***C,*** *Courtesy Dr. Nouna M. Simon;* ***D,*** *from Zitelli BJ, Davis HW: Atlas of Pediatric Physical Diagnosis, 5th ed., St. Louis, Mosby, 2007;* ***F,*** *from Moll JMH: Rheumatology, 2nd ed., London, Churchill Livingstone, 1997.*

15

ANSWERS TO EXERCISES

A

1. osseous
2. osteocytes
3. cartilage
4. osteoblasts
5. osteoclasts
6. calcium and phosphorus
7. sesamoid
8. diaphysis
9. epiphyses
10. epiphyseal plate
11. cancellous or trabecular
12. fat
13. periosteum
14. compact bone
15. haversian
16. articular cartilage
17. medullary cavity
18. orthopedist and osteopath
19. chiropractor
20. physiatrist

B

1. parietal bone
2. ethmoid bone
3. occipital bone
4. frontal bone
5. sphenoid bone
6. temporal bone
7. zygomatic bone
8. nasal bone
9. vomer
10. mandible
11. maxilla
12. lacrimal bones

C

1. neural canal
2. intervertebral disk
3. vertebral arch
4. vertebral body

D

1. cervical
2. thoracic
3. lumbar
4. sacral
5. coccygeal

E

1. scapula
2. humerus
3. sternum
4. femur
5. phalanges
6. metacarpals
7. ulna
8. radius
9. clavicle
10. carpals
11. vertebral column
12. patella
13. tibia
14. fibula
15. ilium, ischium, pubis
16. metatarsals

F

1. opening of the occipital bone through which the spinal cord passes
2. heel bone; largest of the tarsal bones
3. lateral extension of the scapula
4. lower portion of the sternum
5. portion of the vertebral arch
6. the bulge on either side of the ankle joint; the lower end of the fibula is the lateral malleolus, and the lower end of the tibia is the medial malleolus
7. depression in the pelvis into which the femur fits
8. area of convergence of the two pubis bones, at the midline
9. bony process at the proximal end of the ulna; elbow joint
10. soft spot between the bones of the skull in an infant
11. round process on the temporal bone behind the ear
12. pole-like process projecting downward from the temporal bone

G

1. formation of bone; osteogenesis imperfecta is known as brittle bone disease
2. excessive calcium in the blood
3. abnormal condition of the vertebrae; degenerative changes in the spine
4. pertaining to the epiphysis
5. removal of calcium from bones
6. formation of bone
7. inflammation of bone; osteitis deformans (Paget disease) causes deformed bones such as an enlarged skull
8. pertaining to the ribs and clavicle

H

1. scapular
2. craniotome
3. humeral
4. subpatellar
5. chondromalacia
6. phalangeal
7. metacarpectomy
8. tibial
9. calcaneal
10. osteodystrophy
11. laminectomy
12. sacroiliac

I

1. myelopoiesis
2. talipes
3. kyphosis
4. hypercalcemia
5. exostoses
6. osteogenesis imperfecta
7. scoliosis
8. lordosis
9. spondylolisthesis
10. osteotome

J

1. increased porosity in bone; decrease in bone density
2. inflammation of bone and bone marrow
3. cancerous tumor of bone; osteoblasts multiply at the ends of long bones
4. crackling sensation as broken bones move against each other
5. softening of bones; rickets in children due to loss of calcium in bones
6. collection of pus
7. deficiency of bone; precursor of osteoporosis
8. malignant tumor of bone in children, often involving the entire shaft of a long bone
9. malignant tumor that has spread to bone from the breast, lung, kidney, or prostate gland
10. break in bone with wound in skin
11. break in bone without wound in skin
12. bone is put in proper place after incision of the skin

K

1. suture joint; a synovial joint is a freely movable joint
2. tendon
3. articulation
4. ligament
5. synovial fluid
6. synovial membrane
7. bursa
8. articular cartilage
9. arthroplasty
10. periarthritis

L

1. tendinitis or tendonitis
2. chondroma
3. chondrosarcoma
4. arthrotomy
5. chondromalacia
6. hemarthrosis
7. bursitis
8. rheumatologist
9. ankylosis
10. tenorrhaphy

M

1. achondroplasia
2. osteoarthritis
3. gouty arthritis
4. rheumatoid arthritis
5. Lyme disease
6. bunion
7. ganglion cyst
8. ankylosing spondylitis
9. systemic lupus erythematosus
10. tenosynovitis
11. carpal tunnel syndrome
12. dislocation

N

1. partial or incomplete displacement of a bone from the joint
2. surgical fixation of a joint (binding it together by fusing the joint surfaces)
3. fever; increase in body temperature
4. pain in a big toe from gouty arthritis
5. pain radiating from the back to the leg (along the sciatic nerve); most commonly caused by a protruding intervertebral disk
6. protrusion of a disk into the neural canal or the spinal nerves
7. removal of a portion of the vertebral arch (lamina) to relieve pressure from a protruding intervertebral disk
8. trauma to a joint with pain, swelling, and injury to ligaments
9. overstretching of a muscle
10. high levels of uric acid in the bloodstream; present in gouty arthritis
11. incision of fascia

O

1. fascia
2. abduction
3. origin of the muscle
4. insertion of the muscle
5. visceral muscle
6. skeletal muscle
7. polymyalgia
8. myocardial
9. electromyography
10. hypertrophy

P

1. D
2. F
3. G
4. H
5. C
6. A
7. B
8. I
9. E

Q

1. malignant tumor of smooth (involuntary, visceral) muscle
2. benign tumor of striated (voluntary, skeletal) muscle
3. inflammation of many muscles; polymyositis rheumatica is a chronic inflammatory condition causing muscle weakness and pain
4. pain of muscle and fibrous tissue (especially of the back); also called fibrositis or rheumatism
5. group of inherited muscular diseases marked by progressive weakness and degeneration of muscles without nerve involvement
6. loss of strength of muscles (often with paralysis) because of a defect at the connection between the nerve and the muscle cell
7. muscles degenerate (paralysis occurs) owing to degeneration of nerves in the spinal cord and lower region of the brain; Lou Gehrig disease
8. deficiency of flesh (muscle mass)

R

1. G
2. J
3. F
4. C
5. A
6. H
7. E
8. B
9. D
10. I

S

1. carpal tunnel syndrome
2. fasciotomy
3. fibromyalgia
4. arthroscopic surgery
5. SLE
6. ACL; orthopedist
7. sciatica; disk; L5–S1; microdiskectomy
8. antibodies; Lyme disease
9. podagra; hyperuricemia; gouty arthritis
10. CXR; vertebrae; osteoporosis

T

1. range of motion: F
2. nonsteroidal anti-inflammatory drug: H
3. temporomandibular joint: A
4. electromyography: D
5. anterior cruciate ligament: B
6. systemic lupus erythematosus: E
7. first cervical vertebra to fifth cervical vertebra: G
8. first thoracic vertebra to twelfth thoracic vertebra: C
9. total hip replacement: J
10. open reduction, internal fixation: I

15

U

1. D: winged scapulae in muscular dystrophy
2. E: clubfoot—talipes
3. A: rheumatoid arthritis
4. F: hemarthrosis
5. B: bunion
6. C: ganglion cyst

Answers to Practical Applications

Operating Room Schedule

1. D
2. F
3. G
4. B
5. A
6. C
7. H
8. E

PRONUNCIATION OF TERMS

To test your understanding of the terminology in this chapter, write the meaning of each term in the space provided. In addition, you may wish to cover the terms and write them by looking at your definitions. Make sure your spelling is correct. The page number after each term indicates where it is defined or used in the book, so you can easily check your responses. You will find complete definitions for all of these terms and their audio pronunciations on the Evolve website.

Pronunciation Guide

ā as in āpe	ă as in ăpple
ē as in ēven	ĕ as in ĕvery
ī as in īce	ĭ as in ĭnterest
ō as in ōpen	ŏ as in pŏt
ū as in ūnit	ŭ as in ŭnder

Terms Related to Bones

TERM	PRONUNCIATION	MEANING
acetabular (596)	ă-cĕ-TĂB-ū-lăr	
acetabulum (592)	ăs-ĕ-TĂB-ū-lŭm	
acromion (592)	ă-KRŌ-mē-ŏn	
articular cartilage (592)	ăr-TĬK-ū-lăr KĂR-tĭ-lăj	
bone (592)	BŌN	
bone depression (592)	BŌN dē-PRĔ-shŭn	
bone process (592)	BŌN PRŎ-sĕs	
calcaneal (596)	kăl-KĀ-nē-ăl	
calcaneus (596)	kăl-KĀ-nē-ŭs	
calcium (592)	KĂL-sē-ŭm	
cancellous bone (592)	KĂN-sĕ-lŭs bōn	
carpals (596)	KĂR-pălz	
cartilage (592)	KĂR-tĭ-lĭj	
cervical vertebrae (587)	SĔR-vĭ-kăl VĔR-tĕ-brā	
chondrocostal (597)	kŏn-drō-KŎS-tăl	
clavicle (597)	KLĂV-ĭ-kl	
coccyx (587)	KŎK-sĭks	
collagen (592)	KŎL-ă-jĕn	
compact bone (592)	KŎM-păkt bōn	
cranial bones (592)	KRĀ-nē-ăl bōnz	
craniotome (597)	KRĀ-nē-ō-tōm	
craniotomy (597)	krā-nē-ŎT-ō-mē	

15

TERM	PRONUNCIATION	MEANING
crepitus (599)	KRĚP-ĭ-tŭs	
decalcification (594)	dē-kăl-sĭ-fĭ-KĀ-shŭn	
diaphysis (592)	dī-ĂF-ĭ-sĭs	
disk (592)	dĭsk	
epiphyseal plate (592)	ĕp-ĭ-FĬZ-ē-ăl plāt	
epiphysis (592)	ĕ-PĬF-ĭ-sĭs	
ethmoid bone (583)	ĔTH-moyd bōn	
Ewing sarcoma (598)	Ū-ĭng săr-KŌ-mă	
exostosis (598)	ĕk-sŏs-TŌ-sĭs	
facial bones (592)	FĀ-shăl bōnz	
femoral (597)	FĔM-ŏr-ăl	
femur (597)	FĒ-mŭr	
fibula (597)	FĬB-ū-lă	
fibular (597)	FĬB-ū-lăr	
fontanelle (592)	fŏn-tă-NĔL	
foramen magnum (592)	fōr-Ā-mĕn MĂG-nŭm	
fracture (599)	FRĂK-shur	
frontal bone (583)	FRŎN-tăl bōn	
haversian canals (593)	hă-VĔR-zhăn kă-NĂLZ	
humeral (597)	HŪ-mĕr-ăl	
humerus (597)	HŪ-mĕr-ŭs	
hypercalcemia (594)	hī-pĕr-kăl-SĒ-mē-ă	
iliac (597)	ĬL-ē-ăk	
ilium (597)	ĬL-ē-ŭm	
ischial (597)	ĬSH-ē-ăl *or* ĬS-kē-ăl	
ischium (597)	ĬSH-ē-ŭm *or* ĬS-kē-ŭm	
kyphosis (594)	kī-FŌ-sĭs	
lacrimal bones (584)	LĂ-krĭ-măl bōnz	
lamina (586)	LĂM-ĭ-nă	
laminectomy (594)	lăm-ĭ-NĔK-tō-mē	
lordosis (594)	lŏr-DŌ-sĭs	

TERM	PRONUNCIATION	MEANING
lumbar vertebrae (587)	LŬM-băr VĔR-tĕ-brā	______
lumbosacral (595)	lŭm-bō-SĀ-krăl	______
malleolar (597)	mă-LĒ-ō-lăr	______
malleolus (593)	măl-LĒ-ō-lŭs	______
mandible (597)	MĂN-dĭ-bl	______
mandibular (597)	măn-DĬB-ū-lăr	______
manubrium (593)	mă-NOO-brē-ŭm	______
mastoid process (593)	MĂS-toyd PRŎS-ĕs	______
maxilla (597)	măk-SĬL-ă	______
maxillary (597)	măk-sĭ-LĂR-ē	______
medullary cavity (593)	MĔD-ū-lăr-ē KĂ-vĭ-tē	______
metacarpals (597)	mĕt-ă-KĂR-pălz	______
metacarpectomy (597)	mĕt-ă-kăr-PĔK-tō-mē	______
metaphysis (593)	mĕ-TĂ-fĭ-sĭs	______
metatarsalgia (597)	mĕt-ă-tăr-SĂL-jă	______
metatarsals (597)	mĕt-ă-TĂR-sălz	______
myelopoiesis (595)	mī-ĕ-lō-poy-Ē-sĭs	______
nasal bones (584)	NĀ-zăl bōnz	______
occipital bone (583)	ŏk-SĬP-ĭ-tăl bōn	______
olecranal (597)	ō-LĔK-ră-năl	______
olecranon (593)	ō-LĔK-ră-nŏn	______
orthopedics (595)	ŏr-thō-PĒ-dĭks	______
osseous tissue (593)	ŎS-ē-ŭs TĬSH-ū	______
ossification (593)	ŏs-ĭ-fĭ-KĀ-shŭn	______
osteitis (595)	ŏs-tē-Ī-tĭs	______
osteoblast (593)	ŎS-tē-ō-blăst	______
osteoclast (593)	ŎS-tē-ō-klăst	______
osteodystrophy (595)	ŏs-tē-ō-DĬS-trō-fē	______
osteogenesis imperfecta (595)	ŏs-tē-ō-JĔN-ĕ-sĭs ĭm-pĕr-FĔK-tă	______
osteogenic sarcoma (600)	ŏs-tē-ō-JĔN-ĭk săr-KŌ-mă	______

15

TERM	PRONUNCIATION	MEANING
osteomalacia (600)	ŏs-tē-ō-mă-LĀ-shă	____________
osteomyelitis (600)	ŏs-tē-ō-mī-ĕ-LĪ-tĭs	____________
osteopenia (600)	ŏs-tē-ō-PĒ-nē-ă	____________
osteoporosis (600)	ŏs-tē-ō-pŏr-Ō-sĭs	____________
osteotome (596)	ŎS-tē-ō-tōm	____________
parietal bone (583)	pă-RĪ-ĕ-tăl bōn	____________
patella (597)	pă-TĔL-ă	____________
pelvimetry (597)	pĕl-VĬM-ĕ-trē	____________
periosteum (593)	pĕ-rē-ŎS-tē-ŭm	____________
peroneal (598)	pĕr-ō-NĒ-ăl	____________
phalangeal (598)	fă-lăn-JĒ-ăl	____________
phalanges (598)	fă-LĂN-jēz	____________
phosphorus (593)	FŎS-fō-rŭs	____________
physiatrist (593)	fĭ-ZĪ-ă-trĭst	____________
pubic (598)	PŪ-bĭk	____________
pubic symphysis (593)	PŪ-bĭk SĬM-fĭ-sĭs	____________
pubis (598)	PŪ-bĭs	____________
radial (598)	RĀ-dē-ăl	____________
radius (598)	RĀ-dē-ŭs	____________
red bone marrow (593)	rĕd bōn MĂ-rō	____________
reduction (599)	rĕ-DŬK-shŭn	____________
ribs (593)	rĭbz	____________
sacral vertebrae (587)	SĀ-krăl VĔR-tĕ-brā	____________
scapula (598)	SKĂP-ū-lă	____________
scapular (598)	SKĂP-ŭ-lăr	____________
scoliosis (595)	skō-lē-Ō-sĭs	____________
sella turcica (593)	SĔ-lă TŬR-sĭ-kă	____________
sinus (593)	SĪ-nŭs	____________
sphenoid bone (583)	SFĒ-noyd bōn	____________
spondylolisthesis (596)	spŏn-dĭ-lō-lĭs-THĒ-sĭs	____________
spondylosis (596)	spŏn-dĭ-LŌ-sĭs	____________

TERM	PRONUNCIATION	MEANING
sternum (598)	STĔR-nŭm	
styloid process (593)	STĪ-loyd PRŎS-ĕs	
subcostal (597)	sŭb-KŎS-tăl	
supraclavicular (597)	soo-pră-klă-VĬK-ū-lăr	
suture (593)	SŪ-tŭr	
talipes (602)	TĂL-ĭ-pēz	
tarsals (598)	TĂR-sălz	
tarsectomy (598)	tăr-SĔK-tō-mē	
temporal bone (583)	TĔM-pōr-ăl bōn	
temporomandibular joint (593)	tĕm-pŏr-ō-măn-DĬB-ŭ-lăr joynt	
thoracic vertebrae (587)	thō-RĂS-ĭk VĔR-tĕ-brā	
tibia (598)	TĬB-ē-ă	
tibial (598)	TĬB-ē-ăl	
trabeculae (593)	tră-BĔK-ū-lē	
ulna (598)	ŬL-nă	
ulnar (598)	ŬL-năr	
vertebra; vertebrae (593)	VĔR-tĕ-bră; VĔR-tĕ-brā	
vertebroplasty (596)	vĕr-TĒ-brō-plăs-tē	
vomer (584)	VŌ-mĕr	
xiphoid process (593)	ZĬF-oyd PRŎS-ĕs	
yellow bone marrow (593)	YĔ-lō bōn MĂ-rō	
zygomatic bones (584)	zī-gō-MĂ-tĭk bōnz	

Terms Related to Joints and Muscles

TERM	PRONUNCIATION	MEANING
abduction (614)	ăb-DŬK-shŭn	
achondroplasia (604)	ā-kŏn-drō-PLĀ-zē-ă	
adduction (614)	ă-DŬK-shŭn	
amyotrophic lateral sclerosis (616)	ā-mī-ō-TRŌ-fĭk LĂT-ĕr-ăl sklĕ-RŌ-sĭs	

15

TERM	PRONUNCIATION	MEANING
ankylosing spondylitis (606)	ăng-kĭ-LŌ-sĭng spŏn-dĭ-LĪ-tĭs	
ankylosis (604)	ăng-kĭ-LŌ-sĭs	
arthrodesis (605)	ăr-thrō-DĒ-sĭs	
arthrotomy (604)	ăr-THRŎT-ō-mē	
articular cartilage (603)	ăr-TĬK-ū-lăr KĂR-tĭ-lĭj	
articulation (603)	ăr-tĭk-ū-LĀ-shŭn	
atrophy (616)	ĂT-rō-fē	
bunion (607)	BŬN-yŭn	
bursa; bursae (603)	BŬR-să; BŬR-sē	
bursitis (604)	bŭr-SĪ-tis	
carpal tunnel syndrome (608)	KĂR-păl TŬN-nĕl SĬN-drōm	
chondroma (604)	kŏn-DRŌ-mă	
chondromalacia (604)	kŏn-drō-mă-LĀ-shă	
dislocation (608)	dĭs-lō-KĀ-shŭn	
dorsiflexion (614)	dŏr-sē-FLĔK-shŭn	
extension (614)	ĕk-STĔN-shŭn	
fascia (614)	FĂSH-ē-ă	
fasciotomy (615)	făsh-e-ŎT-tō-mē	
fibromyalgia (615)	fī-brō-mī-ĂL-jă	
flexion (614)	FLĔK-shŭn	
ganglion cyst (608)	GĂNG-lē-ŏn sĭst	
gouty arthritis (606)	GŎW-tē ăr-THRĪ-tĭs	
hemarthrosis (604)	hĕm-ăr-THRŌ-sĭs	
herniation of a intervertebral disk (609)	hĕr-nē-Ā-shŭn of a ĭn-tĕr-vĕr-TĒ-brăl dĭsk	
hydrarthrosis (604)	hī-drăr-THRŌ-sĭs	
hypertrophy (616)	hī-PĔR-trō-fē	
hyperuricemia (606)	hī-pĕr-ŭr-ĭ-SĒ-mē-ă	
leiomyoma (615)	lī-ō-mī-Ō-mă	
leiomyosarcoma (615)	lī-ō-mī-ō-săr-KŌ-mă	

15

TERM	PRONUNCIATION	MEANING
ligament (603)	LĬG-ă-mĕnt	
ligamentous (604)	lĭg-ă-MĔN-tŭs	
Lyme disease (610)	līm dĭ-ZĒZ	
meniscus (603)	mĕ-NĬS-kŭs	
muscular dystrophy (617)	MŬS-kū-lăr DĬS-trŏ-fē	
myalgia (616)	mī-ĂL-jă	
myasthenia gravis (616)	mī-ăs-THĒ-nē-ă GRĂ-vĭs	
myopathy (616)	mī-ŎP-ă-thē	
myositis (616)	mī-ō-SĪ-tĭs	
osteoarthritis (606)	ŏs-tē-ō-ăr-THRĪ-tĭs	
plantar flexion (616)	PLĂN-tăr FLĔK-shun	
podagra (606)	pō-DĂG-ră	
polyarthritis (604)	pŏl-ē-ărth-RĪ-tĭs	
polymyalgia (617)	pŏl-ē-mī-ĂL-jă	
polymyositis (617)	pŏl-ē-mī-ō-SĪ-tĭs	
pronation (614)	prō-NĀ-shŭn	
pyrexia (606)	pī-RĔK-sē-ă	
rhabdomyoma (616)	răb-dō-mī-Ō-mă	
rhabdomyosarcoma (606)	răb-dō-mī-ō-săr-KŌ-mă	
rheumatoid arthritis (606)	ROO-mă-toyd ăr-THRĪ-tĭs	
rheumatologist (605)	roo-mă-TŎL-ō-jĭst	
rotation (614)	rō-TĀ-shŭn	
sarcopenia (616)	săr-kō-PĒ-nē-ă	
spinal stenosis (605)	SPĪ-năl stĕ-NŌ-sĭs	
sprain (610)	sprān	
strain (610)	strān	
striated muscle (614)	STRĪ-ā-tĕd MŬS-l	
subluxation (608)	sŭb-lŭk-SĀ-shŭn	
supination (614)	soo-pĭ-NĀ-shŭn	
suture joint (603)	SOO-chŭr joint	
synovial cavity (603)	sĭ-NŌ-vē-ăl KĂV-ĭ-tē	

15

TERM	PRONUNCIATION	MEANING
synovial fluid (603)	sĭ-NŌ-vē-ăl FLOO-ĭd	
synovial joint (603)	sĭ-NŌ-vē-ăl joint	
synovial membrane (603)	sĭ-NŌ-vē-ăl MĔM-brān	
synovitis (605)	sĭn-ō-VĪ-tĭs	
systemic lupus erythematosus (610)	sĭs-TĔM-ĭk LOO-pŭs ĕ-rĭ-thĕ-mă-TŌ-sŭs	
tendinitis (605)	tĕn-dĭ-NĪ-tĭs	
tendon (603)	TĔN-dŭn	
tenorrhaphy (605)	tĕn-ŎR-ă-fē	
tenosynovitis (605)	tĕn-ō-sī-nō-VĪ-tĭs	
visceral muscle (614)	VĬS-ĕr-ăl MŬS-l	

Laboratory Tests and Clinical Procedures

TERM	PRONUNCIATION	MEANING
antinuclear antibody test (617)	ăn-tē-NŪ-klē-ăr ĂN-tĭ-bŏd-ē tĕst	
arthrocentesis (618)	ăr-thrō-sĕn-TĒ-sĭs	
arthrography (618)	ăr-THRŎG-ră-fē	
arthroplasty (618)	ăr-thrō-PLĂS-tē	
arthroscopy (618)	ăr-THRŎS-kō-pē	
bone density test (619)	bōn DĔN-sĭ-tē tĕst	
bone scan (620)	bōn skăn	
diskography (620)	dĭsk-ŎG-ră-fē	
electromyography (620)	ē-lĕk-trō-mī-ŎG-ră-fē	
erythrocyte sedimentation rate (617)	ĕ-RĬTH-rō-sīt sĕd-ĭ-mĕn-TĀ-shŭn rāt	
muscle biopsy (620)	MŬS-l BĪ-ŏp-sē	
rheumatoid factor test (617)	ROO-mă-tŏyd FĂK-tŏr tĕst	
serum calcium (617)	SĔR-ŭm KĂL-sē-ŭm tĕst	
serum creatine kinase (617)	SĔR-ŭm KRĒ-ă-tĭn KĪ-nās	
uric acid test (618)	ŪR-ĭk ĂS-ĭd tĕst	

REVIEW SHEET

Write the meanings of the word parts in the spaces provided. Check your answers with the information in the chapter or in the Glossary (Medical Word Parts—English) at the end of the book.

Combining Forms

COMBINING FORM	MEANING	COMBINING FORM	MEANING
acetabul/o	______	ligament/o	______
ankyl/o	______	lord/o	______
arthr/o	______	lumb/o	______
articul/o	______	malleol/o	______
burs/o	______	mandibul/o	______
calc/o	______	maxill/o	______
calcane/o	______	metacarp/o	______
calci/o	______	metatars/o	______
carp/o	______	my/o	______
cervic/o	______	myel/o	______
chondr/o	______	myocardi/o	______
clavicul/o	______	myos/o	______
coccyg/o	______	olecran/o	______
cost/o	______	orth/o	______
crani/o	______	oste/o	______
fasci/o	______	patell/o	______
femor/o	______	ped/o	______
fibr/o	______	pelv/i	______
fibul/o	______	perone/o	______
humer/o	______	phalang/o	______
ili/o	______	plant/o	______
ischi/o	______	pub/o	______
kyph/o	______	radi/o	______
lamin/o	______	rhabdomy/o	______
leiomy/o	______	rheumat/o	______

COMBINING FORM	MEANING	COMBINING FORM	MEANING
sacr/o	________________	tars/o	________________
sarc/o	________________	ten/o	________________
scapul/o	________________	tendin/o	________________
scoli/o	________________	thorac/o	________________
spondyl/o	________________	tibi/o	________________
stern/o	________________	uln/o	________________
synov/o	________________	vertebr/o	________________

Suffixes

SUFFIX	MEANING	SUFFIX	MEANING
-algia	________________	-penia	________________
-asthenia	________________	-physis	________________
-blast	________________	-plasty	________________
-clast	________________	-porosis	________________
-desis	________________	-stenosis	________________
-emia	________________	-tome	________________
-listhesis	________________	-trophy	________________
-malacia	________________		

Prefixes

PREFIX	MEANING	PREFIX	MEANING
a-, an-	________________	hyper-	________________
ab-	________________	meta-	________________
ad-	________________	peri-	________________
dia-	________________	poly-	________________
dorsi-	________________	sub-	________________
epi-	________________	supra-	________________
exo-	________________	sym-	________________

evolve *Please refer to the Evolve website for additional exercises and images related to this chapter.*

CHAPTER 16

Skin

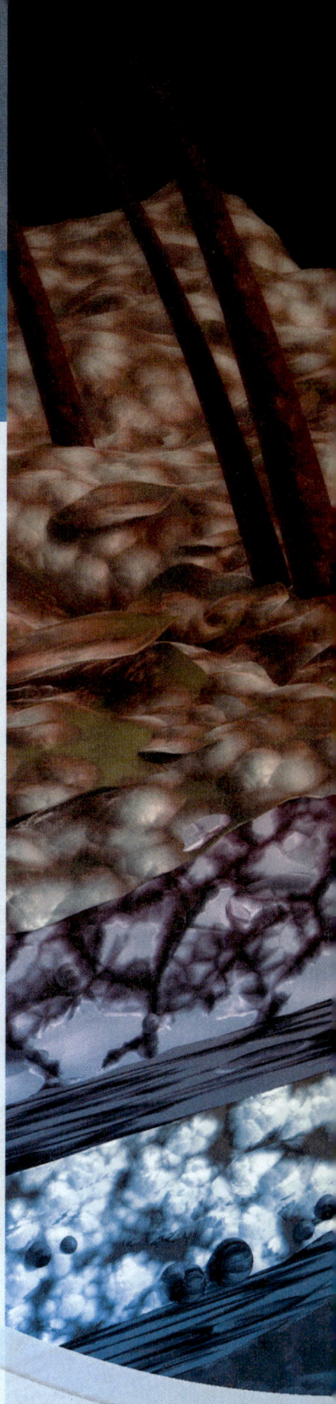

This chapter is divided into the following sections:

CHAPTER GOALS

- Name the layers of the skin and the accessory structures associated with the skin.
- Build medical words using the combining forms that are related to the specialty of dermatology.
- Identify lesions, signs and symptoms, and pathologic conditions that relate to the skin.
- Describe laboratory tests and clinical procedures that pertain to the skin, and recognize relevant abbreviations.
- Apply your new knowledge to understanding medical terms in their proper contexts, such as medical reports and records.

Introduction

The skin and its accessory structures (hair, nails, and glands) make up the **integumentary system** of the body. Integument means covering, and the skin (weighing 8 to 10 pounds and extending over an area of 22 square feet in an average adult) is the outer covering for the body. It is, however, more than a simple body covering. This complex system of specialized tissues contains glands that secrete several types of fluids, nerves that carry impulses, and blood vessels that aid in the regulation of the body temperature.

The skin has many important functions:

First, as a protective membrane over the entire body, the skin guards the deeper tissues of the body against excessive loss of water, salts, and heat and against invasion of pathogens and their toxins. Secretions from the skin are slightly acidic in nature, which contributes to the skin's ability to prevent bacterial invasion. Specialized cells (Langerhans cells) react to the presence of antigens and have an immune function.

Second, the skin contains two types of glands that produce important secretions. These glands in the skin are the **sebaceous glands** and the **sweat glands.** Sebaceous glands produce **sebum,** an oily secretion, and sweat glands produce **sweat,** a watery secretion. Sebum and sweat pass to the outer edges of the skin through ducts and leave the skin through openings, or pores. Sebum lubricates the surface of the skin, and sweat cools the body as it evaporates from the skin surface.

Third, nerve fibers under the skin are receptors for sensations such as pain, temperature, pressure, and touch. Thus, the body's adjustment to the environment depends on sensory messages relayed to the brain and spinal cord by sensitive nerve endings in the skin.

Fourth, different tissues in the skin maintain body temperature (thermoregulation). Nerve fibers coordinate thermoregulation by carrying messages to the skin from heat centers in the brain that are sensitive to increases and decreases in body temperature. Impulses from these fibers cause blood vessels to dilate to bring blood to the surface and cause sweat glands to produce the watery secretion that carries heat away.

Anatomy of the Skin

Figure 16-1A shows three layers of the skin. Label them from the outer surface inward:

Epidermis [1]—a thin, cellular membrane layer; containing keratin
Dermis [2]—dense, fibrous, connective tissue layer; containing collagen
Subcutaneous layer [3]—thick, fat-containing tissue

EPIDERMIS

The epidermis is the outermost, totally cellular layer of the skin. It is composed of **squamous epithelium.** Epithelium is the covering of both the internal and the external surfaces of the body. Squamous epithelial cells are flat and scale-like. In the outer layer of the skin, these cells are arranged in several layers **(strata)** to form **stratified squamous epithelium.**

The epidermis lacks blood vessels, lymphatic vessels, and connective tissue (elastic fibers, cartilage, fat) and is therefore dependent on the deeper dermis layer and its rich network of capillaries for nourishment. In fact, oxygen and nutrients seep out of the capillaries in the dermis, pass through tissue fluid, and supply nourishment to the lower layers of the epidermis.

Figure 16-1B illustrates the multilayered cells of the epidermis. The deepest layer is called the **basal layer** [4]. The cells in the basal layer are constantly growing and multiplying and are the source of all the other cells in the epidermis. As the basal layer cells divide, they

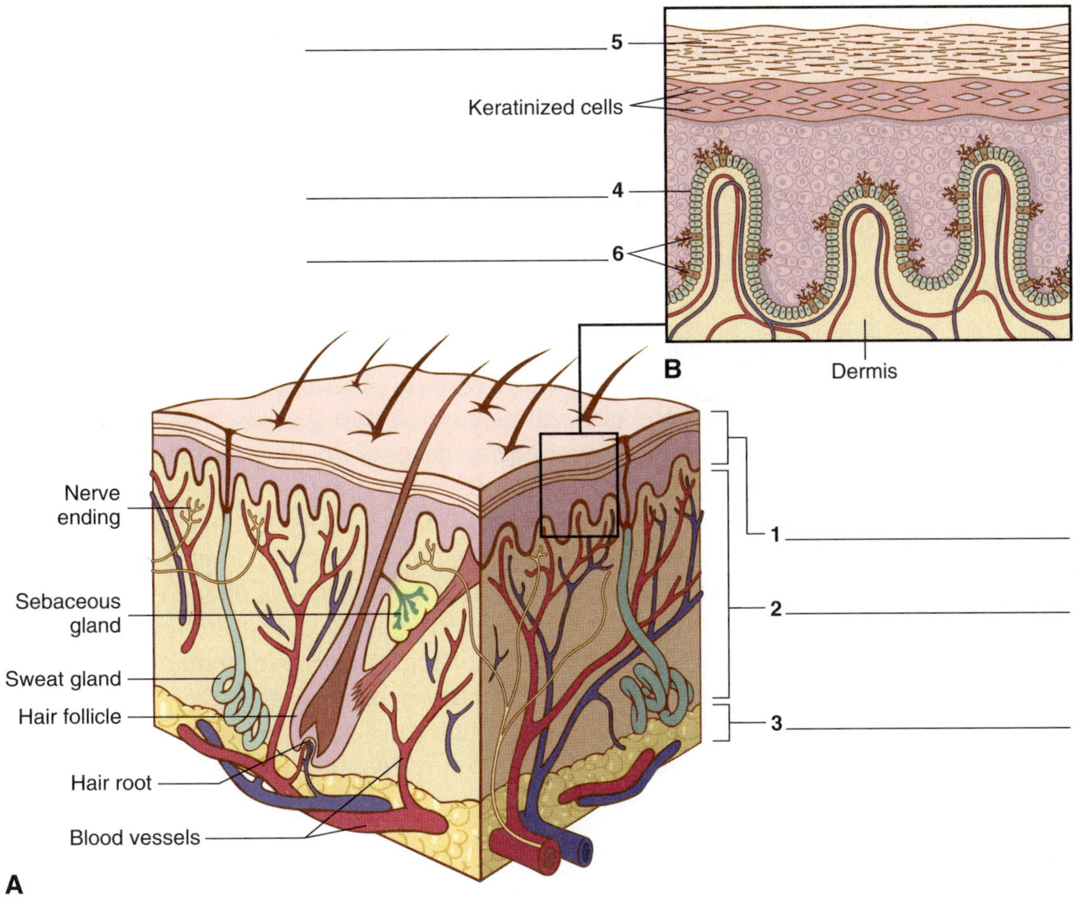

FIGURE 16-1 **Skin. A, Three layers of the skin. B, Epidermis.**

are pushed upward and away from the blood supply of the dermal layer by a steady stream of younger cells. In their movement toward the most superficial layer of the epidermis, called the **stratum corneum** [5], the cells flatten, shrink, lose their nuclei, and die, becoming filled with a hard protein material called **keratin.** The cells are then called keratinocytes, reflecting their composition of keratin. Finally, within 3 to 4 weeks after beginning as a basal cell in the deepest part of the epidermis, the keratinized cell is sloughed off from the surface of the skin. The epidermis is thus constantly renewing itself, with cells dying at the same rate at which they are replaced.

The basal layer of the epidermis contains special cells called **melanocytes** [6]. Melanocytes contain a pigment called **melanin** that is transferred to other epidermal cells and gives color to the skin. The number of melanocytes in all human races is the same, but the amount of melanin within each cell accounts for the color differences among the races. Individuals with darker skin possess more melanin within the melanocytes, not a greater number of melanocytes. Individuals who are incapable of forming melanin are called **albinos.** Skin and hair are white. In albinos, eye color varies from red to blue to brown, depending on the amount of melanin present in the iris (pigmented portion of the eye). Occulocutaneous albinism affects eyes, skin, and hair, while ocular albinism affects the eyes only.

Types of Melanin: Eumelanin and Pheomelanin

Eumelanin (eu- = true) is more common and is a brown-black pigment. **Pheomelanin** (pheo- = dusky) is a red-yellow pigment. People with darker skin have more eumelanin, whereas people with lighter skin have more pheomelanin. Pheomelanin is a photo-sensitizer (doesn't protect the skin from damaging ultraviolet rays) and makes lighter-skinned individuals more susceptible to skin cancer.

16

Melanin production increases with exposure to strong ultraviolet light, and this creates a suntan, which is a protective response. When the melanin cannot absorb all of the ultraviolet rays, the skin becomes sunburned and inflamed (redness, swelling, and pain). Over a period of years, excessive exposure to sun tends to cause wrinkles, permanent pigmentary changes, and even cancer of the skin. Because dark-skinned people have more melanin, they acquire fewer wrinkles and they are less likely to develop the types of skin cancer that are associated with ultraviolet light exposure.

DERMIS

The dermis, directly below the epidermis, is composed of blood and lymph vessels and nerve fibers, as well as the accessory organs of the skin, which are the hair follicles, sweat glands, and sebaceous glands. To support the elaborate system of nerves, vessels, and glands, the dermis contains connective tissue cells and fibers that account for the extensibility and elasticity of the skin.

The dermis is composed of interwoven elastic and **collagen** fibers. Collagen (**colla** = glue) is a fibrous protein material found in bone, cartilage, tendons, and ligaments, as well as in the skin. It is tough and resistant but also flexible. In the infant, collagen is loose and delicate; it becomes harder as the body ages. During pregnancy, overstretching of the skin with weight gain may break the elastic fibers, resulting in linear markings called **striae** ("stretch marks") on the woman's abdomen and elsewhere. Collagen fibers support and protect the blood and nerve networks that pass through the dermis. Collagen diseases affect connective tissues of the body. Examples of these connective tissue collagen disorders are systemic lupus erythematosus and scleroderma.

SUBCUTANEOUS LAYER

The subcutaneous layer (epidermis and dermis are the cutaneous layers) specializes in the formation of fat. **Adipocytes** (fat cells) are predominant in the subcutaneous layer, and they manufacture and store large quantities of fat. Obviously, fat deposition varies in different areas of the body and among individual people. Functionally, this layer of the skin is important in protection of the deeper tissues of the body, as a heat insulator, and for energy storage.

ACCESSORY STRUCTURES OF THE SKIN

HAIR

A hair fiber is composed of a tightly fused meshwork of cells filled with the hard protein called **keratin.** Hair growth is similar to the growth of the epidermal layer of the skin. Deep-lying cells in the hair root (Figure 16-2) produce keratinized cells that move upward through **hair follicles** (sacs within which each hair fiber grows). Melanocytes (see Figure 16-2) are located at the root of the hair follicle, and they donate the melanin pigment to the cells of the hair fiber.

Of the 5 million hairs on the body, about 100,000 are on the head. They grow about ½ inch (1.3 cm) per month. Cutting the hair has no effect on its rate of growth.

What causes hair color?

Concentration of eumelanin and pheomelanin cause the variations in hair color. For example:

- Black hair = high levels of black eumelanin
- Brown hair = high levels of brown eumelanin
- Blond hair = low levels of black eumelanin
- Red hair = high levels of pheomelanin
- Grey hair = low concentration of eumelanin and pheomelanin

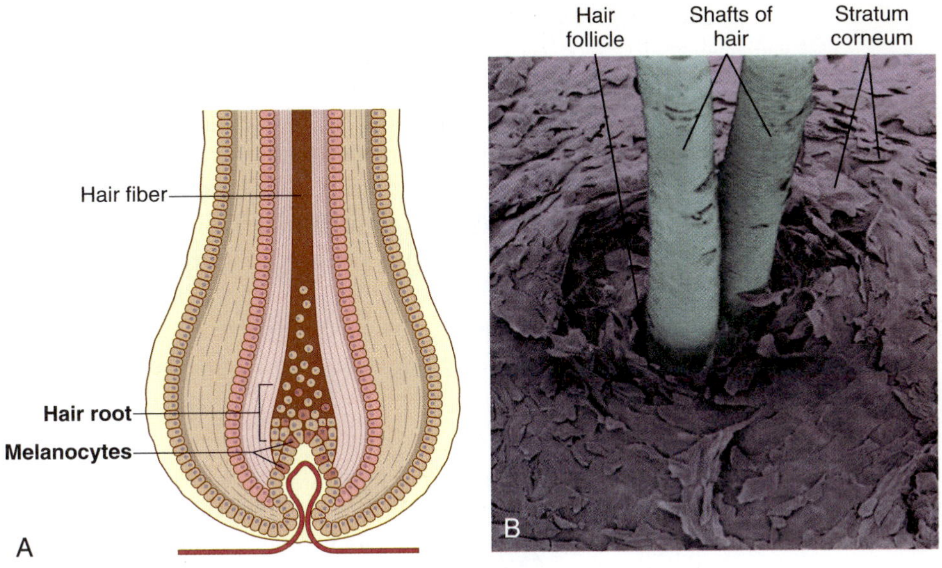

FIGURE 16-2 **A,** Enlargement of a **hair follicle. B,** Scanning electron micrograph of **hair shafts** (visible parts of hair) extending from their hair follicles.

NAILS

Nails are hard keratin plates covering the dorsal surface of the last bone of each toe and finger. They are composed of keratinocytes that are cemented together tightly and can extend indefinitely unless cut or broken. A nail grows in thickness and length as a result of division of cells in the region of the nail matrix, which is at the base (proximal portion) of the nail plate.

Fingernails grow about 1 mm per week, which means that they can regrow in 3 to 5 months. Toenails grow more slowly than fingernails; it takes 12 to 18 months for toenails to be replaced completely.

The **lunula** is a semilunar (half-moon–shaped) whitish region at the base of the nail plate. It generally can be seen in the thumbnail of most people and is evident to varying degrees in other fingernails. Air mixed in with keratin and cells rich in nuclei give the lunula its whitish color. The **cuticle,** a narrow band of epidermis (layer of keratin), is at the base and sides of the nail plate. The **paronychium** is the soft tissue surrounding the nail border. Figure 16-3A illustrates the anatomic structure of a nail.

Nail growth and appearance commonly alter during systemic disease. For example, grooves in nails may occur with high fevers and serious illness, and spoon nails (flattening of the nail plate) develop in iron deficiency anemia. **Onycholysis** (**onych/o** = nail) is the loosening of the nail plate with separation from the nail bed (Figure 16-3B). It may occur with infection of the nail and is often seen in psoriasis.

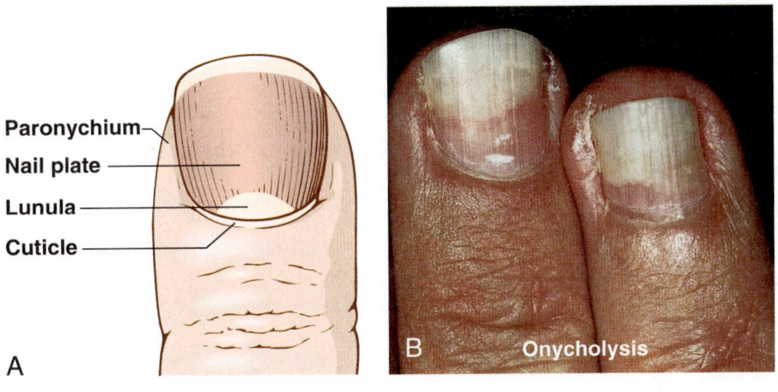

FIGURE 16-3 **A, Anatomic structure of a nail. B, Onycholysis.** Infection or trauma to the nail may be the cause of the detachment of the nail plate from the nail bed.

GLANDS

Sebaceous Glands

Sebaceous glands are located in the dermal layer of the skin over the entire body, with the exception of the palms (hands), soles (feet), and lips. They secrete an oily substance called **sebum.** Sebum, containing lipids, lubricates the skin and minimizes water loss. Sebaceous glands are closely associated with hair follicles, and their ducts open into the hair follicle through which the sebum is released. Figure 16-4 shows the relationship of the sebaceous gland to the hair follicle. The sebaceous glands are influenced by sex hormones, which cause them to hypertrophy at puberty and atrophy in old age. Increased production of sebum during puberty contributes to blackhead (comedo) formation and acne in some people.

Sweat Glands

Sweat glands (the most common type are **eccrine sweat glands**) are tiny, coiled glands found on almost all body surfaces (about 2 million in the body). They are most numerous in the palm of the hand (3000 glands per square inch) and in the sole of the foot. As illustrated in Figure 16-4, the coiled eccrine sweat gland originates deep in the dermis and straightens out to extend up through the epidermis. The tiny opening on the surface is a **pore.**

Sweat, or perspiration, is almost pure water, with dissolved materials such as salt making up less than 1% of the total composition. It is colorless and odorless. The odor produced when sweat accumulates on the skin is caused by the action of bacteria on the sweat.

Sweat cools the body as it evaporates into the air. Perspiration is controlled by the sympathetic nervous system, whose nerve fibers are activated by the heart regulatory center in the hypothalamic region of the brain, which stimulates sweating.

16

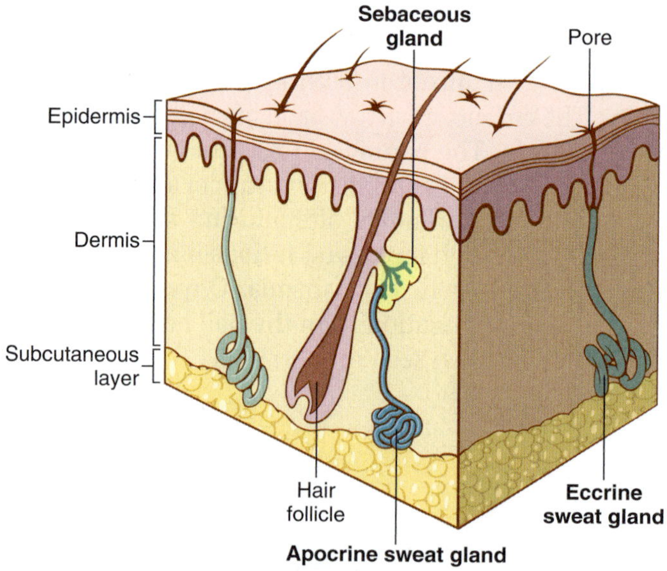

FIGURE 16-4 Sebaceous gland, eccrine sweat gland, and apocrine sweat gland.

A special variety of sweat gland, active only from puberty onward and larger than the ordinary kind, is concentrated in a few areas of the body near the reproductive organs and in the armpits. These glands **(apocrine sweat glands)** secrete an odorless sweat, containing substances easily broken down by bacteria on the skin. The bacterial waste products produce a characteristic human body odor. The milk-producing mammary gland is another type of apocrine gland; it secretes milk after the birth of a child.

VOCABULARY

This list reviews many of the new terms introduced in the text. Short definitions reinforce your understanding of the terms. Refer to the Pronunciation of Terms on page 688 for help with unfamiliar or difficult words.

adipocyte	Fat cell.
albino	Person with skin deficient in pigment (melanin).
apocrine sweat gland	One of the large dermal exocrine glands located in the axilla and genital areas. It secretes sweat that, in action with bacteria, is responsible for human body odor.
basal layer	Deepest region of the epidermis; it gives rise to all the epidermal cells.
collagen	Structural protein found in the skin and connective tissue.
cuticle	Band of epidermis at the base and sides of the nail plate.
dermis	Middle layer of the skin.
eccrine sweat gland	Most numerous sweat-producing exocrine gland in the skin.
epidermis	Outermost layer of the skin.
epithelium	Layer of skin cells forming the outer and inner surfaces of the body.
hair follicle	Sac within which each hair grows.
integumentary system	The skin and its accessory structures such as hair and nails.
keratin	Hard protein material found in the epidermis, hair, and nails. Keratin means horn and commonly is found in the horns of animals.
lunula	The half-moon–shaped, whitish area at the base of a nail.
melanin	Skin pigment. It is formed by melanocytes in the epidermis. **Eumelanin** is brown-black pigment, while **pheomelanin** is red-yellow.
paronychium	Soft tissue surrounding the nail border.
pore	Tiny opening on the surface of the skin.
sebaceous gland	Oil-secreting gland in the dermis that is associated with hair follicles.
sebum	Oily substance secreted by sebaceous glands.
squamous epithelium	Flat, scale-like cells composing the epidermis.
stratified	Arranged in layers.
stratum (plural: strata)	A layer (of cells).
stratum corneum	Outermost layer of the epidermis, which consists of flattened, keratinized cells.
subcutaneous layer	Innermost layer of the skin, containing fat tissue.

16

TERMINOLOGY

Write the meanings of the medical terms in the spaces provided.

COMBINING FORMS

COMBINING FORM	MEANING	TERMINOLOGY	MEANING
adip/o	fat (see **lip/o** and **steat/o**)	adipose	_______________
albin/o	white	albinism *Table 16-1 lists combining forms for colors and examples of terms using those combining forms.*	_______________
caus/o	burn, burning	causalgia *Intensely unpleasant burning sensation in skin and muscles when there is damage to nerves.*	_______________
cauter/o	heat, burn	electrocautery *An instrument containing a needle or blade used during surgery to burn through tissue by means of an electrical current. Electrocauterization is very effective in minimizing blood loss.*	_______________
cutane/o	skin (see **derm/o**)	subcutaneous *Epidermis and dermis are the cutaneous layers of the skin.*	_______________
derm/o, dermat/o	skin	epidermis	_______________
		dermatitis	_______________
		dermatologist	_______________
		dermabrasion *Abrasion means a scraping away. Dermabrasion using a sandpaper-like material removes acne scars and fine wrinkles.*	_______________
		epidermolysis *Loosening of the epidermis with the development of large blisters; occurs after injury, or with blister-producing diseases.*	_______________
diaphor/o	profuse sweating (see **hidr/o**)	diaphoresis *Commonly called sweating.*	_______________
erythem/o, erythemat/o	redness	erythema *Flushing; widespread redness of the skin. Pronunciation is ĕr-ĭ-THĒ-mă.* ***Erythematous*** *means pertaining to erythema.*	_______________
hidr/o	sweat	anhidrosis *Do not confuse hidr/o with hydr/o (water)!*	_______________
ichthy/o	dry, scaly (fish-like)	ichthyosis *This is usually a hereditary condition in which the skin is dry, rough, and scaly (resembling fish scales) because of a defect in keratinization. Ichthyosis also can be acquired, appearing with malignancies such as lymphomas and multiple myeloma. Greek ichthys means fish (Figure 16-5A).*	_______________

TABLE 16-1 COLORS

Combining Form	Meaning	Terminology
albin/o	white	albinism
anthrac/o	black (as coal)	anthracosis
chlor/o	green	chlorophyll
cirrh/o	tawny yellow	cirrhosis
cyan/o	blue	cyanosis
eosin/o	rosy	eosinophil
erythr/o	red	erythrocyte
jaund/o	yellow	jaundice
leuk/o	white	leukoderma
lute/o	yellow	corpus luteum
melan/o	black	melanocyte
poli/o	gray	poliosis (decrease of melanin in hair, eyebrows, and eyelashes)
xanth/o	yellow	xanthoma

COMBINING FORM	MEANING	TERMINOLOGY	MEANING
kerat/o	hard	keratosis *See page 670.*	______
leuk/o	white	leukoplakia *The suffix -plakia means plaques (Figure 16-5B).*	______
lip/o	fat	lipoma	______
		liposuction *Removal of subcutaneous fat tissue through a tube that is introduced into the fatty area via a small incision. The fat is aspirated (suctioned out).*	______
melan/o	black	melanocyte	______
		melanoma *This is a malignant skin tumor. See page 672.*	______

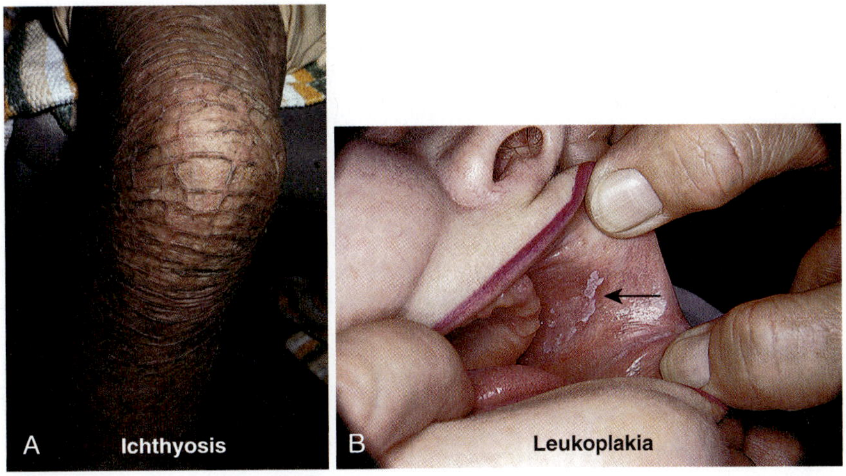

FIGURE 16-5 **A, Ichthyosis. B, Leukoplakia.**

COMBINING FORM	MEANING	TERMINOLOGY	MEANING
myc/o	fungus (fungi include yeasts, molds, and mushrooms)	mycosis *An example of a mycosis (fungal infection) is* ***tinea pedis,*** *commonly called* ***"athlete's foot"*** *(Figure 16-6A). Another fungal infection is tinea corporis (ringworm). See page 669.*	
onych/o	nail (see **ungu/o**)	onycholysis *Separation of the nail plate from the nail bed in fungal infections or after trauma. See Figure 16-3, page 665. Onycholysis is often seen in psoriasis.*	
		onychomycosis *Fungal infection of the nails, which become white, opaque, thick, and brittle.*	
		paronychia *Par- means near or beside. Paronychia is inflammation and swelling of the soft tissue around the nail and is associated with torn cuticles or ingrown nails (Figure 16-6B).*	
phyt/o	plant	dermatophytosis *Examples are fungal infections (mycoses) (see Figure 16-6A).*	
pil/o	hair (see **trich/o**), hair follicle	pilosebaceous *Sebace/o indicates a gland that secretes sebum. The pilosebaceous unit is the combination of the hair follicle and attached sebaceous gland.*	
py/o	pus	pyoderma *Pus within the skin (-derma).* ***Impetigo*** *is a purulent (pus-containing) skin disease caused by bacterial infection. See page 667.*	
rhytid/o	wrinkle	rhytidectomy *Cosmetic plastic surgery to remove wrinkles and excess skin; also called rhytidoplasty or face lift. Laser treatments,* ***Botox Cosmetic*** *(purified botulinum toxin) injections, and injectable fillers are used to soften facial lines and wrinkles.*	
seb/o	sebum (oily secretion from sebaceous glands)	seborrhea *Excessive secretion from sebaceous glands.* ***Seborrheic dermatitis*** *commonly is known as* ***dandruff.***	
squam/o	scale-like	squamous epithelium *Cells are flat and scale-like; pavement epithelium.*	

Is Botox Cosmetic Safe?

Botox Cosmetic (onabotulinumtoxin A) has been FDA approved since 2002, for cosmetic use to the brow and facial frown lines. Over a million patients have been treated with Botox Cosmetic, and there have been no reported fatal or permanent adverse effects related to its use. Botox Cosmetic works by blocking the connection between nerves and muscles. Muscles do not contract, thus preventing lines and wrinkles in the skin. When injected in small doses directly into the muscle, Botox Cosmetic can reduce specific facial lines for several months.

The FDA has also approved injectable dermal fillers for deep facial wrinkles and folds. These include Restylane, Perlane, Juvederm, and Radiesse. New additional neuromodulators similar to Botox Cosmetic are also available: Xeomin (incobotulinumtoxin A) and Dysport (abobotulinumtoxin A).

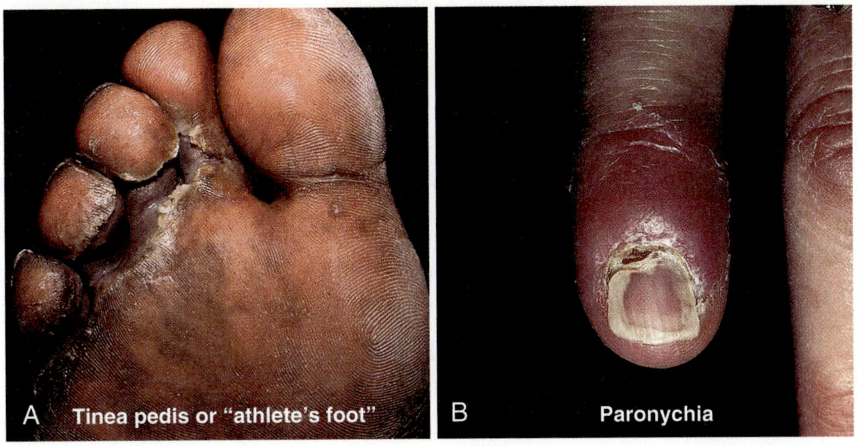

FIGURE 16-6 **A, Mycosis. B, Acute paronychia** most commonly occurs from nail biting, finger sucking, aggressive manicuring, or penetrating trauma. The most common infecting organism is *Staphylococcus aureus.*

COMBINING FORM	MEANING	TERMINOLOGY	MEANING
steat/o	fat	steatoma ____________________ *Cystic collection of sebum (fatty material) that forms in a sebaceous gland and can become infected;* ***sebaceous cyst.*** *See Figure 16-7A.*	
trich/o	hair	hypertrichosis ____________________	
ungu/o	nail	subungual ____________________	
xanth/o	yellow	xanthoma ____________________ *Nodules develop under the skin owing to excess lipid deposits and can be associated with a high cholesterol level. A xanthoma that appears on the eyelids is a* ***xanthelasma*** *(-elasma = a flat plate) (Figure 16-7B).*	
xer/o	dry	xerosis ____________________ *This is very dry skin.*	

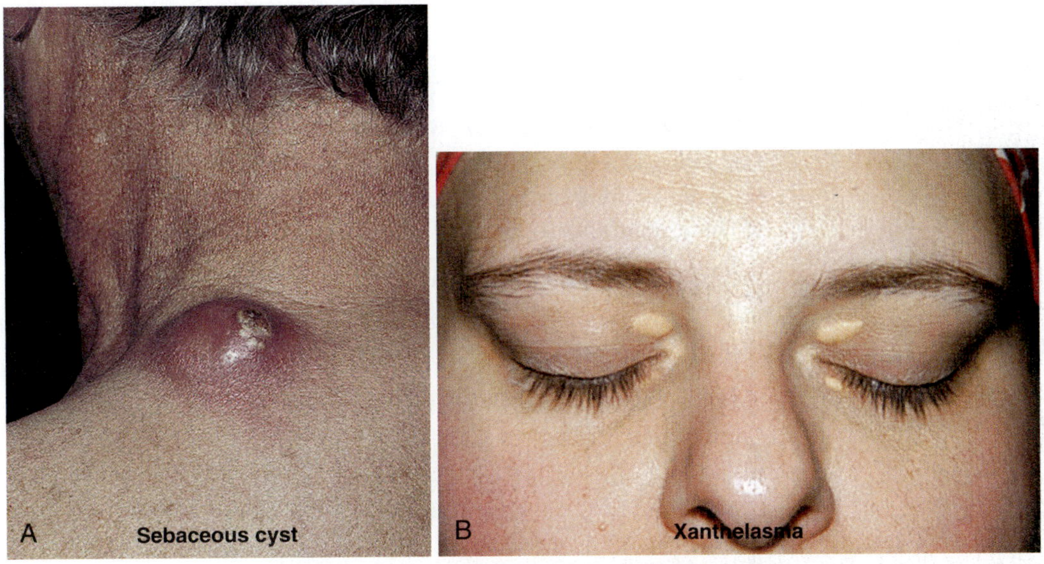

FIGURE 16-7 **A, Sebaceous cyst. B, Xanthelasma.**

PATHOLOGY

CUTANEOUS LESIONS

A **lesion** is an area of abnormal tissue anywhere on or in the body. It may be caused by disease or trauma (external forces). The following terms describe common skin lesions, which are illustrated in Figure 16-8A to L.

A. crust — **Collection of dried serum and cellular debris.**

A scab is a crust. It forms from the drying of a body exudate, as in eczema, impetigo, and seborrhea.

B. cyst — **Thick-walled, closed sac or pouch containing fluid or semisolid material.**

Examples of cysts are the **pilonidal cyst,** which is found over the sacral area of the back in the midline and contains hairs (**pil/o** = hair, **nid/o** = nest); and a **sebaceous cyst,** a collection of yellowish, cheesy sebum commonly found on the scalp, vulva, and scrotum.

C. erosion — **Wearing away or loss of epidermis.**

Erosions do not penetrate below the dermoepidermal junction. They occur as a result of inflammation or injury and heal without scarring.

D. fissure — **Groove or crack-like sore.**

An anal fissure is a break in the skin lining of the anal canal.

E. macule — **Flat lesion measuring less than 1 cm in diameter.**

Freckles, tattoo marks, and flat moles are examples. A **patch** is a large macule, greater than 1 cm in diameter.

16

F. nodule — **Solid, round or oval elevated lesion 1 cm or more in diameter.**

An enlarged lymph node and solid growths are examples.

G. papule — **Small (less than 1 cm in diameter), solid elevation of the skin.**

Pimples are examples of papules. Papules may become confluent (run together) and form **plaques,** which are elevated flat lesions.

H. polyp — **Growth extending from the surface of mucous membrane.**

Polyps (a type of papule) commonly are found in the nose and sinuses, colon, urinary bladder, and uterus.

I. pustule — **Papule containing pus.**

A pustule is a small **abscess** (collection of pus) on the skin.

J. ulcer — **Open sore on the skin or mucous membranes (deeper than an erosion).**

Decubitus ulcers (bedsores) are caused by pressure that results from lying in one position (Latin *decubitus* means lying down). Pressure ulcers usually involve loss of tissue substance and pus or exudate formation.

K. vesicle — **Small collection (papule) of clear fluid (serum); blister.**

Vesicles form in burns, allergies, and dermatitis. A **bulla** (*plural*: bullae) is a large vesicle.

L. wheal — **Smooth, edematous (swollen) papule or plaque that is redder or paler than the surrounding skin.**

Wheals may be papular, as in a mosquito bite, or may involve a wide area, as in allergic reactions. Wheals often are accompanied by itching and are seen in hives, anaphylaxis, and insect bites.

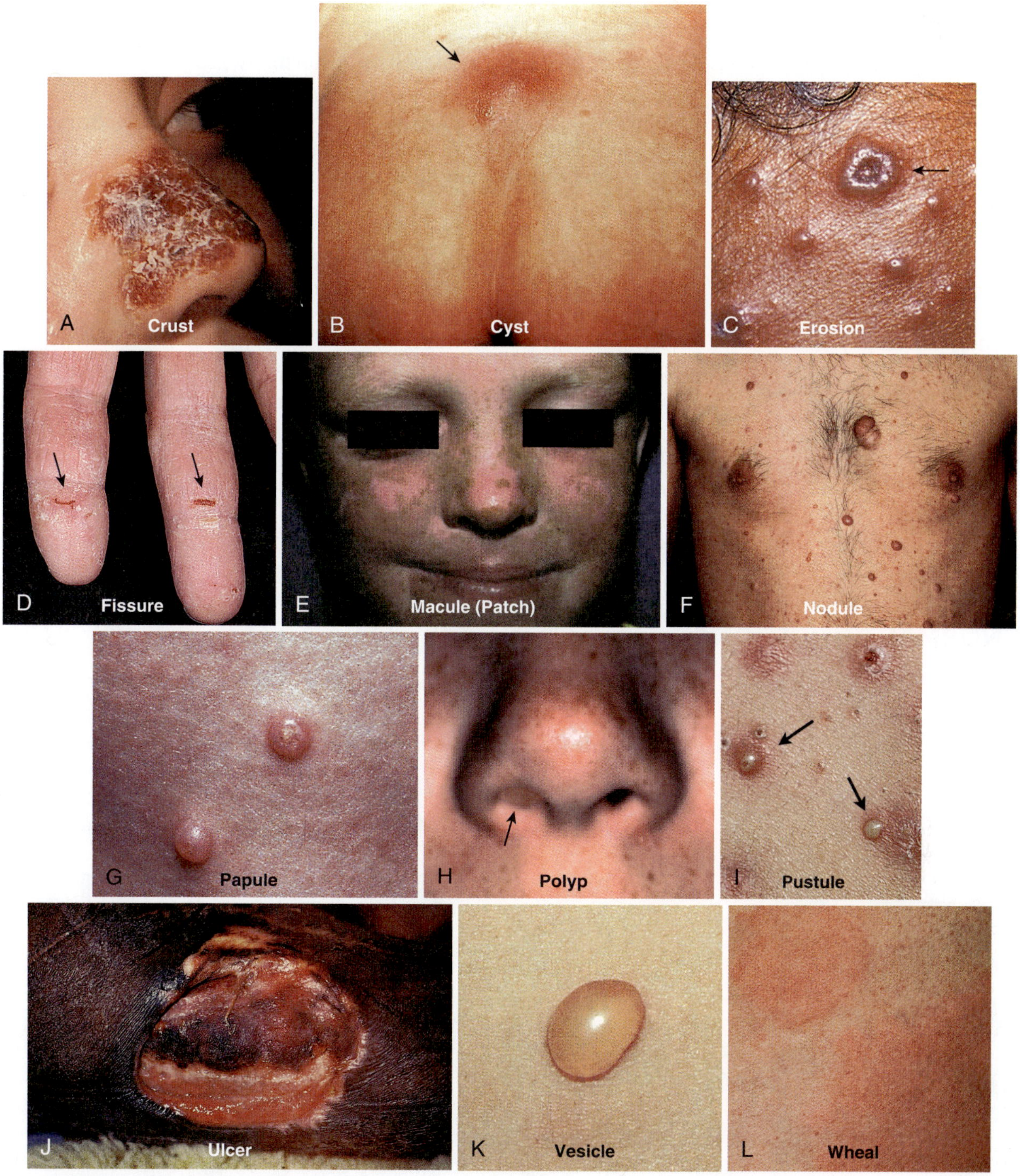

FIGURE 16-8 **Cutaneous lesions. A, Crust**—scab. **B, Cyst**—pilonidal cyst. **C, Erosion**—in varicella (chickenpox after rupture of blister). **D, Fissures. E, Macule**—freckles. **F, Nodules. G, Papules. H, Polyp**—nasal polyp. **I, Pustules**—acne. **J, Ulcer**—decubitus ulcer. **K, Vesicle**—bulla. **L, Wheal**—urticaria.

SIGNS AND SYMPTOMS

alopecia

Absence of hair from areas where it normally grows.

Alopecia, or baldness, may be hereditary (usual progressive loss of scalp hair in men) or it may be caused by disease, injury, or treatment (chemotherapy) or may occur with old age. **Alopecia areata** is an autoimmune disease in which hair falls out in patches without scarring or inflammation (Figure 16-9A).

ecchymosis, ecchymoses

Bluish-purplish mark (bruise) on the skin.

Ecchymoses (**ec-** = out, **chym/o** = pour) are caused by hemorrhages into the skin from injury or spontaneous leaking of blood from vessels (Figure 16-9B).

petechia, petechiae

Small, pinpoint hemorrhage.

Petechiae (pĕ-TĒ-kē-ī) are smaller versions of ecchymoses (Figure 16-9C). Both ecchymoses and petechiae are forms of **purpura** (bleeding into the skin).

pruritus

Itching.

Pruritus is a symptom associated with most forms of dermatitis and with other conditions as well. It arises as a result of stimulation of nerves in the skin by substances released in allergic reactions or by irritation caused by substances in the blood or by foreign bodies.

ABNORMAL CONDITIONS

acne

Chronic papular and pustular eruption of the skin with increased production of sebum.

Acne vulgaris (Latin *vulgaris* means ordinary) is caused by the buildup of sebum and keratin in the pores of the skin. A **blackhead** or open **comedo** (*plural*: **comedones**) is a sebum plug partially blocking the pore (Figure 16-10). If the pore becomes completely blocked, a **whitehead** (closed comedo) forms. Bacteria

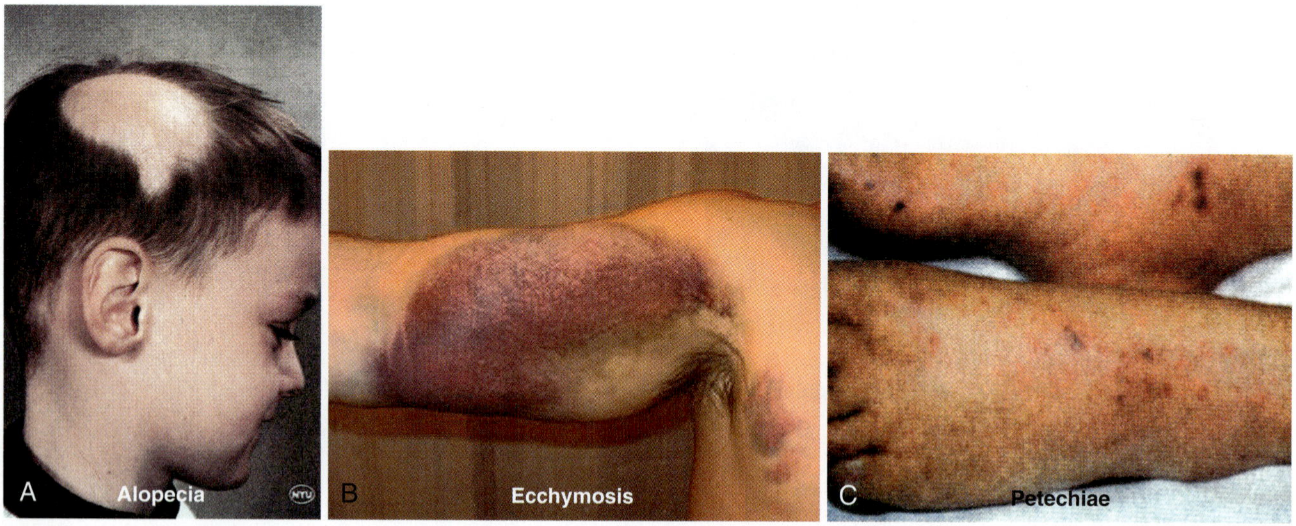

FIGURE 16-9 **A, Alopecia areata. B, Ecchymosis.** High-grade tear at the myotendinous junction at the right pectoralis major muscle. **C, Petechiae.**

Pruritus

Be sure to spell pruritus correctly. It is a condition, not an inflammation (-itis).

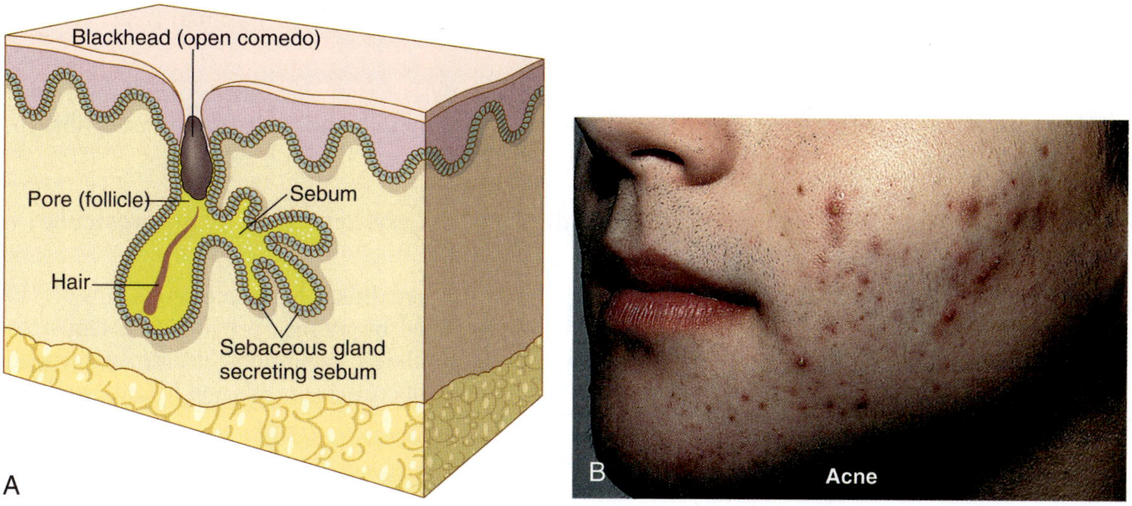

FIGURE 16-10 **A,** Formation of a **blackhead (open comedo)** in a dilated pore filled with oxidized sebum and bacteria. **B, Acne vulgaris** on the face.

in the skin break down the sebum, producing inflammation in the surrounding tissue. Papules, pustules, and cysts can thus form. Treatment consists of long-term antibiotic use and medications to decrease inflammation in the skin. Benzoyl peroxide and tretinoin (Retin-A) are topical medications used to prevent comedo formation; isotretinoin (Accutane) is used in severe cystic or treatment-resistant acne.

burns

Injury to tissues caused by heat contact.

Burns may be caused by dry heat (fire), moist heat (steam or liquid), chemicals, lightning, electricity, or radiation. Burns usually are classified as follows:

first-degree burns—superficial epidermal lesions, erythema, hyperesthesia, and no blisters.

second-degree burns (partial-thickness burn injury)—epidermal and dermal lesions, erythema, blisters, and hyperesthesia (Figure 16-11A).

third-degree burns (full-thickness burn injury)—epidermis and dermis are destroyed (necrosis of skin), and subcutaneous layer is damaged, leaving charred, white tissue (Figure 16-11B).

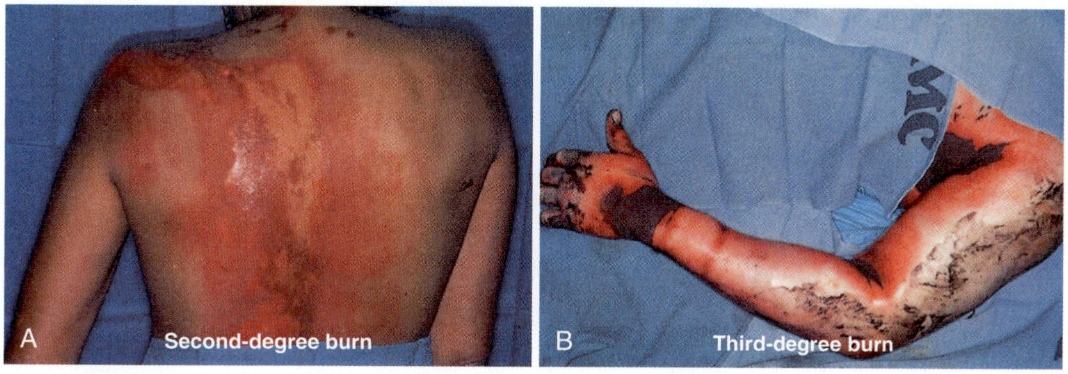

FIGURE 16-11 **Burns. A, Second-degree burn.** Wound is painful and very sensitive to touch and air currents. **B, Third-degree burn** showing variable color (deep-red, white, black, and brown). The wound itself is insensate (patient does not respond to pinprick).

cellulitis

Diffuse, acute infection of the skin marked by local heat, redness, pain, and swelling.

Abscess formation and tissue destruction can occur if appropriate antibiotic therapy is not given. Areas of poor lymphatic drainage are susceptible to this skin infection (Figure 16-12A).

eczema (atopic dermatitis)

Inflammatory skin disease with erythematous, papulovesicular, or papalosquamous lesions.

This is a chronic or acute **atopic dermatitis** (rash often begins on face, hands, elbows, or knees) It is accompanied by intense pruritus and tends to occur in patients with a family history of allergic conditions. Treatment depends on the cause but usually includes the use of corticosteroids and moisturizers. See Figure 16-12B.

exanthematous viral diseases

Rash (exanthem) of the skin due to a viral infection.

Examples are **rubella** (German measles), **rubeola** (measles), and **varicella** (chickenpox). These conditions are no longer as common in children because of vaccination programs. However, **erythema infectiosum** (fifth disease) is a common exanthematous viral disease. See Figure 16-13A. **Hand-foot-and-mouth disease** is another common viral illness in children. See Figure 16-13B.

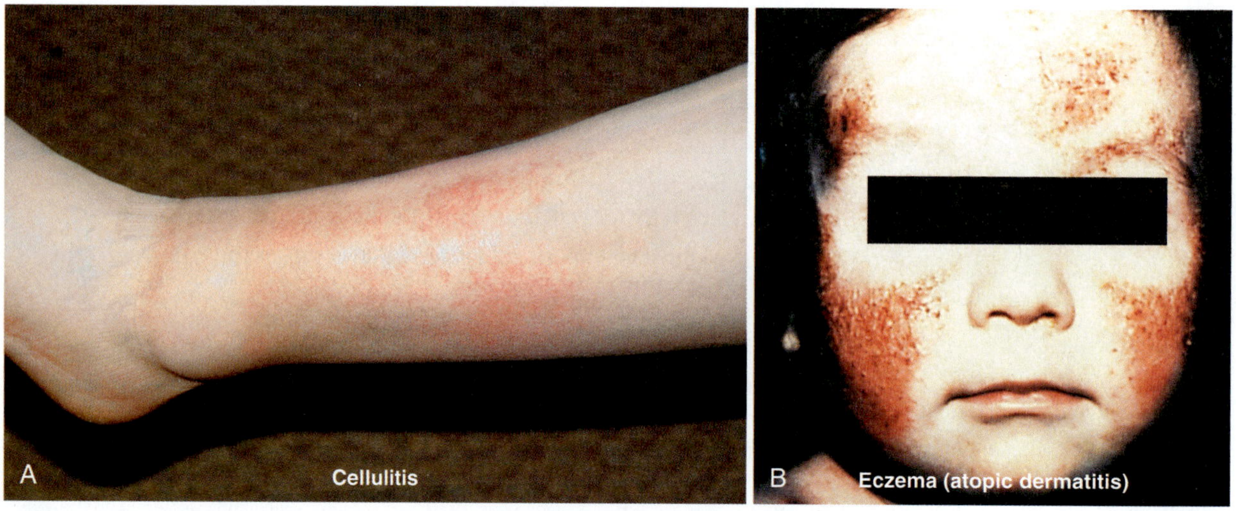

FIGURE 16-12 **A, Cellulitis.** Traveling on a safari in Botswana, a 63-year-old woman noticed swelling, redness, and pain in her lower leg. After a local physician prescribed oral antibiotics, she was advised to interrupt her trip to get IV antibiotics at a major hospital. Her cellulitis cleared in a week. **B, Eczema (atopic dermatitis)** in an infant. Greater than 70% of patients have a family history of other atopic conditions such as allergic rhinitis, hay fever, and asthma.

Atopic dermatitis

Atopic means pertaining to **atopy**, which means out of place or unusual (a = no, top = place). It is a hyperallergic condition that may be hereditary, but contact with an allergen must occur before a hypersensitivity reaction can develop.

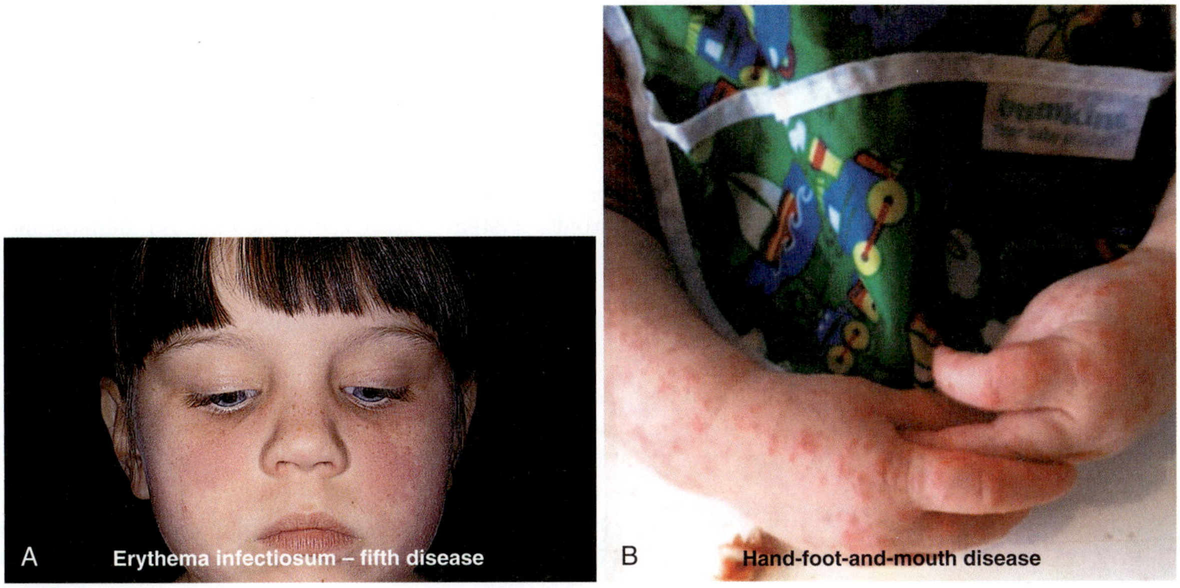

FIGURE 16-13 **A, Erythema infectiosum - fifth disease.** It is marked by fever and an erythematous rash that has a "slapped cheek" appearance on the face and later involving the arms, buttocks, and trunk. It is caused by a parvovirus. **B, Hand-foot-and-mouth disease.** It is caused by an enterovirus.

gangrene

Death of tissue associated with loss of blood supply.

In this condition, ischemia resulting from injury, inflammation, frostbite, diseases such as diabetes, or arteriosclerosis can lead to necrosis of tissue followed by bacterial invasion and putrefaction (proteins are decomposed by bacteria). See Figure 16-14A.

impetigo

Bacterial inflammatory skin disease characterized by vesicles, pustules, and crusted-over lesions.

This is a contagious **pyoderma** (**py/o** = pus) and usually is caused by staphylococci or streptococci. Systemic use of antibiotics combined with proper cleansing of lesions is effective treatment. See Figure 16-14B.

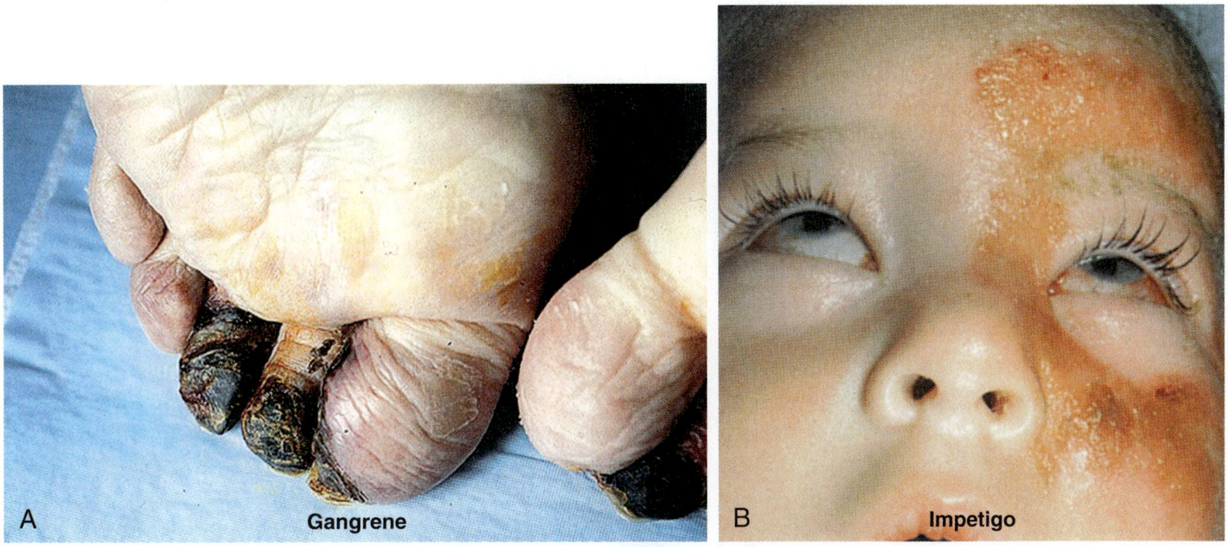

FIGURE 16-14 **A, Gangrene. B, Impetigo.**

psoriasis

Chronic, recurrent dermatosis marked by itchy, scaly, red plaques covered by silvery gray scales (Figure 16-15A).

Psoriasis commonly involves the forearms, knees, legs, and scalp. It is neither infectious nor contagious but is caused by an increased rate of growth of the basal layer of the epidermis. It is an autoinflammatory disease that can run in families. Treatment is **palliative** (relieving but not curing) and includes topical lubricants, keratolytics, and steroids. Systemic treatments include psoralen–ultraviolet A (PUVA) light therapy and immunomodulators.

scabies

Contagious, parasitic infection of the skin with intense pruritus. (Figure 16-15B)

Scabies (from Latin *scabere,* to scratch) commonly affects areas such as the groin, nipples, and skin between the fingers. Treatment is with topical medicated cream to destroy the scabies mites (tiny parasites).

scleroderma

Chronic progressive disease of the skin and internal organs with hardening and shrinking of connective tissue. See Figure 16-16A.

Fibrous scar-like tissue forms in the skin, and the heart, lungs, kidneys, and esophagus may be affected as well. Skin is thick, hard, and rigid, with areas of both depigmented and hyperpigmentation. It is an autoimmune disease for which palliative treatment consists of immunosuppressive and anti-inflammatory agents, antifibrotics, and physical therapy.

systemic lupus erythematosus (SLE)

Chronic autoimmune inflammatory disease of collagen in skin, joints, and internal organs.

Lupus, meaning wolf-like (the shape and color of the skin lesions resembled those in the bite of a wolf), produces a characteristic "butterfly" pattern of redness over the cheeks and nose. See Figure 16-16B. In more severe cases, the extent of erythema increases, and all exposed areas of the skin may be involved. Primarily a disease of females, lupus is an autoimmune disorder. High levels of certain antibodies are found in the patient's blood. Corticosteroids and immunosuppressive drugs are used to control symptoms.

SLE should be differentiated from chronic **discoid lupus erythematosus (DLE),** which is a photosensitive, scaling, plaque-like eruption of the skin confined to the face, scalp, ears, chest, arms, and back, which heals with scarring. SLE should also be differentiated from **lupus vulgaris**, which refers to a cutaneous form of tuberculosis.

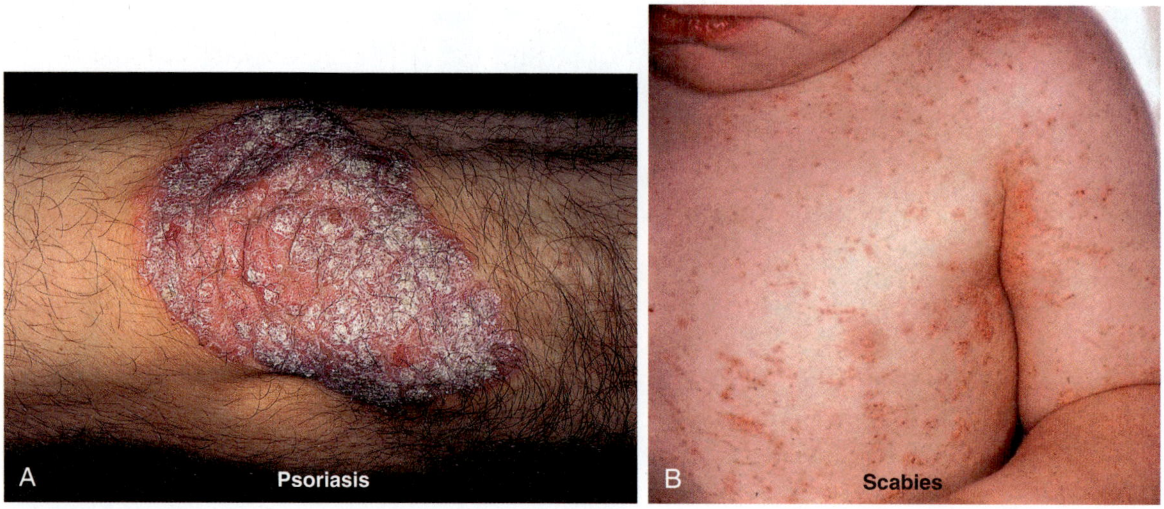

FIGURE 16-15 **A, Psoriasis.** Thick red plaques have a sharply defined border and an adherent silvery scale. **B, Scabies.**

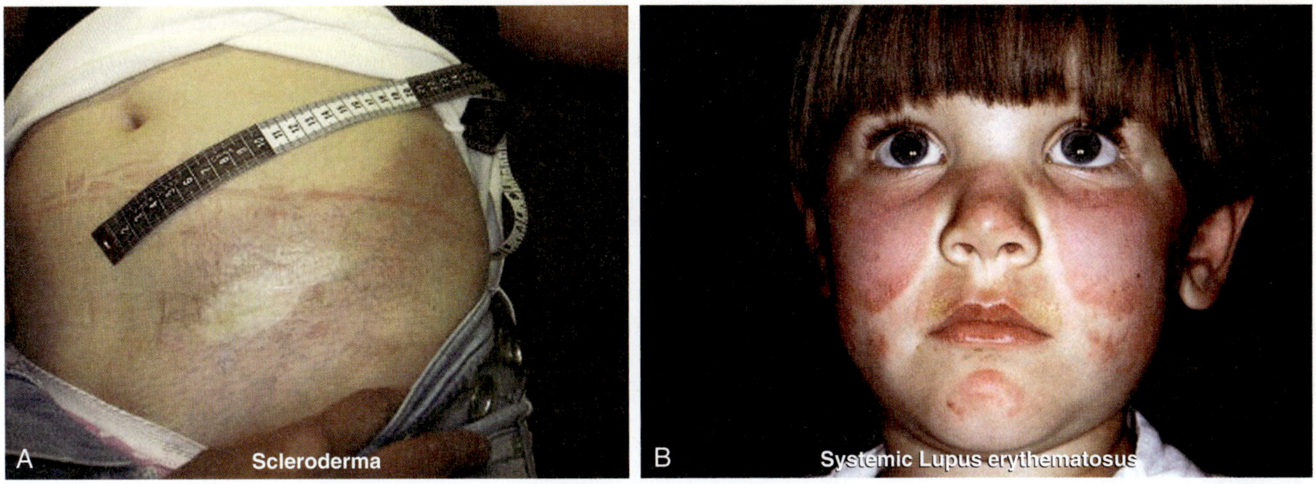

FIGURE 16-16 **A, Scleroderma. B, Systemic lupus erythematosus.**

tinea

Infection of the skin caused by a fungus.

Tinea corporis, or ringworm, so called because the infection is in a ring-like pattern (Figure 16-17A), is highly contagious and causes severe pruritus. Other examples are **tinea pedis** (athlete's foot, which affects the skin between the toes), **tinea capitis** (on the scalp), **tinea barbae** (affecting the skin under a beard), and **tinea unguium** (affecting the nails) (Figure 16-17B). Treatment is with antifungal agents. (Latin *tinea* means worm or moth—apparently the Romans thought that skin affected with tinea looked "moth-eaten.")

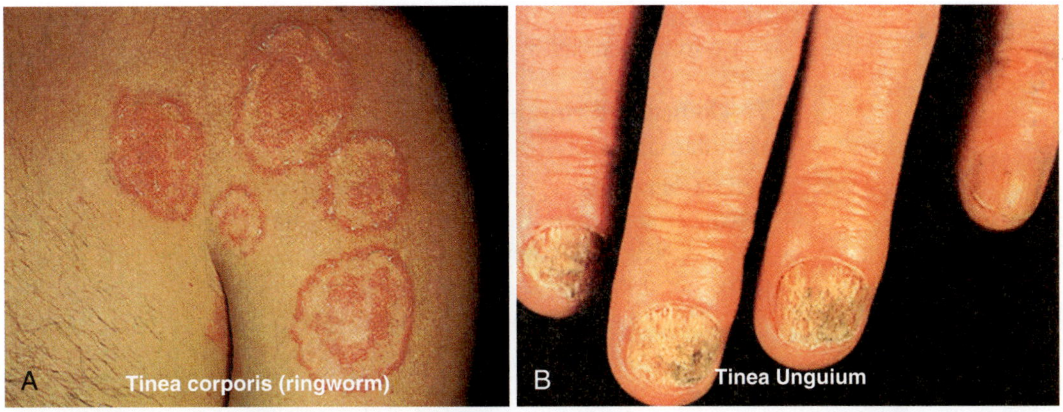

FIGURE 16-17 **A, Tinea corporis (ringworm). B, Tinea unguium.** Fungal infection of the nail (onychomycosis) causes the distal nail plate to turn yellow or white. Hyperkeratotic debris accumulates, causing the nail to separate from the nail bed (**onycholysis**).

urticaria (hives)

Acute allergic reaction in which red, round wheals develop on the skin.

Hives are often a reaction to foods (shellfish, nuts, eggs) or medicine. Histamine is released into the bloodstream, causing **pruritus** and **edema** (swelling). **Angioedema** is swelling around the face. Other substances and events that can trigger hives are animal dander, insect bites, and pollen. See Figure 16-18A.

vitiligo

Loss of pigment (depigmentation) in areas of the skin (milk-white patches).

This is a form of **leukoderma** (Figure 16-18B). The skin changes result from an autoimmune process, and there is an increased association of vitiligo with autoimmune disorders such as thyroiditis, hyperthyroidism, and diabetes mellitus.

SKIN NEOPLASMS

Benign Neoplasms

callus

Increased growth of cells in the keratin layer of the epidermis caused by pressure or friction.

The feet (Figure 16-19A) and the hands are common sites for callus formation. A **corn** is a type of callus that develops a hard core (a whitish, cone-shaped central kernel).

keloid

Excess hypertrophied, thickened scar developing after trauma or surgical incision.

Keloids (Figure 16-19B) result from excessive collagen formation in the skin during connective tissue repair. Keloids extend beyond the boundaries of the original injury. The term comes from the Greek *kelis*, meaning blemish. Surgical excision often is combined with intralesional steroid injections or ablative laser treatments.

A normal scar left by a healed wound is called a **cicatrix** (SĬK-ă-trĭks).

keratosis

Thickened and rough lesion of the epidermis; associated with aging or skin damage.

Actinic keratosis is caused by long-term ultraviolet light exposure and is a precancerous lesion that can evolve into squamous cell carcinoma (Figure 16-20A). **Seborrheic keratosis** is a benign lesion that results from overgrowth of the upper epidermis and is dark in color.

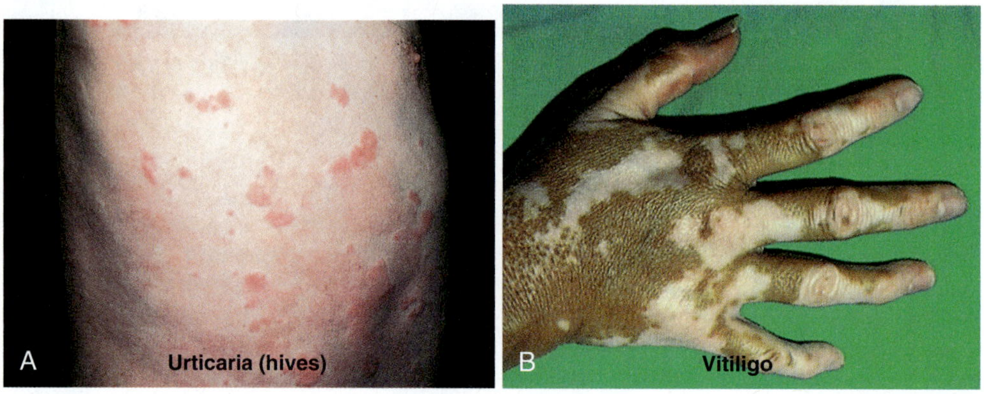

FIGURE 16-18 **A, Urticaria (hives).** Erythematous, edematous, often circular plaques. **B, Vitiligo** on the hand (from Latin *vitium*, blemish). Epidermal melanocytes are completely lost in depigmented areas through an autoimmune process.

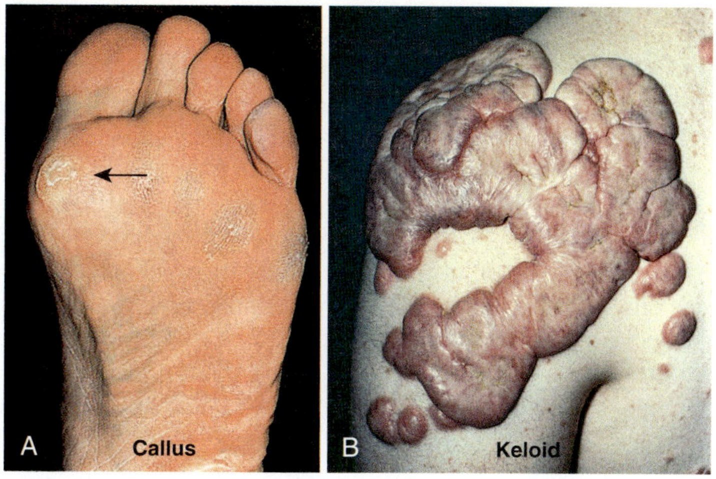

FIGURE 16-19 **A, Callus** on the sole of the foot. **B, Keloid.**

leukoplakia

White, thickened patches on mucous membrane tissue of the tongue or cheek (evolves to squamous cell carcinoma). See Figure 16-5B, page 659.

One type is a precancerous lesion that is common in smokers and may be caused by chronic inflammation.

nevus, nevi

Pigmented lesion of the skin (see Figure 16-20B).

Nevi are commonly known as moles. Many are present at birth, but some are acquired.

Dysplastic nevi are moles that have atypical cells and may progress to form a type of skin cancer called melanoma (see **malignant melanoma**).

verruca, verrucae

Epidermal growth (wart) caused by a virus.

Verruca vulgaris (common wart) is the most frequent type of wart (Figure 16-20C). **Plantar warts** occur on the soles of the feet, juvenile warts occur on the hands and face of children, and venereal warts occur on the genitals and around the anus. Warts are removed with acids, electrocautery, or freezing with liquid nitrogen (cryosurgery). If the virus remains in the skin, the wart frequently regrows.

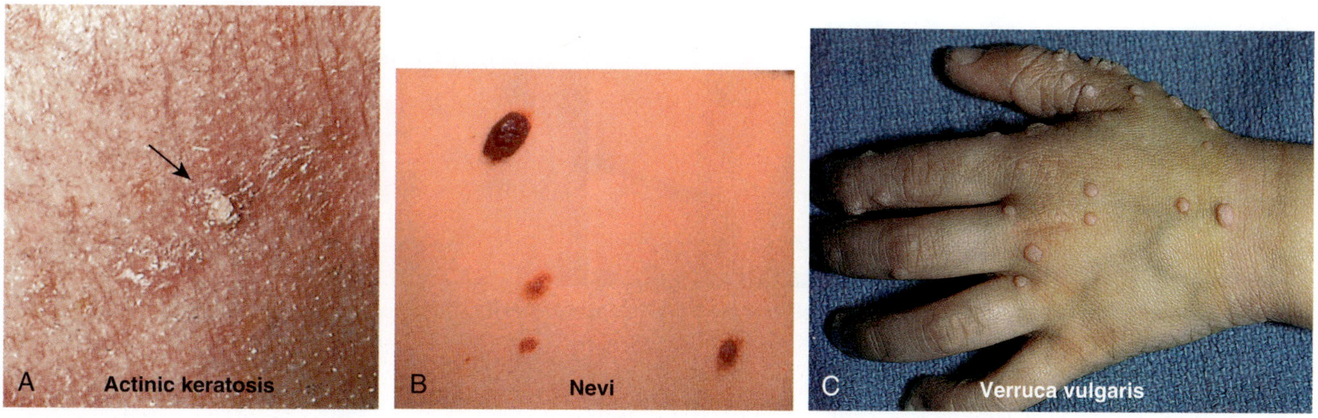

FIGURE 16-20 **A, Actinic (solar) keratosis. B, Nevi. C, Verruca vulgaris.** A wart consists of multiple papules with rough, pebble-like surfaces.

Cancerous Lesions

basal cell carcinoma

Malignant tumor of the basal cell layer of the epidermis.

This is the most frequent type of skin cancer. It is a slow-growing tumor that usually occurs on chronically sun-exposed skin, especially near or on the nose (Figure 16-21A). It almost never metastasizes.

squamous cell carcinoma

Malignant tumor of the squamous epithelial cells in the epidermis.

This tumor may grow in places other than the skin, wherever squamous epithelium is found (mouth, larynx, bladder, esophagus, lungs). **Actinic** (sun-related) **keratoses** are premalignant lesions in people with sun-damaged skin. Progression to squamous cell carcinoma (Figure 16-21B) may occur if lesions are not removed. Treatment is removal by surgical excision, cryotherapy, electrodesiccation and curettage, or radiotherapy.

malignant melanoma

Cancerous growth composed of melanocytes.

This malignancy is attributed to a genetic predisposition and to exposure to ultraviolet light. Melanoma usually begins as a mottled, light brown to black macule with irregular borders (Figure 16-22). The lesion may turn shades of red, blue, and white and may crust on the surface and bleed. Melanomas may arise in preexisting moles (dysplastic nevi) and frequently appear on the upper back, lower legs, arms, head, and neck.

Biopsy is required to confirm the diagnosis of melanoma, and prognosis is best determined by measuring tumor thickness in millimeters.

Melanomas often metastasize to the lung, liver, bone, and brain. Treatment may include excision of the tumor, regional lymphadenectomy, chemotherapy/immunotherapy, or radiotherapy. See the ***In Person*** story on page 677.

Kaposi sarcoma

Malignant, vascular, neoplastic growth characterized by cutaneous nodules.

Frequently arising on the lower extremities, nodules range in color from deep pink to dark blue and purple. One form of this condition is associated with acquired immunodeficiency syndrome (AIDS). See Figure 14-11, page 559.

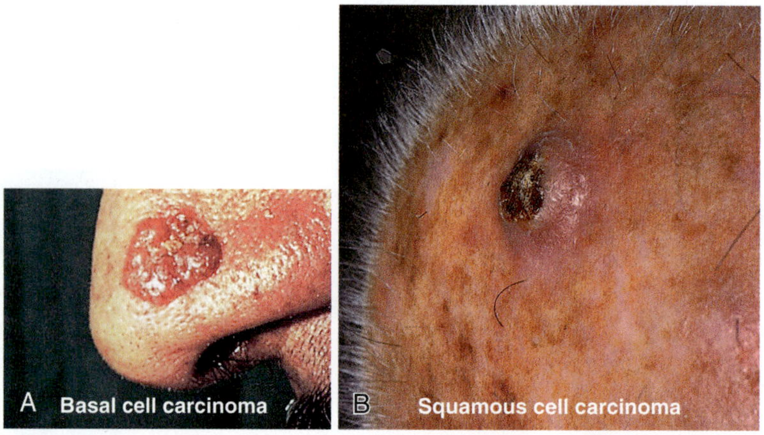

FIGURE 16-21 **A, Basal cell carcinoma. B, Squamous cell carcinoma.** Advanced lesions are often nodular and ulcerated.

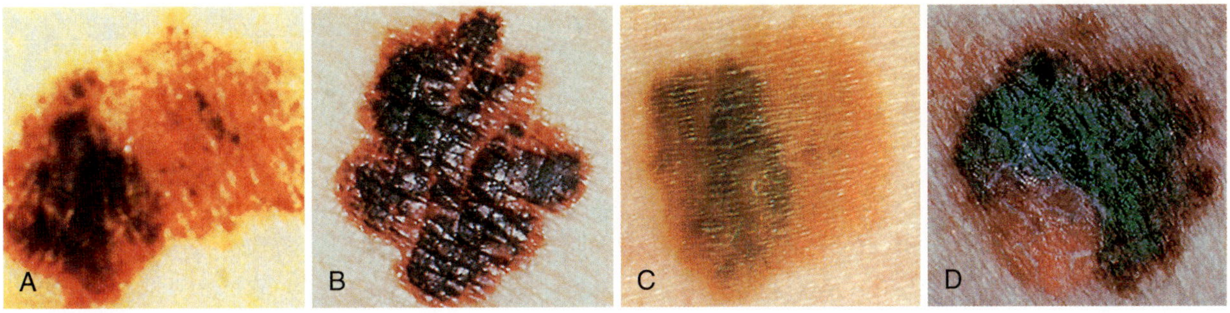

FIGURE 16-22 **The ABCDEs of Melanoma:**
Asymmetry: one half unlike the other half
Border: irregular or poorly circumscribed border
Color: varies from one area to another; shades of tan and brown, black, and sometimes white, red, or blue
Diameter: usually larger than 6 mm (diameter of a pencil eraser)
Evolution: change in the lesion over time

LABORATORY TESTS AND CLINICAL PROCEDURES

LABORATORY TESTS

bacterial analyses

Samples of skin are examined for presence of microorganisms.

Purulent (pus-filled) material or **exudate** (fluid that accumulates) often is taken for examination.

fungal tests

Scrapings from skin lesions, hair specimens, or nail clippings are sent to a laboratory for culture and microscopic examination.

The specimen also may be treated with a potassium hydroxide (KOH) preparation and examined microscopically. A positive result on a KOH test reveals elements that indicate the presence of a fungal infection.

CLINICAL PROCEDURES

cryosurgery

Use of subfreezing temperature achieved with liquid nitrogen application to destroy tissue.

curettage

Use of a sharp dermal curette to scrape away a skin lesion.

A curette is shaped like a spoon or scoop.

electrodesiccation

Tissue is destroyed by burning with an electric spark.

This procedure is used along with curettage to remove and destroy small cancerous lesions with well-defined borders.

Mohs surgery

Thin layers of malignant tissue are removed, and each slice is examined under a microscope to check for adequate extent of the resection.

Mohs surgery (also called Mohs micrographic surgery) is a specialized form of excision to treat basal cell carcinomas, squamous cell carcinomas, and other tumors. See Figure 16-23.

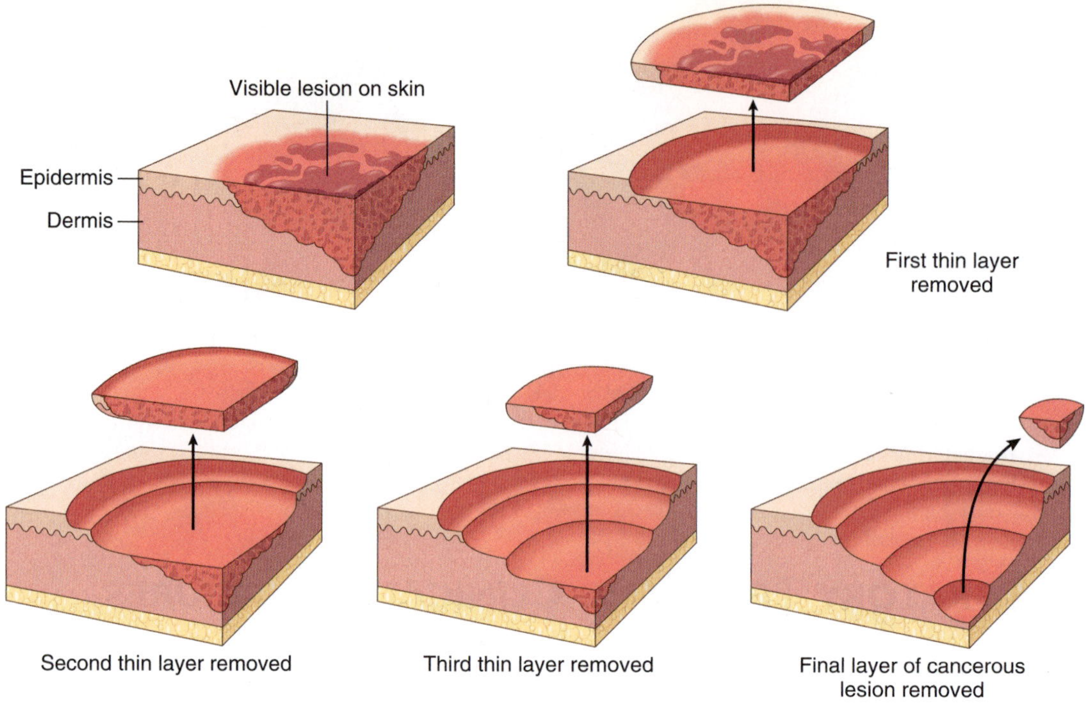

FIGURE 16-23 **Mohs surgery.**

16

skin biopsy

Suspected malignant skin lesions are removed and examined microscopically by a pathologist.

In a **punch biopsy,** a surgical instrument removes a core of tissue obtained by rotation of its sharp, circular edge. In a **shave biopsy,** tissue is excised using a cut parallel to the surface of the surrounding skin.

skin test

Substances are injected intradermally or applied to the skin, and results are observed.

Skin tests are used to diagnose allergies and disease. In the **patch test,** an allergen-treated piece of gauze or filter paper is applied to the skin. If the skin becomes red or swollen, the result is positive. In the **scratch test,** several scratches are made in the skin, and a very minute amount of test material is inserted into the scratches. The Schick test (for diphtheria) and the Mantoux and purified protein derivative (PPD) tests (for tuberculosis) are other skin tests.

ABBREVIATIONS

ABCDE	asymmetry (of shape), border (irregularity), color (variation within one lesion), diameter (greater than 6 mm), evolution (change)—characteristics associated with melanoma	**PPD**	purified protein derivative—used in skin test for tuberculosis
Bx	biopsy	**PUVA**	psoralen–ultraviolet A light therapy; treatment for psoriasis and other skin conditions
Derm	dermatology	**SLE**	systemic lupus erythematosus
DLE	discoid lupus erythematosus	**SC**	subcutaneous

PRACTICAL APPLICATIONS

This section contains disease descriptions, a medical report, and a case report using terms that you have studied in this and previous chapters. Explanations of more difficult terms are added in brackets.

DISEASE DESCRIPTIONS

1. **Candidiasis** (*Candida* is a yeast-like fungus): This fungus is normally found on mucous membranes, skin, and vaginal mucosa. Under certain circumstances (excessive warmth and moisture; administration of antibiotics and corticosteroids; debilitated states; infancy), it can proliferate and cause localized or generalized mucocutaneous disease. Examples are paronychial lesions, lesions in areas of the body where the rubbing of opposed surfaces is common (groin, perianal, axillary, inframammary, and interdigital), thrush (white plaques attached to oral or vaginal mucous membranes), and vulvovaginitis.

2. **Cellulitis:** This is a common nonsuppurative infection of connective tissue with severe inflammation of the dermal and subcutaneous layers of the skin. Cellulitis appears on an extremity as a warm reddish area of tender edematous skin. A surgical wound, puncture, insect bite, skin ulcer, or patch of dermatitis is the usual means of entry for bacteria (most cases are caused by streptococci or Staphylococcus aureus). Therapy includes rest, elevation, hot wet packs, and antibiotics. Any cellulitis on the face should be given special attention because the infection may extend directly to the brain.

3. **Mycosis fungoides (cutaneous T cell lymphoma):** This rare, chronic skin condition is caused by the infiltration of the skin by atypical lymphocytes. Contrary to its name (myc/o = fungus), it is not caused by a fungus but was formerly thought to be of fungal origin. It can manifest with generalized erythroderma or large, reddish, raised tumors that spread and ulcerate. In some cases, the malignant cells may involve lymph nodes and other organs. Treatment with cortisone ointments, topical nitrogen mustard, psoralen–ultraviolet light A (PUVA), and systemic retinoids or immunomodulators can be effective in controlling the disease.

MEDICAL RECORD: FINDINGS ON DERMATOLOGIC EXAMINATION

A wide variety of lesions are seen on the face, shoulders, and back. The predominant lesions are pustules or papules. Many pustules are confluent [running together] over the chin and forehead. Comedones are present on the face, especially along the midface. Inflammatory papules are present on the lower cheeks and chin. Large abscesses and ulcerated cysts are present over the upper shoulder area. Numerous scars are present over the face and upper back.

Questions about the Medical Record

See page 687 for answers.

1. In this skin condition, the primary lesions are
   a. Discolored flat lesions
   b. Grooves or crack-like sores
   c. Small elevations containing pus

2. Comedones are
   a. Sebum plugs partially blocking skin pores
   b. Contagious, infectious plugs of sebum
   c. Small, pinpoint hemorrhages

3. The papules described are known as
   a. Purpura
   b. Pimples
   c. Freckles

4. In the scapular region, lesions are
   a. Large pigmented areas
   b. Numerous collections of blisters
   c. Large collections of sacs containing pus with erosion of skin

5. What is your diagnosis of this skin condition, based on the physical examination?
   a. Acne vulgaris
   b. Leukoplakia
   c. Scabies

CASE REPORT: BASAL CELL CARCINOMA

A 76-year-old woman noticed a 1-inch-diameter flaky patch on her scalp. Over a period of months, the lesion increased in size and became ulcerated, with the skull bone visible (Figure 16-24A). A biopsy was performed and pathologic examination revealed basal cell carcinoma. Mohs micrographic surgery was attempted but a CT study of the head/brain with contrast showed the likelihood of residual tumor extending into the skull (Figure 16-24B).

Major surgery was performed to resect residual malignant tissue. A large portion of skull was removed and replaced with titanium mesh on which muscle from her back and skin from her leg were grafted. The primary surgical area healed well. Pathologic examination confirmed the presence of tumor invading the skull and underlying dura at the surgical margin. The patient is now receiving radiation therapy for 6 weeks to treat the affected area.

Commentary: *Most basal cell carcinomas are small tumors that are easily removed by local surgery, such as Mohs. When treatment is delayed, however, they can become very large and require major surgical procedures with grafting. They can continue to grow locally and invade adjacent tissues, as occurred in this case.*

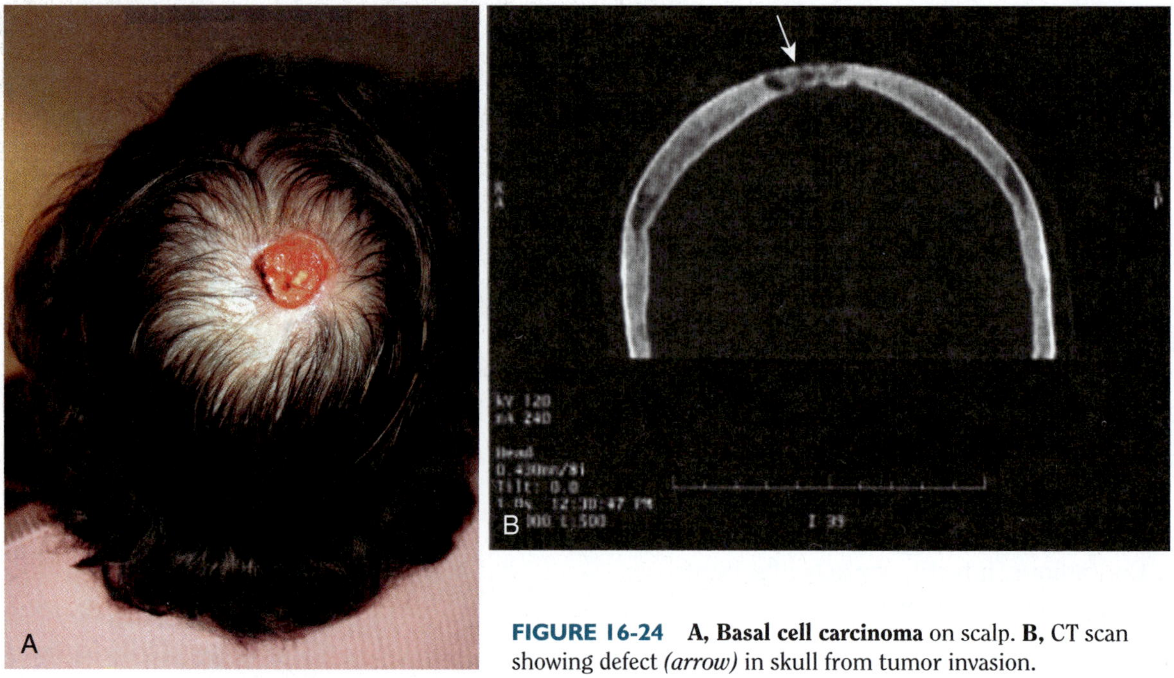

FIGURE 16-24 **A, Basal cell carcinoma** on scalp. **B,** CT scan showing defect *(arrow)* in skull from tumor invasion.

IN PERSON

This is a first-person account describing the course of metastatic melanoma. It is written by the husband of a patient.

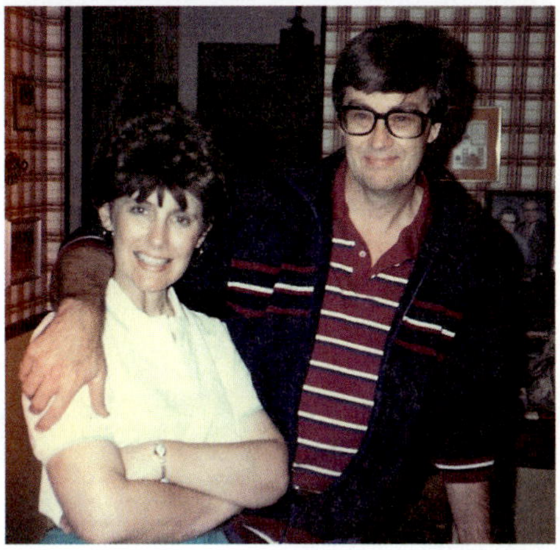

Mary Ann showed me the mole on her arm near her armpit and I knew immediately that this was not going to be a good thing. It was raised, red and black, irregular shape. That was more than 30 years ago, before the Internet, and no way to confirm our fear. Four days later the mole was excised, and within a week, we received confirmation that it was a melanoma.

We had various opinions about the next step, but Mary Ann had always been convinced that you always go to a teaching hospital and find the experts. We selected a surgeon at Georgetown Hospital and she underwent a resection of an area on her arm that was about 3 × 4 inches. The nodes in her armpit were also removed, which I questioned. If the cancer had spread to her nodes then it was already metastatic and, either way, she risked getting edema in her arm. Fortunately, there was no node involvement and she didn't get edema. Again, with no Internet we had to spend several nights at the Library of Medicine trying to educate ourselves with what we were dealing with. We didn't know about the classifications and TNM readings weren't mentioned to us. We only knew the depth of the tumor and, relating that to the charts, we found implied a 30% to 40% five year survival rate.

Living in anticipation of recurrence was extremely stressful. Mary Ann dwelled a lot on her demise despite my and her friends' efforts to put on a happy face and trying to fill the days with distractions. Her 6 month chest x-rays and checkups gradually became less stressful, leaving us with the feeling that it was okay to enjoy life again. Two and a half years after her operation, that changed. A tumor showed up in her lung. Again she found the best thoracic surgeon in the area and had it removed. Six weeks later two small tumors appeared below her ribcage right where the drain from her operation had been. These were the first of many that appeared just below the dermis, in her abdomen, thigh, and back. This was over a period of about 8 months, and during this time Mary Ann entered her first trial in which she received an injectable, specific antigen that was designed to boost her immune system. Remarkably, Mary Ann the fighter began to emerge. With two preteen daughters to nurture, she put tumor removal and weekly injections on her to-do list.

At this time, she was under increased stress dealing with the loss of her mother to a heart attack. During the funeral she complained of severe back pain, and when we returned home tests revealed metastases on her spinal cord. Again, she found the best neurological surgeon and had them removed. She had to relearn how to walk again and had barely begun to recover when her sisters called to tell her that her father had died of a heart attack. She knew even before I told her and, I remember her words: "Bring it on, give me all you've got, I can take it."

Shortly after his funeral she began to have "dancing spots" in her right eye, a sign of a metastatic brain tumor. Her oncologist was adamantly opposed to surgery. His advice was to stick to the protocol, and not put her through an operation because she would be dead in six months. Mary Ann and I believed that the drug protocol alone was not going to give her more time. She was determined to have the surgery and subsequent radiation. Recovery was difficult and she lost her hair in the radiation field, but it was a fortunate time in that she met Davi Chabner, who was to be her best friend and catalyst for enjoying life again. A year later there was another brain tumor, which was removed and followed by more radiation. She then took part in a brief trial using monoclonal antibodies. A couple of more surface tumors were removed, but then: no more! Remission! Life was good. Vacations, golf with friends, visits to college to see our daughters, trips to see Mary Ann's sisters, all was a pleasant blend of what you do with the time you have. Although she had a multitude of friends that she saw often, it was Mary Ann's time with Davi and her husband that kept her enthused over every day.

Five years later Mary Ann woke up with night sweats and a low-grade fever that wouldn't go away. Our worst fears were realized. A large, inoperable tumor was in her spleen. Less than 4 months later she died. Looking back, she went through a lot during her 9-year ordeal, but she beat the odds, and through sheer willpower enjoyed her time to the fullest. That was over 20 years ago, and to this day, I still meet people who remember her fondly and remark that she was one of their best friends. That was Mary Ann. No matter what she was going through she was still interested in *your* life.

Bob Rowe is a retired software engineer and avid golfer.

Note: In the last two years, therapy for metastatic melanoma has been radically improved by a new targeted agent, Vemurafenib, and new monoclonal antibodies that promote an immune response to the tumor.

EXERCISES

Remember to check your answers carefully with the Answers to Exercises, page 686.

A Select from the following terms to complete the sentences below.

adipocyte	dermis	melanin
basal layer	keratin	sebum
collagen	lunula	stratum corneum
cuticle		

1. A fat cell is a/an ______________.
2. The half-moon–shaped white area at the base of a nail is the ______________.
3. A structural protein found in skin and connective tissue is ______________.
4. A pigment found in the epidermis is ______________.
5. The deepest region of the epidermis is the ______________.
6. The outermost layer of the epidermis, which consists of flattened, keratinized cells, is the ______________.
7. An oily substance secreted by sebaceous glands is ______________.
8. The middle layer of the skin is the ______________.
9. A hard, protein material found in epidermis, hair, and nails is ______________.
10. A band of epidermis at the base and sides of the nail plate is the ______________.

B Complete the following terms based on their meanings as given below.

1. the outermost layer of skin: epi______________
2. profuse sweating: dia______________
3. excessive secretion from sebaceous glands: sebo______________
4. inflammation and swelling of soft tissue around a nail: par______________
5. fungal infections of hands and feet: dermato______________
6. burning sensation (pain) in skin: caus______________

C **Match the terms in Column I with the descriptive meanings in Column II. Write the letter of the answer in the space provided.**

COLUMN I

1. squamous epithelium ______
2. sebaceous gland ______
3. albinism ______
4. electrocautery ______
5. subcutaneous tissue ______
6. collagen ______
7. dermis ______
8. melanocyte ______
9. erythema ______
10. dermabrasion ______

COLUMN II

A. connective tissue layer of skin
B. surgical procedure to scrape away tissue
C. flat, scale-like cells
D. connective tissue protein
E. pigment deficiency of the skin
F. contains a dark pigment
G. redness of skin
H. contains lipocytes
I. oil-producing organ
J. knife used to burn through tissue

D **Build medical terms based on the definitions and word parts given.**

1. pertaining to under the skin: sub________________________
2. abnormal condition of lack of sweat: an________________________
3. abnormal condition of proliferation of horny, keratinized cells: kerat________________________
4. abnormal condition of dry, scaly skin:________________________osis
5. loosening of the epidermis: epidermo________________________
6. yellow tumor (nodule under the skin): ________________________oma
7. pertaining to under the nail: sub________________________
8. abnormal condition of excessive hair growth: hyper________________________
9. abnormal condition of nail fungus: onycho________________________
10. removal of wrinkles:________________________ectomy

E Give the meanings for the following combining forms.

1. melan/o ______________________________
2. adip/o ______________________________
3. squam/o ______________________________
4. xanth/o ______________________________
5. myc/o ______________________________
6. onych/o ______________________________
7. pil/o ______________________________
8. xer/o ______________________________
9. trich/o ______________________________
10. erythem/o ______________________________
11. albin/o ______________________________
12. ichthy/o ______________________________
13. hidr/o ______________________________
14. ungu/o ______________________________
15. cauter/o ______________________________
16. steat/o ______________________________
17. rhytid/o ______________________________
18. py/o ______________________________
19. hydr/o ______________________________
20. cutane/o ______________________________

F **Match each of the following lesions with their illustrations below** (Figure 16-25).

crust (scab)	macule	pustule
cyst	nodule	ulcer
erosion	papule	vesicle
fissure	polyp	wheal

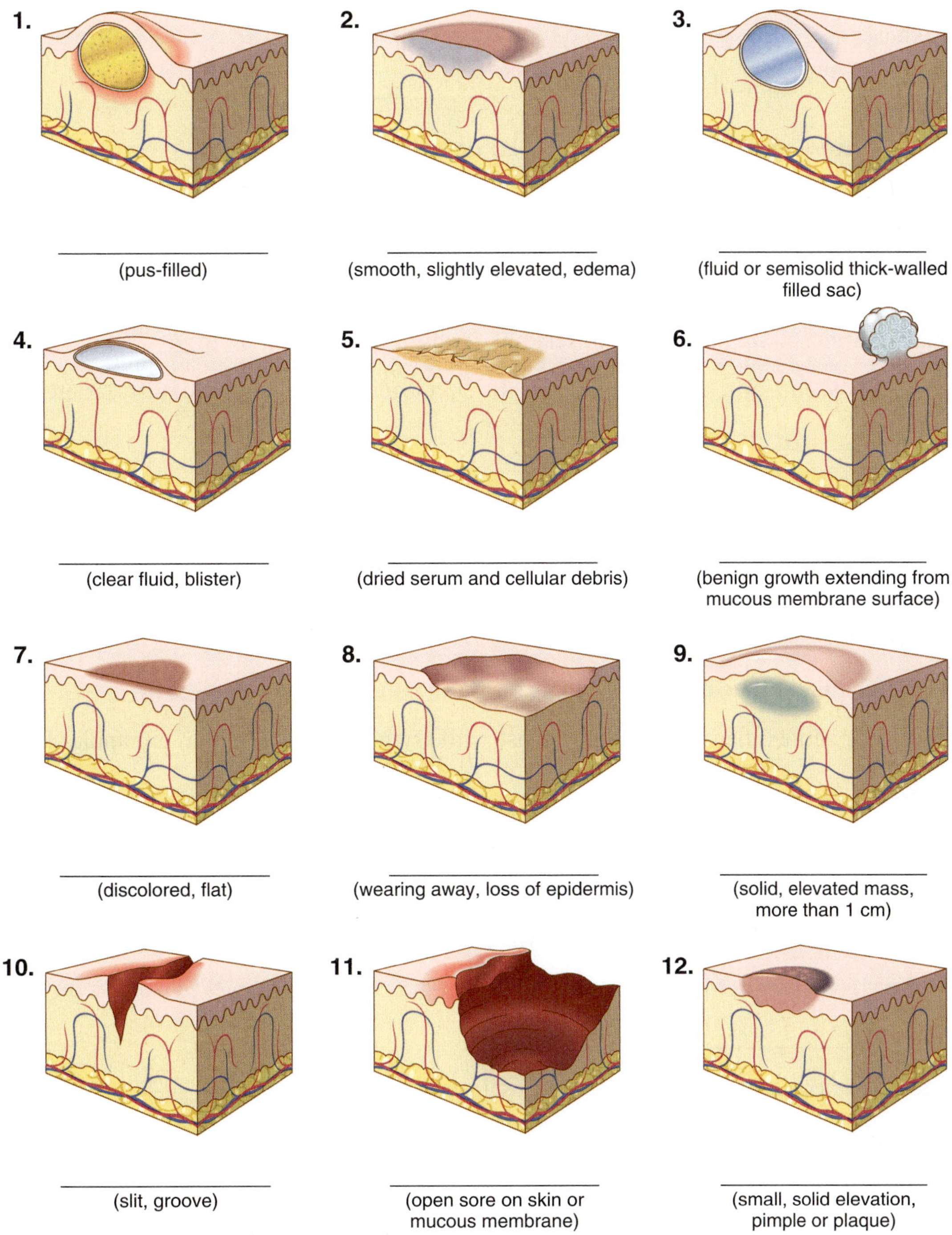

1. ______________ (pus-filled)
2. ______________ (smooth, slightly elevated, edema)
3. ______________ (fluid or semisolid thick-walled filled sac)
4. ______________ (clear fluid, blister)
5. ______________ (dried serum and cellular debris)
6. ______________ (benign growth extending from mucous membrane surface)
7. ______________ (discolored, flat)
8. ______________ (wearing away, loss of epidermis)
9. ______________ (solid, elevated mass, more than 1 cm)
10. ______________ (slit, groove)
11. ______________ (open sore on skin or mucous membrane)
12. ______________ (small, solid elevation, pimple or plaque)

FIGURE 16-25 Cutaneous lesions.

G **Give the medical terms for the following.**

1. baldness ________________
2. bluish black mark (macule) caused by hemorrhages into the skin ________________
3. itching ________________
4. acute allergic reaction in which red, round wheals develop on the skin ________________
5. blackhead ________________
6. small, pinpoint hemorrhages ________________

H **Match the pathologic skin condition with its description below.**

acne vulgaris	gangrene	scleroderma
basal cell carcinoma	impetigo	squamous cell carcinoma
decubitus ulcer	malignant melanoma	systemic lupus erythematosus
eczema	psoriasis	tinea

1. malignant neoplasm originating in scale-like cells of the epidermis ________________
2. buildup of sebum and keratin in pores of the skin leading to papular and pustular eruptions ________________
3. fungal skin infection ________________
4. chronic disease marked by hardening and shrinking of connective tissue in the skin ________________
5. bedsore ________________
6. necrosis of skin tissue resulting from ischemia ________________
7. chronic or acute inflammatory skin disease with erythematous, pustular, or papular lesions ________________
8. widespread inflammatory disease of the joints and collagen of the skin with "butterfly" rash on the face ________________
9. cancerous tumor composed of melanocytes ________________
10. chronic, recurrent dermatosis marked by silvery-gray scales covering red patches on the skin ________________
11. malignant neoplasm originating in the basal layer of the epidermis ________________
12. contagious, infectious pyoderma ________________

I **Circle the term that best fits the definition given.**

1. contagious parasitic infection with intense pruritus: **(scleroderma, scabies)**
2. measles: **(rubella, rubeola)**
3. chickenpox: **(varicella, eczema)**
4. thickened excess cicatrix (scar): **(tinea, keloid)**
5. white patches on mucous membrane of tongue or inner cheek: **(leukoplakia, albinism)**
6. characterized by a rash: **(gangrene, exanthematous)**
7. thickening of epidermis related to sunlight exposure: **(actinic keratosis, callus)**
8. small, pinpoint hemorrhages: **(psoriasis, petechiae)**
9. large blisters: **(bullae, pustules)**
10. hyperpigmented macule or papule of skin (mole): **(nevus, verruca)**
11. sac of fluid and hair over sacral region: **(ecchymosis, pilonidal cyst)**
12. acute allergic reaction in which hives develop: **(vitiligo, urticaria)**

J **Describe the following types of burns.**

1. second-degree burn ______________________________
2. first-degree burn ______________________________
3. third-degree burn ______________________________

K **Match the following medical terms with their more common meanings below.**

alopecia	exanthem	tinea pedis
comedones	nevi	urticaria
decubitus ulcer	pruritus	verrucae
ecchymosis	seborrheic dermatitis	vesicles

1. blackheads ____________________
2. moles ____________________
3. baldness ____________________
4. itching ____________________
5. hives ____________________
6. bedsore ____________________
7. warts ____________________
8. athlete's foot ____________________
9. "black-and-blue" mark ____________________
10. dandruff ____________________
11. blisters ____________________
12. rash ____________________

L **Describe how the following conditions affect the skin.**

1. pyoderma ______________________________
2. xerosis ______________________________
3. leukoderma ______________________________
4. erythema ______________________________
5. callus ______________________________
6. keloid ______________________________
7. gangrene ______________________________

M **Give short answers to complete the following sentences.**

1. Two skin tests for allergy are ______________ and ______________ .
2. The ______________ test is an intradermal test for diphtheria.
3. The ______________ test and the ______________ test are skin tests for tuberculosis.
4. Purulent means ______________ .
5. A surgical procedure to core out a disk of skin for microscopic analysis is a/an ______________ .
6. The procedure in which thin layers of a malignant growth are removed and each is examined under the microscope is ______________ .
7. A type of skin cancer associated with AIDS and marked by dark blue-purple lesions over the skin is ______________ .
8. Abnormal, premalignant moles are ______________ .
9. Removal of skin tissue using a cut parallel to the surface of the surrounding skin is called a/an ______________ .
10. Destruction of tissue using intensely cold temperatures is ______________ .
11. Scraping away skin to remove acne scars and fine wrinkles on the skin is ______________ .
12. Removal of subcutaneous fat tissue by aspiration is ______________ .
13. Destruction of tissue using an electric spark is ______________ .
14. Use of a sharp, spoon-like instrument to scrape away tissue is ______________ .

16

N Circle the term that best completes the meaning of the sentence.

1. Since he was a teenager, Jim had had red, scaly patches on his elbows and the front of his knees. Dr. Horn diagnosed Jim's dermatologic condition as **(vitiligo, impetigo, psoriasis)** and prescribed a special cream.
2. Clarissa noticed a rash across the bridge of her nose and aching in her joints. She saw a rheumatologist, who did some blood work and diagnosed her condition as **(rheumatoid arthritis, systemic lupus erythematosus, scleroderma)**.
3. Bea had large red plaques develop all over her trunk and neck after eating shrimp. The doctor prescribed hydrocortisone cream to relieve her itching **(seborrhea, acne, urticaria)**.
4. The poison ivy Maggie touched caused very uncomfortable **(pruritus, calluses, keratosis)**, and she was scratching her arms raw.
5. Kelly was fair-skinned with red hair. She had many benign nevi on her arms and legs, but Dr. Keefe was especially worried about one pigmented lesion with an irregular, raised border, which he biopsied and found to be malignant **(melanoma, Kaposi sarcoma, pyoderma)**.
6. After 5 days of high fever, 3-year-old Sadie developed a red rash all over her body. The pediatrician described it as a viral **(eczema, purpura, exanthem)** and told her mother it was a case of **(rubeola, impetigo, scabies)**.
7. Several months after her surgery, Mabel's scar became raised and thickened and grew beyond the boundaries of the incision. It had **(atrophied, stratified, hypertrophied)**, and her physician described it as a **(nevus, verruca, keloid)**.
8. Perry had a bad habit of biting his nails and picking at the **(follicle, cuticle, subcutaneous tissue)** surrounding his nails. Often, he developed inflammation and swelling of the soft tissue around the nail, a condition known as **(onychomycosis, onycholysis, paronychia)**.
9. Brenda noticed a small papillomatous wart on her hand. Her **(oncologist, dermatologist, psychologist)** explained that it was a **(pustule, polyp, verruca)** and was caused by a **(bacterium, virus, toxin)**. The doctor suggested removing it by **(Mohs surgery, cryosurgery, dilation and curettage)**.
10. Sarah, a teenager, was self-conscious about the inflammatory lesions of papules and pustules on her face. She noticed blackheads or **(wheals, bullae, open comedones)** and whiteheads (closed comedones). She was advised to begin taking antibiotics and applying topical medications to treat her **(acne vulgaris, scleroderma, gangrene)**.

ANSWERS TO EXERCISES

A

1. adipocyte
2. lunula
3. collagen
4. melanin
5. basal layer
6. stratum corneum
7. sebum
8. dermis
9. keratin
10. cuticle

B

1. epidermis
2. diaphoresis
3. seborrhea
4. paronychia
5. dermatophytosis or dermatomycosis (tinea)
6. causalgia

C

1. C
2. I
3. E
4. J
5. H
6. D
7. A
8. F
9. G
10. B

D

1. subcutaneous
2. anhidrosis
3. keratosis
4. ichthyosis
5. epidermolysis
6. xanthoma
7. subungual
8. hypertrichosis
9. onychomycosis
10. rhytidectomy

E

1. black
2. fat
3. scale-like
4. yellow
5. fungus
6. nail
7. hair
8. dry
9. hair
10. redness
11. white
12. scaly, dry
13. sweat
14. nail
15. heat, burn
16. fat
17. wrinkle
18. pus
19. water
20. skin

F

1. pustule
2. wheal
3. cyst
4. vesicle
5. crust (scab)
6. polyp
7. macule
8. erosion
9. nodule
10. fissure
11. ulcer
12. papule

G

1. alopecia
2. ecchymosis
3. pruritus
4. urticaria
5. comedo
6. petechiae

H

1. squamous cell carcinoma
2. acne vulgaris
3. tinea
4. scleroderma
5. decubitus ulcer
6. gangrene
7. eczema
8. systemic lupus erythematosus
9. malignant melanoma
10. psoriasis
11. basal cell carcinoma
12. impetigo

I

1. scabies
2. rubeola
3. varicella
4. keloid
5. leukoplakia
6. exanthematous
7. actinic keratosis
8. petechiae
9. bullae
10. nevus
11. pilonidal cyst
12. urticaria

J

1. damage to the epidermis and dermis with blisters, erythema, and hyperesthesia
2. damage to the epidermis with erythema and hyperesthesia; no blisters
3. destruction of both epidermis and dermis and damage to subcutaneous layer

K

1. comedones
2. nevi
3. alopecia
4. pruritus
5. urticaria
6. decubitus ulcer
7. verrucae
8. tinea pedis
9. ecchymosis
10. seborrheic dermatitis
11. vesicles
12. exanthem

L

1. collections of pus in the skin
2. dry skin
3. white patches of skin (vitiligo)
4. redness of skin
5. increased growth of epidermal horny-layer cells due to excess pressure or friction
6. thickened, hypertrophied scar tissue
7. necrosis (death) of skin tissue

M

1. scratch test; patch test
2. Schick
3. Mantoux; PPD
4. pus-filled
5. punch biopsy
6. Mohs surgery
7. Kaposi sarcoma
8. dysplastic nevi
9. shave biopsy
10. cryosurgery
11. dermabrasion
12. liposuction
13. electrodesiccation
14. curettage

N

1. psoriasis
2. systemic lupus erythematosus
3. urticaria
4. pruritus
5. melanoma
6. exanthem; rubeola
7. hypertrophied; keloid
8. cuticle; paronychia
9. dermatologist; verruca; virus; cryosurgery
10. open comedones; acne vulgaris

16

Answers to Practical Applications

1. c
2. a
3. b
4. c
5. a

PRONUNCIATION OF TERMS

To test your understanding of the terminology in this chapter, write the meaning of each term in the space provided. In addition, you may wish to cover the terms and write them by looking at your definitions. Make sure your spelling is correct. The page number after each term indicates where it is defined or used in the book, so you can easily check your responses. You will find complete definitions for all of these terms and their audio pronunciations on the Evolve website.

Pronunciation Guide

ā as in āpe	ă as in ăpple
ē as in ēven	ĕ as in ĕvery
ī as in īce	ĭ as in ĭnterest
ō as in ōpen	ŏ as in pŏt
ū as in ūnit	ŭ as in ŭnder

Terminology

TERM	PRONUNCIATION	MEANING
adipocyte (657)	ĂD-ĭ-pō-sīt	
adipose (658)	ĂD-ĭ-pōs	
albinism (658)	ĂL-bĭ-nĭzm	
albino (657)	ăl-BĪ-nō	
anhidrosis (658)	ăn-hī-DRŌ-sĭs	
apocrine sweat gland (657)	ĂP-ō-krĭn swĕt glănd	
basal layer (657)	BĀ-săl LĀ-ĕr	
causalgia (658)	kăw-ZĂL-jă	
collagen (657)	KŎL-ă-jĕn	
cuticle (657)	KŪ-tĭ-kl	
dermabrasion (658)	dĕrm-ă-BRĀ-zhŭn	
dermatitis (658)	dĕr-mă-TĪ-tŭs	
dermatologist (658)	dĕr-mă-TŎL-ō-jĭst	
dermatophytosis (660)	dĕr-mă-tō-fī-TŌ-sĭs	
dermis (657)	DĔR-mĭs	
diaphoresis (658)	dī-ă-fŏr-RĒ-sĭs	
eccrine sweat gland (657)	Ĕ-krĭn swĕt glănd	
electrocautery (658)	ĕ-lĕk-trō-KĂW-tĕr-ē	
epidermis (657)	ĕp-ĭ-DĔR-mĭs	
epidermolysis (658)	ĕp-ĭ-dĕr-MŎL-ĭ-sĭs	
epithelium (657)	ĕp-ĭ-THĒL-ē-ŭm	
erythema (658)	ĕr-ĭ-THĒ-mă	
erythematous (658)	ĕr-ĭ-THĒ-mă-tŭs	
hair follicle (657)	hār FŎL-ĭ-kl	

TERM	PRONUNCIATION	MEANING
hypertrichosis (661)	hī-pĕr-trĭ-KŌ-sĭs	
ichthyosis (658)	ĭk-thē-Ō-sĭs	
integumentary system (657)	ĭn-tĕg-ū-MĔN-tăr-ē SĬS-tĕm	
keratin (657)	KĔR-ă-tĭn	
keratosis (659)	kĕr-ă-TŌ-sĭs	
leukoplakia (659)	lōō-kō-PLĀ-kē-ă	
lipoma (659)	lī-PŌ-mă *or* lĭ-PŌ-mă	
liposuction (659)	lī-pō-SŬK-shun	
lunula (657)	LŪ-nū-lă	
melanin (657)	MĔL-ă-nĭn	
melanocyte (659)	mĕ-LĂN-ō-sīt	
mycosis (660)	mī-KŌ-sĭs	
onycholysis (660)	ŏn-ĭ-KŎL-ĭ-sĭs	
onychomycosis (660)	ŏn-ĭ-kō-mī-KŌ-sĭs	
paronychia (660)	păr-ō-NĬK-ē-ă	
paronychium (657)	păr-ŏn-NĬK-ē-um	
pilosebaceous (660)	pī-lō-sĕ-BĀ-shŭs	
pore (657)	PŎR	
pyoderma (660)	pī-ō-DĔR-mă	
rhytidectomy (660)	rĭt-ĭ-DĔK-tō-mē	
sebaceous gland (657)	sĕ-BĀ-shŭs glănd	
seborrhea (660)	sĕb-ō-RĒ-ă	
seborrheic dermatitis (660)	sĕb-ō-RĒ-ĭk dĕr-mă-TĪ-tĭs	
sebum (657)	SĒ-bŭm	
squamous epithelium (657)	SKWĀ-mŭs ĕp-ĭ-THĒ-lē-ŭm	
steatoma (661)	stē-ă-TŌ-mă	
stratified (657)	STRĂT-ĭ-fīd	
stratum; (*pl.* strata) (657)	STRĂ-tŭm; STRĂ-tă	
stratum corneum (657)	STRĂ-tŭm KŎR-nē-ŭm	
subcutaneous layer (657)	sŭb-kū-TĀ-nē-ŭs LĀ-ĕr	
subungual (661)	sŭb-ŬNG-wăl	
xanthoma (661)	zăn-THŌ-mă	
xerosis (661)	zĕr-Ō-sĭs	

16

Pathology; Laboratory Tests and Clinical Procedures

TERM	PRONUNCIATION	MEANING
abscess (662)	ĂB-sĕs	
acne (664)	ĂK-nē	
alopecia areata (664)	ăl-ō-PĒ-shē-ă ăr-ē-ĂT-ă	
atopic dermatitis (666)	ā-TŎP-ĭk dĕr-mă-TĪ-tĭs	
bacterial analyses (673)	băk-TĒR-ē-ăl ă-NĂL-ĭ-sēz	
basal cell carcinoma (672)	BĀ-săl sĕl kăr-sĭ-NŌ-mă	
bulla; bullae (662)	BŬL-ă; BŬL-ē	
burns (665)	bŭrnz	
callus (670)	KĂL-ŭs	
cellulitis (666)	sĕl-ū-LĪ-tĭs	
cicatrix (670)	SĬK-ă-trĭks	
comedo; comedones (664)	KŎM-ĕ-dō; kŏm-ĕ-DŌNZ	
crust (662)	krŭst	
cryosurgery (673)	krī-ō-SŬR-gĕr-ē	
curettage (673)	kū-rĕ-TĂZH	
cyst (662)	sĭst	
decubitus ulcer (662)	dē-KŪ-bĭ-tŭs ŬL-sĕr	
dysplastic nevi (671)	dĭs-PLĂS-tik NĒ-vī	
ecchymosis; ecchymoses (664)	ĕk-ĭ-MŌ-sĭs; ĕk-ĭ-MŌ-sēz	
eczema (666)	ĔK-zĕ-mă	
electrodesiccation (673)	ĕ-lĕk-trō-dĕ-sĭ-KĀ-shun	
erosion (662)	ĕ-RŌ-zhŭn	
exanthematous viral disease (666)	ĕg-zăn-THĔM-ă-tŭs VĪ-răl dĭ-ZĒZ	
fissure (662)	FĬSH-ŭr	
fungal tests (674)	FŬNG-ăl tĕsts	
gangrene (667)	găng-GRĒN	
impetigo (667)	ĭm-pĕ-TĪ-gō	
Kaposi sarcoma (672)	KĂH-pō-sē săr-KŌ-mă	
keloid (670)	KĒ-loyd	
keratosis (670)	kĕr-ă-TŌ-sĭs	

TERM	PRONUNCIATION	MEANING
macule (662)	MĂK-ūl	
malignant melanoma (672)	mă-LĬG-nănt mĕ-lă-NŌ-mă	
Mohs surgery (673)	mōz SŬR-jĕ-rē	
nevus; nevi (671)	NĒ-vŭs; NĒ-vī	
nodule (662)	NŎD-ūl	
papule (662)	PĂP-ūl	
petechia; petechiae (664)	pĕ-TĒ-kē-ă; pĕ-TĒ-kē-ī	
pilonidal cyst (662)	pī-lō-NĪ-dăl sĭst	
polyp (662)	PŎL-ĭp	
pruritus (664)	proo-RĪ-tŭs	
psoriasis (668)	sō-RĪ-ă-sĭs	
purpura (664)	PŬR-pŭr-ă	
pustule (662)	PŬS-tūl	
rubella (666)	roo-BĔL-ă	
rubeola (666)	roo-bē-Ō-lă	
scabies (668)	SKĀ-bēz	
scleroderma (668)	sklĕr-ō-DĔR-mă	
sebaceous cyst (661)	sĕ-BĀ-shŭs sĭst	
skin biopsy (674)	skĭn BĪ-ŏp-sē	
skin test (674)	skĭn tĕst	
squamous cell carcinoma (672)	SKWĀ-mŭs sĕl kăr-sĭ-NŌ-mă	
systemic lupus erythematosus (668)	sĭs-TĔM-ĭk LOO-pŭs ĕr-ĭ-thē-mă-TŌ-sŭs	
tinea (669)	TĬN-ē-ă	
ulcer (662)	ŬL-sĕr	
urticaria (670)	ŭr-tĭ-KĀ-rē-ă	
varicella (666)	văr-ĭ-SĔL-ă	
verruca; verrucae (671)	vĕ-ROO-kă; vĕ-ROO-kē	
vesicle (662)	VĔS-ĭ-kl	
vitiligo (670)	vĭt-ĭl-Ī-gō	
wheal (662)	wēl	

16

REVIEW SHEET

Write the meanings of the word parts in the spaces provided, and test yourself. Check your answers with the information in the chapter or in the Glossary (Medical Word Parts—English) at the end of the book.

Combining Forms

COMBINING FORM	MEANING	COMBINING FORM	MEANING
adip/o	________	melan/o	________
albin/o	________	myc/o	________
caus/o	________	onych/o	________
cauter/o	________	phyt/o	________
cutane/o	________	pil/o	________
derm/o	________	py/o	________
dermat/o	________	rhytid/o	________
diaphor/o	________	seb/o	________
erythem/o	________	sebace/o	________
erythemat/o	________	squam/o	________
hidr/o	________	steat/o	________
hydr/o	________	trich/o	________
ichthy/o	________	ungu/o	________
kerat/o	________	xanth/o	________
leuk/o	________	xer/o	________
lip/o	________		

Suffixes

SUFFIX	MEANING	SUFFIX	MEANING
-algia	______	-osis	______
-derma	______	-ous	______
-esis	______	-plakia	______
-lysis	______	-plasty	______
-ose	______	-rrhea	______

Give combining forms for the following (first letters are given).

fat	a ______	sweat	d ______
	l ______		h ______
	s ______	yellow	x ______
white	a ______	dry	x ______
	l ______	dry, scaly (fish-like)	i ______
skin	c ______	redness	e ______
	d ______		e ______
nail	o ______	hard	k ______
	u ______	heat, burn	c ______
hair	p ______	black	m ______
	t ______	fungus	m ______
plant	p ______		

16

Identify the following skin conditions:

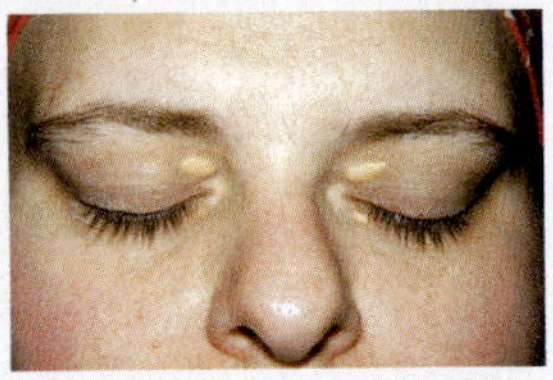

A. ______________________

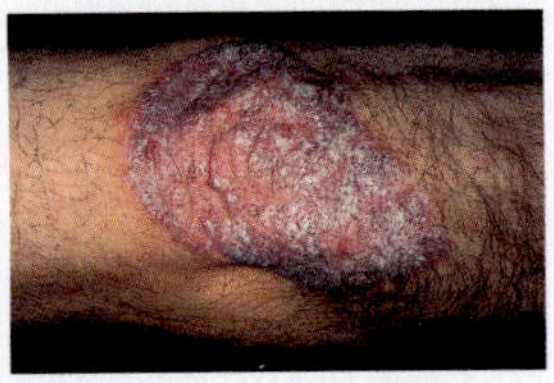

B. ______________________

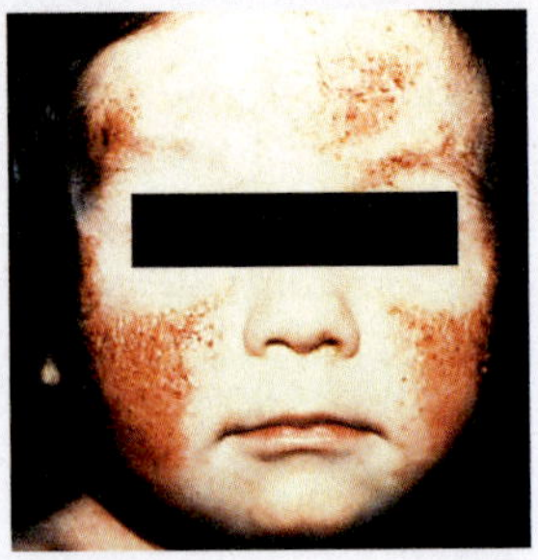

C. ______________________

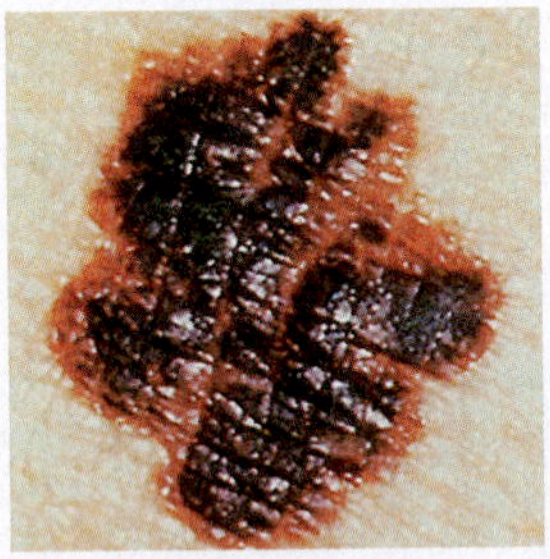

D. ______________________

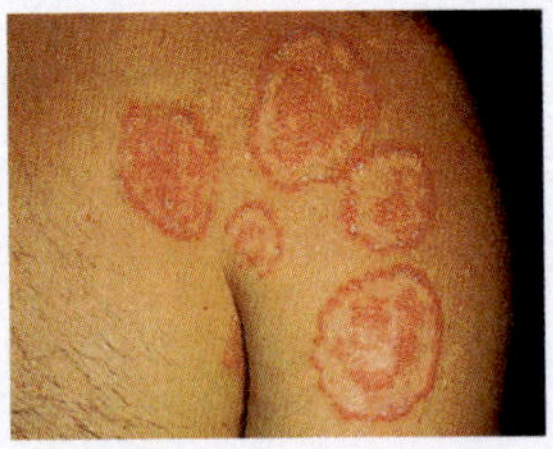

E. ______________________

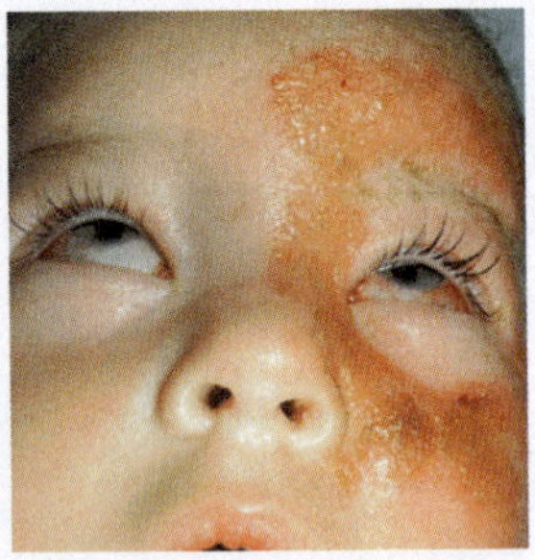

F. ______________________

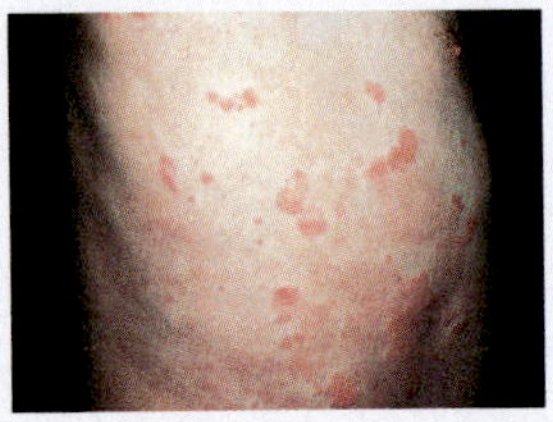

G. ______________________

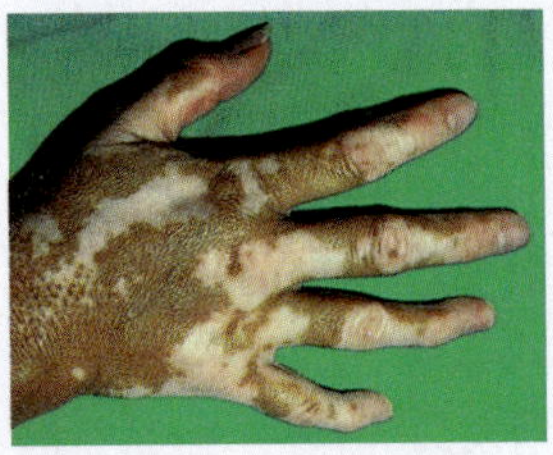

H. ______________________

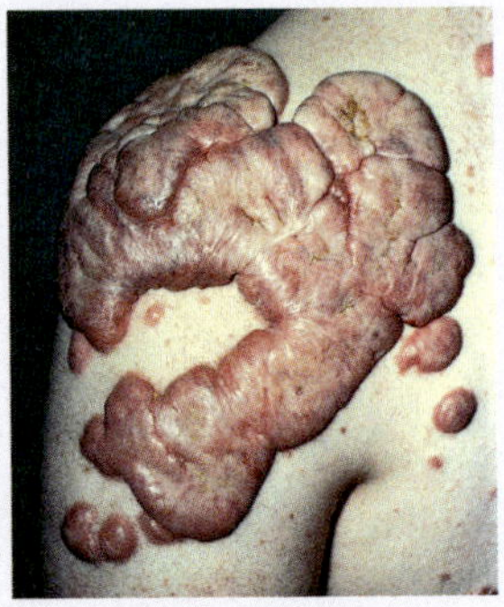

I. ______________________

CHAPTER 17

Sense Organs: The Eye and the Ear

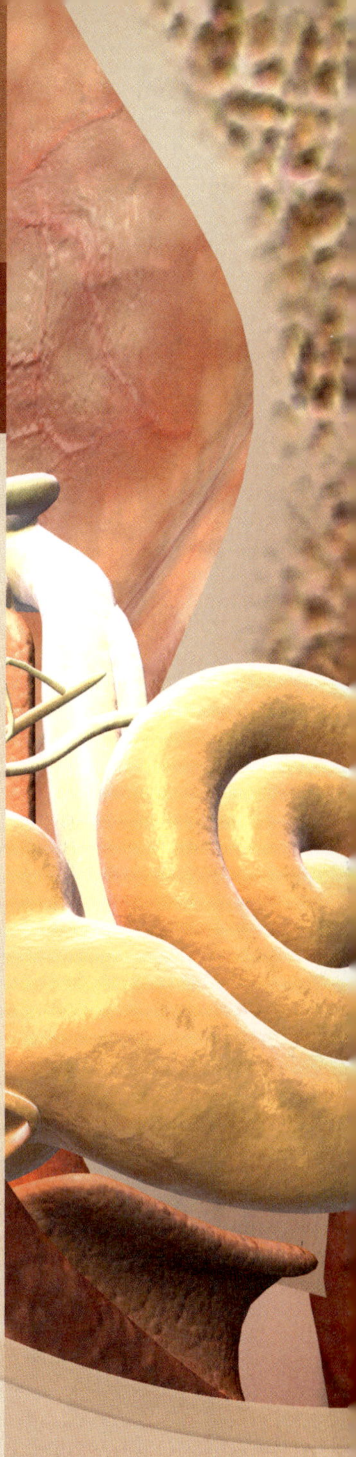

This chapter is divided into the following sections:

CHAPTER GOALS

- Identify locations and functions of the major parts of the eye and the ear.
- Name the combining forms, prefixes, and suffixes most commonly used to describe these organs and their parts.
- Describe the abnormal conditions that may affect the eye and the ear.
- Identify clinical procedures that pertain to ophthalmology and otology.
- Apply your new knowledge to understanding medical terms in their proper contexts, such as medical reports and records.

INTRODUCTION

The **eye** and the **ear** are sense organs, like the skin, taste buds, and **olfactory** (centers of smell in the nose) regions. As such, they are receptors whose sensitive cells may be activated by a particular form of energy or stimulus in the external or internal environment. The sensitive cells in the eye and ear respond to the stimulus by initiating a series of nerve impulses along sensory nerve fibers that lead to the brain.

No matter what stimulus affects a particular receptor, the resulting sensation is determined by regions in the brain connected to that receptor. Thus, mechanical injury that stimulates receptor cells in the eye and the ear may produce sensations of vision (flashes of light) and sound (ringing in the ears). If a workable connection could be made between the sensitive receptor cells of the ear and the area in the brain associated with sight, it would be possible to "see" sounds.

Figure 17-1 reviews the general pattern of events when such stimuli as light and sound are applied to sense organs such as the eye and the ear.

THE EYE

ANATOMY AND PHYSIOLOGY

Label Figure 17-2 as you read the following:

Light rays enter the central dark opening of the eye, the **pupil** [1], which is surrounded by the colored portion of the eye, or **iris** (see the photo inset). The **conjunctiva** [2] is a membrane lining the inner surfaces of the eyelids and anterior portion of the eyeball over the white of the eye. The conjunctiva is clear and almost colorless except when blood vessels are dilated. Dust and smoke may cause the blood vessels to dilate, giving the conjunctiva a reddish appearance—commonly known as bloodshot eyes.

Before entering the eye through the pupil, light passes through the **cornea** [3]. The cornea is a fibrous, transparent tissue that extends like a dome over the pupil and iris. The function of the cornea is to bend, or **refract,** the rays of light so they are focused properly on the sensitive receptor cells in the posterior region of the eye. The normal, healthy cornea is avascular (has no blood vessels) but receives nourishment from blood vessels near its junction with the opaque white of the eye, the **sclera** [4]. Corneal transplants for people with scarred or opaque corneas are often successful because antibodies responsible for rejection of foreign tissue usually do not reach the avascular, transplanted corneal tissue. The sclera is a fibrous layer under the conjunctiva. It extends from the cornea on the anterior surface of the eyeball to the optic nerve in the back of the eye.

The **choroid** [5] is a dark brown membrane inside the sclera. It contains many blood vessels that supply nutrients to the eye. The choroid is continuous with the pigment-containing **iris** [6] and the **ciliary body** [7] on the anterior surface of the eye. The choroid, iris, and ciliary body are known as the **uvea** of the eye.

The iris is the colored portion of the eye (it can appear blue, green, hazel, gray, or brown), which has a circular opening in the center that forms the pupil. Muscles of the iris constrict

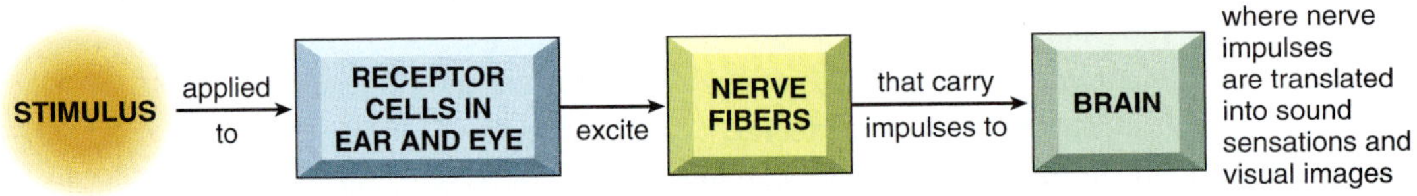

FIGURE 17-1 **Pattern of events in the stimulation of a sense organ.**

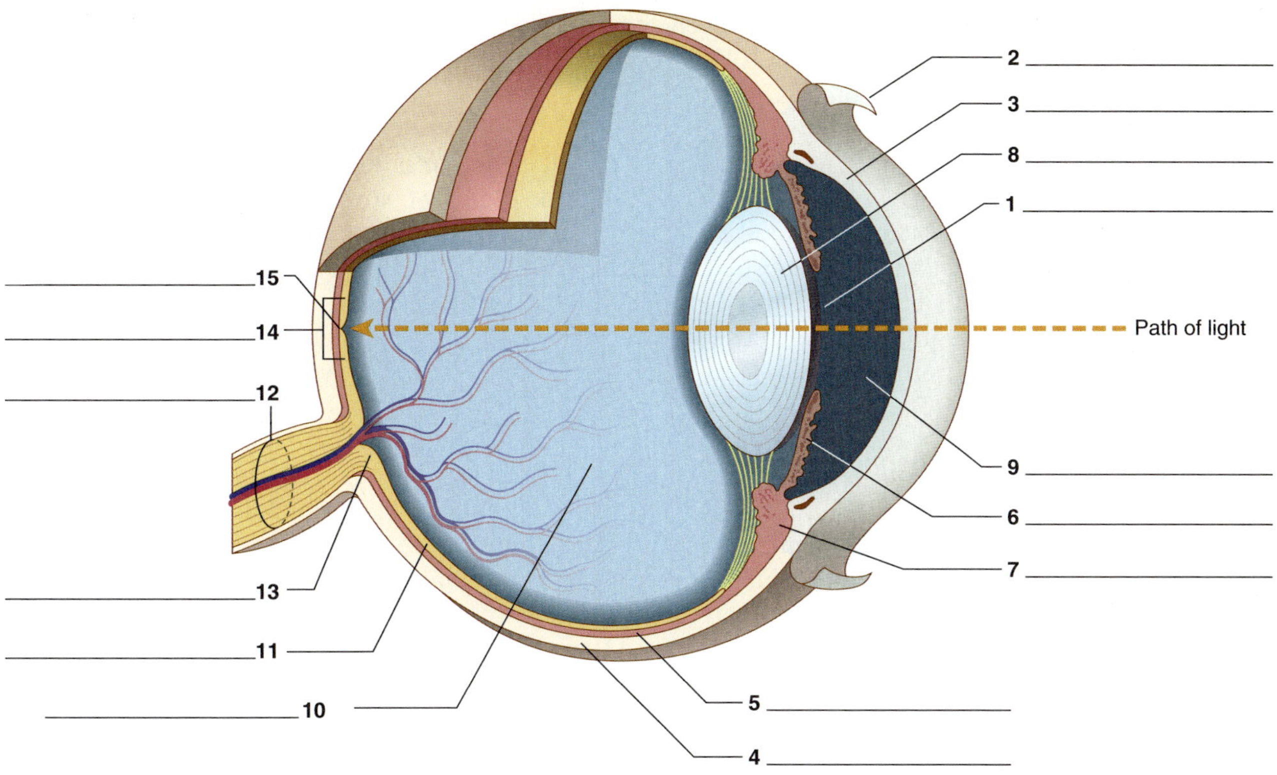

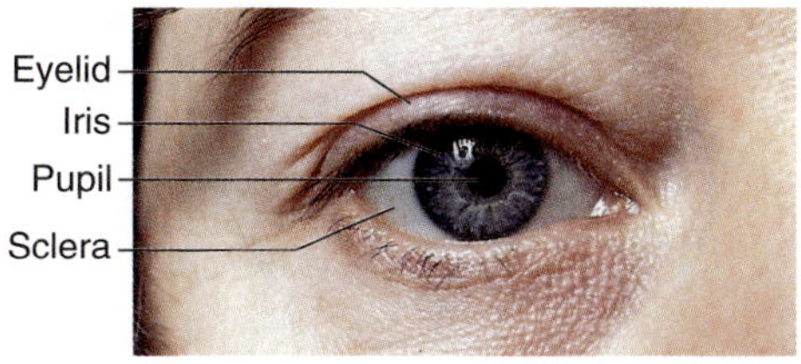

FIGURE 17-2 **The structure of the eye.**

the pupil in bright light and dilate the pupil in dim light, thereby regulating the amount of light entering the eye.

The ciliary body surrounds the outside of the **lens** [8] in a circular fashion for 360 degrees. There are fine thread-like attachments (zonules) that connect the ciliary body and the lens and allow the muscles in the ciliary body to adjust the shape and thickness of the lens. These changes in the shape of the lens cause **refraction** of light rays. Refraction is the bending of rays as they pass through the cornea, lens, and other tissues. Muscles of the ciliary body produce flattening of the lens (for distant vision) and thickening and rounding of the lens (for close vision). This refractory adjustment to focus on an object from far to near is called **accommodation.**

Besides regulating the shape of the lens, the ciliary body also secretes a fluid called **aqueous humor,** which is found in the **anterior chamber** [9] of the eye. Aqueous humor maintains the shape of the anterior portion of the eye and nourishes the structures in that region. The fluid is constantly produced and leaves the eye through a canal that carries it into the bloodstream. Another cavity of the eye is the **vitreous chamber,** which is a large region behind the lens filled with a soft, jelly-like material, the **vitreous humor** [10]. Vitreous humor maintains the shape of the eyeball and is not constantly re-formed. Its escape (due to trauma or surgical damage) may result in significant damage to the eye, leading to possible retinal damage and blindness. Both the aqueous and the vitreous humors further refract light rays.

The **retina** [11] is the thin, delicate, and sensitive nerve layer of the eye. As light energy, in the form of waves, travels through the eye, it is refracted (by the cornea, lens, and fluids), so that it focuses on sensitive receptor cells of the retina called the **rods** and **cones.** There are approximately 6.5 million cones and 120 million rods in the retina. The cones function in bright levels of light and are responsible for color and central vision. There are three types of cones, each stimulated by one of the primary colors in light (red, green, or blue). Most cases of color blindness affect either the green or the red receptors, so that the two colors cannot be distinguished from each other. Rods function at reduced levels of light and are responsible for peripheral vision.

When light rays are focused on the retina, a chemical change occurs in the rods and cones, initiating nerve impulses that then travel from the eye to the brain via the **optic nerve** [12]. The region in the eye where the optic nerve meets the retina is called the **optic disc** [13]. Because there are no light receptor cells in the optic disc, it is known as the blind spot of the eye. The **macula** [14] is a small, oval, yellowish area adjacent to the optic disc. It contains a central depression called the **fovea centralis** [15], which is composed largely of cones and is the location of the sharpest vision in the eye. If a portion of the fovea or macula is damaged, vision is reduced and central-vision blindness occurs. Figure 17-3 shows the retina of a normal eye as seen through an ophthalmoscope. The **fundus** of the eye is this posterior, inner part that is visualized through the ophthalmoscope.

Figure 17-4 illustrates what happens when you look at an object and "see" it. If an object is in your left visual field (purple area), sensitive cells—rods and cones—in the right half of

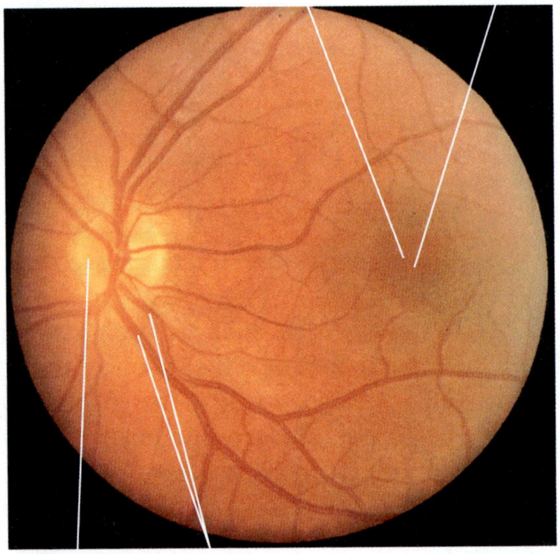

FIGURE 17-3 **The posterior, inner part (fundus) of the eye**, showing the retina as seen through an ophthalmoscope.

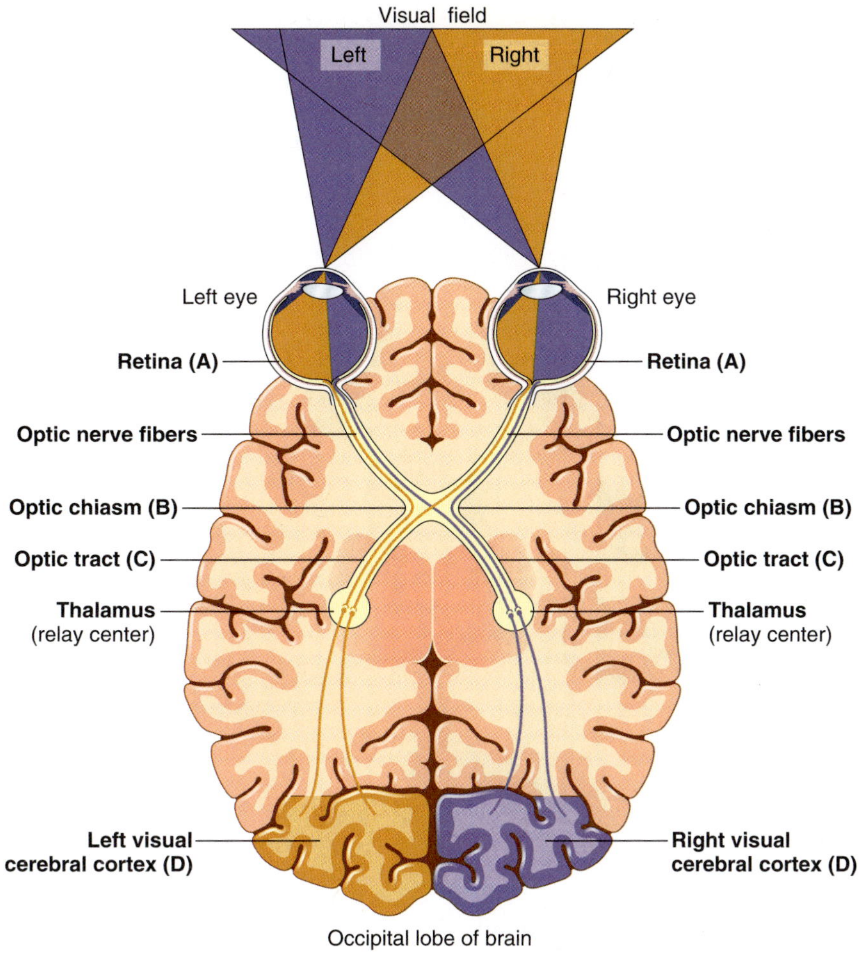

FIGURE 17-4 **Visual pathway from the retina *(A)* to the visual cerebral cortex *(D)*** (occipital lobe of the brain). Objects in the left visual field are "seen" by the right side of the brain, whereas objects in the right visual field are projected into the left visual cerebral cortex.

each **retina** (labeled A in the figure) are stimulated. Similarly, if an object is in your right visual field (orange color), rods and cones are stimulated in the left half of each retina. Nervous impulses then travel along optic nerve fibers from each retina and then merge to form the **optic chiasm** (B). Here, medial or nasal optic nerve fibers cross and temporal fibers do not. Thus, fibers from the right half of each retina (purple color) form an **optic tract** (C) leading, via the **thalamus** (relay center), to the **right visual cerebral cortex** (D). Similarly, fibers from the left half of each retina (orange color) form an optic tract leading to the **left visual cerebral cortex** (D). Images (one from each eye) are then fused in the occipital lobe of the brain, producing a single visual sensation with the three-dimensional effect. This is **binocular vision.**

Brain damage to nerve cells in the right visual cerebral cortex (such as in a stroke) causes loss of vision in the left visual field (purple), whereas damage in the left cerebral cortex causes loss of vision in the right visual field (gold). This loss of vision, which occurs in both eyes, on the contralateral (opposite side) visual field is called **hemianopsia** (**hemi-** means half, **an-** means without, **-opsia** means vision). In the right eye, the loss is on the left nasal visual field, and in the left eye, the loss is on the left temporal visual field.

Figure 17-5 reviews the pathway of light rays from the cornea to the cerebral cortex of the brain.

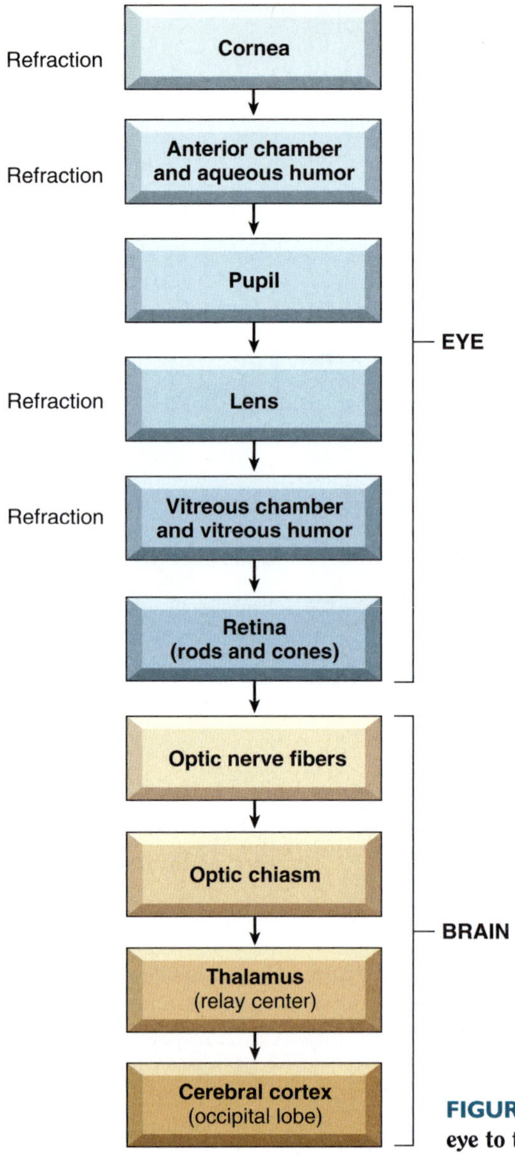

FIGURE 17-5 **Pathway of light rays from the cornea of the eye to the cerebral cortex of the brain.**

VOCABULARY—THE EYE

This list reviews many new terms related to the eye introduced in the text. Short definitions reinforce your understanding of the terms. Refer to the Pronunciation of Terms on page 740 for help with unfamiliar or difficult words.

accommodation	Normal adjustment of the eye to focus on objects from far to near. The ciliary body adjusts the lens (rounding it) and the pupil constricts. When the eye focuses from near to far, the ciliary body flattens the lens and the pupil dilates.
anterior chamber	Area behind the cornea and in front of the lens and iris. It contains aqueous humor.
aqueous humor	Fluid produced by the ciliary body and found in the anterior chamber. A humor (Latin *humidus* means moist) is any body fluid, including blood and lymph.

biconvex	Consisting of two surfaces that are rounded, elevated, and curved evenly, like part of a sphere. The lens of the eye is a biconvex body.
choroid	Middle, vascular layer of the eye, between the retina and the sclera.
ciliary body	Structure surrounding the lens that connects the choroid and iris. It contains ciliary muscles, which control the shape of the lens, and it secretes aqueous humor.
cone	Photoreceptor cell in the retina that transforms light energy into a nerve impulse. Cones are responsible for color and central vision.
conjunctiva	Delicate membrane lining the undersurface of the eyelids and covering the anterior eyeball.
cornea	Fibrous transparent layer of clear tissue that extends over the anterior portion of the eyeball. Derived from Latin *corneus*, meaning horny, perhaps because as it protrudes outward, it was thought to resemble a horn.
fovea centralis	Tiny pit or depression in the retina that is the region of clearest vision.
fundus of the eye	Posterior, inner part of the eye.
iris	Pigmented (colored) layer that opens and closes to allow more or less light into the eye. The central opening of the iris is the pupil.
lens	Transparent, biconvex body behind the pupil of the eye. It bends (refracts) light rays to bring them into focus on the retina.
macula	Yellowish region on the retina lateral to and slightly below the optic disc; contains the fovea centralis, which is the area of clearest vision.
optic chiasm	Point at which optic nerve fibers cross in the brain (Latin *chiasma* means crossing).
optic disc	Region at the back of the eye where the optic nerve meets the retina. It is the blind spot of the eye because it contains only nerve fibers, no rods or cones, and is thus insensitive to light.
optic nerve	Cranial nerve carrying impulses from the retina to the brain (cerebral cortex).
pupil	Central opening of the eye, surrounded by the iris, through which light rays pass. It appears dark.
refraction	Bending of light rays by the cornea, lens, and fluids of the eye to bring the rays into focus on the retina. **Refract** means to break (-fract) back (re-).
retina	Light-sensitive nerve cell layer of the eye containing photoreceptor cells (rods and cones).
rod	Photoreceptor cell of the retina essential for vision in dim light and for peripheral vision.
sclera	Tough, white outer coat of the eyeball.
thalamus	Relay center of the brain. Optic nerve fibers pass through the thalamus on their way to the cerebral cortex.
vitreous humor	Soft, jelly-like material behind the lens in the vitreous chamber; helps maintain the shape of the eyeball.

TERMINOLOGY—THE EYE

Write the meanings of the medical terms related to the eye in the spaces provided.

COMBINING FORMS: STRUCTURES AND FLUIDS

COMBINING FORM	MEANING	TERMINOLOGY	MEANING
aque/o	water	aqueous humor	____________
blephar/o	eyelid (see **palpebr/o**)	blepharitis *Figure 17-6A.*	____________
		blepharoptosis *Pronounced blĕf-ă-rŏp-TŌ-sĭs. Also called* ***ptosis.*** *This condition may be caused by abnormalities of the eyelid muscle or by nerve damage.*	____________
conjunctiv/o	conjunctiva	conjunctivitis *Commonly called* ***pinkeye*** *(Figure 17-6B). Conjunctivitis occurs when blood vessels dilate from allergens like pollen (allergic conjunctivitis), bacterial infection (bacterial conjunctivitis), or virus (viral conjunctivitis).*	____________
cor/o	pupil (see **pupill/o**)	anisocoria *Anis/o means unequal. Anisocoria may be an indication of neurologic injury or disease (Figure 17-7A).*	____________

17

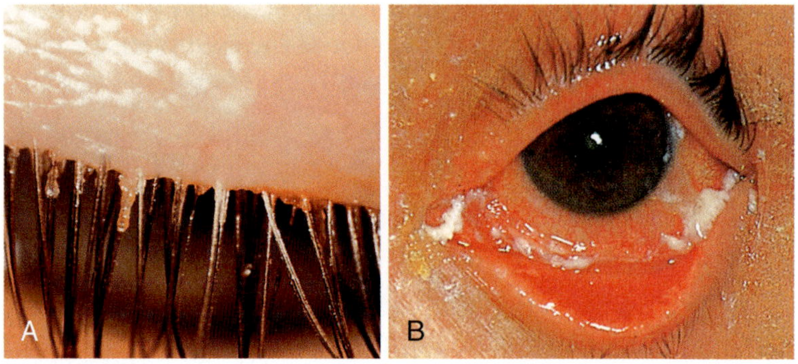

FIGURE 17-6 **A, Blepharitis.** Notice the crusting on the eyelid and eyelashes. **B, Acute bacterial conjunctivitis.** Notice the discharge of pus characteristic of this highly contagious infection of the conjunctiva.

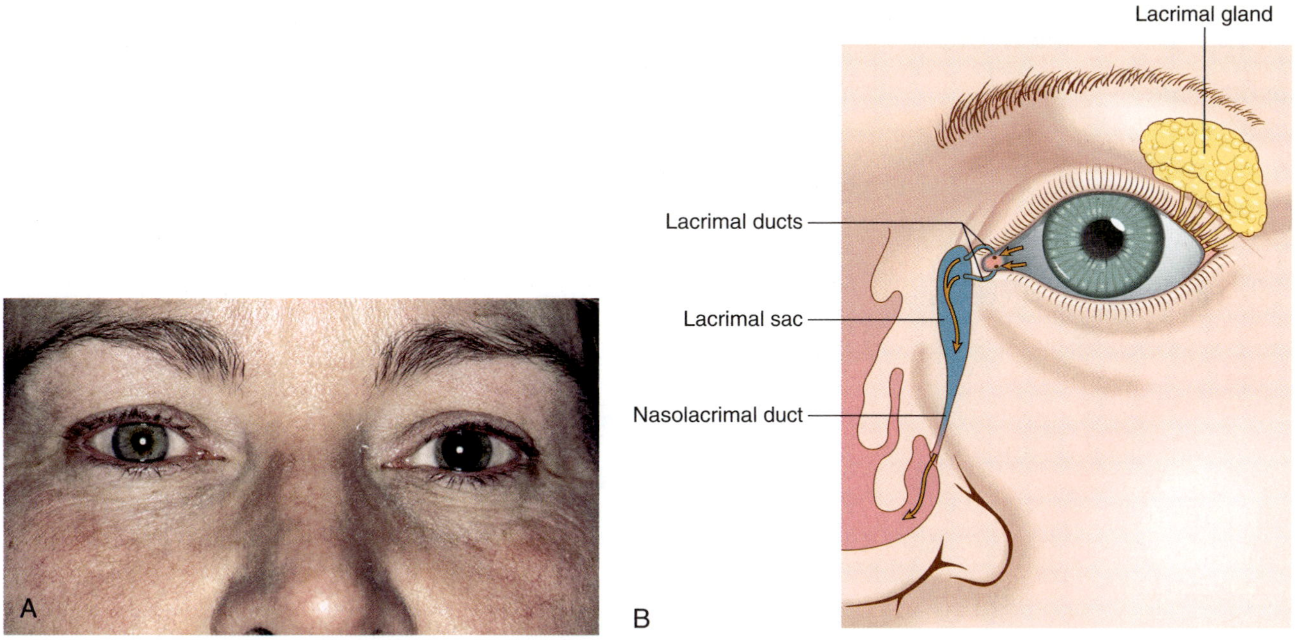

FIGURE 17-7 A, Anisocoria. B, Lacrimal (tear) gland and ducts.

COMBINING FORM	MEANING	TERMINOLOGY	MEANING
corne/o	cornea (see **kerat/o**)	corneal abrasion	
cycl/o	ciliary body or muscle of the eye	cycloplegic	
dacry/o	tears, tear duct (see **lacrim/o**)	dacryoadenitis *Figure 17-7B shows the lacrimal gland and lacrimal ducts.*	
ir/o, irid/o	iris (colored portion of the eye around the pupil)	iritis *Characterized by pain, sensitivity to light, and lacrimation. A corticosteroid is prescribed to reduce inflammation.*	
		iridic	
		iridectomy *A portion of the iris is removed to improve drainage of aqueous humor or to extract a foreign body.*	
kerat/o	cornea	keratitis *Note that kerat/o here does not refer to keratin (protein in skin tissue).*	
lacrim/o	tears	lacrimal	
		lacrimation	
ocul/o	eye	intraocular	

COMBINING FORM	MEANING	TERMINOLOGY	MEANING
ophthalm/o	eye	ophthalmologist	____________
		Medical doctor who specializes in treating disorders of the eye.	
		ophthalmic	____________
		ophthalmoplegia	____________
opt/o, optic/o	eye, vision	optic	____________
		optometrist	____________
		Nonmedical professional who can examine eyes to determine vision problems and prescribe lenses; a doctor of optometry (OD).	
		optician	____________
		Nonmedical professional who grinds lenses and fits glasses but cannot prescribe lenses.	
palpebr/o	eyelid	palpebral	____________
papill/o	optic disc; nipple-like	papilledema	____________
		The suffix -edema means swelling. This condition is associated with increased intracranial pressure and hyperemia (increased blood flow) in the region of the optic disc.	
phac/o, phak/o	lens of the eye	phacoemulsification	____________
		Technique of cataract extraction using ultrasonic vibrations to fragment (emulsify) the lens and aspirate it from the eye.	
		aphakia	____________
		This may be congenital, but most often it is the result of extraction of a cataract (clouded lens) without placement of an artificial lens (pseudophakia).	
pupill/o	pupil	pupillary	____________
retin/o	retina	retinitis	____________
		***Retinitis pigmentosa** is a genetic disorder (pigmented scar forms on the retina) that destroys retinal rods. Decreased vision and night blindness (nyctalopia) occur.*	
		hypertensive retinopathy	____________
		*Lesions such as narrowing of arterioles, microaneurysms, hemorrhages, and **exudates** (fluid leakage) are found on examination of the fundus.*	
scler/o	sclera (white of the eye); hard	corneoscleral	____________
		scleritis	____________

Palpebral/Palpable

Don't confuse *palpebral* with *palpable*, which means detectable or distinguishable by touch.

scler/o

The combining form scler/o also means hard, as in **scler**oderma (a hardening and thickening of the skin) and arterio**scler**osis (hardening of arteries with collection of plaque).

COMBINING FORM	MEANING	TERMINOLOGY	MEANING
uve/o	uvea; vascular layer of the eye (iris, ciliary body, and choroid)	uveitis	______________
vitre/o	glassy	vitreous humor	______________

COMBINING FORMS: CONDITIONS

COMBINING FORM	MEANING	TERMINOLOGY	MEANING
ambly/o	dull, dim	amblyopia ______________ *The suffix -opia means vision. Amblyopia is unilateral or bilateral reduction of visual acuity. Early in life (before age 7 to 10) ocular misalignment, such as with strabismus, uncorrected errors of refraction, or other eye disorders, can lead to amblyopia (also known as lazy eye).*	
dipl/o	double	diplopia ______________	
glauc/o	gray	glaucoma ______________ *Here, -oma means mass or collection of fluid (aqueous humor). The term comes from the dull gray-green color of the affected eye in advanced cases.* *See page 709.*	
mi/o	smaller, less	miosis ______________ *Contraction of the pupil. A* ***miotic*** *is a drug (such as pilocarpine) that causes the pupil to contract.*	
mydr/o	widen, enlarge	mydriasis ______________ *Enlargement of pupils. Tropicamide, atropine, and cocaine cause dilation, or enlargement, of pupils.*	
nyct/o	night	nyctalopia ______________ *-opia means vision; -al comes from Greek ala, meaning blindness. Night blindness is poor vision at night but good vision on bright days. Deficiency of vitamin A leads to nyctalopia.*	
phot/o	light	photophobia ______________ *Sensitivity to light.*	
presby/o	old age	presbyopia ______________ *See page 707.*	
scot/o	darkness	scotoma ______________ *Area of decreased vision surrounded by an area of normal vision; a blind spot. This can result from damage to the retina or the optic nerve.*	
xer/o	dry	xerophthalmia ______________	

17

SUFFIXES

SUFFIX	MEANING	TERMINOLOGY	MEANING
-opia	vision	hyperopia	____________ *Hypermetropia (farsightedness).*
-opsia	vision	hemianopsia	____________ *Absence of vision in half of the visual field (space of vision of each eye). Stroke victims frequently have damage to the brain on one side of the visual cortex and experience hemianopsia (the visual loss is in the right or the left visual field of both eyes).*
-tropia	to turn	esotropia	____________ *Inward (eso-) turning of an eye.* ***Exotropia*** *is an outward turning of an eye. These conditions are examples of* ***strabismus*** *(defect in eye muscles so that both eyes cannot be focused on the same point at the same time).*

ERRORS OF REFRACTION

astigmatism

Defective curvature of the cornea or lens of the eye.

This problem results from one or more abnormal curvatures of the cornea or lens. This causes light rays to be unevenly and not sharply focused on the retina, so that the image is distorted. A cylindrical lens placed in the proper position in front of the eye can correct this problem (Figure 17-8A).

hyperopia (hypermetropia)

Farsightedness.

As Figure 17-8B illustrates, the eyeball in this condition is too short or the refractive power of the lens is too weak. Parallel rays of light tend to focus behind the retina, which results in a blurred image. A convex lens (thicker in the middle than at the sides) bends the rays inward before they reach the cornea, and thus the rays can be focused properly on the retina.

myopia

Nearsightedness.

In myopia the eyeball is too long (front to back) or the refractive power of the lens so strong that light rays do not properly focus on the retina. The image perceived is blurred because the light rays are focused in front of the retina. Concave glasses (thicker at the periphery than in the middle) correct this condition because the lenses spread the rays out before they reach the cornea, so that they can be properly focused directly on the retina (Figure 17-8C).

Myopia/Miotic

In this term, my- comes from Greek *myein*, meaning to shut, referring to the observation that myopic persons frequently peer through half-closed eyelids. Don't confuse **myopia** with **miotic,** which is a drug that contracts the pupil of the eye.

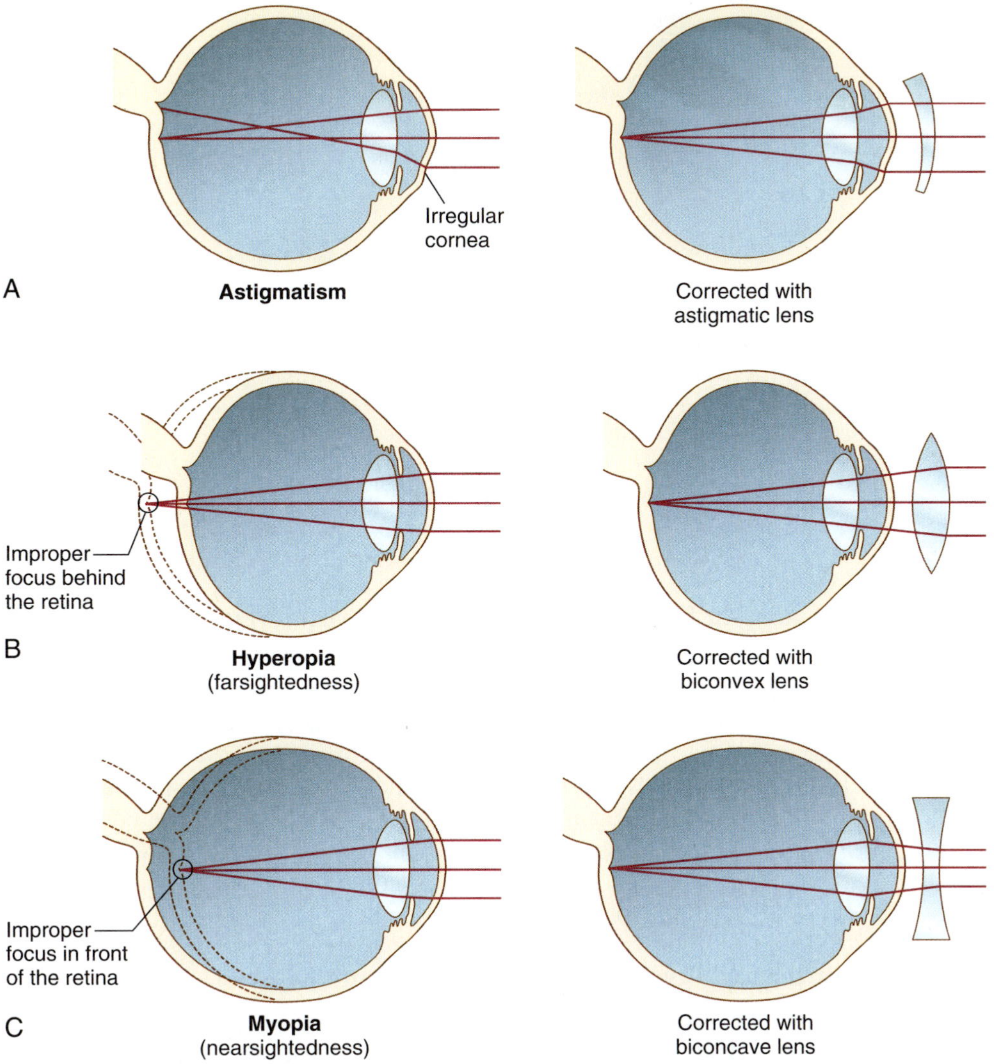

FIGURE 17-8 **Errors of refraction. A, Astigmatism** and its correction. **B, Hyperopia** and its correction. **C, Myopia** and its correction. *Dashed lines* in **B** and **C** indicate the contour and size of the normal eye.

presbyopia

Impairment of vision as a result of old age.

With increasing age, loss of elasticity of the ciliary body impairs its ability to adjust the lens for accommodation to near vision. The lens of the eye cannot become fat to bend the rays coming from near objects (less than 20 feet). The light rays focus behind the retina, as in hyperopia. Therefore, a convex lens is needed to refract the rays coming from objects closer than 20 feet.

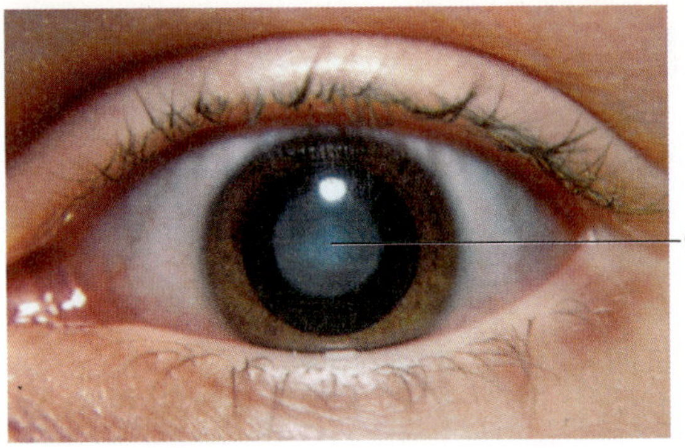

FIGURE 17-9 **Cataract.** The lens appears cloudy. *(Courtesy Ophthalmic Photography at the University of Michigan, WK Kellogg Eye Center, Ann Arbor. From Black JM, Hawks JH: Medical-Surgical Nursing: Clinical Management for Positive Outcomes, 7th ed., Philadelphia, Saunders, 2005.)*

PATHOLOGY—THE EYE

cataract

Clouding of the lens, causing decreased vision (Figure 17-9).

A cataract is a type of degenerative eye disease (protein in the lens aggregates and clouds vision) and is linked to the process of aging (senile cataracts). Some cataracts, however, are present at birth, and others occur with diabetes mellitus, ocular trauma, and prolonged high-dose corticosteroid administration. Vision appears blurred as the lens clouds over and becomes opaque. Lens cloudiness can be seen with an ophthalmoscope or the naked eye. Surgical removal of the lens with implantation of an artificial lens behind the iris (the preferred position) is the method of treatment. If an intraocular lens cannot be inserted, the patient may wear eyeglasses or contact lenses to help refraction.

chalazion

Small, hard, cystic mass (granuloma) on the eyelid.

Chalazions (kă-LĀ-zē-ŏnz) are formed as a result of chronic inflammation of a sebaceous gland (meibomian gland) along the margin of the eyelid (Figure 17-10). They often require incision and drainage.

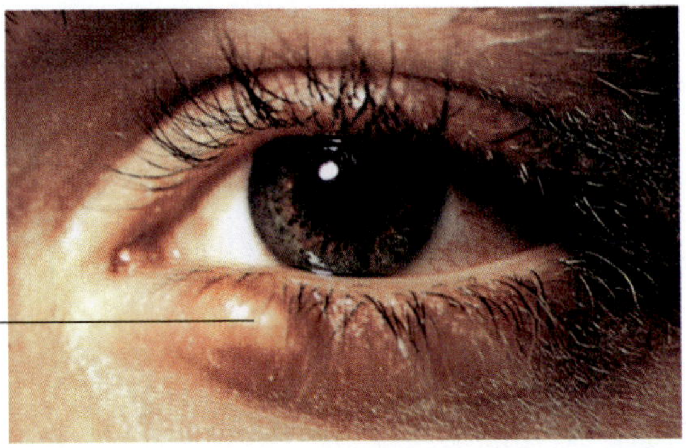

FIGURE 17-10 **Chalazion.** *(Courtesy Ophthalmic Photography at the University of Michigan, WK Kellogg Eye Center, Ann Arbor. From Black JM, Hawks JH, Keene AM: Medical-Surgical Nursing, 5th ed., Philadelphia, Saunders, 1997.)*

diabetic retinopathy

Retinal effects of diabetes mellitus include microaneurysms, hemorrhages, dilation of retinal veins, and neovascularization (new blood vessels form in the retina).

Macular edema occurs as fluid leaks from blood vessels into the retina and vision is blurred. **Exudates** (fluid leaking from the blood) appear in the retina as yellow-white spots. Laser photocoagulation and vitrectomy (see pages 715 and 716) are helpful for patients in whom hemorrhaging has been severe. The latest treatment for diabetic macular edema involves injecting medications into the vitreous jelly. Corticosteroids and agents that promote regression of abnormal blood vessels are used to decrease fluid leakage and neovascularization.

glaucoma

Increased intraocular pressure results in damage to the retina and optic nerve with loss of vision.

Intraocular pressure is elevated because of the inability of aqueous humor to drain from the eye and enter the bloodstream. Normally, aqueous humor is formed by the ciliary body, flows into the anterior chamber, and leaves the eye at the angle where the cornea and the iris meet. If fluid cannot leave or too much fluid is produced, pressure builds up in the anterior chamber (Figure 17-11).

Glaucoma is diagnosed by means of **tonometry** (see page 713), with an instrument applied externally to the eye after administration of local anesthetic. Acute glaucoma is marked by extreme ocular pain, blurred vision, redness of the eye, and dilation of the pupil. If untreated, it causes blindness. Chronic glaucoma may produce no symptoms initially. A patient with glaucoma may experience a gradual loss of peripheral vision, with headaches, blurred vision, and halos around bright lights.

Administration of drugs to lower intraocular pressure can control the condition. Sometimes, laser therapy is used to treat narrow-angle glaucoma by creating a hole in the periphery of the iris (iridotomy), which allows aqueous humor to flow more easily out of the anterior chamber and reduces intraocular pressure. Laser therapy **(trabeculoplasty)** for chronic open-angle glaucoma causes scarring in the drainage angle, which improves aqueous humor outflow and reduces intraocular pressure.

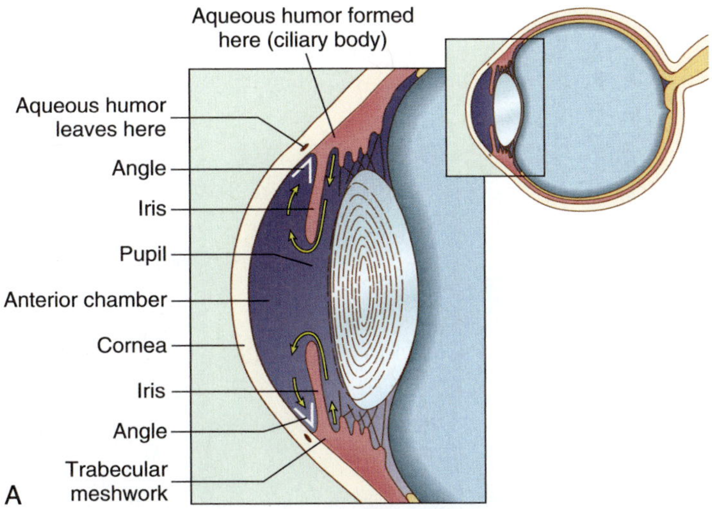

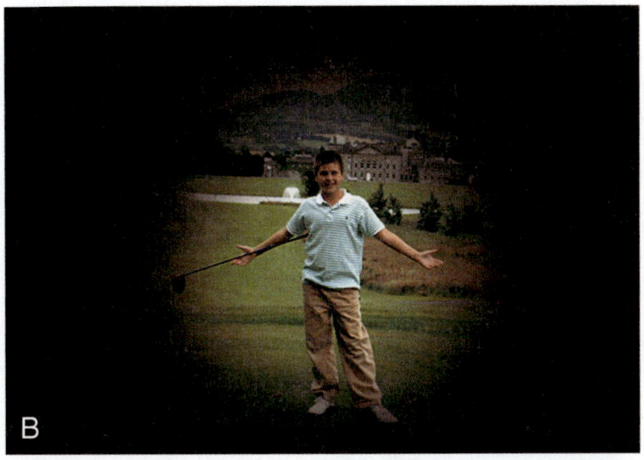

FIGURE 17-11 **A, Glaucoma and circulation of aqueous humor.** Circulation is impaired in glaucoma, so that aqueous fluid builds up in the anterior chamber. The most common type of glaucoma is **open-angle glaucoma,** in which there are open chamber angles but resistance to the flow of aqueous humor. **B,** How a person with glaucoma would see an image. Damage to the optic nerve usually starts as loss of peripheral vision. *(**B,** Courtesy Solomon J. Thompson.)*

TABLE 17-1 EYELID ABNORMALITIES

Abnormality	Description
Blepharitis	Inflammation of eyelid, causing redness, crusting, and swelling along lid margins
Chalazion	Granuloma formed around an inflamed sebaceous gland
Dacryocystitis	Blockage, inflammation, and infection of a nasolacrimal duct and lacrimal sac, causing redness and swelling in the region between the nose and the lower lid
Ectropion	Outward sagging and eversion of the eyelid, leading to improper lacrimation and corneal drying and ulceration
Entropion	Inversion of the eyelid, causing the lashes to rub against the eye; corneal abrasion may result
Hordeolum (stye)	Infection of a sebaceous gland producing a small, superficial white nodule along lid margin
Ptosis	Drooping of upper lid margin as a result of neuromuscular problems or trauma
Xanthelasma	Raised yellowish plaque on eyelid caused by lipid disorder (xanth/o = yellow, -elasma = plate)

hordeolum (stye *or* sty)

Localized, purulent, inflammatory staphylococcal infection of a sebaceous gland in the eyelid.

Hot compresses may help localize the infection and promote drainage. In some cases, surgical incision may be necessary. Latin *hordeolum* (hŏr-DĒ-ō-lŭm) means barley corn. See Table 17-1 for a list of common eyelid abnormalities.

macular degeneration

Progressive damage to the macula of the retina.

Macular degeneration is one of the leading causes of blindness in the elderly. It causes severe loss of central vision (Figure 17-12). Peripheral vision (using the part of the retina that is outside the macular region) is retained.

Macular degeneration occurs in both a "dry" and a "wet" form. The dry form (affecting about 85% of patients) is marked by atrophy and degeneration of retinal cells and deposits of clumps of extracellular debris, or **drusen.** The wet form results from development of new (neovascular) and leaky (exudative) blood vessels close to the macula.

There is no treatment for the dry form of macular degeneration except attempting to slow the progression of the disease by taking vitamin and mineral supplements, and actions such as smoking cessation. Wet macular degeneration may be treated with laser photocoagulation of the leaking vessels and injection of medication into the vitreous jelly that promotes regression of abnormal blood

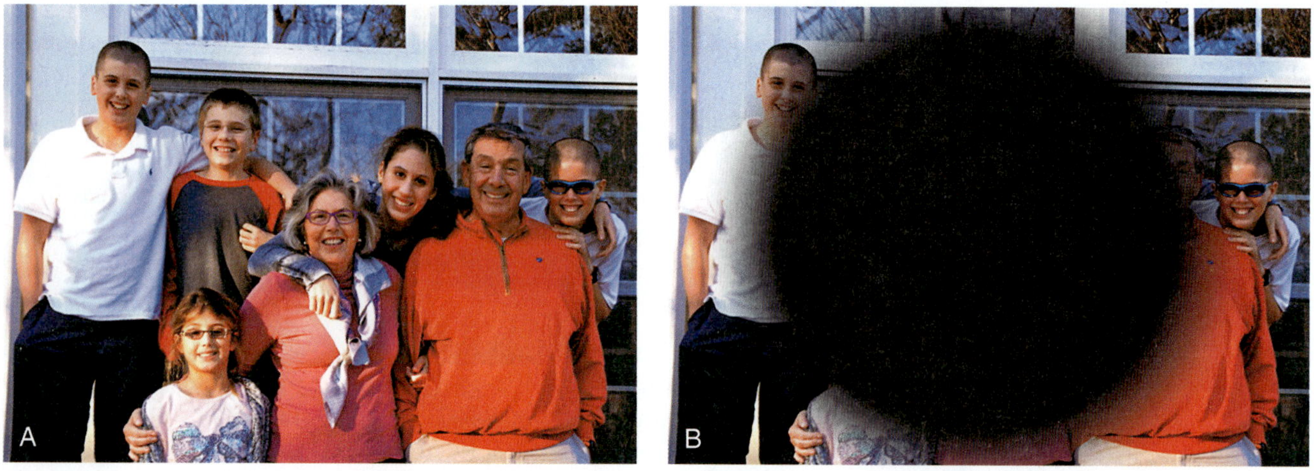

FIGURE 17-12 **(A)** Picture as seen with **normal vision.** **(B)** The same picture as it would appear to someone with **macular degeneration.** *(Photograph shows Solomon, Ben, Bebe, Gus, and Louisa with proud grandparents.)*

vessels. Unfortunately, in many cases, patients with wet macular degeneration have more severe vision loss, and success of treatment is limited.

nystagmus

Repetitive rhythmic movements of one or both eyes.

Brain tumors or diseases of the inner ear may cause nystagmus. Nystagmus is normal in newborns.

retinal detachment

Two layers of the retina separate from each other.

Trauma to the eye, head injuries, bleeding, scarring from infection, or shrinkage of the vitreous humor can produce holes or tears in the retina and result in the separation of layers. Patients often experience **photopsia** (bright flashes of light) and **floaters** (black spots or filmy shapes), which are vitreous clumps that detach from the retina. Later, they notice a shadow or curtain falling across the field of vision. In some cases, floaters may be a sign of a retinal hole, tear, or detachment caused by pigmented cells from the damaged retina or bleeding that has occurred as a result of a detachment. See the ***In Person*** story on page 726.

Photocoagulation (making pinpoint burns to form scar tissue and seal holes) and cryotherapy (creating a "freezer burn" that forms a scar and knits a tear together) are used to repair smaller retinal tears. For larger retinal detachments, a **scleral buckle** (see page 715) made of silicone is sutured to the sclera directly over the detached portion of the retina to push the two retinal layers together. In selected retinal detachments, a procedure called **pneumatic retinopexy** is performed. A gas bubble is injected into the vitreous cavity to put pressure on the area of retinal tear until the retina is reattached.

strabismus

Abnormal deviation of the eye.

A failure of the eyes to look in the same direction because of weakness of a muscle controlling the position of one eye (Figure 17-13). Different forms of strabismus include **esotropia** (one eye turns inward; cross-eyed), **exotropia** (one eye turns outward; wall-eyed), **hypertropia** (upward deviation of one eye), and **hypotropia** (downward deviation of one eye). Treatment may include medications in the form of eye drops, corrective lenses, eye exercises with patching of the normal eye, or surgery to restore muscle balance.

In children, strabismus may lead to **amblyopia** (partial loss of vision or lazy eye). Amblyopia is reversible until the retina is fully developed, at the age of 7 to 10 years. When strabismus develops in an adult, **diplopia** (double vision) is a common problem.

17

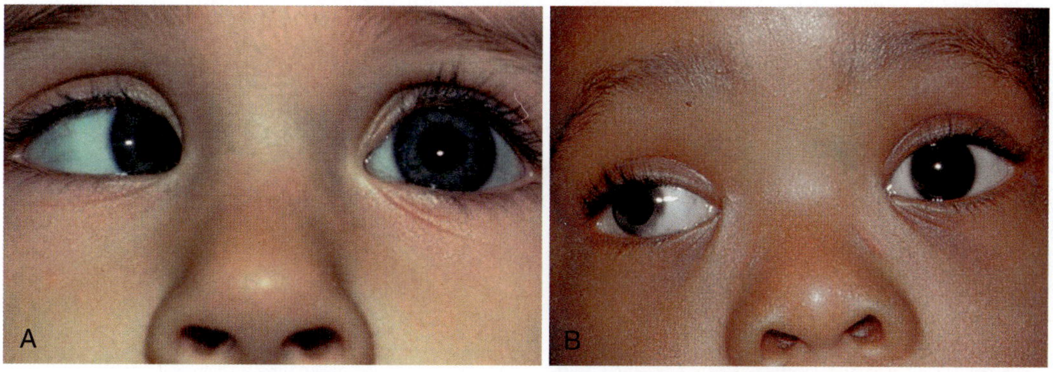

FIGURE 17-13 Strabismus. A, Esotropia. B, Exotropia.

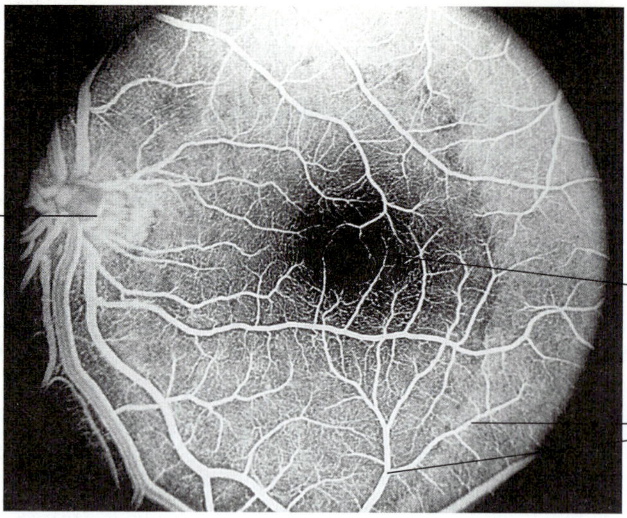

FIGURE 17-14 **Normal eye seen on fluorescein angiogram.**

Clinical Procedures—The Eye

Diagnostic

fluorescein angiography

Intravenous injection of fluorescein (a dye) followed by serial photographs of the retina through dilated pupils.

This test provides diagnostic information about blood flow in the retina, detects vascular changes in diabetic and hypertensive retinopathy, and identifies lesions in the macular area of the retina (Figure 17-14).

17

ophthalmoscopy

Visual examination of the interior of the eye.

Ideally, the pupil is dilated and the physician holds the ophthalmoscope close to the patient's eye, shining the light into the back of the eye (Figure 17-15). Ophthalmologists may also use special lenses in conjunction with a hand lamp or a slit lamp (Figure 17-16).

slit lamp microscopy

Examination of anterior ocular structures under microscopic magnification.

This procedure provides a magnified view of the conjunctiva, sclera, cornea, anterior chamber, iris, lens, and vitreous. Devices attached to a slit lamp expand

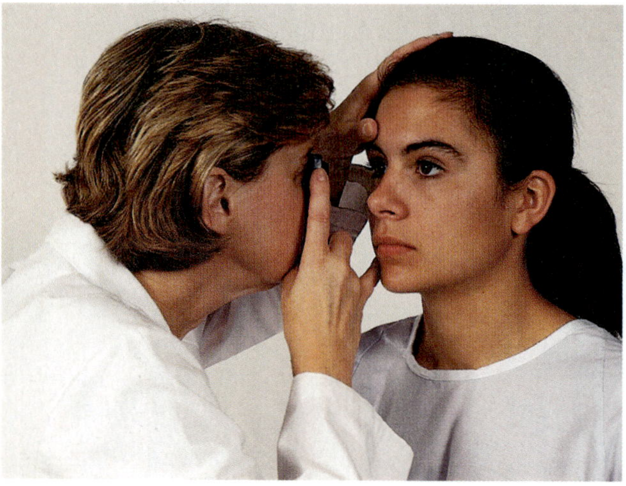

FIGURE 17-15 **Ophthalmoscopy.** In addition to examining the cornea, lens, and vitreous humor for opacities (cloudiness), the examiner can see the blood vessels at the back of the eye (fundus) and note degenerative changes in the retina.

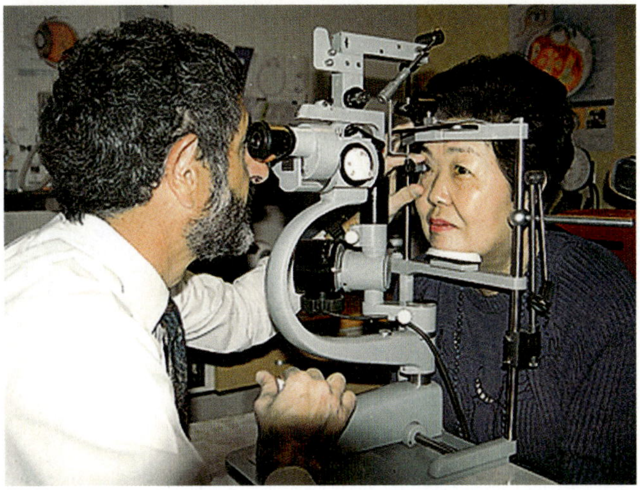

FIGURE 17-16 **Slit lamp examination measuring intraocular pressure by tonometry.**

the scope of the examination. **Tonometry** (ton/o = tension) measures intraocular pressure to detect glaucoma (see Figure 17-16). Special magnifying lenses also permit examination of the fundus, as with a direct ophthalmoscope.

visual acuity test

Clarity of vision is assessed (Figure 17-17A).

A patient reads from a **Snellen chart** at 20 feet (distance vision test). Visual acuity is expressed as a ratio, such as 20/20. The first number is the distance the patient is standing from the chart. The second number is the distance at which a person with normal vision could read the same line of the chart. If the best a patient can see is the 20/200 line, then at 20 feet the patient can see what a "healthy" eye sees at 200 feet.

Mirrors are used so that measurements can be taken at less than 20 feet and still be equivalent to those for vision measured at 20 feet.

visual field test

Measurement of the area (peripheral and central) within which objects are seen when the eyes are fixed, looking straight ahead without movement of the head (Figure 17-17B).

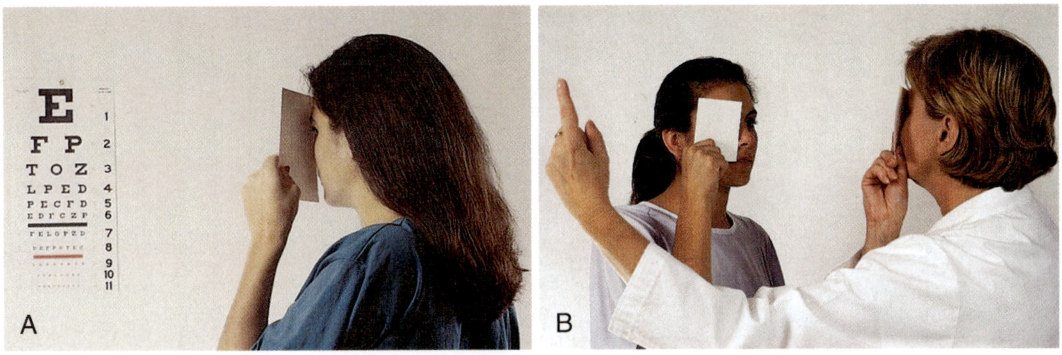

FIGURE 17-17 **A, The Snellen chart** assesses visual acuity. **B, Visual fields** are examined by comparing the patient's field of vision with that of the examiner's (assuming the examiner's is normal).

Direct Ophthalmoscopy and Slit Lamp Microscopy

As part of a visual examination, both of these procedures are often used. **Direct ophthalmoscopy** examines the fundus and interior of the eye, whereas **slit lamp microscopy** visualizes the anterior part of the eye.

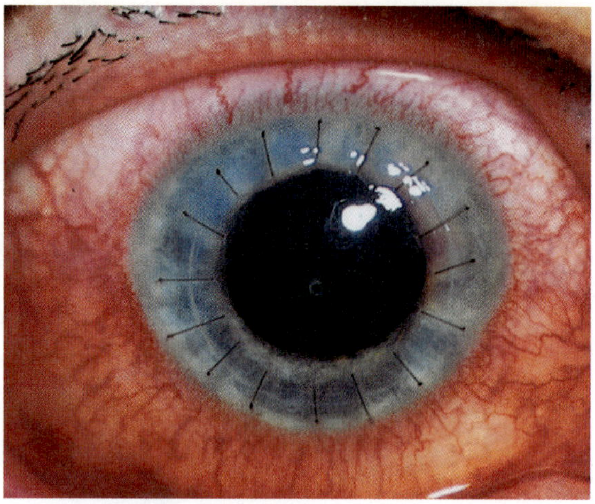

FIGURE 17-18 **Clinical appearance of the eye after keratoplasty.** *(Courtesy Ophthalmic Photography at the University of Michigan, WK Kellogg Eye Center, Ann Arbor. From Black JM, Hawks JH: Medical-Surgical Nursing: Clinical Management for Positive Outcomes, 7th ed., Philadelphia, Saunders, 2005, p. 1958.)*

TREATMENT

enucleation

Removal of the entire eyeball.

This surgical procedure is necessary to treat tumors such as ocular melanoma (malignant tumor of pigmented cells in the choroid layer) or if an eye has become blind and painful from trauma or disease, such as glaucoma.

keratoplasty

Surgical repair of the cornea.

Also known as a **corneal transplant** procedure **(penetrating keratoplasty).** The ophthalmic surgeon removes the patient's scarred or opaque cornea and replaces it with a donor cornea ("button" or graft), which is sutured into place (Figure 17-18).

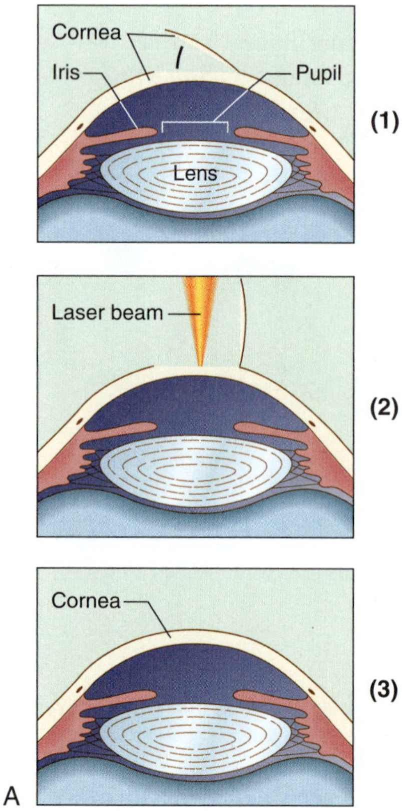

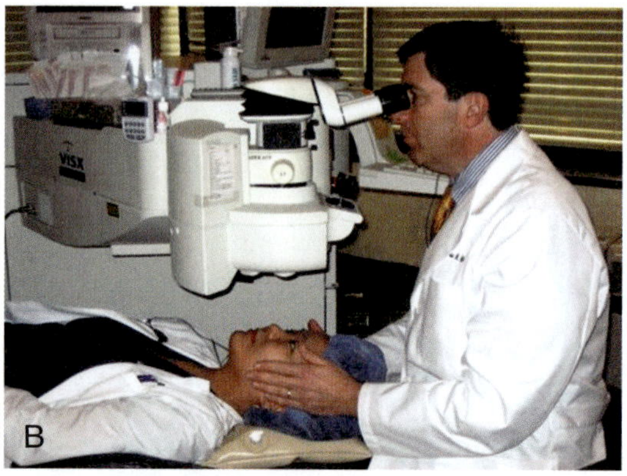

FIGURE 17-19 **A, LASIK refractive surgery:** (1). An instrument to cut the cornea (microkeratome) creates a hinged cap of tissue, which then is lifted off the corneal surface. (2). An excimer laser vaporizes and reshapes the cornea to correct the refraction. (3). The corneal flap is replaced. **B,** Ophthalmologists typically perform LASIK surgery as an office procedure. The patient with corrected vision returns home that day and is visually functioning normally or close to it the next day. *(**B,** Courtesy Eric R. Mandel, MD, Mandel Vision, New York.)*

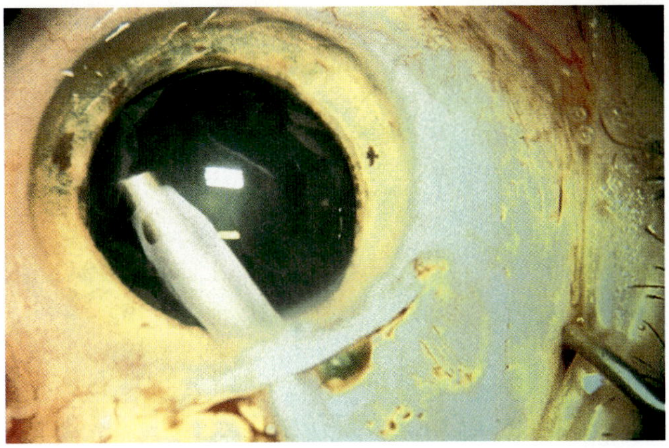

FIGURE 17-20 **Phacoemulsification of a cataractous lens through a small scleral tunnel incision.**

laser photocoagulation

Intense, precisely focused light beam (argon laser) creates an inflammatory reaction that seals retinal tears and leaky retinal blood vessels.

This procedure is useful to treat retinal tears, diabetic retinopathy, and macular degeneration. Laser is an acronym for light amplification by stimulated emission of radiation.

LASIK

Use of an excimer laser to correct errors of refraction (myopia, hyperopia, and astigmatism).

Performed as an outpatient procedure with use of local anesthesia. The surgeon lifts the top layer of the cornea (a flap is made) and uses a laser to sculpt the cornea. The corneal flap is then repositioned. LASIK is an acronym for laser in situ keratomileusis (shaping the cornea) (Figure 17-19).

phacoemulsification

Ultrasonic vibrations break up the lens, which then is aspirated through the ultrasonic probe (Figure 17-20).

This is the typical surgery for cataract removal. The ophthalmic surgeon uses a small, scleral tunnel or self-sealing corneal incision. In most patients, a foldable intraocular lens (IOL) is implanted at the time of surgery.

scleral buckle

Suture of a silicone band to the sclera over a detached portion of the retina.

The band pushes the two parts of the retina against each other to bring together the two layers of the detached retina (Figure 17-21).

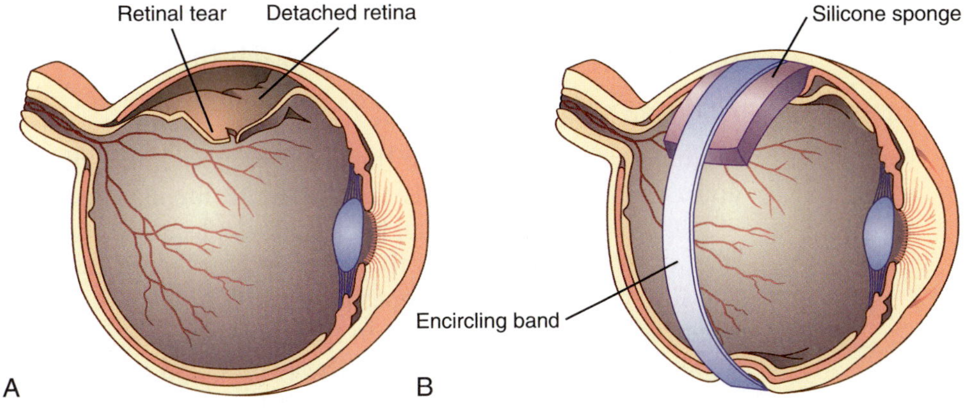

FIGURE 17-21 **A, Detached retina. B, Scleral buckling procedure** to repair retinal detachment.

17

vitrectomy — **Removal of the vitreous humor.**

The vitreous is replaced with a clear solution. This is necessary when blood and scar tissue accumulate in the vitreous humor (a complication of diabetic retinopathy).

ABBREVIATIONS—THE EYE

AMD	age-related macular degeneration
HEENT	head, eyes, ears, nose, and throat
IOL	intraocular lens
IOP	intraocular pressure
LASIK	laser in situ keratomileusis
OD	right eye (Latin, *oculus dexter*); doctor of optometry (optometrist)
OS	left eye (Latin, *oculus sinister*)
OU	both eyes (Latin, *oculus uterque*, "each eye")
PERRLA	pupils equal, round, reactive to light and accommodation
POAG	primary open-angle glaucoma
PRK	photorefractive keratectomy—a laser beam flattens the cornea to correct myopia
VA	visual acuity
VF	visual field

THE EAR

ANATOMY AND PHYSIOLOGY

Sound waves are received by the outer ear, conducted to special receptor cells within the ear, and transmitted by those cells to nerve fibers that lead to the auditory region of the brain in the cerebral cortex. Sensations of sound are perceived within the nerve fibers of the cerebral cortex.

Label Figure 17-22 as you read the following paragraphs describing the anatomy and physiology of the ear.

The ear can be divided into three separate regions: outer ear, middle ear, and inner ear. The outer and middle ears function in the conduction of sound waves through the ear, and the inner ear contains structures that receive the auditory waves and relay them to the brain.

Outer Ear

Sound waves enter the ear through the **pinna,** or **auricle** [1], which is the projecting part, or flap, of the ear. The **external auditory meatus (auditory canal)** [2] leads from the pinna and is lined with numerous glands that secrete a yellowish brown, waxy substance called **cerumen.** Cerumen lubricates and protects the ear.

Middle Ear

Sound waves travel through the auditory canal and strike a membrane between the outer and the middle ear. This is the **tympanic membrane,** or **eardrum** [3]. As the eardrum vibrates, it moves three small bones, or **ossicles,** that conduct the sound waves through the middle ear. These bones, in the order of their vibration, are the **malleus** [4], the **incus** [5], and the **stapes** [6]. As the stapes moves, it touches a membrane called the **oval window** [7], which separates the middle from the inner ear.

Before proceeding with the pathway of sound conduction and reception into the inner ear, an additional structure that affects the middle ear should be mentioned. The **auditory** or **eustachian tube** [8] is a canal leading from the middle ear to the pharynx. It normally is closed but opens on swallowing. In an efficient way, this tube can prevent damage to the eardrum and shock to the middle and inner ears. Normally the pressure of air in the middle ear is equal to the pressure of air in the external environment; however, if you ascend in the atmosphere, as in flying in an airplane, climbing a high mountain, or riding a fast elevator, the atmospheric pressure, along with that in the outer ear, drops, while the pressure in the middle ear remains the same—greater than in the outer ear. This inequality of air pressure on the inside and outside of the eardrum forces the eardrum to bulge outward and potentially burst if the difference in pressures increases. Swallowing opens the eustachian tube so that air can leave the middle ear and enter the throat until the atmospheric and middle ear pressures are balanced. The eardrum then relaxes, and the danger of its bursting is averted.

Inner Ear

Sound vibrations, having been transmitted by the movement of the eardrum to the bones of the middle ear, reach the inner ear via the fluctuations of the oval window that separates the middle and inner ears. The inner ear is also called the **labyrinth** because of its circular, maze-like structure. The part of the labyrinth that leads from the oval window is a bony, snail shell–shaped structure called the **cochlea** [9]. The cochlea contains special auditory liquids called **perilymph** and **endolymph** through which the vibrations travel. Also present in the cochlea is a sensitive auditory receptor area called the **organ of Corti.** In the organ of Corti, tiny hair cells receive vibrations from the auditory liquids and relay the sound waves to **auditory nerve fibers** [10], which end in the auditory center of the cerebral cortex, where these impulses are interpreted and "heard."

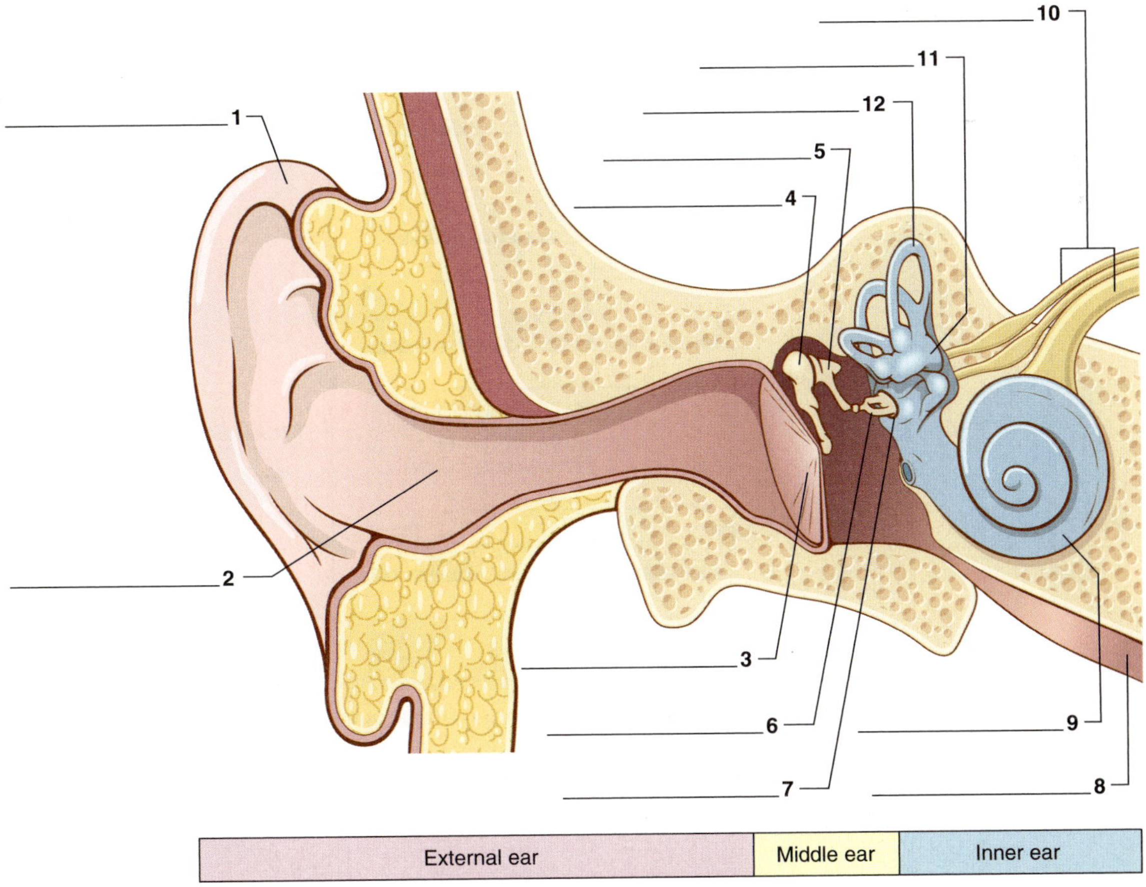

FIGURE 17-22 Anatomy of the ear.

Study Figure 17-23, which is a schematic representation of the pathway of sound vibrations from the outer ear to the brain.

The ear is an important organ of equilibrium (balance), as well as an organ for hearing. Refer back to Figure 17-22. The **vestibule** [11] connects the cochlea (for hearing) to three **semicircular canals** [12] (for balance). The semicircular canals (containing two membranous sacs called the saccule and utricle) contain a fluid, endolymph, as well as sensitive hair cells. In an intricate manner, the fluid and hair cells fluctuate in response to the movement of the head. This sets up impulses in nerve fibers that lead to the brain. Messages are then sent to muscles in all parts of the body to ensure that equilibrium is maintained.

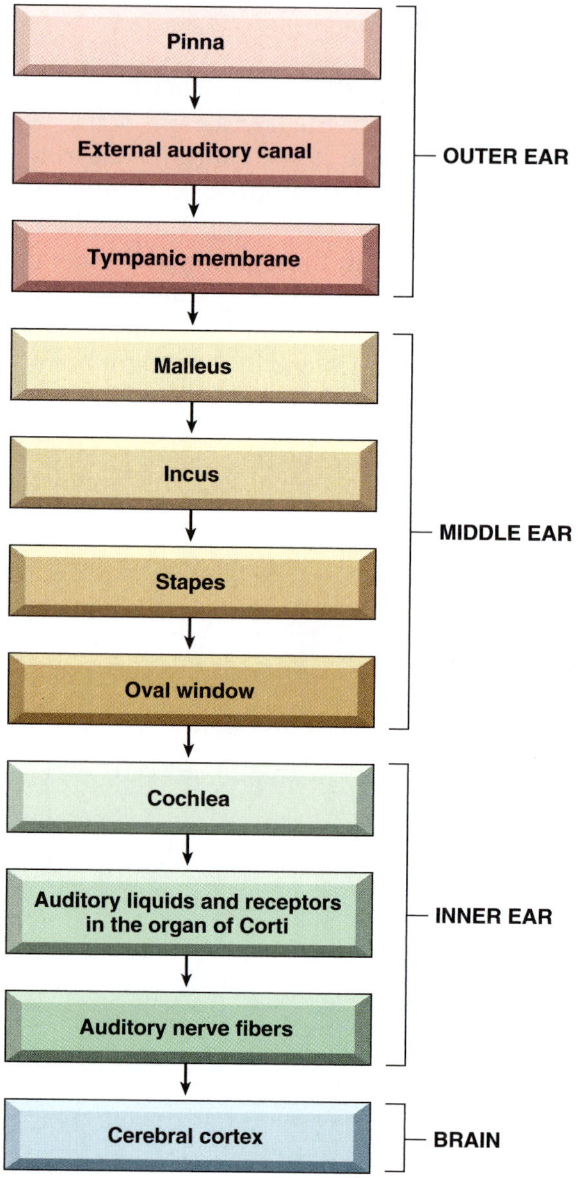

FIGURE 17-23 Pathway of sound vibrations from the outer ear to the brain (cerebral cortex.)

17

VOCABULARY—THE EAR

This list reviews many new terms related to the ear introduced in the text. Short definitions reinforce your understanding of the terms. Refer to the Pronunciation of Terms on page 743 for help with unfamiliar or difficult words.

auditory canal	Channel that leads from the pinna to the eardrum.
auditory meatus	Auditory canal.
auditory nerve fibers	Carry impulses from the inner ear to the brain (cerebral cortex). These fibers compose the vestibulocochlear nerve (cranial nerve VIII).
auditory tube	Channel between the middle ear and the nasopharynx; **eustachian tube.**
auricle	Flap of the ear; the protruding part of the external ear, or **pinna.**
cerumen	Waxy substance secreted by the external ear; also called **earwax.**
cochlea	Snail shell–shaped, spirally wound tube in the inner ear; contains hearing-sensitive receptor cells.
endolymph	Fluid within the labyrinth of the inner ear.
eustachian tube	Auditory tube.
incus	Second ossicle (bone) of the middle ear; incus means **anvil.**
labyrinth	Maze-like series of canals of the inner ear. This includes the cochlea, vestibule, and semicircular canals.
malleus	First ossicle of the middle ear; malleus means **hammer.**
organ of Corti	Sensitive auditory receptor area found in the cochlea of the inner ear.
ossicle	Small bone of the ear; includes the malleus, incus, and stapes.
oval window	Membrane between the middle ear and the inner ear.
perilymph	Fluid contained in the labyrinth of the inner ear.
pinna	Auricle; flap of the ear.
semicircular canals	Passages in the inner ear associated with maintaining equilibrium.
stapes	Third ossicle of the middle ear. Stapes means **stirrup.**
tympanic membrane	Membrane between the outer and the middle ear; also called the **eardrum.**
vestibule	Central cavity of the labyrinth, connecting the semicircular canals and the cochlea. The vestibule contains two structures, the **saccule** and **utricle,** that help to maintain equilibrium.

TERMINOLOGY—THE EAR

Write the meanings of the medical terms related to the ear in the spaces provided.

COMBINING FORMS

COMBINING FORM	MEANING	TERMINOLOGY	MEANING
acous/o	hearing	acoustic	
audi/o	hearing; the sense of hearing	audiogram	
		audiologist *A health care professional specializing in the evaluation and rehabilitation of people with hearing loss.*	
audit/o	hearing	auditory	
aur/o, auricul/o	ear (see **ot/o**)	aural	
		postauricular	
cochle/o	cochlea	cochlear	
mastoid/o	mastoid process	mastoiditis *The **mastoid process** is the posterior portion of the temporal bone extending downward behind the external auditory meatus. Mastoiditis, caused by bacterial infection, spreads from the middle ear.*	
myring/o	eardrum, tympanic membrane (see **tympan/o**)	myringotomy	
		myringitis	
ossicul/o	ossicle	ossiculoplasty	
ot/o	ear	otic	
		otomycosis	
		otopyorrhea	
		otolaryngologist *An otolaryngologist is a medical doctor specializing in the ear, nose, and throat.*	
salping/o	eustachian tube, auditory tube	salpingopharyngeal *In the context of female reproductive anatomy, salping/o means the fallopian tubes.*	

Audiogram/Audiometry

An audiogram is the record (chart) produced when an individual's hearing is tested by **audiometry** (see page 724).

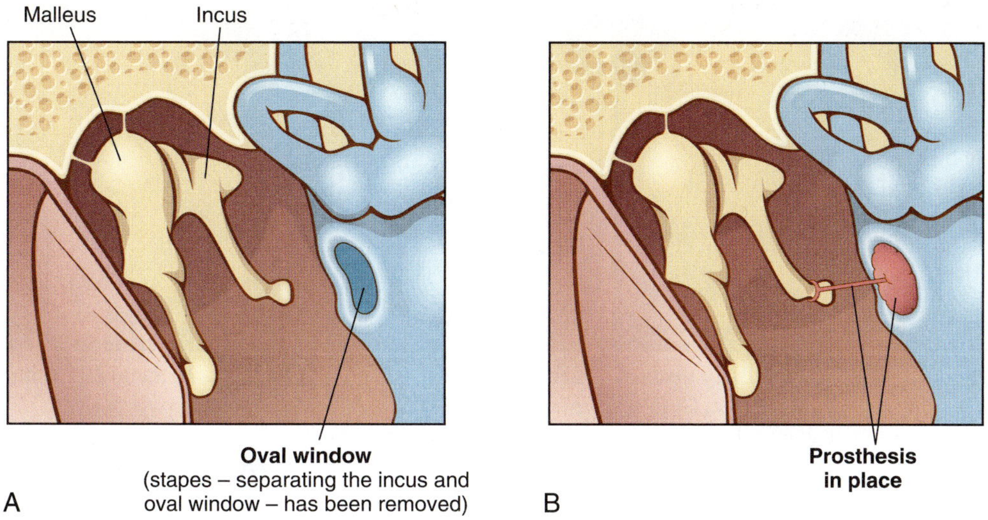

FIGURE 17-24 **A, Stapedectomy.** Using microsurgical technique and a laser, the stapes bone is removed from the middle ear. **B,** A **prosthetic device** (wire, Teflon, or metal) is placed into the incus and attached to a hole in the oval window.

COMBINING FORM	MEANING	TERMINOLOGY	MEANING
staped/o	stapes (third bone of the middle ear)	stapedectomy	______________ *After stapedectomy a prosthetic device is used to connect the incus and the oval window (Figure 17-24). Also see otosclerosis, page 723.*
tympan/o	eardrum, tympanic membrane	tympanoplasty	______________ *Surgical reconstruction of the bones of the middle ear with reconnection of the eardrum to the oval window. Figure 17-25A shows a normal tympanic membrane (eardrum).*
vestibul/o	vestibule	vestibulocochlear	______________

SUFFIXES

SUFFIX	MEANING	TERMINOLOGY	MEANING
-acusis *or* **-cusis**	hearing	hyperacusis	______________ *Abnormally acute sensitivity to sounds.*
		presbycusis	______________ *This type of nerve deafness occurs with the process of aging.*
-meter	instrument to measure	audiometer	______________
-otia	ear condition	macrotia	______________ *Abnormally large ears; congenital anomaly.*

17

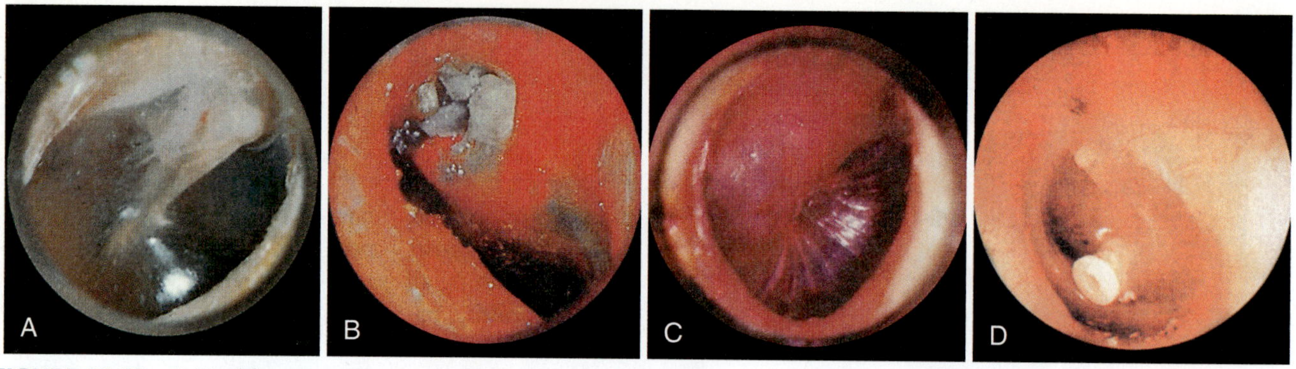

FIGURE 17-25 **A, Healthy tympanic membrane. B, Tympanic membrane with cholesteatoma. C, Tympanic membrane with acute otitis media. D, Myringotomy with tympanostomy tube.** (***A** to **C**, Courtesy Richard A. Buckingham, Clinical Professor, Otolaryngology, Abraham Lincoln School of Medicine, University of Illinois, Chicago. From Barkauskas VH et al: Health and Physical Assessment, 3rd ed., St. Louis, Mosby, 2002, pp. 278 and 290; **D**, from Fireman P, Slavin RG: Atlas of Allergies, 2nd ed., London, Glower Medical Publishing, 1996.*)

PATHOLOGY—THE EAR

acoustic neuroma

Benign tumor arising from the acoustic vestibulocochlear nerve (eighth cranial nerve) in the brain.

Initially, this tumor causes tinnitus (ringing in the ears), vertigo (dizziness), and decreased hearing. Small tumors are resected by microsurgical techniques or ablated (removed) by radiosurgery (using powerful and precise x-ray beams rather than a surgical incision).

17

cholesteatoma

Collection of skin cells and cholesterol in a sac within the middle ear.

These cyst-like masses produce a foul-smelling discharge and are most often the result of chronic otitis media. They are associated with perforations of the tympanic membrane (Figure 17-25B).

deafness

Loss of the ability to hear.

Nerve deafness (sensorineural hearing loss) results from impairment of the cochlea or auditory (acoustic) nerve. **Conductive deafness** results from impairment of the middle ear ossicles and membranes transmitting sound waves into the cochlea. Hearing aids help people with conductive or sensorineural hearing loss. These devices have a microphone to pick up sounds, an amplifier to increase their volume, and a speaker to transmit amplified sounds. See Figure 17-26.

Meniere disease

Disorder of the labyrinth of the inner ear; elevated endolymph pressure within the cochlea (cochlear hydrops) and semicircular canals (vestibular hydrops).

Signs and symptoms are tinnitus, heightened sensitivity to loud sounds, progressive loss of hearing, headache, nausea, and vertigo. Attacks last minutes or continue for hours. The cause is unknown, and treatment is bed rest, sedation, and drugs to combat nausea and vertigo. Surgery may be necessary to relieve accumulation of fluid from the inner ear.

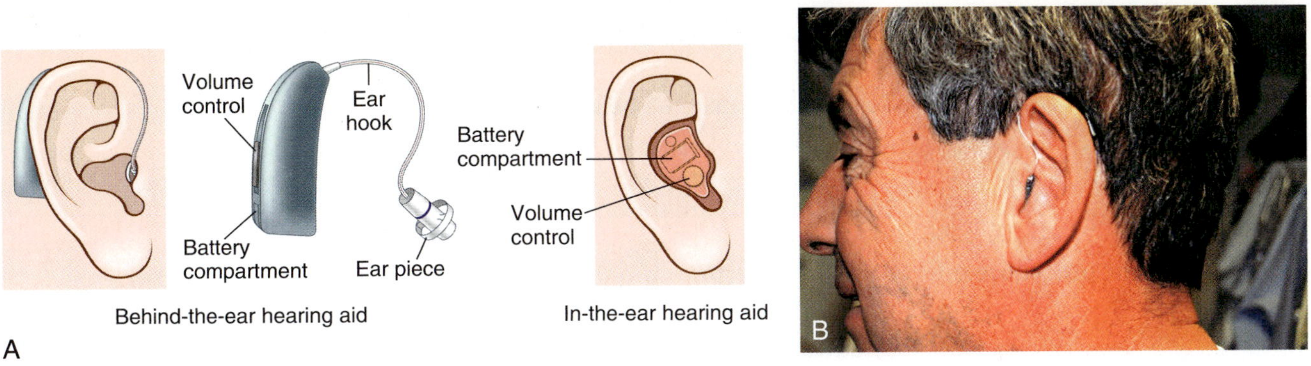

FIGURE 17-26 **Hearing aids: A,** Two types of hearing aid devices. **B,** Behind the ear hearing aid device in place.

otitis media

Inflammation of the middle ear.

Acute otitis media is infection of the middle ear, often following an upper respiratory infection (URI). Pain and fever with redness and loss of mobility of the tympanic membrane occur (Figure 17-25C). As bacteria invade the middle ear, pus formation occurs **(suppurative otitis media).** It is treated with antibiotics, but if the condition becomes chronic, myringotomy may be required to ventilate the middle ear.

Serous otitis media is a noninfectious inflammation with accumulation of serous fluid. It often results from a dysfunctional or obstructed auditory tube. Treatment includes myringotomy to aspirate fluid and placement of tympanostomy tubes in the eardrum to allow ventilation of the middle ear (Figure 17-25D).

otosclerosis

Hardening of the bony tissue of the middle ear.

The result of this hereditary condition is that bone forms around the oval window and causes fixation or **ankylosis** (stiffening) of the stapes bone (ossicle). Conduction deafness occurs, as the ossicles cannot pass on vibrations when sound enters the ear. Stapedectomy with replacement by a **prosthesis** (artificial part) is effective in restoring hearing (see Figure 17-24 on page 721). In order to perform this operation, the oval window must be **fenestrated** (opened) using a laser.

tinnitus

Sensation of noises (ringing, buzzing, whistling, booming) in the ears.

Caused by irritation of delicate hair cells in the inner ear, this disease symptom may be associated with presbycusis, Meniere disease, otosclerosis, chronic otitis, labyrinthitis, and other disorders. Tinnitus can be persistent and severe and can interfere with the affected person's daily life. Treatment includes biofeedback to help the patient relax and exert control over stress and anxiety if these are contributing factors. Tinnitus, a Latin-derived term, means tinkling.

vertigo

Sensation of irregular or whirling motion either of oneself or of external objects.

Vertigo can result from disease in the labyrinth of the inner ear or in the nerve that carries messages from the semicircular canals to the brain. Equilibrium and balance are affected, and nausea may occur as well.

Tinnitus

Note the spelling! Tinnitus is a condition (-itus), not an inflammation (-itis).

CLINICAL PROCEDURES—THE EAR

audiometry

Testing the sense of hearing.

An **audiometer** is an electrical device that delivers acoustic stimuli of specific frequencies to determine a patient's hearing loss for each frequency (Figure 17-26A). Results are shown on a chart or **audiogram** (Figure 17-26B).

cochlear implant procedure

Surgical insertion of a device that allows sensorineural hearing–impaired persons to understand speech.

Electrical signals are sent directly into the auditory nerve by means of multiple electrodes inserted into the cochlea. An external microphone and speech processor pick up sound signals and convert them to electrical impulses (Figure 17-28A).

ear thermometry

Measurement of the temperature of the tympanic membrane by detection of infrared radiation from the eardrum.

A device is inserted into the auditory canal, and results, which reflect the body's temperature, are obtained within 2 seconds.

otoscopy

Visual examination of the ear canal with an otoscope (see Figure 17-28B).

tuning fork test

Test of ear conduction using a vibration source (tuning fork).

To perform the **Rinne test,** the examiner places the base of the vibrating fork against the patient's mastoid bone (bone conduction) and in front of the auditory meatus (air conduction). In the **Weber test,** the tuning fork is placed on the center of the forehead. The loudness of sound is equal in both ears if hearing is normal.

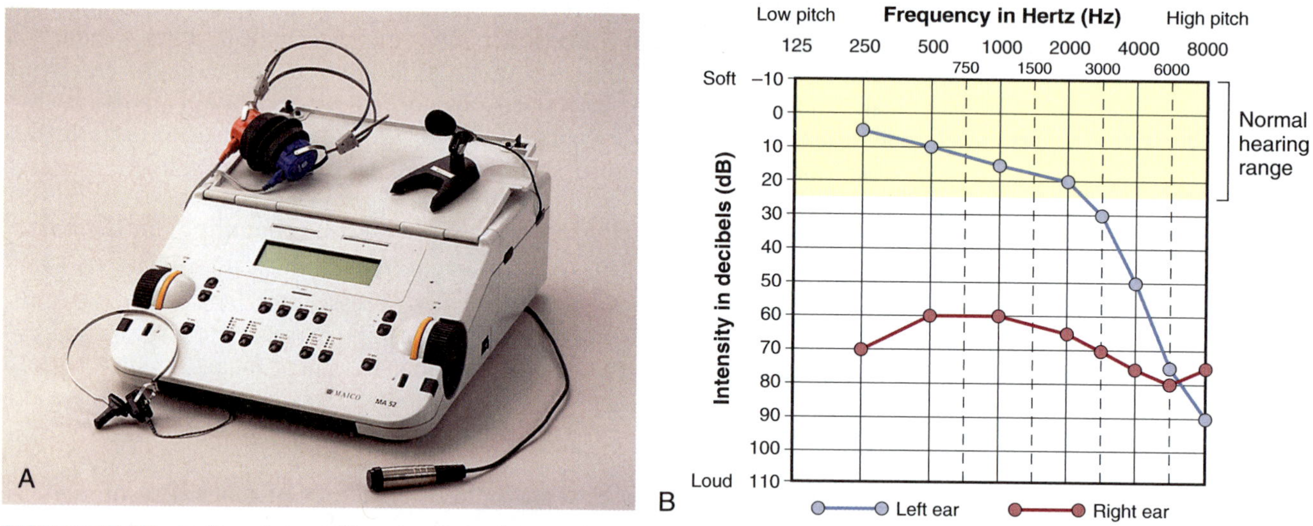

FIGURE 17-27 **A, Pure-tone audiometer. B, Audiogram** for a person with normal hearing in the left ear only for low frequencies (pitch). Notice the *blue line* sloping downward, showing severe high-frequency hearing loss in the left ear. There is moderate to severe hearing loss in the right ear. The decibel (dB) level of the softest sound you are able to hear is called your threshold. Thresholds of 0 to 25 dB *(yellow area)* are considered normal (for adults). *(**A,** Courtesy Maico, Inc., Minneapolis. In Ignatavicius DD, Workman ML: Medical-Surgical Nursing: Critical Thinking for Collaborative Care, 5th ed., Philadelphia, Saunders, 2005, p. 1120.)*

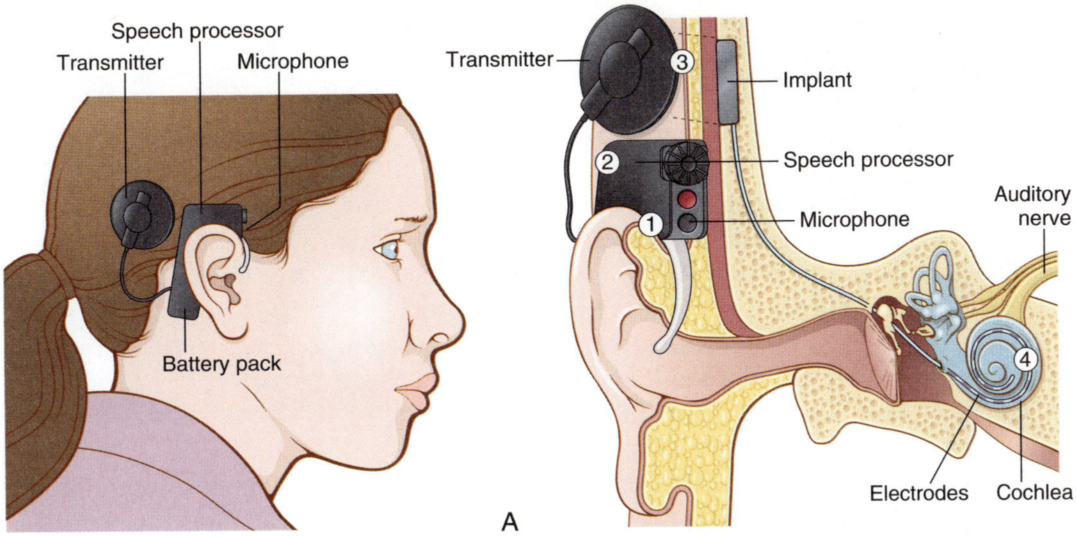

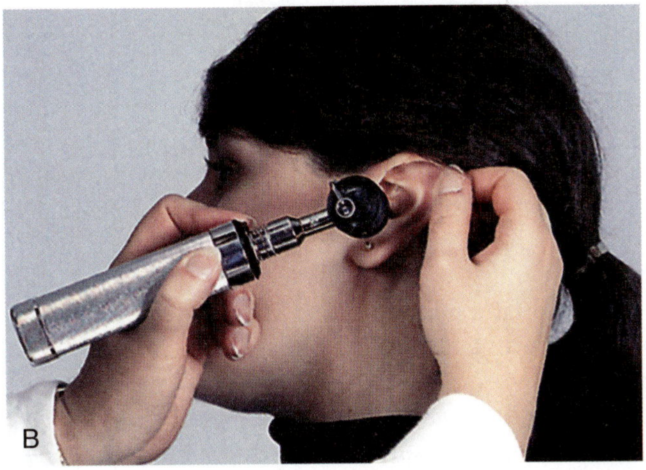

FIGURE 17-28 **A, Cochlear implant.** (1). Microphone receives sound. (2). Speech processor converts sounds into digital signals. (3). Signals are sent to a transmitter that relays them to an implant, where they are converted to electrical impulses. (4). Impulses are sent to electrodes that stimulate nerve cells in the cochlea, which sends them to the auditory nerve and brain. **B, Otoscopic examination.** The auricle is pulled up and back. The hand holding the otoscope is braced against the patient's face for stabilization.

ABBREVIATIONS—THE EAR

AD	right ear (Latin, *auris dextra*)
AOM	acute otitis media
AS	left ear (Latin, *auris sinistra*)
EENT	eyes, ears, nose, and throat
ENG	electronystagmography—a test of the balance mechanism of the inner ear by assessing eye movements (**nystagmus** is rapidly twitching eye movements)
ENT	ears, nose, and throat
ETD	eustachian tube dysfunction
HEENT	head, eyes, ears, nose, and throat
PE tube	pressure-equalizing tube—a polyethylene ventilating tube placed in the eardrum (to treat recurrent episodes of acute otitis media)
SOM	serous otitis media

IN PERSON

This first person story is written by a man with retinal detachment.

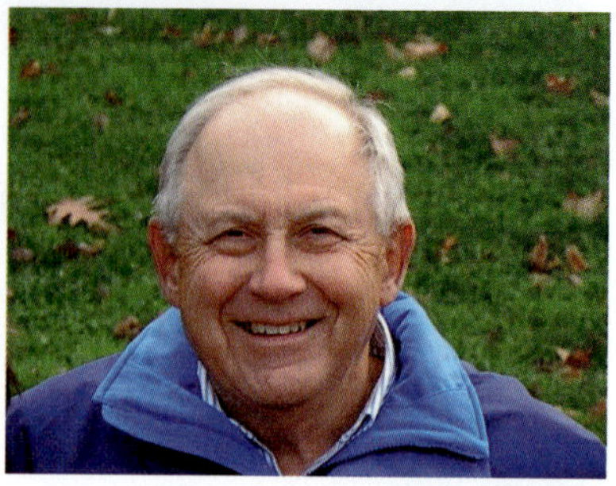

One day, while out for my usual walk, I sneezed due to the higher pollen we were experiencing. It was not an easy sneeze, and I was aware of the result immediately. I noticed some new floaters in my left eye. No pain, but a little feeling that something wasn't right. I did not see flashes of bright light (a good thing).

I hoped that the floaters would minimize and when they did not, I called my optometrist for an appointment. My appointment was at 10:30 and by 11:00 he had discovered a possible tear in my left retina. He walked me down the hall to an ophthalmologist, who confirmed the tear and suggested cryopexy, which involves numbing the eye, inserting a probe into the area, and freezing the tear back to the back of the eye. I was through all of this by 11:30. Timing is everything.

The ophthalmologist explained that waiting 2-3 days may allow the tear to progress to a detachment which, if not caught, could cause more serious problems.

If you think about a sneeze, it involves the head moving forward and stopping abruptly. As we get older, the clear jell (vitreous) inside the eye may pull away from the retina at the back of the eye. If this pulls away gradually, usually there is no problem. However, if there is a hard pull and a tear, the vitreous can pass through the tear lifting the retina off the back of eye, much like wallpaper can peel off a wall. There are a number of conditions that may lead to the chance of retinal problems such as nearsightedness, cataract surgery, glaucoma, family history, etc.

17

As explained to me, if you are going to sneeze, grasp your head with both hands (perhaps while holding a tissue to your nose) to prevent the head from moving radically. That may stop the sudden front to back movement of your head.

The bad news is that I couldn't play golf for a couple of weeks after the cryopexy. My left eye looked horrible (itching and swollen) and I had a bunch of dark floaters in it. It was like trying to dodge 3-4 gnats right in front of my eyes. The good news is that my vision is intact.

My doctor told me that once you have had one episode there is a 15% chance of developing the same problem in the other eye. Right on schedule, a year later, my right eye had a tear/separation. This time though, the separation was located on the nasal side of the eye which precluded using the cryogenic method of sealing the retina. My choice, in his office at least, was for a laser correction. I asked about the particulars: including safety, whether it would correct the problem, and how long would the procedure take. I was given assurances for my first two concerns, and told the procedure might take 5 minutes. I agreed to do it, but had concerns about how I could stay still for 5 minutes while he fired laser shots through my eye to stitch up the tear. After numbing the eye and putting me in the correct position, the doctor proceeded to light up my eye with 30 very bright flashes. He finished in 15 seconds. While I was pulling back from the head rest, I asked why had he told me that it would take five minutes. He said, with a little smile, that he didn't want me to starting figuring his fee based on a per second basis while I was undergoing the treatment. Pretty clever, and worth the smile that I gave him.

Needless to say, both eyes are fine. I still have floaters in both eyes and occasionally swipe at nonexistent gnats.

It may have no relation, but my golf handicap has dropped 4 shots lower since last spring and two below my historical prior low. Isn't technology great or what?

Mac McGinnis is a retired businessman and dedicated golfer.

PRACTICAL APPLICATIONS

This section contains an operating room schedule and an operative report. Explanations of more difficult terms are added in brackets. Answers to the matching questions are on page 739.

OPERATING ROOM SCHEDULE: Eye and Ear Procedures

Match the operation in Column I with a diagnosis/surgical indication in Column II.

COLUMN I		COLUMN II
1. phacoemulsification with IOL; OS	______	A. scarred and torn cornea
2. blepharoplasty	______	B. ptosis of eyelid skin
3. scleral buckle	______	C. retinal detachment
4. vitrectomy	______	D. diabetic retinopathy
5. radical mastoidectomy	______	E. macular degeneration
6. keratoplasty	______	F. chronic stye
7. cochlear implant	______	G. chronic infection of a bone behind the ear
8. laser photocoagulation of the macula	______	H. severe deafness
9. incision and drainage of hordeolum	______	I. cataracts

OPERATIVE REPORT

Preoperative Diagnosis. Bilateral chronic serous otitis media; tonsilloadenoiditis.

Operation. Bilateral myringotomies and ventilation tube insertion; T&A.

Procedure. With the patient in the supine position and under general endotracheal anesthesia, inspection of AD was made under the operating microscope. The external canal was clear; tympanic membrane was divided. A purulent discharge appeared to be present. This drainage was suctioned out and the ear thoroughly lavaged [washed out]. A ventilating tube was put in place and otic drops were administered. Same procedure for AS.

The patient was placed in the Rose position [supine with the head over the table edge in full extension] and the adenoids were removed with adenoid curettes and adenoid biopsy forceps. A nasopharyngeal sponge was put in place. The right tonsil was then grasped with tonsil forceps, dissected free, and removed with snare. Bleeding was controlled with suction cautery. The nasopharyngeal sponge was removed and no further bleeding noted. The patient tolerated the procedure well and left the OR in good condition.

EXERCISES

Remember to check your answers carefully with the Answers to Exercises, page 737.

A Match the structure of the eye with its description below. Write the letter of the description in the space provided.

COLUMN I		COLUMN II
1. pupil	_____	A. Contains sensitive cells called rods and cones that transform light energy into nerve impulses.
2. conjunctiva	_____	B. Contains muscles that control the shape of the lens and secretes aqueous humor.
3. cornea	_____	C. Transparent structure behind the iris and in front of the vitreous humor; it refracts light rays onto the retina.
4. sclera	_____	D. Jelly-like material behind the lens that helps maintain the shape of the eyeball.
5. choroid	_____	E. Open center of the iris through which light rays enter.
6. iris	_____	F. Vascular layer of the eyeball that is continuous with the iris.
7. ciliary body	_____	G. Delicate membrane lining the eyelids and covering the anterior eyeball.
8. lens	_____	H. Fibrous layer of clear tissue that extends over the anterior portion of the eyeball.
9. retina	_____	I. Colored portion of the eye; surrounds the pupil.
10. vitreous humor	_____	J. Tough, white outer layer of the eyeball.

B Supply the terms that complete the following sentences.

1. The region at the back of the eye where the optic nerve meets the retina is the ____________________.
2. The normal adjustment of the lens (becoming fatter) to bring an object into focus for near vision on the retina is ____________________.
3. A yellowish region on the retina lateral to the optic disc is the ____________________.
4. The tiny pit or depression in the retina that is the region of clearest vision is the ____________________.
5. The bending of light rays by the cornea, lens, and fluids of the eye is ____________________.
6. The point at which the fibers of the optic nerve cross in the brain is the ____________________.
7. The photoreceptor cells in the retina that make the perception of color possible are the ____________________.

8. The photoreceptor cells in the retina that make vision in dim light possible are the

    ____________________.

9. The ____________________ is the area behind the cornea and in front of the lens and iris. It contains aqueous humor.

10. The posterior, inner part of the eye is the ____________________.

C Arrange the following terms in proper sequence to show the pathway of light rays to the visual region of the brain.

anterior chamber and aqueous humor
cerebral cortex (occipital lobe)
cornea
lens
optic chiasm
optic nerve fibers
pupil
retina
thalamus
vitreous chamber and vitreous humor

1. ____________________ fibrous transparent layer of clear tissue over the eyeball
2. ____________________ space and fluid in the front of the eye
3. ____________________ central opening of the iris
4. ____________________ transparent, biconvex body that refracts light rays
5. ____________________ space and soft, jelly-like material in the posterior (back) of eye
6. ____________________ light-sensitive inner nerve cell layer; rods and cones
7. ____________________ cranial nerve
8. ____________________ area of brain where optic nerve fibers cross
9. ____________________ relay center of the brain
10. ____________________ visual region of the brain

D Give the meanings of the following terms.

1. optic nerve ____________________
2. biconvex ____________________
3. anisocoria ____________________
4. cycloplegic ____________________
5. palpebral ____________________
6. mydriasis ____________________
7. miosis ____________________
8. papilledema ____________________
9. photophobia ____________________
10. scotoma ____________________

E **Complete the medical terms based on their meanings and the word parts given.**

1. inflammation of an eyelid: ______________________itis
2. inflammation of the conjunctiva: ______________________itis
3. inflammation of a tear gland: ______________________itis
4. inflammation of the iris: ______________________itis
5. inflammation of the cornea: ______________________itis
6. inflammation of the white of the eye: ______________________itis
7. inflammation of the retina: ______________________itis
8. prolapse of the eyelid: blephar ______________________
9. pertaining to tears: ______________________al
10. pertaining to within the eye: intra ______________________

F **Select from the following terms to match the meanings below.**

aphakia	hemianopsia	optometrist
corneal ulcer	ophthalmologist	uveitis
esotropia	optician	xerophthalmia
exotropia		

1. fibrous layer of clear tissue over the front of the eyeball has a defect resulting from infection ______________________
2. inflammation of the vascular layer of the eye (iris, ciliary body, and choroid) ______________________
3. condition of dry eyes ______________________
4. absence of vision in half of the visual field ______________________
5. eye abnormally turns outward ______________________
6. medical doctor who treats diseases of the eyes ______________________
7. nonmedical professional who can examine eyes and prescribe glasses ______________________
8. nonmedical professional who grinds lenses and fits glasses ______________________
9. absence of the lens of the eye ______________________
10. eye abnormally turns inward ______________________

G **Describe the following visual conditions.**

1. amblyopia ____
2. hyperopia ____
3. presbyopia ____
4. myopia ____

5. nyctalopia ______________________________

6. diplopia ______________________________

7. astigmatism ______________________________

H Complete the following sentences.

1. In the myopic eye, light rays do not focus properly on the ______________.
   Either the eyeball is too ______________ or the refractive power of the lens is too ______________, so that the image is blurred and comes to a focus in ______________ of the retina. The type of lens used to correct this refractive error is called a/an ______________ lens.
2. In the hyperopic eye, the eyeball is too ______________ or the refractive power of the lens too ______________, so that the image is blurred and focused in ______________ of the retina. The type of lens used to correct this refractive error is called a/an ______________ lens.
3. A miotic is a drug that ______________ the pupil of the eye.
4. A mydriatic is a drug that ______________ the pupil of the eye.

I Match the following abnormal conditions of the eye with their meanings as given below.

cataract	hordeolum (stye)	retinal detachment
chalazion	macular degeneration	retinitis pigmentosa
diabetic retinopathy	nystagmus	strabismus
glaucoma		

1. retinal microaneurysms, hemorrhages, dilation of retinal veins, and neovascularization occur secondary to an abnormal endocrine condition ______________
2. two layers of the retina separate from each other ______________
3. abnormal deviations of the eye occur (esotropia and exotropia) ______________
4. clouding of the lens causes decreased vision ______________
5. loss of central vision caused by deterioration of the macula of the retina ______________
6. localized, purulent infection of a sebaceous gland in the eyelid ______________
7. small, firm, cystic mass on the eyelid; formed as a result of chronic inflammation of a sebaceous gland ______________
8. increased intraocular pressure results in optic nerve damage ______________
9. pigmented scarring forms throughout the retina ______________
10. repetitive rhythmic movements of one or both eyes ______________

J **Label the following figure of the eye using the list of terms below.**

anterior chamber	fovea centralis	optic nerve
choroid	iris	pupil
ciliary body	lens	retina
conjunctiva	macula	sclera
cornea	optic disc	vitreous humor

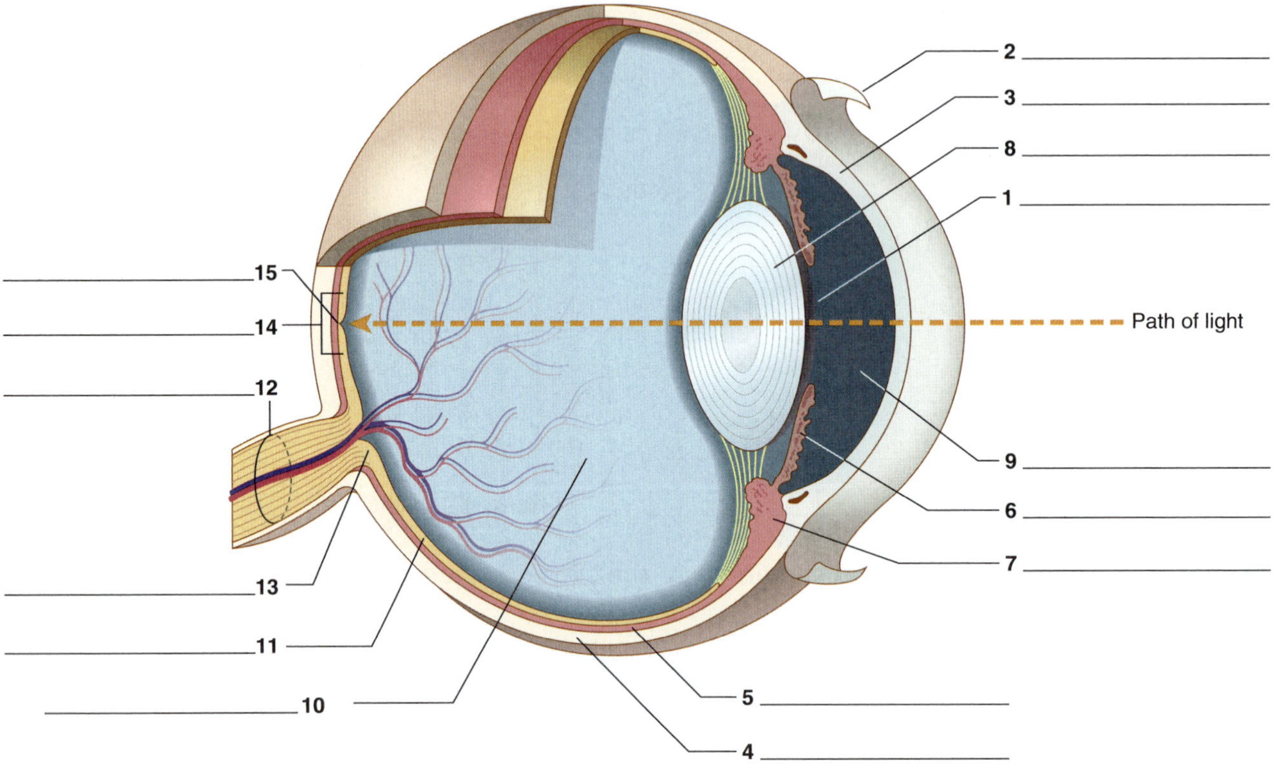

K **Match the following conditions with the images shown below.**

1. stroke (hemianopsia) ________ 2. glaucoma ________ 3. cataract ________

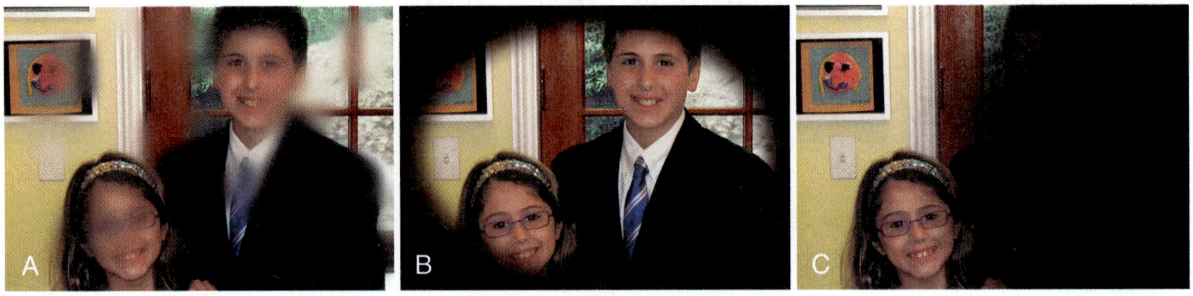

L **Give the meaning of the following combining forms.**

1. lacrim/o ______
2. dacry/o ______
3. kerat/o ______
4. corne/o ______
5. blephar/o ______
6. palpebr/o ______
7. cor/o ______
8. pupill/o ______
9. phac/o ______
10. phak/o ______
11. ocul/o ______
12. ophthalm/o ______
13. opt/o ______
14. scot/o ______

M **Give the meanings of the following abbreviations.**

1. OU ______
2. VA ______
3. OD ______
4. OS ______
5. VF ______
6. IOL ______
7. IOP ______
8. PERRLA ______

N Match the following clinical procedures with their meanings as given below.

fluorescein angiography	ophthalmoscopy	tonometry
keratoplasty	phacoemulsification	visual acuity test
laser photocoagulation	scleral buckle	visual field test
LASIK	slit lamp microscopy	vitrectomy

1. ultrasonic vibrations break up the lens, and it is aspirated from the eye ______________
2. test of clearness of vision ______________
3. measurement of tension or pressure within the eye; glaucoma test ______________
4. high-energy light radiation beams are used to stop retinal hemorrhaging ______________
5. a laser removes corneal tissue (sculpts it) to correct myopia ______________
6. intravenous injection of dye followed by photographs of the eye through dilated pupils ______________
7. suture of a silicone band to the sclera to correct retinal detachment ______________
8. test to measure central and peripheral vision (area within which objects are seen) when the eyes are looking straight ahead ______________
9. removal (and replacement) of diseased fluid in the chamber behind the lens of the eye ______________
10. visual examination of the interior of the eye after dilation of the pupil ______________
11. use of an instrument for microscopic examination of parts of the eye ______________
12. corneal transplant surgery ______________

17

O Arrange the following terms in the correct order to indicate their sequence in the transmission of sound waves to the brain from the outer ear. **See page 718.**

auditory liquids and receptors	external auditory canal	pinna (auricle)
auditory nerve fibers	incus	stapes
cerebral cortex	malleus	tympanic membrane
cochlea	oval window	

1. ______________
2. ______________
3. ______________
4. ______________
5. ______________
6. ______________
7. ______________
8. ______________
9. ______________
10. ______________
11. ______________

P **Give short definitions for the following medical terms.**

1. labyrinth ______________________________
2. semicircular canals ______________________________
3. auditory (eustachian) tube ______________________________
4. stapes ______________________________
5. organ of Corti ______________________________
6. perilymph and endolymph ______________________________
7. cerumen ______________________________
8. vestibule ______________________________
9. oval window ______________________________
10. tympanic membrane ______________________________

Q **Complete the following terms based on their definitions.**

1. instrument to examine the ear: ____________________scope
2. removal of the third bone of the middle ear: ____________________ectomy
3. pertaining to the auditory tube and throat: ____________________pharyngeal
4. flow of pus from the ear: oto____________________
5. instrument to measure hearing: ____________________meter
6. incision of the eardrum: ____________________tomy
7. surgical repair of the eardrum: ____________________plasty
8. deafness due to old age: ____________________cusis
9. small ear: micr____________________
10. inflammation of the middle ear: ot____________________

R **Give short definitions for the following medical terms.**

1. vertigo ______________________________
2. Meniere disease ______________________________
3. otosclerosis ______________________________
4. tinnitus ______________________________
5. labyrinthitis ______________________________
6. cholesteatoma ______________________________
7. suppurative otitis media ______________________________
8. acoustic neuroma ______________________________
9. mastoiditis ______________________________
10. myringitis ______________________________

S **Give the meanings of the following abbreviations relating to otology.**

1. ENG ______________________________
2. AS ______________________________
3. AD ______________________________
4. EENT ______________________________
5. ENT ______________________________
6. PE tube ______________________________

T **Circle the correct term(s) to complete each sentence.**

1. Dr. Jones specializes in pediatric ophthalmology. His examination of children with poor vision often leads to the diagnosis of **(cataract, amblyopia, glaucoma)**, or lazy eye.
2. Stella's near vision became progressively worse as she aged. Her physician told her that she had a common condition called **(presbyopia, detached retina, anisocoria)**, which often develops beginning in middle age.
3. Matthew rubbed his itchy eyes constantly and thus spread his "pinkeye" or **(conjunctivitis, blepharitis, myringitis)** from one eye to the other. Dr. Chang prescribed antibiotics for this common condition, because Matthew had a purulent discharge suggestive of an infection.
4. As Paul's **(mastoiditis, otitis media, tinnitus)** became progressively worse, his doctor worried that this ringing in his ears might be caused by a benign brain tumor, a/an **(cholesteatoma, acoustic neuroma, glaucoma)**.
5. Before her second birthday, Sally had so many episodes of **(vertigo, otosclerosis, suppurative otitis media)** that Dr. Sills recommended the placement of PE tubes.
6. Sixty-eight-year-old Bob experienced blurred vision in the central portion of his visual field. After careful examination of his **(cornea, sclera, retina)**, his **(ophthalmologist, optician, optometrist)** diagnosed his condition as **(glaucoma, iritis, macular degeneration)**. The doctor explained that the form of this condition was atrophic or **(dry, wet)**, causing photoreceptor rods and cones to die.
7. If Bob's condition had been diagnosed as the **(dry, wet)** form, it might have been treated with **(cryotherapy, intraocular lenses, laser photocoagulation)** to seal leaky blood vessels.
8. Sarah suddenly experienced bright flashes of light in her right eye. She also told her physician that she had a sensation of a curtain being pulled over part of the visual field in that eye. Her doctor examined her eye with **(keratoplasty, ophthalmoscopy, tonometry)** and determined that she had **(retinal refraction, retinal detachment, diabetic retinopathy)**. Corrective surgery, known as **(enucleation, vitrectomy, scleral buckling),** was recommended.
9. Carol awakened with a sensation of dizziness or **(vertigo, tinnitus, presbycusis)** as she tried to get out of bed. She was totally incapacitated for several days and noticed hearing loss in her left ear. Her physician explained that fluid called **(pus, endolymph, mucus)** had accumulated in her **(auditory tube, middle ear, cochlea)** and her condition was **(otosclerosis, cholesteatoma, Meniere disease)**. He prescribed drugs to control her dizziness and nausea.
10. Patients with conductive hearing loss are helped by reconstruction of the **(labyrinth, tympanic membrane, auditory tube)**, a procedure known as **(myringoplasty, audiometry, otoscopy)**. Patients with sensorineural hearing loss may be helped by a **(hearing aid, cochlear implant, stapedectomy)**.

ANSWERS TO EXERCISES

A

1. E
2. G
3. H
4. J
5. F
6. I
7. B
8. C
9. A
10. D

B

1. optic disc
2. accommodation
3. macula
4. fovea centralis
5. refraction
6. optic chiasm
7. cones
8. rods
9. anterior chamber
10. fundus

C

1. cornea
2. anterior chamber and aqueous humor
3. pupil
4. lens
5. vitreous chamber and vitreous humor
6. retina
7. optic nerve fibers
8. optic chiasm
9. thalamus
10. cerebral cortex (occipital lobe)

D

1. cranial nerve that carries impulses from the retina to the brain
2. having two sides that are rounded, elevated, and curved evenly
3. condition of pupils of unequal (anis/o) size
4. pertaining to paralysis of the ciliary muscles
5. pertaining to the eyelid
6. condition of enlargement of the pupil
7. condition of constriction of the pupil
8. swelling in the region of the optic disc
9. condition of sensitivity to ("fear of") light
10. blind spot; area of darkened (diminished) vision surrounded by clear vision

E

1. blepharitis
2. conjunctivitis
3. dacryoadenitis
4. iritis
5. keratitis
6. scleritis
7. retinitis
8. blepharoptosis
9. lacrimal
10. intraocular

F

1. corneal ulcer
2. uveitis
3. xerophthalmia
4. hemianopsia
5. exotropia
6. ophthalmologist
7. optometrist
8. optician
9. aphakia
10. esotropia

G

1. decreased (dim) vision; lazy eye (resulting from strabismus and uncorrected refractive errors in childhood)
2. farsightedness
3. decreased vision at near, resulting from old age
4. nearsightedness
5. night blindness; decreased vision at night
6. double vision
7. defective curvature of the lens and cornea leading to blurred vision

H

1. retina; long; strong; front; concave
2. short; weak; back; convex
3. constricts
4. dilates

17

I

1. diabetic retinopathy
2. retinal detachment
3. strabismus
4. cataract
5. macular degeneration
6. hordeolum (stye)
7. chalazion
8. glaucoma
9. retinitis pigmentosa
10. nystagmus

J

1. pupil
2. conjunctiva
3. cornea
4. sclera
5. choroid
6. iris
7. ciliary body
8. lens
9. anterior chamber
10. vitreous humor
11. retina
12. optic nerve
13. optic disc
14. macula
15. fovea centralis

K

1. C. Stroke (hemianopsia)—loss of half of the visual field caused by a stroke affecting the left visual cortex
2. B. Glaucoma—loss of peripheral vision first (darkness around the edges of the picture)
3. A. Cataract—causes blurred vision

L

1. tears
2. tears
3. cornea
4. cornea
5. eyelid
6. eyelid
7. pupil
8. pupil
9. lens
10. lens
11. eye
12. eye
13. eye
14. darkness

M

1. both eyes
2. visual acuity
3. right eye
4. left eye
5. visual field
6. intraocular lens
7. intraocular pressure
8. pupils equal, round, reactive to light and accommodation

N

1. phacoemulsification
2. visual acuity test
3. tonometry
4. laser photocoagulation
5. LASIK
6. fluorescein angiography
7. scleral buckle
8. visual field test
9. vitrectomy
10. ophthalmoscopy
11. slit lamp microscopy
12. keratoplasty

O

1. pinna (auricle)
2. external auditory canal
3. tympanic membrane
4. malleus
5. incus
6. stapes
7. oval window
8. cochlea
9. auditory liquids and receptors
10. auditory nerve fibers
11. cerebral cortex

P

1. cochlea and organs of equilibrium (semicircular canals and vestibule)
2. organ of equilibrium in the inner ear
3. passageway between the middle ear and the throat
4. third ossicle (little bone) of the middle ear
5. region in the cochlea that contains auditory receptors
6. auditory fluids circulating within the inner ear
7. wax in the external auditory meatus
8. central cavity of the inner ear that connects the semicircular canals and the cochlea
9. delicate membrane between the middle and the inner ears
10. eardrum

Q

1. otoscope
2. stapedectomy
3. salpingopharyngeal
4. otopyorrhea
5. audiometer
6. myringotomy (tympanotomy)
7. tympanoplasty (myringoplasty)
8. presbycusis
9. microtia
10. otitis media

R

1. sensation of irregular or whirling motion either of oneself or of external objects
2. disorder of the labyrinth marked by elevation of ear fluids and pressure within the cochlea (tinnitus, vertigo, and nausea result)
3. hardening in the bony tissue of the ossicles of the middle ear
4. noise (ringing, buzzing) in the ears
5. inflammation of the labyrinth of the inner ear
6. collection of skin cells and cholesterol in a sac within the middle ear
7. inflammation of the middle ear with bacterial infection and pus collection
8. benign tumor arising from the acoustic nerve in the brain
9. inflammation of the mastoid process (behind the ear)
10. inflammation of the eardrum

S

1. electronystagmography; a test of balance
2. left ear
3. right ear
4. eyes, ears, nose, and throat
5. ears, nose, and throat
6. pressure-equalizing tube; ventilating tube placed in the eardrum

T

1. amblyopia
2. presbyopia
3. conjunctivitis
4. tinnitus; acoustic neuroma
5. suppurative otitis media
6. retina; ophthalmologist; macular degeneration; dry
7. wet; laser photocoagulation
8. ophthalmoscopy; retinal detachment; scleral buckling
9. vertigo; endolymph; cochlea; Meniere disease
10. tympanic membrane; myringoplasty; cochlear implant

Answers to Practical Applications

Operating Room Schedule: Eye and Ear Procedures

1. I
2. B
3. C
4. D
5. G
6. A
7. H
8. E
9. F

PRONUNCIATION OF TERMS

To test your understanding of the terminology in this chapter, write the meaning of each term in the space provided. In addition, you may wish to cover the terms and write them by looking at your definitions. Make sure your spelling is correct. The page number after each term indicates where it is defined or used in the book, so you can easily check your responses. You will find complete definitions for all of these terms and their audio pronunciations on the Evolve website.

Pronunciation Guide

ā as in āpe	ă as in ăpple
ē as in ēven	ĕ as in ĕvery
ī as in īce	ĭ as in ĭnterest
ō as in ōpen	ŏ as in pŏt
ū as in ūnit	ŭ as in ŭnder

Vocabulary and Terminology: Eye

TERM	PRONUNCIATION	MEANING
accommodation (700)	ă-kŏm-ō-DĀ-shŭn	
amblyopia (705)	ăm-blē-Ō-pē-ă	
anisocoria (702)	ăn-ī-sō-KŌ-rē-ă	
anterior chamber (700)	ăn-TĒ-rē-ŏr CHĀM-bĕr	
aphakia (704)	ă-FĀ-kē-ă	
aqueous humor (700)	ĂK-wē-ŭs *or* Ā-kwē-ŭs HŪ-mŏr	
astigmatism (706)	ă-STĬG-mă-tĭzm	
biconvex (701)	bī-KŎN-vĕks	
blepharitis (702)	blĕf-ă-RĪ-tĭs	
blepharoptosis (702)	blĕf-ă-rŏp-TŌ-sĭs	
cataract (708)	KĂT-ă-răkt	
chalazion (708)	kă-LĀ-zē-ŏn	
choroid (701)	KŎR-oyd	
ciliary body (701)	SĬL-ē-ăr-ē BŎD-ē	
cone (701)	kōn	
conjunctiva (701)	kŏn-jŭnk-TĪ-vă	
conjunctivitis (702)	kŏn-jŭnk-tĭ-VĪ-tĭs	
cornea (701)	KŎR-nē-ă	
corneal abrasion (703)	KŎR-nē-ăl ă-BRĀ-zhŭn	
corneoscleral (704)	kŏr-nē-ō-SKLĔ-răl	
cycloplegic (703)	sī-klō-PLĒ-jĭk	
dacryoadenitis (703)	dăk-rē-ō-ăd-ĕ-NĪ-tĭs	
diabetic retinopathy (709)	dī-ă-BĔT-ĭk rĕ-tĭn-NŎP-ă-thē	

17

TERM	PRONUNCIATION	MEANING
diplopia (705)	dĭp-LŌ-pē-ă	
enucleation (714)	ē-nū-klē-Ā-shun	
esotropia (706)	ĕs-ō-TRŌ-pē-ă	
exotropia (711)	ĕk-sō-TRŌ-pē-ă	
fluorescein angiography (712)	floo-ō-RĔS-ē-ĭn ăn-jē-ŎG-ră-fē	
fovea centralis (701)	FŌ-vē-ă sĕn-TRĂ-lĭs	
fundus of the eye (701)	FŬN-dŭs of the ī	
glaucoma (709)	glaw-KŌ-mă	
hemianopsia (706)	hĕ-mē-ă-NŎP-sē-ă	
hordeolum (710)	hŏr-DĒ-ō-lŭm	
hyperopia (706)	hī-pĕr-Ō-pē-ă	
hypertensive retinopathy (704)	hī-pĕr-TĔN-sĭv rĕ-tĭ-NŎP-ă-thē	
intraocular (703)	ĭn-tră-ŎK-ū-lăr	
iridectomy (703)	ĭr-ĭ-DĔK-tō-mē	
iridic (703)	ĭ-RĪD-ĭk	
iris (701)	Ī-rĭs	
iritis (703)	ī-RĪ-tĭs	
keratitis (703)	kĕr-ă-TĪ-tĭs	
keratoplasty (714)	kĕr-ă-tō-PLĂS-tē	
lacrimal (703)	LĂK-rĭ-măl	
lacrimation (703)	lă-krĭ-MĀ-shŭn	
laser photocoagulation (715)	LĀ-zĕr fō-tō-kō-ăg-ū-LĀ-shŭn	
lens (701)	lĕnz	
macula (701)	MĂK-ū-lă	
macular degeneration (710)	MĂK-ū-lăr dē-jĕn-ĕ-RĀ-shŭn	
miosis (705)	mī-Ō-sĭs	
miotic (705)	mī-ŎT-ĭk	
mydriasis (705)	mĭ-DRĪ-ă-sĭs	
myopia (706)	mī-Ō-pē-ă	
nyctalopia (705)	nĭk-tă-LŌ-pē-ă	
nystagmus (711)	nĭ-STĂG-mŭs	

17

TERM	PRONUNCIATION	MEANING
ophthalmic (704)	ŏf-THĂL-mĭk	
ophthalmologist (704)	ŏf-thăl-MŎL-ō-jĭst	
ophthalmoplegia (704)	ŏf-thăl-mō-PLĒ-jă	
ophthalmoscopy (712)	ŏf-thăl-MŎS-kō-pē	
optic chiasm (701)	ŎP-tĭk KĪ-ăzm	
optic disc (701)	ŎP-tĭk dĭsk	
optician (704)	ŏp-TĬSH-ăn	
optic nerve (701)	ŎP-tĭk nĕrv	
optometrist (704)	ŏp-TŎM-ĕ-trĭst	
palpebral (704)	PĂL-pĕ-brăl	
papilledema (704)	păp-ĕ-lĕ-DĒ-mă	
phacoemulsification (715)	făk-ō-ĕ-mŭl-sĭ-fĭ-KĀ-shŭn	
photophobia (705)	fō-tō-FŌ-bē-ă	
presbyopia (707)	prĕz-bē-Ō-pē-ă	
pupil (701)	PŪ-pĭl	
pupillary (704)	PŪ-pĭ-lăr-ē	
refraction (701)	rē-FRĂK-shŭn	
retina (701)	RĔT-ĭ-nă	
retinal detachment (711)	RĔ-tĭ-năl dē-TĂCH-mĕnt	
retinitis pigmentosa (704)	rĕt-ĭ-NĪ-tĭs pĭg-mĕn-TŌ-să	
rod (701)	rŏd	
sclera (701)	SKLĔ-ră	
scleral buckle (715)	SKLĔ-răl BŬ-kl	
scleritis (704)	sklĕ-RĪ-tĭs	
scotoma (705)	skō-TŌ-mă	
slit lamp microscopy (712)	slĭt lămp mī-KRŎS-kō-pē	
strabismus (711)	stră-BĬZ-mŭs	
thalamus (701)	THĂL-ă-mŭs	
tonometry (713)	tō-NŎM-ĕ-trē	
uveitis (705)	ū-vē-Ī-tĭs	
visual acuity test (713)	VĬZ-ū-ăl ă-KŪ-ĭ-tē tĕst	

17

TERM	PRONUNCIATION	MEANING
visual field test (713)	VĬZ-ū-ăl fēld tĕst	________
vitrectomy (716)	vĭ-TRĔK-tō-mē	________
vitreous humor (701)	VĬT-rē-ŭs HŪ-mŏr	________
xerophthalmia (705)	zĕr-ŏf-THĂL-mē-ă	________

Vocabulary and Terminology: Ear

TERM	PRONUNCIATION	MEANING
acoustic (720)	ă-KOOS-tĭk	________
acoustic neuroma (722)	ă-KOOS-tĭk nū-RŌ-mă	________
audiogram (724)	ĂW-dē-ō-grăm	________
audiologist (720)	ăw-dē-ŎL-ō-gĭst	________
audiometer (724)	ăw-dē-ŎM-ĕ-tĕr	________
audiometry (724)	ăw-dē-ŎM-ĕ-trē	________
auditory canal (719)	ĂW-dĭ-tō-rē kă-NĂL	________
auditory meatus (719)	ĂW-dĭ-tō-rē mē-Ā-tŭs	________
auditory nerve fibers (719)	ĂW-dĭ-tō-re nĕrv FĪ-bĕrz	________
auditory tube (719)	ĂW-dĭ-tō-rē toob	________
aural (720)	ĂW-răl	________
auricle (719)	ĂW-rĭ-kl	________
cerumen (719)	sĕ-ROO-mĕn	________
cholesteatoma (722)	kō-lē-stē-ă-TŌ-mă	________
cochlea (719)	KŎK-lē-ă	________
cochlear (720)	KŎK-lē-ăr	________
deafness (722)	DĔF-nĕs	________
ear thermometry (724)	ēr thĕr-MŎM-ĕ-trē	________
endolymph (719)	ĔN-dō-lĭmf	________
eustachian tube (719)	ū-STĀ-shŭn toob	________
hyperacusis (721)	hī-pĕr-ă-KŪ-sis	________
incus (719)	ĬNG-kŭs	________
labyrinth (719)	LĂB-ĭ-rĭnth	________
macrotia (721)	măk-RŌ-shē-ă	________

TERM	PRONUNCIATION	MEANING
malleus (719)	MĂL-ē-ŭs	
mastoiditis (720)	măs-toy-DĪ-tĭs	
Meniere disease (722)	mĕn-ē-ĀR dĭ-ZĒZ	
myringitis (720)	mĭr-ĭn-JĪ-tĭs	
myringotomy (720)	mĭr-ĭn-GŎT-ō-mē	
organ of Corti (719)	ŎR-găn of CŎR-tē	
ossicle (719)	ŎS-ĭ-kl	
ossiculoplasty (720)	ŏs-ĭ-kū-lō-PLĂS-tē	
otic (720)	Ō-tĭk	
otitis media (723)	ō-TĪ-tĭs MĒ-dē-ă	
otolaryngologist (720)	ō-tō-lă-rĭn-GŎL-ō-jĭst	
otomycosis (720)	ō-tō-mī-KŌ-sĭs	
otopyorrhea (720)	ō-tō-pī-ō-RĒ-ă	
otosclerosis (723)	ō-tō-sklĕ-RŌ-sĭs	
otoscopy (724)	ō-TŎS-kō-pē	
oval window (719)	Ō-văl WĪN-dō	
perilymph (719)	PĔR-ĭ-lĭmf	
pinna (719)	PĬN-ă	
postauricular (720)	pōst-aw-RĬK-ū-lăr	
presbycusis (721)	prĕz-bē-KŪ-sĭs	
salpingopharyngeal (720)	săl-pĭng-gō-fă-RĬN-gē-ăl	
semicircular canals (719)	sĕ-mē-SĔR-kū-lăr kă-NĂLZ	
stapedectomy (721)	stā-pĕ-DĔK-tō-mē	
stapes (719)	STĀ-pēz	
tinnitus (723)	TĬN-nĭ-tŭs	
tuning fork test (724)	TOO-nĭng fŏrk tĕst	
tympanic membrane (719)	tĭm-PĂN-ĭk MĔM-brān	
tympanoplasty (721)	tĭm-pă-nō-PLĂS-tē	
vertigo (723)	VĔR-tĭ-gō	
vestibule (719)	VĔS-tĭ-būl	
vestibulocochlear (721)	vĕs-tĭb-ū-lō-KŌK-lē-ăr	

REVIEW SHEET

Write the meaning of the word parts in the spaces provided and test yourself. Check your answers with the information in the chapter or in the Glossary (Medical Word Parts—English) at the end of the book.

Combining Forms

COMBINING FORM	MEANING	COMBINING FORM	MEANING
acous/o	______	myring/o	______
ambly/o	______	nyct/o	______
anis/o	______	ocul/o	______
aque/o	______	ophthalm/o	______
audi/o	______	opt/o	______
audit/o	______	optic/o	______
aur/o	______	ossicul/o	______
auricul/o	______	ot/o	______
blephar/o	______	palpebr/o	______
cochle/o	______	papill/o	______
conjunctiv/o	______	phac/o	______
cor/o	______	phak/o	______
corne/o	______	phot/o	______
cycl/o	______	presby/o	______
dacry/o	______	pupill/o	______
dipl/o	______	retin/o	______
glauc/o	______	salping/o	______
ir/o	______	scler/o	______
irid/o	______	scot/o	______
kerat/o	______	staped/o	______
lacrim/o	______	tympan/o	______
mastoid/o	______	uve/o	______
mi/o	______	vestibul/o	______
myc/o	______	vitre/o	______
mydr/o	______	xer/o	______

Suffixes

SUFFIX	MEANING	SUFFIX	MEANING
-acusis	________________	-opsia	________________
-cusis	________________	-otia	________________
-meter	________________	-phobia	________________
-metry	________________	-plegic	________________
-opia	________________	-tropia	________________

Use the following terms to label the diagram below.

auditory nerve fibers
cochlea
eustachian tube
external auditory meatus
incus
malleus
oval window
pinna (auricle)
semicircular canals
stapes
tympanic membrane (eardrum)
vestibule

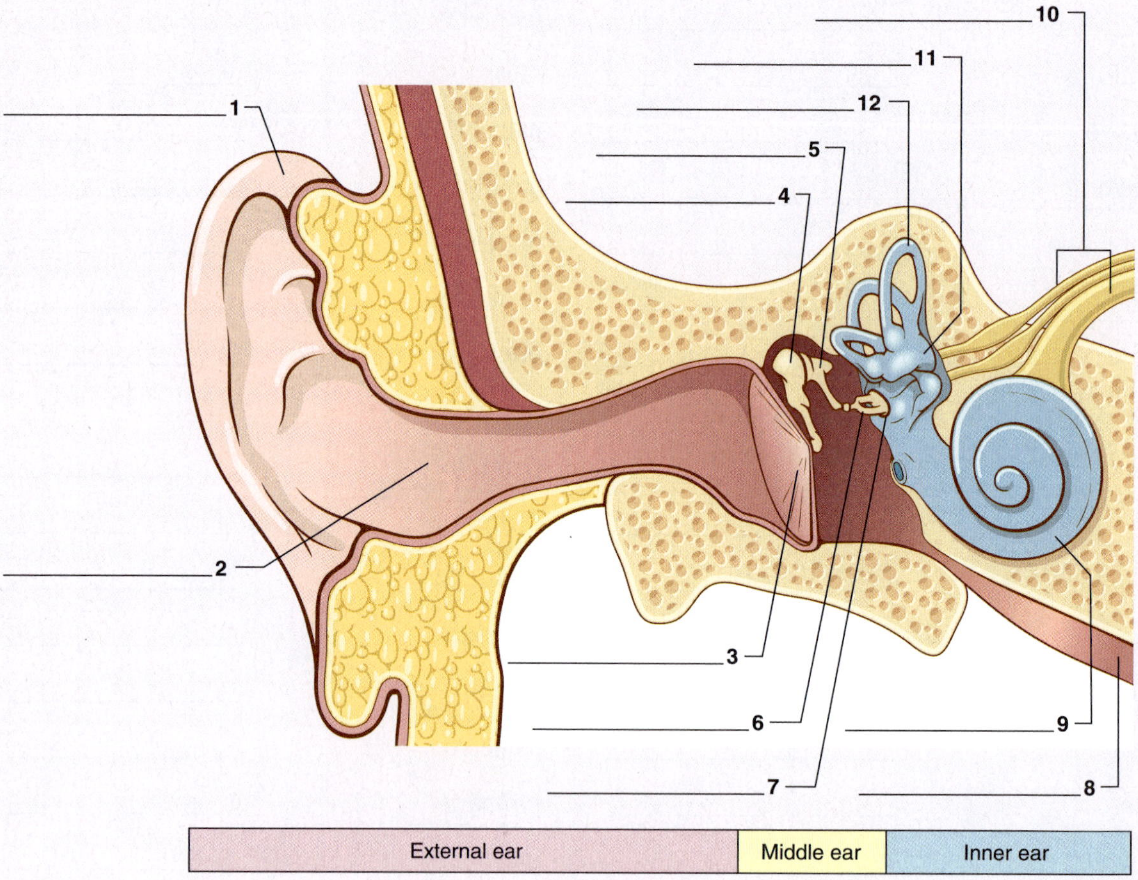

evolve *Please refer to the Evolve website for additional exercises and images related to this chapter.*

CHAPTER 18

Endocrine System

This chapter is divided into the following sections:

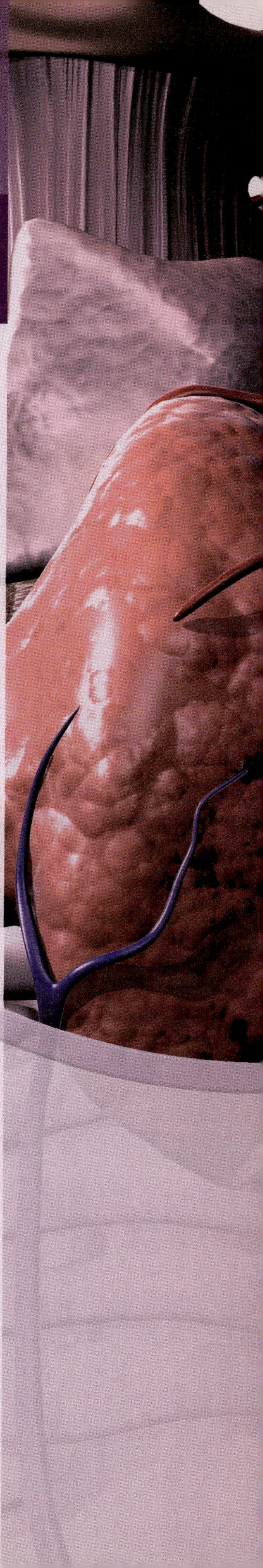

CHAPTER GOALS

- Identify the endocrine glands and their hormones.
- Gain an understanding of the functions of these hormones in the body.
- Analyze medical terms related to the endocrine glands and their hormones.
- Identify the abnormal conditions resulting from excessive and deficient secretions of the endocrine glands.
- Describe laboratory tests and clinical procedures related to endocrinology, and recognize relevant abbreviations.

INTRODUCTION

The endocrine system is an information signaling system much like the nervous system. However, the nervous system uses nerves to conduct information, whereas the endocrine system uses blood vessels as information channels. **Glands** located in many regions of the body release into the bloodstream specific chemical messengers called **hormones** (from the Greek word *hormōn*, meaning urging on) that regulate the many and varied functions of an organism. For example, one hormone stimulates the growth of bones, another causes the maturation of sex organs and reproductive cells, and another controls the metabolic rate (metabolism) within all the individual cells of the body. In addition, one powerful endocrine gland below the brain secretes a wide variety of different hormones that travel through the bloodstream and regulate the activities of other endocrine glands.

Hormones produce their effects by binding to **receptors,** which are recognition sites in the various **target tissues** on which the hormones act. The receptors initiate specific biologic effects when the hormones bind to them. Each hormone has its own receptor, and binding of a receptor by a hormone is much like the interaction of a key and a lock.

Endocrine glands, no matter which hormones they produce, secrete their hormones directly into the bloodstream. **Exocrine glands** send chemical substances (tears, sweat, milk, saliva) via ducts to the outside of the body. Examples of exocrine glands are sweat, mammary, mucous, salivary, and lacrimal (tear) glands.

The ductless, internally secreting **endocrine glands** are listed as follows. Locate these glands on Figure 18-1.

[1] thyroid gland
[2] parathyroid glands (four glands)
[3] adrenal glands (one pair)
[4] pancreas (islets of Langerhans)
[5] pituitary gland
[6] ovaries in female (one pair)
[7] testes in male (one pair)
[8] pineal gland

The last two glands on this list, the pineal and the thymus glands, are included as endocrine glands because they are ductless, although little is known about their endocrine function in the human body. The **pineal gland,** located in the central portion of the brain, secretes melatonin. **Melatonin** functions to support the body's "biological clock" and is thought to induce sleep. The pineal gland has been linked to a mental condition, seasonal affective disorder (SAD), in which the person suffers depression in winter months. Melatonin secretion increases with deprivation of light and is inhibited by sunlight. Calcification of the pineal gland can occur and can be an important radiologic landmark when x-rays of the brain are examined.

Hormones are also secreted by endocrine tissue in other organs apart from the major endocrine glands. Examples are **erythropoietin** (kidney), **human chorionic gonadotropin** (placenta), and **cholecystokinin** (gallbladder). **Prostaglandins** are hormone-like substances that affect the body in many ways. First found in semen (produced by the prostate gland) but now recognized in cells throughout the body, prostaglandins (1) stimulate the contraction of the uterus; (2) regulate body temperature, platelet aggregation, and acid secretion in the stomach; and (3) have the ability to lower blood pressure.

Endocrine tissue (apart from the major glands) is reviewed in Table 18-1. Use it as a reference.

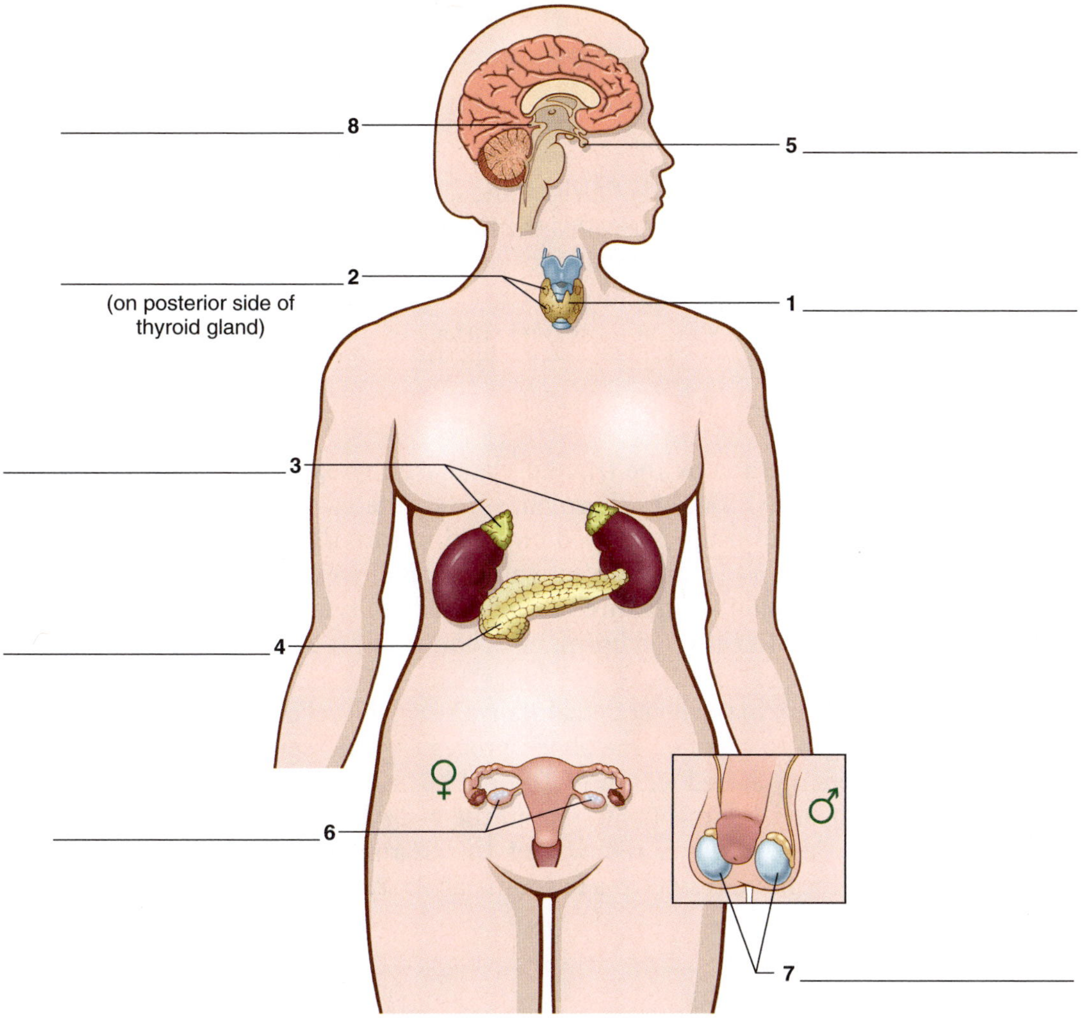

FIGURE 18-1 The endocrine system.

TABLE 18-1 ENDOCRINE TISSUE (APART FROM MAJOR GLANDS): LOCATION, SECRETION, AND ACTION

Location	Secretion	Action
Body cells	Prostaglandins	Aggregation of platelets Contract uterus Lower acid secretion in stomach Lower blood pressure
Gastrointestinal tract	Cholecystokinin Gastrin Secretin	Contracts gallbladder Stimulates gastric secretion Stimulates pancreatic enzymes
Kidney	Erythropoietin	Stimulates erythrocyte production
Pineal gland	Melatonin	Induces sleep and affects mood
Placenta	Human chorionic gonadotropin	Sustains pregnancy
Skin	Vitamin D	Affects absorption of calcium

THYROID GLAND

LOCATION AND STRUCTURE

Label Figure 18-2.

The **thyroid gland** [1] is composed of a right and a left lobe on either side of the **trachea** [2], just below a large piece of cartilage called the **thyroid cartilage** [3]. The thyroid cartilage covers the larynx and produces the prominence on the neck known in men as the "Adam's apple." The **isthmus** [4] of the thyroid gland is a narrow strip of glandular tissue that connects the two lobes on the ventral (anterior) surface of the trachea.

FUNCTION

Two of the hormones secreted by the thyroid gland are **thyroxine** or **tetraiodothyronine (T4)** and **triiodothyronine (T3).** These hormones are synthesized in the thyroid gland from **iodine,** which is picked up from the blood circulating through the gland, and from an amino acid called tyrosine. T4 (containing four atoms of iodine) is much more concentrated in the blood, whereas T3 (containing three atoms of iodine) is far more potent in affecting the metabolism of cells. Most thyroid hormone is bound to protein molecules as it travels in the bloodstream.

T4 and T3 are necessary in the body to maintain a normal level of metabolism in all body cells. Cells need oxygen to carry on metabolic processes, one aspect of which is burning food to release the energy stored within it. Thyroid hormone aids cells in their uptake of oxygen and thus supports the metabolic rate in the body. Injections of thyroid hormone raise the metabolic rate, whereas removal of the thyroid gland, diminishing thyroid hormone content in the body, results in a lower metabolic rate, heat loss, and poor physical and mental development.

18

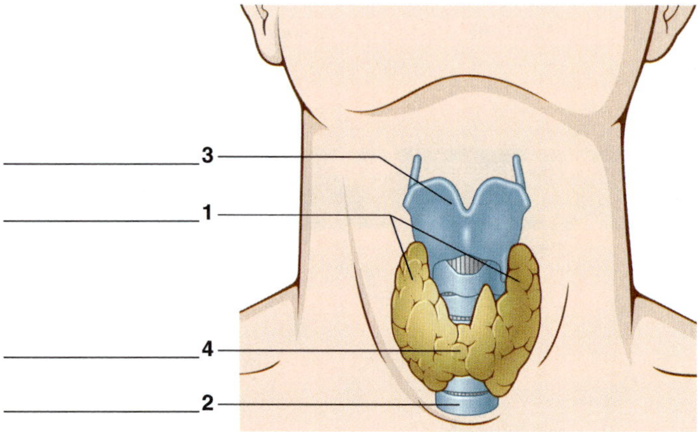

FIGURE 18-2 The thyroid gland, anterior view. Notice how the thyroid gland covers the trachea like a shield *(thyr/o = shield).*

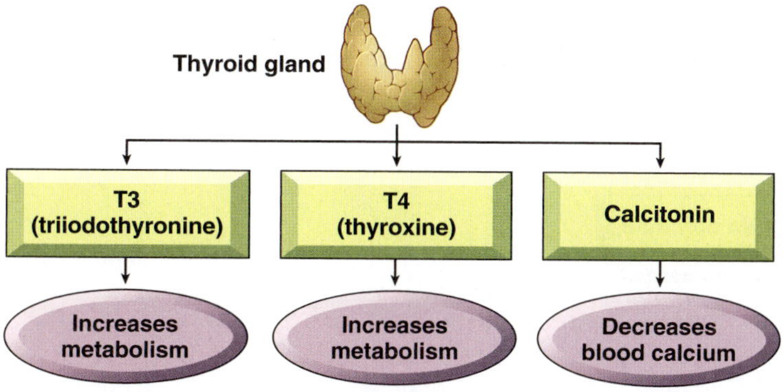

FIGURE 18-3 **The thyroid gland: its hormones and actions.**

A more recently discovered hormone produced by the thyroid gland is **calcitonin.** Calcitonin is secreted when calcium levels in the blood are high. It stimulates calcium to leave the blood and enter the bones, thus lowering blood calcium back to normal. Calcitonin contained in a nasal spray may be used for treatment of osteoporosis (loss of bone density). By increasing calcium storage in bone, calcitonin strengthens weakened bone tissue and prevents spontaneous bone fractures. Figure 18-3 summarizes the hormones secreted by the thyroid gland.

PARATHYROID GLANDS

LOCATION AND STRUCTURE

Label Figure 18-4.

The **parathyroid glands** [1] are four small oval bodies located on the dorsal aspect of the **thyroid gland** [2].

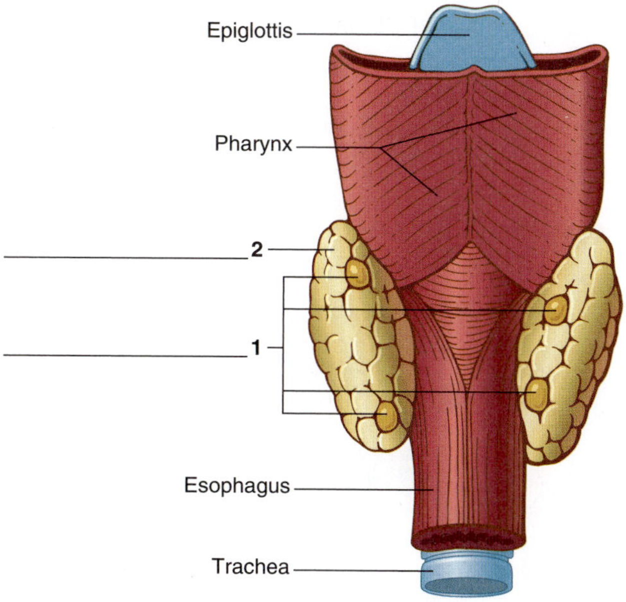

FIGURE 18-4 **The parathyroid glands,** posterior view. The prefix, para-, means near, or alongside.

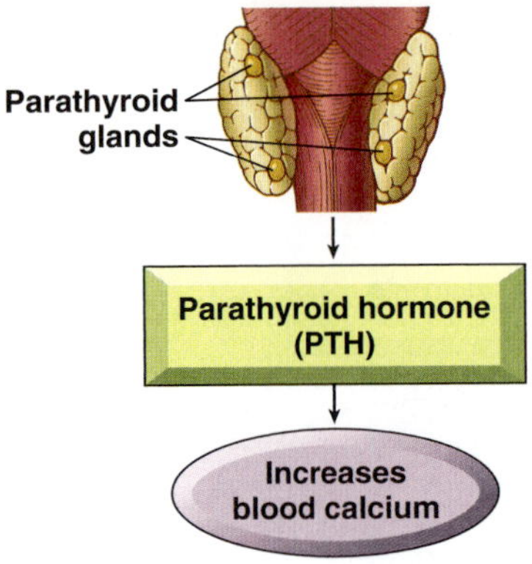

FIGURE 18-5 **The parathyroid glands: their hormones and action.**

FUNCTION

Parathyroid hormone (PTH) is secreted by the parathyroid glands. This hormone (also known as **parathormone**) mobilizes **calcium** (a mineral substance) from bones into the bloodstream, where calcium is necessary for proper functioning of body tissues, especially muscles. Normally, calcium in the food we eat is absorbed from the intestine and carried by the blood to the bones, where it is stored. The adjustment of the level of calcium in the blood is a good example of the way hormones in general control the **homeostasis** (equilibrium or constancy in the internal environment) of the body. If blood calcium decreases (as in pregnancy or in vitamin D deficiency), parathyroid hormone secretion increases, causing calcium to leave bones and enter the bloodstream. In this way, blood calcium levels are brought back to normal (Figure 18-5).

18

ADRENAL GLANDS

LOCATION AND STRUCTURE

Label Figure 18-6.

The **adrenal glands** are two small glands, one on top of each **kidney** [1]. Each gland consists of two parts: an outer portion, the **adrenal cortex** [2], and an inner portion, the **adrenal medulla** [3]. The adrenal cortex and adrenal medulla are two glands in one, secreting different hormones. The adrenal cortex secretes **steroids** or **corticosteroids** (complex

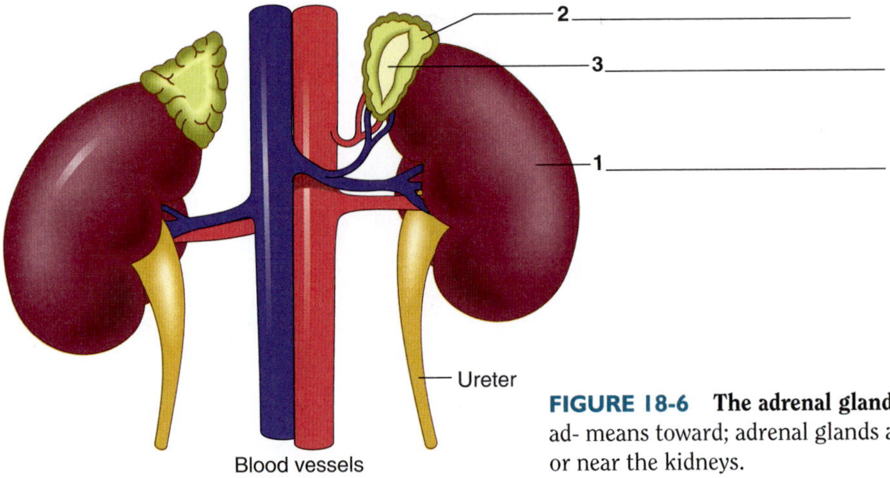

FIGURE 18-6 **The adrenal glands.** The prefix ad- means toward; adrenal glands are located "toward" or near the kidneys.

chemicals derived from cholesterol); the adrenal medulla secretes **catecholamines** (chemicals derived from amino acids).

FUNCTION

The **adrenal cortex** secretes three types of **corticosteroids.**

1. **Glucocorticoids**—These steroid hormones have an important influence on the metabolism of sugars, fats, and proteins within all body cells and have a powerful anti-inflammatory effect.

   Cortisol helps regulate glucose, fat, and protein metabolism. It raises blood glucose as part of a response to stress. **Cortisone** is a hormone very similar to cortisol and can be prepared synthetically. Cortisone is useful in treating inflammatory conditions such as rheumatoid arthritis.
2. **Mineralocorticoids**—The major mineralocorticoid is **aldosterone.** It regulates the concentration of mineral **salts (electrolytes)** in the body. Aldosterone acts on the kidney to reabsorb **sodium** (an important **electrolyte**) and water and to excrete **potassium** (another major **electrolyte**). Thus, it regulates blood volume and blood pressure and electrolyte concentration.
3. **Sex hormones**—**Androgens** (testosterone) and **estrogens** are secreted in small amounts and influence secondary sex characteristics, such as pubic and axillary hair in boys and girls. In females, the masculinizing effects of adrenal androgens (increased body hair), may appear when levels of ovarian estrogen decrease after menopause.

Think of the "three S's" to recall the main adrenal cortex hormones that influence **sugar** (cortisol), **salt** (aldosterone), and **sex** (androgens and estrogens).

The **adrenal medulla** secretes two types of **catecholamine** hormones:

1. **Epinephrine (adrenaline)**—Increases heart rate and blood pressure, dilates bronchial tubes, and releases glucose (sugars) from glycogen (storage substance) when the body needs it for more energy.
2. **Norepinephrine (noradrenaline)**—Constricts blood vessels to raise blood pressure.

Both epinephrine and norepinephrine are **sympathomimetic** agents because they mimic, or copy, the actions of the sympathetic nervous system. They are released to help the body meet the challenges of stress in response to stimulation by the sympathetic nervous system.

Figure 18-7 summarizes hormones secreted by the adrenal glands and their actions.

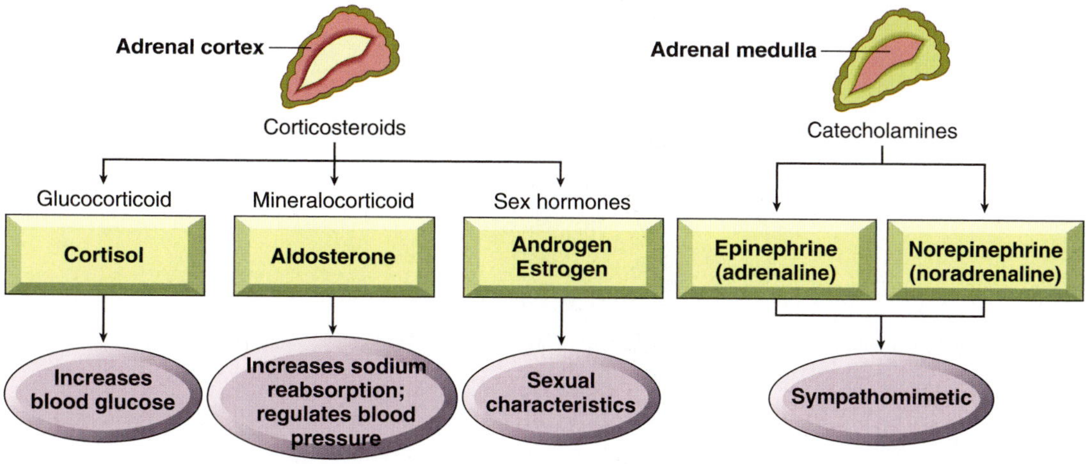

FIGURE 18-7 The adrenal cortex and adrenal medulla: their hormones and actions.

PANCREAS

LOCATION AND STRUCTURES

Label Figure 18-8.

The **pancreas** [1] is located near and partly behind the **stomach** [2] in the region of the first and second lumbar vertebrae. The endocrine tissue of the pancreas consists of specialized hormone-producing cells called the **islets of Langerhans** [3] or **islet cells.** More than 98% of the pancreas consists of exocrine cells (glands and ducts). These cells secrete digestive enzymes into the gastrointestinal tract.

FUNCTION

The islets of Langerhans produce **insulin** (produced by beta cells) and **glucagon** (produced by alpha cells). Both play a role regulating blood **glucose** (sugar) levels. When blood glucose rises, insulin lowers blood sugar by helping it enter body cells. Insulin also lowers blood sugar by causing conversion of **glucose** to **glycogen** (a starch storage form of sugar) in the liver. If blood glucose levels fall too low, glucagon raises blood sugar by acting on liver cells to promote conversion of glycogen back to glucose. Thus, the endocrine function of the pancreas is another example of **homeostasis,** the body's ability to regulate its inner environment to maintain stability.

Figure 18-9 reviews the secretions of the islet cells and their actions.

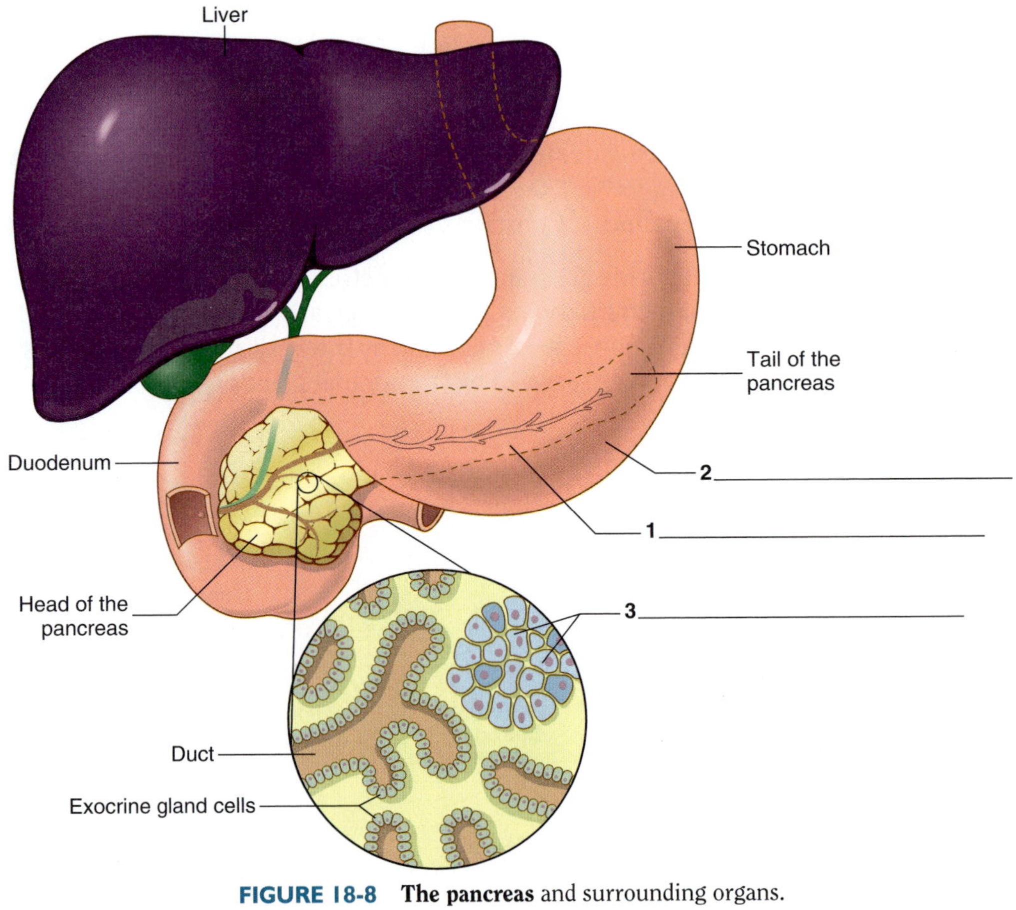

FIGURE 18-8 **The pancreas** and surrounding organs.

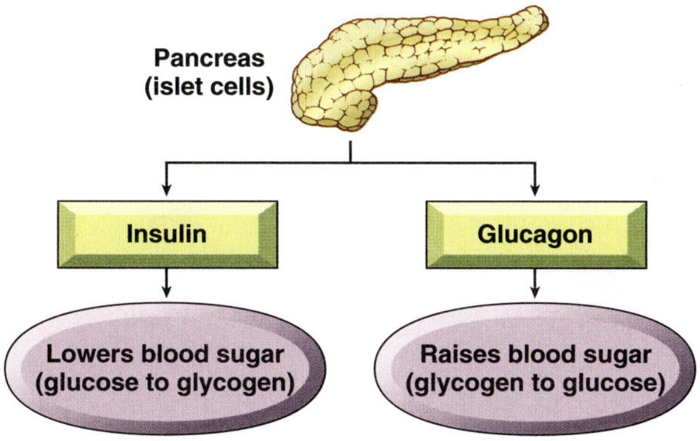

FIGURE 18-9 The pancreas (islet cells): its hormones and actions. Insulin is the only hormone that lowers blood sugar levels.

Pituitary Gland

LOCATION AND STRUCTURE

Label Figure 18-10.

The **pituitary gland,** also called the **hypophysis,** is a small pea-sized gland located at the base of the brain in a small pocket-like depression of the skull called the **sella turcica.** It is a well-protected gland, with the entire mass of the brain above it and the nasal cavity below. The ancient Greeks incorrectly imagined that its function was to produce *pituita,* or nasal secretion.

The pituitary consists of two distinct parts: an **anterior lobe** or **adenohypophysis** [1], composed of glandular epithelial tissue, and a **posterior lobe** or **neurohypophysis** [2], composed of nervous tissue. The **hypothalamus** [3] is a region of the brain under the thalamus and above the pituitary gland. Signals transmitted from the hypothalamus control secretions by the pituitary gland. Special secretory neurons in the hypothalamus send releasing and inhibiting factors (hormones) via capillaries to the anterior pituitary gland.

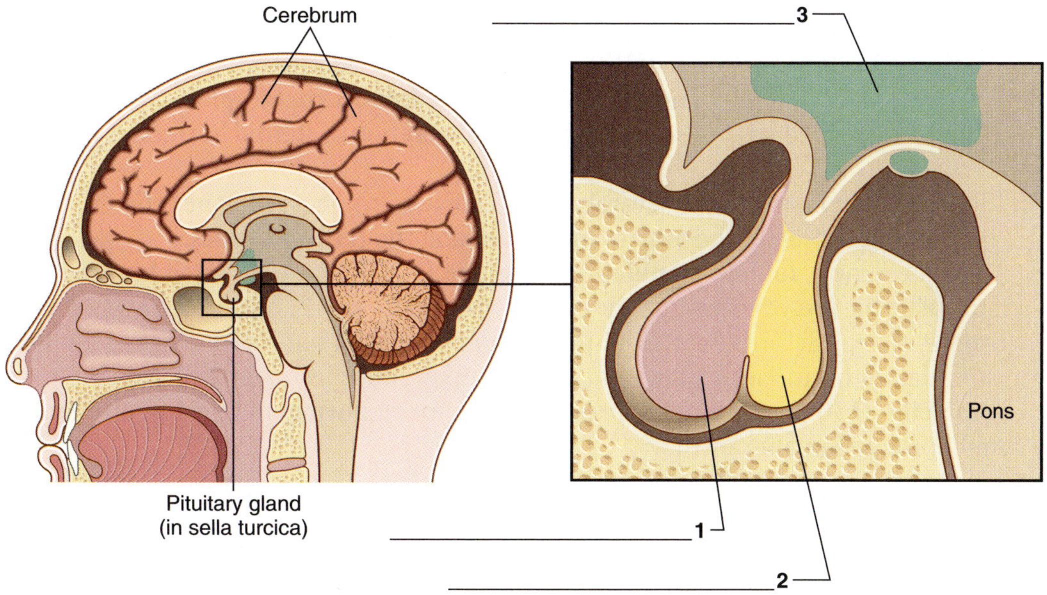

FIGURE 18-10 The pituitary gland.

18

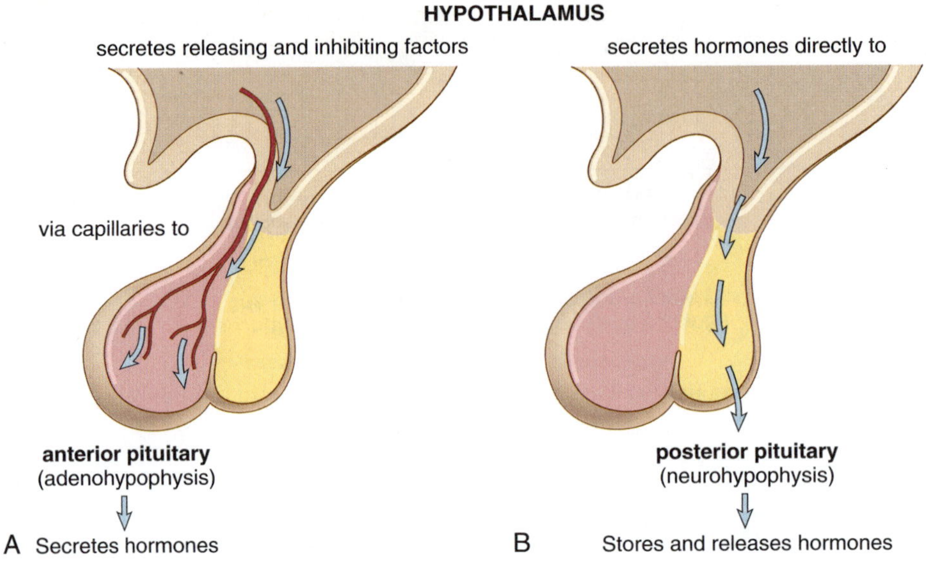

FIGURE 18-11 **A, The relationship of the hypothalamus to the anterior pituitary gland. B, The relationship of the hypothalamus to the posterior pituitary gland.**

These factors stimulate or inhibit secretion of hormones from the anterior pituitary (Figure 18-11A). The hypothalamus also produces and secretes hormones directly to the posterior pituitary gland, where the hormones are stored and then released (Figure 18-11B).

FUNCTION

Although no bigger than a pea, the **pituitary gland** is often called the **"master gland"** because it makes hormones that control several other endocrine glands.

The major hormones of the **anterior pituitary gland** are:

1. **Growth hormone (GH),** or **somatotropin (STH)**—Promotes protein synthesis that results in the growth of bones, muscles, and other tissues. GH also stimulates the liver to make insulin-like growth factor, which stimulates the growth of bones. It increases blood glucose levels and is secreted during exercise, sleep, and hypoglycemia.
2. **Thyroid-stimulating hormone (TSH),** or **thyrotropin**—Stimulates the growth of the thyroid gland and secretion of thyroxine (T4) and triiodothyronine (T3).
3. **Adrenocorticotropic hormone (ACTH),** or **adrenocorticotropin**—Stimulates the growth of the adrenal cortex and increases its secretion of steroid hormones (primarily cortisol).
4. **Gonadotropic hormones**—Several gonadotropic hormones influence the growth and hormone secretion of the ovaries in females and the testes in males.

   In the female, **follicle-stimulating hormone (FSH)** and **luteinizing hormone (LH)** stimulate the growth of eggs in the ovaries, the production of hormones, and ovulation. In the male, FSH influences the production of sperm, and LH (an interstitial cell–stimulating hormone) stimulates the testes to produce testosterone.
5. **Prolactin (PRL)**—Stimulates breast development during pregnancy and sustains milk production after birth.

The **posterior pituitary gland** stores and releases two important hormones that are synthesized in the hypothalamus:

1. **Antidiuretic hormone (ADH),** also called **vasopressin**—Stimulates the reabsorption of water by the kidney tubules. In addition, ADH also increases blood pressure by constricting arterioles.

2. **Oxytocin (OT)**—Stimulates the uterus to contract during childbirth and maintains labor during childbirth. Oxytocin is also secreted during suckling and causes the production of milk from the mammary glands.

Figure 18-12 summarizes hormones secreted by the pituitary gland and their functions.

OVARIES

LOCATION AND STRUCTURE

The **ovaries** are two small glands located in the lower abdominal region of the female. The ovaries produce the female gamete, the ovum, as well as hormones that are responsible for female sex characteristics and regulation of the menstrual cycle.

FUNCTION

The ovarian hormones are **estrogens** (**estradiol** and estrone) and **progesterone.** Estrogens stimulate development of ova (eggs) and development of female secondary sex characteristics. Progesterone is responsible for the preparation and maintenance of the uterus in pregnancy.

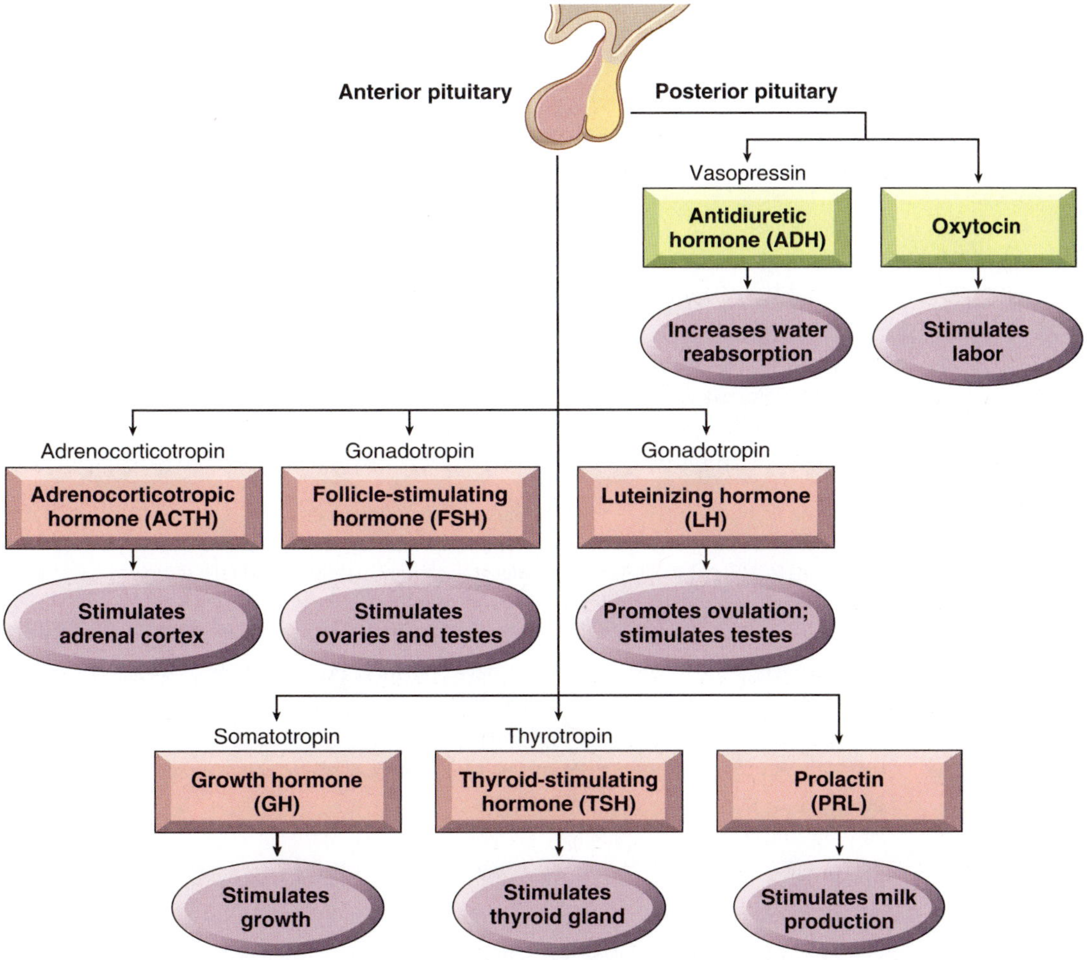

FIGURE 18-12 **The pituitary gland: its hormones and actions.**

TESTES

LOCATION AND STRUCTURE

The **testes** are two small ovoid glands suspended from the inguinal region of the male by the spermatic cord and surrounded by the scrotal sac. The testes produce the male gametes, spermatozoa, as well as the male hormone called **testosterone.**

FUNCTION

Testosterone is an **androgen** (male steroid hormone) that stimulates development of sperm and secondary sex characteristics in the male (development of beard and pubic hair, deepening of voice, and distribution of fat).

Figure 18-13 reviews the hormones secreted by the ovaries and testes.

Table 18-2 lists the major endocrine glands, their hormones, and the actions they produce.

TABLE 18-2 MAJOR ENDOCRINE GLANDS: THE HORMONES THEY PRODUCE AND THEIR ACTIONS

Endocrine Gland	Hormone	Action
Thyroid	• Thyroxine (T4); triiodothyronine (T3)	• Increases metabolism in body cells
	• Calcitonin	• Decreases blood calcium
Parathyroids	• Parathyroid hormone	• Increases blood calcium
Adrenals		
Cortex	• Cortisol (glucocorticoid)	• Increases blood sugar
	• Aldosterone (mineralocorticoid)	• Increases reabsorption of sodium
	• Androgens, estrogens (sex hormones)	• Secondary sex characteristics
Medulla	• Epinephrine (adrenaline)	• Sympathomimetic
	• Norepinephrine (noradrenaline)	• Sympathomimetic
Pancreas		
Islet cells	• Insulin	• Decreases blood sugar (glucose to glycogen)
	• Glucagon	• Increases blood sugar (glycogen to glucose)
Pituitary		
Anterior lobe	• Growth hormone (GH) (somatotropin)	• Increases bone and tissue growth
	• Thyroid-stimulating hormone (TSH)	• Stimulates thyroid gland and thyroxine secretion
	• Adrenocorticotropic hormone (ACTH)	• Stimulates adrenal cortex, especially cortisol secretion
	• Gonadotropins	
	Follicle-stimulating hormone (FSH)	• Oogenesis and spermatogenesis
	Luteinizing hormone (LH)	• Promotes ovulation; testosterone secretion
	• Prolactin (PRL)	• Promotes growth of breast tissue and milk secretion
Posterior lobe	• Antidiuretic hormone (ADH) (vasopressin)	• Stimulates reabsorption of water by kidney tubules
	• Oxytocin	• Stimulates contraction of the uterus during labor and childbirth
Ovaries	• Estrogens	• Promote development of ova and female secondary sex characteristics
	• Progesterone	• Prepares and maintains the uterus in pregnancy
Testes	• Testosterone	• Promotes development of sperm and male secondary sex characteristics

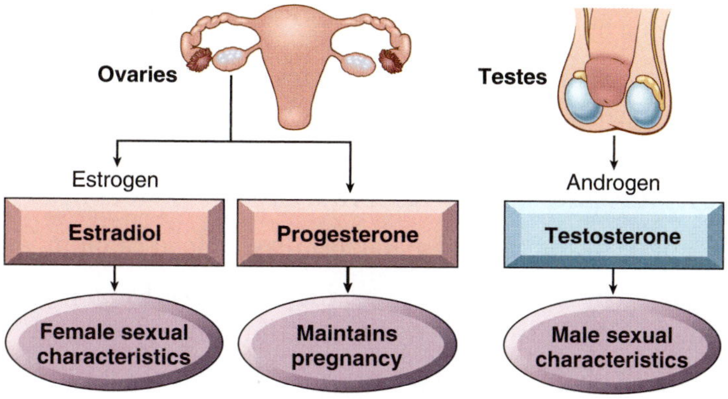

FIGURE 18-13 **The ovaries and testes: their hormones and actions.**

VOCABULARY

This list reviews many new terms introduced in the text. Short definitions reinforce your understanding of the terms. Refer to the Pronunciation of Terms on page 790 for help with unfamiliar or difficult words.

MAJOR ENDOCRINE GLANDS	
adrenal cortex	Outer section (cortex) of each adrenal gland; secretes cortisol, aldosterone, and sex hormones.
adrenal medulla	Inner section (medulla) of each adrenal gland; secretes epinephrine and norepinephrine.
ovaries	Located in the lower abdomen of a female; responsible for egg production and estrogen and progesterone secretion.
pancreas	Located behind the stomach. Islet (alpha and beta) cells (islets of Langerhans) secrete hormones from the pancreas. The pancreas also contains cells that are exocrine in function. They secrete enzymes, via a duct, into the small intestine to aid digestion.
parathyroid glands	Four small glands on the posterior of the thyroid gland. Some people may have three or five parathyroid glands.
pituitary gland (hypophysis)	Located at the base of the brain in the sella turcica; composed of an anterior lobe **(adenohypophysis)** and a posterior lobe **(neurohypophysis).** It weighs only 1⁄16 of an ounce and is a half-inch across.
testes	Two glands enclosed in the scrotal sac of a male; responsible for sperm production and testosterone secretion.
thyroid gland	Located in the neck on either side of the trachea; secretes thyroxine, triiodothyronine, and calcitonin.
HORMONES	
adrenaline (epinephrine)	Secreted by the adrenal medulla; increases heart rate and blood pressure.
adrenocorticotropic hormone (ACTH)	Secreted by the anterior lobe of the pituitary gland (adenohypophysis); also called **adrenocorticotropin**. ACTH stimulates the adrenal cortex.

18

aldosterone	Secreted by the adrenal cortex; increases salt (sodium) reabsorption.
androgen	Male hormone secreted by the testes and to a lesser extent by the adrenal cortex; testosterone is an example.
antidiuretic hormone (ADH)	Secreted by the posterior lobe of the pituitary gland (neurohypophysis). ADH **(vasopressin)** increases reabsorption of water by the kidney.
calcitonin	Secreted by the thyroid gland; decreases blood calcium levels.
cortisol	Secreted by the adrenal cortex; increases blood sugar. It is secreted in times of stress and has an anti-inflammatory effect.
epinephrine (adrenaline)	Secreted by the adrenal medulla; increases heart rate and blood pressure and dilates airways (sympathomimetic). It is part of the body's "fight or flight" reaction.
estradiol	Estrogen (female hormone) secreted by the ovaries.
estrogen	Female hormone secreted by the ovaries and to a lesser extent by the adrenal cortex. Examples are estradiol and estrone.
follicle-stimulating hormone (FSH)	Secreted by the anterior lobe of the pituitary gland (adenohypophysis). FSH stimulates hormone secretion and egg production by the ovaries and sperm production by the testes.
glucagon	Secreted by alpha islet cells of the pancreas; increases blood sugar by conversion of glycogen (starch) to glucose.
growth hormone (GH); somatotropin	Secreted by the anterior lobe of the pituitary gland (adenohypophysis); stimulates growth of bones and soft tissues.
insulin	Secreted by beta islet cells (Latin *insula* means island) of the pancreas. Insulin helps glucose (sugar) to pass into cells, and it promotes the conversion of glucose to glycogen.
luteinizing hormone (LH)	Secreted by the anterior lobe of the pituitary gland (adenohypophysis); stimulates ovulation in females and testosterone secretion in males.
norepinephrine	Secreted by the adrenal medulla; increases heart rate and blood pressure (sympathomimetic). Nor- in chemistry means a parent compound from which another is derived. Also called noradrenaline.
oxytocin (OT)	Secreted by the posterior lobe of the pituitary gland (neurohypophysis); stimulates contraction of the uterus during labor and childbirth.
parathormone (PTH)	Secreted by the parathyroid glands; increases blood calcium.
progesterone	Secreted by the ovaries; prepares the uterus for pregnancy.
prolactin (PRL)	Secreted by the anterior lobe of the pituitary gland (adenohypophysis); promotes milk secretion.
somatotropin (STH)	Secreted by the anterior lobe of the pituitary gland (adenohypophysis); **growth hormone.**
testosterone	Male hormone secreted by the testes.
thyroid-stimulating hormone (TSH); thyrotropin	Secreted by the anterior lobe of the pituitary gland (adenohypophysis). TSH acts on the thyroid gland to promote its functioning. Note: TSH is not secreted by the thyroid gland.

thyroxine (T4)	Secreted by the thyroid gland; also called **tetraiodothyronine.** T4 increases metabolism in cells.
triiodothyronine (T3)	Secreted by the thyroid gland; T3 increases metabolism in cells. Note: The extra n in -thyronine (pronounced THĪ-rō-nēn) avoids the combination of two vowels (o and i).
vasopressin	Secreted by the posterior lobe of the pituitary gland (neurohypophysis); **antidiuretic hormone (ADH).** Vasopressin increases water reabsorption and raises blood pressure.
RELATED TERMS	
catecholamines	Hormones derived from an amino acid and secreted by the adrenal medulla. Epinephrine is a catecholamine.
corticosteroids	Hormones (steroids) produced by the adrenal cortex. Examples are cortisol (raises sugar levels), aldosterone (raises salt reabsorption by kidneys), and androgens and estrogens (sex hormones).
electrolyte	Mineral salt found in the blood and tissues and necessary for proper functioning of cells; potassium, sodium, and calcium are electrolytes.
glucocorticoid	Steroid hormone secreted by the adrenal cortex; regulates glucose, fat, and protein metabolism. Cortisol raises blood sugar and is part of the stress response.
homeostasis	Tendency of an organism to maintain a constant internal environment.
hormone	Substance, secreted by an endocrine gland, that travels through the blood to a distant organ or gland where it influences the structure or function of that organ or gland.
hypothalamus	Region of the brain lying below the thalamus and above the pituitary gland. It secretes releasing factors and hormones that affect the pituitary gland.
mineralocorticoid	Steroid hormone secreted by the adrenal cortex to regulate mineral salts (electrolytes) and water balance in the body. Aldosterone is an example.
receptor	Cellular or nuclear protein that binds to a hormone so that a response can be elicited.
sella turcica	Cavity in the skull that contains the pituitary gland.
sex hormones	Steroids (androgens and estrogens) produced by the adrenal cortex to influence male and female sexual characteristics.
steroid	Complex substance related to fats (derived from a sterol, such as cholesterol), and of which many hormones are made. Examples of steroids are estrogens, androgens, glucocorticoids, and mineralocorticoids. **Ster/o** means solid; **-ol** means oil.
sympathomimetic	Pertaining to mimicking or copying the effect of the sympathetic nervous system. Adrenaline (epinephrine) is a sympathomimetic hormone (it raises blood pressure and heart rate and dilates airways).
target tissue	Cells of an organ that are affected or stimulated by specific hormones.

TERMINOLOGY

Write the meanings of the medical terms in the spaces provided.

COMBINING FORMS: GLANDS

COMBINING FORM	MEANING	TERMINOLOGY	MEANING
aden/o	gland	adenectomy	
adrenal/o	adrenal gland	adrenalectomy	
gonad/o	sex glands (ovaries and testes)	gonadotropin *Here, -tropin means to act on. Gonadotropins act on (stimulate) gonads. Examples of gonadotropins are FSH and LH, secreted by the pituitary gland.*	
		hypogonadism *Deficiency of gonadotropins can produce hypogonadism.*	
pancreat/o	pancreas	pancreatectomy	
parathyroid/o	parathyroid gland	parathyroidectomy	
pituitar/o	pituitary gland; hypophysis	hypopituitarism *Pituitary dwarfism (see page 774) is caused by hypopituitarism.*	
thyr/o, thyroid/o	thyroid gland	thyrotropic hormone *Thyroid-stimulating hormone (TSH) is a thyrotropic hormone secreted by the pituitary gland.*	
		thyroiditis *May result from bacterial or viral infection, or an autoimmune reaction. Symptoms are throat pain, swelling, tenderness, and signs of hyperthyroidism. The condition may progress to destruction of the thyroid gland and hypothyroidism. In* ***Hashimoto disease,*** *or* ***autoimmune thyroiditis,*** *antibodies trigger lymphocytes to destroy follicular cells in the thyroid gland, producing hypothyroidism.*	

COMBINING FORMS: RELATED TERMS

COMBINING FORM	MEANING	TERMINOLOGY	MEANING
andr/o	male	androgen *Androgens are produced by the testes in males and by the adrenal cortex in males and females.*	
calc/o, calci/o	calcium	hypercalcemia	
		hypocalcemia	
		hypercalciuria	

COMBINING FORM	MEANING	TERMINOLOGY	MEANING
cortic/o	cortex, outer region	corticosteroid	
crin/o	secrete	endocrinologist	
dips/o	thirst	polydipsia *Poly- means many or increased. Uncontrolled diabetes (mellitus or insipidus) causes increased thirst. See page 771.*	
estr/o	female	estrogenic	
gluc/o	sugar	glucagon *In this term, -agon means to assemble or gather together. Glucagon raises blood sugar by stimulating its release from glycogen into the bloodstream.*	
glyc/o	sugar	hyperglycemia	
		glycemic *A patient with diabetes mellitus requires glycemic control.*	
		glycogen *Glycogen is animal starch that can be converted to glucose by the liver. Glucagon promotes glycogenolysis.*	
home/o	sameness	homeostasis *The suffix -stasis means to control.*	
hormon/o	hormone	hormonal	
kal/i	potassium	hypokalemia *This condition can occur in dehydration and with excessive vomiting and diarrhea. The heart is particularly sensitive to potassium loss.*	
lact/o	milk	prolactin *The suffix -in means a substance.*	
myx/o	mucus	myxedema *Mucus-like material accumulates under the skin. See page 767.*	
natr/o	sodium	hyponatremia *Occurs with hyposecretion of the adrenal cortex as salts and water leave the body.*	

Potassium and Sodium

In patient charts, potassium is abbreviated as **K** and sodium is abbreviated as **Na**. As electrolytes, they are written as **K^+** and **Na^+**.

COMBINING FORM	MEANING	TERMINOLOGY	MEANING
phys/o	growing	hypophysectomy ____________ *The hypophysis is the pituitary gland, which is so named because it grows from the undersurface (hypo-) of the brain (Figure 18-14).*	
somat/o	body	somatotropin ____________ *Growth hormone.*	
ster/o	solid structure	steroid ____________ *This complex, solid, ring-shaped molecule resembles a sterol (such as cholesterol); many hormones (androgens, estrogens, glucocorticoids, and mineralocorticoids) are steroids.*	
toc/o	childbirth	oxytocin ____________ *Oxy- means rapid.*	
toxic/o	poison	thyrotoxicosis ____________ *Condition caused by excessive thyroid gland activity and oversecretion of thyroid hormone. Signs and symptoms are sweating, weight loss, tachycardia, and nervousness.*	
ur/o	urine	antidiuretic hormone ____________ *Posterior pituitary hormone that affects the kidneys and reduces water loss.*	

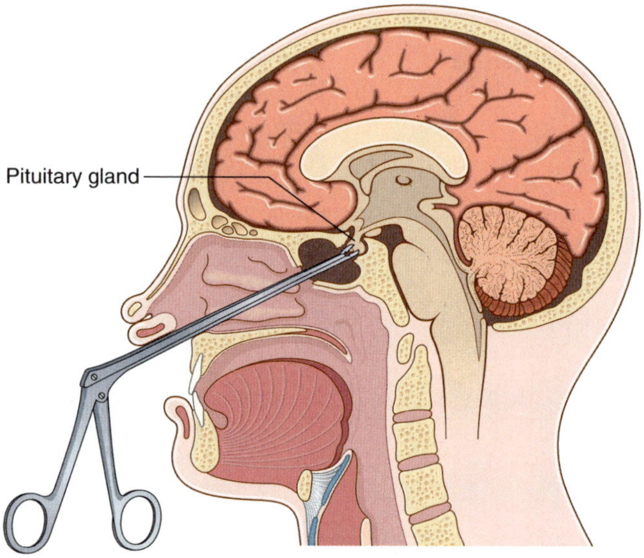

FIGURE 18-14 **Hypophysectomy.** Abnormal pituitary gland tissue is removed with instruments passed through the nasal passages and an opening created in the sphenoid bone (transsphenoidal hypophysectomy). The gland is removed to slow the growth of endocrine-dependent malignant tumors or to excise a pituitary tumor. Other treatments to destroy pituitary tissue include radiation therapy, radioactive implants, and cryosurgery.

SUFFIXES

SUFFIX	MEANING	TERMINOLOGY	MEANING
-agon	assemble, gather together	glucagon	
-emia	blood condition	hypoglycemia	
-in, -ine	substance	epinephrine	
-tropin	stimulating the function of (to turn or act on)	adrenocorticotropin *The ending -tropic is the adjective form (adrenocorticotropic hormone).*	
-uria	urine condition	glycosuria *Sign of diabetes mellitus.*	

PREFIXES

PREFIX	MEANING	TERMINOLOGY	MEANING
eu-	good, normal	euthyroid	
hyper-	excessive; above	hyperkalemia *Seen in acute renal failure, massive trauma, and major burns.*	
hypo-	deficient; below; under; less than normal	hypoinsulinism *Deficient secretion of insulin by the pancreas.*	
oxy-	rapid, sharp, acid	oxytocin	
pan-	all	panhypopituitarism	
poly-	many or increased	polyuria *This is a sign of uncontrolled diabetes (mellitus and insipidus).*	
tetra-	four	tetraiodothyronine *Iod/o means iodine.*	
tri-	three	triiodothyronine	

Oxy/o Meaning Acid

In 1774, the French scientist Antoine Lavoisier named a new gas **oxygen** because he incorrectly believed that the gas was an essential part of all acids.

PATHOLOGY

THYROID GLAND

Enlargement of the thyroid gland is **goiter** (Figure 18-15A). **Endemic** (**en-** = in; **dem/o** = people) **goiter** occurs in certain regions where there is a lack of **iodine** in the diet. Goiter develops when low iodine levels lead to low T3 and T4 levels. This causes feedback to the hypothalamus and adenohypophysis, stimulating them to secrete releasing factors and TSH. TSH then promotes the thyroid gland to secrete T3 and T4, but because there is no iodine available, the only effect is to increase the size of the gland (goiter). Prevention includes increasing the supply of iodine (as iodized salt) in the diet.

Another type of goiter is **nodular** or **adenomatous goiter,** in which hyperplasia occurs as well as formation of nodules and adenomas. Some patients with nodular goiter develop hyperthyroidism with clinical signs and symptoms such as rapid pulse, tremors, nervousness, and excessive sweating. Treatment is with thyroid-blocking drugs or radioactive iodine to suppress thyroid functioning.

Hypersecretion

hyperthyroidism

Overactivity of the thyroid gland; thyrotoxicosis.

The most common form of this condition is **Graves disease** (resulting from autoimmune processes). Because metabolism is faster, the condition is marked by an increase in heart rate (with irregular beats), higher body temperature, hyperactivity, weight loss, and increased peristalsis (diarrhea occurs). In addition, **exophthalmos** (protrusion of the eyeballs, or **proptosis**) occurs as a result of swelling of tissue behind the eyeball, pushing it forward. Treatment of Graves disease includes management with antithyroid drugs to reduce the amount of thyroid hormone produced by the gland and administration of radioactive iodine, which destroys the overactive glandular tissue. Figure 18-15B shows a patient with Graves disease.

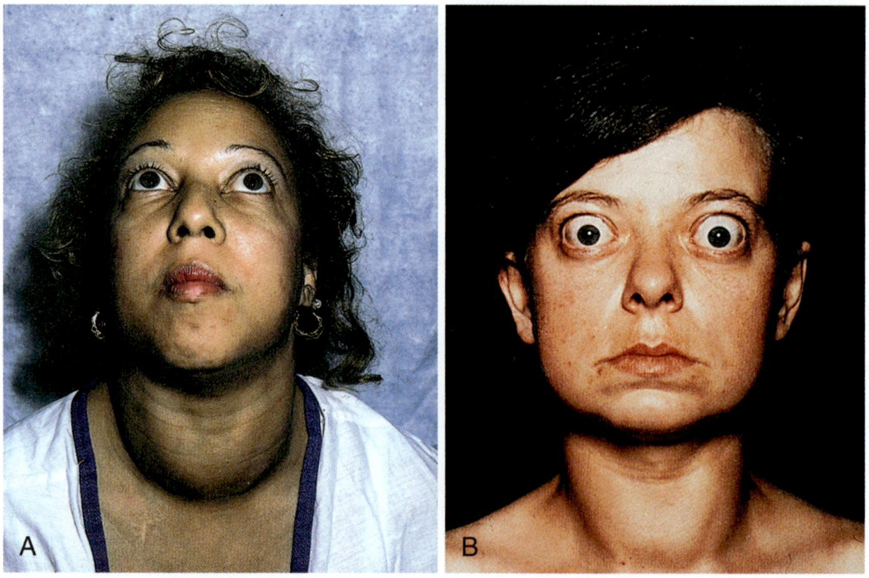

FIGURE 18-15 **A, Goiter.** Notice the wide neck, indicating enlargement of the thyroid gland. Goiter comes from the Latin guttur, meaning throat. **B, Exophthalmos** in **Graves disease.** Note the staring or startled expression resulting from periorbital edema (swelling of tissue around the eyeball or orbit of the eye). Exophthalmos usually persists despite treatment of Graves disease.

Hyposecretion

hypothyroidism

Underactivity of the thyroid gland.

Any of several conditions can produce hypothyroidism (thyroidectomy, thyroiditis, endemic goiter, destruction of the gland by irradiation), but all have similar physiologic effects. These include fatigue, muscular and mental sluggishness, weight gain, fluid retention, slow heart rate, low body temperature, and constipation. Two examples of hypothyroid disorders are myxedema and cretinism.

Myxedema is advanced hypothyroidism in adulthood. Atrophy of the thyroid gland occurs, and practically no hormone is produced. The skin becomes dry and puffy (edema) because of the collection of mucus-like (myx/o = mucus) material under the skin. Many patients also develop atherosclerosis because lack of thyroid hormone increases the quantity of blood lipids (fats). Recovery may be complete if thyroid hormone is given soon after symptoms appear. Figure 18-16A on page 768 shows a patient with myxedema.

In **cretinism,** extreme hypothyroidism during infancy and childhood leads to a lack of normal physical and mental growth. Skeletal growth is more inhibited than soft tissue growth, so the affected person has the appearance of an obese, short, and stocky child. Treatment consists of administration of thyroid hormone, which may be able to reverse some of the hypothyroid effects.

Neoplasms

thyroid carcinoma

Cancer of the thyroid gland.

More than half of thyroid malignancies are slow-growing papillary carcinomas and about one third are slow-growing follicular carcinomas. Others include rapidly growing anaplastic (widely metastatic) tumors. Radioactive iodine scans distinguish hyperfunctioning areas from hypofunctioning areas. "Hot" tumor areas (those collecting more radioactivity than surrounding tissues) usually indicate hyperthyroidism and benign growth; "cold," nonfunctional nodules can be either benign or malignant. Ultimately, fine needle aspiration, surgical biopsy, or excision is required to make the diagnosis. Total or subtotal thyroidectomy with lymph node removal is indicated for most thyroid carcinomas. Postsurgical treatment with radioactive iodine destroys remaining tissue, and high doses of exogenous thyroid hormone are given to suppress TSH, in an effort to cause regression of residual tumor dependent on TSH.

PARATHYROID GLANDS

Hypersecretion

hyperparathyroidism

Excessive production of parathormone.

Hypercalcemia occurs as calcium leaves the bones and enters the bloodstream, where it can produce damage to the kidneys and heart. Bones become decalcified with generalized loss of bone density (osteoporosis) and susceptibility to fractures and formation of cysts. Kidney stones can occur as a result of hypercalcemia and hypercalciuria. The cause is parathyroid hyperplasia or a parathyroid tumor. Treatment is resection of the overactive tissue. Medical therapy is another option for the patient who is not a surgical candidate. Bisphosphonates, such as alendronate (Fosamax), decrease bone turnover and decrease hypercalcemia.

Hyposecretion

hypoparathyroidism

Deficient production of parathyroid hormone.

Hypocalcemia results as calcium remains in bones and is unable to enter the bloodstream. This leads to muscle and nerve weakness with spasms of muscles, a condition called **tetany** (constant muscle contraction). Administration of calcium plus large quantities of vitamin D (to promote absorption of calcium) can control the calcium level in the bloodstream.

ADRENAL CORTEX

Hypersecretion

adrenal virilism

Excessive secretion of adrenal androgens.

Adrenal hyperplasia or more commonly adrenal adenomas or carcinomas can cause **virilization** in adult women. Signs and symptoms include amenorrhea, **hirsutism** (excessive hair on the face and body), acne, and deepening of the voice. Drug therapy to suppress androgen production and adrenalectomy are possible treatments.

Cushing syndrome

Group of signs and symptoms produced by excess cortisol from the adrenal cortex.

A number of signs and symptoms occur as a result of increased cortisol secretion, including obesity, moon-like fullness of the face, excess deposition of fat in the thoracic region of the back (so-called buffalo hump), hyperglycemia, hypernatremia, hypokalemia, osteoporosis, virilization, and hypertension. The cause may be excess ACTH secretion or tumor of the adrenal cortex. Tumors and disseminated cancers can be associated with ectopic secretion of hormone, such as ectopic ACTH produced by nonendocrine neoplasms (lung and thyroid tumors). Figure 18-16B shows a woman with Cushing syndrome. See the ***In Person*** story, page 781, of a woman's journey with Cushing syndrome.

18

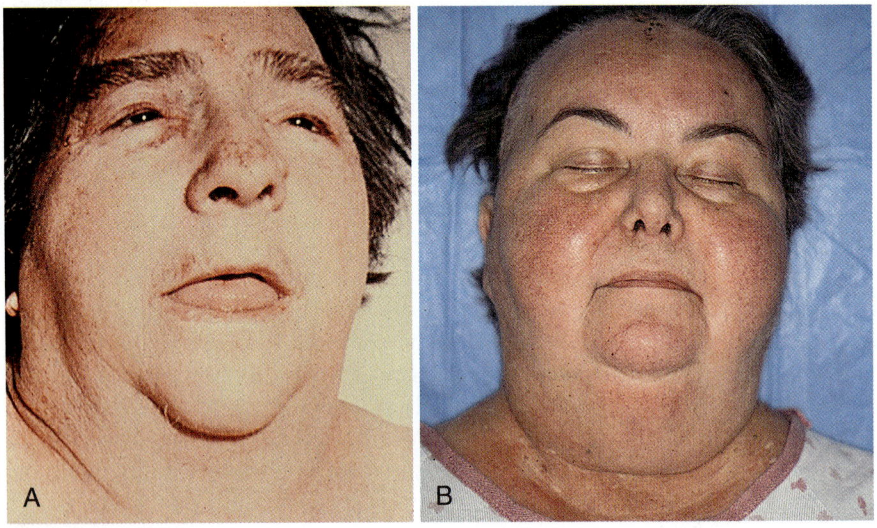

FIGURE 18-16 **A, Myxedema.** Note the dull, puffy, yellowed skin; coarse, sparse hair; prominent tongue. **B, Cushing syndrome.** Elevated plasma levels of cortisol (steroids) produce obesity, rounded facial appearance (moon-face), thin skin that bruises easily, and muscle weakness. *(**A,** Courtesy Paul W. Ladenson, MD, Johns Hopkins University and Hospital, Baltimore)*

Cushing Disease

Cushing disease is one cause of Cushing syndrome. In Cushing disease, a benign tumor of the pituitary gland (pituitary adenoma) increases ACTH secretion, stimulating the adrenal cortex to produce excess cortisol. The cure for Cushing disease is removal of the pituitary adenoma. Dr. Harvey Cushing described the condition in 1932.

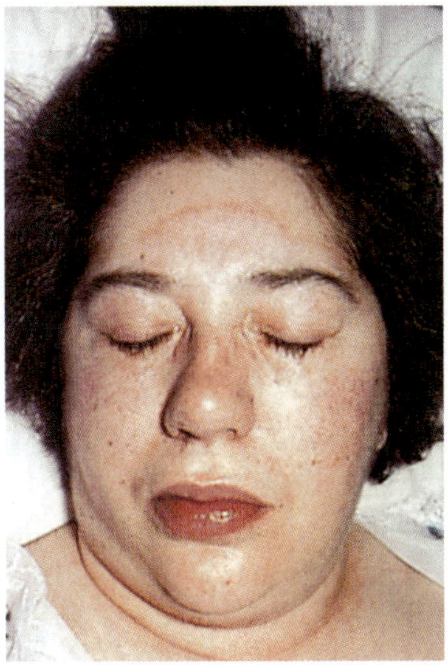

FIGURE 18-17 **Addison disease.** Notice the darker skin discoloration, especially evident on the face.

In clinical practice, most cases of Cushing syndrome result from chronic use of cortisone-like drugs, such as steroids. Examples are the cases in young athletes seeking to improve their performance and in patients treated for autoimmune disorders, asthma, kidney, and skin conditions. Steroids (prednisone is an example) are never discontinued abruptly because the adrenal cortex and pituitary gland (ACTH producer) need time to "restart" after long periods of prescribed cortisol use (the adrenal gland stops producing cortisol when cortisol is given as therapy).

Hyposecretion

Addison disease

Hypofunctioning of the adrenal cortex.

The adrenal cortex is essential to life. When aldosterone and cortisol blood levels are low, the patient experiences generalized malaise, weakness, muscle atrophy, and severe loss of fluids and electrolytes (with hypoglycemia, low blood pressure, and hyponatremia). An insufficient supply of cortisol signals the pituitary to secrete more ACTH, which increases pigmentation of scars, skin folds, and breast nipples (hyperpigmentation) (Figure 18-17).

Primary insufficiency is believed to be due to autoimmune adrenalitis. Treatment consists of daily cortisone administration and intake of salts or administration of a synthetic form of aldosterone.

ADRENAL MEDULLA

Hypersecretion

pheochromocytoma

Benign tumor of the adrenal medulla; tumor cells stain a dark or dusky (phe/o) color (chrom/o).

The tumor cells produce excess secretion of epinephrine and norepinephrine. Signs and symptoms are hypertension, tachycardia, palpitations, severe headaches, sweating, flushing of the face, and muscle spasms. Surgery to remove the tumor and administration of antihypertensive drugs are possible treatments.

PANCREAS

Hypersecretion

hyperinsulinism

Excess secretion of insulin causing hypoglycemia.

The cause may be a tumor of the pancreas (benign adenoma or carcinoma) or an overdose of insulin. Hypoglycemia occurs as insulin draws sugar out of the bloodstream. Fainting spells, convulsions, and loss of consciousness are common because a minimal level of blood sugar is necessary for proper mental functioning.

Hyposecretion

diabetes mellitus (DM)

Lack of insulin secretion or resistance of insulin in promoting sugar, starch, and fat metabolism in cells.

In diabetes mellitus (mellitus means sweet or sugary), insulin insufficiency or ineffectiveness prevents sugar from leaving the blood and entering the body cells, where it is used to produce energy. There are two types of diabetes mellitus.

Type 1 diabetes is an **autoimmune disease.** Autoantibodies against normal pancreatic islet cells are present. Onset is usually in early childhood but can occur in adulthood, and the etiology involves destruction of the beta islet cells, producing complete deficiency of insulin in the body. Patients usually are thin and require frequent injections of insulin to maintain a normal level of glucose in the blood. Type 1 requires patients to monitor their blood glucose levels several times a day using a glucometer. To test sugar levels with this device, the user pricks a finger to draw blood. At a minimum, patients test before each meal and at bedtime, but many test up to 12 times a day. Patients must continually (every day) balance insulin levels with food and exercise (see the ***In Person*** account on pages 779-780). In addition to injecting insulin into the body (buttocks, thighs, abdomen and arms), it is also possible to administer insulin through a portable pump, which infuses the drug continuously through a indwelling needle under the skin (Figure 18-18).

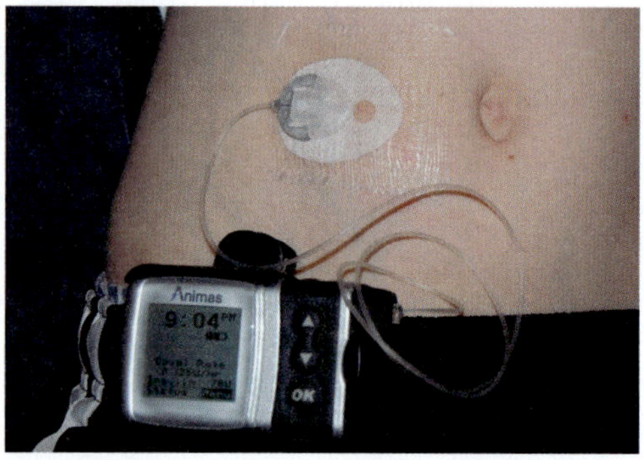

FIGURE 18-18 Insulin pump. This device can be programmed to deliver doses of insulin according to varying body needs. **Basal insulin** is delivered continuously over 24 hours and mimics the normal secretion by the pancreas. **Bolus insulin** is delivered or injected at mealtimes to "cover" a specific amount of sugar or starch ingested. *(Courtesy Ruthellen Sheldon.)*

Insulin

There are many different types of insulin. Insulin can be **rapid-acting** (peak at 30 to 60 minutes and last 3 to 5 hours), **short-acting** (peak at 1½ to 2 hours and last 6 to 8 hours), **intermediate-acting** (peak at 4 to 12 hours and last 14 to 24 hours), or **long-acting** (peak at 1 to 2 hours and last up to 24 hours). The rapid and short-acting insulins are taken before a meal to reduce the blood sugar spike that normally occurs after eating. Intermediate- and long-acting insulins mimic the natural production of insulin by the pancreas.

Type 2 diabetes is a separate disease from type 1. Patients often are older, and usually there is a family history of type 2 diabetes. Obesity is very common. The islet cells are not initially destroyed, and there is a relative deficiency of insulin secretion with a resistance by target tissues to insulin. **Insulin resistance** usually develops 5 to 10 years before type 2 diabetes is diagnosed, and is associated with an increased risk of cardiovascular disease. Often, high blood pressure, high cholesterol, and central abdominal obesity are seen in people who have insulin resistance. Treatment of type 2 diabetes is with diet, weight reduction, exercise, and, if necessary, insulin or oral hypoglycemic agents. Oral hypoglycemic agents stimulate the release of insulin from the pancreas and improve the body's sensitivity to insulin.

Table 18-3 compares the clinical features, symptoms, and treatment of type 1 and type 2 diabetes.

Both type 1 and type 2 diabetes are associated with primary and secondary complications. The **primary complication** of type 1 is **hyperglycemia.** Hyperglycemia can lead to **ketoacidosis** (fats are improperly burned, leading to an accumulation of ketones and acids in the body). Ketoacidosis can also result from illness or infection, and initial symptoms may be upset stomach and vomiting. **Hypoglycemia** occurs when too much insulin is taken by the patient. **Insulin shock** is severe hypoglycemia caused by an overdose of insulin, decreased intake of food, or excessive exercise. Signs and symptoms are sweating, hunger, confusion, trembling, nervousness, and numbness. Treatment of severe hypoglycemia is with either a shot of glucagon or intravenous glucose to restore normal blood glucose levels. Convulsions, coma, and loss of consciousness can result if treatment is not given.

TABLE 18-3 COMPARISON OF TYPE 1 AND TYPE 2 DIABETES MELLITUS

Category	Type 1*	Type 2†
Clinical features	Usually occurs before age 30 Abrupt, rapid onset of symptoms Little or no insulin production Thin or normal body weight at onset Ketoacidosis often occurs	Usually occurs after age 30 Gradual onset; asymptomatic Insulin usually present 85% are obese Ketoacidosis seldom occurs
Symptoms	Polyuria (glycosuria promotes loss of water) Polydipsia (dehydration causes thirst) Polyphagia (tissue breakdown causes hunger)	Polyuria sometimes seen Polydipsia sometimes seen Polyphagia sometimes seen
Treatment	Insulin	Diet (weight loss); oral hypoglycemics or insulin

*Type 1 formerly was called juvenile (juvenile-onset) diabetes.
†Type 2 formerly was called adult-onset diabetes.

18

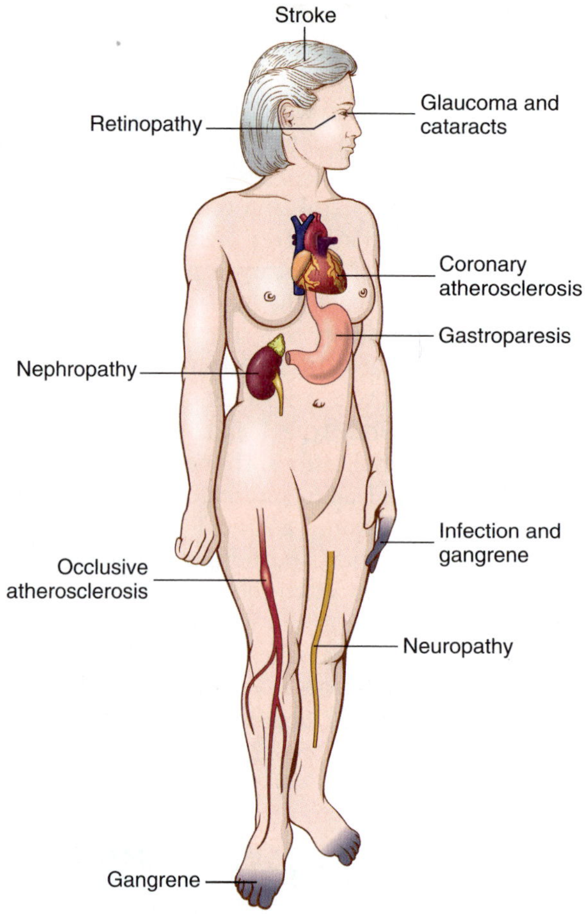

FIGURE 18-19 **Secondary complications of diabetes mellitus.** Many of these complications can be avoided or minimized with optimal glycemic control.

Secondary (long-term) **complications** may appear many years after the patient develops diabetes. These include destruction of retinal blood vessels **(diabetic retinopathy),** causing visual loss and blindness; destruction of the kidneys **(diabetic nephropathy),** causing renal insufficiency and often requiring hemodialysis or renal transplantation; destruction of blood vessels, with **atherosclerosis** leading to stroke, heart disease, and peripherovascular ischemia (gangrene, infection, and loss of limbs); and destruction of nerves **(diabetic neuropathy)** involving pain or loss of sensation, most commonly in the extremities. Loss of gastric motility **(gastroparesis)** also occurs. Figure 18-19 reviews the secondary complications of diabetes mellitus.

As a result of hormonal changes during pregnancy, **gestational diabetes** can occur in women with a predisposition to diabetes during the second or third trimester of pregnancy. After delivery, blood glucose usually returns to normal. Type 2 diabetes may develop in these women later in life.

PITUITARY GLAND: ANTERIOR LOBE

Hypersecretion

acromegaly

Hypersecretion of growth hormone from the anterior pituitary after puberty, leading to enlargement of extremities.

An excess of growth hormone (GH) is produced by adenomas of the pituitary gland that occur during adulthood. This excess GH stimulates the liver to secrete a hormone (somatomedin C, or insulin-like growth factor [IGF]) that causes the clinical manifestations of acromegaly (acr/o in this term means extremities). Bones in the hands, feet, face, and jaw grow abnormally large, producing a characteristic "Frankenstein"-type facial appearance. The pituitary adenoma can be irradiated or surgically removed. Figure 18-20 shows the features of a woman with acromegaly. Measurement of blood levels of somatomedin C as GH fluctuates is a test for acromegaly.

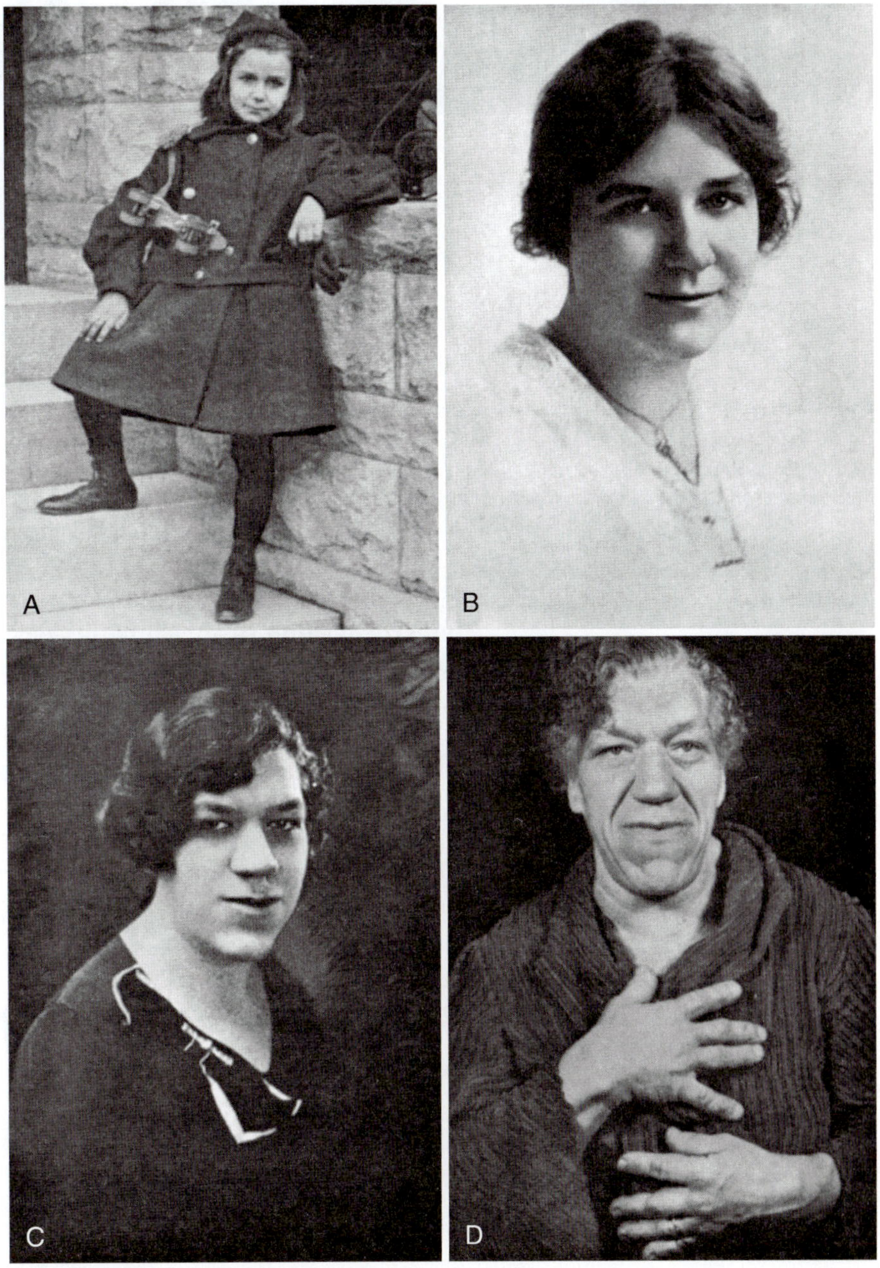

FIGURE 18-20 Progression of acromegaly. A, The patient at age 9 years; **B,** at age 16, with possible early features of acromegaly; **C,** at age 33, with well-established acromegaly; **D,** at age 52, with end-stage acromegaly.

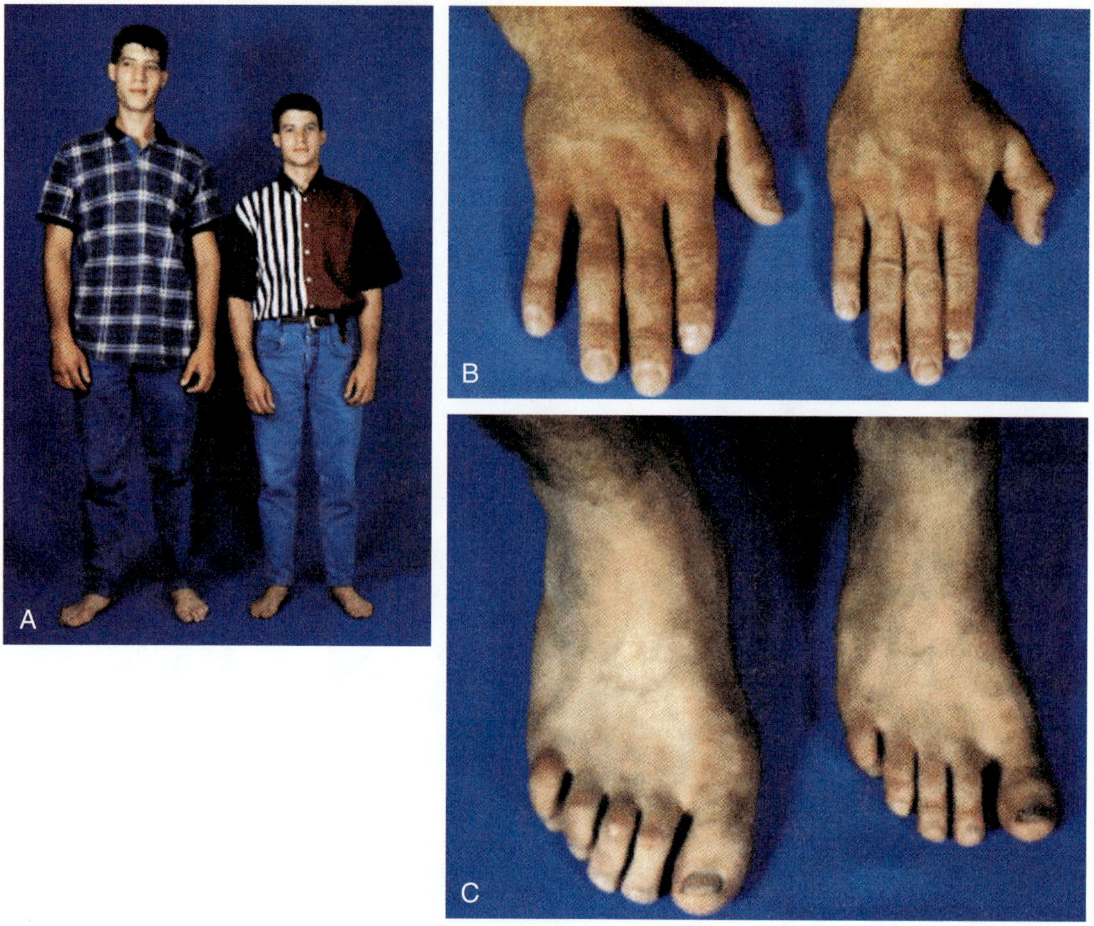

FIGURE 18-21 **Gigantism.** A 22-year-old man with gigantism due to excess growth hormone is shown to the left of his identical twin. The increased height **(A)** and enlarged hand **(B)** and foot **(C)** of the affected twin are apparent. Their height and features began to diverge at the age of approximately 13 years. *(Courtesy Robert F. Gagel, M.D. and Ian E. McCutcheon, M.D., University of Texas, M.D. Anderson Cancer Center, Houston, Texas.)*

gigantism

Hypersecretion of growth hormone from the anterior pituitary before puberty, leading to abnormal overgrowth of body tissues.

Benign adenomas of the pituitary gland that occur before a child reaches puberty produce an excess of growth hormone. See Figure 18-21. Gigantism can be corrected by early diagnosis in childhood, followed by resection of the tumor or irradiation of the pituitary.

Hyposecretion

dwarfism

Congenital hyposecretion of growth hormone; hypopituitary dwarfism.

Children who are affected are normal mentally, but their bones remain small. Treatment consists of administration of growth hormone. Achondroplastic dwarfs differ from hypopituitary dwarfs in that they have a genetic defect in cartilage formation that limits the growth of long bones.

panhypopituitarism

Deficiency of all pituitary hormones.

Tumors of the sella turcica as well as arterial aneurysms may be etiologic factors, causing a failure of the pituitary to secrete hormones that stimulate major glands in the body.

PITUITARY GLAND: POSTERIOR LOBE

Hypersecretion

syndrome of inappropriate ADH (SIADH)

Excessive secretion of antidiuretic hormone.

Hypersecretion of ADH produces excess water retention in the body. Treatment consists of dietary water restriction. Tumor, drug reactions, and head injury are some of the possible causes.

Hyposecretion

diabetes insipidus (DI)

Insufficient secretion of antidiuretic hormone (vasopressin).

Deficiency of antidiuretic hormone causes the kidney tubules to fail to hold back (reabsorb) needed water and salts. Clinical manifestations include polyuria and polydipsia. Synthetic preparations of ADH are administered with nasal sprays or intramuscularly as treatment. **Insipidus** means tasteless, reflecting the condition of dilute urine, as opposed to **mellitus,** meaning sweet or like honey, reflecting the sugar content of urine in diabetes mellitus. The term diabetes comes from the Greek diabainein, meaning to pass through. Both diabetes insipidus and diabetes mellitus are characterized by polyuria.

Table 18-4 reviews the abnormal conditions associated with hypersecretions and hyposecretions of the endocrine glands.

TABLE 18-4 ABNORMAL CONDITIONS OF ENDOCRINE GLANDS

Endocrine Gland	Hypersecretion	Hyposecretion
Adrenal cortex	• Adrenal virilism • Cushing syndrome	• Addison disease
Adrenal medulla	• Pheochromocytoma	
Pancreas	• Hyperinsulinism	• Diabetes mellitus
Parathyroid glands	• Hyperparathyroidism (hypercalcemia, osteoporosis, kidney stones)	• Hypoparathyroidism (tetany, hypocalcemia)
Pituitary—anterior lobe	• Acromegaly • Gigantism	• Dwarfism • Panhypopituitarism
Pituitary—posterior lobe	• Syndrome of inappropriate antidiuretic hormone	• Diabetes insipidus
Thyroid gland	• Exophthalmic goiter (Graves disease, thyrotoxicosis) • Nodular (adenomatous) goiter	• Cretinism (children) • Endemic goiter • Myxedema (adults)

LABORATORY TESTS

fasting plasma glucose (FPG)

Also known as fasting blood sugar test. Measures circulating glucose level in a patient who has fasted at least 8 hours.

This test can diagnose **diabetes** and **pre-diabetes** (blood glucose is higher than normal but not high enough for diagnosis of diabetes). A normal result is 99 mg/dL or lower. Pre-diabetes levels are 100 to 125 mg/dL and diabetes is 126 mg/dL and above. A casual non-fasting plasma glucose level of 200 mg/dL plus the presence of signs and symptoms such as increased urination, increased thirst, and unexplained weight loss can also diagnose diabetes. An oral **glucose tolerance test** is used to diagnose pre-diabetes and gestational diabetes.

The **glycosylated hemoglobin (HbA_{1c}) test** (**A1c** for short), by measuring the percentage of red blood cells with glucose attached, monitors long-term glucose control. A high level indicates poor glucose control in diabetic patients.

serum and urine tests

Measurement of hormones, electrolytes, glucose, and other substances in serum (blood) and urine as indicators of endocrine function.

Serum studies include growth hormone, somatomedin C (insulin-like growth factor), prolactin level, gonadotropin levels, parathyroid hormone, calcium, and cortisol. A high reading on blood glucose testing by **glucometer** in a doctor's office may be the first indication of a diabetes diagnosis (levels may be as high as 750 mg/dL, whereas normal is about 100 mg/dL).

Urine studies include dipstick testing for glucose (Clinistix, Labstix) and ketones (Acetest, Ketostix), and measurement of 17-ketosteroids (to check adrenal and gonadal function). A **urinary microalbumin assay** may detect small quantities of albumin in urine as a marker or harbinger of diabetic nephropathy.

18

thyroid function tests

Measurement of T3, T4, and TSH in the bloodstream.

CLINICAL PROCEDURES

exophthalmometry

Measurement of eyeball protrusion (as in Graves disease) with an exophthalmometer.

computed tomography (CT) scan

X-ray imaging of endocrine glands in cross section and other views, to assess size and infiltration by tumor.

magnetic resonance imaging (MRI)

Magnetic waves produce images of the hypothalamus and pituitary gland to locate abnormalities.

thyroid scan

Scanner detects radioactivity and visualizes the thyroid gland.

Administration of radioactivity is either intravenous (with radioactive technetium) or oral (with radioactive iodine). The latter is called **RAIU (radioactive iodine uptake scan).** Thyroid function is assessed; nodules and tumors can be evaluated.

ultrasound examination

Sound waves show images of endocrine organs.

Thyroid ultrasound is the best method to evaluate thyroid structures and abnormalities (nodules).

ABBREVIATIONS

A1C	blood test that measures glycosylated hemoglobin (HbA_{1c}) to assess glucose control
ACTH	adrenocorticotropic hormone
ADH	antidiuretic hormone—vasopressin
Ca^{++}	calcium, an important electrolyte
CGMS	continuous glucose monitoring system—senses and records blood glucose levels continuously
DI	diabetes insipidus
DKA	diabetic ketoacidosis
DM	diabetes mellitus
FBG	fasting blood glucose
FBS	fasting blood sugar
FSH	follicle-stimulating hormone
GH	growth hormone
GTT	glucose tolerance test—measures ability to respond to a glucose load; a test for diabetes
HbA_{1c} (test) *or* **HBA1C**	test for the presence of glucose attached to hemoglobin (glycosylated hemoglobin test); a high level indicates poor glucose control in diabetic patients
hCG *or* **HCG**	human chorionic gonadotropin
K^+	potassium—an important electrolyte
LH	luteinizing hormone
MDI	multiple daily injection—for delivery of either basal or bolus insulin as basal/bolus. It is a diabetes management regimen.
Na^+	sodium—an important electrolyte
OT, OXT	oxytocin
PRL	prolactin
PTH	parathyroid hormone (parathormone)
RAI	radioactive iodine—treatment for Graves disease
RIA	radioimmunoassay—measures hormone levels in plasma
RAIU	radioactive iodine uptake (imaging test or scan)
SIADH	syndrome of inappropriate antidiuretic hormone (secretion)
SMBG	self-monitoring of blood glucose
STH	somatotropin—growth hormone
T3	triiodothyronine
T4	thyroxine—tetraiodothyronine
TFT	thyroid function test
TSH	thyroid-stimulating hormone—secreted by the anterior pituitary gland

PRACTICAL APPLICATIONS

The following table lists endocrine medicines and how they are used. Answers are found on page 789.

ENDOCRINE MEDICINES (brand names are in parentheses)	
Antidiabetic Medicines	
• **insulin**	Injected synthetic hormone, lowers blood sugar, comes in short-acting and long-acting forms; used in type 1 and type 2 diabetes
• **metformin** (Glucophage)	Oral hypoglycemic medication that reduces glucose production by the liver and increases the body's sensitivity to insulin; used in type 2 diabetes
• **sulfonylureas** **glipizide** (Glucotrol) **glyburide** (Diabeta or Micronase)	Oral hypoglycemic medications that stimulate pancreatic beta cells to produce insulin; used in type 2 diabetes
Thyroid Medicines	
• **levothyroxine** (Synthroid, Levoxyl)	Oral synthetic thyroid hormone (T4); used in hypothyroidism
• **liothyronine** (Cytomel)	Oral synthetic thyroid hormone (T3); used in hypothyroidism
• **thyroid ISP** (Armour thyroid)	Desiccated thyroid extract (combination of T3 and T4); used in hypothyroidism
• **methimazole** (Tapazole)	Inhibits thyroid hormone production; used in Graves hyperthyroidism
• **prophylthiouracil** (PTU)	Inhibits thyroid hormone production; used in Graves hyperthyroidism
• **beta blockers** (atenolol, propranolol)	Reduces the symptoms of hyperthyroidism (palpitations, tachycardia, tremors)
Corticosteroids	
• **prednisone** • **hydrocortisone**	Used in the treatment of hypoadrenalism
Bisphosphonates	
• **alendronate** (Fosamax) • **ibandronate** (Boniva)	Used to build bone strength in osteoporosis and to treat hyperparathyroidism
Diabetes Insipidus Medicine	
• **desmopressin** (DDAVP, Stimate)	Intranasal or oral synthetic form of vasopressin (antidiuretic hormone); used to treat diabetes insipidus

18

Questions:

1. Which endocrine medicine treats hypothyroidism?
   a. prednisone
   b. prophylthiouracil
   c. liothyronine
2. Which endocrine medicine treats type 2 diabetes?
   a. desmopressin
   b. metformin
   c. hydrocortisone
3. Which endocrine medicine treats osteoporosis?
   a. alendronate
   b. beta blockers
   c. insulin

IN PERSON

This first-person account was written by the mother of a 12-year-old boy who was diagnosed with diabetes at age 8.

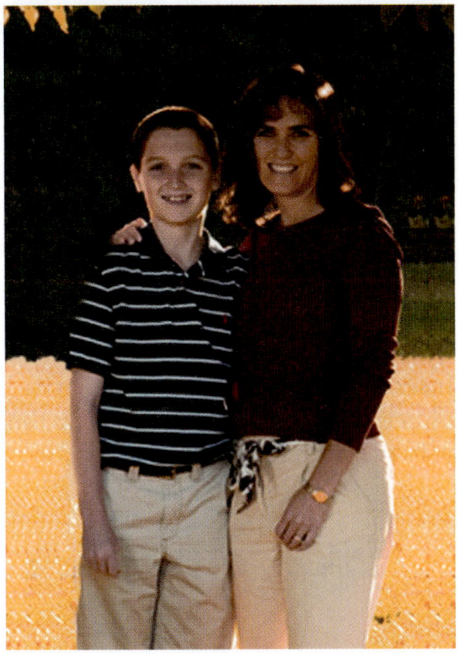

On school days, I wake up Jake at 6:30 AM. He tests his blood sugar by pricking his finger until it bleeds and sticking a test strip into the drop of blood. Then he inserts the strip into a small handheld glucometer and waits 3 to 5 seconds for a reading of his blood sugar. If this is 120 mg/dL or higher, he gives himself insulin 10 to 15 minutes before breakfast. I calculate how many carbohydrates (by reading labels and measuring food quantities precisely) he will have in his breakfast so that he can bolus [give himself enough insulin to cover the food he will eat] correctly. He has an insulin pump, so he types in the amount of carbohydrates he will eat plus his current blood sugar reading. The pump calculates how much insulin he needs to cover the carbs and any extra insulin he may need to bring down a high blood sugar. After he boluses he waits 15 minutes to eat breakfast. If his blood sugar is less than 120 mg/dL he will not bolus until he starts eating, because if the insulin acts too rapidly his blood sugar can drop too low.

As I cook his breakfast, I count carbs exactly—3 eggs (he needs protein to keep his blood sugar stable throughout the morning), 15 carbs of fruit (15 grapes, ½ banana, ½ small apple, or 1½ clementines), one 8-oz cup of low-carb juice, and 3 waffles. If his blood sugar is low, he will eat.

I then count carbs for his lunch and place an index card in his lunch bag to show the nurse before his lunchtime bolus. At school, he visits the nurse if he feels high or low, and at lunch as well… I worry about his exposure to all the sick kids at school when he visits the nurse. At school, if his blood sugar is high, he drinks water and tests his urine for ketones to make sure he does not have ketonuria, which may indicate ketoacidosis. If it is positive for ketones, he is sent home from school (fortunately, this has never happened).

At lunch, he leaves class early to test his blood sugar and does the same calculations as at breakfast. He waits for the nurse to manually compute the amount of insulin he needs to make sure that it matches the calculation of the pump. Then he boluses and goes to lunch. If his blood sugar is less than 70, he can't go to lunch with his friends. He eats or drinks some fast-acting sugar (Skittles, Smarties, or Sprite) and waits for his blood sugar to rise to an acceptable range.

We plan ahead for all field trips and food snacks that are brought into the classroom. If Jake is playing sports, he times his meals with the start of the activity so his blood sugar is around 150. He disconnects his pump during sports. Jake is an avid soccer player. At halftime he tests his blood sugar. If it is low, he needs to eat. If it is high, he needs to reconnect his pump and get more insulin. After sports, his blood sugar usually spikes because of an adrenaline [epinephrine] rush and then crashes down 3 to 10 hours later. This is unpredictable and never consistent, so it takes guesswork to keep him in range after a sports game or practice.

During the night, his dad and I set alarms to wake up every few hours to test him. If his blood sugar is high while he sleeps, we use his pump to give him a correction. If it is low, we wake him and have him drink Sprite or eat Smarties. Sometimes we check him four or five times during the night. Even if his numbers are stable, it's not a guarantee that he won't drop suddenly and have a seizure (this happened once after we had tested him at 11 PM and 2 AM and he was steady). He never complains about all the interruptions to his sleep and does a great job of falling right back to sleep when awakened.

Every 2 days he changes his insertion site for the insulin pump. He can't do this alone. The pump is connected to his body with a small cannula [tube]. It is inserted manually via a needle into his hip region. The needle is then removed and the tiny Teflon cannula remains in his body, delivering fast-acting insulin under the skin. Plastic tubing clips into the cannula and then attaches to the side of his pump. He clips his pump to his waist or places it in his pocket. When he bathes, he disconnects from his pump, and when he sleeps, he places it on the mattress next to his body.

His body naturally rejects the Teflon cannula, so after 2 days his pump site must be changed. We realize this because his blood sugar numbers start rising for no apparent reason. Typically, we will change out the pump site and notice that it is red and sometimes the cannula tip is bent. Although changing the pump site is time-consuming and expensive, a bad site means that not enough insulin is getting into his body, which can quickly spiral into stomach pains, ketonuria, and ketoacidosis (DKA).

Jake has just started to wear a continuous glucose monitoring system (CGMS). This has a small sensor that is inserted into his arm to measure blood sugar in his interstitial fluid every minute. It is new technology that will actually beep at night if his blood sugar is dropping. Jake doesn't like the system because it is painful to insert and is cumbersome to carry. Plus, it doesn't replace fingersticks for blood sugar readings. It is also difficult to calibrate his CGMS, so the readings are not 100% reliable. This is still very new technology; we are very hopeful that future generations will be more reliable!

In general, Jake's diabetes doesn't disrupt his life other than the nighttime checks, wearing an insulin pump, and paying attention to how many carbs he eats. We encourage him to make good nutritional choices (not always easy for a kid) and to limit certain foods (doughnuts, Slurpees, candy) for special occasions. He must also carry a glucometer with him at all times and a sugar to take when his blood glucose is low.

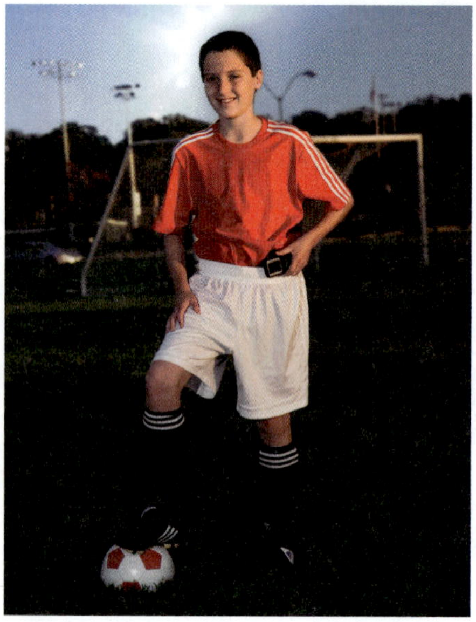

Having a child with diabetes forces me to carefully plan the preparation and timing of meals. I always have certain foods and medical supplies in the house and I carry snacks and sugar sources wherever I go. I am always available to Jake and to the school nurse. I don't always have a good night's sleep. I think I would sleep better if I were not so driven to keep his blood sugar in a healthy range. Right now, my body has adjusted to this new sleep pattern and I'm happy to wake up for him. I try to be at all his sports events to help him manage his blood sugars properly before, during, and after games. He can't go to a friend's house for a sleepover and he cannot attend overnight camp. His dad or I must always be in town. Keeping Jake's blood sugar in tight control hopefully means that he will avoid many of the complications frequently encountered later in life by people with type 1 diabetes.

Ruthellen Sheldon and her son, Jake, live in Maryland.

IN PERSON

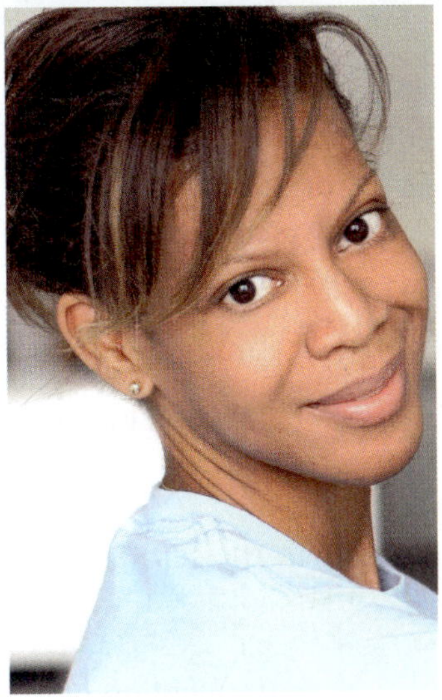

This first-person story is about a young woman's experience with Cushing syndrome.

I've always been a bit of a skinny-mini and had no major health issues. But in 1997 I started having irregular periods. Not only were they irregular, I gained 6 to 9 pounds every month. I knew something was wrong.

This began my year-long journey with Cushing syndrome. Initially, I saw two general practitioners, had blood work done, and was told I was fine. As I gained more weight, Cushing's symptoms became more apparent. I developed striae—purplish marks on my thighs,* a big round moon face, and a hump back.† I also became extremely fatigued when performing simple tasks. At the time, however, I had no idea or clue of what was happening.

Next, I saw my gynecologist. Again more blood work and I was told I'm fine. This process continued on with three other doctors. I pressed on from feeling misunderstood, depressed, and utterly tired and found an endocrinologist. After 3 months of testing, he located the problem: a tumor on my right adrenal gland. A month later I had a right adrenalectomy. Thankfully, my left adrenal works great, and I don't have to take any hormone pills. I was also thrilled that the 72 pounds I gained over the year melted away in a few months.

I'll never forget this experience. Having an unknown medical condition is very stressful. But, in some ways, I was even more stressed and depressed because my doctors seemed to dismiss my symptoms. I didn't own a computer at the time and I remember calling up a friend and asking her to do some research for me. I really felt I had to educate myself. I still don't know what caused the adrenal gland tumor or how I could have prevented it. But, I am better and my Cushing's journey taught me to be a better advocate for myself.

Tanzie Johnson is a professional photographer living in New York City.

18

*The weight gain in Cushing's syndrome stretches the skin, which is thin and weakened, causing it to hemorrhage.
†Fat pads accumulate along the collarbone and on the back of the neck (buffalo hump).

EXERCISES

Remember to check your answers carefully with the Answers to Exercises, page 788.

A Match the endocrine gland with its location.

adrenal cortex	pancreas	testis
adrenal medulla	parathyroid	thyroid
ovary	pituitary (hypophysis)	

1. behind the stomach ________________
2. posterior side of the thyroid gland ________________
3. inner section of glands above each kidney________________
4. in the scrotal sac ________________
5. on either side of the trachea ________________
6. outer section of gland above each kidney ________________
7. lower abdomen of a female ________________
8. below the brain in the sella turcica ________________

18

B Name the endocrine organs (including the appropriate lobe or region) that produce the following hormones.

1. follicle-stimulating hormone ________________
2. vasopressin ________________
3. aldosterone ________________
4. insulin ________________
5. thyroxine ________________
6. cortisol ________________
7. gonadotropic hormones ________________
8. epinephrine ________________
9. oxytocin ________________
10. prolactin ________________
11. growth hormone ________________
12. glucagon ________________
13. adrenocorticotropic hormone ________________
14. estradiol ________________
15. progesterone ________________
16. testosterone ________________
17. thyroid-stimulating hormone ________________

C **Give the meanings of the following abbreviations for hormones.**

1. ADH ____________________
2. ACTH ____________________
3. LH ____________________
4. FSH ____________________
5. TSH ____________________
6. PTH ____________________
7. GH ____________________
8. PRL ____________________
9. T4 ____________________
10. T3____________________
11. OT ____________________
12. STH ____________________

D **Match the following hormones with their actions.**

ACTH	epinephrine	parathyroid hormone
ADH	estradiol	testosterone
aldosterone	insulin	thyroxine
cortisol		

1. sympathomimetic; raises heart rate and blood pressure ____________________
2. promotes growth and maintenance of male sex characteristics ____________________
3. stimulates water reabsorption by kidney tubules; decreases urine output ____________________
4. increases metabolism in body cells ____________________
5. raises blood calcium ____________________
6. increases reabsorption of sodium by kidney tubules ____________________
7. stimulates secretion of hormones from the adrenal cortex ____________________
8. increases blood sugar ____________________
9. helps transport glucose to cells; decreases blood sugar ____________________
10. develops and maintains female sex characteristics ____________________

E **Indicate whether the following conditions are related to hypersecretion or hyposecretion. Also, select from the following the endocrine glands and hormones involved in each disease.**

Glands

adenohypophysis
adrenal cortex
adrenal medulla
neurohypophysis
ovaries
pancreas
parathyroid gland
testes
thyroid

Hormones

ADH
aldosterone
cortisol
epinephrine
GH
insulin
parathyroid hormone
thyroxine

Condition	***Hypo or Hyper***	***Gland and Hormone***
1. Cushing syndrome	____________	______________________________
2. tetany	____________	______________________________
3. Graves disease	____________	______________________________
4. diabetes insipidus	____________	______________________________
5. acromegaly	____________	______________________________
6. myxedema	____________	______________________________
7. diabetes mellitus	____________	______________________________
8. Addison disease	____________	______________________________
9. gigantism	____________	______________________________
10. endemic goiter	____________	______________________________
11. cretinism	____________	______________________________
12. pheochromocytoma	____________	______________________________

18

F **Build medical terms based on the definitions and word parts given.**

1. abnormal condition (poison) of the thyroid gland: thyro________________________
2. removal of the pancreas: ________________________ectomy
3. condition of deficiency or underdevelopment of the sex organs: hypo________________________
4. pertaining to producing female (characteristics): ________________________genic
5. removal of the pituitary gland: ________________________ectomy
6. deficiency of calcium in the blood: hypo________________________
7. excessive sugar in the blood: ________________________emia
8. inflammation of the thyroid gland: ________________________itis
9. specialist in the study of hormone disorders: ________________________ist

G **Give the meanings of the following conditions.**

1. hyponatremia ______________________________
2. polydipsia ______________________________
3. hyperkalemia ______________________________
4. hypercalcemia ______________________________
5. hypoglycemia ______________________________
6. glycosuria ______________________________
7. euthyroid ______________________________
8. hyperthyroidism ______________________________
9. tetany ______________________________
10. ketoacidosis ______________________________

H **The following hormones are all produced by the anterior lobe of the pituitary gland (note that they all have the same suffix, -tropin). Name the target tissue they act on or stimulate in the body.**

1. gonadotropins ______________________________
2. somatotropin ______________________________
3. thyrotropin ______________________________
4. adrenocorticotropin ______________________________

I **Give the meanings of the following medical terms.**

1. steroids ______________________________
2. catecholamines ______________________________
3. adenohypophysis ______________________________
4. tetany ______________________________
5. exophthalmos ______________________________
6. mineralocorticoids ______________________________
7. homeostasis ______________________________
8. sympathomimetic ______________________________
9. glucocorticoids ______________________________
10. epinephrine ______________________________

11. glycogen ___
12. androgen ___
13. corticosteroid ___
14. oxytocin ___
15. tetraiodothyronine ___
16. adrenal virilism ___
17. thyroid carcinoma ___
18. hirsutism ___
19. acromegaly ___
20. estradiol ___

J **Give the meanings of the following terms related to diabetes mellitus.**

1. type 1 ___
2. diabetic neuropathy ___
3. ketoacidosis ___
4. hypoglycemia ___
5. type 2 ___
6. diabetic retinopathy ___
7. diabetic coma ___
8. diabetic nephropathy ___
9. atherosclerosis ___
10. hyperglycemia ___
11. gastroparesis ___
12. insulin shock ___

K **Explain the following laboratory tests or clinical procedures related to the endocrine system.**

1. thyroid scan ___
2. fasting plasma glucose ___
3. exophthalmometry ___
4. thyroid function test ___

L **Circle the term that best completes the meaning of the sentence.**

1. Phyllis was diagnosed with Graves disease when her husband noticed her **(panhypopituitarism, hirsutism, exophthalmos)**. Her eyes seemed to be bulging out of their sockets.

2. Helen had a primary brain tumor called a **(pituitary, thyroid, adrenal)** adenoma. Her entire endocrine system was disrupted, and her physician recommended surgery and radiation therapy to help relieve her symptoms.

3. Bessie's facial features gradually became "rough" in her late thirties and forties. By the time she was 50, her children noticed her very large hands and recommended that she see an endocrinologist, who diagnosed her chronically progressive condition as **(hyperinsulism, gigantism, acromegaly)**.

4. Bobby was brought into the emergency department because he was found passed out in the kitchen. He had forgotten his insulin and had developed **(Cushing disease, hyperparathyroidism, diabetic ketoacidosis)**.

5. Because her 1-hour test of blood sugar was slightly abnormal, Selma's obstetrician ordered a **(glucose tolerance test, thyroid function test, Pap smear)** to rule out gestational **(hyperthyroidism, chlamydial infection, diabetes)**.

6. Bill noticed that he was passing his urine more frequently, a condition known as **(polyphagia, polyuria, hyperglycemia)**, and was experiencing increased thirst, manifested as **(polydipsia, hypernatremia, polyphagia)**. His wife urged him to see a physician, who performed a **(serum calcium test, urinalysis, serum sodium test)** that revealed inappropriately dilute **(blood, sweat, urine)**. Measurement of the hormone **(PTH, ADH, STH)** in his blood showed low levels. His diagnosis was **(DI, DM, SIADH)**. Treatment with **(oxytocin, cortisol, vasopressin)** was prescribed via nasal spray, and his condition improved.

7. Mary noticed that she had gained weight recently and that her face had a moon-like fullness with new heavy hair growth. Blood and urine tests showed excessive secretion of adrenal **(mineralocorticoids, catecholamines, glucocorticoids)**. Her diagnostic work-up included a/an **(CT scan of the abdomen, MRI study of the head, chest x-ray)**, which revealed enlargement of both **(kidneys, adrenal glands, lobes of the brain)**. Her doctor made the diagnosis of **(Graves disease, Cushing syndrome, Addison disease)**.

8. Jack had several fractures of ribs and vertebrae in a skiing accident. X-ray images of his bones revealed a generalized decrease in bone density, a condition known as **(osteoporosis, tetany, acromegaly)**. A blood test showed high serum **(sodium, calcium, growth hormone)** and high levels of **(mineralocorticoids, somatotropin, parathyroid hormone)**. An ultrasound scan of the neck revealed a **(thymus, parathyroid, thyroid)** adenoma, which was removed surgically, and he recovered fully. His bone disease and other abnormalities were all related to **(hypoparathyroidism, hyperparathyroidism, hypothyroidism)**.

ANSWERS TO EXERCISES

A

1. pancreas
2. parathyroid
3. adrenal medulla
4. testis
5. thyroid gland
6. adrenal cortex
7. ovary
8. pituitary (hypophysis)

B

1. anterior pituitary gland (adenohypophysis)
2. posterior pituitary gland (neurohypophysis)
3. adrenal cortex
4. beta islet cells of the pancreas
5. thyroid gland
6. adrenal cortex
7. anterior pituitary gland; these hormones are FSH and LH
8. adrenal medulla
9. posterior pituitary gland
10. anterior pituitary gland
11. anterior pituitary gland
12. alpha islet cells of the pancreas
13. anterior pituitary gland
14. ovaries
15. ovaries
16. testes
17. anterior pituitary gland

C

1. antidiuretic hormone
2. adrenocorticotropic hormone
3. luteinizing hormone
4. follicle-stimulating hormone
5. thyroid-stimulating hormone
6. parathyroid hormone
7. growth hormone
8. prolactin
9. thyroxine; tetraiodothyronine
10. triiodothyronine
11. oxytocin
12. somatotropin (growth hormone)

D

1. epinephrine
2. testosterone
3. ADH
4. thyroxine
5. parathyroid hormone
6. aldosterone
7. ACTH
8. cortisol
9. insulin
10. estradiol

E

1. hypersecretion; adrenal cortex; cortisol
2. hyposecretion; parathyroid gland; parathyroid hormone
3. hypersecretion; thyroid gland; thyroxine
4. hyposecretion; neurohypophysis; ADH
5. hypersecretion; adenohypophysis; GH
6. hyposecretion; thyroid gland; thyroxine
7. hyposecretion; pancreas; insulin
8. hyposecretion; adrenal cortex; aldosterone and cortisol
9. hypersecretion; adenohypophysis; GH
10. hyposecretion; thyroid gland; thyroxine
11. hyposecretion; thyroid gland; thyroxine
12. hypersecretion; adrenal medulla; epinephrine

F

1. thyrotoxicosis
2. pancreatectomy
3. hypogonadism
4. estrogenic
5. hypophysectomy
6. hypocalcemia
7. hyperglycemia
8. thyroiditis
9. endocrinologist

G

1. deficient sodium in the blood
2. condition of excessive thirst
3. excessive potassium in the blood
4. excessive calcium in the blood
5. deficient sugar in the blood
6. condition of sugar in the urine
7. normal thyroid function
8. condition of increased secretion from the thyroid gland
9. constant muscle contraction (result of hypoparathyroidism)
10. condition of excessive ketones (acids) in the blood as a result of diabetes mellitus

H

1. the male and female sex organs (ovaries and testes); examples of gonadotropins are FSH and LH
2. bones; another name for somatotropin is growth hormone
3. thyroid gland; another name for thyrotropin is thyroid-stimulating hormone (TSH)
4. adrenal cortex; another name for adrenocorticotropin is adrenocorticotropic hormone (ACTH)

I

1. complex substances derived from cholesterol; hormones from the adrenal cortex and sex hormones are steroids
2. complex substances derived from an amino acid; epinephrine (adrenaline) and norepinephrine (noradrenaline) are examples
3. anterior lobe of the pituitary gland
4. continuous contractions of muscles associated with low levels of parathyroid hormone
5. eyeballs that bulge outward; associated with hyperthyroidism
6. steroid hormones from the adrenal cortex (outer region of the adrenal gland) that influence salt (minerals such as sodium and potassium) metabolism
7. tendency of an organism to maintain a constant internal environment
8. a substance that mimics the action of the sympathetic nerves; epinephrine (adrenaline) is an example
9. steroid hormones from the adrenal cortex that influence sugar metabolism in the body
10. catecholamine hormone from the adrenal medulla; adrenaline
11. animal starch; storage form of glucose
12. male hormone; testosterone is an example
13. hormone secreted by the adrenal cortex; cortisol is an example
14. hormone from the posterior lobe of the pituitary that stimulates contraction of the uterus during labor
15. major hormone from the thyroid gland; thyroxine (contains four iodine atoms)
16. abnormal secretion of androgens from the adrenal cortex produces masculine characteristics in a female
17. cancerous tumor of the thyroid gland
18. excessive hair on the body (result of excessive secretion of androgens)
19. enlargement of extremities (excessive secretion of growth hormone after puberty)
20. female hormone; an estrogen

J

1. destruction of the beta cells (islets of Langerhans); insulin is not produced
2. destruction of nerves as a secondary complication of diabetes mellitus
3. abnormal condition of high levels of ketones (acids) in the blood as a result of improper burning of fats; fats are burned because the cells do not have sugar available as a result of lack of insulin or inability of insulin to act
4. too little sugar in the blood; this can occur if too much insulin is taken by a diabetic patient
5. insulin deficiency and resistance by target tissue to the action of insulin
6. destruction of blood vessels in the retina as a secondary complication of diabetes mellitus
7. unconsciousness caused by high levels of sugar in the blood; water leaves cells to balance the large amounts of sugar in the blood, leading to cellular dehydration
8. destruction of the kidneys as a secondary complication of diabetes mellitus
9. collection of fatty plaque in arteries
10. high level of sugar in the blood; insulin is unavailable or unable to transport sugar from the blood into cells
11. decreased gastric motility (-paresis means slight paralysis); secondary complication of diabetes
12. hypoglycemic shock caused by an overdose of insulin, decreased intake of food, or excessive exercise

K

1. Radioactive compound is given, and the thyroid gland is imaged using a scanning device.
2. Measurement of blood sugar levels in a fasting patient (at least 4 hours) and after intervals of 30 minutes and 1, 2, and 3 hours after ingestion of glucose.
3. Measurement of eyeball protrusion (symptom of Graves disease)
4. Measurement of T3, T4, and TSH in the bloodstream

L

1. exophthalmos
2. pituitary
3. acromegaly
4. diabetic ketoacidosis
5. glucose tolerance test; diabetes
6. polyuria; polydipsia; urinalysis; urine; ADH; DI; vasopressin
7. glucocorticoids; CT scan of the abdomen; adrenal glands; Cushing syndrome
8. osteoporosis; calcium; parathyroid hormone; parathyroid; hyperparathyroidism

Answers to Practical Applications

Endocrine Medicines

1. c
2. b
3. a

18

PRONUNCIATION OF TERMS

To test your understanding of the terminology in this chapter, write the meaning of each term in the space provided. In addition, you may wish to cover the terms and write them by looking at your definitions. Make sure your spelling is correct. The page number after each term indicates where it is defined or used in the book, so you can easily check your responses. You will find complete definitions for all of these terms and their audio pronunciations on the Evolve website.

Pronunciation Guide

ā as in āpe	ă as in ăpple
ē as in ēven	ĕ as in ĕvery
ī as in īce	ĭ as in ĭnterest
ō as in ōpen	ŏ as in pŏt
ū as in ūnit	ŭ as in ŭnder

Vocabulary and Terminology

TERM	PRONUNCIATION	MEANING
adenectomy (762)	ăd-ĕ-NĔK-tō-mē	______
adenohypophysis (759)	ăd-ĕ-nō-hī-PŎF-ĭ-sĭs	______
adrenal cortex (759)	ă-DRĒ-năl KŎR-tĕks	______
adrenalectomy (762)	ă-drē-năl-ĔK-tō-mē	______
adrenaline (759)	ă-DRĔN-ă-lĭn	______
adrenal medulla (759)	ă-DRĒ-năl mĕ-DŪ-lă	______
adrenocorticotropic hormone (759)	ă-drē-nō-kŏr-tĭ-kō-TRŌP-ĭk HŎR-mōn	______
adrenocorticotropin (765)	ă-drē-nō-kŏr-tĭ-kō-TRŌ-pĭn	______
aldosterone (760)	ăl-DŎS-tĕ-rōn	______
androgen (760)	ĂN-drō-jĕn	______
antidiuretic hormone (760)	ăn-tĭ-dī-ū-RĔT-ĭk HŎR-mōn	______
calcitonin (760)	kăl-sĭ-TŌ-nĭn	______
catecholamines (761)	kăt-ĕ-KŌL-ă-mēnz	______
corticosteroids (761)	kŏr-tĭ-kō-STĒ-roydz	______
cortisol (760)	KŎR-tĭ-sōl	______
electrolyte (761)	ĕ-LĔK-trō-līt	______
endocrinologist (763)	ĕn-dō-krĭ-NŎL-ō-jĭst	______
epinephrine (760)	ĕp-ĭ-NĔF-rĭn	______
estradiol (760)	ĕs-tră-DĪ-ŏl	______
estrogen (760)	ĔS-trō-jĕn	______
estrogenic (763)	ĕs-trō-JĔN-ĭk	______
euthyroid (765)	ū-THĪ-royd	______

18

TERM	PRONUNCIATION	MEANING
follicle-stimulating hormone (760)	FŎL-ĭ-kl STĬM-ū-lā-tĭng HŎR-mōn	____________
glucagon (760)	GLOO-kă-gŏn	____________
glucocorticoid (761)	gloo-kō-KŎR-tĭ-koyd	____________
glycemic (763)	glī-SĒ-mĭk	____________
glycogen (763)	GLĪ-kō-jĕn	____________
glycosuria (765)	glī-kōs-Ū-rē-ă	____________
gonadotropin (762)	gō-năd-ō-TRŌ-pĭn	____________
growth hormone (760)	grōth HŎR-mōn	____________
homeostasis (761)	hō-mē-ō-STĀ-sĭs	____________
hormonal (763)	hŏr-MŌ-năl	____________
hormone (761)	HŎR-mōn	____________
hypercalcemia (762)	hī-pĕr-kăl-SĒ-mē-ă	____________
hypercalciuria (762)	hī-pĕr-kăl-sē-ŪR-ē-ă	____________
hyperglycemia (763)	hī-pĕr-glī-SĒ-mē-ă	____________
hyperkalemia (763)	hī-pĕr-kā-LĒ-mē-ă	____________
hypocalcemia (762)	hī-pō-kăl-SĒ-mē-ă	____________
hypoglycemia (765)	hī-pō-glī-SĒ-mē-ă	____________
hypogonadism (762)	hī-pō-GŌ-năd-ĭzm	____________
hypoinsulinism (765)	hī-pō-ĬN-sū-lĭn-ĭzm	____________
hypokalemia (763)	hī-pō-kā-LĒ-mē-ă	____________
hyponatremia (763)	hī-pō-nā-TRĒ-mē-ă	____________
hypophysectomy (764)	hī-pō-fĭ-ZĔK-tō-mē	____________
hypophysis (759)	hī-PŎF-ĭ-sĭs	____________
hypopituitarism (762)	hī-pō-pĭ-TOO-ĭ-tă-rĭzm	____________
hypothalamus (761)	hī-pō-THĂL-ă-mŭs	____________
insulin (760)	ĬN-sū-lĭn	____________
luteinizing hormone (760)	LOO-tē-ĭn-īz-ĭng HŎR-mōn	____________
mineralocorticoid (761)	mĭn-ĕr-ăl-ō-KŎR-tĭ-koyd	____________
neurohypophysis (759)	noo-rō-hī-PŎF-ĭ-sĭs	____________
norepinephrine (760)	nŏr-ĕp-ĭ-NĔF-rĭn	____________

18

TERM	PRONUNCIATION	MEANING
ovaries (759)	ō-vă-rēz	
oxytocin (760)	ŏk-sĕ-TŌ-sĭn	
pancreas (759)	PĂN-krē-ăs	
pancreatectomy (762)	păn-krē-ă-TĔK-tō-mē	
parathormone (760)	păr-ă-THŎR-mōn	
parathyroidectomy (762)	păr-ă-thī-roy-DĔK-tō-mē	
parathyroid glands (759)	păr-ă-THĪ-royd glănz	
pineal gland (748)	pī-NĒ-ăl glănd	
pituitary gland (759)	pĭ-TOO-ĭ-tĕr-ē glănd	
polydipsia (763)	pŏl-ē-DĬP-sē-ă	
polyuria (765)	pŏl-ē-Ū-rē-ă	
progesterone (760)	prō-JĔS-tĕ-rōn	
prolactin (760)	prō-LĂK-tĭn	
receptor (761)	rē-SĔP-tŏr	
sella turcica (761)	SĔL-ă TŬR-sĭ-kă	
sex hormones (761)	sĕx HŎR-monz	
somatotropin (760)	sō-mă-tō-TRŌ-pĭn	
steroid (761)	STĔR-oyd	
sympathomimetic (761)	sĭm-pă-thō-mĭ-MĔT-ĭk	
target tissue (761)	TĂR-gĕt TĬS-ū	
testes (759)	TĔS-tēz	
testosterone (760)	tĕs-TŎS-tĕ-rōn	
tetraiodothyronine (765)	tĕ-tră-ī-ō-dō-THĪ-rō-nēn	
thyroid gland (759)	THĪ-royd glănd	
thyroiditis (762)	thī-royd-Ī-tĭs	
thyrotropin (760)	thī-rō-TRŌ-pĭn	
thyroxine (761)	thī-RŎK-sĭn	
triiodothyronine (761)	trī-ī-ō-dō-THĪ-rō-nēn	
vasopressin (761)	văz-ō-PRĔS-ĭn	

Pathology, Laboratory Tests, and Clinical Procedures

TERM	PRONUNCIATION	MEANING
acromegaly (773)	ăk-rō-MĔG-ă-lē	______
Addison disease (769)	ĂD-ĭ-sŏn dĭ-ZĒZ	______
adrenal virilism (768)	ă-DRĒ-năl VĬR-ĭ-lĭzm	______
cretinism (767)	KRĒ-tĭn-ĭzm	______
Cushing syndrome (768)	KŬSH-ĭng SĬN-drōm	______
diabetes insipidus (775)	dī-ă-BĒ-tēz ĭn-SĬP-ĭ-dŭs	______
diabetes mellitus (770)	dī-ă-BĒ-tēz MĔL-ĭ-tŭs	______
dwarfism (774)	DWĂRF-ĭzm	______
endemic goiter (766)	ĕn-DĔM-ĭk GOY-tĕr	______
exophthalmometry (776)	ĕk-sŏf-thăl-MŎM-ĕ-trē	______
exophthalmos (766)	ĕk-sŏf-THĂL-mōs	______
fasting plasma glucose (776)	FĂS-tĭng PLĂS-măh GLŪ-kōs	______
gastroparesis (772)	găs-trō-păr-Ē-sĭs	______
gigantism (774)	JĪ-găn-tĭzm	______
glucose tolerance test (776)	GLOO-kōs TŎL-ĕr-ăns tĕst	______
goiter (766)	GOY-tĕr	______
Graves disease (766)	GRĀVZ dĭ-ZĒZ	______
hirsutism (768)	HĔR-soot-ĭzm	______
hyperinsulinism (770)	hī-pĕr-ĬN-sū-lĭn-ĭzm	______
hyperparathyroidism (767)	hī-pĕr-pă-ră-THĪ-royd-ĭzm	______
hyperthyroidism (766)	hī-pĕr-THĪ-royd-ĭsm	______
hypoparathyroidism (768)	hī-pō-pă-ră-THĪ-royd-ĭzm	______
hypothyroidism (767)	hī-pō-THĪ-royd-ĭzm	______
ketoacidosis (771)	kē-tō-ă-sĭ-DŌ-sĭs	______
myxedema (767)	mĭk-sĕ-DĒ-mă	______
nodular goiter (766)	NŎD-ū-lăr GOY-tĕr	______
panhypopituitarism (774)	păn-hī-pō-pĭ-TOO-ĭ-tăr-ĭzm	______
pheochromocytoma (769)	fē-ō-krō-mō-sī-TŌ-mă	______

18

TERM	PRONUNCIATION	MEANING
syndrome of inappropriate ADH (775)	SĬN-drōm ŏf ĭn-ă-PRŌ-prē-ĭt ADH	____________
tetany (768)	TĔT-ă-nē	____________
thyroid carcinoma (767)	THĪ-royd kăr-sĭ-NŌ-mă	____________
thyroid function tests (776)	THĪ-royd FŬNK-shŭn tĕsts	____________
thyroid scan (776)	THĪ-royd skăn	____________
thyrotoxicosis (766)	thī-rō-tŏk-sĭ-KŌ-sĭs	____________

REVIEW SHEET

Write the meanings of the word parts in the spaces provided and test yourself. Check your answers with the information in the chapter or in the Glossary (Medical Word Parts—English) at the end of the book.

Combining Forms

COMBINING FORM	MEANING	COMBINING FORM	MEANING
aden/o	______________	lact/o	______________
adrenal/o	______________	myx/o	______________
andr/o	______________	natr/o	______________
calc/o, calci/o	______________	pancreat/o	______________
cortic/o	______________	parathyroid/o	______________
crin/o	______________	phys/o	______________
dips/o	______________	pituitar/o	______________
estr/o	______________	somat/o	______________
gluc/o	______________	ster/o	______________
glyc/o	______________	thyr/o	______________
gonad/o	______________	thyroid/o	______________
home/o	______________	toc/o	______________
hormon/o	______________	toxic/o	______________
insulin/o	______________	ur/o	______________
kal/i	______________		

Suffixes

SUFFIX	MEANING	SUFFIX	MEANING
-agon	______________	-osis	______________
-ectomy	______________	-physis	______________
-emia	______________	-stasis	______________
-genic	______________	-tocin	______________
-in, -ine	______________	-tropin	______________
-megaly	______________	-uria	______________
-oid	______________		

Prefixes

PREFIX	MEANING	PREFIX	MEANING
eu-	______	pan-	______
hyper-	______	poly-	______
hypo-	______	tetra-	______
oxy-	______	tri-	______

Complete the following table and check your answers with Table 18-4 on p. 775.

Endocrine Gland	Hypersecretion	Hyposecretion
Adrenal cortex	______ ______	______
Adrenal medulla	______	
Pancreas	______	______
Parathyroid glands	______	______
Pituitary—anterior lobe	______ ______	______ ______
Pituitary—posterior lobe	______	______
Thyroid gland	______ ______	______ ______ ______

18

evolve *Please refer to the Evolve website for additional exercises, games, and images related to this chapter.*

CHAPTER 19

Cancer Medicine (Oncology)

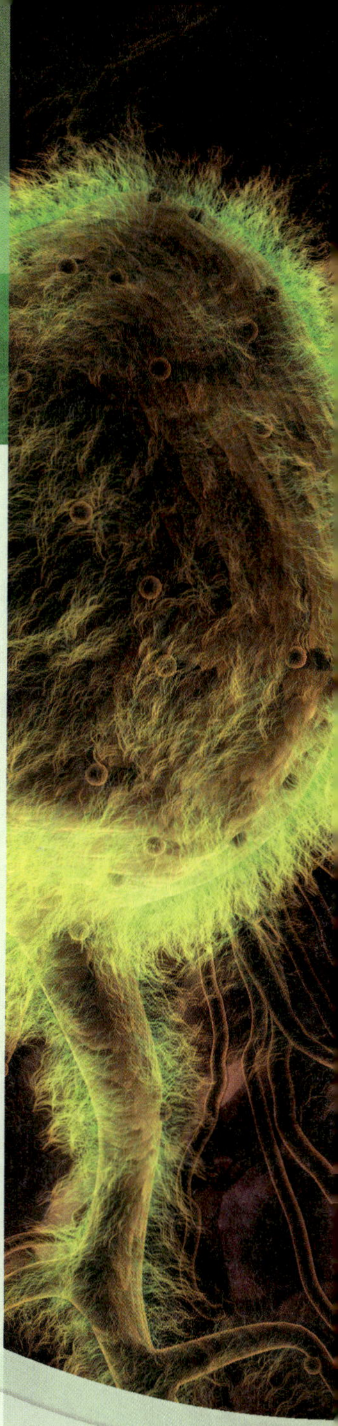

This chapter is divided into the following sections:

CHAPTER GOALS

- Identify medical terms that describe the growth and spread of tumors.
- Recognize terms related to the causes, diagnosis, and treatment of cancer.
- Review how tumors are classified and described by pathologists.
- Describe x-ray studies, laboratory tests, and other procedures used by physicians for determining the presence and extent of spread (staging) of tumors.
- Apply your new knowledge to understanding medical terms in their proper contexts, such as medical reports and records.

INTRODUCTION

Cancer is a disease caused by abnormal and excessive growth of cells in the body. It may occur in any tissue and at any time of life, although cancer occurs most frequently in older people. Cancer cells accumulate as growths called **malignant tumors** that compress, invade, and ultimately destroy the surrounding normal tissue. In addition to their local growth, cancerous cells spread throughout the body by way of the bloodstream or lymphatic vessels. In some patients the spread of cancers from their site of origin to distant organs occurs early in the course of tumor growth and ultimately results in death.

Although more than half of all patients who develop cancer are cured of their disease, about 550,000 people die of cancer each year. Lung cancers, followed by breast and colorectal cancers, are the most common causes of cancer death for women, whereas lung, colorectal, and prostate cancers are the leading causes of death due to cancer in men. This chapter explores the terminology related to this common and often fatal group of diseases.

CHARACTERISTICS OF TUMORS

Tumors (neoplasms) are new growths that arise from normal tissue. They may be either **malignant** (capable of invasion and spread to surrounding or more distant sites) or **benign** (noninvasive and not spreading to other sites). There are several differences between benign and malignant tumors. Some of these differences are:

1. Benign tumors **grow slowly,** and malignant tumor cells **multiply rapidly.**
2. Benign tumors are often **encapsulated** (contained within a fibrous capsule or cover), so that the tumor cells do not invade the surrounding tissue. Malignant tumors characteristically are **invasive** and **infiltrative,** extending into neighboring normal tissue.
3. Benign tumors are composed of organized and specialized **(differentiated)** cells that closely resemble the normal, mature tissue from which they are derived. For example,

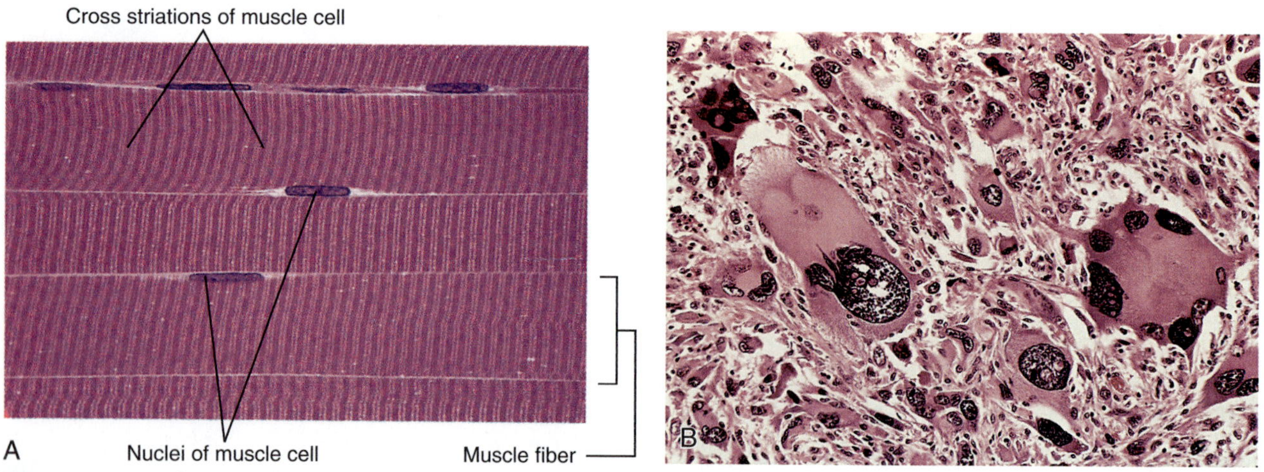

FIGURE 19-1 **A, Photomicrograph of normal skeletal muscle cells (fibers).** Note the orderly arrangement and the long, narrow, threadlike shape of the cells. There are many nuclei per cell and many cross striations. **B, Anaplastic tumor cells of the skeletal muscle (rhabdomyosarcoma).** Note the variation in size and shape of the nuclei (pleomorphism; pleo = many, morph/o = shape), hyperchromatic (intensely staining) nuclei, and large tumor cells (which may possess more than one nucleus). ***(B,** courtesy Trace Worrell, MD, Department of Pathology, University of Texas Southwestern Medical School, Dallas.)*

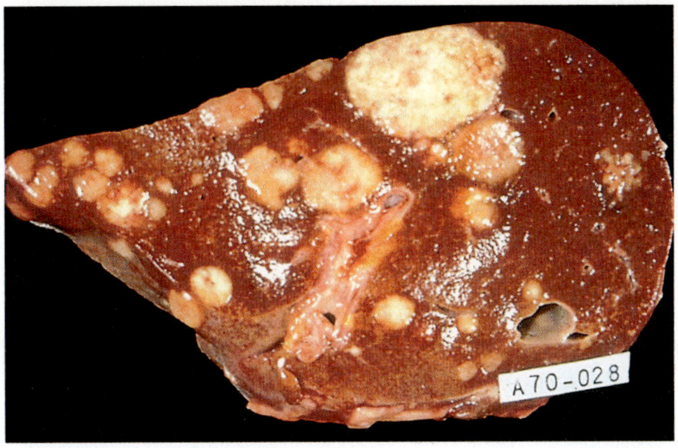

FIGURE 19-2 A liver studded with metastatic cancer.

benign tumors derived from epithelial cells that line the wall of the gastrointestinal tract look very much like their normal counterparts. Malignant tumors are composed of cancerous cells that resemble primitive cells and lack the capacity to perform mature cell functions. This characteristic of malignant tumors is called **anaplasia.** Anaplasia (ana- means backward and -plasia means growth) indicates that the cancerous cells are **dedifferentiated,** or **undifferentiated** (reverting to a less specialized state), in contrast with the normal, differentiated tissue of their origin. Anaplastic cells lack an orderly arrangement. Thus, tumor cells vary in size and shape and are piled one on top of the other in a disorganized fashion. The nuclei in these cells are large and **hyperchromatic** (stain excessively with dyes that recognize genetic material, DNA). Figure 19-1A and B shows normal skeletal muscle and anaplastic malignant muscle tumor cells.

4. Cells from benign tumors do not spread or **metastasize** to form secondary tumor masses in distant places in the body. Cells from malignant tumors, however, can detach themselves from the primary tumor site, penetrate a blood vessel or lymphatic vessel, travel through the bloodstream or lymphatic system, and establish a new tumor site at a distant tissue, such as the lung, liver, or bone marrow. The secondary growth is called a **metastasis.** Figure 19-2 shows metastatic tumors within the liver.

Figure 19-3 reviews the differences between benign and malignant tumors.

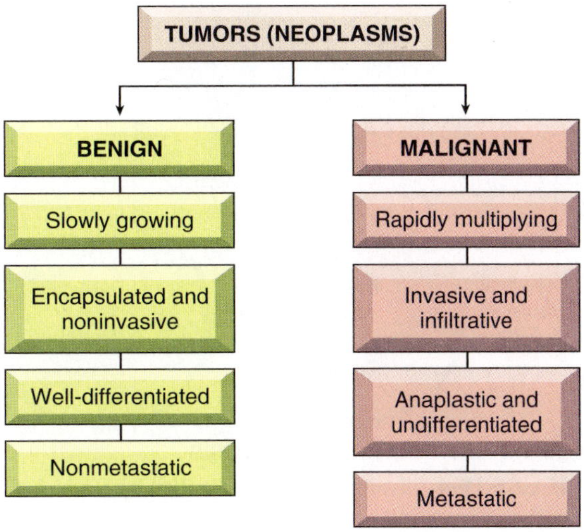

FIGURE 19-3 Differences between benign and malignant tumors.

CARCINOGENESIS

WHAT CAUSES CANCER?

The causes of transformation from a normal cell to a cancerous one **(carcinogenesis)** are only partly understood. What is clear is that malignant transformation results from damage to the genetic material, or **DNA (deoxyribonucleic acid),** of the cell. Strands of DNA in the cell nucleus form **chromosomes,** which become readily visible under a microscope when a cell is preparing to divide into two (daughter) cells. In order to understand what causes cancer, it is necessary to learn more about DNA and its functions in a normal cell.

DNA has two main functions in a normal cell. First, DNA controls the production of new cells (cell division). When a cell divides, the DNA material in each chromosome copies itself so that exactly the same DNA is passed to the two new daughter cells that are formed. This process of cell division is called **mitosis** (Figure 19-4A).

Second, DNA contains the master code for all proteins produced in the cell. Between cycles of mitosis, DNA controls the production of new proteins **(protein synthesis)** in the cell. DNA contains about 20,000 to 30,000 separate and distinct **genes** that direct the production of all proteins, which in turn control all aspects of cell function. Genes are composed of an arrangement of units called **nucleotides** (containing a sugar, phosphate, and a base, such as adenine, guanine, thymine, or cytosine). DNA (as a string of coded nucleotides) sends a molecular message outside the nucleus to the cytoplasm of the cell, directing the synthesis of specific proteins (such as hormones and enzymes) essential for normal cell function and growth. This message is transmitted in the following way. In the nucleus, the coded message with instructions for making a specific protein is copied from DNA onto another molecule called **RNA (ribonucleic acid).** Then RNA travels from the nucleus to the cytoplasm of the cell, carrying the coded message that directs the formation of specific proteins (Figure 19-4B).

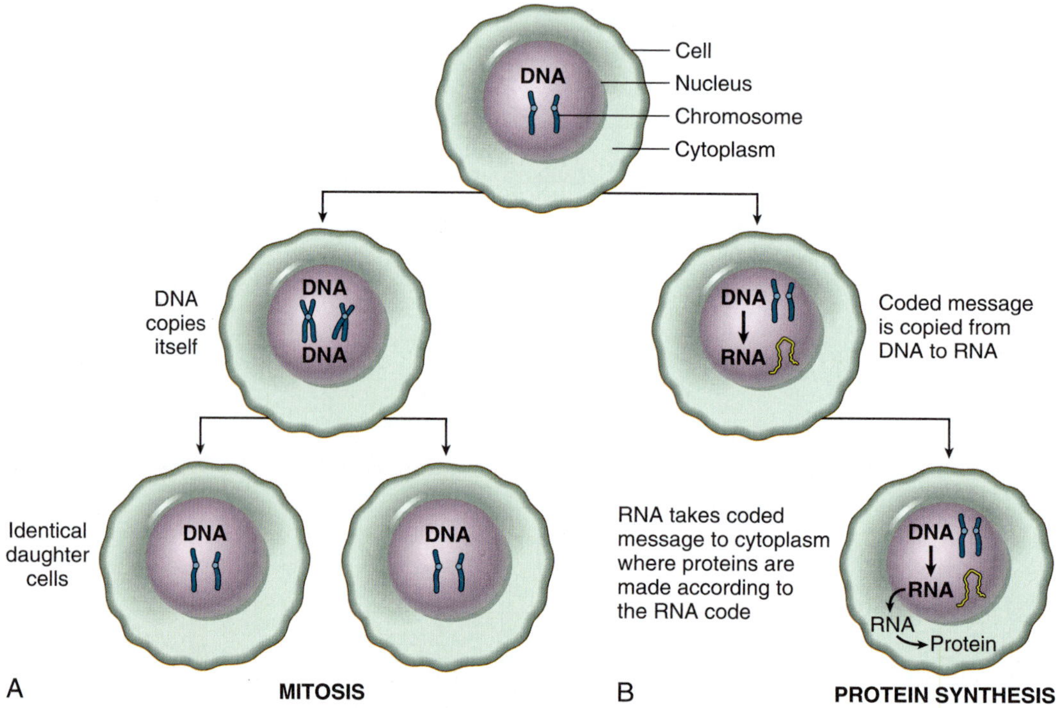

FIGURE 19-4 **Two processes controlled by DNA. A, Mitosis** (the process of cell division). **B, Protein synthesis** (creating new proteins for cellular growth).

When a cell becomes malignant, however, the processes of mitosis and protein synthesis are disturbed. Cancer cells reproduce almost continuously, and abnormal proteins are made. Malignant cells are **anaplastic;** that is, their DNA stops making codes that allow the cells to carry on the function of mature cells. Instead, altered DNA and altered cellular programs make new signals that lead to cell proliferation, movement of cells, invasion of adjacent tissue, and metastasis.

Various kinds of damage to DNA results in malignancy; DNA damage may be caused by environmental factors, such as toxic chemicals, sunlight, tobacco smoke, and viruses. The specific damage usually involves chemical changes in the nucleotide components of DNA. These changes interfere with the accurate coding for new protein synthesis. Once these changes are established in a cell, they are passed on to daughter cells. Such an inheritable change in DNA is called a **mutation.** Mutations, particularly those that stimulate cell growth or block DNA repair, lead to formation of malignant tumors.

Although most DNA changes, or mutations, lead to higher-than-normal rates of growth, some mutations found in cancer cells actually prevent the cells from dying. In recent years, scientists have recognized that in some types of cancers, the normal blueprints that direct aging or damaged cells to die are missing. Normal cells undergo spontaneous disintegration by a process known as **apoptosis,** or programmed cell death. Some cancer cells have lost elements of this program and thus can live indefinitely.

ENVIRONMENTAL AGENTS

Agents from the environment, such as chemicals, drugs, tobacco smoke, radiation, and viruses, can cause damage to DNA and thus produce cancer. These environmental agents are called **carcinogens.**

Chemical carcinogens are found in a variety of products and drugs, including **hydrocarbons**—in cigarette, cigar, and pipe smoke and automobile exhaust—insecticides, dyes, industrial chemicals, insulation, and hormones. For example, the hormone diethylstilbestrol (DES) causes a malignant tumor, carcinoma of the vagina, in daughters of women treated with DES during pregnancy. Drugs such as estrogens can cause cancer by stimulating the proliferation of cells in target organs such as the lining of the uterus.

Radiation, whatever its source—sunlight, x-rays, radioactive substances—consists of waves of energy. When this energy interacts with DNA, it causes DNA damage and mutations that lead to cancer. Thus, leukemia (a cancerous condition of white blood cells) may be an occupational hazard of radiologists, who are routinely exposed to x-rays. There is a high incidence of leukemia and other cancers among survivors of atomic bomb explosions, as at Hiroshima and Nagasaki. Ultraviolet radiation in sunlight can cause skin cancer, especially in persons with lightly pigmented, or fair, skin.

Some **viruses** are carcinogenic. For example, the human T cell leukemia virus (HTLV) causes a form of leukemia in adults. Kaposi sarcoma is caused by another virus, herpesvirus type 8. Other viruses are known to cause cervical cancer (papillomavirus) and a tumor of lymph nodes called Burkitt lymphoma (Epstein-Barr virus). These tumor-producing viruses, called **oncogenic viruses,** fall into two categories: **RNA viruses** (composed of RNA and known as retroviruses) and **DNA viruses** (composed of DNA).

In addition to transmission of cancer by whole viruses, pieces of normal DNA called **oncogenes** can cause normal cells to become malignant if they are activated by mutations. An oncogene (cancer-causing gene) is a piece of DNA whose activation is associated with the conversion of a normal cell into a cancerous cell. Some examples of oncogenes are ***ras*** (colon cancer), ***myc*** (lymphoma), and ***abl*** (chronic myelogenous leukemia [CML]).

In chronic myelogenous leukemia, the oncogene *abl* is activated when pieces from two different chromosomes switch locations. This genetic change (mutation) is called a **translocation.** The oncogene *abl* on chromosome 9 moves to a new location on the base of

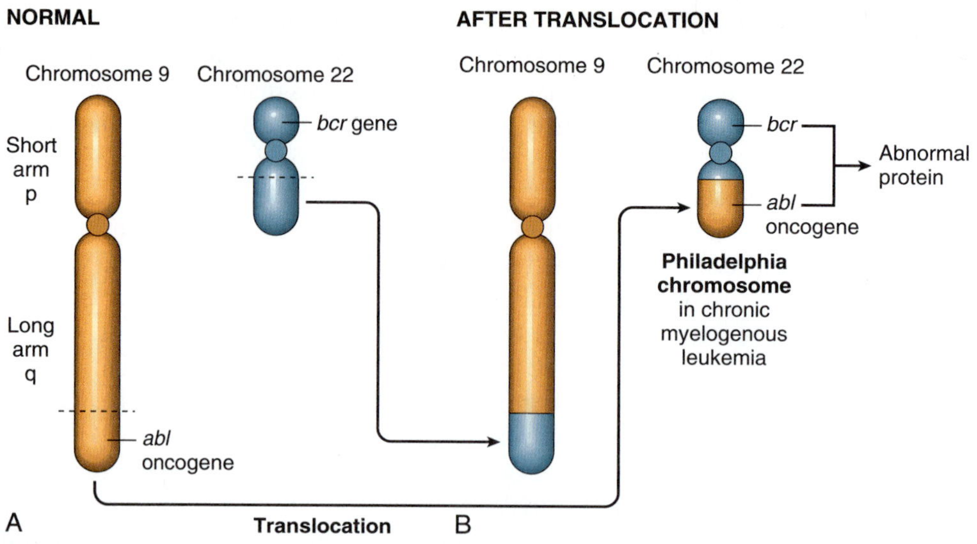

FIGURE 19-5 Chromosomal (oncogene) translocation resulting in the Philadelphia chromosome, associated with chronic myelogenous leukemia (CML). **A,** Normal chromosomes 9 and 22. **B, Translocation** of the *abl* oncogene from the long arm (q) of chromosome 9 to the long arm of chromosome 22 (next to the *bcr* gene). This forms a combination oncogene *bcr-abl* that produces an abnormal protein (tyrosine kinase), which leads to malignant transformation (in this case, CML).

chromosome 22, in a chromosome region called ***bcr*** (**b**reakpoint **c**luster **r**egion). When *bcr* and *abl* are near each other, they cause the production of an abnormal protein that makes the leukocyte divide and causes a malignancy (chronic myelogenous leukemia). The new chromosome formed from the translocation and containing the ***bcr-abl*** gene fragments is called the **Philadelphia chromosome** (it was discovered in 1970 in Philadelphia) (Figure 19-5).

HEREDITY

Cancer may be caused by not only environmental factors but also inherited factors. Susceptibility to some forms of cancer is transmitted from parents to offspring through defects in the DNA of the egg or sperm cells. Examples of known inherited cancers are **retinoblastoma** (tumor of the retina of the eye), **adenomatous polyposis coli syndrome** (premalignant polyps that grow in the colon and rectum), and certain other inherited forms of colon, breast, and kidney cancer.

Each of these diseases is caused by loss of a segment of DNA or by a change in the coding sequence of DNA. Detection of these changes in the DNA code is possible by analysis of genes on the chromosomes from any cell, such as a blood cell, taken from an affected individual. Such inherited defects are detected by DNA sequencing, a step-by-step analysis of the nucleotide sequence of the affected gene, or by small DNA probes that test the overall fit of a person's gene to a normal gene sequence.

In many cases, it is believed that these tumors arise because of inherited or acquired abnormalities in certain genes called **suppressor genes.** In normal persons, these suppressor genes regulate growth, promote differentiation, and suppress oncogenes from causing cancer. Loss of a normal suppressor gene takes the brake off the process of cell division and leads to cancer. Examples of suppressor genes are the **retinoblastoma (Rb) type 1 gene *(RB1)*** and the **TP53** (p53 is the protein it encodes). A loss or mutation of TP53 (located on chromosome 17) can lead to human cancers, such as brain tumors or breast cancer.

TABLE 19-1 EXAMPLES OF GENES IMPLICATED IN HEREDITARY CANCERS

Cancer	Gene	Chromosomal Location*
Breast; ovarian	*BRCA1*	17q21
Breast; ovarian	*BRCA2*	3q12-13
HNPCC (hereditary non-polyposis colon cancer)	*MLH 1* *MSH 2*	8q23.3 11q.23.1
Leukemia	*MLL*	11q23
Li-Fraumeni syndrome (multiple cancers)	*TP53*	17p13
Polyposis coli syndrome	*APC*	5q21
Renal cell carcinoma	*VHL*	3p21-26
Retinoblastoma	*RB1*	13q14
Wilms tumor	*WT1*	11p13

*The first number is the chromosome; p is the short arm of the chromosome, and q is the long arm of the chromosome. The second number is the region (band) of the chromosome.

Because inherited changes can be detected by analyzing DNA in any tissue of the body, not simply cancerous cells, blood cells from family members may be tested to determine whether a person has inherited the cancer-causing gene. This is known as **genetic screening.** Affected patients may be watched carefully to detect tumors at an early stage. Table 19-1 lists several hereditary cancers and the name of the responsible gene. Figure 19-6 reviews the role of environmental agents and heredity in carcinogenesis.

CLASSIFICATION OF CANCEROUS TUMORS

Almost half of all cancer deaths are caused by malignancies that originate in lung, breast, or colon; however, in all there are more than 100 distinct types of cancer, each having a unique set of symptoms and requiring a specific type of therapy. It is possible to divide these types of cancer into three broad groups on the basis of **histogenesis**—that is, by identifying the particular type of tissue **(hist/o)** from which the tumor cells arise **(-genesis).** These major groups are **carcinomas, sarcomas,** and **mixed-tissue tumors.**

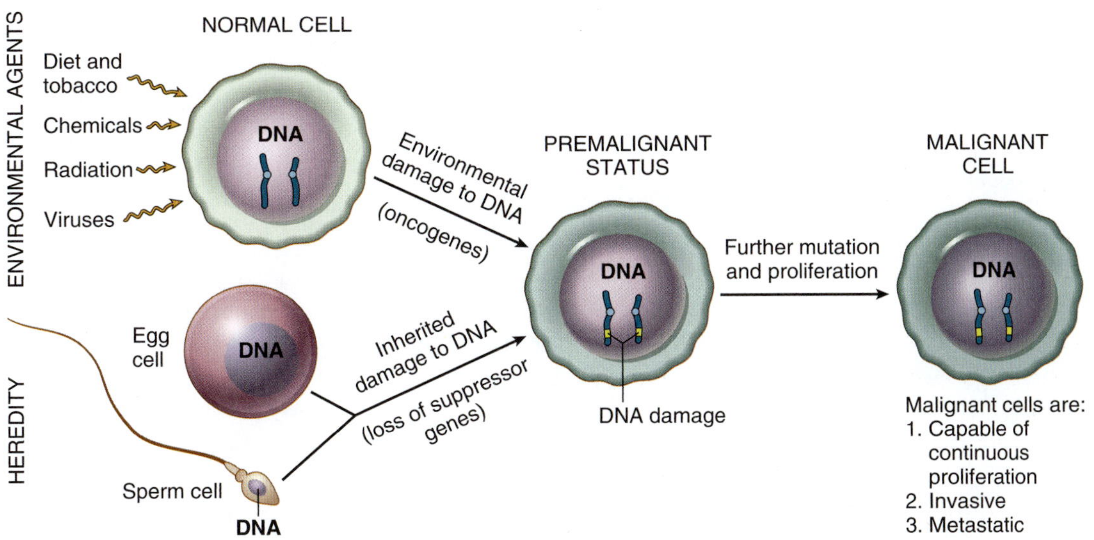

FIGURE 19-6 The role of environmental agents and heredity in carcinogenesis (transformation of a normal to a malignant cell).

19

CARCINOMAS

Carcinomas, the largest group, are solid tumors that are derived from epithelial tissue that lines external and internal body surfaces, including skin, glands, and digestive, urinary, and reproductive organs. Approximately 90% of all malignancies are carcinomas.

Table 19-2 gives examples of specific carcinomas and the epithelial tissue from which they derive. Benign tumors of epithelial origin are usually designated by the term **adenoma,** which indicates that the tumor is of epithelial or glandular **(aden/o)** origin. For example, a gastric adenoma is a benign tumor of the glandular epithelial cells lining the stomach. Malignant tumors of epithelial origin are named by using the term **carcinoma** and adding the type of tissue in which the tumor occurs. Thus, a **gastric adenocarcinoma** is a cancerous tumor arising from glandular cells lining the stomach.

TABLE 19-2 CARCINOMAS AND THE EPITHELIAL TISSUES FROM WHICH THEY DERIVE

Type of Epithelial Tissue	Malignant Tumor (Carcinomas)
Gastrointestinal tract	
Colon	Adenocarcinoma of the colon
Esophagus	Esophageal carcinoma
Liver	Hepatocellular carcinoma (hepatoma)
Stomach	Gastric adenocarcinoma
Glandular tissue	
Adrenal glands	Carcinoma of the adrenals (adrenocortical carcinoma)
Breast	Carcinoma of the breast
Pancreas	Carcinoma of the pancreas (pancreatic adenocarcinoma)
Prostate	Carcinoma of the prostate
Salivary glands	Adenoid cystic carcinoma
Thyroid	Carcinoma of the thyroid
Kidney and bladder	
	Renal cell carcinoma (hypernephroma) Transitional cell carcinoma of the bladder
Lung	
	Adenocarcinoma (bronchioloalveolar) Large cell carcinoma Small (oat) cell carcinoma Squamous cell (epidermoid)
Reproductive organs	
	Adenocarcinoma of the uterus Carcinoma of the penis Choriocarcinoma of the uterus or testes Cystadenocarcinoma (mucinous or serous) of the ovaries Seminoma and embryonal cell carcinoma (testes) Squamous cell (epidermoid) carcinoma of the vagina or cervix
Skin	
Basal cell layer	Basal cell carcinoma
Melanocyte	Malignant melanoma
Squamous cell layer	Squamous cell carcinoma

SARCOMAS

Sarcomas also are malignant tumors but are less common than carcinomas. They derive from connective tissues in the body, such as bone, fat, muscle, cartilage, and bone marrow and from cells of the lymphatic system. Often, the term **mesenchymal tissue** is used to describe embryonic connective tissue from which sarcomas are derived. The middle, or mesodermal, layer of the embryo gives rise to the connective tissues of the body as well as to blood and lymphatic vessels.

Table 19-3 gives examples of specific types of sarcomas and the connective tissues from which they derive. Benign tumors of connective tissue origin are named by adding the suffix **-oma** to the type of tissue in which the tumor occurs. For example, a benign tumor of bone is called an **osteoma.** Malignant tumors of connective tissue origin are frequently named using the term **sarcoma** (**sarc/o** = flesh). For example, an **osteosarcoma** is a malignant tumor of bone.

TABLE 19-3 SARCOMAS AND THE CONNECTIVE TISSUES FROM WHICH THEY DERIVE

Type of Connective Tissue	Malignant Tumor
Bone	
	Osteosarcoma (osteogenic sarcoma) Ewing sarcoma
Muscle	
Smooth (visceral) muscle	Leiomyosarcoma
Striated (skeletal) muscle	Rhabdomyosarcoma
Cartilage	
	Chondrosarcoma
Fat	
	Liposarcoma
Fibrous tissue	
	Fibrosarcoma
Blood vessel tissue	
	Angiosarcoma
Blood-forming tissue	
All leukocytes	Leukemias
Lymphocytes	Lymphomas Hodgkin disease Non-Hodgkin lymphomas: 1. follicular 2. diffuse large cell 3. Burkitt 4. anaplastic large cell
Plasma cells (bone marrow)	Multiple myeloma
Nerve tissue	
Embryonic nerve tissue	Neuroblastoma
Glial tissue	Astrocytoma (tumor of glial cells called astrocytes) Glioblastoma multiforme
Nerve cells of the gastrointestinal tract	Gastrointestinal stromal tumor (GIST)

19

TABLE 19-4	MIXED-TISSUE TUMORS
Type of Tissue	**Malignant Tumor**
Kidney	**Wilms tumor (embryonal adenosarcoma)**
Ovaries and testes	**Teratoma (tumor composed of bone, muscle, skin, gland cells, cartilage, etc.)** **Germ cell tumor**

In addition to the solid tumors of connective tissue origin, sarcomas include tumors arising from blood-forming tissue. **Leukemias** are tumors derived from bone marrow, and **lymphomas** are derived from immune cells of the lymphatic system. Cells within the brain (glial cells) and embryonic tissue of the nervous system give rise to **gliomas** (such as astrocytomas of the brain) and **neuroblastomas,** respectively.

MIXED-TISSUE TUMORS

Mixed-tissue tumors are derived from tissue that is capable of differentiating into both epithelial and connective tissue. These uncommon tumors are thus composed of several different types of cells. Examples of mixed-tissue tumors (Table 19-4) are found in the kidney, ovaries, and testes.

PATHOLOGIC DESCRIPTIONS

The following terms are used to describe the appearance of a malignant tumor, on either gross (visual) or microscopic examination.

GROSS DESCRIPTIONS

cystic — **Forming large open spaces filled with fluid. Mucinous** tumors are filled with mucus (thick, sticky fluid), and **serous** tumors are filled with a thin, watery fluid resembling serum. The most common site of cystic tumors is in ovaries (Figure 19-7A).

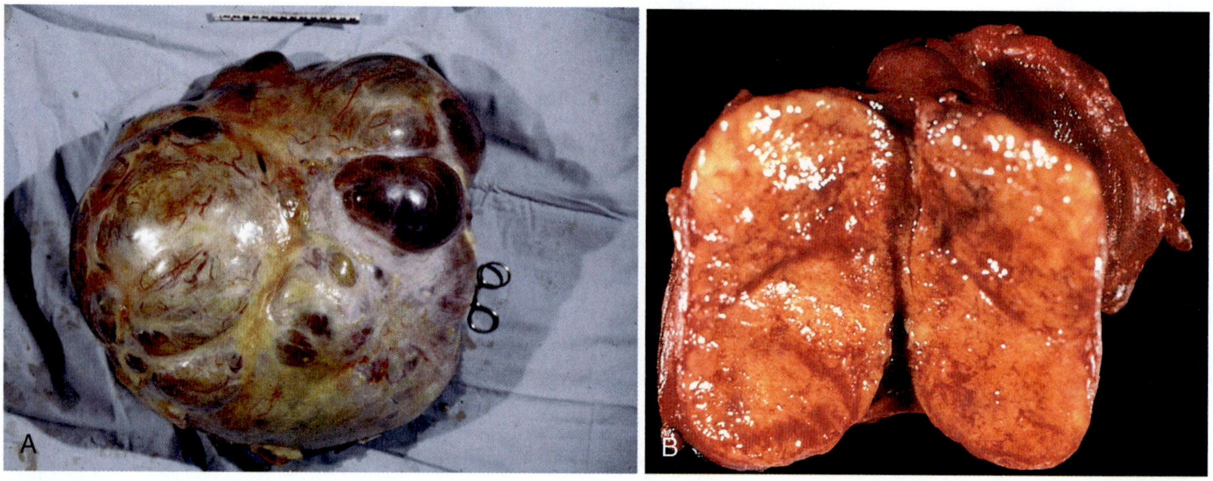

FIGURE 19-7 **A, Cystic ovarian adenocarcinoma.** Note the tumor has formed fluid cysts and blood-filled sacs. **B, Medullary carcinoma** of the thyroid. Tumor shows a solid pattern of growth. *(**A**, Courtesy Dr. Annekathryn Goodman, Massachusetts General Hospital, Boston)*

fungating — **Mushrooming pattern of growth in which tumor cells pile one on top of another and project from a tissue surface.** Tumors found in the colon are often of this type.

inflammatory — **Having the features of inflammation—that is, redness, swelling, and heat.** Inflammatory changes result from tumor blockage of the lymphatic drainage of the skin, as in breast cancer.

medullary — **Large, soft, fleshy tumors.** Thyroid and breast tumors may be medullary (Figure 19-7B).

necrotic — **Containing dead tissue.** Any type of tumor can outgrow its blood supply with resulting cell death and necrosis of part or all of the tumor.

polypoid — **Growths that form projections extending outward from a base. Sessile** polypoid tumors extend from a broad base, and **pedunculated** polypoid tumors extend from a stem or stalk. Both benign and malignant tumors of the colon may grow as polyps. Benign polyps of the colon have a significant risk of becoming malignant over time and should be removed to prevent cancer (Figure 19-8A).

ulcerating — **Characterized by an open, exposed surface resulting from the death of overlying tissue.** Ulcerating tumors often are found in the stomach, breast, colon, and skin (Figure 19-8B).

verrucous — **Resembling a wart-like growth.** Tumors of the gingiva (gum) frequently are verrucous.

MICROSCOPIC DESCRIPTIONS

alveolar — **Tumor cells form patterns resembling small sacs;** commonly found in tumors of muscle, bone, fat, and cartilage.

carcinoma in situ — **Referring to localized tumor cells that have not invaded adjacent structures.** (Latin *in situ* means in place.) Cancer of the cervix may begin as carcinoma in situ.

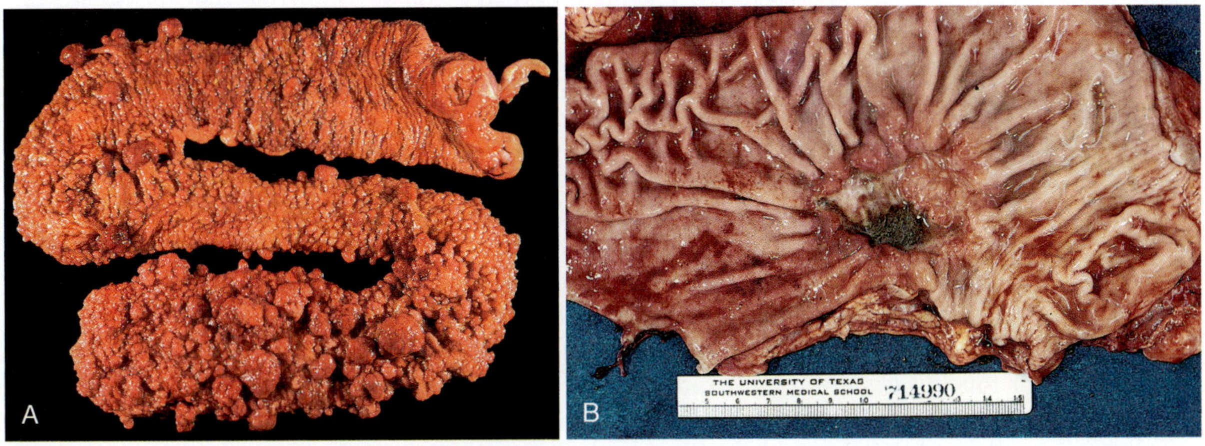

FIGURE 19-8 **A, Adenomatous polyposis of the colon.** These innumerable polypoid adenomas have a strong tendency for progression to colon adenocarcinoma. **B, Gastric (stomach) carcinoma with a large irregular ulcer.**

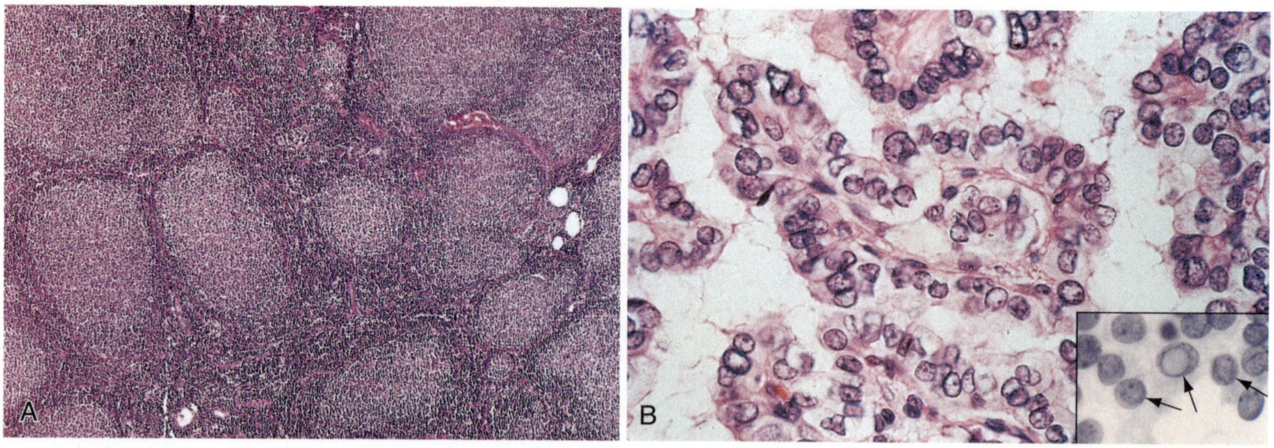

FIGURE 19-9 **A, Follicular non-Hodgkin lymphoma involving a lymph node. B, Papillary carcinoma of the thyroid.**

diffuse — **Spreading evenly throughout the affected tissue.** Malignant lymphomas may display diffuse involvement of lymph nodes.

dysplastic — **Containing abnormal-appearing cells that are not clearly cancerous.** Dysplastic nevi (moles on skin) are an example. They are often forerunners of skin cancers.

epidermoid — **Resembling squamous epithelial cells (thin, plate-like);** often occurring in the respiratory tract.

follicular — **Forming small glandular sacs.** Thyroid gland cancer and lymphomas are examples (Figure 19-9A).

papillary — **Forming small, finger-like or nipple-like projections of cells.** Bladder and thyroid cancers are examples (Figure 19-9B).

pleomorphic — **Composed of a variety of types of cells.** Mixed-cell tumors are examples.

scirrhous — **Densely packed** (scirrhous means hard) **tumors, due to dense bands of fibrous tissue;** commonly found in breast or stomach cancers.

undifferentiated — **Lacking microscopic structures typical of normal mature cells.**

GRADING AND STAGING SYSTEMS

Tumors are classified on the basis of tissue of origin, microscopic appearance, and extent of spread. Of particular importance are the tumor's **grade** (its degree of maturity or differentiation under the microscope) and its **stage** (its extent of spread within the body). These two properties influence the prognosis (the chances of successful treatment and survival) and determine the specific treatment to be used.

When **grading** a tumor, the pathologist is concerned with the microscopic appearance of the tumor cells, specifically with their degree of maturation or differentiation. Often, three or four grades are used. **Grade I** tumors are very well differentiated, so that they closely resemble cells from the normal parent tissue of their origin. **Grade IV** tumors are so undifferentiated or anaplastic that even recognition of the tumor's tissue of origin may be difficult. **Grades II** and **III** are intermediate in appearance, moderately or poorly differentiated, as opposed to well differentiated (grade I) and undifferentiated (grade IV).

Grading is often of value in determining the prognosis of certain types of cancers, such as cancer of the urinary bladder, prostate gland and ovary, and brain tumors (astrocytomas). Patients with grade I tumors have a high survival rate, and patients with grade II, III, and IV tumors have an increasingly poorer survival rate. Grading is also used in evaluating cells obtained from body fluids in preventive screening tests, such as **Papanicolaou (Pap) smears** of the uterine cervix.

The **staging** of cancerous tumors is based on the extent of spread of the tumor. It relies on careful definition of the size and spread of the tumor, using CT, PET/CT, and MRI scans and radionuclide (radioactive) bone scans. See Figure 19-15, page 826, for a PET/CT scan showing lymph node metastases. An example of a staging system is the tumor-node-metastasis **(TNM) International Staging System.** It has been applied to malignancies such as lung cancer, as well as to many other tumors. In this staging system, **T** specifies the size and degree of local extension of the **tumor; N** is the number of regional lymph **nodes** that have been invaded by tumor; and **M** specifies the presence or absence of **metastases** (spreads to distant sites) of the tumor cells. Numbers denote size and degree of involvement: For example, 0 indicates undetectable, and 1, 2, 3, and 4, a progressive increase in size or involvement. TNM staging may be based on clinical data (physical examination and radiologic assessment) or actual histopathologic evaluation of the tumor and adjacent lymph nodes. In some cases, bone marrow, liver, or other tissues are biopsied to confirm metastases. Table 19-5 presents the TNM staging system for non–small cell lung cancer. Once the T, N, and M categories have been assigned, then this information is combined to give an overall stage grouping of I, II, III, or IV.

TABLE 19-5 INTERNATIONAL TNM STAGING SYSTEM FOR NON–SMALL CELL LUNG CANCER

Categories of Stages for T, N, and M

T = primary tumor

Tx Positive cytologic malignant findings; no tumor can be found
Tis Carcinoma in situ; cancer only in top layers of cells; no deep invasion
T1 Tumor is <3 cm (1 1/4 inches) diameter; **T1a** = 2 cm or less; **T1b** = between 2 and 3 cm
T2 Tumor is between 3 and 7 cm across; **T2a** = 5 cm or less; **T2b** = between 5 and 7 cm
T3 Tumor larger than 7 cm across and grown into chest wall, diaphragm, mediastinal pleura, or pericardium
T4 Tumor invades the mediastinum, heart, aorta, trachea, or esophagus

N = regional lymph nodes

N0 No node involvement
N1 Ipsilateral (same side as primary tumor) bronchopulmonary or hilar nodes involved
N2 Ipsilateral mediastinal nodes or ligament involved
N3 Contralateral (opposite side) mediastinal, hilar, supraclavicular (collarbone) nodes involved

M = distant metastases

M0 No metastases
M1 Metastases present with site specified (e.g. brain, liver)

Stage Grouping	TNM Description		U.S. 5-Year Survival Rate
I A	T1, N0, M0	T1a/T1b, N0, M0	75%
I B	T2, N0, M0	T2a, N0, M0	55%
II A	T1, N1, M0 T2a, N1, M0	T1a/T1b, N1, M0 T2b, N0, M0	50%
II B	T2b, N1, M0	T3, N0, M0	40%
III A	T1-3, N2, M0 T4, N0/N1, M0	T3, N1, M0	10–35%
III B	Any T, N3, M0	T4, N2, M0	5%
IV	Any T, any N, M1		<5%

CANCER TREATMENT

Four major approaches to cancer treatment are **surgery, radiation therapy, chemotherapy,** and **biological therapy.** Each method **(modality)** may be used alone, but often they are used together in combined-modality regimens to improve the overall diagnosis and treatment result.

SURGERY

In many patients with cancer, the tumor is discovered before it has spread, and it may be cured by surgical excision. Some common cancers in which surgery may be curative are those of the stomach, breast, colon, lung, and uterus (endometrium). Often, surgical removal of the primary tumor prevents local spread or complications, even in the presence of distant disease. A **debulking procedure** may be used to remove as much of the primary tumor mass as possible, even if the tumor is attached to a vital organ and cannot be completely removed. After removal of the primary tumor, the patient often receives **adjuvant** (assisting) radiation therapy and/or chemotherapy to prevent recurrence at distant sites.

The following is a list of terms that describe surgical procedures used in diagnosing and treating cancer.

cauterization	Process of burning tissue to destroy it. Examples are electrocauterization (using a needle or snare heated by electric current), laser, dry ice, and chemicals.
core needle biopsy	Placement of a large-bore needle that extracts a thin core of tissue.
cryosurgery	Use of subfreezing temperature to destroy tissue.
en bloc resection	Tumor is removed along with a large area of surrounding tissue containing lymph nodes. Modified radical mastectomy, colectomy, and gastrectomy are examples.
excisional biopsy	Removal of tumor and a margin of normal tissue. This procedure provides a specimen for diagnosis and may be curative for small noninvasive tumors.
exenteration	Wide resection involving removal of the tumor, its organ of origin, and all surrounding tissue in the body space. Pelvic exenteration with removal of the uterus, ovaries, bladder, and segments of the large bowel may be performed to treat large primary tumors of the uterus.
fine needle aspiration	Placement of a very thin needle inside the tumor mass and extracting cells for microscopic evaluation.
fulguration	Destruction of tissue by electric sparks generated by a high-frequency current.
incisional biopsy	Piece of tumor is removed for examination to establish a diagnosis. More extensive surgical procedure or other forms of treatment, such as chemotherapy or radiation therapy, are then used to treat the bulk of the tumor.

RADIATION THERAPY (RADIATION ONCOLOGY)

The goal of **radiation therapy (RT)** is to deliver a maximal dose of ionizing radiation to the tumor tissue and a minimal dose to the surrounding normal tissue. High-dose **irradiation** (exposure of tissue to radiation) destroys tumor cells and produces damage to DNA. Newer techniques of irradiation use high-energy beams of **protons** (sub-atomic particles) to improve the uniformity (conformality) of dose and to limit damage to normal tissues.

Terms used in the field of radiation therapy for cancer are as follows:

brachytherapy — Implantation of small, sealed containers or seeds of radioactive material directly into the tumor (interstitial therapy); or in a cavity of the tumor (intracavitary therapy, as in endometrial cancer). An implant may be temporary (as in treatment for tumors of the head and neck or gynecologic malignancies) or permanent (as with prostatic implants, or "seeds," placed into the affected area of the gland).

electron beams — Low-energy beams for treatment of skin or surface tumors.

external beam irradiation (teletherapy) — Radiation therapy applied to a tumor from a distant source (linear accelerator).

fields — Dimensions of the size of radiation area used to treat a tumor from a specific angle.

fractionation — A method of dividing radiation into small, repeated doses rather than fewer large doses. Fractionation allows larger total doses to be given while causing less damage to normal tissue.

gray (Gy) — Unit of absorbed radiation dose. Historically, the unit in use was **rad** (100 rad equal 1 Gy).

linear accelerator — Large electronic device that produces high-energy x-ray (or photon) beams for the treatment of deep-seated tumors (Figure 19-10). Intraoperative radiation therapy (IORT) is direct application of radiation during surgery using a linear accelerator in the operating room.

photon therapy — Radiation therapy using x-rays or gamma rays. A linear accelerator produces photon beams to treat tumors. See the ***In Person*** account of a woman undergoing radiotherapy on page 828.

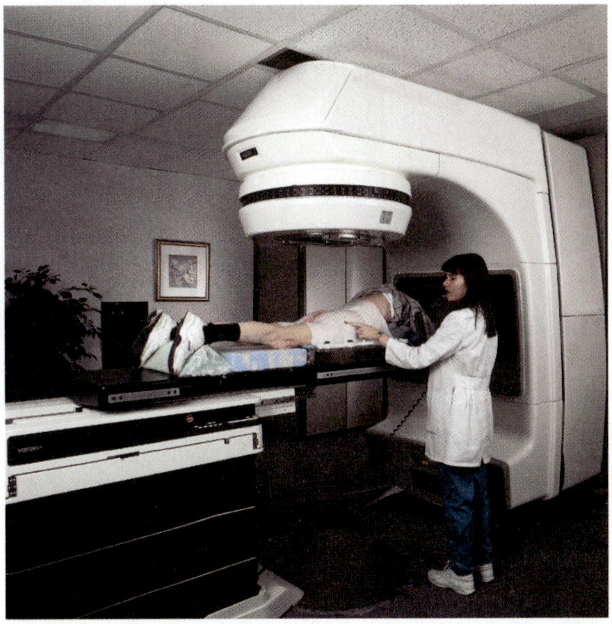

FIGURE 19-10 Linear accelerator. Radiation therapy (photon therapy) delivered to a patient positioned under a linear accelerator. **Intensity-modulated radiation therapy (IMRT)** is an advanced mode of high-precision radiotherapy that uses computer-controlled linear accelerators to deliver precise radiation doses to a malignant tumor. This is a type of **conformal radiation therapy** that uses computer technology to create a three-dimensional image of a tumor so that rotating beams can shape exactly to the contour of the tumor. *(Courtesy Dr. Arthur Brimberg, Riverhill Radiation Oncology, Yonkers, New York.)*

19

proton therapy	Small subatomic positively charged particles (protons) produced by a cyclotron deposit all the absorbed dose at a focused finite point. This reduces the dose affecting normal surrounding tissues by at least 50% (Figure 19-11A).
radiocurable tumor	Tumor that can be completely eradicated by radiation therapy. Usually, this is a localized tumor with no evidence of metastasis. Lymphomas, Hodgkin disease, and seminomas of the testes are examples (Figure 19-12).
radioresistant tumor	Tumor that requires large doses of radiation to produce death of the cells. Melanoma and renal carcinoma are the most radioresistant.
radiosensitive tumor	Tumor in which irradiation can cause the death of cells without serious damage to surrounding tissue **(morbidity).** Tumors of hematopoietic (blood-forming) and lymphatic origins are radiosensitive.
radiosensitizers	Drugs that increase the sensitivity of tumors to x-rays. Many cancer chemotherapy drugs, especially 5-fluorouracil and cisplatin, sensitize tumors and normal tissue to radiation, thereby improving the outcome of treatment.
simulation	Study prior to radiation therapy using CT scan and/or MRI to map treatment. Simulation is required for all patients undergoing RT.
stereotactic radiosurgery	Single large dose of radiation (Gamma Knife surgery) delivered from several different angles under stereotactic (highly precise) guidance to destroy a vascular abnormality (**arteriovenous malformation**, which is a tangle of blood vessels in the brain) or to treat small intracranial tumors (see Figure 19-11B).

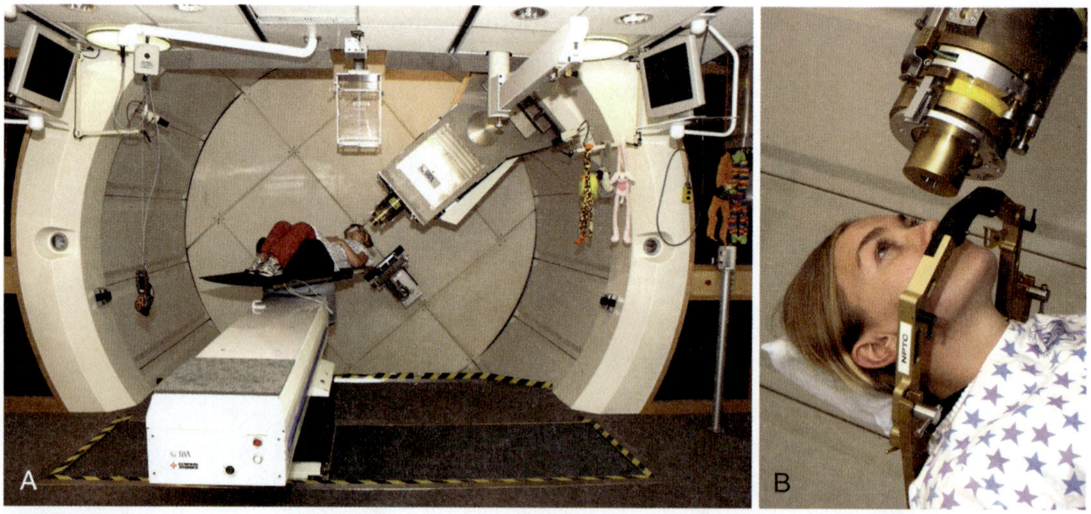

FIGURE 19-11 **A, Proton therapy machine.** Proton beam radiation therapy is useful in treating a variety of cancers including tumors of the head and neck, brain, eye, and prostate. **B, Proton stereotactic radiosurgery.** A model poses to show how a proton beam device is brought near a patient in preparation for stereotactic radiosurgery. *(Courtesy Dr. Jay Loeffler, Radiation Oncology Department, Massachusetts General Hospital, Boston.)*

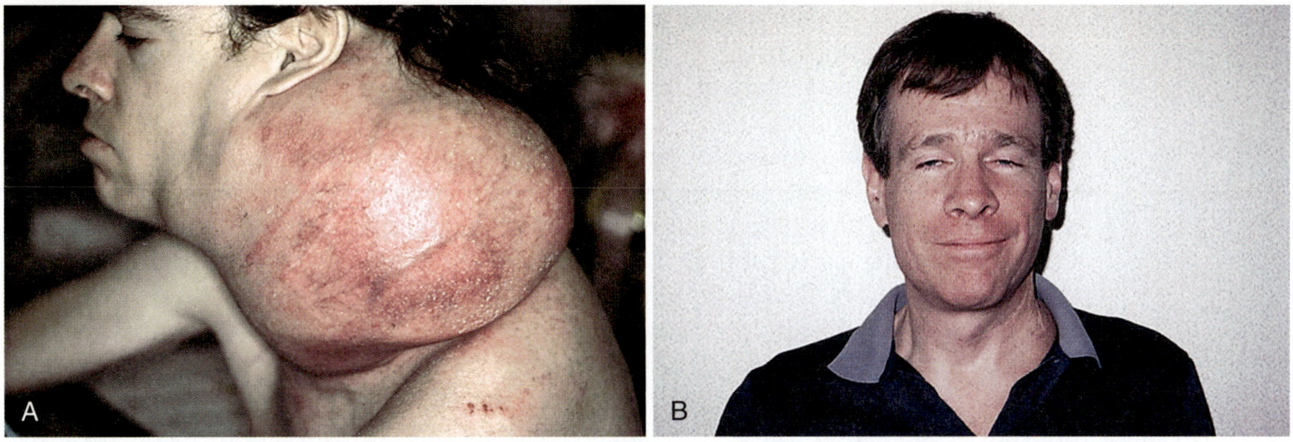

FIGURE 19-12 **A, Patient with Hodgkin disease before radiation therapy. B, The same patient 6 years after radiation therapy.**

Radiotherapy, although it may be either **palliative** (relieving symptoms) or curative, can produce undesirable side effects on normal body tissues that are incidentally irradiated. Some complications due to irradiation of normal tissue surrounding the tumor and in the path of the beam of photons may be reversible with time, and recovery takes place soon after radiotherapy is completed. Side effects include the following:

Alopecia (baldness)—may be permanent or temporary with radiation therapy
Fibrosis (increase in connective tissue) in normal tissues
Infertility (inability to contribute to conception of a child)
Mucositis (inflammation and ulceration of mucous membranes)—in the mouth, pharynx, vagina, bladder, or large or small intestine
Myelosuppression (bone marrow depression)—anemia, leukopenia, and thrombocytopenia
Nausea and vomiting—as reaction to radiation therapy to the brain (vomiting center is located in the brainstem) or gastrointestinal tract (loss of epithelial lining tissue)
Pneumonitis (inflammation of the lungs)
Secondary tumors (new types of tumors, originating at a site separate from the primary tumor)—including sarcomas or carcinomas, or leukemias that may arise from damaged tissue
Xerostomia (dryness of the mouth)—occurs after radiation therapy to the salivary glands

CHEMOTHERAPY, BIOLOGICAL THERAPY, AND DIFFERENTIATING AGENTS

Chemotherapy

Cancer chemotherapy is the treatment of cancer using chemicals (drugs). It is the standard treatment for many types of cancer, and it produces cures in most patients who have testicular cancer, acute lymphocytic leukemia (children), and Hodgkin disease. Chemotherapy may be used alone or in combination with surgery and irradiation to improve cure rates.

The ideal is to administer drugs that kill large numbers of tumor cells without harming normal cells. Because normal cells, such as bone marrow and gastrointestinal lining cells, have a rapidly dividing cell population, they suffer considerable damage from antitumor drugs. Scientists working in the field of pharmacokinetics measure the rate of disappearance of drugs from the bloodstream and tissues. They also use information from animal experiments and clinical trials to design better routes (oral, intravenous) and schedules of administration to achieve the greatest tumor kill with the least toxicity (harm) to normal cells.

Combination chemotherapy is the use of two or more antitumor drugs together to kill a specific type of malignant growth. In chemotherapy, drugs are given according to a written **protocol,** or plan, that details the route, schedule, and frequency of doses administered. Usually, drug therapy is continued until the patient achieves a complete **remission,** the absence of all signs of disease. At times, chemotherapy is an **adjuvant** (aid) to surgery. Drugs are used to kill possible hidden disease in patients who, after surgery, are otherwise free of any evidence of malignancy.

Drugs cause tumor cells to die by damaging their DNA. Tumor cells with damaged DNA undergo **apoptosis,** or self-destruction. They have impaired capacity to repair their DNA and, in general, are less able than normal cells to survive DNA damage due to drugs and radiation.

The following are categories of cancer chemotherapeutic agents. For your reference, Table 19-6 lists the specific drugs in each of these categories and the particular cancers they are used to treat.

1. **Alkylating agents.** These are synthetic compounds containing one or two alkyl groups. The chemicals interfere with the process of DNA synthesis by attaching to DNA molecules. Toxic side effects include nausea and vomiting, diarrhea, bone marrow depression (myelosuppression), and alopecia (hair loss). These are common side effects because cells in the gastrointestinal tract, bone marrow, and scalp are rapidly dividing cells that, along with tumor cells, are susceptible to the lethal effects of chemotherapeutic drugs. Most side effects disappear after treatment is suspended.
2. **Antibiotics.** These drugs are produced by bacteria or fungi. Most act by binding to DNA in the cell, thus promoting DNA strand breaks and preventing the replication or copying of DNA. Toxic side effects include alopecia, stomatitis (inflammation of the mouth), myelosuppression, and gastrointestinal disturbances.
3. **Antimetabolites.** These drugs inhibit the synthesis of nucleotide components of DNA, or they may act as fraudulent copies of normal nucleotides and become incorporated into the DNA strand, where they directly block the replication of DNA. Toxic side effects are myelosuppression with leukopenia, thrombocytopenia, and anemia; and damage to cells that line the mouth and digestive tract, leading to stomatitis, nausea, and vomiting.

Clinical Trials

Clinical trials are research studies designed to find treatments that work for patients. The studies follow a predefined protocol and are divided into four phases:

Phase I: The experimental drug or treatment is tested in a small group of people (20 to 80) for the first time to evaluate its safety. Phase I trials also determine a safe dosage range and schedule of administration (daily or weekly, oral or intravenous, and so on).

Phase II: Experimental treatment is given to a larger group of people (200 to 300) to identify tumor response rate and define safety risks for patients with a specific type of cancer.

Phase III: A larger and more definitive trial is conducted in which hundreds or thousands of subjects take part. Patients are randomly assigned to the new treatment or to a standard, established treatment. The effectiveness and overall risk-versus-benefit ratio for the experimental treatment are compared with those for standard treatment. A new drug may be approved by the FDA (U.S. Food and Drug Administration) based on these results.

Phase IV: Large studies are conducted after the FDA has granted its initial approval of a new treatment for marketing. These trials are designed to monitor safety in large populations and identify new indications beyond those already approved.

TABLE 19-6 SELECTED CANCER CHEMOTHERAPEUTIC AGENTS AND THE CANCERS THEY TREAT

Chemotherapeutic Agent	Type of Cancer
Alkylating Agents	
Bendamustine (Ribomustine)	Non-Hodgkin lymphoma
Carmustine (BCNU)	Brain
Carboplatin (Paraplatin)	Ovarian
Cisplatin (Platinol)	Testicular; ovarian
Cyclophosphamide (Cytoxan)	Lymphoma
Dacarbazine (DTIC-Dome)	Hodgkin lymphoma
Temozolomide (Temodar)	Brain (glioma)
Antibiotics	
Bleomycin (Blenoxane)	Testicular
Daunorubicin (Cerubidine)	Acute myelogenous leukemia (AML)
Doxorubicin (Adriamycin, Doxil)	Breast
Antimetabolites	
Capecitabine (Xeloda)	Breast and colon
Cladribine (Leustatin)	Hairy cell leukemia
Cytarabine (ara-C, Cytosar-U)	Acute myelogenous leukemia (AML)
Fludarabine (Fludara)	Chronic lymphocytic leukemia (CLL)
5-Fluorouracil (5-FU) (various)	Colon
Gemcitabine (Gemzar)	Pancreatic cancer
Methotrexate, MTX (Folex, Mexate)	Acute lymphocytic leukemia (ALL)
Pemetrexed (Alimta)	Lung cancer
Antimitotics	
Docetaxel (Taxotere)	Breast
Paclitaxel (Taxol)	Breast, ovary
Vinblastine (Velban)	Lymphoma
Vincristine (Oncovin)	Lymphoma
Vinorelbine (Navelbine)	Breast
Hormones and Hormone Antagonists	
Abiraterone (Zyliga)	Prostate cancer
Dexamethasone (Decadron)	Lymphoma
Flutamide (Eulexin)	Prostate
Letrozole (Femara)	Breast
Leuprolide (Lupron)	Prostate
Prednisone (various)	Acute lymphocytic leukemia (ALL)
Tamoxifen (Nolvadex)	Breast

Note: Brand names are in parentheses. Often drugs are given in combinations according to carefully planned regimens called **protocols.**

4. **Antimitotics.** These chemicals are derived from bacteria, fungi, or plants or from animals found on coral reefs or in the ocean. **Paclitaxel (Taxol)** and the vinca alkaloids are isolated from plants and block the function of the cell structural protein, the microtubule, which is essential for mitosis. They are used frequently in combination with other chemotherapeutic agents. Side effects include myelosuppression, alopecia, and nerve damage.
5. **Hormonal agents.** Hormones are a class of chemicals made by endocrine glands in the body. Examples are estrogens made in the ovaries and androgens made in the testes and adrenal glands. Hormones attach to receptor proteins in target tissues. The hormone-receptor complex stimulates certain normal tissues, such as breast or uterine lining cells, to divide and grow. Some tumors, such as prostate cancers, depend on the presence of a hormone (in this case, androgens) to grow, and hormone removal (orchiectomy) leads to tumor regression. Steroid (cholesterol-derived) hormones, such as prednisone, have growth-inhibiting effects on leukemias and breast cancer. Other compounds, called hormone antagonists, are designed to block the growth-promoting effects of estrogens or androgens, and are used in breast cancer and prostate cancer, respectively.

Breast cancers have **estrogen receptors.** These tumors respond to the removal of estrogen by oophorectomy or the use of antiestrogen drugs, such as **tamoxifen,** which block estrogenic effects. **Flutamide** blocks androgen action and causes regression of prostate cancer. **Aromatase inhibitors,** such as anastrozole, prevent the conversion of androgen to estrogen, and starve breast tumors of their estrogen supply in postmenopausal women.

Figure 19-13 illustrates the mechanisms of action for various types of cancer chemotherapeutic agents. Often, drugs are administered in combination, according to carefully planned **protocols** (regimens). Consult the Evolve site for Chapter 19 to see examples of cancer chemotheraputic protocols.

A new class of anticancer drugs are **molecularly targeted drugs.** These drugs are designed to block the function of growth factors, their receptors, and abnormal or overactive signaling pathways in tumor cells.

Tumor cells can also grow by establishing a new blood supply via **angiogenesis** (growth of new blood vessels). Tumors secrete specific proteins, such as **vascular endothelial growth factor (VEGF),** which stimulates the formation of new vessels. **Antiangiogenic drugs** interfere with angiogenesis and stop the growth of new blood vessels. An example of this type of drug is **Avastin** (bevacizumab), a monoclonal antibody that destroys VEGF.

Molecularly Targeted Drugs

Examples are:

Gleevec (imatinib mesylate)—blocks Bcr-Abl tyrosine kinase in chronic myelogenous leukemia cells.
Tarceva (erlotinib)—blocks epidermal growth factor (EGFR) in lung cancer cells.
Zelboraf (vemurafenib)—blocks mutated BRAF enzyme in 50% of melanoma patients.

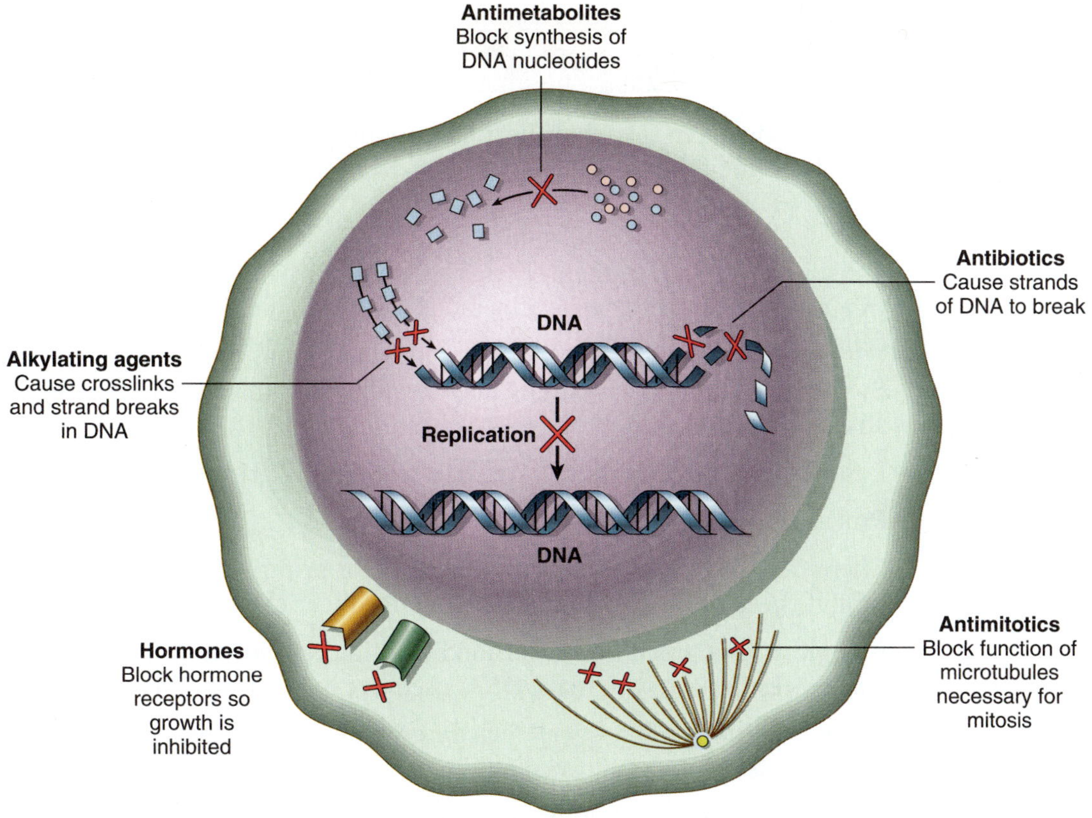

FIGURE 19-13 **Mechanisms of action of cancer chemotherapeutic agents.**

Biological Therapy

Another approach to cancer treatment is to use the body's own defenses to fight tumor cells. Investigators are exploring how the elements of the immune system can be restored, enhanced, mimicked, and manipulated to destroy cancer cells. Substances produced by normal cells that directly block tumor growth or that stimulate the immune system and other body defenses are called **biological response modifiers.** Examples of these substances are **interferons** (made by lymphocytes), **monoclonal antibodies** (made by mouse or human immune cells and capable of binding to human tumors), **colony-stimulating factors (CSFs)** that stimulate blood-forming cells to combat the myelosuppressive side effects of chemotherapy, and **interleukins** that stimulate the immune system to destroy tumors. Consult the Evolve website for Chapter 19 for specific biological agents and their modes of action.

Differentiating Agents

Some new drugs cause tumor cells to differentiate, stop growing, and die. These include **ATRA (all-*trans* retinoic acid),** a vitamin A derivative, that is highly active against acute promyelocytic leukemia (APL), and **arsenic trioxide (Trisenox),** which has similar effects on APL. Consult the Evolve website for Chapter 19 for a list of the newest anticancer drugs with their modes of action.

VOCABULARY

This list reviews many of the new terms introduced in the text. Short definitions reinforce your understanding of the terms. Refer to the Pronunciation of Terms section, p. 841 for help with unfamiliar or difficult words.

adjuvant therapy	Assisting primary treatment. Drugs are given early in the course of treatment, along with surgery or radiation to attack deposits of cancer cells that may be too small to be detected by diagnostic techniques.
alkylating agents	Synthetic chemicals containing alkyl groups that attack DNA, causing strand breaks.
anaplasia	Loss of differentiation of cells; reversion to a more primitive cell type.
angiogenesis	Process of forming new blood vessels.
antibiotics	Chemical substances, produced by bacteria or primitive plants. They inhibit the growth of cells and are used in cancer chemotherapy.
antimetabolites	Chemicals that prevent cell division by inhibiting formation of substances necessary to make DNA; used in cancer chemotherapy.
antimitotics	Drugs that block mitosis (cell division). Taxol is an antimitotic used to treat breast and ovarian cancers.
apoptosis	Programmed cell death. (Apo- means off, away; -ptosis means to fall.) Normal cells undergo apoptosis when damaged or aging. Some cancer cells have lost the ability to undergo apoptosis, and they live forever.
benign tumor	Noncancerous growth (neoplasm).
biological response modifiers	Substances produced by normal cells that either directly block tumor growth or stimulate the immune system to fight cancer.
biological therapy	Use of the body's own defenses to destroy tumor cells.
brachytherapy	Radiotherapy that uses insertion of sealed containers into body cavities or radioactive seeds directly into the tumor.
carcinogens	Agents that cause cancer: chemicals and drugs, radiation, and viruses.
carcinoma	Cancerous tumor made up of cells of epithelial origin.
cellular oncogenes	Pieces of DNA that, when activated by mutations or by dislocation, can cause a normal cell to become malignant.
chemotherapy	Treatment with drugs.
combination chemotherapy	Use of several chemotherapeutic agents together for the treatment of tumors.
dedifferentiation	Loss of differentiation of cells; reversion to a more primitive, embryonic cell type; anaplasia or undifferentiation.
deoxyribonucleic acid (DNA)	Genetic material within the nucleus of a cell; controls cell division and protein synthesis.
differentiating agents	Drugs that promote tumor cells to differentiate, stop growing, and die.
differentiation	Specialization of cells.

electron beams	Low-energy beams of radiation for treatment of skin or surface tumors.
encapsulated	Surrounded by a capsule; benign tumors are encapsulated.
external beam irradiation	Applying radiation to a tumor from a source outside the body.
fields	Dimensions of the area of the body undergoing irradiation.
fractionation	Giving radiation in small, repeated doses.
genetic screening	Family members are tested to determine whether they have inherited a cancer-causing gene.
grading of tumors	Evaluating the degree of maturity of tumor cells or indication of malignant transformation.
gray (Gy)	Unit of absorbed radiation dose.
gross description of tumors	Visual appearance of tumors to the naked eye: cystic, fungating, inflammatory, medullary, necrotic, polypoid, ulcerating, or verrucous.
infiltrative	Extending beyond normal tissue boundaries into adjacent tissues.
invasive	Having the ability to enter and destroy surrounding tissue.
irradiation	Exposure to any form of radiant energy such as light, heat, or x-rays.
linear accelerator	Large electronic device that produces high-energy x-ray beams for treatment of deep-seated tumors.
malignant tumor	A tumor having the characteristics of continuous growth, invasiveness, and metastasis.
mesenchymal	Embryonic connective tissue (mes = middle, enchym/o = to pour). This is the tissue from which connective tissues (bone, muscle, fat, cartilage) arise.
metastasis	Spread of a malignant tumor to a secondary site; literally, beyond (meta-) control (-stasis).
microscopic description of tumors	Appearance of tumors when viewed under a microscope: alveolar, carcinoma in situ, diffuse, dysplastic, epidermoid, follicular, papillary, pleomorphic, scirrhous, or undifferentiated.
mitosis	Replication of cells; a stage in a cell's life cycle involving the production of two identical cells from a parent cell.
mixed-tissue tumors	Tumors composed of different types of tissue (epithelial as well as connective tissue).
modality	Method of treatment, such as surgery, chemotherapy, or irradiation.
molecularly targeted drugs	Anticancer drugs designed to block the function of growth factors, their receptors, and signaling pathways in specific tumor cells.
morbidity	Condition of being unwell or deficient in normal function.
mucinous	Containing mucus.
mutation	Change in the genetic material (DNA) of a cell; may be caused by chemicals, radiation, or viruses or may occur spontaneously.
neoplasm	New growth; benign or malignant tumor.
nucleotide	Unit of DNA (gene) composed of a sugar, phosphate, and a base. The sequence or arrangement of nucleotides on a gene is the genetic code.

oncogene	Region of DNA in tumor cells (cellular oncogene) or in viruses that cause cancer (viral oncogene). Oncogenes are designated by a three-letter name, such as *abl*, *erb*, *jun*, *myc*, *ras*, and *src*.
palliative	Relieving but not curing symptoms.
pedunculated	Possessing a stem or stalk (peduncle); characteristic of some polypoid tumors.
photon therapy	Radiation therapy using energy in the form of x-rays or gamma rays.
protocol	Detailed plan for treatment of an illness.
proton therapy	Subatomic positively charged particles (protons) produced by a cyclotron deposit a dose of radiation at a tightly focused point in the body.
radiation	Energy carried by a stream of particles.
radiocurable tumor	Tumor that is destroyed by radiation therapy.
radioresistant tumor	Tumor that requires large doses of radiation to be destroyed.
radiosensitive tumor	Tumor in which radiation can cause the death of cells without serious damage to surrounding tissue.
radiosensitizers	Drugs that increase the sensitivity of tumors to x-rays.
radiotherapy	Treatment of tumors using doses of radiation; radiation oncology.
relapse	Recurrence of tumor after treatment.
remission	Partial or complete disappearance of symptoms of disease.
ribonucleic acid (RNA)	Cellular substance that represents a copy of DNA and directs the formation of new protein inside cells.
sarcoma	Cancerous tumor derived from connective or flesh tissue.
serous	Having the appearance of a thin, watery fluid (serum).
sessile	Having no stem; characteristic of some polypoid tumors.
simulation	Study using CT scan or MRI to map treatment before with radiotherapy is given.
solid tumor	Tumor composed of a mass of cells.
staging of tumors	System of evaluating the extent of spread of tumors. An example is the TNM (tumor-node-metastasis) system.
stereotactic radiosurgery	Delivery of dose of radiation under stereotactic (highly precise) guidance (Gamma Knife surgery).
steroids	Complex, naturally occurring chemicals derived from cholesterol. Some are used in cancer chemotherapy.
surgical procedures to treat cancer	Methods of removing cancerous tissue: cryosurgery, cauterization, en bloc resection, excisional biopsy, exenteration, fulguration, incisional biopsy.
viral oncogenes	Pieces of DNA from viruses that infect a normal cell and cause it to become malignant.
virus	An infectious agent that reproduces by entering a host cell and using the host's genetic material to make copies of itself.

TERMINOLOGY

Write the meanings of the medical terms in the spaces provided.

COMBINING FORMS

COMBINING FORM	MEANING	TERMINOLOGY	MEANING
alveol/o	small sac	alveolar *Microscopic description of tumor cell arrangement (found in connective tissue tumors).*	
cac/o	bad	cachexia *General ill health and malnutrition (wasting of muscle and emaciation) associated with chronic, severe disease (-hexia means state or condition).*	
carcin/o	cancer, cancerous	carcinoma in situ *Localized cancer; confined to the site of origin.*	
cauter/o	burn, heat	electrocauterization	
chem/o	chemical, drug	chemotherapy	
cry/o	cold	cryosurgery	
cyst/o	sac of fluid	cystic tumor	
fibr/o	fibers	fibrosarcoma	
follicul/o	small glandular sacs	follicular *A microscopic description of cellular arrangement in glandular tumors.*	
fung/i	fungus, mushroom	fungating tumor	
medull/o	soft, inner part	medullary tumor	
mucos/o	mucous membrane	mucositis	
mut/a	genetic change	mutation *-tion means process.*	
mutagen/o	causing genetic change	mutagenic	
necr/o	death	necrotic tumor	

19

COMBINING FORM	MEANING	TERMINOLOGY	MEANING
neur/o	nerve	neurofibromatosis *Fibromas are tumors of fibrous connective tissue. Tumors begin in supporting cells of nerves and the myelin sheath around nerve cells. Most tumors are benign but some may become cancerous. It is a genetic disorder occurring in 1 in 3000 births, but some cases arise via spontaneous mutation.*	______
onc/o	tumor	oncology	______
papill/o	nipple-like	papillary *A microscopic description of tumor cell growth.*	______
plas/o	formation	dysplastic *Microscopic description of cells that are highly abnormal but not clearly cancerous. The suffix -tic means pertaining to.*	______
ple/o	many, more	pleomorphic *Microscopic description of tumors that are composed of a variety of cells.*	______
polyp/o	polyp	polypoid tumor *The suffix -oid means resembling.*	______
prot/o	first	protocol *The ending -col, from Latin kolla, means glued page. A protocol is a written plan detailing the procedures to be followed in research or treatment.*	______
radi/o	rays	radiation *Use of radioactive substances in the diagnosis and treatment of disease.* ***Irradiation*** *is exposure to any form of radiation (ionizing, heat, light, or x-rays).*	______
sarc/o	flesh, connective tissue	osteosarcoma	______
scirrh/o	hard	scirrhous *Microscopic description of densely packed, fibrous tumor cell composition.*	______
xer/o	dry	xerostomia	______

19

SUFFIXES

SUFFIX	MEANING	TERMINOLOGY	MEANING
-blastoma	immature tumor	retino<u>blastoma</u> *Childhood cancer arising from immature cells in the retina (posterior, light-sensitive area of the eye).*	___
		neuro<u>blastoma</u> *This sarcoma of nervous system origin affects infants and children up to the age of 10 years, usually arising in immature tissues of the autonomic nervous system or adrenal medulla.*	___
-genesis	formation	angio<u>genesis</u>	___
-oma	mass, tumor	adenocarcin<u>oma</u>	___
-plasia	formation, growth	hyper<u>plasia</u>	___
-plasm	formation, growth	neo<u>plasm</u>	___
-suppression	to stop	myelo<u>suppression</u>	___
-therapy	treatment	radio<u>therapy</u> *Ionizing radiation is used to treat malignancies.*	___

19

PREFIXES

PREFIX	MEANING	TERMINOLOGY	MEANING
ana-	backward	<u>ana</u>plasia	___
apo-	off, away	<u>apo</u>ptosis	___
brachy-	short (distance)	<u>brachy</u>therapy *Radiation delivered in close range to tumor site.*	___
epi-	upon	<u>epi</u>dermoid *Microscopic description of tumor cells that resemble epidermal tissue.*	___
meta-	beyond; change	<u>meta</u>stasis	___
		<u>meta</u>plasia *Abnormal transformation of adult differentiated cells to differentiated tissue of another kind. This change is reversible. An example is the change (from columnar epithelial cells to squamous epithelial cells) that occurs in the respiratory epithelium of habitual cigarette smokers.*	___
tele-	far	<u>tele</u>therapy *Also called **external beam radiotherapy.***	___

LABORATORY TESTS

cytogenetic analysis

Chromosomes of normal or tumor cells are examined for breaks, translocations, or deletions of DNA.

The results of cytogenetic analysis can help confirm the diagnosis of a particular form of leukemia or other cancer.

immunohistochemistry

Localizing antigens or proteins in tissues using labeled (colored or fluorescent) antibodies.

This technique allows for evaluation of the presence and amount of specific molecules in normal and tumor cells.

protein marker tests

Measure the level of proteins in the blood or on the surface of tumor cells.

These tests diagnose cancer or detect its recurrence after treatment. Examples are:

Protein	Where Measured	Type of Cancer
acid phosphatase	blood	prostate
alpha-fetoprotein (AFP)	blood	liver, testicular
beta-hCG	blood	choriocarcinoma, testicular
CA-125	blood	ovarian
CEA (carcinoembryonic antigen)	blood	colorectal, GI
estrogen receptor	tumor cells	breast
PSA (prostate-specific antigen)	blood	prostate
15.3 and 29.7	blood	breast
19.9	blood	pancreatic

CLINICAL PROCEDURES

The following are specialized procedures used to detect or treat malignancies. X-rays, CT scans, MRI, and ultrasound imaging (described throughout the text and specifically in Chapter 20) also are important diagnostic procedures in oncology.

bone marrow biopsy

Aspiration of bone marrow tissue and examination under a microscope for evidence of malignant cells.

bone marrow or stem cell transplantation

Bone marrow or stem cells are infused intravenously into a patient.

In **autologous marrow transplantation,** marrow previously obtained from the patient and stored is reinfused when needed. In **allogeneic marrow transplantation** (all/o = other), marrow is obtained from a living donor other than the recipient. In **peripheral blood stem cell transplantation,** immature blood cells called stem cells are selected and harvested from the blood of a patient instead of from the bone marrow. After undergoing chemotherapy, the patient gets a reinfusion of the stem cells to repopulate the bone marrow with blood cells.

core needle biopsy — **Insertion of a large-bore needle into tissue to remove a core of cells for microscopic examination.**

A needle (aspiration) biopsy is the insertion of a fine needle and aspiration (extraction) of a sample from a fluid-filled cavity or solid mass of tumor.

exfoliative cytology — **Cells are scraped from the region of suspected disease and examined under a microscope.**

The Pap test (smear) to detect carcinoma of the cervix and vagina is an example (Figure 19-14).

fiberoptic colonoscopy — **Visual examination of the colon using a fiberoptic instrument.**

This is an important screening procedure using an endoscope to detect cancer and remove premalignant polyps.

laparoscopy — **Visual examination of the abdominal cavity using small incisions and a laparoscope. Also known as peritoneoscopy.**

mammography — **X-ray examination of the breast to detect breast cancer.**

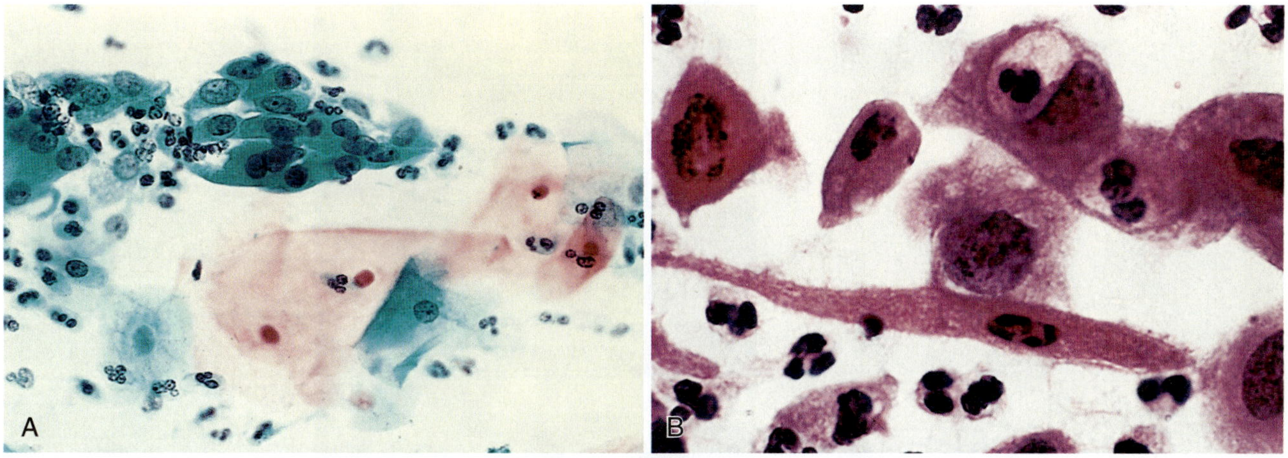

FIGURE 19-14 **A, Normal exfoliative cytological smear (Pap smear) from the cervicovaginal region.** It shows flattened squamous cells and some neutrophils as well. **B, Abnormal cervicovaginal smear** shows numerous malignant cells that have pleomorphic (irregularly shaped) and hyperchromatic (stained) nuclei. *(**A** and **B**, Courtesy Dr. P.K. Gupta, Department of Pathology and Laboratory Medicine, University of Pennsylvania Medical Center, Philadelphia.)*

PET/CT scan

Diagnostic procedure combining CT (computed tomography) and PET (positron emission tomography).

The combination provides a more complete picture of a tumor's location and growth or spread than either done independently. See Figure 19-15. PET/CT uses a combination of two machines: one to examine chemical reactions (PET scan) and the other to examine physical structures (CT scan).

radionuclide scans

Radioactive substances (radionuclides) are injected intravenously, and scans (images) of organs are obtained.

These tests detect tumor and metastases. Examples of radionuclides are gallium-67 (whole-body scan), rose Bengal (liver), and technetium-99m (liver and spleen).

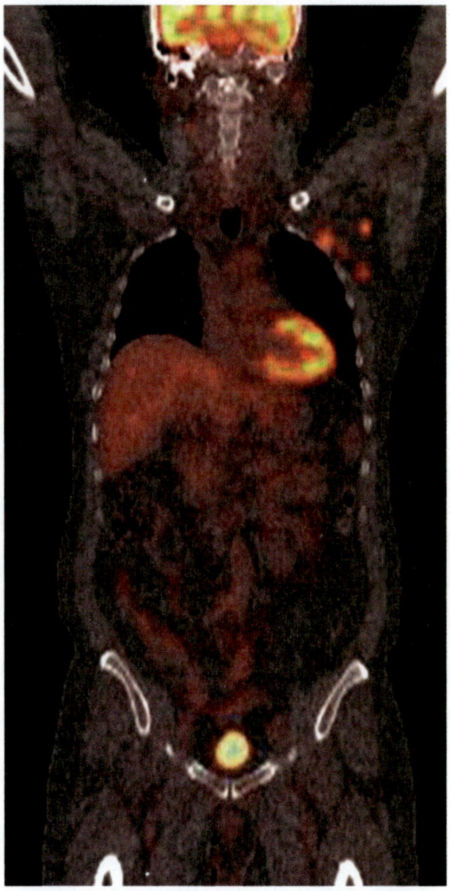

FIGURE 19-15 PET/CT scan. The PET/CT scan captures three areas of increased radioactivity, in the lymph nodes of the left axilla (armpit). By overlaying PET and CT images, physicians can identify spread of malignancy or metastasis. *(Courtesy Massachusetts General Hospital, Boston, Massachusetts.)*

ABBREVIATIONS

AFP	alpha-fetoprotein
ATRA	all-*trans* retinoic acid—treatment for acute myelogenous leukemia
BMT	bone marrow transplantation
bx	biopsy
CA	cancer
CEA	carcinoembryonic antigen
cGy	centigray (one hundredth of a gray) or rad
chemo	chemotherapy
CR	complete response—disappearance of all tumor
CSF	colony-stimulating factor—examples: G-CSF (granulocyte colony-stimulating factor) and GM-CSF (granulocyte-macrophage colony-stimulating factor)
DES	diethylstilbestrol
DNA	deoxyribonucleic acid
EGFR	epidermal growth factor receptor
ER	estrogen receptor
EPO	erythropoietin; promotes growth of red blood cells
FNA	fine needle aspiration
5-FU	5-fluorouracil
Ga	gallium
GIST	gastrointestinal stromal tumor
Gy	gray—unit of absorbed radiation dose
H&E	hematoxylin and eosin—a dye combination used to stain pathology specimens
HER2-neu	growth factor gene highly activated in cells of certain types of breast cancer
HNPCC	hereditary non-polyposis colorectal cancer
IGRT	intensity-modulated gated radiation therapy—use of imaging mechanism attached to linear accelerator is added to IMRT to gate (track) a tumor moving during respiration
IHC	immunohistochemistry
IMRT	intensity-modulated radiation therapy—high doses of radiation are delivered directly to cancer cells in a targeted way, more precisely than in conventional radiotherapy
IORT	intraoperative radiation therapy
Mets	metastases
MoAb	monoclonal antibody
NED	no evidence of disease
NF	neurofibromatosis
NHL	non-Hodgkin lymphoma
NSCLC	non–small cell lung cancer
Pap smear	Papanicolaou smear
PD	progressive disease—tumor increases in size
PR	partial response—tumor is one half its original size
prot.	protocol
PSA	prostate-specific antigen
PSCT	peripheral stem cell transplantation
PSRS	proton stereotactic radiosurgery
RNA	ribonucleic acid
RT	radiation therapy
SD	stable disease—tumor does not shrink but does not grow
TNM	tumor-nodes-metastases
VEGF	vascular endothelial growth factor
XRT, RT	radiation therapy

IN PERSON: RADIOTHERAPY

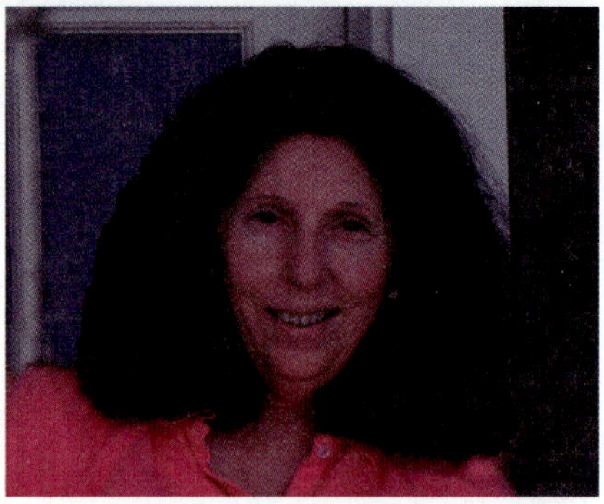

This first-person narrative describes a woman experiencing radiation therapy for breast cancer.

THE GOOD, THE BAD AND THE UGLY

My life changed forever when I got that phone call that no one wants to hear, "your biopsy is malignant." (See Mary's In Person piece in Chapter 8 describing the biopsy procedure.) So after they tell you that you have cancer, you are scared to death, begin to contemplate your mortality, and wonder how to break the news to your husband, children, loved ones and friends. You settle down, and marshal up your strength to fight this beast that attacks too many of us.

After my biopsy, I met with a team that included my surgeon, my radiation oncologist and my medical oncologist. It was decided that the best course of action was to perform a lumpectomy to remove the malignant tissue in my breast. At the same time, I would also have a sentinel node biopsy to check for lymphatic invasion. Surgery would be followed by a course of radiation therapy and then a 5-year regimen of the drug Tamoxifen.

Approximately three weeks after the surgery, which went very well thanks to my breast surgeon, I met with my radiation oncologist. She explained all the benefits and risks associated with radiation. She and her assistant exemplified one of the nicest things you can say about your doctors: their bedside manner. It was calming, supportive, and reassuring. We had a brief conversation as to the mechanics of beginning this phase of my treatment. Then I signed a very scary 4-page list of the minor and major side effects that could occur as a consequence of treatment.

19

I left their office and went home to clear my calendar, because every week for the next few weeks I would have to show up at the same time, same place, five days a week. For those of you who work full time as I do, it is a major disruption to your life. Even if you don't work full time, it is a hassle driving to the hospital, waiting for treatment and dealing with delays because the machines malfunction, etc. On my first appointment I did not receive any radiation. Instead, the technicians (with whom you will develop a close relationship), create your cradle. This is a mold that will hold you in the exact position for all of your treatments. After extensive calculations, I was marked on both sides of my body with a special kind of indelible ink. It was sort of a circle with an "x" in the middle, vaguely resembling an ancient hieroglyph. I also received a small permanent tattoo on the middle of my breast bone, which enables the machine to correctly target the beams.

THE FIRST TIME

Ever since I was a small child I have loved science fiction books and movies. My first experience with radiation reminded me of a true classic in that genre. Radiation treatment is very regimented; by that I mean they are on a very strict schedule. My daily time was 10:30 AM. This means that each day you should arrive 15 minutes early so that you can check in (they make a little plastic credit card for you to swipe when you come into to the main room and then go into the waiting area). Once you are in the waiting area, one of the technicians will come over and take your card, you will go to a locker room and change into a gown and come back and wait your turn to enter the chamber of horrors.

I had no idea what to expect as I was led into this cavernous room. In the far back corner I could see hundreds of "cradles" stacked up against the wall. They positioned me into my cradle on this bed; then they started to calibrate the machine against the markings on my body. When all the bodily GPS was in sync, they all scurried out of the room and went behind the giant lead walls (the cowards). When I was first ushered into the room the door was open. Now the door slowly started sliding shut and it sounded like a hundred heavy garage doors grinding across the floor. That door must have weighed several tons. After what seemed an eternity, a series of strange clicking noises commenced and the giant circular machine that hovered over me began to move closer, gyrating slowly back and forth until it was properly fixed. Suddenly a red sign began flashing on the wall warning that radiation was in progress. A huge pulse of light shot out and a humming sound began. The machine gradually rotated, irradiating different sections of my body. It only lasted about ten minutes, which was quite a relief. I was afraid I would be in there a long time. The technicians scattered back in, helped me out of my cradle and off I went to the locker room to change.

THE UGLY

As you can imagine this routine begins to wear on you. Fatigue from the radiation began to increase slowly, and redness appeared like a mild sunburn on the irradiated areas. Starting with the second week of treatment, my skin became extremely itchy and I developed folliculitis (inflammation of hair follicles). I applied cream twice a day, which helped, but didn't offer much relief.

I must say that the most disconcerting aspect of radiation treatment involved the daily routine and not the actual radiation itself. Patients must adhere to a strict schedule, and this means that you get to know the patients ahead of and behind you. They were my radiation buddies. During the course of my treatment, I met several very brave men and women, most of them with cancers more serious than my own. Sadly, at least two of my friends are no longer with us. One was a young woman in her mid-thirties with two small children. She suffered from bone cancer and was having palliative radiation. The cruelty and unfairness of life sat next to me every day. After my first week of treatment, I left the hospital and said to my friend, "I may have breast cancer, but after meeting all these people, I feel like one of the luckiest people in the world."

TREATMENT ENDS

It seemed like forever, but finally the day came for me to ring the bell. At Hopkins, on the last day of your treatment, you walk into the main hall and ring what looks like a small fire bell. Then you have your picture taken with one of your technicians. I thought it was over, but not quite! My oncologist explained to me that although the treatments were over, the effects of the radiation would keep working in my body. I called it the "gift that just keeps giving." Two weeks after my procedure ended, my skin broke down with blisters and bleeding in the worst possible places, the skin under my breast. Being a large breasted woman this was a horrid complication. Trying to wear a bra was out of the question until it finally healed. I didn't want to go to my office braless and my collection of underwire brassieres would have rubbed right against the raw part of my skin. I bought some very loose fitting tops and did a lot of work from home. Shooting pains would occur from the radiation, setting off nerve fibers, subsiding each month.

I am amazed at what my journey revealed. Most of all, it taught me about how wonderful friends can be, how much of a difference support groups can make, and why dedicated medical professionals deserve so much thanks and praise. A very lovely woman I met along the way shared some wisdom that I will pass along to all of you reading my story. She said, "At first cancer is your whole world, then it becomes a room, then it becomes a drawer in that room, and then it becomes a box in the drawer." I still take that box out once in a while, but not as often.

Mary Braun is Vice President, Investments at Chapin Davis, Baltimore, MD.

PRACTICAL APPLICATIONS

Answers to questions are on page 840.

FYI: OTHER MALIGNANT TUMORS

A number of malignant tumors do not contain the combining form carcin/o or sarc/o in their names:

MALIGNANT TUMOR	DESCRIPTION
glioma	primary brain tumor
hepatoma	liver tumor (hepatocellular carcinoma)
hypernephroma	kidney tumor
lymphoma	lymph node tumor
melanoma	tumor of pigmented skin cells
mesothelioma	tumor of cells within the pleura
multiple myeloma	bone marrow cell tumor
thymoma	thymus gland tumor

QUESTIONS ABOUT FYI: OTHER MALIGNANT TUMORS

1. Which tumor develops from a dysplastic nevus? ____________________
2. Which tumor arises from an organ located within the mediastinum? ____________________
3. Which tumor arises from an organ in the RUQ of the abdomen? ____________________
4. Which tumor has types called astrocytoma, ependymoma, glioblastoma multiforme?

   ____
5. Which tumor is also known as a renal cell carcinoma? ____________________
6. Which tumor is characterized by large numbers of plasma cells (bone marrow antibody-producing cells)? ____________________
7. Which tumor arises from membrane cells surrounding the lungs? ____________________
8. Which tumor has a type known as Hodgkin disease? ____________________

CASE STUDY: SUSPECTED BREAST CANCER

A 52-year-old married woman presented to her physician with a painless mass in her left breast. During breast examination a 1.0-cm, firm, nontender mass was palpated in the upper outer quadrant located at the 2 o'clock position, 3 cm from the areola. The mass was not fixed to the skin, and there was no cutaneous erythema or edema. No axillary or supraclavicular lymphadenopathy was noted.

An excisional biopsy of the mass was performed. The pathology report described a gross specimen of fatty breast tissue. Microscopic evaluation of the nodule revealed an invasive ductal carcinoma. The margins of the lumpectomy specimen were free of tumor. Sentinel node biopsy revealed no tumor involvement.

A portion of the specimen was sent for estrogen receptor assay and proved to be positive. The patient was informed of the diagnosis and underwent additional studies, including chest x-ray, liver chemistries, CBC, and bone scan; all results were negative.

The patient was staged as having a T1N0M0, stage I carcinoma of the left breast. She was referred to a radiation oncologist for primary radiation therapy. After completion of radiotherapy, she was treated with tamoxifen. Prognosis is excellent for cure.

Questions about the Case Study

1. Where was the primary breast lesion located?
   a. Under the pigmented area of the breast
   b. About an inch and a half above and to the left of the nipple and pigmented area
   c. Near the axilla and under the shoulder blade

2. Other associated findings were
   a. Redness and swelling
   b. Enlarged lymph nodes under the armpit
   c. None of the above

3. The tumor was composed of
   a. Dense connective tissue surrounding the tumor cells, giving it a hard structure
   b. Glandular tumor with invasion of surrounding tissue
   c. Cells that had extended into the skin overlying the tumor

4. What procedure gave evidence that the tumor had not yet metastasized?
   a. Estrogen receptor assay
   b. Excisional biopsy of the mass
   c. Sentinel node biopsy

5. What additional therapy was undertaken?
   a. Bone scan, liver chemistries, CBC, and chest x-ray
   b. Radiation to the breast
   c. Radiation to the breast and then treatment with an estrogen blocker

6. Tamoxifen was prescribed because
   a. The tumor was found to be nonresponsive to estrogen
   b. The tumor was found to be stimulated by estrogen, and tamoxifen is an antiestrogen
   c. The tumor was at an advanced stage

CHART ROUNDS REVIEW: CENTER FOR RADIATION ONCOLOGY

Patient A has metastatic lung carcinoma, with severe chest pain on deep breathing, and is being treated palliatively with 3000 cGy to the mid- and upper thorax.

Patient B is being treated for esophageal carcinoma. Because of previous treatment for breast cancer, the radiation dose to the recurrent field is limited to 3000 cGy.

Patient C is being treated for a pathologic stage IIB Hodgkin disease following the mantle [upper chest and neck]-only protocol.

Patient D is being treated for a GBM [glioblastoma multiforme]. The plan needs to be signed. The films look fine.

Questions about the Chart Rounds Review

1. Which patient is being treated for a brain tumor?
2. Which patient is being treated for lesions in the ribs?
3. Which patient has disease in cervical and thoracic lymph nodes?
4. Which patient is being treated for gastrointestinal cancer?

PATHOLOGY REPORT: RESECTED SPLEEN, GROSS DESCRIPTION

The spleen weighs 127 grams and measures 13.0 × 9.2 cm. External surface is smooth, leathery, homogeneous, and dark purplish brown. There are no defects in the capsule. The blood vessels of the hilum of the spleen are patent, with no thrombi or other abnormalities. On section of the spleen at 2- to 3-mm intervals, there are three well-defined, pale gray nodules on the cut surface, ranging from 0.5 to 1.1 cm in greatest dimension. The remainder of the cut surface is homogeneous and dark purple, and the tissue consistency is firm. *Possible diagnosis:* Hodgkin disease.

Question about the Pathology Report

1. Which information leads the pathologist to the diagnosis of metastatic cancer?
   a. Blood clots in patent blood vessels
   b. Capsular defects
   c. Uniform, smooth surface
   d. Examination of the spleen showed abnormal growth

19

SHORT HISTORIES

As you read these actual patient histories, congratulate yourself on your understanding of medical terms!

1. A 28-year-old man feels a hard, non-tender mass in his right testicle. He goes to his doctor, who checks his serum human chorionic gonadotropin and alpha fetoprotein levels and finds both quite elevated. The tentative diagnosis is a germ cell tumor of the testis. A CT scan of the abdomen reveals extensive lymphadenopathy. A chest CT shows nodes in both lungs suggestive of tumor. An orchiectomy confirms the diagnosis of testicular cancer. He is given four cycles of chemotherapy with vinblastine, cisplatin, and bleomycin and his serum AFP and HCG markers return to normal. His CT scans reveal no evidence of residual tumor.

2. A 42-year-old woman notices repeated episodes of red blood in her stool with each bowel movement. A colonoscopy reveals a 4-cm mass arising from the epithelium of the rectum. A biopsy demonstrates a rectal adenocarcinoma. An abdominal CT shows two large metastases in the liver and enlarged lymph nodes. She first receives 4 cycles of chemotherapy, which cause the liver lesions to shrink significantly and the lymph nodes to regress. The remaining liver lesions are surgically resected. Radiation therapy with chemotherapy (5-fluorouracil) is then administered to shrink the rectal tumor and lymph nodes, after which the rectal mass shrinks to a small 1-cm nodule. This is resected surgically. The lymph nodes are removed and contain no tumor.

3. A 62-year-old man has a routine PSA drawn. It is elevated at 5.8 (normal is less than 4.0). A transrectal biopsy of the prostate reveals a Gleason grade 6 adenocarcinoma in 4 of 12 biopsy pieces. He chooses to be treated with brachytherapy. Treatment causes dysuria, cystitis, and proctitis, but these symptoms disappear three weeks after therapy ends, and his PSA is now undetectable.

EXERCISES

Remember to check your answers carefully with those given in the Answers to Exercises, page 839.

A Identify the following characteristics of malignant tumors based on their definitions as given below. Word parts are given as clues.

1. loss of differentiation of cells and reversion to a more primitive cell type:

   ana ______________________
2. extending beyond the normal tissue boundaries: in ______________________
3. having the ability to enter and destroy surrounding tissue: in ______________________
4. spreading to a secondary site: meta ______________________

B Match the following terms or abbreviations with their meanings below.

chemical carcinogen	mitosis	RNA
DNA	mutation	ultraviolet radiation
ionizing radiation	oncogene	virus

1. replication of cells; two identical cells are produced from a parent cell ______________________
2. change in the genetic material of a cell ______________________
3. genetic material within the nucleus that controls replication and protein synthesis

   ____
4. cellular substance (ribonucleic acid) that is important in protein synthesis

   ____
5. rays given off by the sun; can be carcinogenic ______________________
6. energy carried by a stream of particles from a radioactive source; can be carcinogenic

   ____
7. infectious agent that reproduces by entering a host cell and using the host's genetic material to make copies of itself ______________________
8. a region of genetic material found in tumor cells and in viruses that cause cancer

   ____
9. an agent (hydrocarbon, insecticide, hormone) that causes cancer ______________________

C Give the meanings of the following terms.

1. solid tumor ______________________
2. adenoma ______________________
3. adenocarcinoma ______________________
4. osteoma ______________________

5. osteosarcoma ______________________________
6. mixed-tissue tumor ______________________________
7. neoplasm ______________________________
8. neurofibromatosis ______________________________
9. benign ______________________________
10. differentiation ______________________________

D Name the terms that describe tumor growth as seen through a microscope. Definitions and word parts are given.

1. small nipple-like projections: pap______________
2. abnormal formation of cells: dys______________
3. localized growth of cells: carcin______________
4. densely packed; containing fibrous tissue:______________ous
5. pattern resembling small, microscopic sacs: alv______________
6. small, round, gland-type clusters: foll______________
7. variety of cell types: pleo______________
8. lacking structures typical of mature cells: un______________
9. spreading evenly throughout the tissue: di______________
10. resembling epithelial cells: epiderm______________

E Match the following gross descriptions of tumors with their meanings as given below.

cystic	medullary	ulcerating
fungating	necrotic	verrucous
inflammatory	polypoid	

1. containing dead tissue ______________
2. mushrooming pattern of growth: tumor cells pile on top of each other ______________
3. characterized by large, open, exposed surfaces ______________
4. characterized by redness, swelling, and heat ______________
5. growths are projections from a base; sessile and pedunculated tumors are examples ______________
6. tumors form large, open spaces filled with fluid; serous and mucinous tumors are examples ______________
7. tumors resemble wart-like growths ______________
8. tumors are large, soft, and fleshy ______________

F Circle or supply the appropriate medical terms.

1. A (**carcinoma/sarcoma**) is a cancerous tumor composed of cells of epithelial tissue. An example of such a cancerous tumor is a/an ______________________.
2. A (**carcinoma/sarcoma**) is a cancerous tumor composed of connective tissue. An example of such a cancerous tumor is a/an ______________________.
3. Retinoblastoma and adenomatous polyposis coli syndrome are examples of (**chemical carcinogens/inherited cancers**).
4. The assessment of a tumor's degree of maturity or microscopic differentiation is (**grading/staging**) of the tumor.
5. The assessment of a tumor's extent of spread within the body is known as (**grading/staging**).
6. In the TNM staging system, T stands for (**tissue/tumor**), N stands for (**node/necrotic**), and M stands for (**mitotic/metastasis**).
7. The transformation of adult, differentiated tissue to differentiated tissue of another type is called (**metaplasia/anaplasia**).
8. The formation of new blood vessels is known as (**apoptosis/angiogenesis**).

G Match the surgical procedure in Column I with its meaning in Column II. Write the letter of the meaning in the space provided.

COLUMN I		COLUMN II
1. fulguration	______	A. removal of tumor and a margin of normal tissue for diagnosis and possible cure of small tumors
2. en bloc resection	______	B. burning a lesion to destroy tumor cells
3. incisional biopsy	______	C. wide resection involving removal of tumor, its organ of origin, and surrounding tissue in the body space
4. excisional biopsy	______	D. destruction of tissue by electric sparks generated by a high-frequency current
5. cryosurgery	______	E. removal of entire tumor and regional lymph nodes
6. cauterization	______	F. freezing a lesion to kill tumor cells
7. exenteration	______	G. cutting into a tumor and removing a piece to establish a diagnosis

H Give medical terms for the following.

1. The method of treating cancer using high-energy radiation is ______________________.
2. If tumor tissue requires large doses of radiation to kill cells, it is a/an ______________ tumor.
3. If radiation can cause loss of tumor cells without serious damage to surrounding regions, the tumor is ______________________.
4. A tumor that can be completely eradicated by RT is a/an ______________________ tumor
5. The method of giving radiation in small, repeated doses is ______________________.
6. Drugs that increase the sensitivity of tumors to x-rays are ______________________.

7. Treatment of cancerous tumors with drugs is ________________________.
8. Benign tumors of supportive cells in nervous system are ________________________.
9. The use of two or more drugs to kill tumor cells is ________________________.
10. A large electronic device that produces high-energy x-ray or photon beams for treatment of deep-seated tumors is a/an ________________________.
11. Alkylating agents, antimetabolites, hormones, antibiotics, and antimitotics all are types of ________________________ agents.
12. Implantation of seeds of radioactive material directly into a tumor is ________________________.
13. The unit of absorbed radiation dose is ________________________.
14. Radiation applied to a tumor from a distant source is ________________________.
15. Technique in which subatomic positively charged particles produced by a cyclotron deposit a dose of radiation at a tightly focused point is ________________________.
16. The dimension of the area of the body that receives radiation is a/an ________________________.
17. Study performed before RT using CT or MRI to map treatment is ________________________.
18. Technique in which a single large dose of radiation is delivered under precise 3D guidance to destroy vascular abnormalities and small brain tumors is ________________________.

I Match each of the following side effects of radiotherapy and chemotherapy with its description or treatment described below.

alopecia	myelosuppression	pneumonitis
fibrosis	nausea	secondary tumors
infertility	oral mucositis	xerostomia

1. Ulceration of lining cells in the mouth caused by radiation to the jaw ________________________
2. Radiation to the lungs causes inflammation of the lungs ________________________
3. Chemotherapy for ovarian cancer causes loss of hair on the head ________________________
4. Bone marrow destruction with leukopenia, anemia, and thrombocytopenia ________________________
5. Radiation to the lungs causes increase in connective tissue ________________________
6. Radiation of salivary glands causes dryness of the mouth ________________________
7. Chemotherapy may cause this sensation leading to vomiting ________________________
8. New type of growths arise at a site separate from the primary tumor ________________________
9. Inability to contribute to conception of a child ________________________

J **Give the meanings of the following medical terms.**

1. modality ______________________________
2. adjuvant therapy ______________________________
3. protocol ______________________________
4. remission ______________________________
5. relapse ______________________________
6. morbidity ______________________________
7. biological therapy ______________________________
8. biological response modifiers ______________________________
9. interferon ______________________________
10. monoclonal antibodies ______________________________
11. apoptosis ______________________________
12. cachexia ______________________________
13. differentiating agents ______________________________
14. molecularly targeted drugs ______________________________
15. nucleotide ______________________________

K **Match the test or procedure with its description below.**

beta-HCG test
bone marrow biopsy
CA-125
CEA test
core needle biopsy
estrogen receptor assay
exfoliative cytology
laparoscopy
PSA test
stem cell transplant

1. test for the presence of a portion of human chorionic gonadotropin hormone (a marker for testicular cancer) ____________________
2. protein marker for ovarian cancer detected in the blood ____________________
3. visual examination of the abdominal cavity; peritoneoscopy ____________________
4. test for the presence of a hormone receptor on breast cancer cells ____________________
5. removal of bone marrow tissue for microscopic examination ____________________
6. obtaining a plug of tissue for microscopic examination ____________________
7. blood test for the presence of an antigen related to prostate cancer ____________________
8. blood test for carcinoembryonic antigen (marker for GI cancer) ____________________
9. cells are scraped off tissue and microscopically examined ____________________
10. an intravenous infusion of blood-forming cells ____________________

L **Circle the correct term to complete each sentence.**

1. Pauline was diagnosed with a meningioma, which is usually a/an (**benign, anaplastic, necrotic**) tumor. The doctor told her that it was not malignant, but that it should be removed because of the pressure it was causing on the surrounding tissues.

2. Marlene underwent surgical resection of her breast mass. Dr. Smith recommended (**dedifferentiated, modality, adjuvant**) therapy because her tumor was large and she had one positive lymph node.

3. Unfortunately, at the time of diagnosis, the tumor had spread to distant sites because it was (**pleomorphic, metastatic, mutagenic**). The oncologist recommended beginning chemotherapy as soon as possible.

4. The polyp in Lisa's colon was **not** pedunculated, and Dr. Sidney described it as flat and (**fungating, scirrhous, sessile**).

5. Mr. Elder had difficulty urinating and had an elevated PSA test. Dr. Jones examined him and found a hard prostate gland. (**Laparoscopy, Electrocauterization, Biopsy**) demonstrated adenocarcinoma.

6. During the days following her chemotherapy for breast cancer, Doris experienced loss of appetite and (**fibrosis, nausea, xerostomia**). Blood tests revealed low levels of blood cells, indicating (**hematopoiesis, myeloma, myelosuppression**). Her physician prescribed (**EPO, VEGF, DES**) for anemia and (**Ca, cGy, G-CSF**) for leukopenia.

7. After Mr. Smith was diagnosed with lung cancer, his tumor was staged IIIA (**T1N0M0, T3N0M0, T1-3N2M0**). This indicated findings of (**tumor <3 cm diameter, distant metastases, tumor with involvement of ipsilateral hilar lymph nodes but no metastases**).

8. Mr. Smith's doctor told him he needed (**CA-125, XRT, PSA**) because his tumor was nonoperable and could not be (**resected, irradiated, electrocauterized**).

19

ANSWERS TO EXERCISES

A

1. anaplasia
2. infiltrative
3. invasive
4. metastasis

B

1. mitosis
2. mutation
3. DNA
4. RNA
5. ultraviolet radiation
6. ionizing radiation
7. virus
8. oncogene
9. chemical carcinogen

C

1. tumor composed of a mass of cells
2. tumor of glandular tissue (benign)
3. cancerous (malignant) tumor of glandular tissue
4. tumor of bone (benign)
5. flesh (connective tissue) tumor of bone (malignant)
6. tumor composed of different types of tissue (both epithelial and connective tissues)
7. new formation (tumor)
8. benign tumors of supportive tissue (neurofibromatosis)
9. noncancerous
10. specialization of cells

D

1. papillary
2. dysplastic
3. carcinoma in situ
4. scirrhous
5. alveolar
6. follicular
7. pleomorphic
8. undifferentiated
9. diffuse
10. epidermoid

E

1. necrotic
2. fungating
3. ulcerating
4. inflammatory
5. polypoid
6. cystic
7. verrucous
8. medullary

F

1. carcinoma; thyroid adenocarcinoma, squamous cell carcinoma
2. sarcoma; liposarcoma, chondrosarcoma, osteogenic sarcoma
3. inherited cancers
4. grading
5. staging
6. tumor; node; metastasis
7. metaplasia
8. angiogenesis

G

1. D
2. E
3. G
4. A
5. F
6. B
7. C

H

1. radiation therapy
2. radioresistant
3. radiosensitive
4. radiocurable
5. fractionation
6. radiosensitizers
7. chemotherapy
8. neurofibromatosis
9. combination chemotherapy
10. linear accelerator
11. chemotherapeutic agents
12. brachytherapy
13. gray
14. external beam radiation (teletherapy)
15. proton therapy
16. field
17. simulation
18. stereotactic radiosurgery

I

1. oral mucositis
2. pneumonitis
3. alopecia
4. myelosuppression
5. fibrosis
6. xerostomia
7. nausea
8. secondary tumors
9. infertility

J

1. method of treatment
2. assisting treatment
3. report or plan of steps taken in an experiment or disease case
4. absence of all signs of disease
5. symptoms of disease return
6. conditions of damage to normal tissue; disease
7. treatment that uses the body's own defense mechanisms to fight tumor cells
8. substances produced by normal cells that directly block tumor growth or that stimulate the immune system
9. a biological response modifier that is made by lymphocytes
10. biological response modifiers that are made by mouse or human immune cells and are able to bind to tumor cells
11. programmed cell death
12. malnutrition marked by weakness and emaciation; usually associated with later stages of cancer
13. drugs that promote tumor cells to differentiate (mature), stop growing, and die
14. anticancer drugs designed to block the function of growth factors, their receptors, and signaling pathways in tumor cells
15. unit of DNA composed of a sugar, phosphate, and base (adenine, cytosine, guanine, or thymine)

K

1. beta-HCG test
2. CA-125
3. laparoscopy
4. estrogen receptor assay
5. bone marrow biopsy
6. core needle biopsy
7. PSA test
8. CEA test
9. exfoliative cytology
10. stem cell transplant

L

1. benign
2. adjuvant
3. metastatic
4. sessile
5. biopsy
6. nausea; myelosuppression; EPO; G-CSF
7. T1-3N2M0, tumor with involvement of ipsilateral hilar lymph nodes but no metastases to the chest wall
8. XRT; resected

Answers to Practical Applications

FYI: Other Malignant Tumors

1. melanoma (a nevus is a benign pigmented lesion or mole)
2. thymoma
3. hepatoma
4. glioma
5. hypernephroma
6. multiple myeloma
7. mesothelioma
8. lymphoma (previously known as lymphosarcoma)

Case Study

1. b
2. c
3. b
4. c
5. c
6. b

Chart Rounds Review

1. patient D
2. patient A
3. patient C
4. patient B

Pathology Report

1. d

PRONUNCIATION OF TERMS

To test your understanding of the terminology in this chapter, write the meaning of each term in the space provided. In addition, you may wish to cover the terms and write them by looking at your definitions. Make sure your spelling is correct. The page number after each term indicates where it is defined or used in the book, so you can easily check your responses. You will find complete definitions for all of these terms and their audio pronunciations on the Evolve website.

Pronunciation Guide

ā as in āpe	ă as in ăpple
ē as in ēven	ĕ as in ĕvery
ī as in īce	ĭ as in ĭnterest
ō as in ōpen	ŏ as in pŏt
ū as in ūnit	ŭ as in ŭnder

Vocabulary and Terminology

TERM	PRONUNCIATION	MEANING
adenocarcinoma (823)	ăd-ĕ-nō-kăr-sĭ-NŌ-mă	
adjuvant therapy (818)	ĂD-jū-vănt THĔR-ă-pē	
alkylating agents (818)	ĂL-kĭ-lā-tĭng Ā-jents	
alopecia (813)	ăl-ō-PĒ-shē-ă	
alveolar (821)	ăl-vē-Ō-lăr *or* ăl-VĒ-ō-lăr	
anaplasia (818)	ăn-ă-PLĀ-zē-ă	
angiogenesis (818)	ăn-jē-ō-GĔN-ĕ-sĭs	
antibiotics (818)	ăn-tĭ-bī-ŎT-ĭks	
antimetabolites (818)	ăn-tĭ-mĕ-TĂB-ō-līts	
antimitotics (818)	ăn-tĭ-mī-TŎT-ĭks	
apoptosis (818)	ăp-ō-TŌ-sĭs *or* ā-pŏp-TŌ-sĭs	
benign tumor (818)	bē-NĪN TOO-mŏr	
biological response modifiers (818)	bī-ō-LŎJ-ĭ-kăl rĕ-SPŎNS MŎD-ĭ-fī-ĕrz	
biological therapy (818)	bī-ō-LŎJ-ĭ-kăl THĔR-ă-pē	
bone marrow biopsy (824)	bōn MĂ-rō BĪ-ŏp-sē	
bone marrow transplantation (824)	bōn MĂ-rō trănz-plănt-Ā-shŭn	
brachytherapy (818)	brā-kē-THĔ-ră-pē	
cachexia (821)	kă-KĔK-sē-ă	
carcinogens (818)	kăr-SĬN-ō-jĕnz	
carcinoma (818)	kăr-sĭ-NŌ-ma	
carcinoma in situ (821)	kăr-sĭ-NŌ-ma ĭn SĪ-too	

TERM	PRONUNCIATION	MEANING
cauterization (810)	kăw-tĕr-ĭ-ZĀ-shŭn	
cellular oncogenes (818)	SĔL-ū-lăr ŎNGK-ō-jēnz	
chemotherapy (818)	kē-mō-THĔR-ă-pē	
combination chemotherapy (818)	KŎM-bĭ-NĀ-shŭn kē-mō-THĔR-ă-pē	
core needle biopsy (810)	kŏr NĒ-dl BĪ-ŏp-sē	
cryosurgery (810)	krī-ō-SŬR-jĕr-ē	
cystic tumor (821)	SĬS-tĭk TOO-mŏr	
cytogenetic analysis (824)	sī-tō-jĕ-NĔT-ĭk ă-NĂL-ĕ-sĭs	
dedifferentiation (818)	dē-dĭf-ĕr-ĕn-shē-Ā-shŭn	
deoxyribonucleic acid (818)	dē-ŏx-ē-rī-bō-noo-KLĒ-ĭk ĂS-ĭd	
differentiating agents (818)	dĭf-ĕr-ĔN-shē-ā-tĭng Ā-gĕnts	
differentiation (818)	dĭf-ĕr-ĕn-shē-Ā-shŭn	
dysplastic (822)	dĭs-PLĂS-tĭk	
electrocauterization (821)	ē-lĕk-trō-kaw-tĕr-ĕ-ZĀ-shun	
electron beams (818)	ē-LĔK-trŏn bēmz	
en bloc resection (810)	ĕn blŏk rē-SĔK-shŭn	
encapsulated (819)	ĕn-KĂP-sū-lāt-ĕd	
epidermoid (823)	ĕp-ĭ-DĔR-moyd	
excisional biopsy (810)	ek-SIZH-ŭn-ăl BĪ-ŏp-sē	
exenteration (810)	ĕks-ĕn-tĕ-RĀ-shŭn	
exfoliative cytology (825)	ĕks-FŌ-lē-ā-tĭv sī-TŎL-ō-jē	
external beam radiation (819)	ĕks-TĔR-năl bēm rā-dē-Ā-shŭn	
fiberoptic colonoscopy (825)	fī-bĕr-ŎP-tĭk kō-lŏn-ŎS-kō-pē	
fibrosarcoma (821)	fī-brō-săr-KŌ-ma	
fibrosis (813)	fī-BRŌ-sĭs	
fields (819)	fēldz	
fine needle aspiration (810)	FĪN NĒ-dl ăs-pĕ-RĀ-shŭn	
follicular (821)	fō-LĬK-ū-lăr	
fractionation (819)	frăk-shă-NĀ-shŭn	

TERM	PRONUNCIATION	MEANING
fulguration (810)	fŭl-gū-RĀ-shŭn	______
fungating tumor (821)	fŭng-GĀ-tĭng *or* FŬNG-gā-tĭng TOO-mŏr	______
genetic screening (819)	jĕ-NĔT-ĭk SCRĒ-nĭng	______
grading of tumors (819)	GRĀ-dĭng of TOO-mŏrz	______
gray (Gy) (819)	grā	______
gross description of tumors (819)	GRŌS dĕ-SKRĬP-shŭn of TOO-mŏrz	______
hyperplasia (823)	hī-pĕr-PLĀ-zē-ă	______
immunohistochemistry (824)	ĭm-ū-nō-hĭs-tō-KĔM-ĭs-trē	______
incisional biopsy (810)	ĭn-SĬZH-ŭn-ăl BĪ-ŏp-sē	______
infertility (813)	ĭn-fĕr-TĬL-ĭ-tē	______
infiltrative (819)	ĬN-fĭl-trā-tĭv	______
invasive (819)	ĭn-VĀ-sĭv	______
irradiation (819)	ĭr-rā-dē-Ā-shŭn	______
laparoscopy (825)	lă-păr-ŎS-kō-pē	______
linear accelerator (819)	LĬN-ē-ăr ăk-sĕl-ĕ-RĀ-tŏr	______
malignant tumor (819)	mă-LĬG-nănt TOO-mŏr	______
mammography (825)	mă-MŎG-ră-fē	______
medullary tumor (821)	MĔD-ū-lār-ē TOO-mŏr	______
mesenchymal (819)	mĕs-ĕn-KĪ-măl	______
metaplasia (823)	mĕ-tă-PLĀ-zē-ă	______
metastasis (819)	mĕ-TĂS-tă-sĭs	______
microscopic description of tumors (819)	mī-krō-SKŎP-ĭk dĕ-SKRĬP-shŭn of TOO-mŏrz	______
mitosis (819)	mī-TŌ-sĭs	______
mixed-tissue tumors (819)	MĬKSD TĬ-shū TOO-mŏrz	______
modality (819)	mō-DĂL-ĭ-tē	______
molecularly targeted drugs (819)	mō-LĔK-ū-lăr-lē TĂR-gĕt-ĕd drŭgz	______
morbidity (819)	mŏr-BĬD-ĭ-tē	______
mucinous (819)	MŪ-sĭ-nŭs	______

TERM	PRONUNCIATION	MEANING
mucositis (821)	mū-kō-SĪ-tĭs	
mutagenic (821)	mū-tă-JĔN-ĭk	
mutation (819)	mū-TĀ-shŭn	
myelosuppression (823)	mī-ĕ-lō-sū-PRĔ-shŭn	
necrotic tumor (821)	nĕ-KRŎT-ĭk TOO-mŏr	
neoplasm (819)	NĒ-ō-plăzm	
neuroblastoma (823)	nōō-rō-blăs-TŌ-mă	
neurofibromatosis (822)	nōō-rō-fī-brō-mă-TŌ-sĭs	
nucleotide (819)	NOO-klē-ō-tīd	
oncogene (820)	ŎNGK-ō-jēn	
oncology (822)	ŏn-KŎL-ō-jē	
osteosarcoma (822)	ŏs-tē-ō-săr-KŌ-mă	
palliative (820)	PĂL-ē-ă-tĭv	
papillary (822)	PĂP-ĭ-lăr-ē	
pedunculated (820)	pĕ-DŬNG-kū-lāt-ĕd	
PET/CT scan (826)	PĔT/CT skăn	
photon therapy (820)	FŌ-tŏn THĔR-ă-pē	
pleomorphic (822)	plē-ō-MŎR-fĭk	
pneumonitis (813)	noo-mō-NĪ-tĭs	
polypoid tumor (822)	PŎL-ĭ-poyd TOO-mŏr	
protein marker tests (824)	PRŌ-tēn MĂRK-ĕr tĕsts	
protocol (820)	PRŌ-tō-kŏl	
proton therapy (820)	PRŌ-tŏn THĔR-ă-pē	
radiation (820)	rā-dē-Ā-shŭn	
radiocurable tumor (820)	rā-dē-ō-KŪR-ă-bl TOO-mŏr	
radionuclide scans (826)	rā-dē-ō-NOO-klīd skănz	
radioresistant tumor (820)	rā-dē-ō-rĕ-ZĬS-tănt TOO-mŏr	
radiosensitive tumor (820)	rā-dē-ō-SĔN-sĭ-tĭv TOO-mŏr	
radiosensitizers (820)	rā-dē-ō-SĔN-sĭ-tī-zĕrz	
radiotherapy (820)	rā-dē-ō-THĔR-ă-pē	
relapse (820)	rē-LĂPS	

TERM	PRONUNCIATION	MEANING
remission (820)	rē-MĬSH-ŭn	
retinoblastoma (823)	rĕt-ĭ-nō-blăs-TŌ-mă	
ribonucleic acid (RNA) (820)	rī-bō-noo-KLĒ-ik ĂS-ĭd	
sarcoma (820)	săr-KŌ-mă	
scirrhous (822)	SKĬR-ŭs	
secondary tumors (813)	SĔ-kŏn-dă-rē TOO-mŏrz	
serous (820)	SĒ-rŭs	
sessile (820)	SĔS-ĭl	
simulation (820)	sĭm-ū-LĀ-shŭn	
solid tumor (820)	SŎL-ĭd TOO-mŏr	
staging of tumors (820)	STĀ-jĭng of TOO-mŏrz	
stem cell transplantation (824)	stĕm sĕl trănz-plănt-Ā-shŭn	
stereotactic radiosurgery (820)	stĕ-rē-ō-TĂK-tĭc rā-dē-ō-SŬR-jĕr-ē	
steroids (820)	STĔR-oydz	
surgical procedures to treat cancer (820)	SŬRG-ĭ-kăl prō-SĒ-jŭrz to trēt KĂN-sĕr	
teletherapy (823)	tĕl-ē-THĔ-ră-pē	
ulcerating tumor (807)	ŬL-sĕ-rā-tĭng TOO-mŏr	
verrucous tumor (807)	vĕ-ROO-kŭs TOO-mŏr	
viral oncogenes (820)	VĪ-răl ŎNGK-ō-jēnz	
virus (820)	VĪ-rŭs	
xerostomia (822)	zĕr-ō-STŌ-mē-ă	

REVIEW SHEET

Write the meanings of the combining forms in the spaces provided and test yourself. Check your answers with the information in the chapter or in the Glossary (Medical Word Parts—English) at the end of the book.

Combining Forms

COMBINING FORM	MEANING	COMBINING FORM	MEANING
aden/o	________________	mutagen/o	________________
alveol/o	________________	necr/o	________________
cac/o	________________	neur/o	________________
carcin/o	________________	onc/o	________________
cauter/o	________________	papill/o	________________
chem/o	________________	pharmac/o	________________
cry/o	________________	plas/o	________________
cyst/o	________________	ple/o	________________
fibr/o	________________	polyp/o	________________
follicul/o	________________	radi/o	________________
fung/i	________________	sarc/o	________________
medull/o	________________	scirrh/o	________________
mucos/o	________________	xer/o	________________
mut/a	________________		

19

Suffixes

SUFFIX	MEANING	SUFFIX	MEANING
-ary	________________	-ptosis	________________
-blastoma	________________	-stasis	________________
-oid	________________	-stomia	________________
-oma	________________	-suppression	________________
-plasia	________________	-therapy	________________
-plasm	________________	-tion	________________

Prefixes

PREFIX	MEANING	PREFIX	MEANING
ana-	________	epi-	________
anti-	________	hyper-	________
apo-	________	meta-	________
brachy-	________	tele-	________
dys-	________		

Write the terms used in cancer medicine next to their meanings below:

adjuvant treatment
brachytherapy
cachexia
carcinoma
carcinoma in situ
exenteration
external beam radiotherapy
fine needle aspiration
metastasis
myelosuppression
protein markers
protocol
sarcoma
simulation

1. Cancerous tumor composed of cells of epithelial origin ________
2. Assisting primary treatment ________
3. Detailed plan of treatment ________
4. Study using CT scan or MRI to map treatment before radiation therapy ________
5. Wide and complete resection of tumor in a cavity of the body ________
6. Cancerous tumor derived from connective (flesh) tissue ________
7. Chemicals in the blood that measure the presence of tumor in the body ________
8. General ill health and malnutrition associated with disease ________
9. Teletherapy ________
10. Insertion of radioactive seeds or sealed containers into tumor ________
11. Malignancy that is localized and not invasive ________
12. Cancerous tumor that has spread to lymph nodes and other organs ________
13. Stopping the growth of cells in the bone marrow ________
14. Extraction of cells for microscopic (biopsy) evaluation ________

evolve *Please refer to the Evolve website for additional exercises, games, and images related to this chapter.*

CHAPTER 20

Radiology and Nuclear Medicine

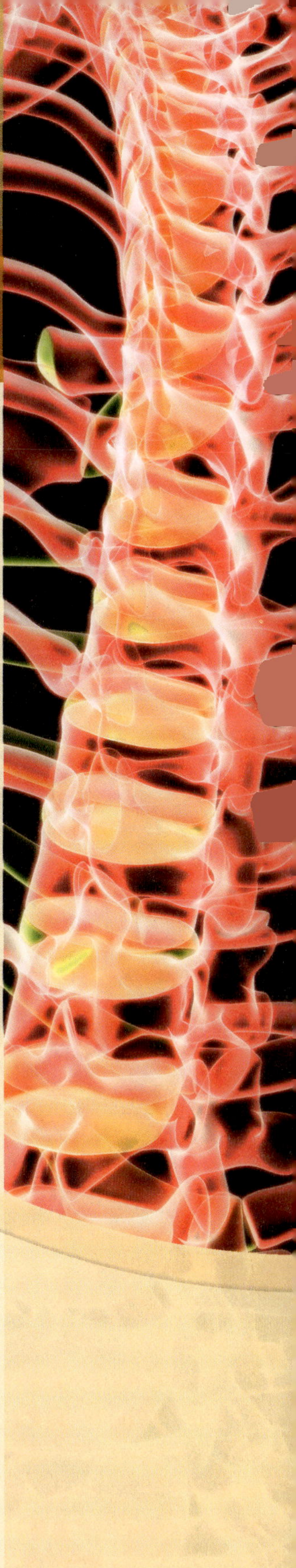

This chapter is divided into the following sections:

CHAPTER GOALS

- List the physical properties of x-rays.
- Identify diagnostic techniques used by radiologists and nuclear physicians.
- Name the x-ray views and patient positions used in x-ray examinations.
- Describe the role of radioactivity in the diagnosis of disease.
- Recognize medical terms used in the specialties of radiology and nuclear medicine.
- Apply your new knowledge to understanding medical terms in their proper contexts, such as medical reports and records.

INTRODUCTION

Radiology is the medical specialty concerned with the study and application of x-rays and other technologies (such as ultrasound and magnetic resonance) to produce and interpret images of the human body for the diagnosis of disease. **X-rays** are invisible waves of energy that are produced by an energy source (such as an x-ray machine or cathode ray tube) and are useful in the diagnosis and treatment of disease.

Nuclear medicine is the medical specialty that uses **radioactive substances** in the diagnosis and treatment of disease. These radioactive substances **(radionuclides)** are materials that emit high-speed particles and energy-containing rays from the interior of their matter. The emitted particles and rays are called **radioactivity** and can be of three types: **alpha particles, beta particles,** and **gamma rays. Gamma rays** are used effectively as a diagnostic label to trace the path and uptake of chemical substances in the body.

The professionals involved in these medical fields are varied. A **radiologist** is a physician who specializes in the practice of diagnostic radiology. A **nuclear medicine physician** specializes in diagnostic radionuclide scanning procedures.

Allied health care professionals who work with physicians in the fields of radiology and nuclear medicine are **radiologic technologists.** Different radiologic technologists called **radiographers** aid physicians in administering diagnostic x-ray procedures, **nuclear medicine technologists** attend to patients undergoing nuclear medicine procedures and operate devices under the direction of a nuclear physician, and **sonographers** aid physicians in performing ultrasound procedures.

RADIOLOGY

CHARACTERISTICS OF X-RAYS

Several characteristics of x-rays are useful to physicians in the diagnosis and treatment of disease. Some of these characteristics are the following:

1. **Ability to cause exposure of a photographic plate.** If a photographic plate is placed in front of a beam of x-rays, the x-rays, traveling unimpeded through the air, will expose the silver coating of the plate and cause it to blacken.
2. **Ability to penetrate different substances to varying degrees.** X-rays pass through the different types of substances in the human body (air in the lungs, water in blood vessels and lymph, fat around muscles, and metal such as calcium in bones) with varying ease. Air is the least dense substance and allows the greatest transmission. Fat is denser, water is next, followed by hard materials, such as calcium in bone, which is the densest and transmits least. If the x-rays are absorbed (stopped) by the denser body substance (e.g., calcium in bones), they do not reach the photographic plate held behind the patient, and white areas are left in the x-ray detector (plate). Figure 20-1 is an example of an x-ray photograph.

   A substance is said to be **radiolucent** if it permits passage of most of the x-rays. Lung tissue (containing air) is an example of a radiolucent substance, and it appears black on an x-ray image. **Radiopaque** substances (bones) are those that absorb most of the x-rays they are exposed to, allowing only a small fraction of the x-rays to reach the x-ray plate. Thus, normally radiopaque, calcium-containing bone appears white on an x-ray image.
3. **Invisibility.** X-rays cannot be detected by sight, hearing, or touch. Workers exposed to x-rays must wear a **film badge** to detect and record the amount of radiation to which they have been exposed. The film badge contains a special film that reacts when

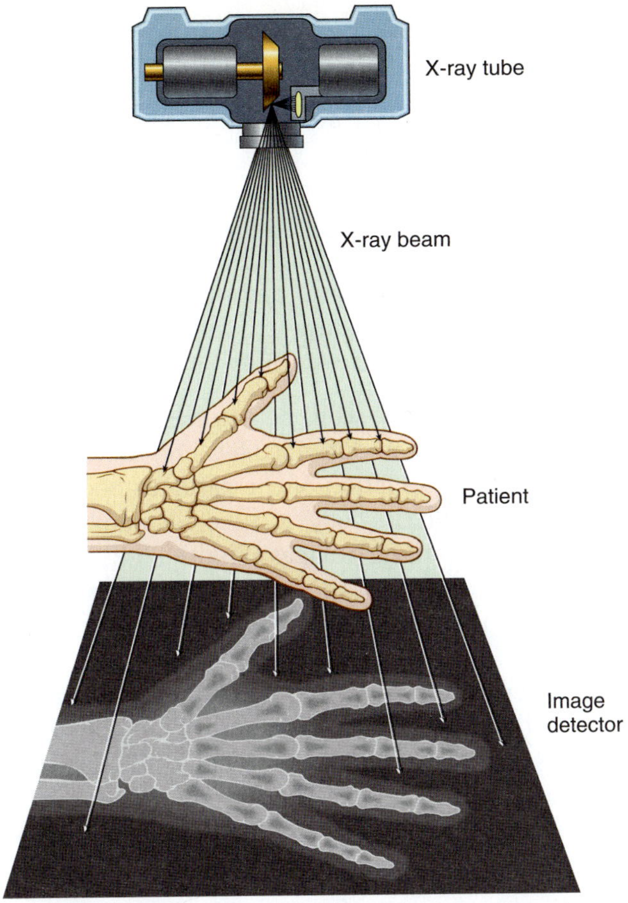

FIGURE 20-1 **X-ray photograph (radiograph) of the hand.** Relative position of x-ray tube, patient (hand), and image detector necessary to make the x-ray photograph is shown. Bones tend to stop (absorb) diagnostic x-rays, but absorption of the x-ray energy occurs to a lesser degree with soft tissue. This results in the light and dark regions that form the image.

exposed to x-rays. The amount of blackness on the film is an indication of the amount of x-rays or gamma rays received by the wearer.

4. **Travel in straight lines.** This property allows the formation of precise shadow images on the x-ray plate and also permits x-ray beams to be directed accurately at a tissue site during radiotherapy.
5. **Scattering of x-rays.** Scattering occurs when x-rays come into contact with any material. Greater scatter occurs with dense objects and less scatter with those substances that are radiolucent. In addition, because scatter can cause blurring (radiographic density that serves no useful purpose) on images, a grid (containing thin lead strips arranged parallel to the x-ray beams) is placed in front of the image detector to absorb scattered radiation before it strikes the x-ray film. In digital imaging, an image receptor replaces film.
6. **Ionization.** X-rays have the ability to ionize substances through which they pass. Ionization is a chemical process in which the energy of an x-ray beam causes rearrangement and disruption within a substance, so that previously neutral particles are changed to charged particles called **ions.** This strongly ionizing ability of x-rays is a double-edged sword. In x-ray or radiation therapy, the ionizing effect of high-energy x-ray beams can help kill cancerous cells and stop tumor growth; however, ionizing x-rays in even small doses can affect normal body cells, leading to tissue damage and malignant changes. Thus, persons exposed to high doses of x-rays are at risk for the development of leukemia, thyroid tumors, breast cancer, or other malignancies.

DIAGNOSTIC TECHNIQUES

X-Ray Studies

X-ray imaging is used in a variety of ways to detect pathologic conditions. **Digital radiography** is a form of x-ray imaging in which digital x-ray sensors are used instead of traditional photographic film. Thus images can be enhanced and transferred easily, and less radiation can be used than in conventional radiology. The most common use of diagnostic x-ray studies is in dental practice, to locate cavities in teeth (dental caries). Other areas examined include the digestive, nervous, reproductive, and endocrine systems and the chest and bones. **Mammography** uses low-dose x-rays to visualize breast tissue. Some special diagnostic x-ray techniques are described next.

Computed Tomography (CT). The CT scan, sometimes called "CAT scan" (because the technique originally was known as "computerized axial tomography"), is made by beaming x-rays at multiple angles through a section of the patient's body. The absorption of all of these x-rays, after they pass through the body, is detected and used by a computer to create multiple views, especially cross-sectional images (Figure 20-2). The ability of a CT scanner to detect abnormalities (the sensitivity of the scanner) is increased with the use of iodine-containing contrast agents, which outline blood vessels and confer additional density to soft tissues.

CT scanners are highly sensitive in detecting disease in bones and can actually provide images of internal organs that are impossible to visualize with ordinary x-ray technique. Figure 20-3 shows a series of CT scans through various regions of the body. New ultrafast CT scanners can produce a three-dimensional (3D) image of a beating heart and surrounding blood vessels. State-of-the-art scanners produce images in 64, 128, 256, and 320 slices and are called **multidetector CT** or **MDCT scanners.**

20

Contrast Studies. In x-ray film, the natural differences in the density of body tissues (e.g., from air in lung or from calcium in bone) produce contrasting shadow images on the x-ray film; however, when x-rays pass through two adjacent body parts composed of substances of the same density (e.g., different digestive organs in the abdomen), their images cannot be distinguished from one another on the film or on the screen. It is necessary, then, to inject a **contrast medium** into the structure or fluid to be visualized so that a specific part, organ, tube, or liquid can be visualized as a negative imprint on the dense contrast agent.

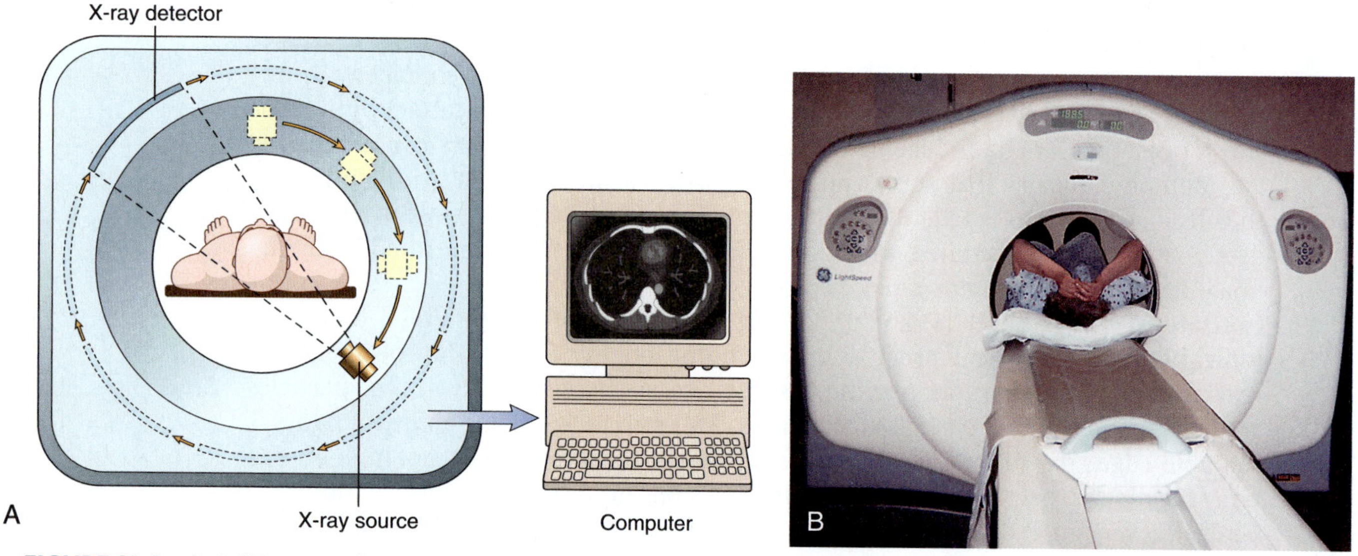

FIGURE 20-2 A, A CT scanner has a rotating x-ray source and a fixed ring of detectors. B, A patient in a CT scanner. This patient has her arms above her head during a chest CT examination.

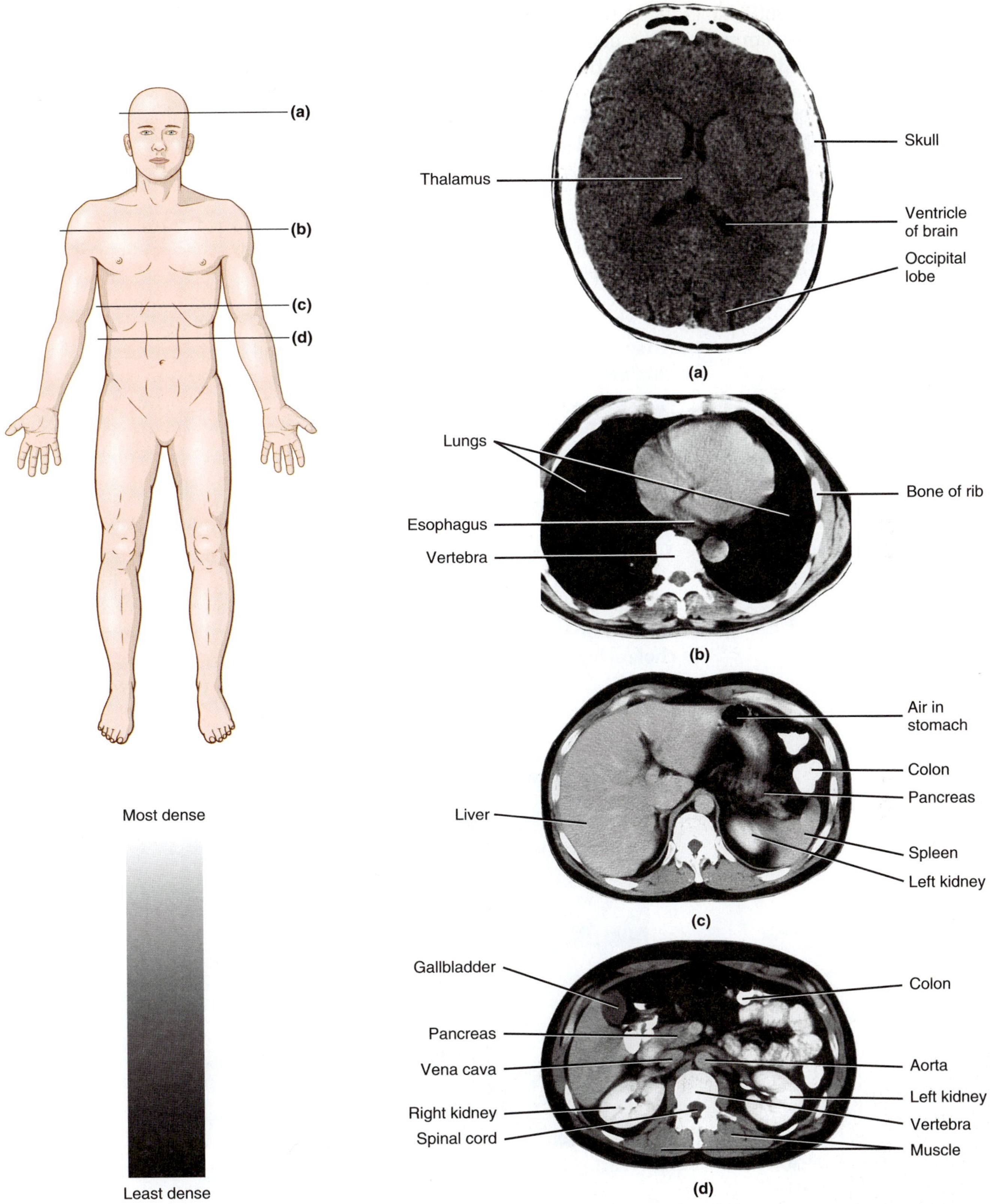

FIGURE 20-3 **CT scans through various regions of the body.** The level of the scan is indicated on the figure of the body. The bar below the figure indicates the gradient of structure density as represented by black (least dense, such as air) and white (most dense, such as bone).

The following are contrast materials used in diagnostic radiologic studies:

Barium Sulfate. Barium sulfate is a radiopaque medium that is mixed in water and used for examination of the upper and lower GI (gastrointestinal) tract. An **upper GI series (UGI)** involves oral ingestion of barium sulfate so that the esophagus, stomach, and duodenum can be visualized. A **small bowel follow-through (SBFT)** series traces the passage of barium in a sequential manner as it passes through the small intestine. A **barium enema (BE)** study is a lower GI series that opacifies the lumen (passageway) of the large intestine using an enema containing barium sulfate. This test has largely been replaced by endoscopy, which allows visualization of the inside of the bowel.

A **double-contrast study** uses both a radiopaque and a radiolucent contrast medium. For example, the walls of the stomach or intestine are coated with barium and the lumen is filled with air. These radiographs show the pattern of mucosal ridges.

Iodine Compounds. Radiopaque fluids containing up to 50% iodine are used in the following tests:

angiography — **X-ray image (angiogram) of blood vessels and heart chambers is obtained after contrast is injected through a catheter into the appropriate blood vessel or heart chamber.** In clinical practice, the terms angiogram and arteriogram are used interchangeably. Figure 20-4 shows **coronary angiography,** which determines the degree of obstruction of the arteries that supply blood to the heart. Figure 20-5A and B shows coronary angiograms before and after stenting of the artery.

cholangiography — **X-ray imaging after injection of contrast into bile ducts.** This is typically accomplished by injecting contrast directly into the common bile duct via a procedure called **endoscopic retrograde cholangiopancreatography (ERCP)** or after surgery of the gallbladder or biliary tract **(intraoperative cholangiography).** An alternative route for injection of contrast is via a needle through the skin and into the liver. This is **percutaneous transhepatic cholangiography** (Figure 20-6).

20

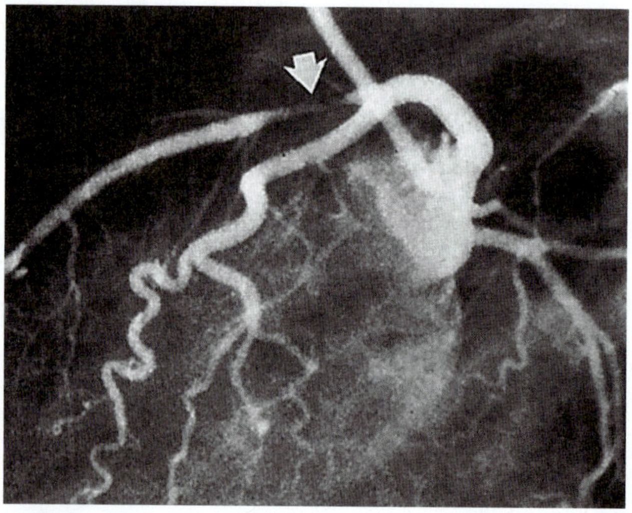

FIGURE 20-4 **Coronary angiography shows stenosis *(arrow)* of the left anterior descending coronary artery.**

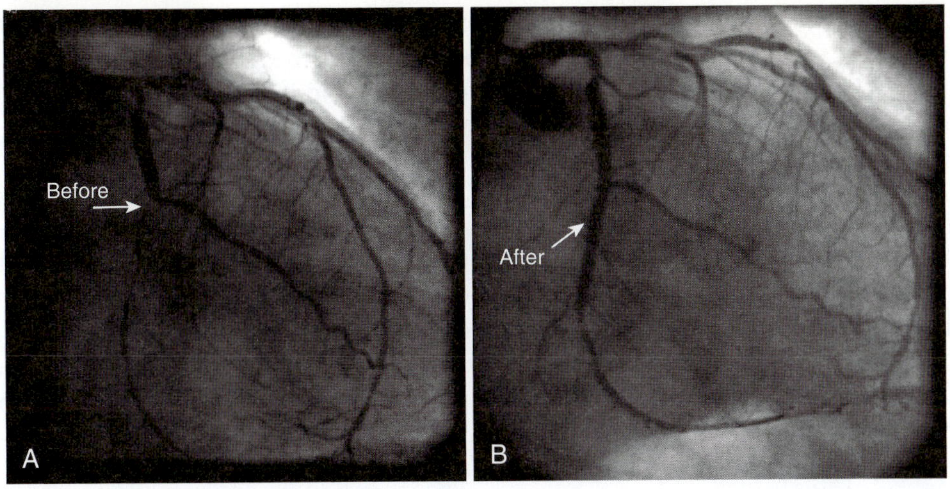

FIGURE 20-5 **Coronary angiograms before and after stenting. A,** Coronary angiogram before stenting shows narrowed coronary artery *(arrow)* preventing blood flow to heart muscle. **B,** Coronary angiogram after stenting shows opening of coronary artery *(arrow)* and increased blood flow to heart muscle. *(Courtesy Dr. Daniel Simon and Mr. Paul Zampino.)*

digital subtraction angiography (DSA) — **X-ray image of contrast-injected blood vessels is produced by taking two x-ray pictures (the first without contrast) and using a computer to subtract obscuring shadows from the second image.**

hysterosalpingography — **X-ray record of the endometrial cavity and fallopian tubes is obtained after injection of contrast material through the vagina and into the endocervical canal.** This procedure determines the patency of the fallopian tubes.

myelography — **X-ray imaging of the spinal cord (myel/o) after injection of contrast agent into the subarachnoid space surrounding the spinal cord.** It usually is performed in patients who cannot undergo MRI (magnetic resonance imaging). After injection of contrast, x-ray films and a CT scan are obtained. This procedure is **CT myelography.**

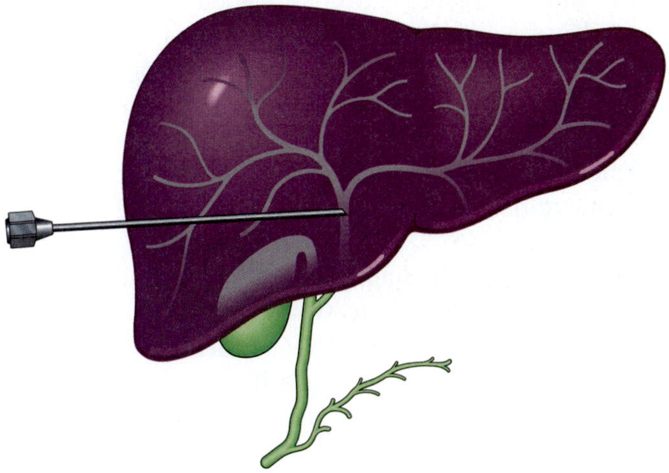

FIGURE 20-6 **Percutaneous transhepatic cholangiography.** The needle is passed through the abdominal wall into liver tissue until the tip penetrates the hepatic duct. Contrast medium is introduced, and x-ray pictures are taken to visualize the biliary tree.

pyelography **X-ray imaging of the renal pelvis and urinary tract.** Contrast is injected into a vein **(intravenous pyelography)** or through a catheter placed through the urethra, bladder, or ureter and into the renal pelvis **(retrograde pyelography). Urography** also describes the process of recording x-ray images of the urinary tract after the introduction of contrast.

Patients may experience side effects caused by iodine-containing contrast substances. These effects can range from mild reactions such as flushing, nausea, warmth, or tingling sensations to severe, life-threatening reactions characterized by airway spasm, hives, laryngeal edema (swelling of the larynx), vasodilation, and tachycardia. Treatment involves immediate establishment of an airway and ventilation followed by injections of epinephrine (adrenaline), corticosteroids, or antihistamines.

Digital imaging techniques can be used to enhance conventional and fluoroscopic x-ray images. A lower dose of x-ray is used to achieve higher-quality images, and digital images can be sent via networks to other locations and computer monitors so that many people can share information and assist in the diagnostic process.

Interventional Radiology. Interventional radiologists perform invasive procedures (therapeutic or diagnostic) usually under CT guidance or fluoroscopy. **Fluoroscopy** is the use of x-rays and a fluorescent screen to produce real-time video images. Procedures include percutaneous biopsy, placement of drainage catheters, drainage of abscesses, occlusion of bleeding vessels, and catheter instillation of antibiotics or chemotherapy agents. In addition, interventional radiologists perform **radiofrequency ablation** (removal) of tumors and tissues (liver, kidney, adrenals). Neurointerventional radiologists perform endovascular procedures including intracranial thrombolysis, head, neck, and intracranial tumor embolizations, extracranial angioplasty and stenting. They also perform nonvascular procedures, such as intervertebral facet injections, nerve root blocks, and vertebroplasties. Vascular interventional radiologists perform laser treatments for varicose veins and uterine fibroid embolization.

Ultrasound Imaging

Ultrasound imaging, or **ultrasonography,** uses high-frequency inaudible sound waves that bounce off body tissues and are then recorded to give information about the anatomy of an internal organ. An instrument called a **transducer** or **probe** is placed near or on the skin, which is covered with a thin coating of gel to ensure good transmission of sound waves. The transducer emits sound waves in short, repetitive pulses. The ultrasound waves move through body tissues and detect interfaces between tissues of different densities. An echo reflection of the sound waves is formed as the waves hit the various body tissues and bounce back to the transducer.

These ultrasonic echoes are then recorded as a composite picture of the area of the body over which the instrument has passed. The record produced by ultrasound is called a **sonogram.**

Ultrasound imaging is used as a diagnostic tool not only by radiologists but also by neurosurgeons and ophthalmologists to detect intracranial and ophthalmic lesions. Cardiologists use ultrasound techniques to detect heart valve and blood vessel disorders **(echocardiography),** and gastroenterologists use it to locate abdominal masses outside the digestive organs. Similarly, pulmonologists use ultrasound procedures for locating and sampling lesions outside the bronchial tubes. Obstetricians and gynecologists use ultrasound imaging to differentiate single from multiple pregnancies, as well as to help in performing amniocentesis. Other uses are to image benign and malignant tumors and

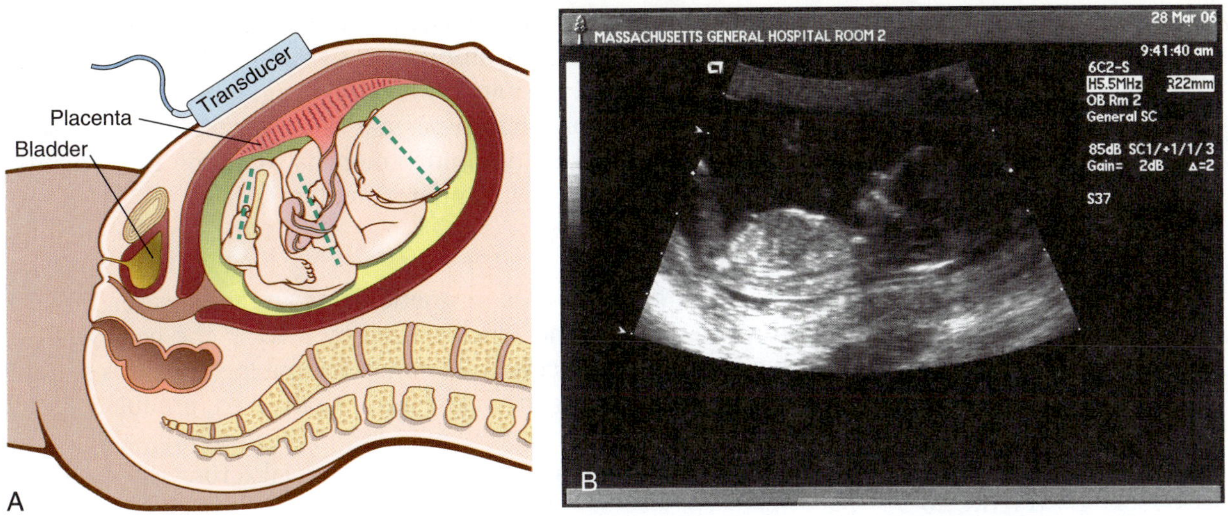

FIGURE 20-7 **A, Fetal measurements taken with ultrasound imaging.** Dashed lines indicate the image planes for measurements of the fetal head, abdomen, and femur. **B, Fetal ultrasound scan** at 13 weeks of pregnancy. *(B, Courtesy Joelle Reidy.)*

determine the size and development of the fetus. Measurements of the head, abdomen, and femur are made from ultrasound images obtained in various fetal planes (Figure 20-7).

Ultrasound imaging has several advantages in that the sound waves are not ionizing and do not injure tissues at the energy ranges used for diagnostic purposes. Because water is an excellent conductor of the ultrasound beams, patients are requested to drink large quantities of water before examination so that the urinary bladder will be distended, allowing better viewing of pelvic and abdominal organs.

Two ultrasound techniques, **Doppler ultrasound** and **color flow imaging,** make it possible to record blood flow velocity (speed). These techniques are used to image major blood vessels to detect obstructions caused by atherosclerotic plaques in patients at risk for stroke. Figure 20-8A and B shows Doppler ultrasound scanning and color flow imaging.

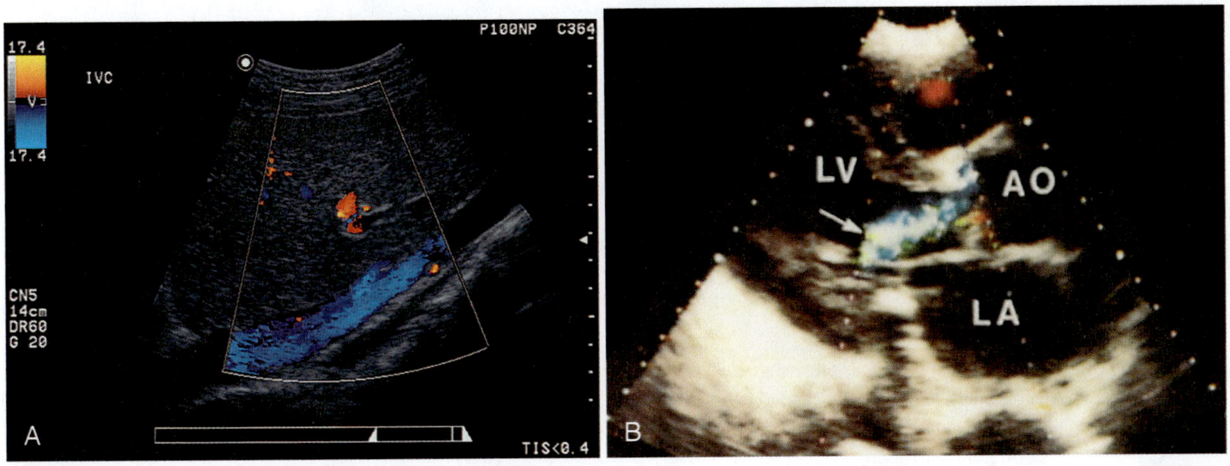

FIGURE 20-8 **A, Doppler ultrasound scan** showing an image of the vena cava (in blue). **B, Color flow imaging in a patient with aortic regurgitation.** The brightly colored, high-velocity jet *(arrow)* can be seen passing from the aorta (AO) to the left ventricle (LV). The center of the jet is white, and the edges are shades of blue.

Ultrasonography is used in interventional radiology to guide needle biopsy for the puncture of cysts, for placing needles during amniocentesis, and for inserting radioactive seeds into the prostate (brachytherapy). In **endoscopic ultrasonography,** a small ultrasound transducer is attached to the tip of an endoscope that is inserted into the body. This technique is used by gastroenterologists and pulmonologists to obtain high-quality and accurate detailed images of the digestive and respiratory systems.

Magnetic Resonance Imaging

Magnetic resonance imaging (MRI) uses magnetic fields and radiowaves rather than x-rays. Hydrogen protons are aligned and synchronized by placing the body in a strong magnetic field. Then the hydrogen molecules relax when the magnetic field is shut down. The rates of alignment and relaxation vary from one tissue to the next, producing a sharply defined picture. Because bone is virtually devoid of water, it does not image well on MRI. The MR technique produces sagittal, coronal (frontal), and axial (cross-sectional) images (Figure 20-9).

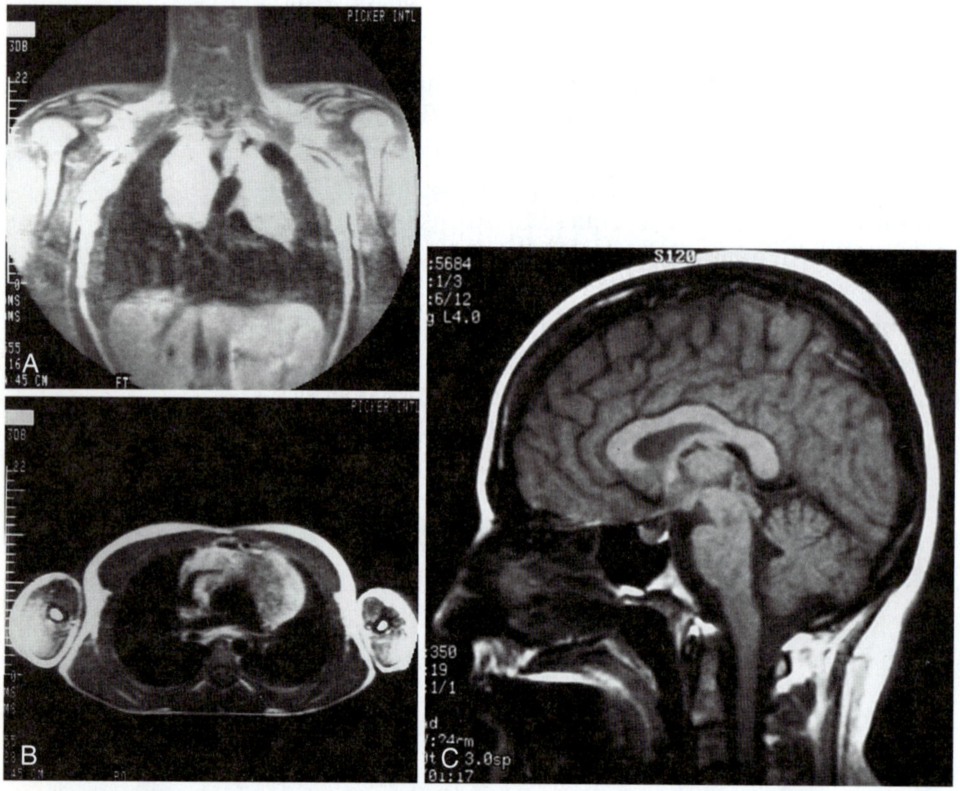

FIGURE 20-9 Magnetic resonance images. A, Frontal (coronal) view of the upper body. White masses in the chest are Hodgkin disease lesions. **B,** Transverse view of the upper body in the same patient, who had a chest mass. **C,** Image obtained in the sagittal plane of the head (the usual MRI view) showing cerebrum, ventricles, cerebellum, and medulla oblongata.

MRI versus CT Scanning

Why do doctors choose MRI or CT scanning? Differences in use depend on the part of the body viewed. In general, CT is useful for visualizing bony structures and solid masses of the chest and abdomen, whereas MRI is better at giving detail in soft tissues that have more water molecules.

CT

1. bones
2. chest lesions and pneumonia
3. bleeding in the brain from head trauma and ruptured arteries

MRI

1. spinal cord and brain tumors
2. joints, tendons, and ligaments
3. liver masses
4. head and neck lesions

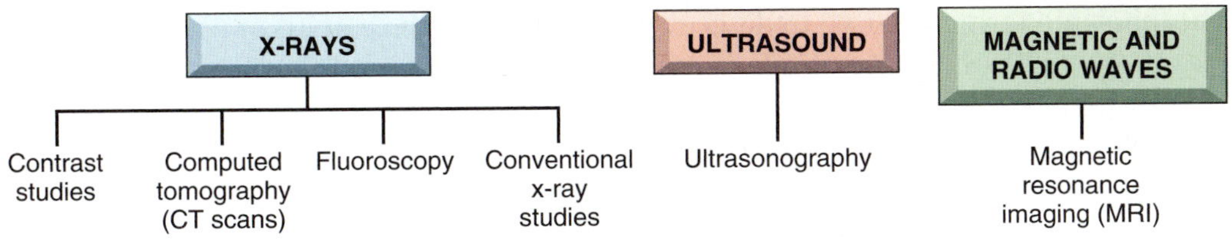

FIGURE 20-10 **Summary of radiologic diagnostic techniques.**

MRI examinations are performed with and without contrast. The contrast agent most commonly used is **gadolinium (Gd).** As iodine contrast does with CT, gadolinium enhances vessels and tissues, increases the sensitivity for lesion detection, and helps differentiate between normal and abnormal tissues and structures. MRI provides excellent soft tissue images, detecting edema in the brain, providing direct imaging of the spinal cord, detecting tumors in the chest and abdomen, and visualizing the cardiovascular system.

MRI is contraindicated for patients with pacemakers or metallic implants because the powerful magnet can alter position and functioning of such devices. However, the Food and Drug Administration (FDA) has recently approved new pacemakers that can be safely used with MRI. The sounds (loud tapping) heard during the test are caused by the pulsing of the magnetic field as the device scans the body. See the ***In Person*** story on page 868.

Figure 20-10 summarizes radiologic diagnostic techniques.

X-RAY POSITIONING

In order to take the best picture of the part of the body being radiographed, the patient, detector, and x-ray tube must be positioned in the most favorable alignment possible. Radiologists use special terms to refer to the direction of travel of the x-ray through the patient. X-ray Terms describing the direction of the x-ray beam follow and are illustrated in Figure 20-11:

1. **Posteroanterior (PA) view.** In this most commonly requested chest x-ray view, x-rays travel from a posteriorly placed source to an anteriorly placed detector.
2. **Anteroposterior (AP) view.** X-rays travel from an anteriorly placed source to a posteriorly placed detector.
3. **Lateral view.** In a left lateral view, x-rays travel from a source located to the right of the patient to a detector placed to the left of the patient.
4. **Oblique view.** X-rays travel in a slanting direction at an angle from the perpendicular plane. Oblique views show regions or structures ordinarily hidden and superimposed in routine PA and AP views.

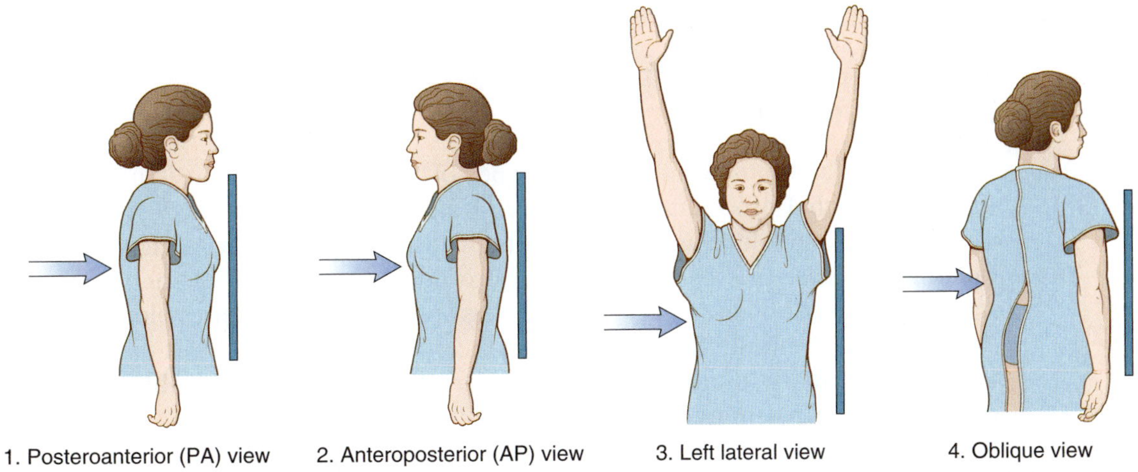

FIGURE 20-11 **Positions for x-ray views.** The arrow denotes the direction of the x-ray beam through the patient.

The following terms are used to describe the position of the patient or part of the body in the x-ray examination:

abduction	Movement away from the midline of the body.
adduction	Movement toward the midline of the body.
eversion	Turning outward.
extension	Lengthening or straightening a flexed limb.
flexion	Bending a part of the body.
inversion	Turning inward.
lateral decubitus	Lying down on the side (with the x-ray beam horizontally positioned).
prone	Lying on the belly (face down).
recumbent	Lying down (may be prone or supine).
supine	Lying on the back (face up).

NUCLEAR MEDICINE

RADIOACTIVITY AND RADIONUCLIDES

The spontaneous emission of energy in the form of particles or rays coming from the interior of a substance is called **radioactivity.** A **radionuclide** (or **radioisotope**) is a substance that gives off high-energy particles or rays as it disintegrates. Radionuclides are produced in either a nuclear reactor or a charged-particle accelerator (cyclotron) or by irradiating stable substances, causing disruption and instability. **Half-life** is the time required for a radioactive substance (radionuclide) to lose half of its radioactivity by disintegration. Knowledge of a radionuclide's half-life is important in determining how long the radioactive substance will emit radioactivity when in the body. The half-life must be long enough to allow for diagnostic imaging but as short as possible to minimize patient exposure to radiation.

Radionuclides emit three types of radioactivity: **alpha particles, beta particles,** and **gamma rays.** Gamma rays, which have greater penetrating ability than alpha and beta particles, and more ionizing power, are especially useful to physicians in both the diagnosis and the treatment of disease. **Technetium-99m** (Tc-99m) is essentially a pure gamma emitter with a half-life of 6 hours. Its properties make it the most frequently used radionuclide in diagnostic imaging.

NUCLEAR MEDICINE TESTS: IN VITRO AND IN VIVO PROCEDURES

Nuclear medicine physicians use two types of tests in the diagnosis of disease: **in vitro** (in the test tube) procedures and **in vivo** (in the body) procedures. **In vitro** procedures involve analysis of blood and urine specimens using radioactive chemicals. For example, a **radioimmunoassay (RIA)** is an in vitro procedure that combines the use of radioactive chemicals and antibodies to detect hormones and drugs in a patient's blood. The test allows the detection of minute amounts of substances or compounds. RIA is used to monitor the amount of digitalis, a drug used to treat heart disease, in a patient's bloodstream and can detect hypothyroidism in newborn infants.

In vivo tests trace the amounts of radioactive substances within the body. They are given directly to the patient to evaluate the function of an organ or to image it. For example, in **tracer studies** a specific radionuclide is incorporated into a chemical substance and administered to a patient. The combination of the radionuclide and a drug or chemical is called a **radiopharmaceutical** (or **radiolabeled compound**). Each radiopharmaceutical is designed to concentrate in a certain organ. The organ can then be imaged using the radiation given off by the radionuclide.

A sensitive, external detection instrument called a **gamma camera** is used to determine the distribution and localization of the radiopharmaceutical in various organs, tissues, and fluids (Figure 20-12). The amount of radiopharmaceutical at a given location is proportional to the rate at which the gamma rays are emitted. Nuclear medicine studies depict the physiologic behavior (how the organ works) rather than the specific anatomy of an organ.

The procedure of making an image by tracking the distribution of radioactive substance in the body is **radionuclide scanning. Uptake** refers to the rate of absorption of the radiopharmaceutical into an organ or tissue.

Radiopharmaceuticals are administered by different routes to obtain a scan of a specific organ in the body. For example, in the case of a **lung scan,** the radiopharmaceutical is given intravenously (for **perfusion studies,** which rely on passage of the radioactive compound through the capillaries of the lungs) or by inhalation of a gas or aerosol (for **ventilation studies**), which fills the air sacs (alveoli). The combination of these tests permits sensitive and specific diagnosis of clots in the lung (pulmonary emboli).

Other diagnostic procedures that use radionuclides include the following:

1. **Bone scan.** Technetium-99m (Tc-99m) is used to label phosphate substances and then is injected intravenously. The phosphate compound is taken up preferentially by bone, and the skeleton is imaged in 2 or 3 hours. Waiting 2 to 3 hours allows much of the radiopharmaceutical to be excreted in urine and allows for better visualization of the radioactive material remaining in the skeleton. The scan detects infection, inflammation, or tumors involving the skeleton, which appear as areas of high uptake ("hot spots") on the scan. See Figure 15-36 on page 620.

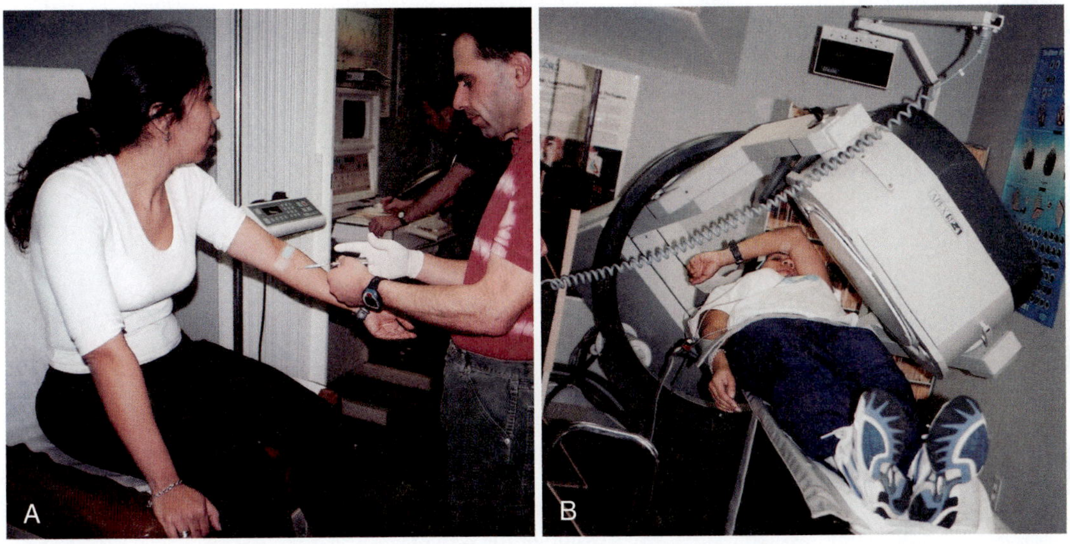

FIGURE 20-12 **A, Patient receiving intravenous injection of radionuclide for detection of heart function. B, Gamma camera** moves around the patient, detecting radioactivity in heart muscle.

2. **Lymphoscintigraphy.** This type of nuclear medicine imaging provides pictures (scintigrams) of the lymphatic system. A **radiotracer** (radioactive isotope) is injected under the skin or deeper using a small needle. A gamma camera then takes a series of images of an area of the body. Physicians perform lymphoscintigraphy to identify a **sentinel lymph node** (the first lymph node to receive lymph drainage from a tumor), identify areas of lymph node blockage, or evaluate lymphedema (accumulation of fluid in soft tissues leading to swelling).
3. **Positron emission tomography (PET scan).** This radionuclide technique produces images of the distribution of radioactivity (through emission of positrons) in a region of the body. It is similar to the CT scan, but radioisotopes are used instead of contrast and x-rays. The radionuclides are incorporated (by intravenous injection) into the tissues to be scanned, and an image is made showing where the radionuclide is or is not being metabolized. The most common radionuclide is radiolabeled fluorodeoxyglucose (18F-FDG), but others are in use. PET scanning has determined that schizophrenics do not metabolize glucose equally in all parts of the brain and that drug treatment can bring improvement to these regions. Areas of metabolic deficiency can be pinpointed by PET, making it helpful in diagnosing and treating other neurologic disorders such as stroke, epilepsy, and Alzheimer disease. Alternatively, areas of infection, inflammation, and tumor demonstrate increased metabolic activity, highlighted as hot spots on the PET scan (Figure 20-13).
4. **PET/CT scan.** This scan combines PET and CT techniques to produce a more accurate image than PET or CT alone. See Figure 20-14. It is often used to detect cancer and metastases, especially to determine if the cancer is responding to treatment.
5. **Single photon emission computed tomography (SPECT).** This technique involves an intravenous injection of radioactive tracer (such as Tc-99m) and the computer reconstruction of a 3D image based on a composite of many views. Clinical applications include detecting liver tumors, detecting cardiac ischemia, and evaluating bone disease of the spine.

20

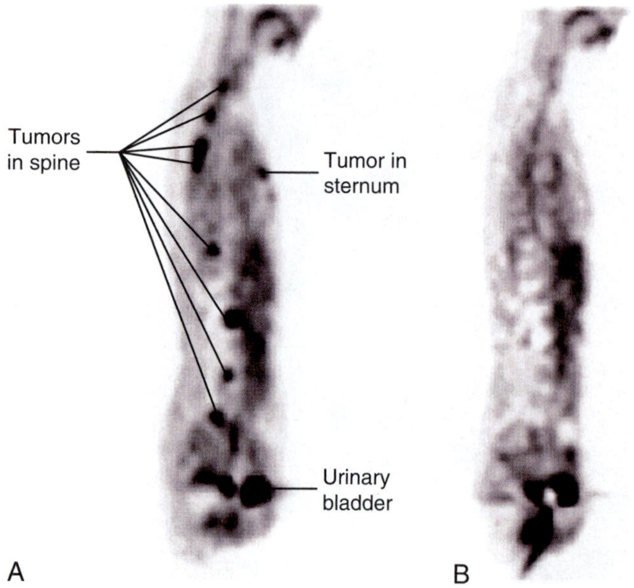

FIGURE 20-13 **Whole-body PET images. A, 18F-FDG sagittal image** obtained in a patient with breast cancer metastases. Numerous tumors (dark spots) are seen along with spine and sternum. **B, Image obtained after chemotherapy** shows regression of the cancer.

Scintigraphy

Scintigraphy is the process of obtaining an image using a radioisotope. The term is derived from Latin *scintilla,* meaning spark. Bone scintigraphy is commonly called a bone scan, and lung scintigraphy is commonly called a lung scan.

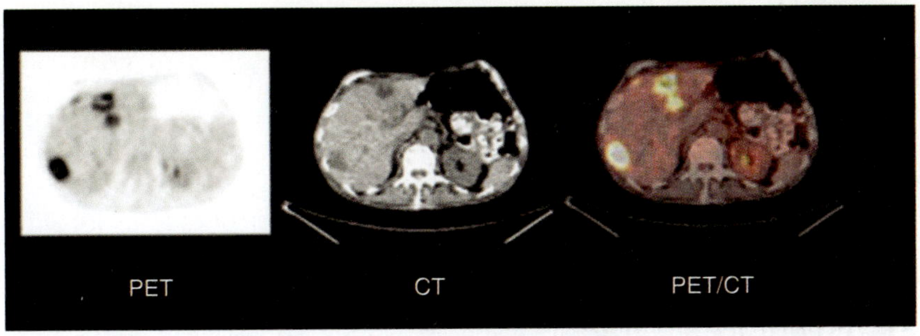

FIGURE 20-14 **PET scan, CT scan, and PET/CT scan.** *(Courtesy UPMC, University of Pittsburgh.)*

6. **Technetium Tc 99m Sestamibi (Cardiolite) scan.** This radiopharmaceutical is injected intravenously and traced to heart muscle. An exercise tolerance test (ETT) is used with it for an ETT-MIBI scan. In a **mu**ltiple **g**ated **a**cquisition **(MUGA)** scan, Tc-99m is injected intravenously to study the motion of the heart wall muscle and the ventricle's ability to eject blood (ejection fraction).
7. **Thallium scan.** Thallium-201 (TL-201) is injected intravenously to evaluate myocardial perfusion. A high concentration of TL-201 is present in well-perfused heart muscle cells, but infarcted or scarred myocardium does not take up any thallium, showing up as "cold spots." If the defective area is ischemic, the cold spots fill in (become "warm") on delayed images (obtained later).
8. **Thyroid scan.** In a thyroid scan, an iodine radionuclide, usually iodine-123 (I-123), is administered orally, and the scan reveals the size, shape, and position of the thyroid gland. Alternatively, radioactive technetium can be administered intravenously. Hyperfunctioning thyroid nodules (adenomas) accumulate higher amounts of radioactivity and are termed "hot." Thyroid carcinoma does not concentrate radioiodine well and is seen as a "cold" spot on the scan. Figure 20-15 shows thyroid scans.

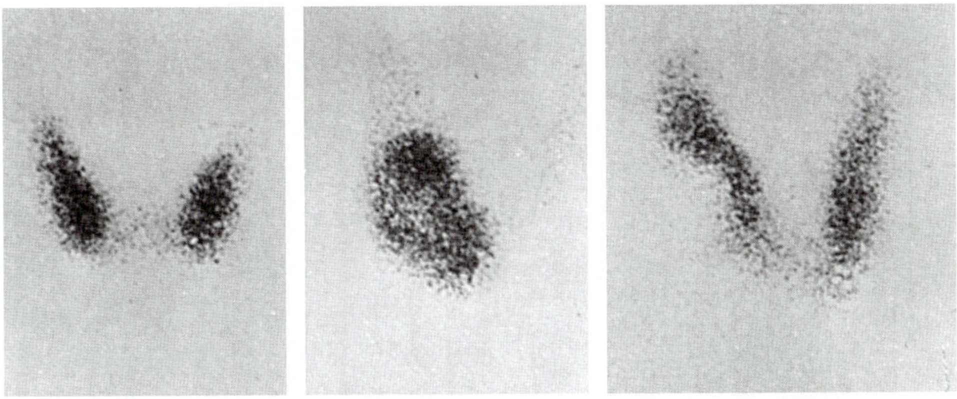

FIGURE 20-15 **I-123 thyroid scans.** The scan of a "hot nodule" shows a darkened area of increased uptake of iodine, which indicates an active nodule. Chances are very good that the nodule is benign. The scan of a "cold nodule" shows an area of decreased uptake, which indicates a nonfunctioning region, a common occurrence when normal tissue is replaced by malignancy.

NUCLEAR MEDICINE TESTS

IN VITRO	**Radioimmunoassay**
IN VIVO	**Tracer Studies:** Bone scan Lung scan (ventilation-perfusion) Lymphoscintigraphy PET/CT scan Positron emission tomography (PET) Radioactive iodine uptake (RAIU) Single photon emission computed tomography (SPECT) Technetium Tc 99m-sestamibi scan Thallium-201 scan Thyroid scan

FIGURE 20-16 In vitro and in vivo nuclear medicine diagnostic tests.

A **radioactive iodine uptake (RAIU)** study is performed to assess the function of the thyroid gland (such as hyperthyroidism). The patient is given radioactive iodine (in this case, I-131), also called radioiodine, in liquid or capsule form, and then a sensor is placed over the thyroid gland. It detects gamma rays emitted from the radioactive tracer, which is taken up by the thyroid more readily than by other tissues. Radioiodine also is used to treat hyperthyroidism, thyroid nodules, or thyroid cancer. After the patient swallows the I-131, it is absorbed into the bloodstream and then travels to the thyroid gland, where it destroys overactive thyroid tissue.

Figure 20-16 reviews in vitro and in vivo nuclear medicine diagnostic tests.

VOCABULARY

This list reviews many of the new terms introduced in the text. Short definitions reinforce your understanding of the terms. Refer to the Pronunciation of Terms on page 876 for help with unfamiliar or difficult words.

computed tomography (CT)	Diagnostic x-ray procedure whereby a cross-sectional image of a specific body segment is produced. Newer CT scanners can create 3D images as well.
contrast studies	Radiopaque materials (contrast media) are injected to obtain contrast with surrounding tissue when shown on the x-ray film.
gamma camera	Machine to detect gamma rays emitted from radiopharmaceuticals during scanning for diagnostic purposes.
gamma rays	High-energy rays emitted by radioactive substances in tracer studies.
half-life	Time required for a radioactive substance to lose half its radioactivity by disintegration.
interventional radiology	Therapeutic or diagnostic procedures performed by a radiologist. Examples are needle biopsy of a mass and drainage of an abscess, typically under the guidance of CT or fluoroscopy.
in vitro	Process, test, or procedure is performed, measured, or observed outside a living organism, often in a test tube.
in vivo	Process, test, or procedure is performed, measured, or observed within a living organism.

ionization	Transformation of electrically neutral substances into electrically charged particles. X-rays cause ionization of particles within tissues.
magnetic resonance imaging (MRI)	Magnetic field and radio waves produce sagittal, coronal, and axial images of the body.
nuclear medicine	Medical specialty that uses radioactive substances (radionuclides) in the diagnosis of disease.
positron emission tomography (PET)	Positron-emitting radioactive substances given intravenously create a cross-sectional image of cellular metabolism based on local concentration of the radioactive substance. PET scans give information about metabolic activity.
radioimmunoassay	Test combines radioactive chemicals and antibodies to detect minute quantities of substances in a patient's blood.
radioisotope	Radioactive form of an element substance; radionuclide.
radiolabeled compound	Radiopharmaceutical; used in nuclear medicine studies.
radiology	Medical specialty concerned with the study of x-rays and their use in the diagnosis of disease. It includes other forms of energy, such as ultrasound and magnetic waves. Also called **diagnostic radiology**.
radiolucent	Permitting the passage of x-rays. Radiolucent structures appear black on x-ray images.
radionuclide	Radioactive form of an element that gives off energy in the form of radiation; radioisotope.
radiopaque	Obstructing the passage of x-rays. Radiopaque structures appear white on the x-ray images.
radiopharmaceutical	Radioactive drug (radionuclide plus chemical) that is administered safely for diagnostic and therapeutic purposes; a radiotracer. An example is technetium 99m, which combines with albumin (for lung perfusion) and DTPA (for renal imaging).
scan	Image of an area, organ or tissue of the body obtained from ultrasonography, radioactive tracer studies, computed tomography, or magnetic resonance imaging.
scintigraphy	Diagnostic nuclear medicine test using radiopharmaceuticals and gamma cameras to create images.
single photon emission computed tomography (SPECT)	Radioactive tracer is injected intravenously and a computer reconstructs a 3D image based on a composite of many views.
tagging	Attaching a radionuclide to a chemical and following its path in the body.
tracer studies	Radionuclides are used as tags, or labels, attached to chemicals and followed as they travel through the body.
ultrasonography (US, U/S)	Diagnostic technique that projects and retrieves high-frequency sound waves as they echo off parts of the body.
ultrasound transducer	Handheld device that sends and receives ultrasound signals.
uptake	Rate of absorption of a radionuclide into an organ or tissue.
ventilation-perfusion studies	Radiopharmaceutical is inhaled (ventilation) and injected intravenously (perfusion) followed by imaging its passage through the respiratory tract.

TERMINOLOGY

Write the meanings of the medical terms in the spaces provided.

COMBINING FORMS

COMBINING FORM	MEANING	TERMINOLOGY	MEANING
is/o	same	radioisotope *Top/o means place; isotopes of an element have similar structures but different weights and stability. A radioisotope (radionuclide) is an unstable form of an element that emits radioactivity.*	______
pharmaceut/o	drug	radiopharmaceutical *In this term, radi/o stands for radioactive.*	______
radi/o	x-rays	radiographer	______
		radiology	______
son/o	sound	hysterosonogram *Saline solution is injected through a catheter inserted into the vagina and cervical canal to the uterus, which is then examined by ultrasound imaging.*	______
therapeut/o	treatment	therapeutic	______
vitr/o	glass	in vitro	______
viv/o	life	in vivo	______

20

SUFFIXES

SUFFIX	MEANING	TERMINOLOGY	MEANING
-gram	record	angiogram	______
		hysterosalpingogram	______
		pyelogram	______
-graphy	process of recording	computed tomography *Tom/o means to cut, as in viewing in slices.*	______
-lucent	to shine	radiolucent *Radiolucent (indicating that x-rays pass through easily) areas on x-ray images appear dark.*	______
-opaque	obscure	radiopaque *Radiopaque (indicating that x-rays do not penetrate) areas on x-ray images appear white/light.*	______

PREFIXES

PREFIX	MEANING	TERMINOLOGY	MEANING
echo-	a repeated sound	echocardiography	______
ultra-	beyond	ultrasonography *Sound waves are beyond the normal range of those that a human can hear.*	______

ABBREVIATIONS

Angio	angiography
AP	anteroposterior
Ba	barium
BE	barium enema
C-spine	cervical spine
CT	computed tomography
CXR	chest x-ray (film)
Decub	decubitus—lying down
DICOM	digital image communication in medicine—standard protocol for transmission between imaging devices (e.g., CT scans and PACS workstations)
DI	diagnostic imaging
DSA	digital subtraction angiography
ECHO	echocardiography
EUS	endoscopic ultrasonography
18F-FDG	fluorodeoxyglucose—radiopharmaceutical used in PET scanning
Gd	gadolinium—MRI contrast agent
I-123	isotope of radioactive iodine—used in thyroid scans
I-131	isotope of radioactive iodine—used in diagnosis (thyroid scan) and treatment for thyroid cancer
IVP	intravenous pyelogram
KUB	kidneys-ureters-bladder (series)—x-ray imaging of these organs without contrast medium
LAT	lateral
LS films	lumbosacral (spine) films
L-spine	lumbar spine
MDCT	multidetector CT scanner
MR, MRI	magnetic resonance, magnetic resonance imaging
MRA	magnetic resonance angiography
MRV	magnetic resonance venography
MUGA	multiple-gated acquisition (scan)—radioactive test to show heart function
PA	posteroanterior
PACS	picture archival and communications system—replacement of traditional films with digital equivalents that can be accessed from several places and retrieved more rapidly
PET	positron emission tomography
PET/CT	positron emission tomography/computed tomography—both studies are performed using a single machine
RAIU	radioactive iodine uptake (test)—evaluates the function of the thyroid gland
RFA	radiofrequency ablation
SBFT	small bowel follow-through
SPECT	single photon emission computed tomography—radioactive substances and a computer are used to create 3D images
Tc-99m	radioactive technetium—used in heart, brain, thyroid, liver, bone, and lung scans
TL-201	thallium-201—radioisotope used in scanning heart muscle
T-spine	thoracic spine
UGI	upper gastrointestinal (series)
US, U/S	ultrasound; ultrasonography
V/Q scan	ventilation-perfusion scan of the lungs (Q stands for rate of blood flow or blood volume)

IN PERSON: CT AND MRI

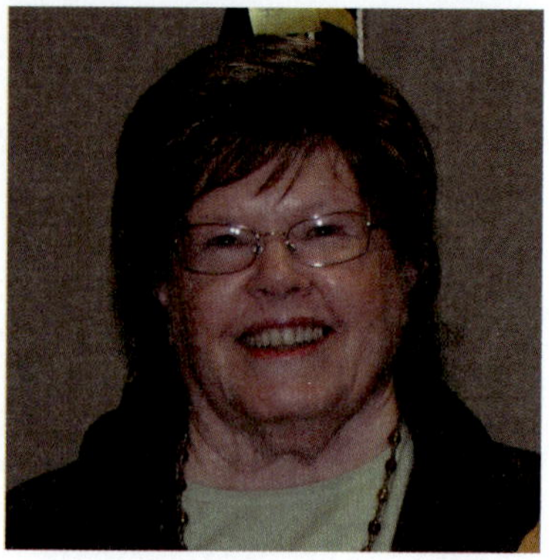

The following first-person narrative provides a detailed look at two common diagnostic procedures-CT and MRI-from the perspective of the patient. It was written by a 77-year-old woman with head and neck cancer.

CT—COMPUTED TOMOGRAPHY

Before an upcoming surgical procedure, I was told that I would need to have a CT scan. The doctors wanted to see if the cancer on my scalp had spread into the bones in my skull. They explained that these images of my head would be in thin "slices," taken as the CT camera rotated around me.

When I arrived in the room, I saw the CT machine. It was a large, circular hollow tube about 18 inches wide. There was a narrow table through the center. It was clear to me immediately that I would not have to worry about feeling "closed in." I lay down on the table, and the technician explained he would add contrast through an intravenous (IV) line halfway through the procedure.

The table was rolled into the machine to a specific spot where a series of pictures were taken. There were several short periods when I was asked to stay as still as possible and hold my breath. The noise was minimal, just soft whirring and clicking. Halfway through the procedure, I was slid out of the machine on the table so that the contrast could be added to the IV line. Once I was back in the machine, more pictures were taken and the test was completed with a minimum of discomfort, much to my grateful surprise.

MRI-MAGNETIC RESONANCE IMAGING

Before yet another surgery procedure, my doctors requested an MRI exam. This time, they wanted to get the best possible image of my malignant tumor and the surrounding area. They explained that the MRI and CT procedures are similar in that they both produce images in thin slices, but that MRI shows more detail, especially of soft tissue.

The technician confirmed I had nothing metal (such as a pacemaker or surgical screws) inside or on my body. The magnet that is used in the MRI machine is so strong that it could cause any metal objects to shift. This movement could disrupt the imaging process or cause damage to tissue in my body.

The MRI machine is a 6 foot-long round tube, open on both ends. Because the body part to be examined was my head, a rubber shield was placed over and very close to my face to hold me in the correct position. I was then rolled inside to the middle of the tube. This was really uncomfortable for me because I have mild claustrophobia. I took deep breaths to relax myself.

Although the technicians had told me the procedure would be loud, I was still taken aback by just how loud it was inside the tube. Even though I was wearing earplugs, the sound was like the pounding of huge hammers held by giant arms, or of heavy-duty jackhammers. At the same time, there was an abrupt shaking of the entire machine from side to side. I knew immediately that this could be an overwhelming experience, so I used the "relax-substitution" method to replace these violent sounds with more familiar ones. I remembered a very loud time as my family and I made our way to Nantucket Island on a ferry for a brief vacation. Now the previously strident and threatening sound was replaced by the welcoming sound of the ferry horn bellowing a happy welcome to the visitors' smiling faces as they came onto the ferry with straw hats, sunscreen, backpacks, and duffel bags. This relaxation method was extremely effective for me. I was then rolled out of the machine for addition of the IV contrast, and the process was repeated.

I am still amazed that the doctors could get such detailed information on what was going on inside my body using these two tests.

PRACTICAL APPLICATIONS

Answers to the questions are found on page 876.

CASE STUDY: MELANOMA FOLLOW-UP

Bill Smith, a 51-year-old sales representative, was initially diagnosed with stage III melanoma 4 years ago. He underwent surgery and received interferon treatment at that time. At his 3-month follow-up CT evaluation last year, Mr. Smith received bad news. The CT scan indicated a small 1-cm nodule that could be a melanoma metastasis. To confirm the diagnosis, Mr. Smith underwent a PET scan.

He was admitted to the nuclear medicine unit of the hospital on the morning of the scan. He had been instructed to fast (no food or beverage 12 hours before the scan). The nuclear medicine physician had told him especially not to eat any type of sugar, which would compete with the radiopharmaceutical 18F-FDG (radiolabeled fluorodeoxyglucose), a radioactive glucose molecule that travels to every cell in the body.

The PET scan began with an injection of a trace amount of 18F-FDG by the physician. Bill was asked to lie still for about an hour in a dark, quiet room and to avoid talking to prevent the compound from concentrating in the tongue and vocal cords. The waiting time allowed the 18F-FDG to be absorbed and released from normal tissue. After emptying his bladder, Bill reclined on a bed that moved slowly and quietly through a PET scanner, a large tube similar to a CT scanner. The radioactive glucose emits charged particles called positrons, which interact with electrons, producing gamma rays that are in turn detected by the scanner. Color-coded images indicate the intensity of metabolic activity throughout the body. Cancerous cells absorb more radioactive glucose than noncancerous cells. The malignant cells show up brighter on the PET scan.

Bill's PET scan proved the CT wrong. His melanoma had not metastasized. He returned home quite relieved.

Questions

1. In CT scanning
   a. A radioactive tracer is used
   b. Magnetic images reveal images in all three planes of the body
   c. A nuclear physician performs the ultrasound procedure
   d. X-rays and a computer produce images in the axial plane

2. In PET scanning
   a. A radioactive tracer is used
   b. X-ray images reveal images in all three planes of the body
   c. A nuclear physician performs the ultrasound procedure
   d. Doppler ultrasound is used

3. Bill's case showed that
   a. CT scanning and PET scanning are equally effective in diagnosis of metastases
   b. PET scanning is useful in cancer diagnosis and staging
   c. Melanoma never progresses to stage IV
   d. A diet high in glucose helps concentrate the radioactive 18F-FDG before the PET scan

GENERAL HOSPITAL: NUCLEAR MEDICINE DEPARTMENT

Available Radionuclides

Radionuclide	Radiopharmaceutical	Administration Route	Target Organ
Xe-133	xenon gas	inhaled	lungs
Tc-99m	albumin microspheres	IV	lungs
Sr-87m (strontium)	solution	IV	bone
Tc-99m	diphosphonate	IV	bone
Tc-99m	pertechnetate	IV	brain
Tc-99m	sulfur colloid	IV	liver/spleen
Tc-99m	HIDA	IV	gallbladder
Tc-99m	DTPA	IV	kidney
Tc-99m	DMSA	IV	kidney
I-123	sodium iodide	PO	thyroid
I-131	sodium iodide	PO	thyroid
TL-201 (thallium)	thallium chloride	IV	heart
Tc-99m	sestamibi	IV	heart
Ga-67 (gallium)	gallium citrate	IV	tumors and abscesses

DMSA, dimercaptosuccinic acid; DTPA, diethylenetriaminepentaacetic acid; HIDA, *N*-(2,6-dimethyl)iminodiacetic acid; IV, intravenous, PO, oral.

20

Questions about the General Hospital: Nuclear Medicine Department

1. Which radionuclide is used with sestamibi in an ETT of heart function?
   a. Thallium-201
   b. Iodine-131
   c. Gallium-67
   d. Technetium-99m

2. Which radionuclide would be used to diagnose disease in an endocrine gland?
   a. Ga-67
   b. I-123
   c. Xe-123
   d. Sr-87m

EXERCISES

Remember to check your answers carefully with the Answers to Exercises, page 875.

A Complete the medical terms based on the definitions and word parts given.

1. Obstructing the passage of x-rays: radio________________
2. Permitting the passage of x-rays: radio________________
3. Aids physicians in performing ultrasound procedures: ________________grapher
4. Transformation of stable substances into charged particles: ________________ization
5. Radioactive drug administered for diagnostic purposes: radio________________
6. Radioactive chemical that gives off energy in the form of radiation: radio________________
7. A physician who specializes in diagnostic radiology: radi________________
8. Study of the uses of radioactive substances in the diagnosis of disease: ____________ medicine

B Match the special diagnostic techniques below with their definitions.

computed tomography
contrast studies
interventional radiology
magnetic resonance imaging
ultrasonography

1. Radiopaque substances are given and conventional x-rays taken ________________.
2. Use of echoes of high-frequency sound waves to diagnose disease ________________.
3. A magnetic field and radio waves are used to form images of the body ________________.
4. X-ray pictures are taken circularly around an area of the body, and a computer synthesizes the information into composite images ________________.
5. Therapeutic procedures are performed by a radiologist under the guidance of CT, MRI, or ultrasonography ________________.

C Match the diagnostic x-ray test in Column I with the part of the body that is imaged in Column II.

COLUMN I

1. myelography ______
2. retrograde pyelography ______
3. angiography ______
4. upper GI series ______
5. cholangiography ______
6. barium enema ______
7. hysterosalpingography ______

COLUMN II

A. spinal cord
B. uterus and fallopian tubes
C. blood vessels
D. esophagus, stomach, and small intestine
E. lower gastrointestinal tract
F. urinary tract
G. bile vessels (ducts)

D **Match the x-ray views or positions in Column I with their meanings in Column II. Write the letter of the answer in the space provided.**

COLUMN I		COLUMN II
1. PA	_____	A. on the side
2. supine	_____	B. turned inward
3. prone	_____	C. movement away from the midline
4. AP	_____	D. lying on the belly
5. lateral	_____	E. x-ray tube positioned on an angle
6. oblique	_____	F. bending a part
7. lateral decubitus	_____	G. straightening a limb
8. adduction	_____	H. lying on the back
9. inversion	_____	I. lying down on the side
10. abduction	_____	J. lying down; prone or supine
11. recumbent	_____	K. anteroposterior view (front to back)
12. eversion	_____	L. turning outward
13. flexion	_____	M. posteroanterior view (back to front)
14. extension	_____	N. movement toward the midline

20

E **Give the meanings of the following medical terms.**

1. in vitro ______________________________
2. in vivo ______________________________
3. radiopharmaceutical ______________________________
4. tracer studies ______________________________
5. uptake ______________________________
6. perfusion lung scan ______________________________
7. ventilation lung scan ______________________________
8. bone scan ______________________________
9. thyroid scan ______________________________
10. technetium Tc 99m Sestamibi scan ______________________________

F Give the meanings of the following terms.

1. gamma camera ______
2. positron emission tomography (PET) ______
3. radioisotope ______
4. transducer ______
5. echocardiography ______
6. lymphoscintigraphy ______
7. radioactive iodine uptake test ______
8. PET/CT scan ______

G Give the meanings of the following word parts.

1. -gram ______
2. ultra- ______
3. vitr/o ______
4. viv/o ______
5. pharmaceut/o ______
6. son/o ______
7. therapeut/o ______

H Give the meanings of the abbreviations in Column I and then select from Column II the best association for each.

COLUMN I

1. MRI ______ ______
2. SPECT ______ ______
3. PACS ______ ______
4. UGI ______ ______
5. CXR ______ ______
6. DSA ______ ______
7. IVP ______ ______
8. LAT ______ ______
9. U/S ______ ______
10. Tc-99m ______ ______

COLUMN II

A. X-ray examination of the kidney after injection of contrast
B. Diagnostic procedure frequently used to assess fetal size and development
C. X-ray examination of the esophagus, stomach, and intestines
D. X-ray of blood vessels made by taking two images (with and without contrast) and subtracting the digitized data for one from the data for the other
E. Radioisotope used in nuclear medicine (tracer studies)
F. Radioactive substances and a computer used to create 3D images
G. Diagnostic procedure produces magnetic resonance images of all three planes of the body and visualizes soft tissue in the nervous and musculoskeletal systems
H. Replacement of traditional films with digital equivalents
I. X-ray view from the side
J. Diagnostic procedure (x-rays are used) necessary to investigate thoracic disease

20

I Circle the correct term to complete each sentence.

1. Mr. Jones was scheduled for ultrasound-guided thoracentesis. He was sent to the (**interventional radiology, radiation oncology, nuclear medicine**) department for the procedure.
2. In order to better visualize Mr. Smith's small intestine, Dr. Wong ordered a (**perfusion study, SBFT, hysterosalpingography**). She hoped to determine why he was having abdominal pain and diarrhea.
3. After a head-on automobile collision, Sam was taken to the emergency department in an unconscious state. The paramedics suspected head trauma, and the doctors ordered an emergency (**PET scan, U/S, CT scan**) of his head.
4. In light of Sue's symptoms of fever, cough, and malaise, the doctors thought that the consolidated, hazy (**radioisotope, radiolucent, radiopaque**) area on the chest x-ray represented a pneumonia.
5. Fred, a lung cancer patient, experienced a seizure recently. His oncologist ordered a brain (**ultrasound, pulmonary angiogram, MRI**) that showed a tumor involving the left frontal lobe of the brain. Fred was treated with Gamma Knife irradiation, and the tumor decreased in size. He has had no further seizures.
6. Tom recently developed a cough and fever. A chest x-ray and (**CT, myelogram, IVP**) of the chest show that a (**pelvic, spinal, mediastinal**) mass is present. (**Mediastinoscopy, Cystoscopy, Lumbar puncture**) and biopsy of the mass reveal Hodgkin disease on histopathologic examination. He is treated with chemotherapy, and his symptoms disappear. A repeat x-ray shows that the mass has decreased remarkably, and a (**SPECT, MRI, PET**) scan shows no uptake of 18F-FDG in the chest, indicating that the mass is fibrosis and not tumor.

7. Paola, a 50-year-old woman with diabetes, experiences chest pain during a stress test, and her (**U/S, ECG, EEG**) shows evidence of ischemia. A (**contrast agent, transducer, radiopharmaceutical**) called technetium Tc 99m sestamibi (Cardiolite) is injected IV, and uptake is assessed with a (**probe, CT scanner, gamma camera**), which shows an area of poor perfusion in the left ventricle.
8. Sally has a routine pelvic examination, and her (**neurologist, gynecologist, urologist**) feels an irregular area of enlargement in the anterior wall of the uterus. A pelvic (**angiogram, U/S study, PET scan**) is performed, which demonstrates the presence of fibroids in the uterine wall. The examination involves placing a gel over her abdominopelvic area and applying a (**ultrasound transducer, radionuclide, MRI scanner**) to send/receive sound vibrations to/from the pelvic region.
9. Sally was having palpitations in the early evening. An ECG revealed possible left ventricular hypertrophy. Her physician ordered an **(ECHO, EUS, UGI)** to rule out valvular heart disease.
10. Joe, a 75-year-old man with a long smoking history, noticed blood in his sputum. His primary care physician ordered a/an **(abdominal CT, chest CT, ultrasound of his heart)** to make the diagnosis.

ANSWERS TO EXERCISES

A

1. radiopaque
2. radiolucent
3. sonographer
4. ionization
5. radiopharmaceutical
6. radioisotope or radionuclide
7. radiologist
8. nuclear

B

1. contrast studies
2. ultrasonography
3. magnetic resonance imaging
4. computed tomography
5. interventional radiology

C

1. A
2. F
3. C
4. D
5. G
6. E
7. B

D

1. M
2. H
3. D
4. K
5. A
6. E
7. I
8. N
9. B
10. C
11. J
12. L
13. F
14. G

E

1. process, test, or procedure in which something is measured or observed outside a living organism
2. process, test, or procedure in which something is measured or observed in a living organism
3. radioactive drug (radionuclide plus chemical) that is given for diagnostic or therapeutic purposes
4. tests in which radioactive substance (radioisotopes) are administered with chemicals and followed as they travel throughout the body
5. the rate of absorption of a radionuclide into an organ or tissue
6. imaging technique in which a radiopharmaceutical is injected intravenously and traced within the blood vessels of the lung scanned
7. imaging technique in which a radiopharmaceutical is inhaled and its passage through the respiratory tract is traced on a scan
8. imaging technique in which a radiopharmaceutical is given intravenously and taken up by bone tissue, followed by scanning to detect the amount of the radioactive substance in the bone
9. imaging technique in which a radioactive substance is given orally and a scan (image) is made to assess its uptake in the thyroid gland
10. test of heart muscle function

F

1. machine that detects rays emitted by radioactive substances
2. radioactive glucose is injected and traced to body cells
3. a radioactive form (radionuclide) of a substance; gives off radiation
4. handheld device that sends and receives ultrasound signals
5. ultrasound is used to create an image of the heart
6. nuclear medicine imaging of the lymphatic system
7. nuclear medicine test to evaluate the function of the thyroid gland
8. combination of a PET scan and a CT scan to show both structure and function of the body

G

1. record
2. beyond
3. glass
4. life
5. drug
6. sound
7. treatment

20

H

1. magnetic resonance imaging: G
2. single photon emission computed tomography: F
3. picture archival and communications system: H
4. upper gastrointestinal (series): C
5. chest x-ray: J
6. digital subtraction angiography: D
7. intravenous pyelogram: A
8. lateral: I
9. ultrasound: B
10. radioactive technetium: E

I

1. interventional radiology
2. SBFT (small bowel follow-through)
3. CT scan
4. radiopaque
5. MRI
6. CT, mediastinal, mediastinoscopy, PET
7. ECG, radiopharmaceutical, gamma camera
8. gynecologist, U/S, transducer
9. ECHO
10. chest CT

Answers to Practical Applications

Case Study: Melanoma Follow-up

1. d
2. a
3. b

General Hospital: Nuclear Medicine Department

1. d
2. b

PRONUNCIATION OF TERMS

To test your understanding of the terminology in this chapter, write the meaning of each term in the space provided. In addition, you may wish to cover the terms and write them by looking at your definitions. Make sure your spelling is correct. The page number after each term indicates where it is defined or used in the book, so you can easily check your responses. You will find complete definitions for all of these terms and their audio pronunciations on the Evolve website.

Pronunciation Guide

ā as ināpe	ă as in ăpple
ē as in ēven	ĕ as in ĕvery
ī as in īce	ĭ as in ĭnterest
ō as in ōpen	ŏ as in pŏt
ū as in ūnit	ŭ as in ŭnder

TERM	PRONUNCIATION	MEANING
abduction (860)	ăb-DŬK-shŭn	
adduction (860)	ă-DŬK-shŭn	
angiogram (866)	ĂN-jē-ō-grăm	
anteroposterior (859)	ăn-tĕr-ō-pōs-TĒ-rē-ŏr	
bone scan (861)	bōn skăn	
cholangiography (854)	kō-lăn-jē-ŎG-ră-fē	
computed tomography (864)	kŏm-PŪ-tĕd tō-MŎG-ră-fē	
contrast studies (864)	KŎN-trăst STŬD-ēz	
echocardiography (867)	ĕk-ō-kăr-dē-ŎG-ră-fē	
eversion (860)	ē-VĔR-zhŭn	
extension (860)	ĕk-STĔN-shŭn	
flexion (860)	FLĔK-shŭn	

TERM	PRONUNCIATION	MEANING
fluoroscopy (856)	floo-RŎS-kō-pē	
gamma camera (864)	GĂ-mă KĂM-ĕr-ă	
gamma rays (864)	GĂ-mă rāz	
half-life (860)	HĂF-līf	
hysterosalpingogram (866)	hĭs-tĕr-ō-săl-PĬNG-gō-grăm	
hysterosonogram (866)	hĭs-tĕr-ō-SŎN-ō-grăm	
interventional radiology (864)	ĭn-tĕr-VĔN-shŭn-ăl rā-dē-ŎL-ō-jē	
inversion (860)	ĭn-VĔR-zhŭn	
in vitro (864)	ĭn VĒ-trō	
in vivo (864)	ĭn VĒ-vō	
ionization (865)	ī-ŏn-ĭ-ZĀ-shŭn	
lateral decubitus (860)	LĂ-tĕr-ăl dĕ-KŪ-bĭ-tŭs	
lymphoscintigraphy (862)	lĭm-fō-sĭn-TĬG-ră-fē	
magnetic resonance imaging (865)	măg-NĔT-ĭk RĔZ-ō-năns ĬM-ă-jĭng	
myelography (855)	mī-ĕ-LŎG-ră-fē	
nuclear medicine (865)	NOO-klē-ăr MĔD-ĭ-sĭn	
oblique (859)	ō-BLĒK	
PET/CT scan (862)	PĔT-CT scăn	
positron emission tomography (865)	PŎS-ĭ-trŏn ē-MĬSH-ŭn tō-MŎG-ră-fē	
posteroanterior (859)	pōs-tĕr-ō-ăn-TĒ-rē-ŏr	
prone (860)	prōn	
pyelogram (866)	PĪ-ē-lō-grăm	
radiographer (866)	rā-dē-ŎG-ră-fĕr	
radioimmunoassay (865)	rā-dē-ō-ĭ-mū-nō-ĂS-ā	
radioisotope (865)	rā-dē-ō-Ī-sō-tōp	
radiolabeled compound (865)	rā-dē-ō-LĀ-bĕld KŎM-pownd	
radiology (865)	rā-dē-ŎL-ō-gē	
radiolucent (865)	rā-dē-ō-LO͞O-sĕnt	
radionuclide (865)	rā-dē-ō-NO͞O-klīd	

TERM	PRONUNCIATION	MEANING
radiopaque (865)	rā-dē-ō-PĀK	
radiopharmaceutical (865)	rā-dē-ō-făr-mă-SŪ-tĭ-kăl	
recumbent (860)	rē-KŬM-bĕnt	
scan (865)	scăn	
scintigraphy (865)	SĬN-tĕ-gră-fē	
single photon emission computed tomography (865)	SĬNG-l PHŌ-tŏn ē-MĬ-shŭn kŏm-PŪ-tĕd tō-MŎG-ră-fē	
sonogram (856)	SŎN-ō-grăm	
supine (860)	SOO-pīn	
tagging (865)	TĂG-ĭng	
technetium Tc 99m sestamibi scan (863)	tĕk-NĒ-shē-ŭm Tc 99m sĕs-tă-MĬ-bē skăn	
thallium scan (863)	THĂL-ē-ŭm skăn	
therapeutic (866)	thĕr-ă-PŪ-tik	
thyroid scan (863)	THĪ-rŏyd skăn	
tracer studies (865)	TRĀ-sĕr STŬ-dēz	
ultrasonography (865)	ŭl-tră-sō-NŎG-ră-fē	
ultrasound transducer (865)	ŭl-tră-SOWND trănz-DOO-sĕr	
uptake (865)	ŬP-tāk	
urography (856)	ū-RŎG-ră-fē	
ventilation-perfusion studies (865)	vĕn-tĭ-LĀ-shŭn-pĕr-FŪ-shŭn STŬ-dēz	

REVIEW SHEET

Write the meanings of the combining forms in the spaces provided, and test yourself. Check your answers with the information in the text or in the Glossary (Medical Word Parts—English) at the end of the book.

Combining Forms

COMBINING FORM	MEANING	COMBINING FORM	MEANING
ion/o	________________	son/o	________________
is/o	________________	therapeut/o	________________
myel/o	________________	vitr/o	________________
pharmaceut/o	________________	viv/o	________________
radi/o	________________		

Suffixes

SUFFIX	MEANING	SUFFIX	MEANING
-gram	________________	-lucent	________________
-graphy	________________	-opaque	________________

Prefixes

PREFIX	MEANING	PREFIX	MEANING
echo-	________________	ultra-	________________

evolve *Please refer to the Evolve website for additional exercises, games, and images related to this chapter.*

CHAPTER 21

Pharmacology

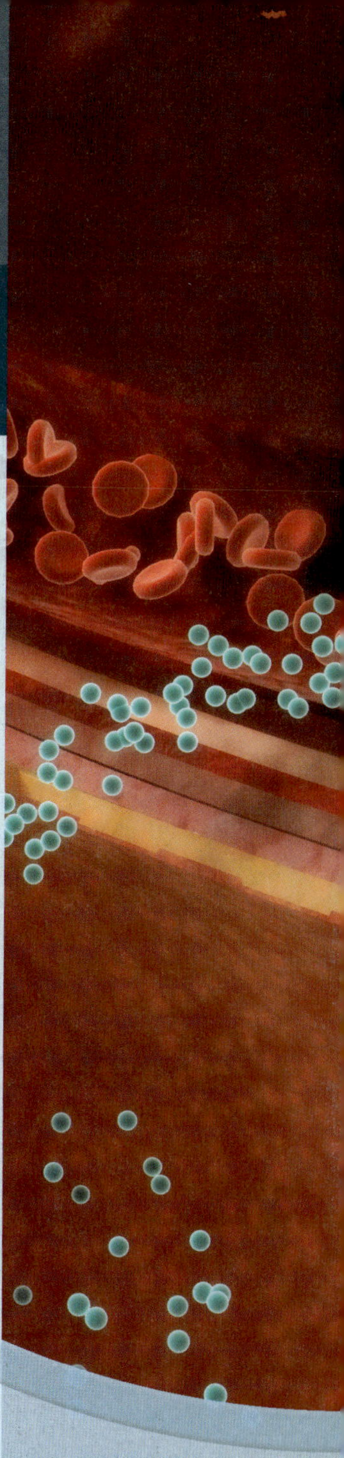

This chapter is divided into the following sections:

CHAPTER GOALS

- Describe the various subspecialty areas of pharmacology.
- Identify the various routes of drug administration.
- Differentiate among the various classes of drugs and name their primary actions and side effects.
- Define medical terms using combining forms and prefixes that relate to pharmacology.
- Apply your new knowledge to understanding medical terms in their proper contexts, such as medical reports and records.

INTRODUCTION

Drugs (medicines) are substances used to prevent or treat a condition or disease. Some drugs are obtained from parts of **plants,** such as the roots, leaves, and fruit. An example of a plant-derived drug is a cardiac medicine, digitalis (from the foxglove plant). Other drugs (antibiotics such as penicillin) are obtained from yeast, molds, and fungi. Drugs also are obtained from **animals;** for example, hormones are secretions from the glands of animals. Some drugs are **synthesized** in a laboratory. Anticancer drugs such as methotrexate and 5-fluorouracil are laboratory-synthesized drugs. **Vitamins** are drugs that are isolated from plant or animal sources and are contained in foods.

A **pharmacist** prepares and dispenses drugs through a **pharmacy** (drugstore) on a written order from a physician. The order is called a **prescription.** Currently, most schools or colleges of pharmacy offer a PharmD (doctor of pharmacy) degree after 6 or 7 years of study. As a health care professional, a pharmacist cooperates with, consults with, and sometimes advises licensed practitioners concerning drugs. In addition, the pharmacist answers patients' questions about their prescription. A **pharmacy technician** helps licensed pharmacists provide medication and other health care products to patients.

Pharmacology is the study of the discovery, properties, uses, and actions of drugs. A **pharmacologist** is either an MD (doctor of medicine) or a PhD (doctor of philosophy) who specializes in the study of medicines. Pharmacology contains many subdivisions of study: **medicinal chemistry, pharmacodynamics, pharmacokinetics, molecular pharmacology, chemotherapy,** and **toxicology.**

Medicinal chemistry is the study of new drug synthesis and the relationship between chemical structure and biological effects. **Pharmacodynamics** involves the study of a drug's effects in the body. **Pharmacokinetics** is the study of a drug's absorption (how drugs pass into the bloodstream), distribution into body compartments, metabolism (changes that drugs undergo within the body), and excretion (removal of the drug from the body) over a period of time.

Molecular pharmacology involves the interaction of drugs and subcellular entities, such as DNA, RNA, and enzymes. It provides important information about the mechanism of action of drugs.

Chemotherapy is the study of drugs that destroy microorganisms, parasites, or malignant cells within the body. Chemotherapy includes treatment of infectious diseases and cancer.

Toxicology is the study of the harmful effects of drugs and chemicals on the body. Toxicologic studies in animals are required by law before new drugs can be tested in humans. A toxicologist also is interested in finding proper **antidotes** to any harmful effects of drugs. Antidotes are substances given to neutralize unwanted effects of drugs.

Figure 21-1 reviews the subspecialty areas of pharmacology.

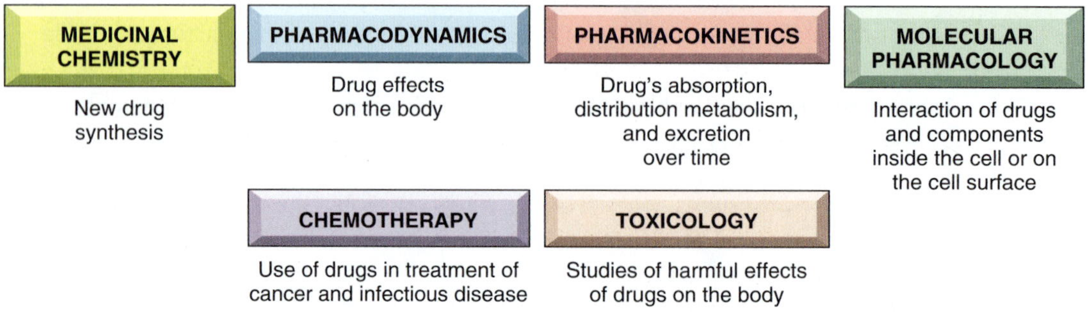

FIGURE 21-1 Subspecialty areas of pharmacology.

DRUG NAMES, STANDARDS, AND REFERENCES

NAMES

A drug can have three different names. The **chemical name** specifies the exact chemical makeup of the drug. This name often is long and complicated.

The **generic name,** typically shorter and less complicated, identifies the drug legally and scientifically. The generic name becomes public property after 17 years of use by the original manufacturer, and any drug manufacturer may use it thereafter. There is only one generic name for each drug.

The **brand name** or trademark is the private property of the individual drug manufacturer, and no competitor may use it. A brand name (also called trade name) often has the superscript ® after or before the name, indicating that it is a registered brand name. Drugs can have several brand names, because each manufacturer producing the drug gives it a different name. When a specific brand name is ordered on a prescription by a physician, it must be dispensed by the pharmacist; no other brand name may be substituted. It is usual practice to capitalize the first letter of a brand name.

The following example shows the chemical, generic, and brand names for the antibiotic drug amoxicillin; note that the drug has several brand names but only one generic, or official, name:

CHEMICAL NAME	GENERIC NAME	BRAND NAMES
[2*S*,5*R*,6*R*]-6-[(*R*)-(–)-2-amino-2-(*p*-hydroxyphenyl) acetamido]-3,3-dimethyl-7-oxo-4-thia-1-azabicyclo[3.2.0] heptane-2-carboxylic acid	amoxicillin	Amoxil Polymox Trimox

STANDARDS

The U.S. **Food and Drug Administration (FDA)** has the legal responsibility for deciding whether a drug may be disseminated and sold. It sets strict standards for efficacy (effectiveness) and purity and requires extensive experimental testing in animals and people before it approves a new drug for sale for a specific medical use, or indication, such as for treatment of tuberculosis. An independent committee of physicians, pharmacologists, pharmacists, and manufacturers, called the **United States Pharmacopeia (USP),** reviews the available commercial drugs and continually reappraises their effectiveness. Three important standards of the USP are that the drug must be safe, clinically useful (effective for patients), and available in pure form (made by good manufacturing methods). If a drug has USP after its name, it has met with the standards of the Pharmacopeia.

REFERENCES

Two large reference listings of drugs are available at libraries and hospitals. The most complete and up-to-date listing is the **hospital formulary,** which gives information about the characteristics of drugs and their clinical usage (application to patient care) as approved by that particular hospital.

The ***Physicians' Desk Reference*** **(PDR)** is published by a private firm, and drug manufacturers pay to have their products listed. The PDR is a useful reference with several different indices to identify drugs, along with a complete description of the drug's properties and approved indications. It also gives precautions, warnings about side effects, and information about the recommended dosage and administration of each drug.

ADMINISTRATION OF DRUGS

The route of administration of a drug (how it is taken into the body) determines how well it is absorbed into the blood, and its speed and duration of action.

Various methods of administering drugs are:

Oral Administration. Drugs given by mouth are slowly absorbed into the bloodstream through the stomach or intestinal wall. This method, although convenient for the patient, has several disadvantages. If the drug is destroyed in the digestive tract by digestive juices, or if the drug is unable to pass through the intestinal wall, it will be ineffective. Oral administration is also a disadvantage if a rapid onset of action is desired. It takes several hours for oral medication to be fully absorbed into the bloodstream.

Sublingual Administration. Drugs placed under the tongue dissolve in the saliva. For some agents, absorption may be rapid. Nitroglycerin tablets are administered in this way to treat attacks of angina (chest pain).

Rectal Administration. Suppositories (cone-shaped objects containing drugs) and aqueous solutions are inserted into the rectum. Drugs are given by rectum when oral administration presents difficulties, as when the patient is nauseated and vomiting.

Parenteral Administration. Injection of drug from a **syringe** (tube) through a hollow needle placed under the skin, into a muscle, vein, or body cavity. There are several types of parenteral injections and instillations:

21

1. **Intracavitary instillation.** This injection is made into a body cavity, such as the peritoneal or pleural cavity. For example, drugs may be introduced into the pleural cavity in people who have pleural effusions due to malignant disease. The drug causes the pleural surfaces to adhere, thereby obliterating the pleural space and preventing the accumulation of fluid. This procedure is known as **pleurodesis.**
2. **Intradermal injection.** This shallow injection is made into the upper layers of the skin and is used chiefly in skin testing for allergic reactions.
3. **Subcutaneous (hypodermic) injection (subQ).** A small hypodermic needle is introduced into the subcutaneous tissue under the skin, usually on the upper arm, thigh, or abdomen. Insulin is injected daily via this route.
4. **Intramuscular injection (IM).** The buttock or upper arm is the usual site for this injection into muscle. When drugs are irritating to the skin or when a large volume of solution must be administered, IM injections are used.
5. **Intrathecal instillation.** This instillation occurs in the space under the membranes (meninges) surrounding the spinal cord and brain. Methotrexate (a cancer chemotherapeutic drug) is introduced intrathecally for treatment of leukemia involving the spinal canal.
6. **Intravenous injection (IV).** This injection is given directly into a vein. It is used when an immediate effect from the drug is desired or when the drug cannot be safely introduced into other tissues. Good technical skill is needed with intravenous injections because leakage of a drug into surrounding tissues may result in irritation and inflammation. Some medicines, such as anticancer drugs, are dissolved in a large volume of saline (sterile salt solution) and given by a several-hour-long intravenous infusion.
7. **Pumps.** Battery-powered pumps may be used for continuous administration of drugs by the subcutaneous or intravenous route.

Inhalation. Vapors, or gases, taken into the nose or mouth are absorbed into the bloodstream through the thin walls of air sacs in the lungs. **Aerosols** (particles of drug suspended in air) are administered by inhalation, as are many anesthetics. Examples of aerosols

TABLE 21-1	ROUTES OF DRUG ADMINISTRATION				
Oral	**Sublingual**	**Rectal**	**Parenteral**	**Inhalation**	**Topical**
Caplets Capsules Tablets	Tablets	Suppositories	Injections and instillations Intracavitary Intradermal Intramuscular Intrathecal Intravenous Pumps Subcutaneous	Aerosols	Lotions Creams Ointments Transdermal patches

are pentamidine, used to prevent a form of pneumonia associated with acquired immunodeficiency syndrome (AIDS), and various aerosolized medicines used to treat asthma (spasm of the lung airways).

Topical Application. Drugs are applied locally on the skin or mucous membranes of the body. **Antiseptics** (against infection) and **antipruritics** (against itching) commonly are used as ointments, creams, and lotions. **Transdermal patches** are used to deliver drugs (such as estrogen for hormone replacement therapy, pain medications, and nicotine for smoking cessation programs) continuously through the skin.

Table 21-1 summarizes the various routes of drug administration. Figure 21-2 illustrates examples of vehicles for drug administration.

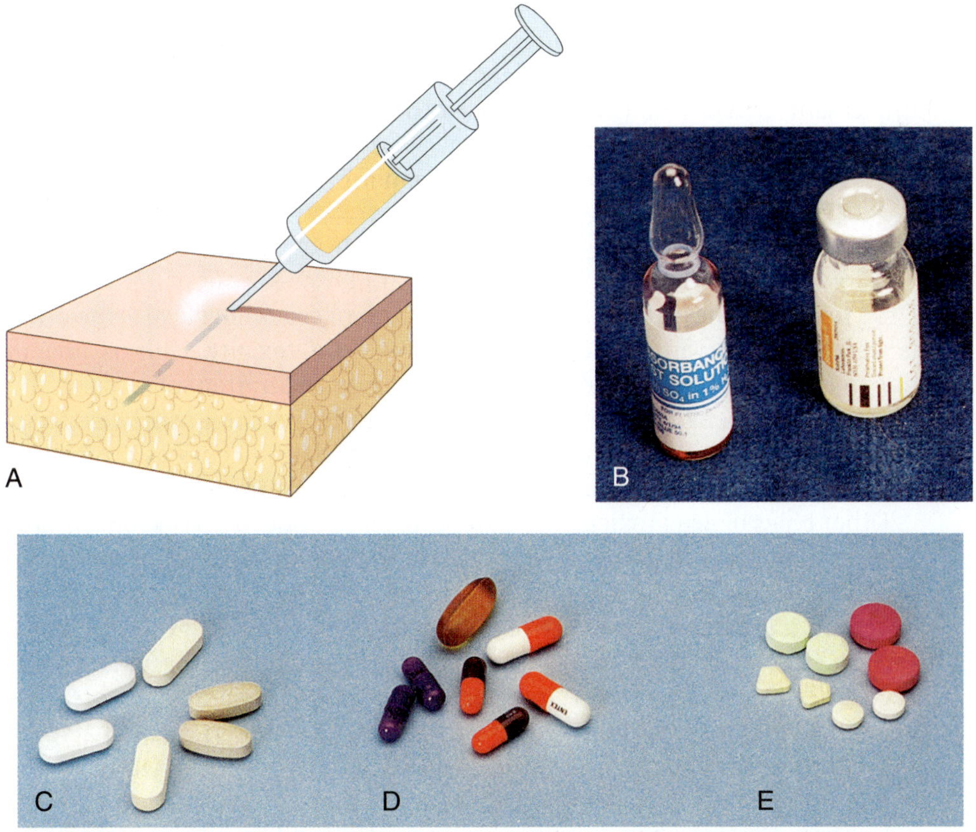

FIGURE 21-2 **Examples of vehicles for drug administration. A, Hypodermic syringe. B, Ampule** (small, sterile glass or plastic container containing a single dose of drug) and **vial** (glass container with a metal-enclosed rubber seal.) **C, Caplets** (coated like a capsule, but solid like a tablet). **D, Capsules** (small soluble containers, usually made of gelatin, used for a dose of medication for swallowing). **E, Tablets** (small solid pills containing a dose of medication).

Drug Actions and Interactions

When a drug enters the body, the target substance with which the drug interacts to produce its effects is called a **receptor.** A drug may cross the cell membrane to reach its intracellular receptor or may react with a receptor on the cell's surface. The **dose** of a drug is the amount of drug administered, usually measured in milligrams or grams. **Schedule** is the exact timing and frequency of drug administration.

Various actions and interactions of drugs in the body can occur after they have been absorbed into the bloodstream.

Additive Action. If the combination of two similar drugs is equal to the **sum** of the effects of each, then the drugs are called additive. For example, if drug A gives 10% tumor kill as a chemotherapeutic agent and drug B gives 20% tumor kill, using A and B together would give 30% tumor kill.

If two drugs give less than an additive effect, they are called **antagonistic.** If they produce greater than additive effects, they are **synergistic** (as described next).

Synergism. A combination of two drugs sometimes can cause an effect that is **greater** than the sum of the individual effects of each drug given alone. For example, INH (isoniazid) and rifampin, two antibiotic drugs, are given together in the treatment of tuberculosis because of their synergistic effect.

Response. This is a desired and beneficial effect of a drug. Lowering blood pressure by antihypertensive drugs is an example.

21

Tolerance. For some drugs, the effects of a given dose diminish as treatment continues, and increasing amounts are needed to produce the same effect. Tolerance is a feature of addiction to drugs such as morphine and meperidine hydrochloride (Demerol). **Addiction** is the physical and psychological **dependence** on and craving for a drug and the presence of clearly unpleasant effects when that drug or other agent is withdrawn. **Controlled substances** are drugs that produce dependence and have potential for abuse or addiction. See pages 905-906 in the Practical Applications section for information about these drugs.

Drug Toxicity

Drug toxicity is the unwanted and potentially dangerous effects of some drugs. **Idiosyncrasy** is an example of an unpredictable type of drug toxicity. This is any unexpected and uncommon side effect that develops after administration of a drug. For example, in some people, penicillin causes an **idiosyncratic reaction,** such as **anaphylaxis** (acute hypersensitivity with asthma and shock). Anaphylaxis occurs as a result of exposure to a previously encountered drug or foreign substance (antigen).

Other types of drug toxicity are more predictable and are based on the dosage of the drug given. Physicians are trained to be aware of the potential toxic effects of all drugs that they prescribe. **Iatrogenic** (produced by treatment) disorders can occur, however, as a result of mistakes in drug use or because of individual sensitivity to a given agent.

Side effects are toxic effects that routinely result from the use of a drug. They often occur with the usual therapeutic dosage of a drug and generally are tolerable and reversible when the drug is discontinued. For example, nausea, vomiting, and alopecia are common side effects of the chemotherapeutic drugs used to treat cancer. Other, rare side effects may be life-threatening, such as severe allergic reactions.

Contraindications are factors in a patient's condition that make the use of a drug dangerous and ill advised. For example, in the presence of kidney failure, it is unwise to administer a drug, such as methotrexate, that is normally eliminated by the kidneys because excess drug will accumulate in the body and cause adverse effects.

Resistance is a lack of beneficial response, and it is seen when drugs that used to be effective are unable to control the disease process in a particular patient. It is often seen in serious bacterial infection or cancer.

CLASSES OF DRUGS

The following are major classes of drugs with indications for their use. Specific drugs in each class are included in tables for your reference (note that the brand names are capitalized). Appendix IV is a complete list of these drugs and their class or type. Notice that many drug types end with the adjectival suffix -ic, meaning pertaining to, although they are used as nouns.

ANALGESICS

An analgesic (alges/o = sensitivity to pain) is a drug that lessens pain. Mild analgesics relieve mild to moderate pain, such as myalgias, headaches, and toothaches. More potent analgesics are **narcotics** or **opioids,** which are derived from opium. These drugs may induce stupor (a condition of near-unconsciousness and reduced mental and physical activity). They are used only to relieve severe pain because they may produce dependence.

Some non-narcotic analgesics reduce fever, pain, and inflammation and are used for joint disorders (osteoarthritis and rheumatoid arthritis), painful menstruation, and acute pain due to minor injuries or infection. These agents are not steroid hormones (such as cortisone) and are known as **nonsteroidal anti-inflammatory drugs (NSAIDs).** NSAIDs act on tissues to inhibit prostaglandins (hormone-like substances that sensitize peripheral pain receptors). A newer class of NSAIDs is the COX-2 (cyclooxygenase-2) inhibitors. These agents block prostaglandin production. They relieve pain and inflammation as do traditional NSAIDs, but produce fewer gastrointestinal side effects than NSAIDs. However, they may increase the risk of clots and heart attacks. Examples of COX-2 inhibitors are Celebrex and Bextra, which are listed in Table 21-2 with other analgesics.

TABLE 21-2 ANALGESICS AND ANESTHETICS

ANALGESICS	ANESTHETICS
Mild	**General**
acetaminophen (Tylenol)	ether
Narcotic (Opioid)	halothane (Fluothane)
codeine	nitrous oxide
hydrocodone w/APAP* (Lortab, Vicodin)	propofol (Diprivan)
hydromorphone (Dilaudid)	thiopental (Pentothal)
meperidine (Demerol)	**Local**
morphine	lidocaine (Xylocaine)
oxycodone (OxyContin, Roxicodone)	lidocaine-prilocaine (EMLA—eutectic mixture of local anesthetics)
oxycodone with APAP* (Percocet, Roxicet, Endocet)	procaine (Novocain)
tramadol (Ultram)	
Nonsteroidal Anti-Inflammatory Drugs [NSAIDs]	
aspirin (Anacin, Ascriptin, Excedrin)	
celecoxib (Celebrex)	
diclofenac sodium (Voltaren)	
ibuprofen (Motrin, Advil)	
ketorolac (Toradol)	
naproxen (Naprosyn)	
valdecoxib (Bextra)	

Note: Brand names are in parentheses.
*APAP, acetyl-*p*-aminophenol—acetaminophen (Tylenol, others).

ANESTHETICS

An anesthetic is an agent that reduces or eliminates sensation. This effect may occur in all tissues of the body **(general anesthetic)** and puts a patient asleep, or may be limited to a particular region **(local anesthetic).** General anesthetics are used for surgical procedures. They depress the activity of the central nervous system, producing loss of consciousness, and block the perception of pain. Local anesthetics inhibit the conduction of pain impulses in sensory nerves in the region in which they are injected or applied. An example is dental anesthesia with a local Novocain injection.

Table 21-2 gives examples of specific anesthetics.

ANTIBIOTICS AND ANTIVIRALS

An antibiotic is a chemical substance produced by a microorganism (bacterium, yeast, or mold) that inhibits **(bacteriostatic)** or kills **(bactericidal)** bacteria, fungi, or parasites. The use of antibiotics (penicillin was first in general use in 1945) has made it possible to cure many conditions such as pneumonia, urinary tract infection, and streptococcal pharyngitis ("strep throat"). Caution about the use of antibiotics is warranted because they are powerful agents. Like all drugs, they have side effects. Also, with indiscriminate use of antibiotics, bacteria and fungi can develop resistance to a particular agent. Infections caused by these resistant bacteria can spread and may be difficult or impossible to cure.

Antifungal medications treat fungal infections. These infections commonly occur in the skin (ringworm), vagina (moniliasis or candidiasis), mouth, bloodstream, and other organs. Antitubercular drugs treat tuberculosis, a chronic and often drug-resistant infection. Antiviral drugs are used against infections due to viruses, such as herpesviruses, Epstein-Barr virus, cytomegalovirus (CMV), and human immunodeficiency virus (HIV).

Table 21-3 lists types of antibiotics (such as antifungal and antitubercular drugs) and antiviral drugs and gives specific examples of each.

ANTICOAGULANTS AND ANTIPLATELET DRUGS

Anticoagulants prevent clotting (coagulation) of blood. They prevent formation of clots or break up clots in blood vessels in conditions such as thrombosis and embolism. They also are used to prevent coagulation in preserved blood used for transfusions. **Heparin** is a natural anticoagulant purified from pig intestine or bovine (cow) lung. It is found in the granules of certain white blood cells. A more easily administered form of heparin called low-molecular-weight heparin (Fragmin, Lovenox) is self-injected on a daily basis and requires no monitoring of blood clotting ability, as is done with regular heparin. Other anticoagulants, including **warfarin (Coumadin),** are manufactured. Coumadin blocks the formation of a number of clot-forming factors in the blood. Its action is reversed by vitamin K. **Tissue-type plasminogen activator (tPA)** dissolves clots and is used to open vessels after myocardial infarction.

TABLE 21-3 ANTIBIOTICS AND ANTIVIRALS

ANTIFUNGAL DRUGS

amphotericin B (Fungilin)
clotrimazole (Lotrimin, Mycelex)
econazole topical (Spectazole)
fluconazole (Diflucan)
itraconazole (Sporanox)
miconazole (Monistat)
nystatin (Nilstat)
terbinafine (Lamisil)

ANTITUBERCULAR DRUGS

ethambutol (Myambutol)
isoniazid [INH] (Nydrazid)
p-aminosalicylic acid granules (PASER)
rifampin (Rifadin)

ANTIVIRAL DRUGS

acyclovir (Zovirax)
efavirenz (Sustiva)*
indinavir (Crixivan)†
interferon alfa-n1 (Wellferon)
lamivudine (Epivir)‡
ribavirin (Copegus, Rebetol)
zidovudine *or* azidothymidine [AZT] (Retrovir)‡
zidovudine plus lamivudine (Combivir)‡

CEPHALOSPORINS—bactericidal and similar to penicillins

cefprozil (Cefzil)
ceftazidime (Fortaz)
cephalexin (Keflex)
cefuroxime axetil (Ceftin)

ERYTHROMYCINS—bacteriostatic

azithromycin (Zithromax)
clarithromycin (Biaxin)
erythromycin (Ery-Tab)

PENICILLINS—bactericidal

amoxicillin trihydrate (Amoxil, Trimox)
amoxicillin with clavulanate (Augmentin)
nafcillin (Unipen)
oxacillin (Bactocill)

QUINOLONES—bactericidal and wide-spectrum

ciprofloxacin (Cipro)
levofloxacin (Levaquin)
ofloxacin (Floxin)

SULFONAMIDES OR SULFA DRUGS—bactericidal

sulfamethoxazole with trimethoprim (Bactrim)
sulfisoxazole (Gantrisin)

TETRACYCLINES—bacteriostatic

doxycycline
tetracycline

Note: Brand names are in parentheses.
*Anti-HIV—non-nucleoside reverse transcriptase inhibitor (NNRTI).
†Anti-HIV—protease inhibitor.
‡Anti-HIV—nucleoside reverse transcriptase inhibitor (NRTI).

Antiplatelet drugs reduce the tendency of platelets to stick together. Aspirin is an example of an antiplatelet drug; daily aspirin prophylaxis is recommended for patients with coronary artery disease and for those who have had heart attacks. Clopidogrel bisulfate (Plavix) inhibits clumping of platelets and is used to prevent clotting after heart attacks and blood vessel procedures, such as angioplasty.

Table 21-4 lists anticoagulants and antiplatelet drugs.

ANTICONVULSANTS

An anticonvulsant prevents or reduces the frequency of convulsions in various types of seizure disorders or epilepsy. Ideally, anticonvulsants depress abnormal spontaneous activity of the brain arising from areas of scar or tumor, without affecting normal brain function. Table 21-4 lists examples of anticonvulsants.

TABLE 21-4 ANTICOAGULANTS, ANTICONVULSANTS, ANTIDEPRESSANTS, AND ANTIDIABETICS

ANTICOAGULANTS AND ANTIPLATELET DRUGS	ANTI-ALZHEIMER DRUGS
aspirin clopidogrel bisulfate (Plavix) dabigatran (Pradaxa) dalteparin (Fragmin)* enoxaparin sodium (Lovenox)* lepirudin (Refludan)† prasugrel (Effient) rivaroxaban (Xarelto) ticagrelor (Brilinta) tissue plasminogen activator [tPA] warfarin (Coumadin) **ANTICONVULSANTS** carbamazepine (Tegretol) felbamate (Felbatol) gabapentin (Neurontin) levetiracetam (Keppra) phenobarbital phenytoin sodium (Dilantin) valproic acid (Depakote) **ANTIDEPRESSANTS** amitriptyline (Elavil)‡ bupropion (Wellbutrin SR) citalopram hydrobromide (Celexa)§ escitalopram (Lexapro)§ fluoxetine (Prozac)§ nortriptyline (Pamelor)‡ paroxetine (Paxil)§ sertraline (Zoloft)§ trazodone (Desyrel)§	donepezil (Aricept) memantine (Namenda) **ANTIDIABETICS** **Insulins** *Rapid-acting* insulin aspart (NovoLog) insulin glulisine (Apidra) insulin lispro (Humalog) *Short-acting* insulin regulator (Humulin R) *Intermediate-acting* insulin NPH (Humulin N) *Long-acting* insulin detemir (Levemir) insulin glargine (Lantus) insulin zinc suspension (Ultralente) **Other Drugs—Oral** acarbose (Precose)—alpha-glucosidase inhibitor glipizide (Glucotrol XL)—sulfonylurea glyburide (Diabeta, Micronase)—sulfonylurea metformin (Glucophage)—biguanide pioglitazone (Actos)—thiazolidinedione repaglinide (Prandin)—meglitinide rosiglitazone (Avandia)—thiazolidinedione

Note: Brand names are in parentheses.
*Low molecular weight heparin.
†Derived from the saliva of the medicinal leech.
‡Tricyclic antidepressant drug.
§Selective serotonin reuptake inhibitor (SSRI).

ANTIDEPRESSANTS AND ANTI-ALZHEIMER DRUGS

Antidepressants treat symptoms of depression. They can elevate mood, increase physical activity and mental alertness, and improve appetite and sleep patterns. Many antidepressants also are mild sedatives and treat mild forms of depression associated with anxiety.

The largest class of antidepressants increases the action of neurotransmitters by blocking their removal (reuptake) from the synapses (spaces between nerve cells). These drugs include **tricyclic antidepressants (TCAs)** and **selective serotonin reuptake inhibitors (SSRIs).** Other antidepressants are **monoamine oxidase inhibitors (MAOIs),** which increase the length of time neurotransmitters work by blocking monoamine oxidase, an enzyme that normally inactivates neurotransmitters.

Lithium is a drug that is used to stabilize the mood swings and unpredictable behavior of people with bipolar disorder (manic-depressive illness).

Anti-Alzheimer drugs, used to treat symptoms of Alzheimer disease, act by aiding brain neurotransmitters (acetylcholine) or shielding brain cells from glutamate, a neurotransmitter that at high levels contributes to death of brain cells. Table 21-4 lists examples of antidepressants and anti-Alzheimer drugs.

ANTIDIABETICS

Antidiabetics are used to treat diabetes mellitus (condition in which either the hormone insulin is not produced, or the body's tissues have developed insensitivity to insulin). Patients with type 1 diabetes have lost the ability to produce insulin as children or young adults and must receive daily injections of **insulin.** Human insulin and synthetic derivations produced by recombinant DNA research have largely replaced animal-derived insulin in the management of diabetes. Rapid-acting insulins start working in 15 to 30 minutes and last 3 to 5 hours. Short-acting insulin begins working within 30 minutes to an hour and lasts 5 to 8 hours. Long-acting insulins have a time to onset of 1 to 3 hours and last between 24 and 36 hours.

Patients with type 2 diabetes usually develop diabetes later in life and have insensitivity to insulin. Their disease may be well controlled on **oral antidiabetic drugs.** These include **sulfonylureas** (lower the levels of glucose in the blood by stimulating the production of insulin), **biguanides** (increase the body's sensitivity to insulin and reduce the production of glucose by the liver), **alpha-glucosidase inhibitors** (temporarily block enzymes that digest sugars), **thiazolidinediones** (enhance glucose uptake into tissues), and **meglitinides** (stimulate the beta cells in the pancreas to produce insulin).

An **insulin pump** is a device strapped to the patient's waist that periodically delivers (via subcutaneous needle in the abdomen) the desired amount of insulin.

Table 21-4 lists antidiabetic drugs.

ANTIHISTAMINES

These drugs block the action of histamine, which is normally released in the body in allergic reactions. Histamine causes allergic symptoms such as hives, bronchial asthma, hay fever, and in severe cases, **anaphylactic shock** (dyspnea, hypotension, and loss of consciousness). Antihistamines cannot cure the allergic reaction, but they relieve its symptoms. Many antihistamines have strong **antiemetic** (prevention of nausea) activity and are used to prevent motion sickness. The most common side effects of antihistamines are drowsiness, blurred vision, tremors, digestive upset, and lack of motor coordination.

Table 21-5 lists common antihistamines.

TABLE 21-5 ANTIHISTAMINES AND ANTIOSTEOPOROSIS DRUGS

ANTIHISTAMINES	ANTIOSTEOPOROSIS DRUGS
	Bisphosphonates (Prevents Bone Loss)
cetirizine (Zyrtec)	alendronate (Fosamax)
chlorpheniramine maleate (Chlor-Trimeton)	denosumab (Prolia)*
diphenhydramine (Benadryl)	ibandronate sodium (Boniva)
fexofenadine (Allegra)	pamidronate disodium (Aredia)
loratadine (Claritin)	teriparatide (Forteo)†
meclizine (Antivert)	zoledronic acid (Zometa)
promethazine (Phenergan)	**Selective Estrogen Receptor Modulators (SERMs)**
	raloxifene (Evista)
	tamoxifen (Nolvadex)

Note: Brand names are in parentheses.
*Monoclonal antibody against a protein that signals bone removal.
†Hormone that stimulates bone formation.

ANTIOSTEOPOROSIS DRUGS

Osteoporosis is a disorder marked by abnormal loss of bone density. Calcium, vitamin D, and estrogen are prescribed to increase calcium deposition in bone. Several different drugs are used to treat osteoporosis. **Bisphosphonates** prevent bone loss, and hormone-like drugs called selective estrogen receptor modulators **(SERMs)** increase bone formation. See Table 21-5.

CARDIOVASCULAR DRUGS

Cardiovascular drugs act on the heart or the blood vessels to treat hypertension, angina (pain due to decreased oxygen delivery to heart muscle), myocardial infarction (heart attack), congestive heart failure, and arrhythmias. Often, before other drugs are used, daily aspirin therapy (to prevent clots in blood vessels) and sublingual **nitroglycerin** (to dilate coronary blood vessels) are prescribed. **Digoxin (Lanoxin)** helps the heart pump more forcefully in heart failure. Other cardiovascular drugs include:

Angiotensin-converting enzyme (ACE) inhibitors—dilate blood vessels to lower blood pressure, improve the performance of the heart, and reduce its workload. They prevent the conversion of angiotensin I into angiotensin II, which is a powerful vasopressor (vasoconstrictor). ACE inhibitors reduce the risk of heart attack, stroke, and death even if a patient is not hypertensive.

Angiotensin II receptor blockers (ARBs)—lower blood pressure by preventing angiotensin from acting on receptors in blood vessels. They are used in patients who do not tolerate ACE inhibitors because of cough or angioedema (swelling of tissues).

Antiarrhythmics—reverse abnormal heart rhythms. They slow the response of heart muscle to nervous system stimulation or slow the rate at which nervous system impulses are carried through the heart.

Beta-blockers—decrease muscular tone in blood vessels (leading to vasodilation), slow heart rate, decrease output of the heart, and reduce blood pressure by blocking the action of epinephrine at receptor sites in the heart muscle and in blood vessels. Beta-blockers are prescribed for angina, hypertension, arrhythmias (such as fibrillation), and prevention of a second heart attack.

Calcium channel blockers—dilate blood vessels and lower blood pressure and are used to treat angina and arrhythmias. They inhibit the entry of calcium (necessary for blood vessel contraction) into the muscles of the heart and blood vessels.

Cardiac glycosides—made from digitalis (foxglove plant). These drugs increase the force of contraction of the heart and are used to treat heart failure and atrial fibrillation.

Cholesterol-binding drugs—bind to dietary cholesterol and prevent its uptake from the gastrointestinal tract.

Cholesterol-lowering drugs (statins)—control hypercholesterolemia (high levels of cholesterol in the blood), which is a major factor in the development of heart disease. These drugs lower cholesterol by reducing its production in the liver.

Diuretics—reduce the volume of blood in the body by promoting the kidney to remove water and salt through urine. They treat hypertension (high blood pressure) and congestive heart failure.

Table 21-6 gives examples of cardiovascular drugs.

ENDOCRINE DRUGS

Endocrine preparations act in much the same manner as the naturally occurring (endogenous) hormones discussed in Chapter 18. **Androgens,** normally made by the testes

TABLE 21-6 CARDIOVASCULAR DRUGS

ANGIOTENSIN-CONVERTING ENZYME (ACE) INHIBITORS	**CALCIUM CHANNEL BLOCKERS**
enalapril maleate (Vasotec) lisinopril (Prinivil, Zestril) quinapril (Accupril) ramipril (Altace)	amlodipine amlodipine besylate (Norvasc) diltiazem (Cardizem CD) nifedipine (Adalat CC, Procardia)
ANGIOTENSIN II RECEPTOR BLOCKERS	**CARDIAC GLYCOSIDES**
irbesartan (Avapro) losartan (Cozaar) valsartan (Diovan)	digoxin (Lanoxin)
ANTIARRHYTHMICS	**CHOLESTEROL-BINDING DRUGS (RESINS)**
amiodarone (Cordarone) ibutilide (Corvert) sotalol (Betapace)	cholestyramine (Questran) colestipol (Colestid)
BETA-BLOCKERS	**CHOLESTEROL-LOWERING DRUGS (STATINS)**
atenolol (Tenormin) carvedilol (Coreg) metoprolol (Lopressor, Toprol-XL) propranolol (Inderal)	atorvastatin calcium (Lipitor) lovastatin (Mevacor) pravastatin (Pravachol) rosuvastatin calcium (Crestor) simvastatin sodium (Zocor)
	DIURETICS
	furosemide (Lasix) hydrochlorothiazide (HydroDiuril) spironolactone (Aldactone) triamterene (Dyazide)

Note: Brand names are in parentheses.

and adrenal glands, are used for male hormone replacement and to treat endometriosis and anemia. **Antiandrogens** interfere with the production of androgens or with their binding in tissues. They are prescribed for prostate cancer. **Estrogens** are female hormones, normally produced by the ovaries, that are used for symptoms associated with menopause (estrogen replacement therapy) and to prevent postmenopausal osteoporosis. **Aromatase inhibitors** also reduce the amount of estrogen (estradiol) in the blood and are effective against breast cancer.

Selective estrogen receptor modulators (SERMs) have estrogen-like effects on bone (increase in bone density) and on lipid metabolism (decrease in cholesterol levels). However, they lack estrogenic effects on uterus and breast tissue. SERMs are used to treat postmenopausal osteoporosis and breast cancer. Tamoxifen and raloxifene are SERMs. **Progestins** are prescribed for abnormal uterine bleeding caused by hormonal imbalance and, together with estrogen, in hormone replacement therapy and oral contraceptives.

Thyroid hormone is administered when there is a low output of hormone from the thyroid gland. **Calcitonin** (a thyroid hormone) is used to treat osteoporosis. It increases calcium in the blood and promotes bone deposition. **Glucocorticoids** (adrenal corticosteroids) are prescribed for reduction of inflammation and a wide range of other disorders, including arthritis, severe skin and allergic conditions, respiratory and blood disorders, gastrointestinal ailments, and malignant conditions.

A fragment of human **parathyroid hormone (PTH)** has been approved for osteoporosis treatment. This agent stimulates new bone formation. **Growth hormone release–inhibiting factor (somatostatin)** can be manufactured and given to treat gastrointestinal symptoms associated with acromegaly and other tumors. It inhibits the production of natural growth hormone.

Table 21-7 gives examples of endocrine drugs.

TABLE 21-7 ENDOCRINE DRUGS

ANDROGENS

fluoxymesterone (Halotestin)
methyltestosterone (Virilon)

ANTIANDROGENS

abiraterone (Zytiga)
flutamide (Eulexin)
goserelin (Zoladex)
leuprolide (Lupron)
nilutamide (Casodex)

AROMATASE INHIBITORS

anastrozole (Arimidex)
exemestane (Aromasin)
fulvestrant (Faslodex)
letrozole (Femara)

ESTROGENS

estrogens (Premarin, Prempro)

GLUCOCORTICOIDS

dexamethasone (Decadron)
prednisone (Deltasone)
triamcinolone (Aristocort)

GROWTH HORMONE–RELEASE INHIBITING FACTOR

octreotide (Sandostatin)

PARATHYROID HORMONE FRAGMENT

teriparatide (Forteo)

PROGESTINS

medroxyprogesterone acetate (Cycrin, Provera)
megestrol (Megace)

SERMs

raloxifene (Evista)
tamoxifen (Nolvadex)

THYROID HORMONES

calcitonin (Cibacalcin)
levothyroxine (Levothroid, Levoxyl, Synthroid)
liothyronine (Cytomel)
thyroid ISP (Armour Thyroid)

Note: Brand names are in parentheses.
SERMs, selective estrogen receptor modulators.

21

GASTROINTESTINAL DRUGS

Gastrointestinal drugs often are used to relieve uncomfortable and potentially dangerous symptoms, rather than as cures for specific diseases. **Antacids** neutralize the hydrochloric acid in the stomach to relieve symptoms of peptic ulcer, esophagitis, and reflux. **Antiulcer** drugs block secretion of acid by cells in the lining of the stomach and are prescribed for patients with gastric and duodenal ulcers and **gastroesophageal reflux disease (GERD).** Histamine H_2 receptor antagonists such as **ranitidine (Zantac)** and **cimetidine (Tagamet)** turn off histamine, which promotes secretion of stomach acid. Another drug, **omeprazole (Prilosec),** works by stopping acid production by a different method (proton pump inhibition).

Antidiarrheal drugs relieve diarrhea and decrease the rapid movement (peristalsis) in the muscular walls of the colon. **Cathartics** relieve constipation and promote defecation for diagnostic and operative procedures and are used to treat disorders of the gastrointestinal tract. Some cathartics increase the intestinal salt content to cause fluid to fill the intestines; others increase the bulk of the feces to promote peristalsis. Another type of cathartic lubricates the intestinal tract to produce soft stools. **Laxatives** are mild cathartics, and **purgatives** are strong cathartics.

Antinauseants (antiemetics) relieve nausea and vomiting and overcome vertigo, dizziness, motion sickness, and similar symptoms due to labyrinthitis (inflammation of the inner ear).

Anti-TNF (tumor necrosis factor) drugs are used to treat **autoimmune diseases** such as **Crohn's.** These drugs are also used against rheumatoid arthritis.

Table 21-8 lists the various types of gastrointestinal drugs and examples of each.

TABLE 21-8 GASTROINTESTINAL DRUGS

ANTACIDS	**ANTI-TNF DRUGS**
aluminum and magnesium antacid (Gaviscon) magnesium antacid (milk of magnesia) aluminum antacid (Rolaids)	adalimumab (Humira) certolizumab pegol (Cimzia) etanercept (Enbrel) infliximab (Remicade)
ANTIDIARRHEALS	**ANTIULCER AND ANTI–GASTROINTESTINAL REFLUX DISEASE (GERD) DRUGS**
diphenoxylate and atropine (Lomotil) loperamide (Imodium) paregoric	cimetidine (Tagamet) esomeprazole (Nexium) famotidine (Pepcid) lansoprazole (Prevacid) omeprazole (Prilosec) ranitidine (Zantac)
ANTINAUSEANTS (ANTIEMETICS)	**CATHARTICS**
metoclopramide (Reglan) ondansetron (Zofran) promethazine (Phenergan) prochlorperazine maleate (Compazine)	casanthranol plus docusate sodium (Peri-Colace)

Note: Brand names are in parentheses.

RESPIRATORY DRUGS

Respiratory drugs are prescribed for the treatment of asthma, emphysema, chronic bronchitis, and bronchospasm. **Bronchodilators** open bronchial tubes and are administered by injection or aerosol inhalers. **Steroid drugs** are inhaled or given intravenously and orally to reduce chronic inflammation in respiratory passageways. **Leukotriene modifiers** are recent additions to the anti-inflammatory therapy of asthma. They prevent asthma attacks by blocking leukotriene (a bronchoconstrictor) from binding to receptors in respiratory tissues. Table 21-9 gives examples of respiratory drugs.

TABLE 21-9 RESPIRATORY DRUGS

BRONCHODILATORS	**STEROIDS: INHALERS**
albuterol (Proventil, Ventolin)* epinephrine (Primatene) formoterol (Foradil)† formoterol plus budesonide (Symbicort)† ipratropium bromide (Atrovent)‡ ipratropium plus albuterol (Combivent)* levalbuterol (Xopenex)* metaproterenol (Alupent)* pirbuterol (Maxair)* salmeterol (Serevent)† salmeterol plus fluticasone (Advair)† theophylline (Theo-Dar) tiotropium bromide (Spiriva)‡	budesonide (Pulmicort) flunisolide (AeroBid) fluticasone propionate (Flovent) mometasone (Asmanex) triamcinolone (Azmacort) **STEROIDS: INTRAVENOUS OR ORAL** dexamethasone (Decadron) methylprednisolone (Medrol) prednisone
LEUKOTRIENE MODIFIERS	
montelukast sodium (Singulair) zafirlukast (Accolate) zileuton (Zyflo)	

Note: Brand names are in parentheses.
*Short-acting; inhaled.
†Long-acting.
‡Anticholinergic; bronchodilator enhancers.

21

SEDATIVE-HYPNOTICS

Sedative-hypnotics are medications that depress the central nervous system and promote drowsiness (sedatives) and sleep (hypnotics). They are prescribed for insomnia and sleep disorders. These products have a very high abuse potential and should be used only for short periods of time and under close supervision. **Barbiturates** and **benzodiazepines** are the two major categories of sedative-hypnotics.

Low doses of **benzodiazepines** (which influence the part of the brain responsible for emotions) may act as sedatives. In higher doses, benzodiazepines may act as hypnotics (to promote sleep).

Table 21-10 gives examples of sedative-hypnotics.

STIMULANTS

Stimulants are drugs that act on the brain to speed up vital processes (heart and respiration) in cases of shock and collapse. They also increase alertness and inhibit hyperactive behavior in children. High doses can produce restlessness, insomnia, and hypertension. Examples of stimulants are **amphetamines**—used to prevent narcolepsy (seizures of sleep), to suppress appetite, and to calm hyperkinetic children. **Caffeine** also is a cerebral stimulant. It is used in drugs to relieve certain types of headache by constricting cerebral blood vessels. Table 21-10 lists examples of stimulants.

TRANQUILIZERS

Tranquilizers are useful for controlling anxiety. Minor tranquilizers **(benzodiazepines)** control minor symptoms of anxiety. Major tranquilizers **(phenothiazines)** control more severe disturbances of behavior. Table 21-10 lists examples of minor and major tranquilizers.

TABLE 21-10 SEDATIVE-HYPNOTICS, STIMULANTS, TRANQUILIZERS

SEDATIVE-HYPNOTICS	TRANQUILIZERS
butabarbital (Butisol)	**Minor**
methaqualone (Quaalude)	alprazolam (Xanax)*
phenobarbital (Luminal)	buspirone (BuSpar)
temazepam (Restoril)*	diazepam (Valium)*
triazolam (Halcion)*	lorazepam (Ativan)*
zolpidem tartrate (Ambien)	**Major**
STIMULANTS	aripiprazole (Abilify)
caffeine	chlorpromazine (Thorazine)†
dextroamphetamine sulfate (Dexedrine)	haloperidol (Haldol)
dextroamphetamine and amphetamine (Adderall)	lithium carbonate (Eskalith)
methylphenidate (Ritalin)	olanzapine (Zyprexa)
modafinil (Provigil)	risperidone (Risperdal)
	thioridazine (Mellaril)†
	trifluoperazine (Stelazine)†

Note: Brand names are in parentheses.
*Benzodiazepine.
†Phenothiazine.

VOCABULARY

This list reviews many of the new terms introduced in the text. Short definitions reinforce your understanding of the terms. Refer to the Pronunciation of Terms on page 915 for help with unfamiliar or difficult words.

GENERAL TERMS	
addiction	Physical and psychological dependence on and craving for a drug.
additive action	Drug action in which the combination of two similar drugs is equal to the sum of the effects of each.
aerosol	Particles of drug suspended in air.
anaphylaxis	Exaggerated hypersensitivity reaction to a previously encountered drug or foreign protein.
antagonistic action	Combination of two drugs gives less than an additive effect (action).
antidote	Agent given to counteract an unwanted effect of a drug.
brand name	Commercial name for a drug; trademark or trade name.
chemical name	Chemical formula for a drug.
contraindications	Factors that prevent the use of a drug or treatment.
controlled substances	Drugs that produce tolerance and dependence and have potential for abuse or addiction. See page 905.
dependence	Physiologic need for a drug due to prolonged use.
dose	Amount of drug administered, usually measured in milligrams.
Food and Drug Administration (FDA)	U.S. government agency having the legal responsibility for enforcing proper drug manufacture and clinical use.
generic name	Legal noncommercial name for a drug.
iatrogenic	Condition caused by treatment (drugs or procedures) given by physicians or medical personnel.
idiosyncratic reaction	Unexpected effect produced in a particularly sensitive patient but not seen in most people.
inhalation	Administration of drugs in gaseous or vapor form through the nose or mouth.
medicinal chemistry	Study of new drug synthesis; relationship between chemical structure and biological effects.
molecular pharmacology	Study of interaction of drugs and their target molecules such as enzymes, or cell surface receptors.
oral administration	Drugs are given by mouth.
parenteral administration	Drugs are given by injection into the skin, muscles, or veins (any route other than through the digestive tract). Examples are subcutaneous, intradermal, intramuscular, intravenous, intrathecal, and intracavitary injections.

pharmacist	Specialist in preparing and dispensing drugs.
pharmacy	Location for preparing and dispensing drugs; also the study of preparing and dispensing drugs.
pharmacodynamics	Study of drug effects within the body.
pharmacokinetics	Study of drug absorption, distribution, metabolism, and excretion over a period of time.
pharmacologist	Specialist in the study of the properties, uses, and side effects of drugs.
pharmacology	Study of the preparation, properties, uses, and side effects of drugs.
***Physicians' Desk Reference* (PDR)**	Reference book that lists drug products.
receptor	Target substance with which a drug interacts in the body.
rectal administration	Drugs are inserted through the anus into the rectum.
resistance	Lack of beneficial response; seen when drugs are unable to control the disease process.
response	Desired and beneficial effect of a drug.
schedule	Exact timing and frequency of drug administration.
side effect	Adverse reaction, usually minor, that routinely results from the use of a drug.
sublingual administration	Drugs are given by placement under the tongue.
synergism	Combination of two drugs causes an effect that is greater than the sum of the individual effects of each drug alone.
syringe	Instrument (tube) for introducing or withdrawing fluids from the body.
tolerance	Larger and larger drug doses must be given to achieve the desired effect. The patient becomes resistant to the action of a drug as treatment progresses.
topical application	Drugs are applied locally on the skin or mucous membranes of the body; ointments, creams, and lotions are applied topically.
toxicity	Harmful effects of a drug.
toxicology	Study of harmful chemicals and their effects on the body.
transport	Movement of a drug across a cell membrane into body cells.
United States Pharmacopeia (USP)	Authoritative list of drugs, formulas, and preparations that sets a standard for drug manufacturing and dispensing.
vitamin	Substance found in foods and essential in small quantities for growth and good health.

CLASSES OF DRUGS AND RELATED TERMS	
ACE inhibitor	Lowers blood pressure. Angiotensin-converting enzyme (ACE) inhibitors block the conversion of angiotensin I to angiotensin II (a powerful vasoconstrictor).
amphetamine	Central nervous system stimulant.
analgesic	Relieves pain.
androgen	Male hormone.
anesthetic	Reduces or eliminates sensation; general and local.
angiotensin II receptor blocker	Lowers blood pressure by preventing angiotensin from acting on receptors in blood vessels.
antacid	Neutralizes acid in the stomach.
antiandrogen	Slows the uptake of androgens or interferes with their effect in tissues.
antiarrhythmic	Treats abnormal heart rhythms.
antibiotic	Chemical substance, produced by a plant or microorganism, that has the ability to inhibit or destroy foreign organisms in the body. Examples are antifungals, cephalosporins, erythromycin, tetracycline, antituberculars, penicillins, quinolones, and sulfonamides.
anticoagulant	Prevents blood clotting.
anticonvulsant	Prevents convulsions (abnormal brain activity).
antidepressant	Relieves symptoms of depression.
antidiabetic	Drug given to prevent or treat diabetes mellitus.
antidiarrheal	Prevents diarrhea.
antiemetic	Prevents nausea and vomiting.
antihistamine	Blocks the action of histamine and helps prevent symptoms of allergy.
antinauseant	Relieves nausea and vomiting; antiemetic.
antiplatelet	Reduces the tendency of platelets to stick together and form a clot.
antiulcer	Inhibits the secretion of acid by cells lining the stomach.
antiviral	Acts against viruses such as herpesviruses and HIV.
aromatase inhibitor	Reduces estrogen in the blood by blocking the enzyme aromatase.
bactericidal	Kills bacteria (-cidal means able to kill).
bacteriostatic	Inhibits bacterial growth (-static means stopping or controlling).
beta-blocker	Blocks the action of epinephrine at sites on receptors of heart muscle cells, the muscle lining of blood vessels, and bronchial tubes; antiarrhythmic, antianginal, and antihypertensive.
bisphosphonate	Prevents bone loss in osteoporosis.
caffeine	Central nervous system stimulant (found in coffee and tea).
calcium channel blocker	Blocks the entrance of calcium into heart muscle and muscle lining of blood vessels; used as an antiarrhythmic, antianginal, and antihypertensive; also called **calcium antagonist.**

cardiac glycoside	Increases the force of contraction of the heart.
cardiovascular drug	Acts on the heart and blood vessels. This category of drug includes ACE inhibitors, beta-blockers, calcium channel blockers, cholesterol-lowering drugs or statins, and diuretics.
cathartic	Relieves constipation.
cholesterol-binding drug	Binds to dietary cholesterol and prevents its uptake from the gastrointestinal tract.
cholesterol-lowering drug	Lowers cholesterol by preventing its production by the liver; statin.
diuretic	Increases the production of urine and thus reduces the volume of fluid in the body; antihypertensive.
emetic	Promotes vomiting.
endocrine drug	A hormone or hormone-like drug. Examples are androgens, estrogens, progestins, SERMs, thyroid hormones, and glucocorticoids.
estrogen	Female hormone that promotes development of secondary sex characteristics and supports reproductive tissues.
gastrointestinal drug	Relieves symptoms of diseases in the gastrointestinal tract. Examples are antacids, antiulcer drugs, antidiarrheal drugs, cathartics, laxatives, purgatives, and antinauseants (antiemetics).
glucocorticoid	Hormone from the adrenal cortex that raises blood sugar and reduces inflammation.
hypnotic	Produces sleep or a trance-like state.
laxative	Weak cathartic.
narcotic	Habit-forming drug (potent analgesic) that relieves pain by producing stupor or insensibility; morphine and opium are examples.
progestin	Female hormone that stimulates the uterine lining during pregnancy and is also used in treatment of abnormal uterine bleeding and for hormone replacement therapy.
purgative	Relieves constipation; strong cathartic.
respiratory drug	Treats asthma, emphysema, and infections of the respiratory system. Bronchodilators are examples.
sedative	A mildly hypnotic drug that relaxes without necessarily producing sleep. **Benzodiazepines** are examples.
stimulant	Excites and promotes activity. Caffeine and amphetamines are examples.
thyroid hormone	Stimulates cellular metabolism.
tranquilizer	Controls anxiety and severe disturbances of behavior.

TERMINOLOGY

Write the meaning of the medical term in the space provided.

COMBINING FORMS

COMBINING FORM	MEANING	TERMINOLOGY	MEANING
aer/o	air	aerosol *The suffix -sol means solution.*	
alges/o	sensitivity to pain	analgesic	
bronch/o	bronchial tube	bronchodilator *Theophylline is a smooth muscle relaxant used to treat asthma, emphysema, and chronic bronchitis.*	
chem/o	drug	chemotherapy	
cras/o	mixture	idiosyncrasy *Idi/o means individual, peculiar; syn- means together. An idiosyncrasy is an abnormal, unexpected effect of a drug that is peculiar to an individual.*	
cutane/o	skin	subcutaneous	
derm/o	skin	hypodermic	
erg/o	work	synergism	
esthes/o	feeling, sensation	anesthesia	
hist/o	tissue	antihistamine *The suffix -amine indicates a nitrogen-containing compound.* ***Histamine*** *is a substance found in all body tissues (it causes capillary dilation and gastric acid secretion and constricts bronchial tube smooth muscle); an excess of histamine is released when the body comes into contact with substances to which it is sensitive.*	
hypn/o	sleep	hypnotic	
iatr/o	treatment	iatrogenic	
lingu/o	tongue	sublingual	
myc/o	mold, fungus	erythromycin	
narc/o	stupor	narcotic	
or/o	mouth	oral	
pharmac/o	drug	pharmacology	
prurit/o	itching	antipruritic	
pyret/o	fever	antipyretic	
thec/o	sheath (of brain and spinal cord)	intrathecal	

COMBINING FORM	MEANING	TERMINOLOGY	MEANING
tox/o	poison	toxic	______
toxic/o	poison	toxicology	______
vas/o	vessel	vasodilator	______
ven/o	vein	intravenous	______
vit/o	life	vitamin *The first vitamins discovered were nitrogen-containing substances called amines. Table 21-11 lists vitamins, their medical names, and foods that are a major source of each.*	______

PREFIXES

PREFIX	MEANING	TERMINOLOGY	MEANING
ana-	upward, excessive, again	anaphylaxis *The suffix -phylaxis means protection.*	______
anti-	against	antidote *The suffix -dote comes from Greek, meaning what is given.*	______
		antibiotic	______
contra-	against, opposite	contraindication *Alternatively, drug* ***indications*** *are reasons to prescribe a medication; a bacterial infection may be an indication to prescribe a specific antibiotic.*	______
par-	other than, apart from	parenteral *Enter/o means intestine.*	______
syn-	together, with	synergistic	______

TABLE 21-11 VITAMINS

Vitamin	Chemical Name(s)	Food Sources
vitamin A	retinol; dehydroretinol	leafy, green and yellow vegetables; liver, eggs, cod liver oil
vitamin B1	thiamine	yeast, ham, liver, peanuts, milk
vitamin B2	riboflavin	milk, liver, green vegetables
vitamin B3	niacin (nicotinic acid)	yeast, liver, peanuts, fish, poultry
vitamin B6	pyridoxine	liver, fish, yeast
vitamin B9	folic acid	vegetables, liver, yeast, sunflower seeds, cereals
vitamin B12	cyanocobalamin	milk, eggs, liver
vitamin C	ascorbic acid	citrus fruits, vegetables
vitamin D	calciferol	cod liver oil, milk, egg yolk
vitamin E	alpha-glucosidase	wheat germ oil, cereals, egg yolk
vitamin K	phytonadione; menaquinone; menadione	alfalfa, spinach, cabbage

ABBREVIATIONS

Many of the notations used by physicians in writing prescriptions are abbreviations for Latin phrases, which appear in italics within parentheses. See Practical Applications for a list of official "do not use" abbreviations and what to use instead.

a.c., ac	before meals *(ante cibum)*
ACE	angiotensin-converting enzyme
ad lib	freely, as desired *(ad libitum)*
APAP	acetaminophen (tylenol)
ARB	angiotensin II receptor blocker
b.i.d., bid	two times a day *(bis in die)*
c̄	with
Caps	capsules
cc	cubic centimeter
FDA	U.S. Food and Drug Administration
gm, g	gram
gtt	drops *(guttae)*
h	hour *(hora)*
h.s., hs	at bedtime *(hora somni)*
H2 blocker	histamine H_2 receptor antagonist
HRT	hormone replacement therapy
IM	intramuscular
INH	isoniazid—antituberculosis agent
IV	intravenous
MAOI	monoamine oxidase inhibitor—an antidepressant
mg	milligram
ml, mL	milliliter
NPO	nothing by mouth *(nil per os)*
NSAID	nonsteroidal anti-inflammatory drug
p̄	after *(post)*
p.c., pc	after meals *(post cibum)*
PCA	patient-controlled analgesia
PDR	*Physicians' Desk Reference*
PO, p.o., po	by mouth *(per os)*
p.r.n., prn	as needed; as necessary (*pro re nata,* as the occasion arises)
Pt	patient
q	every *(quaque)*
q.h., qh	every hour *(quaque hora)*
q2h	every 2 hours
q.i.d., qid	four times a day *(quater in die)*
q.s., qs	sufficient quantity *(quantum satis)*
qAM	every morning
qPM	every evening
Rx	prescription
s̄	without *(sine)*
SERM	selective estrogen receptor modulator
Sig.	directions—how to take medication
SL	sublingual
s.o.s.	if it is necessary *(si opus sit)*
SSRI	selective serotonin reuptake inhibitor—an antidepressant
subQ	subcutaneous
tab	tablet
TCA	tricyclic antidepressant
t.i.d., tid	three times daily *(ter in die)*

PRACTICAL APPLICATIONS

See the Evolve website for this chapter, where you can find a list of the top 100 prescribed drugs for 2010.

OFFICIAL "DO NOT USE" LIST[1]

Do Not Use	*Potential Problem*	Use Instead
U, u (unit)	Mistaken for "0" (zero), the number "4" (four) or "cc"	Write "unit"
IU (International Unit)	Mistaken for "IV" (intravenous) or the number "10" (ten)	Write "International Unit"
Q.D., QD, q.d., qd (daily) Q.O.D., QOD, q.o.d., qod (every other day)	Mistaken for each other Period after the Q mistaken for "I" and "O" mistaken for "I"	Write "daily" Write "every other day"
Trailing zero (X.0 mg)* Lack of leading zero (.X mg)	Decimal point is missed	Write X mg Write 0.X mg
MS MSO_4 and $MgSO_4$	Can mean morphine sulfate or magnesium sulfate Confused for one another	Write "morphine sulfate" Write "magnesium sulfate"

[1]Applies to all orders and all medication-related documentation that is handwritten (including free-text computer entry) or on pre-printed forms.

***Exception:** A "trailing zero" may be used only where required to demonstrate the level of precision of the value being reported, such as for laboratory results, imaging studies that report size of lesions, or catheter/tube sizes. It may not be used in medication orders or other medication-related documentation.

Additional Abbreviations, Acronyms and Symbols

(For possible future inclusion in the Official "Do Not Use" List)

Do Not Use	*Possible Problem*	Use Instead
> (greater than) < (less than)	Misinterpreted as the number "7" (seven) or the letter "L" Confused for one another	Write "greater than" Write "less than"
Abbreviations for drug names	Misinterpreted due to similar abbreviations for multiple drugs	Write drug names in full
Apothecary units	Unfamiliar to many practitioners Confused with metric units	Use metric units
@	Mistaken for the number "2" (two)	Write "at"
cc	Mistaken for U (units) when poorly written	Write "mL" or "ml" or "milliliters" ("mL" is preferred)
μg	Mistaken for mg (milligrams) resulting in one thousand-fold overdose	Write "mcg" or "micrograms"

PRESCRIPTIONS

The usual order of drug prescription information is as follows: name of the drug, dosage, route of administration, time of administration. Frequently, the physician will include a qualifying phrase to indicate why the prescription is being written. Not all information is listed with every prescription.

Exercise: Answers are found on page 914.

Match the following prescriptions with their explanations below.

a. Fluoxetine (Prozac) 20 mg PO b.i.d.
b. Lisinopril (Zestril) 20 mg 1 cap qAM
c. Ondansetron (Zofran) 4 mg 1 tab/cap t.i.d. p.r.n. for nausea
d. Ranitidine (Zantac) 300 mg 1 tab p.c. t.i.d.
e. Olanzapine (Zyprexa) 5 mg 1 tab qPM
f. Acetaminophen (300 mg) & codeine (30 mg) 1 tab q.i.d. p.r.n. for pain

1. anti-GERD drug taken after meals 3 times a day ______
2. Tylenol with a narcotic taken 4 times a day as needed ______
3. antidepressant taken by mouth twice a day ______
4. antiemetic taken 3 times a day as needed ______
5. antihypertensive taken every morning ______
6. antipsychotic, one tablet every evening ______

CONTROLLED SUBSTANCES

Controlled substances are drugs regulated under existing federal law. The substances are divided into five classes (schedules) based on the substance's medicinal value, harmfulness, and potential for abuse or addiction. Schedule I includes the most dangerous drugs that have no recognized medicinal use, and Schedule V includes the least dangerous drugs. The following table lists examples of drugs in each class with their type, trade and/or "street" names, and medical uses.

DRUG	TYPE	TRADE OR OTHER NAME(S)	MEDICAL USE(S)
Class (Schedule) I			
heroin	narcotic	diacetylmorphine, horse, smack	None
LSD (lysergic acid diethylamide)	hallucinogen	acid, microdot	None
mescaline, peyote	hallucinogen	mesc, buttons, cactus	None
methaqualone	depressant	Quaalude*, Parest	sedative-hypnotic

*Quaaludes have been discontinued in the United States but their (ab)use continues due to Internet availability.

Class (Schedule) II

Dangerous substances with general medical indications and high potential for abuse and addiction.

hydromorphone	narcotic	Dilaudid	analgesic
marijuana	cannabis	pot, Acapulco, grass, reefer	under investigation
meperidine	narcotic	Demerol	analgesic

DRUG	TYPE	TRADE OR OTHER NAME(S)	MEDICAL USE(S)
cocaine	stimulant	coke, flake, snow	local anesthetic
methylphenidate	stimulant	Ritalin	hyperkinesis
oxycodone	narcotic	Tylox, Percodan, OxyContin, OC, OX, Oxy	analgesic, pain management
crystal methamphetamine	stimulant	crystal meth, ice	weight control
phencyclidine	hallucinogen	PCP, angel dust, hog	veterinary anesthetic
opium	narcotic	Dover's powder, paregoric	analgesic, antidiarrheal
morphine	narcotic	morphine, pectoral syrup	analgesic, antitussive
barbiturates	depressant	amobarbital (Amytal), pentobarbital (Nembutal), secobarbital (Seconal)	anesthetic, anticonvulsant, sedative-hypnotic
amphetamines	stimulant	Dexedrine, Desoxyn	weight control, narcolepsy

Class (Schedule) III

Carries less potential for abuse, but casual use can lead to psychological addiction and dependence.

anabolic steroids	male sex hormones	testosterone, Anavar, Winstrol, Dianabol	hormone deficiency, increasing muscle mass
barbiturates	depressant	aprobarbital (Alurate), butalbital (Fiorinal), butabarbital (Butisol)	anesthetic, anticonvulsant, sedative-hypnotic
codeine	narcotic	codeine	analgesic, antitussive

Class (Schedule) IV

Carries low potential for abuse but a risk of psychological or limited physical dependence.

barbiturates	depressant	phenobarbital	anesthetic, anticonvulsant, sedative-hypnotic
benzodiazepines	minor tranquilizer	lorazepam (Ativan), diazepam (Valium), chlordiazepoxide (Librium), clonazepam (Klonopin), triazolam (Halcion), alprazolam (Xanax)	antianxiety, sedative-hypnotic, anticonvulsant
nonbenzodiazepine agent	hypnotic	eszopiclone (Lunesta)	insomnia

Class (Schedule) V

This class includes codeine preparations (Robitussin A-C), opium preparations (Kapectolin PG—antidiarrheal), Lomotil (antidiarrheal), and Motofen (antidiarrheal).

EXERCISES

Remember to check your answers carefully with the Answers to Exercises, page 913.

A Name the pharmacologic specialty based on its description as given.

1. use of drugs in the treatment of disease ______________________
2. study of new drug synthesis ______________________
3. study of how drugs interact with their target molecules ______________________
4. study of the harmful effects of drugs ______________________
5. study of drug effects in the body ______________________
6. measurement of drug absorption, distribution, metabolism, and excretion over a period of time

   ____

B Match the following terms with their meanings below.

antidote	pharmacist	toxicologist
chemical name	pharmacologist	trade (brand) name
Food and Drug Administration	*Physicians' Desk Reference*	United States Pharmacopeia
generic name		

1. Specialist in the study of the harmful effects of drugs on the body is a/n

   ______________________.
2. Agent given to counteract harmful effects of a drug is a/an ______________________.
3. Government agency with legal responsibility for enforcing proper drug manufacture and clinical use is ______________________.
4. The ______________________ is the commercial name for a drug.
5. The ______________________ is the complicated chemical formula for a drug.
6. The ______________________ is the legal noncommercial name for a drug.
7. Professional who prepares and dispenses drugs is a/an ______________________.
8. Specialist (MD or PhD) who studies the properties, uses, and side effects of drugs is a/an

   ______________________.
9. Reference book listing drug products is ______________________.
10. Authoritative listing of drugs, formulas, and preparations that sets a standard for drug manufacturing and dispensing is ______________________.

C **Name the route of drug administration based on its description as given below.**

1. administered via suppository or fluid into the anus ____________
2. administered via vapor or gas into the nose or mouth ____________
3. administered under the tongue ____________
4. applied locally on skin or mucous membrane ____________
5. injected via syringe under the skin or into a vein, muscle, or body cavity ____________
6. given by mouth and absorbed through the stomach or intestinal wall ____________

D **Give the meanings of the following terms.**

1. intravenous ____________
2. intrathecal ____________
3. antiseptic ____________
4. antipruritic ____________
5. aerosol ____________
6. intramuscular ____________
7. subcutaneous ____________
8. intracavitary ____________
9. addiction ____________
10. dose ____________
11. resistance ____________
12. response ____________
13. schedule ____________
14. dependence ____________

E **Match the routes of drug administration in Column I with the medications or procedures in Column II. Write the letter of the answer in the space provided.**

COLUMN I		COLUMN II
1. intravenous	_____	A. lotions, creams, ointments
2. rectal	_____	B. tablets and capsules
3. oral	_____	C. skin testing for allergy
4. topical	_____	D. lumbar puncture
5. inhalation	_____	E. deep injection, usually in buttock
6. intrathecal	_____	F. suppositories
7. intramuscular	_____	G. blood transfusions
8. intradermal	_____	H. aerosol medications

F **The following are descriptions of drug actions. Supply the word that fits the description.**

1. combination of two drugs is greater than the total effects of each drug by itself ________________
2. combination of two drugs that is equal to the sum of the effects of each ________________
3. effects of a given drug dose become less as treatment continues, and larger and larger doses must be given to achieve the desired effect ________________
4. an unexpected effect that may appear in a patient following administration of a drug ________________
5. two drugs give less than an additive effect (action) ________________

G **Give the meanings of the following terms that describe classes of drugs.**

1. antibiotic ________________
2. antidepressant ________________
3. antihistamine ________________
4. analgesic ________________
5. anticoagulant ________________
6. anesthetic ________________
7. antidiabetic ________________
8. sedative ________________
9. stimulant ________________
10. tranquilizer ________________

H **Match the term in Column I with the associated term in Column II. Write the letter of the answer in the space provided.**

COLUMN I		COLUMN II
1. antihistamine	______	A. caffeine or amphetamines
2. analgesic	______	B. penicillin or erythromycin
3. antidiabetic	______	C. insulin
4. anticoagulant	______	D. benzodiazepine
5. antibiotic	______	E. heparin
6. stimulant	______	F. nonsteroidal anti-inflammatory drug
7. sedative-hypnotic	______	G. phenothiazine
8. tranquilizer	______	H. anaphylactic shock

I Give the meanings of the following terms.

1. beta-blocker ______
2. androgen ______
3. glucocorticoid ______
4. calcium channel blocker ______
5. estrogen ______
6. antacid ______
7. cathartic ______
8. antiemetic ______
9. bronchodilator ______
10. hypnotic ______
11. diuretic ______
12. cholesterol-lowering drug ______

J Match the type of drug in Column I with the condition it treats in Column II. Write the letter of the answer in the space provided.

COLUMN I

1. anticonvulsant ______
2. anticoagulant ______
3. antacid ______
4. progestins ______
5. antibiotic ______
6. ACE inhibitor ______
7. bronchodilator ______
8. antihistamine ______
9. tranquilizer ______
10. analgesic ______

COLUMN II

A. abnormal uterine bleeding caused by hormonal imbalance
B. severe behavior disturbances and anxiety
C. epilepsy
D. congestive heart failure and hypertension
E. epigastric discomfort
F. myalgia and neuralgia
G. anaphylactic shock
H. thrombosis and embolism
I. streptococcal pharyngitis
J. asthma

K **Complete the following terms based on definitions given.**

1. agent that reduces fever: anti________________________
2. agent that reduces itching: anti________________________
3. habit-forming analgesic: ________________________tic
4. two drugs cause an effect greater than the sum of each alone: syn________________________
5. antibiotic derived from a red mold: ________________________mycin
6. legal nonproprietary name of a drug: ________________________ name
7. factor in a patient's condition that prevents the use of a particular drug:
   contra________________________
8. drug that produces an absence of sensation or feeling: an________________________

L **Using the terms listed below, complete the following sentences.**

ACE inhibitor	antidepressant	diuretic
anesthetic	antiestrogen	NSAID
antibiotic	antihistamine	oral antidiabetic
anticonvulsant	antiviral	SERM

1. Cephalosporins (such as cefuroxime and cefprozil) and penicillins are examples of a/an ________________________ drug.
2. Advil (ibuprofen) is an example of a/an ________________________.
3. Carbamazepine (Tegretol) and phenytoin (Dilantin) are examples of a/an ________________________ drug.
4. Zovirax (acyclovir) and Crixivan (indinavir) are both types of a/an ________________________ drug.
5. Nolvadex (tamoxifen), used to treat estrogen receptor–positive breast cancer in women, is an example of a/an ________________________ drug.
6. Patients with high blood pressure may need Vasotec (enalapril) or Zestril (lisinopril). Both of these are examples of a/an ________________________.
7. Metformin (Glucophage) and rosiglitazone (Avandia) are two types of ________________________ drugs.
8. Evista (raloxifene), used to treat osteoporosis in postmenopausal women, is an example of a selective estrogen receptor modulator or ________________________.
9. Amitriptyline (Elavil) and fluoxetine (Prozac) are two types of a/an ________________________ drug.
10. If you have an allergy, your doctor may prescribe Allegra (fexofenadine), which is a/an ________________________ drug.
11. Two agents that reduce the amount of fluid in the blood and thus lower blood pressure are Lasix (furosemide) and Aldactone (spironolactone). These are ________________________ drugs.
12. Xylocaine (lidocaine) and Pentothal (thiopental) are examples of a/an ________________________ drug.

M Give the meanings of the following abbreviations.

1. NSAID ______
2. p.r.n. ______
3. q.i.d. ______
4. ad lib ______
5. t.i.d. ______
6. mg ______
7. c̄ ______
8. s̄ ______
9. NPO ______
10. p.c. ______
11. b.i.d. ______
12. q.h. ______
13. PO ______
14. q ______

N Translate the following prescription orders.

1. 1 tab PO q.i.d. p.c. and h.s. ______
2. 15-60 mg IM q4-6h ______
3. 2 caps p.o. h.s. ______
4. 1 tab SL p.r.n. ______
5. Apply topically qhs prn ______

O Circle the term that best completes the meaning of the sentence.

1. After his heart attack, Bernie was supposed to take many drugs, including diuretics and a/an (**progestin, laxative, anticoagulant**) to prevent blood clots.
2. Estelle was always anxious and had a hard time sleeping. Dr. Max suggested that a mild (**antacid, anticonvulsant, tranquilizer**) would help her relax and concentrate on her work.
3. During chemotherapy Helen was very nauseated. Dr. Cohen prescribed an (**antihypertensive, antiemetic, antianginal**) to relieve her symptoms of queasy stomach.
4. The two antibiotics worked together and were therefore (**idiosyncratic, generic, synergistic**) in killing the bacteria in Susan's bloodstream.
5. The label warned that the drug might impair fine motor skills. It listed the (**side effects, antidote, pharmacodynamics**) of the sedative.
6. After receiving the results of Judy's sputum culture, her physician, an expert in (**endocrinology, cardiology, infectious disease**), recommended Biaxin and other (**antihistamines, antibiotics, antidepressants**) to combat the *Mycobacterium avium* complex disease in her (**heart, thyroid gland, lungs**).

7. Our dog, Eli, has had seizures since he was hit by a car last year. The veterinarian currently prescribes phenobarbital, an (**anticoagulant, antinauseant, anticonvulsant**), 45 mg b.i.d. (**every other day, twice a day, every evening**).

8. To control his type 1 (**heart disease, asthma, diabetes**), David gives himself daily injections of (**oral drugs, insulin, aromatase inhibitors**).

9. Many students who want to stay awake to study are taking (**stimulants, sedatives, tranquilizers**) containing (**lithium, caffeine, butabarbital**).

10. Shelly's wheezing, coughing, and shortness of breath when she is stressed and exposed to animal dander all pointed to a diagnosis of (**pneumonia, asthma, heart disease**), which required treatment with steroids and (**antivirals, diuretics, bronchodilators**).

ANSWERS TO EXERCISES

A

1. chemotherapy
2. medicinal chemistry
3. molecular pharmacology
4. toxicology
5. pharmacodynamics
6. pharmacokinetics

B

1. toxicologist
2. antidote
3. Food and Drug Administration
4. trade (brand) name
5. chemical name
6. generic name
7. pharmacist
8. pharmacologist
9. *Physicians' Desk Reference*
10. United States Pharmacopeia

C

1. rectal
2. inhalation
3. sublingual
4. topical
5. parenteral
6. oral

D

1. within a vein
2. within a sheath (membranes around the spinal cord or brain)
3. an agent that works against infection
4. an agent that works against itching
5. a solution of particles (drug) in air (vapor or gas)
6. within a muscle
7. under the skin
8. within a cavity
9. physical and psychological dependence on a drug
10. amount of drug administered
11. lack of beneficial response
12. desired and beneficial effect of a drug
13. exact timing and frequency of drug administration
14. prolonged use of a drug that may lead to physiologic need for its actions in the body

E

1. G
2. F
3. B
4. A
5. H
6. D
7. E
8. C

F

1. synergism (potentiation)
2. additive action
3. tolerance
4. idiosyncrasy
5. antagonistic

G

1. an agent that inhibits or kills germ life (microorganisms)
2. an agent that relieves the symptoms of depression
3. an agent that blocks the action of histamine and relieves allergic symptoms
4. an agent that relieves pain
5. an agent that prevents blood clotting
6. an agent that reduces or eliminates sensation
7. an agent used to prevent diabetes mellitus
8. an agent (mildly hypnotic) that relaxes and calms nervousness
9. an agent that excites and promotes activity
10. a drug used to control anxiety and severe disturbances of behavior

H

1. H
2. F
3. C
4. E
5. B
6. A
7. D
8. G

I

1. drug that blocks the action of epinephrine at sites of receptors of heart muscles, blood vessels, and bronchial tubes (antihypertensive, antianginal, and antiarrhythmic)
2. a drug that produces male sexual characteristics
3. a hormone from the adrenal glands that reduces inflammation and raises blood sugar
4. a drug that blocks the entrance of calcium into heart muscle and blood vessel walls (antianginal, antiarrhythmic, and antihypertensive)
5. a hormone that produces female sexual characteristics
6. a drug that neutralizes acid in the stomach
7. a drug that relieves constipation
8. a drug that prevents nausea and vomiting
9. a drug that opens air passages
10. an agent that produces sleep
11. a drug that reduces the volume of blood and lowers blood pressure
12. a drug that reduces cholesterol levels (treats hypercholesterolemia)

J

1. C
2. H
3. E
4. A
5. I
6. D
7. J
8. G
9. B
10. F

K

1. antipyretic
2. antipruritic
3. narcotic
4. synergism
5. erythromycin
6. generic
7. contraindication
8. anesthetic

L

1. antibiotic
2. NSAID
3. anticonvulsant
4. antiviral
5. antiestrogen
6. ACE inhibitor
7. oral antidiabetic for type 2 diabetes
8. SERM
9. antidepressant
10. antihistamine
11. diuretic
12. anesthetic

M

1. nonsteroidal anti-inflammatory drug
2. as needed
3. four times a day
4. freely as desired
5. three times a day
6. milligram
7. with
8. without
9. nothing by mouth
10. after meals
11. twice a day
12. every hour
13. by mouth
14. every

N

1. take one tablet by mouth, four times a day, after meals and at bedtime
2. administer 15-60 milligrams intramuscularly, every 4-6 hours
3. take two capsules by mouth at bedtime
4. place one tablet under the tongue, as needed
5. apply to the skin, at bedtime as needed

O

1. anticoagulant
2. tranquilizer
3. antiemetic
4. synergistic
5. side effects
6. infectious disease, antibiotics, lungs
7. anticonvulsant, twice a day
8. diabetes, insulin
9. stimulants, caffeine
10. asthma, bronchodilators

Answers to Practical Applications

Prescriptions

1. d
2. f
3. a
4. c
5. b
6. e

PRONUNCIATION OF TERMS

To test your understanding of the terminology in this chapter, write the meaning of each term in the space provided. In addition, you may wish to cover the terms and write them by looking at your definitions. Make sure your spelling is correct. The page number after each term indicates where it is defined or used in the book, so you can easily check your responses. You will find complete definitions for all of these terms and their audio pronunciations on Evolve website.

Pronunciation Guide

ā as in āpe	ă as in ăpple
ē as in ēven	ĕ as in ĕvery
ī as in īce	ĭ as in ĭnterest
ō as in ōpen	ŏ as in pŏt
ū as in ūnit	ŭ as in ŭnder

TERM	PRONUNCIATION	MEANING
ACE inhibitor (899)	ĀCE ĭn-HĬB-ĭ-tŏr	
addiction (897)	ă-DĬK-shŭn	
additive action (897)	ĂD-ĭ-tĭv ĂK-shŭn	
aerosol (897)	ĀR-ō-sōl	
amphetamine (899)	ăm-FĔT-ă-mēn	
analgesic (899)	ăn-ăl-JĒ-zĭk	
anaphylaxis (897)	ăn-ă-fĭ-LĂK-sĭs	
androgen (899)	ĂN-drō-jĕn	
anesthesia (901)	ăn-ĕs-THĒ-zē-ă	
anesthetic (899)	ăn-ĕs-THĔ-tĭk	
angiotensin II receptor blocker (899)	ăn-jē-ō-TĔN-sĭn II rē-CĔP-tŏr BLŎK-ĕr	
antacid (899)	ănt-ĂS-ĭd	
antagonistic action (897)	ăn-tă-gŏn-NĬS-tĭk ĂK-shŭn	
antiandrogen (899)	ăn-tē-ĂN-drō-jĕn	
antiarrhythmic (899)	ăn-tē-ā-RĬTH-mĭk	
antibiotic (899)	ăn-tĭ-bī-ŎT-ĭk	
anticoagulant (899)	ăn-tĭ-kō-ĂG-ū-lănt	
anticonvulsant (899)	ăn-tĭ-kŏn-VŬL-sănt	
antidepressant (899)	ăn-tĭ-dĕ-PRĔS-ănt	
antidiabetic (899)	ăn-tĭ-dī-ă-BĔT-ĭk	
antidiarrheal (899)	ăn-tĭ-dī-ă-RĒ-ăl	
antidote (897)	ĂN-tĭ-dōt	
antiemetic (899)	ăn-tĭ-ĕ-MĔ-tĭk	

TERM	PRONUNCIATION	MEANING
antihistamine (899)	ăn-tĭ-HĬS-tă-mēn	
antinauseant (899)	ăn-tĭ-NAW-zē-ănt	
antiplatelet (899)	ăn-tĭ-PLĀT-lĕt	
antipruritic (901)	ăn-tĭ-proo-RĬT-ĭk	
antipyretic (901)	ăn-tĭ-pī-RĔT-ĭk	
antiulcer (899)	ăn-tĭ-ŬL-sĕr	
antiviral (899)	ăn-tē-VĪ-răl	
aromatase inhibitor (899)	ă-RŌ-mă-tās ĭn-HĬB-ĭ-tŏr	
bactericidal (899)	băk-tĕ-rĭ-SĪ-dăl	
bacteriostatic (899)	băk-tĕ-rē-ō-STĂ-tĭk	
beta-blocker (899)	BĀ-tă BLŎK-ĕr	
bronchodilator (901)	brŏng-kō-DĪ-lā-tŏr	
bisphosphonate (899)	bĭs-FŎS-fō-nāt	
brand name (897)	brănd nām	
caffeine (899)	kăf-ĒN	
calcium channel blocker (899)	KĂL-sē-ŭm CHĂN-ĕl BLŎK-ĕr	
cardiac glycoside (900)	KĂR-dē-ăk GLĪ-kō-sīd	
cardiovascular drug (900)	kăr-dē-ō-VĂS-kū-lăr drŭg	
cathartic (900)	kă-THĂR-tĭk	
chemical name (897)	KĔM-ĭ-kal nām	
chemotherapy (901)	kē-mō-THĔR-ă-pē	
cholesterol-binding drug (900)	kō-LĔS-tĕr-ŏl BĪN-dĭng drŭg	
cholesterol-lowering drug (900)	kō-LĔS-tĕr-ŏl LŌ-wĕr-ĭng drŭg	
contraindications (897)	kŏn-tră-ĭn-dĭ-KĀ-shŭnz	
controlled substances (897)	kŏn-TRŌLD SŬB-stăn-sĕz	
dependence (897)	dĭ-PEN-dents	
diuretic (900)	dī-ū-RĔT-ĭk	
dose (897)	dōs	
emetic (900)	ĕ-MĔT-ĭk	
erythromycin (901)	ĕ-rĭth-rō-MĪ-sĭn	
endocrine drug (900)	ĔN-dō-krĭn drŭg	

TERM	PRONUNCIATION	MEANING
estrogen (900)	ĔS-trō-jĕn	______
gastrointestinal drug (900)	găs-trō-ĭn-TĔS-tĭ-năl drŭg	______
generic name (897)	jĕ-NĔR-ĭk nām	______
glucocorticoid (900)	gloo-kō-KŎR-tĭ-koyd	______
hypnotic (900)	hĭp-NŎT-ĭk	______
hypodermic (901)	hī-pō-DĔR-mĭk	______
iatrogenic (897)	ī-ăt-rō-JĔN-ĭk	______
idiosyncrasy (901)	ĭd-ē-ō-SĬN-kră-sē	______
idiosyncratic reaction (897)	ĭd-ē-ō-sĭn-KRĂ-tĭk rē-ĂK-shŭn	______
inhalation (897)	ĭn-hă-LĀ-shŭn	______
intrathecal (901)	ĭn-tră-THĒ-kăl	______
intravenous (902)	ĭn-tră-VĒ-nŭs	______
laxative (900)	LĂK-să-tĭv	______
medicinal chemistry (897)	mĕ-DĬ-sĭ-năl KĔM-ĭs-trē	______
molecular pharmacology (897)	mō-LĔK-ū-lăr făr-mă-KŎL-ō-jē	______
narcotic (900)	năr-KŎT-ĭk	______
oral administration (897)	ŎR-ăl ăd-mĭn-ĭs-TRĀ-shŭn	______
parenteral administration (897)	pă-RĔN-tĕr-ăl ăd-mĭn-ĭs-TRĀ-shŭn	______
pharmacist (898)	FĂR-mă-sĭst	______
pharmacy (898)	FĂR-mă-sē	______
pharmacodynamics (898)	făr-mă-kō-dī-NĂM-ĭks	______
pharmacokinetics (898)	făr-mă-kō-kĭ-NĔT-ĭks	______
pharmacologist (898)	făr-mă-KŎL-ō-gĭst	______
pharmacology (898)	făr-mă-KŎL-ō-gē	______
progestin (900)	prō-JĔS-tĭn	______
purgative (900)	PŬR-gă-tĭv	______
receptor (898)	rē-SĔP-tŏr	______
rectal administration (898)	RĔK-tăl ăd-mĭn-ĭs-TRĀ-shŭn	______
resistance (898)	rē-SĬS-tăns	______
respiratory drug (900)	rĕs-pĭr-ă-TŎR-ē drŭg	______

TERM	PRONUNCIATION	MEANING
response (898)	rĕ-SPŌNS	
schedule (898)	SKĔD-ūl	
sedative (900)	SĔD-ă-tĭv	
side effect (898)	sīd ĕ-FĔKT	
stimulant (900)	STĬM-ū-lănt	
subcutaneous (901)	sŭb-kū-TĀ-nē-ŭs	
sublingual administration (898)	sŭb-LĬNG-wăl ăd-mĭn-ĭs-TRĀ-shŭn	
synergism (898)	SĬN-ĕr-jĭzm	
synergistic (902)	sĭn-ĕr-JĬS-tĭk	
syringe (898)	sĭ-RĬNJ	
thyroid hormone (900)	THĪ-royd HŎR-mōn	
tolerance (898)	TŎL-ĕr-ănz	
topical application (898)	TŎP-ĭ-kl ăp-lĭ-KĀ-shŭn	
toxic (902)	TŎK-sĭk	
toxicity (898)	tŏk-SĬS-ĭ-tē	
toxicology (898)	tŏk-sĭ-KŎL-ō-jē	
tranquilizer (900)	TRĂN-kwĭ-lī-zĕr	
transport (898)	TRĂNZ-pŏrt	
vasodilator (902)	văz-ō-DĪ-lā-tŏr	
vitamin (898)	VĪ-tă-mĭn	

REVIEW SHEET

Write the meanings of the word parts in the spaces provided, and test yourself. Check your answers with the information in the chapter or in the Glossary (Medical Word Parts—English) at the end of the book.

Combining Forms

COMBINING FORM	MEANING	COMBINING FORM	MEANING
aer/o	____________	lingu/o	____________
alges/o	____________	myc/o	____________
bronch/o	____________	narc/o	____________
chem/o	____________	or/o	____________
cras/o	____________	pharmac/o	____________
cutane/o	____________	prurit/o	____________
derm/o	____________	pyret/o	____________
enter/o	____________	thec/o	____________
erg/o	____________	tox/o	____________
esthes/o	____________	toxic/o	____________
hist/o	____________	vas/o	____________
hypn/o	____________	ven/o	____________
iatr/o	____________	vit/o	____________

Suffixes

SUFFIX	MEANING	SUFFIX	MEANING
-amine	____________	-in	____________
-dote	____________	-phylaxis	____________
-genic	____________	-sol	____________

Prefixes

PREFIX	MEANING	PREFIX	MEANING
ana-	____________	par-	____________
anti-	____________	syn-	____________
contra-	____________		

evolve *Please refer to the Evolve website for additional exercises, games, and images related to this chapter.*

CHAPTER 22

Psychiatry

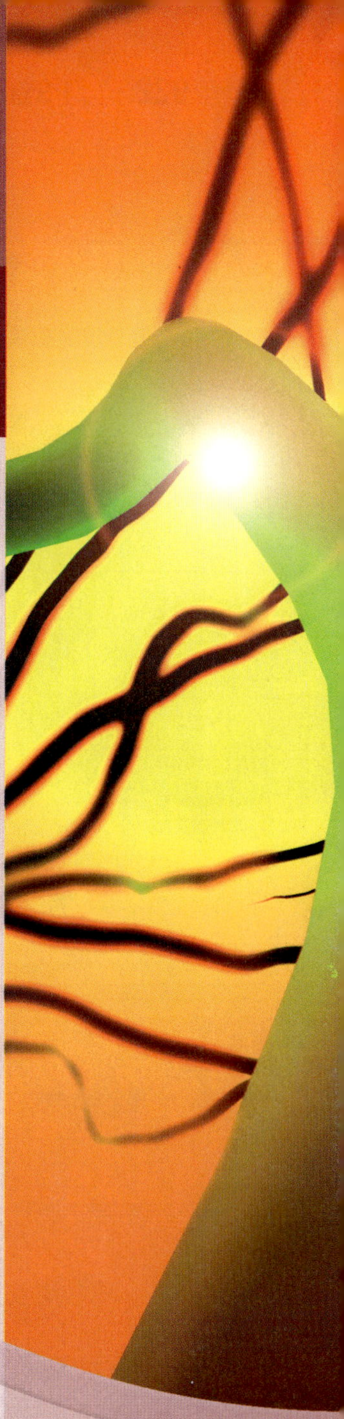

This chapter is divided into the following sections:

CHAPTER GOALS

- Differentiate among a psychiatrist, a psychologist, and other mental health specialists.
- Describe tests used by clinical psychologists to evaluate a patient's mental health and intelligence.
- Define terms that describe major psychiatric disorders.
- Identify terms that describe psychiatric symptoms.
- Compare different types of therapy for psychiatric disorders.
- Identify the categories of psychiatric drugs, and name commonly used drugs in each category.
- Define combining forms, suffixes, prefixes, and abbreviations related to psychiatry.
- Apply your new knowledge to understanding medical terms in their proper contexts, such as medical reports and records.

INTRODUCTION

You will find this chapter different from others in the book. Some, but not all, psychiatric disorders are not readily explainable in terms of abnormalities in the structure or chemistry of an organ or tissue, as are other illnesses. In addition, the causes of mental disorders are complex and include significant psychological and social as well as chemical and structural elements. This chapter provides a simple outline of psychiatric disorders and definitions of major psychiatric terms. For more extensive and detailed information, you may wish to consult the ***Diagnostic and Statistical Manual of Mental Disorders,* fourth edition, text revision (DSM-IV-TR),** published by the American Psychiatric Association (Washington, DC), as well as other textbooks of psychiatry.

Psychiatry (**psych/o** = mind, **iatr/o** = treatment) is the branch of medicine that deals with the diagnosis, treatment, and prevention of mental illness. It is a specialty of clinical medicine like surgery, internal medicine, pediatrics, and obstetrics.

Psychiatrists complete the same medical training (4 years of medical school) as for other physicians and receive an MD (doctor of medicine) degree. Then they spend a variable number of years training in the methods and practice of **psychotherapy** (psychological techniques for treating mental disorders) and **psychopharmacology** (drug therapy). Psychiatrists complete 4 years of residency training and then extra years of fellowship training to specialize in various aspects of psychiatry. **Child psychiatrists** specialize in the treatment of children; **forensic psychiatrists** specialize in the legal aspects of psychiatry, such as the determination of mental competence in criminal cases. **Psychoanalysts** complete 3 to 5 additional years of training in a special psychotherapeutic technique called **psychoanalysis** in which the patient freely relates her or his thoughts and associations to the analyst, who does not interfere with the process. Interpretations are offered at appropriate times.

A **psychologist** is a nonmedical professional who is trained in methods of psychological testing, psychotherapy, analysis, and research and completes a doctor of philosophy (PhD) or doctor of education (EdD) degree program in a specific field of interest, such as **clinical** (patient-oriented) **psychology, experimental research,** or **social psychology** (focusing on social interaction and the ways the actions of others influence the behavior of the individual). A **clinical psychologist,** like a psychiatrist, can use various methods of psychotherapy to treat patients but, unlike a psychiatrist, cannot prescribe drugs or electroconvulsive therapy. Other nonphysicians trained in the treatment of mental illness include licensed clinical social workers, psychiatric nurses, and licensed mental health clinicians (LMHCs).

Clinical psychologists are trained in the use of tests to evaluate various aspects of a patient's mental health and intelligence. Examples are **intelligence (IQ) tests** such as the **Wechsler Adult Intelligence Scale (WAIS)** and the **Stanford-Binet Intelligence Scale.** Two projective **(personality) tests** are the use of **Rorschach technique,** in which inkblots, as shown in Figure 22-1, are used to bring out associations, and the **Thematic Apperception Test (TAT),** in which pictures are used as stimuli for making up stories (Figure 22-2). Both tests are revealing of personality structure. Examples of **graphomotor projection tests** are the **Draw a Person Test,** in which the patient is asked to copy a body, and the **Bender-Gestalt Test,** in which the patient is asked to draw certain geometric designs. The Bender-Gestalt Test picks up deficits in mental processing and memory caused by brain damage and is used to screen children for developmental delays. The **Minnesota Multiphasic Personality Inventory (MMPI)** contains true-false questions that reveal aspects of personality, such as sense of duty or responsibility, ability to relate to others, and dominance (assertiveness, resourcefulness). This test is widely used as a measure of psychological health in adolescents and adults. The patient's responses to questions are compared with responses made by patients with diagnoses of schizophrenia, depression, and so on.

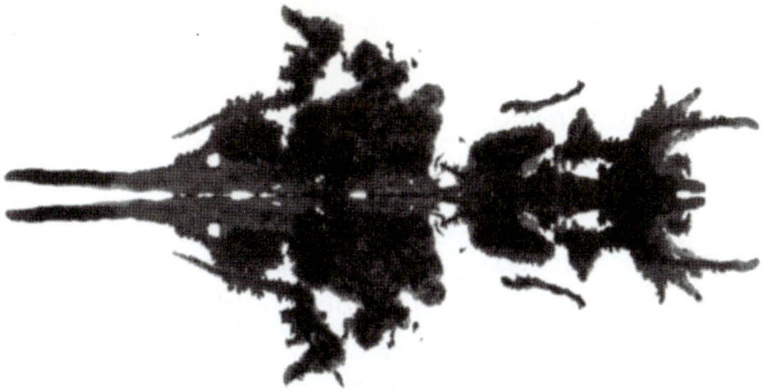

FIGURE 22-1 **Inkblots** like this one are presented on 10 cards in the Rorschach test. The patient describes images seen in the blot.

Psychiatric Clinical Symptoms

The following terms describe abnormalities that are evident to an examining mental health professional. Familiarity with these terms will help you understand the next section, Psychiatric Disorders.

amnesia Loss of memory.

anxiety Varying degrees of uneasiness, apprehension, or dread often accompanied by palpitations, tightness in the chest, breathlessness, and choking sensations.

apathy Absence of emotions; lack of interest, emotional involvement, or motivation.

compulsion Uncontrollable urge to perform an act repeatedly.

conversion Anxiety becomes a bodily symptom, such as blindness, deafness, or paralysis, that does not have a physical basis.

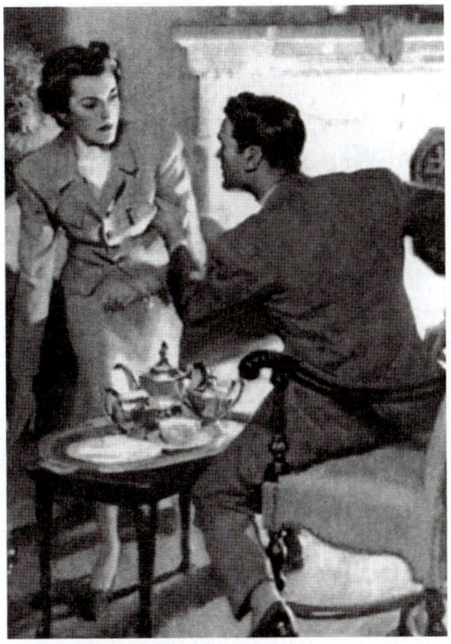

FIGURE 22-2 A sample picture from the **Thematic Apperception Test.** The patient is asked to tell the story that the picture illustrates.

delusion A fixed, false belief that cannot be changed by logical reasoning or evidence.

dissociation Uncomfortable feelings are separated from their real object. In order to avoid mental distress, the feelings are redirected toward a second object or behavior pattern.

dysphoria Sadness, hopelessness; depressive mood, or feeling "low."

euphoria Exaggerated feeling of well-being ("high").

hallucination False or unreal sensory perception as, for example, hearing voices when none are present; an **illusion** is a false perception of an actual sensory stimulus.

labile Variable; undergoing rapid emotional change.

mania Elation or irritability, associated with distractibility, hyperactivity, talkativeness, injudicious acts, flight of ideas, and racing thoughts.

mutism Non-reactive state with inability to speak.

obsession An involuntary, persistent idea or emotion; the suffix -mania indicates a strong obsession with something (e.g., pyromania is an obsession with fire).

paranoia Overly suspicious system of thinking; fixed delusion that one is being harassed, persecuted, or unfairly treated.

PSYCHIATRIC DISORDERS

Sigmund Freud's ideas of personality structure play an important role in the understanding of many types of psychiatric disorders. Freud believed that personality is made up of three major parts: the **id,** the **ego,** and the **superego.** The **id** represents the unconscious instincts and psychic energy present from birth. The id contains basic drives that, operating according to the pleasure principle, seek immediate gratification regardless of the reality of the situation.

The **ego** is the central coordinating branch of the personality. It is the mediator between the id and the outside world. It is the part of the personality that evaluates and assesses the reality of a situation **(reality testing)** and, if necessary, postpones the gratification of a need or drive (id) until a satisfactory object or situation arises. The ego is perceived as being "self" by the individual.

The **superego** is the internalized conscience and moral part of the personality. It encompasses the sense of discipline derived from parental authority and society. Guilt feelings, for example, arise from behavior and thoughts that do not conform to the standards of the superego.

Freud believed that certain psychological disorders occur when conflicts arise between two or more of these aspects of the personality. **Defense mechanisms,** such as denial, are techniques people use to ward off the anxiety produced by these conflicts. For example, a person afflicted with a serious illness may avoid confronting his or her present or future problems by denial. Thus, he or she may refuse to believe the diagnosis, may miss appointments, may neglect medication, or may ignore symptoms. All individuals use defense mechanisms to cope with difficult problems. The use of these mechanisms may be regarded as abnormal or normal according to whether that use makes a constructive or destructive contribution to the individual's personality.

The term **psychosis** is frequently used to describe mental illness. A **psychosis** involves significant impairment of reality testing, with symptoms such as **delusions** (false beliefs), **hallucinations** (false sensory perceptions), and bizarre behavior. Schizophrenic disorders are examples of psychoses. Patients exhibit a disturbed sense of self, inappropriate affect (emotional reactions), and withdrawal from the external world.

Psychiatric disorders that are discussed in this section are **anxiety disorders, delirium** and **dementia, dissociative disorders, eating disorders, mood disorders, personality disorders, pervasive developmental disorders, schizophrenia, sexual** and **gender identity disorders, somatoform disorders,** and **substance-related disorders.**

ANXIETY DISORDERS

Anxiety disorders are characterized by the experience of unpleasant tension, distress, troubled feelings, and avoidance behavior. A **panic attack** is a defined period of intense fear or discomfort in which symptoms develop abruptly and reach a peak within 10 minutes. Symptoms and clinical signs may include the following:

- Palpitations
- Sweating
- Trembling
- Smothering or shortness of breath
- Feeling of choking
- Chest pain
- Nausea
- Feeling dizzy or faint
- Feelings of unreality or depersonalization
- Fear of losing control or going crazy
- Fear of dying
- Numbness or tingling
- Hot flashes

Panic disorder is a condition characterized by recurrent, unexpected panic attacks and persistent concern about having another panic attack in between episodes. A panic attack can occur in the context of other anxiety disorders, such as phobic, obsessive-compulsive, post-traumatic stress, and generalized anxiety disorders.

Phobic disorders are characterized by irrational or debilitating fears associated with a specific object or situation. The patient with a phobic disorder goes to extreme lengths to avoid the object of her or his fear. The object that is feared often is symbolic of an unconscious conflict that is the cause of the phobia and thus diverts the patient's attention from the conflict, keeping it unconscious. Panic attacks (periods of intense apprehension and fear) can occur in anticipation of the phobic situation.

Agoraphobia (agora- = marketplace) is the fear of being in open, crowded, public places from which escape would be difficult or in which help might not be available, or of going out alone in "unsafe" places. Persons with agoraphobia limit their normal activities to avoid situations that trigger their anxiety. Thus, they may feel comfortable only when at home or in the company of a friend or relative.

A **social phobia (social anxiety disorder)** is the fear of situations in which the affected person is open to public scrutiny, which could result in possible embarrassment and humiliation. For example, the fear may focus on speaking in public, using public lavatories, or eating in public.

Other specific phobias are **claustrophobia** (fear of closed-in places; **claustr/o** = barrier), **acrophobia** (fear of heights; in this term, **acr/o** = a high point), and **zoophobia** (fear of animals; **zo/o** = animals).

Obsessive-compulsive disorder (OCD) involves recurrent thoughts **(obsessions)** and repetitive acts **(compulsions)** that dominate the patient's life. The patient experiences anxiety if he or she is prevented from performing special rituals. Often the OCD consumes time and interferes with the individual's social or occupational functioning. Several antidepressant drugs, including clomipramine, have been used to treat OCD, with considerable success, particularly when combined with cognitive behavioral therapy.

Post-traumatic stress disorder (PTSD) is the development of symptoms (intense fear, helplessness, insomnia, nightmares, and diminished responsiveness to the external world) following exposure to a traumatic event. Flashbacks, bothersome thoughts, and anxiety often triggered by reminders occur in episodes long after a life-threatening or major emotional event. People avoid situations with reminders. Many survivors of the September 11, 2001, attack on the World Trade Center towers and the Pentagon experienced post-traumatic stress disorder.

Generalized anxiety disorder (GAD) is characterized by chronic anxiety and exaggerated worry and tension even when there is little or nothing to provoke such feelings.

DELIRIUM AND DEMENTIA

Delirium and **dementia** are disorders of **cognition** (mental processes of thinking, perception, reasoning, and judgment).

Delirium is an acute, temporary disturbance of consciousness characterized by mental confusion and often psychotic symptoms. The affected person usually presents with rambling, irrelevant, or incoherent speech, sensory misperceptions, and disorientation as to time, place, or person and with memory impairment. Delirium is caused by a variety of conditions, including drug intoxication or withdrawal, seizures or head trauma, and metabolic disturbances such as hypoxia, hypoglycemia, electrolyte imbalances, or hepatic or renal failure. **Delirium tremens** is brought on by stopping alcohol consumption suddenly after prolonged periods of heavy alcohol ingestion.

Dementia is impairment of judgment, memory, and abstract thinking that involves a general, more gradual loss of intellectual abilities as well as changes in personality. It also includes difficulty with language and with simple acts like dressing or brushing the teeth. Dementia may be caused by conditions, some reversible and some progressive, involving damage to the brain. The most common cause is Alzheimer disease, but other causes are cerebrovascular disease (stroke), central nervous system (CNS) infection, medications and drugs, brain trauma, tumors, and Parkinson and Huntington diseases. Depression also can manifest as (pseudo)dementia. It is important to identify treatable causes of dementia.

DISSOCIATIVE DISORDER

A **dissociative disorder** is a condition involving breakdown in memory, identity, or perception. People with dissociative disorder escape reality through amnesia, **fugue** (sudden travel away from home or work), or alternate identities.

EATING DISORDERS

Eating disorders are severe disturbances in eating behavior. Examples are **anorexia nervosa** and **bulimia nervosa.** Anorexia nervosa is characterized by refusal to maintain a minimal normal body weight. The affected person is intensely afraid of gaining weight and has a disturbance in perception of the shape or size of her or his body. (The term **anorexia,** meaning "lack of appetite," is a misnomer because lack of appetite is rare.) The condition predominantly affects adolescent females, and its principal symptom is a conscious, relentless attempt to diet along with excessive, compulsive overactivity, such as exercise, running, or gymnastics. Most postmenarchal females with this disorder are amenorrheic.

Bulimia nervosa (**bulimia** means abnormal increase in hunger) is characterized by binge eating (uncontrolled indulgence in food) followed by purging (eliminating food from the body). Persons with bulimia maintain normal or nearly normal weight because after bingeing they engage in inappropriate purging. Examples of purging are self-induced vomiting and the misuse of laxatives or enemas.

MOOD DISORDERS

A mood disorder is a condition of prolonged, intense abnormal mood, like sadness, that dominates the patient's entire mental life for some time. Examples of mood disorders are **bipolar disorder** and **depressive disorder.**

Bipolar disorders (**bi-** = two; **pol/o** = extreme) are characterized by one or more **manic** episodes alternating with depressive episodes. A manic episode is a period during which the predominant mood is excessively elevated (euphoria), expansive, or irritable. Associated symptoms include inflated self-esteem, or grandiosity, decreased need for sleep, a nearly continuous flow of rapid speech with quick changes of topic, distractibility, an increase in goal-directed activity, and excessive involvement in pleasurable activities that have a high potential for painful consequences. Often there are increased sociability and participation in multiple activities marked by intrusive, domineering, and demanding behavior. **Hypomania** (in this term, **hypo-** = decrease) describes a mood resembling mania, but of lesser intensity. **Bipolar disorder I** is characterized by one or more manic episodes, often alternating with major depressive episodes. **Bipolar disorder II** is characterized by recurrent major depressive episodes alternating with hypomanic episodes.

Cyclothymic disorder (**cycl/o** = cycle, **thym/o** = mind) is a mild form of bipolar disorder characterized by at least 2 years of hypomania and numerous depressive episodes that do not meet the criteria that define a major depressive episode.

Depressive disorders are marked by the occurrence of one or more major depressive episodes without a history of mania or hypomania. **Major depression** involves episodes of severe **dysphoria** (sadness, hopelessness, worry, discouragement). Other signs and symptoms are appetite disturbances (increase or decrease) and changes in weight; sleep disorders such as insomnia or hypersomnia; fatigue or low energy; feelings of worthlessness, hopelessness, or excessive or inappropriate guilt; difficulty thinking or concentrating; and recurrent thoughts of death or suicide. **Dysthymia** (or **dysthymic disorder**) is a depressive disorder involving depressed mood (feeling sad or "down in the dumps") that persists over a 2-year period but is not as severe as major depression. Also, there are no psychotic features (delusions, hallucinations, incoherent thinking) as are sometimes found in major depression.

Researchers have noted a relationship between the onset of an episode of depressive disorder and a particular period of the year. A regular appearance of depression may occur within approximately 60 days, between the beginning of October and the end of November, every year. This is referred to as **seasonal affective** (mood) **disorder (SAD).** A change from depression to mania or hypomania also may occur within a 60-day period from mid-February to mid-April.

PERSONALITY DISORDERS

Personality traits are established patterns of thinking and ways of relating to and perceiving the environment and the self; however, when these traits become inflexible and rigid or are the source of impaired functioning, distress, and conflict with others, they constitute **personality disorders.** Types of personality disorders include the following:

antisocial	No loyalty to or concern for others, and without moral standards; acts only in response to desires and impulses; cannot tolerate frustration and blames others when he or she is at fault.
borderline	Instability in interpersonal relationships and sense of self; characterized by alternating involvement with and rejection of people. Frantic efforts are made to avoid real or imagined abandonment.
histrionic	Emotional, attention-seeking, immature, and dependent; irrational outbursts and tantrums; flamboyant and theatrical; having general dissatisfaction with the self and angry feelings about the world.
narcissistic	Grandiose sense of self-importance or uniqueness and preoccupation with fantasies of success and power. **Narcissism** is a pervasive interest in the self with a lack of empathy for others.
paranoid	Continually suspicious and mistrustful of other people but not to a psychotic or delusional degree; jealous and overly concerned with hidden motives of others; quick to take offense.
schizoid	Emotionally cold and aloof; indifferent to praise or criticism or to the feelings of others; few friendships and rarely appears to experience strong emotions, such as anger or joy.

PERVASIVE DEVELOPMENTAL DISORDERS

Pervasive developmental disorders are a group of childhood disorders characterized by delays in the development of socialization and communication skills. Examples are **autism** and **Asperger syndrome. Autism,** commonly becoming evident during the first 3 years of life, is marked by difficulties in verbal and nonverbal communication and in social and play interactions. It is a spectrum disorder, affecting each individual differently and at varying degrees. Persons with autism may exhibit some of the following traits:

- Resistance to change; insistence on sameness
- Using gestures or pointing instead of words to communicate needs
- Repeating words or phrases
- Preference for being alone; aloof in manner
- Tantrums
- Difficulty in interacting with others
- Not wanting to be touched
- Little or no eye contact
- Uneven gross/fine motor skills
- Sensitivity to sound
- Obsessive attachment to objects

Symptoms of autism may lessen as the child develops and receives treatment. See the ***In Person*** feature on page 943.

Asperger syndrome is often referred to as a less severe type of autism. Children with Asperger syndrome frequently have normal language skills and normal intelligence. They usually want to interact with others but don't know how to do it. They may have fine rote memory skills but have difficulty with abstract concepts. Repetitive and restricted patterns of behavior may also be part of the picture.

SCHIZOPHRENIA

Schizophrenia is a chronic psychotic disorder characterized by disturbed thinking and disorganized speech. It includes the following symptoms:

Delusions such as "people are out to get me" or thought broadcasting (belief that internal thoughts are broadcast to the external world so that others can hear them).

Hallucinations involving voices or sounds that do not exist but seem real.

Thought disorder, such as loosening of associations (ideas shift from one subject to another, completely unrelated or only obliquely connected). This may result in incoherent, incomprehensible speech.

Disorders of movement, including involuntary movements and mannerisms or clumsiness or uncoordination.

Flat affect marked by monotonous voice, immobile face, and no signs of expression. **Affect** (external expression of emotion) also may be inappropriate (smiling and laughing when the subject is serious).

Impaired interpersonal functioning and relationship to the external world, such as emotional detachment and social withdrawal.

Positive symptoms of schizophrenia are thought disorder, hallucinations, and delusions. **Negative symptoms** include flat affect (apathy), social withdrawal, and inability to experience pleasure.

Psychiatrists describe subtypes types of schizophrenia, such as **catatonic type** (the patient is mute and does not move or react to the outside environment); **disorganized type** (the patient exhibits disorganized speech and bizarre behavior); and **paranoid type** (the patient experiences prominent delusions of grandeur or persecution and auditory hallucinations).

SEXUAL AND GENDER IDENTITY DISORDERS

Sexual disorders are divided into two types: **paraphilias** and **sexual dysfunctions. Paraphilias** (**para-** = abnormal, **-philia** = attraction to or love) are characterized by recurrent intense sexual urges, fantasies, or behaviors that involve unusual objects, activities, or situations. **Sexual dysfunctions** are disturbances in sexual desire or changes in sexual response, such as premature ejaculation and dyspareunia (painful sexual intercourse) that are not the result of a general medical condition.

Examples of paraphilias are:

exhibitionism	Compulsive need to expose one's body, particularly the genitals, to an unsuspecting stranger.
fetishism	The use of nonliving objects (articles of clothing) as substitutes for a human sexual love object.
pedophilia	Sexual urges and fantasies involving sexual activity with a prepubescent child (age 13 or younger).
sexual masochism	Sexual gratification is gained by being humiliated, beaten, bound, or otherwise made to suffer by another person.
sexual sadism	Sexual gratification is gained by inflicting physical or psychological pain or humiliation on others.
transvestic fetishism	Cross-dressing; wearing clothing of the opposite sex. This disorder has been described in heterosexual males who have intense sexually arousing fantasies, urges, or behaviors involving cross-dressing.
voyeurism	Sexual excitement is achieved by observing unsuspecting people who are naked, undressing, or engaging in sexual activity.

A **gender identity disorder** is likely to be reclassified as **gender dysphoria** in the next edition of the DSM. In DSM-IV-TR, this condition is defined as a strong and persistent cross-gender identification with the opposite sex manifested in preference for cross-dressing and cross-gender roles in make-believe play or in persistent fantasies of being the other sex.

SOMATOFORM DISORDERS

In somatoform disorders, the patient's mental conflicts are expressed as physical symptoms. The physical signs and symptoms, such as abdominal or chest pain, nausea, vomiting, diarrhea, palpitations, deafness, blindness, and paralysis, are not adequately explained by a physical or other mental disorder or by injury and are not side effects of medication, drugs, or alcohol. There is no diagnosable medical condition such as depression that fully accounts for a physical symptom.

Examples of somatoform (**somat/o** = body) disorders are **conversion disorder** and **hypochondriasis.**

Conversion disorder is a loss of physical functioning that suggests a physical disorder but that instead is an expression of a psychological conflict or need. The patient usually has a feared or unconscious conflict that threatens to escape from **repression** (a defense mechanism in which a person removes unacceptable ideas or impulses from consciousness), but the energies associated with this conflict are experienced as a physical symptom. The conversion symptom (examples are paralysis, blindness, seizures, paresthesias, and dyskinesia) enables the affected person to avoid the conflict and get support from the surrounding environment. For example, a person with repressed anger and desire to physically harm a family member may suddenly develop paralysis of the arm (conversion symptom). Another example of a conversion symptom might be paralysis of the finger used to pull the trigger of a gun if there was internal conflict about firing the weapon.

Hypochondriasis is a preoccupation with body aches, pains, and discomforts in the absence of real illness. Appropriate physical evaluation and diagnostic testing do not support the diagnosis of any physical disorder that can account for the symptoms or the person's interpretation of them. Ruling out a physical abnormality does not reassure the person with hypochondriasis.

SUBSTANCE-RELATED DISORDERS

Substance-related disorders are characterized by symptoms and behavioral changes associated with regular use or discontinuation of substances that affect the central nervous system. Continued or periodic use of certain drugs produces a state of dependence. **Psychological dependence** is a compulsion to continue taking a drug despite adverse consequences, and **physiologic dependence** is characterized by the onset of withdrawal symptoms when the drug is discontinued abruptly. A significant feature of physiologic dependence is **tolerance.** Tolerance is the declining effect of the drug so that the dose must be increased to give the same effect.

Examples of substances that are associated with drug abuse (use of a drug for purposes other than those for which it is prescribed) and dependence are:

Alcohol. Alcohol dependence often is associated with the use and abuse of other psychoactive drugs (cannabis, cocaine, heroin, amphetamines). Signs of alcohol dependence and intoxication include slurred speech, incoordination, unsteady gait, nystagmus (rapid, rhythmic movement of the eyeball), impairment in attention or memory, stupor, or coma. It also is associated with depression, as either a cause or a consequence of the drinking.

Amphetamines. These central nervous system stimulants are taken orally or administered intravenously. Examples are amphetamine (Benzedrine), dextroamphetamine (Dexedrine), methamphetamine (Desoxyn, or "speed"), and methylphenidate (Ritalin). Some appetite suppressants (diet pills) are amphetamine-like drugs. Psychological and behavioral changes associated with amphetamine dependence include anger, tension or anxiety, impaired judgment, inability to enjoy what was previously pleasurable, and social isolation. Physical signs and symptoms include tachycardia or bradycardia, pupillary dilation, nausea, elevated or low blood pressure, and muscular weakness. Serious depression can occur during withdrawal.

Cannabis. This class of drugs includes all substances with psychoactive properties derived from the cannabis plant plus chemically similar synthetic substances. Examples are **marijuana,** hashish, and purified delta-9-tetrahydrocannabinol (THC), the major psychoactive ingredient in these substances. Psychological and physical signs and symptoms after the smoking of cannabis include euphoria, impaired motor coordination, anxiety, sensation of slowed time, social withdrawal, and impaired memory and judgment. Other signs of cannabis intoxication are increased appetite, dry mouth, tachycardia, and paranoia.

Cocaine. Cocaine is a stimulant drug that produces euphoria as well as vasoconstriction, tachycardia, and hypertension. It comes from the leaves of the coca tree that grows in Central and South America. The form of cocaine most commonly used in the United States is cocaine hydrochloride powder, which is inhaled through the nostrils and then absorbed into the bloodstream through mucous membranes. It also can be injected intravenously, either alone or mixed with heroin (speedball). This mixture is particularly dangerous because cocaine and heroin act synergistically to depress respiratory function. If the cocaine is separated from its powdered salt form and combined with ether, ammonia, or baking soda, the resulting cocaine alkaloid is commonly called freebase. This form can be smoked and is known as crack or rock. Often, the user of cocaine also is dependent on alcohol or sedatives, which are taken in an attempt to alleviate the unpleasant aftereffects (anxiety, depression, and fatigue) of cocaine intoxication.

Hallucinogens. These drugs produce a state of central nervous system excitement, hyperactivity, hallucinations, delusions, hypertension, and mood changes. Examples of hallucinogens are **lysergic acid diethylamide (LSD), mescaline (peyote),** and **phencyclidine (PCP).** The use of hallucinogens generally is episodic because their psychoactive effects are highly potent; frequent use may lead to marked tolerance.

Opioids. This group of drugs includes **heroin** and **morphine** and synthetic drugs with morphine-like action, such as **codeine,** meperidine (Demerol), and oxycodone (OxyContin is sustained-release oxycodone). These compounds are prescribed as analgesics (painkillers), anesthetics, or cough suppressants. Typical signs and symptoms of opioid intoxication are pupillary constriction, euphoria, slowness in movement, drowsiness, and slurred speech. Effects of overdose are slow and shallow breathing, convulsions, coma, and possible death. Signs and symptoms of opioid withdrawal are watery eyes, rhinorrhea (runny nose), pupillary dilation, abdominal cramps and diarrhea, and muscle and joint pain.

Sedatives, Hypnotics, or Anxiolytics. These drugs have a soothing, relaxing, euphoric effect and also can produce sleep (hypnotics). Sleeping pills include **barbiturates** such as phenobarbital and secobarbital. Other drugs that produce a barbiturate-like effect are **benzodiazepines,** including temazepam (Restoril), clonazepam (Klonopin), alprazolam (Xanax), and diazepam (Valium). Intoxication is characterized by slurred speech and disorientation. Effects of overdose are shallow respiration, cold and clammy skin, dilated pupils, weak and rapid pulse, coma, and possibly death. Sudden cessation of these drugs can result in seizures.

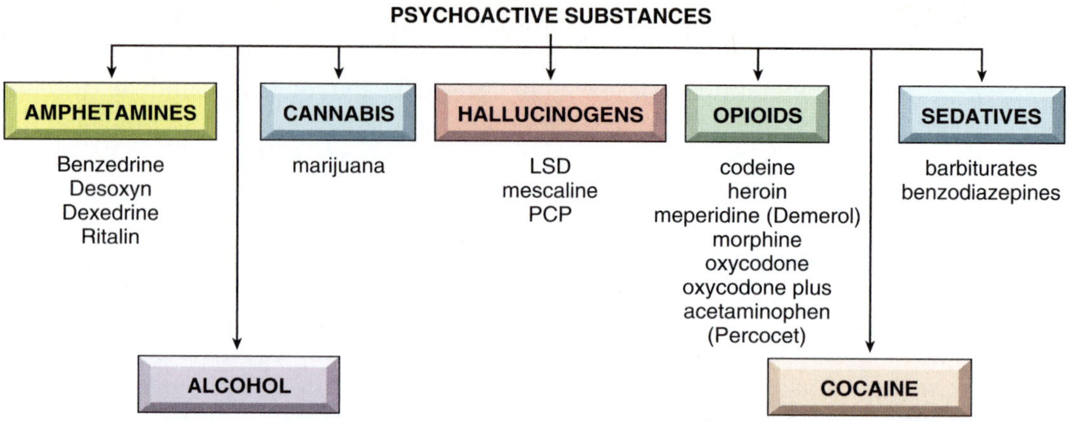

FIGURE 22-3 **Psychoactive substances** that if abused can lead to drug dependence.

Figure 22-3 reviews the types of psychoactive substances that lead to drug dependence and abuse.

Table 22-1 reviews psychiatric disorders and gives examples of each type.

TABLE 22-1 PSYCHIATRIC DISORDERS

Category	Example(s)
Anxiety disorders	• Panic disorder • Phobic disorders • Obsessive-compulsive disorder • Post-traumatic stress disorder • Generalized anxiety disorder
Delirium	• Delirium tremens • Toxic delirium
Dementia	• Alzheimer disease • Multi-infarct dementia
Dissociative disorders	• Dissociative identity disorder, amnesia, fugue, multiple personality disorder
Eating disorders	• Anorexia nervosa • Bulimia nervosa
Mood disorders	• Bipolar I • Bipolar II • Cyclothymic disorder • Depressive disorders • Dysthymia • Seasonal affective disorder (SAD)
Personality disorders	• Antisocial, borderline, histrionic, narcissistic, paranoid, schizoid
Pervasive developmental disorders	• Autism, Asperger syndrome
Schizophrenia	• Positive and negative symptoms; paranoid, disorganized, catatonic, and residual types
Sexual and gender identity disorders	• Paraphilias • Sexual dysfunction • Gender identity disorder
Somatoform disorders	• Conversion disorder • Hypochondriasis • Pain disorder
Substance-related disorders	• Alcohol, amphetamines, cannabis, cocaine, hallucinogens, opioids, sedatives

THERAPEUTIC MODALITIES

Some major therapeutic techniques that are used to treat psychiatric disorders are **psychotherapy, electroconvulsive therapy,** and **drug therapy (psychopharmacology).**

PSYCHOTHERAPY

Psychotherapy is the treatment of emotional problems and disorders using psychological techniques. The following are psychotherapeutic techniques used by psychiatrists, psychologists, and other mental health professionals.

Cognitive Behavioral Therapy (CBT). This is a relatively short-term, focused psychotherapy for a wide range of psychological problems, including depression, anxiety, anger, marital conflict, fears, and substance abuse. The focus is on how the person who is experiencing difficulty is thinking, behaving, and communicating today, rather than on early childhood experiences. Because CBT is based on the idea that thoughts cause feelings and behaviors (not people, situations, or events), if the person can change established ways of thinking, then he or she can feel better even if the situation does not change. CBT techniques often are used to lower anxiety.

Family Therapy. Treatment of an entire family can help the members resolve and understand their conflicts and problems.

Group Therapy. In a group with a mental health professional leader as a neutral moderator, patients with similar problems gain insight into their own personalities through discussions and interaction with each other. In **psychodrama,** patients express their feelings by acting out family and social roles along with other patient-actors on a stage. After a scene has been presented, the audience (composed of other patients) is asked to make comments and offer interpretations about what they have observed.

Hypnosis. A **trance** (state of altered consciousness) is created to help in recovery of deeply repressed memories. Hypnotic techniques are also used for anxiety reduction, creating a sense of psychological safety and for problem solving.

Insight-Oriented Psychotherapy. This type of psychotherapy uses face-to-face discussion of life problems and associated feelings. The aim is to increase understanding of underlying conflicts, themes, thoughts, and behavior patterns to improve mood (depressive feelings).

Play Therapy. In this form of therapy, the child uses play with toys to express conflicts and feelings that he or she is unable to communicate in a direct manner.

Psychoanalysis. This long-term and intense form of psychotherapy seeks to influence behavior and resolve internal conflicts by allowing patients to bring their unconscious emotions to the surface. Through techniques such as **free association** (the patient speaks his or her thoughts one after another without censorship), **transference** (the patient relates to the therapist as to a person who figured prominently in early childhood, such as a parent or sibling), and **dream interpretation,** the patient is able to bring unconscious emotional conflicts to awareness and thus can overcome these problems.

Sex Therapy. This form of therapy can help people overcome sexual dysfunctions such as **frigidity** (inhibited sexual response in women), **impotence** (inability of a man to achieve and/or maintain an erection), and **premature ejaculation** (release of semen before coitus can be achieved).

Supportive Psychotherapy. The therapist offers encouragement, support, and hope to patients facing difficult life transitions and events.

ELECTROCONVULSIVE THERAPY

In **electroconvulsive therapy (ECT),** an electrical current is applied to the brain (usually to one hemisphere) while the patient is anesthetized, with assisted ventilation. Actual physical convulsions are imperceptible. This therapy is used chiefly for serious depression and the depressive phase of bipolar (manic-depressive) disorder. With the introduction of antidepressant drugs, there are fewer indications for electroconvulsive therapy, although it can be life-saving when a rapid response is needed.

DRUG THERAPY

The following are categories of drugs used to treat psychiatric disorders. Figure 22-4 reviews these groups and lists specific drugs in each category.

- **Antianxiety and antipanic agents.** These drugs lessen anxiety, tension, and agitation, especially when they are associated with panic attacks. Examples are **benzodiazepines (BZDs),** which act as antianxiety agents, sedatives, or anticonvulsants (clonazepam). Benzodiazepines directly affect the brain to slow down the transmission of nerve impulses. Other antianxiety and antipanic agents are **selective serotonin reuptake inhibitors (SSRIs).** These agents prevent the reuptake of serotonin (a neurotransmitter) into nerve endings, allowing it to linger in the space between it and the next nerve cell.
- **Antidepressants.** These drugs gradually reverse depressive symptoms and return the patient to a more even state, with less persistent and less severe depressive symptoms. The basis of depression is thought to be an imbalance in the levels of neurotransmitters in the brain. Several groups of drugs are used as antidepressants. These include:
    1. **SSRIs (selective serotonin reuptake inhibitors)** such as fluoxetine (Prozac). They improve mood, mental concentration, physical activity, and sleep patterns.
    2. **Monoamine oxidase (MAO) inhibitors.** These drugs suppress an enzyme, monoamine oxidase, that normally degrades neurotransmitters. MAO inhibitors are not as widely prescribed as other antidepressants because serious cardiovascular and liver complications can occur with their use.
    3. **Tricyclic antidepressants.** These drugs contain three fused rings (tricyclic) in their chemical structure. They block the reuptake of neurotransmitters at nerve endings. **Tetracyclic antidepressants** such as mirtazapine (Remeron) are also used to treat depression symptoms.
    4. **Atypical antidepressants.** These are antidepressants that do not fit in the previous categories. **Serotonin-norepinephrine reuptake inhibitors (SNRIs)** are antidepressant drugs that increase the levels of the two neurotransmitters serotonin and norepinephrine in the brain. Examples are venlafaxine (Effexor), desvenlafaxine (Pristiq), and duloxetine (Cymbalta).
- **Anti–obsessive-compulsive disorder (OCD) agents.** These drugs are prescribed to relieve the symptoms of OCD. Tricyclic antidepressants and SSRIs are examples of these agents.
- **Antipsychotics (neuroleptics).** These drugs modify psychotic symptoms and behavior. **Atypical antipsychotics** are the major examples. They are used to treat schizophrenia, bipolar disorder, and other mental illness. They reduce the anxiety, tension, agitation, and aggressiveness associated with psychoses and modify psychotic symptoms such as delusions and hallucinations. Other drugs, such as **phenothiazines** and haloperidol (Haldol), are still used as well. An important potential adverse effect of taking neuroleptic drugs is **tardive dyskinesia (TD);** tardive means late and dyskinesias are abnormal movements. This is a potentially irreversible condition marked by involuntary movements. Early detection is important. The AIMS (abnormal involuntary movement scale) is used to monitor

Category	Class	Drugs
ANTIANXIETY AND ANTIPANIC AGENTS	Benzodiazepines (BZDs)	alprazolam (Xanax) clonazepam (Klonopin) diazepam (Valium) lorazepam (Ativan)
	Selective serotonin reuptake inhibitors (SSRIs)	citalopram (Celexa) escitalopram (Lexapro) paroxetine (Paxil) sertraline (Zoloft)
	Other	buspirone (BuSpar)
ANTIDEPRESSANTS	SSRIs	citalopram (Celexa) escitalopram (Lexapro) fluoxetine (Prozac) paroxetine (Paxil) sertraline (Zoloft)
	Monoamine oxidase (MAO) inhibitors	phenelzine (Nardil) isocarboxazid (Marplan) selegiline (Deprenyl) tranylcypromine (Parnate)
	Tricyclics	amitriptyline (Elavil) imipramine (Tofranil) nortriptyline (Aventyl, Pamelor)
	Atypicals and serotonin-norepinephrine reuptake inhibitors (SNRIs)	bupropion (Wellbutrin) duloxetine (Cymbalta) desvenlafaxine (Pristiq) mirtazapine (Remeron) trazodone (Desyrel) venlafaxine (Effexor)
ANTIOBSESSIVE-COMPULSIVE DISORDER AGENTS	Tricyclic	clomipramine (Anafranil)
	SSRIs	fluvoxamine (Luvox) sertraline (Zoloft)
ANTIPSYCHOTICS (NEUROLEPTICS)	Atypicals	aripiprazole (Abilify) haloperidol (Haldol) olanzapine (Zyprexa) quentiapine (Seroquel) risperidone (Risperdal) ziprasidone (Geodon)
	Phenothiazines	chlorpromazine (Thorazine) thiothixene (Navane)
HYPNOTICS	Sedative	zaleplon (Sonata) zolpidem (Ambien)
	BZDs	lorazepam (Ativan) temazepam (Restoril) triazolam (Halcion)
MOOD STABILIZERS	Antimanic	lithium (Eskalith, Lithane)
	Anticonvulsants	carbamazepine (Tegretol) lamotrigine (Lamictal) topiramate (Topamax) valproate (Depakene, Depakote)
STIMULANTS	Anti-ADHDs	dextroamphetamine (Dexedrine) methylphenidate (Ritalin, Concerta)

FIGURE 22-4 Psychiatric drug categories and specific drugs.

patients for signs of TD. Weight gain and increased risk for developing diabetes also are important side effects of atypical antipsychotics.

- **Hypnotics.** These drugs are used to produce sleep (hypn/o = sleep) and relieve insomnia. Examples are sedatives and benzodiazepines.
- **Mood stabilizers.** These drugs are used primarily to treat patients with the mania-predominant forms of bipolar disease. **Lithium** (Eskalith, Lithane) is commonly used to reduce the levels of manic symptoms, such as rapid speech, hyperactive movements, grandiose ideas, agitation and irritability, and decreased need for sleep. It also is used as an adjunct in the treatment of depression. Lithium is a simple salt that is thought to stabilize nerve membranes. **Anticonvulsant drugs** also are used as mood stabilizers.
- **Stimulants.** These drugs **(amphetamines)** are prescribed for **attention-deficit hyperactivity disorder (ADHD)** in children. Common manifestations of ADHD are a short attention span and easy distractibility, emotional unstability, impulsivity, and moderate to severe hyperactivity.

VOCABULARY

This list reviews many of the new terms introduced in the text. Short definitions reinforce your understanding of the terms. Refer to the Pronunciation of Terms on page 956 for help with unfamiliar or difficult words.

GENERAL TERMINOLOGY, SYMPTOMS, AND DISORDERS	
affect	External expression of emotion, or emotional response.
amnesia	Loss of memory.
anorexia nervosa	Eating disorder with excessive dieting and refusal to maintain a normal body weight.
anxiety disorders	Characterized by unpleasant tension, distress, and avoidance behavior; examples are panic disorder, phobias, obsessive-compulsive disorder, post-traumatic stress disorder, and generalized anxiety disorder.
apathy	Absence of emotions; lack of interest or emotional involvement.
autism	Pervasive developmental disorder characterized by inhibited social interaction and communication and by restricted, repetitive behavior.
bipolar disorder	Mood disorder with alternating periods of mania and depression.
bulimia nervosa	Eating disorder with binge eating followed by vomiting, purging, and depression.
cannabis	Plant substance from which marijuana is obtained.
compulsion	Uncontrollable urge to perform an act repeatedly.
conversion disorder	Condition marked by physical symptoms with no organic basis, appearing as a result of anxiety and unconscious inner conflict.
defense mechanism	Unconscious technique (coping mechanism) used to resolve or conceal conflicts and anxiety. It protects the individual against anxiety and stress; examples are acting out, denial, and repression.
delirium	Confused thinking, disorientation, changes in alertness, difficulty paying attention, and fearfulness. This is usually a reversible impairment in thinking. **Delirium tremens** is associated with alcohol withdrawal.

delusion	Fixed, false belief that cannot be changed by logical reasoning or evidence.
dementia	Loss of intellectual abilities with impairment of memory, judgment, and reasoning as well as changes in personality.
depression	Major mood disorder with chronic sadness, loss of energy, hopelessness, worry, and discouragement and, commonly, suicidal impulses and thoughts.
dissociative disorder	Chronic or sudden disturbance in memory, identity, or consciousness; examples are multiple personality disorder, psychogenic disorders, amnesia, and fugue.
ego	Central coordinating branch of the personality or mind.
fugue	Flight from customary surroundings; dissociative disorder.
gender identity disorder	Strong and persistent cross-gender identification with the opposite sex.
hallucination	False sensory perception (hearing voices and seeing things).
id	Major unconscious part of the personality; energy from instinctual drives and desires.
labile	Unstable; undergoing rapid emotional change.
mania	Extreme excitement, hyperactive elation, and agitation. Don't confuse with the suffix -mania (see page 940), meaning obsession.
mood disorders	Prolonged emotion dominates a person's life; examples are bipolar and depressive disorders.
mutism	Nonreactive state with inability to speak.
obsessive-compulsive disorder	Anxiety disorder in which recurrent thoughts and repetitive acts dominate behavior.
paranoia	Overly suspicious system of thinking with fixed delusions of being harassed, persecuted, or unfairly treated.
paraphilia	Recurrent intense sexual urge, fantasy, or behavior that involves unusual objects, activities, or situations.
personality disorders	Lifelong personality patterns marked by inflexibility and impairment of social functioning.
pervasive developmental disorders	Group of childhood disorders characterized by delays in socialization and communication skills; autism and Asperger syndrome are examples.
phobia	Irrational or disabling fear (avoidance) of an object or situation.
post-traumatic stress disorder	Anxiety-related symptoms appear after personal experience of a traumatic event.
projective (personality) test	Diagnostic personality test using stimuli (inkblots, pictures, abstract patterns, incomplete sentences) to evoke responses that reflect aspects of an individual's personality.
psychiatrist	Physician (MD) with medical training in the diagnosis, prevention, and treatment of mental disorders. Examples are a **child psychiatrist** (diagnosing and treating children) and a **forensic psychiatrist** (specializing in legal considerations such as criminal responsibility, guardianship, and competence to stand trial). Forensic comes from the Latin *forum*, meaning public place.

psychologist	Nonmedical professional (often a PhD or an EdD) specializing in mental processes and how the brain functions in health and disease. Areas of interest are **clinical psychology** (providing testing and counseling services to patients with mental and emotional disorders), **experimental psychology** (performing laboratory tests and experiments in a controlled environment to study mental processes), and **social psychology** (study of the effects of group membership on behavior and attitudes of individuals).
psychosis	A disorder marked by loss of contact with reality often associated with delusions and hallucinations.
reality testing	Psychological process that distinguishes fact from fantasy; severely impaired in psychosis.
repression	Defense mechanism by which unacceptable thoughts, feelings, and impulses are automatically pushed into the unconscious, out of awareness.
schizophrenia	Chronic psychotic disorder that may include hallucinations, disorganized speech and behavior, flat affect, and lack of initiative.
sexual disorders	Paraphilias and sexual dysfunctions.
somatoform disorder	Presence of physical symptoms that cannot be explained by an actual physical disorder or other well-described mental disorder such as depression.
substance-related disorder	Regular overuse of psychoactive substances (alcohol, amphetamines, cannabis, cocaine, hallucinogens, opioids, and sedatives) that affect the central nervous system.
superego	Internalized conscience and moral aspect of the personality.
THERAPY	
amphetamines	Central nervous system stimulants that may be used to treat attention deficit-hyperactivity disorder and depression.
atypical antipsychotics	Drugs that treat psychotic symptoms and behavior (schizophrenia, bipolar disease, and other mental illness).
benzodiazepines	Drugs that lessen anxiety, tension, agitation, and panic attacks.
cognitive behavioral therapy	Focuses on the connection between behavior and thoughts. Conditioning (changing behavior patterns by training and repetition) is used to relieve anxiety and improve symptoms of illness.
electroconvulsive therapy	Electric current is used to produce convulsions and loss of consciousness; effective in the treatment of major depression. Modern techniques use anesthesia, so the convulsion is not observable.
family therapy	Treatment of an entire family to resolve and shed light on conflicts.
free association	Psychoanalytic technique in which the patient verbalizes, without censorship, the passing contents of his or her mind.
group therapy	Group of patients with similar problems gain insight into their personalities through discussion and interaction with each other.
hypnosis	Induced trance (state of altered consciousness).

insight-oriented therapy	Face-to-face discussion of life problems and associated feelings. The patient tells his or her story and has the opportunity to connect emotional patterns in his or her life history with present concerns. Also called psychodynamic therapy.
lithium	Medication used to treat the manic stage of bipolar illness.
neuroleptic drug	Any drug that favorably modifies psychotic symptoms. Examples are phenothiazines such as chlorpromazine (Thorazine).
phenothiazines	Antipsychotic (neuroleptic) drugs.
play therapy	Treatment in which a child, through use of toys in a playroom setting, expresses conflicts and feelings that cannot be communicated in a direct manner.
psychoanalysis	Treatment that allows the patient to explore inner emotions and conflicts so as to understand and change current behavior.
psychodrama	Group therapy in which a patient expresses feelings by acting out family and social roles with other patients.
psychopharmacology	Treatment of psychiatric disorders with drugs.
sedatives	Drugs that lessen anxiety.
supportive psychotherapy	Offering encouragement, support, and hope to patients facing difficult life transitions and events.
transference	Psychoanalytic process in which the patient relates to the therapist as though the therapist were a prominent childhood figure.
tricyclic antidepressants	Drugs used to treat severe depression; three-ringed fused structure.

TERMINOLOGY

Write the meanings of the medical terms in the spaces provided.

COMBINING FORMS

COMBINING FORM	MEANING	TERMINOLOGY	MEANING
anxi/o	uneasy, anxious, distressed	anxiolytic *This type of drug relieves anxiety.*	______________
aut/o	self	autism	______________
hallucin/o	hallucination, to wander in the mind	hallucinogen *A **hallucination** is a sensory perception in the absence of any external stimuli, and an **illusion** is an error in perception in which sensory stimuli are present but incorrectly interpreted.*	______________
hypn/o	sleep	hypnosis *The Greek god of sleep (Hypnos) put people to sleep by touching them with his magic wand or by fanning them with his dark wings.*	______________

COMBINING FORM	MEANING	TERMINOLOGY	MEANING
iatr/o	treatment	psychiatrist	______
		iatrogenic	______
ment/o	mind	mental	______
neur/o	nerve	neurotransmitter *Examples of neurotransmitters are serotonin and norepinephrine.*	______
phil/o	attraction to, love	paraphilia *Para- means abnormal.*	______
phren/o	mind	schizophrenia *Schiz/o means split.*	______
psych/o	mind	psychosis *Loss of contact with reality associated with symptoms such as delusions, hallucinations, and bizarre behavior.*	______
		psychopharmacology	______
		psychotherapy	______
schiz/o	split	schizoid *Used to describe a mild form of schizophrenia or a withdrawn, introverted personality.*	______
somat/o	body	psychosomatic	______
		somatoform disorder *The suffix -form means resembling. Symptoms of these disorders resemble those of actual physical disease, but the origins are in the mind (psychogenic).*	______

22

SUFFIXES

SUFFIX	MEANING	TERMINOLOGY	MEANING
-genic	produced by	psychogenic	______
-leptic	to seize hold of	neuroleptic drug	______
-mania	obsessive preoccupation	kleptomania *Klept/o means to steal.*	______
		pyromania *Pyr/o means fire, heat.*	______
-phobia	fear (irrational and often disabling)	agoraphobia *Agora- means marketplace. Agoraphobics fear leaving home or a safe place.*	______
		xenophobia *Xen/o means stranger. Table 22-2 lists other phobias.*	______

TABLE 22-2 PHOBIAS

Source of Fear/ Anxiety	Medical Term	Source of Fear/ Anxiety	Medical Term
air	aerophobia	**heights**	acrophobia
animals	zoophobia	**insects**	entomophobia
bees	apiphobia, melissophobia	**light**	photophobia
blood or bleeding	hematophobia, hemophobia	**marriage**	gamophobia
books	bibliophobia	**men**	androphobia
cats	ailurophobia	**needles**	belonephobia
corpses	necrophobia	**pain**	algophobia
crossing a bridge	gephyrophobia	**sexual intercourse**	coitophobia, cypridophobia
darkness	nyctophobia, scotophobia	**sleep**	hypnophobia
death	thanatophobia	**snakes**	ophidiophobia
dogs	cynophobia	**spiders**	arachnophobia
drugs	pharmacophobia	**traveling**	hodophobia
eating	phagophobia	**vomiting**	emetophobia
enclosed places	claustrophobia	**women**	gynephobia, gynophobia
hair	trichophobia, trichopathophobia	**worms**	helminthophobia
		writing	graphophobia

SUFFIX	MEANING	TERMINOLOGY	MEANING
-phoria	feeling, bearing	eu<u>phoria</u> *The prefix eu- means good.*	______
		dys<u>phoria</u> *The prefix dys- means bad or unpleasant.*	______
-thymia	mind	cyclo<u>thymia</u> *cycl/o means circle or recurring. Alternating periods of hypomania and depression; lesser intensity than in bipolar disorder.*	______
		dys<u>thymia</u> *Depressed mood that is not as severe as in major depression.*	______
		eu<u>thymic</u> *Feeling well.*	______

PREFIXES

PREFIX	MEANING	TERMINOLOGY	MEANING
a-, an-	no, not	<u>an</u>orexia nervosa *-orexia means appetite.*	______
cata-	down	<u>cata</u>tonia *Ton/o means tension. A state of psychologically induced immobility with muscular rigidity.*	______

22

PREFIX	MEANING	TERMINOLOGY	MEANING
hypo-	deficient, less than, below	hypomania	______
		hypochondriasis *Chondr/o means cartilage. The Greeks believed that the liver and spleen (under the cartilage of the ribs) were the seat of melancholy or sadness.*	______
para-	abnormal	paranoia *The no- in this term comes from the Greek word nous, meaning mind.*	______

ABBREVIATIONS

AD	Alzheimer disease—a form of dementia
ADHD	attention-deficit hyperactivity disorder
ADLs	activities of daily living
AIMS	abnormal involuntary movement scale—used to monitor signs of tardive dyskinesia
ASD	autism spectrum disorder
BZD	benzodiazepine
CA	chronological age
CBT	cognitive behavioral therapy
CNS	central nervous system
DSM-IV-TR	*Diagnostic and Statistical Manual of Mental Disorders, Fourth* edition, *Text Revision*
DT	delirium tremens
ECT	electroconvulsive therapy
GAD	generalized anxiety disorder
IQ	intelligence quotient An IQ test is a standardized test to determine mental age of an individual. The average person is considered to have an IQ of between 90 and 110. Those who score below 70 are considered mentally retarded.
LSD	lysergic acid diethylamide—a hallucinogen
MA	mental age—as determined by psychological tests
MAOI	monoamine oxidase inhibitor; an example is phenelzine (Nardil)
MDD	major depressive disorder
MMPI	Minnesota Multiphasic Personality Inventory
MR	mental retardation
OCD	obsessive-compulsive disorder
PDD	pervasive developmental disorder—includes autism and Asperger syndrome
PTSD	post-traumatic stress disorder
Rx	therapy
SAD	seasonal affective disorder
SNRI	serotonin-norepinephrine reuptake inhibitor; an example is duloxetine (Cymbalta)
SSRI	selective serotonin reuptake inhibitor; an example is fluoxetine (Prozac)
TAT	Thematic Apperception Test
TCA	tricyclic antidepressants
TD	tardive dyskinesia
THC	delta-9-tetrahydrocannabinol—active ingredient in marijuana
WAIS	Wechsler Adult Intelligence Scale
WISC	Wechsler Intelligence Scale for Children
Ψ	symbol for psych-
ΨRx	psychotherapy

22

IN PERSON: LIVING WITH AUTISM

The following feature was written by the mother of a young boy diagnosed with autism.

"What you do from now on will determine whether your son will be able to live on his own as an adult or whether he will have to live in a facility."

I was told this by a physician when my son, Jeff, was diagnosed with autism.

It began early on. For the first year of his life Jeff had difficulty tolerating many situations and often cried. Loud noises such as barking dogs, motorcycles, and the trash truck sent him into a crying frenzy. If he was in a quiet room, in a swing or being held he was comfortable. Most other situations he could only tolerate for 60-90 minutes after which he would cry for 20-30 minutes as if relieving stress. As Jeff aged his tolerance slowly increased but even at four years old overstimulation caused him to cry daily.

Jeff experienced numerous other challenges as well. His ability to play was impaired. If a toy did not light up or play music he was not interested in it. The exception was Matchbox cars, which he did enjoy. However, he did not play with them appropriately. He merely lined them up. Jeff never engaged in imaginative play nor could he carry on a back-and-forth conversation. His speech was rote and he had extreme difficulty communicating and relating to peers.

After visiting several doctors in search of a diagnosis, we were told Jeff was autistic. We also learned that his discomfort and crying were a result of sensory integration challenges that children on the autism spectrum experience. Sensory integration is the process of organizing useful perceptions, emotions and thoughts. When sensory integration is whole and balanced, body movements are highly adaptive and good behavior is a natural outcome. This was not the case with Jeff.

It was difficult to accept the diagnosis, but we had to move on. The next step was finding proper treatment for Jeff. After much consideration we decided on DIR/Floortime Therapy ("Floortime"), supplemented with Occupational Therapy ("OT") to address Jeff's sensory integration needs.

Floortime is a play-based treatment, focusing on helping children master the building blocks of relating, communicating and thinking. Guided interactions between the child and parent, sibling, grandparent or caregiver, move the child through six Floortime developmental stages which are:

1 Self-Regulation and Shared Attention
2 Engagement and Relating
3 Two-way Intentional Communication
4 Purposeful Complex Problem Solving Communication
5 Creating Ideas
6 Logical Reasoning, Thinking Logically

I was taught Floortime by a professional and spent nights watching instructional videos and reading Floortime books. I worked with Jeff each day, including Saturday and Sunday. We did Floortime constantly even during meals, riding in the car and during bath time. I was working for my son's future. The more therapy he received, the better his chances of "recovery." No opportunity was missed.

Each week, over the course of several years, our program leader would assess Jeff's development and determine when he had mastered a skill and when further interventions were needed.

Over several years, Floortime was resolving Jeff's developmental issues, and OT was helping his sensory integration issues, but another problem was becoming more extreme. By first grade, Jeff had developed anxiety that was so irrational and overwhelming that it impaired his school, social and family life. He was very fearful and always thinking about the worst things that could happen. Conversations often would "spin out of control" as Jeff worried irrationally about things that might happen to him. During these times, I would attempt to distract him only to have the anxiety recur.

As time went on Jeff was not only verbalizing his anxiety, but manifested other unconscious behaviors such as eye and verbal tics, chewing on his shirt, and pulling on his hair.

Our team of doctors did not have a specific answer for Jeff's anxiety. We tried numerous treatments including psychotherapy, de-sensitization therapy, applied behavioral therapy, occupational body regulating therapy, and cognitive behavioral therapy. None had much effect on reducing anxiety.

Finally, one of our doctors suggested a study at a nearby university which was funded by the National Institute of Mental Health. The program was specifically designed for children on the autism spectrum suffering from very high anxiety. It was a treatment protocol based on a collaborative, family-based intervention approach using targeted cognitive behavioral therapy techniques. It took into consideration Jeff's spectrum-based deficits and taught him how his anxiety could be managed by using a coping plan and actively facing his fears. The program lasted nearly a year. But we used it regularly for months after it ended. It made a noticeable positive impact on Jeff's anxiety.

By his fourth grade year Jeff's physical size of 5'0" and 80 pounds allowed our child psychiatrist to prescribe anxiety medication. This made a noticeable positive impact on his anxiety.

Today Jeff is in a mainstream fifth grade classroom at a public elementary school. He is able to relate to others with real warmth. He has many friends, a great imagination and a mischievous sense of humor. His anxiety has decreased to the point that it does not drastically interfere with his life. It continues to lessen each month.

Through it all, my family and I have learned that with the proper therapies and treatments, we can define an autistic child's potential not by assumed limitations, but by their own growth.

PRACTICAL APPLICATIONS

CASE REPORTS

CASE REPORT 1: MAJOR DEPRESSION

Mrs. Carr, a 58-year-old widow, was brought to an emergency department by her daughter, who found her at home in bed in the middle of the day. For a period of months, Mrs. Carr had become increasingly withdrawn and dysphoric, without any precipitating events. She had become progressively less active and even required encouragement to eat and perform her daily tasks. Her daughter and son-in-law became alarmed but did not know what to do. Mrs. Carr's medical history was unremarkable, but her psychiatric history revealed an episode of postpartum depression following the birth of one of her children.

On examination, the ER physician noted that Mrs. Carr was withdrawn and negativistic, refusing to cooperate with the examination, and even refusing to open her mouth. There were signs of acute dehydration and decline in personal hygiene and grooming.

Further questioning of her daughter revealed that Mrs. Carr had become increasingly paranoid and had delusions of sinfulness and guilt. Recently, she had shown signs of increasing mutism.

The physician recognized signs of major depression and arranged for immediate hospitalization. Mrs. Carr responded favorably to combined use of an antipsychotic and an antidepressant drug. An alternative treatment would have been a course of electroconvulsive therapy, which also produces favorable results.

CASE REPORT 2: SOMATOFORM DISORDER

A 35-year-old man presented with a 6-year history of abdominal pain that he was convinced was cancer. For most of his life, the patient had been dominated by a tyrannical father who never gave him the love he craved. When the patient was 29, his father died of carcinoma of the colon, and soon afterward, the patient developed abdominal pain. His complaints gradually increased as his identification with his father, as well as his unconscious hostility toward him, increased. The patient came to the clinic almost daily with complaints of bloody stools (the feces were found to be free of blood) and the belief that he had cancer. He felt that none of the clinic doctors listened to him, just as his father had not.

Treatment included development of a long-standing, trusting, positive relationship with one of the clinic physicians, who allowed the patient time to talk about the illness. His hypochondriasis gradually subsided during a 12-month period of a supportive physician-patient relationship.

CASE REPORT 3: BIPOLAR DISORDER

A 30-year-old woman first presented with depression at age 26. Her depression was characterized by sadness lasting most of the day, crying spells, severe irritability, hypersomnia with some periods of insomnia, anergia (low energy), severe inappropriate guilt feelings, and absence of libido (sex drive). The patient described periods of high energy when her "mind ran away," and her mood was irritable with a decreased need for sleep. Initially, she stated that these times would last 1 or 2 days at the most. Her family would avoid confrontations with her during those periods of energy and activity. The patient was initially diagnosed as suffering from dysthymic disorder with major depression. A bipolar illness was suspected based on her 1- or 2-day bursts of energy and activity. History from family members confirmed that she had experienced expanded mood states lasting up to a week that met the DSM-IV-TR criteria for hypomanic episodes. Her diagnosis was changed to bipolar II disorder. She was placed on a regimen of bupropion (Wellbutrin), and the dose was increased to 300 mg/day. Her mood improved in a general way with less irritability, more energy, and less sadness. She continued to have rather pronounced premenstrual worsening of her mood, however, that did not respond to an increase in the dose of bupropion. In the meantime, her physician added lithium to her medical regimen of fluoxetine (Prozac) with robust and stable augmentation. Lithium improved the quality of the patient's response to the bupropion by eliminating the premenstrual worsening of mood and fully normalizing her sleep pattern. Lithium was then replaced with valproate (Depakote) and the dose titrated to 1000 mg/day. Her robust, stable antidepressant response returned without side effects beyond mild weight gain, for which regular exercise was prescribed.

CASE REPORT 4: SCHIZOPHRENIA

Mike is a 33-year-old divorced man with two children ages 8 and 10, he rarely ever sees. He has never been evaluated by a psychiatrist. His family physician has tried to get him to see a local psychiatrist, but Mike refuses to go. Mike says he knows someone has removed his brain and replaced it with someone else's. He believes that this brain is controlling him and that he is not responsible for his actions. He works every day and has been on his current job for 15 years. He says he has lots of friends but sometimes he thinks it's one of them who did this to him. He reports incidents in which he has been injected with something while shopping and speaks of a government conspiracy to kill him. He has a college education and has a degree in computer science. His family physician ordered an MRI study, which showed negative findings, and he also had an EEG. The EEG results came back normal.

EXERCISES

Remember to check your answers carefully with the Answers to Exercises, page 952.

A Give the terms for the following definitions.

1. physician specializing in treating mental illness ______________________
2. nonphysician professionals trained in the treatment of mental illness ______________________
3. therapist who practices psychoanalysis ______________________
4. branch of psychiatry dealing with legal matters ______________________
5. unconscious part of the personality ______________________
6. conscious, coordinating part of the personality ______________________
7. conscience or moral part of the personality ______________________
8. psychological process used to distinguish fact from fantasy testing ______________________
9. unconscious technique used to resolve or conceal conflicts and anxiety ______________________ mechanism.
10. branch of psychology dealing with patient care ______________________

22

B Match each of the following psychiatric symptoms with its best meaning from the list below.

amnesia	conversion	mania
anxiety	delusion	mutism
apathy	dissociation	obsession
compulsion	hallucination	

1. nonreactive state marked by inability to speak ______________________
2. state of excessive excitability; agitation ______________________
3. loss of memory ______________________
4. uncontrollable urge to perform an act repeatedly ______________________
5. persistent idea, emotion, or urge ______________________
6. feelings of apprehension, uneasiness, dread ______________________
7. uncomfortable feelings are separated from their real object and redirected toward a second object or behavior pattern ______________________
8. anxiety becomes a bodily symptom that has no organic basis ______________________
9. absence of emotions; lack of motivation or emotional involvement ______________________
10. fixed false belief that cannot be changed by logical reasoning or evidence ______________________
11. false or unreal sensory perception ______________________

C Give the meanings of the following terms.

1. dysphoria ____________________
2. euphoria ____________________
3. amnesia ____________________
4. paranoia ____________________
5. psychosis ____________________
6. iatrogenic ____________________
7. phobia ____________________
8. agoraphobia ____________________
9. labile ____________________
10. affect ____________________

D Select from the following terms to complete the sentences below.

anxiety disorder	eating disorder	sexual disorder
delirium	mood disorder	somatoform disorder
dementia	personality disorder	substance-related disorder
dissociative disorder		

1. Disturbance of memory and identity that hides the anxiety of unconscious conflicts is ____________________.
2. Troubled feelings, unpleasant tension, distress, and avoidance behavior describe a/an ____________________.
3. An illness related to regular use of drugs and alcohol is a/an ____________________.
4. Bulimia nervosa is an example of a/an ____________________.
5. A disorder involving paraphilias is a/an ____________________.
6. An illness marked by prolonged emotions (mania and depression) is a/an ____________________.
7. A mental disorder in which physical symptoms cannot be explained by an actual physical disorder is a/an ____________________.
8. A lifelong personality pattern that is inflexible and causes distress, conflict, and impairment of social functioning is a/an ____________________.
9. Loss of intellectual abilities with impairment of memory, judgment, and reasoning is ____________________.
10. Confusion in thinking with faulty perceptions and irrational behavior is ____________________.

E **Give the meanings of the following terms.**

1. obsessive-compulsive disorder ______________________
2. post-traumatic stress disorder ______________________
3. bipolar disorder ______________________
4. fugue ______________________
5. paranoia ______________________
6. amphetamines ______________________
7. cannabis ______________________
8. schizophrenia ______________________
9. sexual sadism ______________________
10. hypochondriasis ______________________

F **Match the general psychiatric disorder in Column I with an association in Column II. Write the letter of the answer in the space provided.**

COLUMN I

1. somatoform disorder ______
2. sexual disorder ______
3. anxiety disorder ______
4. mood disorder ______
5. substance-related disorder ______
6. schizophrenia ______
7. dissociative disorder ______
8. personality disorder ______
9. pervasive developmental disorder ______

COLUMN II

A. conversion disorder
B. cocaine abuse
C. phobia
D. positive and negative symptoms
E. pedophilia
F. autism
G. bipolar I and II
H. narcissism
I. fugue

G **Give the meanings of the following terms.**

1. anorexia nervosa ______________________
2. bulimia nervosa ______________________
3. repression ______________________
4. dementia ______________________
5. hypomania ______________________
6. hallucinogen ______________________
7. opioids ______________________
8. cocaine ______________________
9. cyclothymic disorder ______________________
10. dysthymia ______________________

H Identify the personality disorder based on its description as given.

1. flamboyant, theatrical, emotionally immature ______________________
2. no loyalty or concern for others; does not tolerate frustration and blames others when he or she is at fault ______________________
3. fantasies of success and power and a grandiose sense of self-importance ______________________
4. pervasive, unwarranted suspiciousness and mistrust of people ______________________
5. emotionally cold, aloof, indifferent to praise or criticism or to the feelings of others ______________________
6. instability in personal relationships and sense of self; alternating overinvolvement with and rejection of people ______________________

I Identify the psychotherapeutic technique based on its description as given below.

1. Patients express feelings by acting out roles with other patients ______________________
2. A trance helps patients recover deeply repressed feelings ______________________
3. Long-term and intense exploration of unconscious feelings uses techniques such as transference and free association ______________________
4. Toys help a child express conflicts and feelings ______________________
5. Conditioning changes actual behavior patterns rather than focusing on subconscious thoughts and feelings ______________________
6. Techniques help patients overcome sexual dysfunctions ______________________
7. Electrical current is applied to the brain to reverse major depression ______________________
8. Agents (chemicals) relieve symptoms of psychiatric disorders ______________________
9. Face-to-face discussion of life's problems and associated feelings ______________________
10. offering encouragement, support, and hope to patients facing difficult life transitions and events ______________________

J Match the following terms with their meanings below.

agoraphobia
amphetamines
benzodiazepines
cyclothymia
dysthymia
kleptomania
lithium
MAO inhibitors
phenothiazines
pyromania
tricyclic and tetracyclic antidepressants
xenophobia

1. Fear of strangers is ______________________.
2. Obsessive preoccupation with stealing is ______________________.
3. Antidepressant agents that work by blocking the action of a specific enzyme are ______________________.
4. Mood disorder marked by depressive periods milder than major depression is ______________________.
5. Antipsychotic (neuroleptic) tranquilizers such as Thorazine are ______________________.
6. Fear of being left alone in unfamiliar surroundings is ______________________.
7. Stimulants used as therapy for mood disorders or for treatment of children with attention-deficit hyperactivity disorder are ______________________.
8. Mild form of bipolar disorder in which hypomanic episodes alternate with depression is ______________________.
9. Obsessive preoccupation with fire is ______________________.
10. Drugs (containing three fused rings) used to elevate mood and increase physical activity and mental alertness are ______________________.
11. Anxiolytic agents that lessen the anxiety associated with panic attacks are ______________________.
12. Drug that treats the manic episodes of bipolar disorder is ______________________.

22

K Give the meanings of the following word parts.

1. phren/o ______________________
2. hypn/o ______________________
3. somat/o ______________________
4. phil/o ______________________
5. iatr/o ______________________
6. schiz/o ______________________
7. -mania ______________________
8. -phobia ______________________
9. -thymia ______________________
10. -tropic ______________________
11. -genic ______________________
12. para- ______________________
13. hypo- ______________________
14. cata- ______________________

L **Match the following psychiatric drugs with their type and the conditions they treat (consult Figure 22-4 on page 935).**

alprazolam (Xanax)
amitriptyline (Elavil)
aripiprazole (Abilify)
escitalopram (Lexapro)
lamotrigine (Lamictal)
methylphenidate (Ritalin, Concerta)
thiothixene (Navane)
zolpidem (Ambien)

1. SSRI; treats anxiety and depression ______________________
2. atypical antipsychotic; treats schizophrenia and bipolar disorder ______________________
3. stimulant; treats attention-deficit hyperactivity disorder ______________________
4. tricyclic antidepressant; treats depression ______________________
5. benzodiazepine; treats anxiety and panic attacks ______________________
6. sedative; treats insomnia ______________________
7. anticonvulsant; treats mood disorders (such as bipolar illness) ______________________
8. phenothiazine; treats schizophrenia ______________________

M **Circle the term that best completes the meaning of the sentence.**

1. Robin fluctuated between bouts of depression and mania and finally was diagnosed as having a (**xenophobic, histrionic, bipolar**) disorder.
2. Although the root of Jon's problems could hardly be addressed simply with medication, his personality disorder and his depression were treated with a selective serotonin reuptake inhibitor (SSRI) called (**lithium, Prozac, Valium**).
3. Hillary had an enormous fear of open-air markets, shopping malls, and stadiums. She was diagnosed as having (**agoraphobia, xenophobia, pyromania**).
4. When Sam was admitted to the hospital after his automobile accident, his physicians were told of his alcoholism. They needed to know Sam's history so that they could prevent (**dementia, dysthymia, delirium tremens**).
5. Hanna was afraid of everyone she met. She had the (**paranoid, narcissistic, schizoid**) delusion that everyone was out to get her.
6. Bill was told that an important potential side effect of taking neuroleptic drugs such as phenothiazines was (**amnesia, gender identity disorder, tardive dyskinesia**).
7. Ever since she was trapped in an elevator for 3 hours, Lil experienced a (**social phobia, panic attack, somatoform disorder**) marked by palpitations, sweating, and trembling when she was unable to get out of an enclosed space.
8. The few survivors of the nightclub fire were diagnosed with (**OCD, dissociative fugue, post-traumatic stress disorder**). They regularly experienced insomnia, nightmares, and feelings of helplessness.

9. Sarah couldn't stop herself from eating a gallon of ice cream and box of cookies every evening. She would then feel very anxious and guilty about overeating and induce vomiting. Her mother took her to a/an (**endocrinologist, psychiatrist, gastroenterologist**), who diagnosed her condition as (**anorexia nervosa, hypochondriasis, bulimia nervosa**) and prescribed (**sex therapy, ECT, psychotherapy**).
10. Bill felt depressed during the months of November through February. In March his (**OCD, ADHD, SAD**) changed and his mood was characterized by (**hypomania, dysphoria, paranoia**).

ANSWERS TO EXERCISES

A

1. psychiatrist
2. psychologist, psychiatric nurse, licensed clinical social worker
3. psychoanalyst
4. forensic psychiatry
5. id
6. ego
7. superego
8. reality
9. defense
10. clinical

B

1. mutism
2. mania
3. amnesia
4. compulsion
5. obsession
6. anxiety
7. dissociation
8. conversion
9. apathy
10. delusion
11. hallucination

C

1. sadness, hopelessness, unpleasant feeling
2. exaggerated feeling of well-being ("high")
3. loss of memory
4. suspicious system of thinking; fixed delusion that one is being treated unfairly or harassed
5. loss of contact with reality; often delusions and hallucinations
6. pertaining to a disorder caused by a treatment
7. irrational fear (avoidance) of an object or a situation
8. fear of leaving one's home or a safe place
9. unstable; undergoing rapid emotional change; fluctuating
10. expression of emotion

D

1. dissociative disorder
2. anxiety disorder
3. substance-related disorder
4. eating disorder
5. sexual disorder
6. mood disorder
7. somatoform disorder
8. personality disorder
9. dementia
10. delirium

E

1. recurrent thoughts and repetitive acts that dominate a person's behavior
2. anxiety-related symptoms appear after exposure to personal experience of a traumatic event
3. alternating periods of mania and depression
4. amnesia with flight from customary surroundings
5. delusions of persecution or grandeur
6. CNS stimulants
7. marijuana, hashish; active substance in marijuana; THC
8. psychosis marked by a split from reality; disorganized thinking and behavior
9. achievement of sexual gratification by inflicting physical or psychological pain
10. preoccupation with bodily aches, pains, and discomforts (in the absence of real illness)

F

1. A
2. E
3. C
4. G
5. B
6. D
7. I
8. H
9. F

22

G

1. eating disorder marked by excessive dieting because of emotional factors
2. eating disorder characterized by binge eating followed by vomiting, purging, and depression
3. a defense mechanism by which unacceptable thoughts, feelings, and impulses are pushed into the unconscious
4. loss of higher mental functioning, memory, judgment, and reasoning
5. mood disorder resembling mania (exaggerated excitement, hyperactivity) but of lesser intensity
6. drug that produces hallucinations (false sensory perceptions)
7. drugs that are derived from opium (morphine and heroin)
8. stimulant drug that causes euphoria and hallucinations
9. alternating periods of hypomania and depressive episodes of lesser intensity than with bipolar illness
10. depressed mood persisting over a 2-year period but not as severe as a major depression

H

1. histrionic
2. antisocial
3. narcissistic
4. paranoid
5. schizoid
6. borderline

I

1. psychodrama
2. hypnosis
3. psychoanalysis
4. play therapy
5. behavioral therapy
6. sexual therapy
7. electroconvulsive therapy
8. psychopharmacology, or drug therapy
9. insight-oriented psychotherapy
10. supportive psychotherapy

J

1. xenophobia
2. kleptomania
3. MAO inhibitors
4. dysthymia
5. phenothiazines
6. agoraphobia
7. amphetamines
8. cyclothymia
9. pyromania
10. tricyclic and tetracyclic antidepressants
11. benzodiazepines
12. lithium

K

1. mind
2. sleep
3. body
4. love, attraction to
5. treatment
6. split
7. obsessive preoccupation
8. fear
9. mind; mood
10. to influence, turn
11. produced by
12. abnormal
13. deficient, less than, below
14. down

L

1. escitalopram (Lexapro)
2. aripiprazole (Abilify)
3. methylphenidate (Ritalin, Concerta)
4. amitriptyline (Elavil)
5. alprazolam (Xanax)
6. zolpidem (Ambien)
7. lamotrigine (Lamictal)
8. thiothixene (Navane)

M

1. bipolar
2. Prozac
3. agoraphobia
4. delirium tremens
5. paranoid
6. tardive dyskinesia
7. panic attack
8. post-traumatic stress disorder
9. psychiatrist; bulimia nervosa; psychotherapy
10. SAD; hypomania

PRONUNCIATION OF TERMS

To test your understanding of the terminology in this chapter, write the meaning of each term in the space provided. In addition, you may wish to cover the terms and write them by looking at your definitions. Make sure your spelling is correct. The page number after each term indicates where it is defined or used in the book, so you can easily check your responses. You will find complete definitions for all of these terms and their audio pronunciations on the Evolve website.

Pronunciation Guide

ā as in āpe	ă as in ăpple
ē as in ēven	ĕ as in ĕvery
ī as in īce	ĭ as in ĭnterest
ō as in ōpen	ŏ as in pŏt
ū as in ūnit	ŭ as in ŭnder

TERM	PRONUNCIATION	MEANING
affect (936)	ĂF-fĕkt	
agoraphobia (940)	ăg-ŏ-ră-FŌ-bē-ă	
amnesia (936)	ăm-NĒ-zē-ă	
amphetamines (938)	ăm-FĔT-ă-mēnz	
anorexia nervosa (936)	ăn-ō-RĔK-sē-ă nĕr-VŌ-să	
antisocial personality (928)	ăn-tē-SŌ-shăl pĕr-sŏ-NĂL-ĭ-tē	
anxiety disorders (936)	ăng-ZĪ-ĕ-tē dĭs-ŎR-dĕrz	
anxiolytic (939)	ăng-zī-ō-LĬT-ik	
apathy (936)	ĂP-ă-thē	
Asperger syndrome (928)	ĂS-pĕr-gĕr SĬN-drōm	
atypical antipsychotics (938)	ā-TĬP-ĭ-kăl ăn-tĭ-sī-KŎT-ĭks	
autism (936)	AW-tĭzm	
benzodiazepines (938)	bĕn-zō-dī-ĂZ-ĕ-pēnz	
bipolar disorder (936)	bī-PŌ-lăr dĭs-ŎR-dĕr	
borderline personality (928)	BŎR-dĕr-līn pĕr-sŏ-NĂL-ĭ-tē	
bulimia nervosa (936)	bū-LĒ-mē-ă nĕr-VŌ-să	
cannabis (936)	KĂ-nă-bis	
catatonia (941)	kăt-ă-TŌN-ē-ă	
claustrophobia (925)	klaws-trō-FŌ-bē-ă	
cognitive behavioral therapy (938)	KŎG-nĭ-tĭv bē-HĀV-yŏr-ăl THĔR-ă-pē	
compulsion (923)	kŏm-PŬL-shŭn	
conversion disorder (936)	kŏn-VĔR-zhŭn dĭs-ŎR-dĕr	

22

TERM	PRONUNCIATION	MEANING
cyclothymia (941)	sī-klō-THĪ-mē-ă	______
defense mechanism (936)	dē-FĔNS mĕ-kăn-NĬZM	______
delirium (936)	dĕ-LĬR-ē-ŭm	______
delirium tremens (926)	dĕ-LĬR-ē-ŭm TRĔ-mĕnz	______
delusion (937)	dĕ-LOO-zhŭn	______
dementia (937)	dē-MĔN-shē-ă	______
depression (927)	dē-PRĔ-shŭn	______
dissociative disorder (937)	dĭs-SŌ-shē-ă-tĭv dĭs-ŎR-der	______
dysphoria (941)	dĭs-FŎR-ē-ă	______
dysthymia (941)	dĭs-THĪ-mē-ă	______
ego (937)	Ē-gō	______
electroconvulsive therapy (938)	ē-lĕk-trō-kŏn-VŬL-sĭv THĔR-ă-pē	______
euphoria (941)	ū-FŎR-ē-ă	______
euthymic (941)	ū-THĪ-mĭk	______
exhibitionism (929)	ĕk-sĭ-BĬSH-ŭ-nĭzm	______
family therapy (938)	FĂM-ĭ-lē THĔR-ă-pē	______
fetishism (929)	FĔT-ĭsh-ĭzm	______
free association (938)	frē ă-sō-shē-Ā-shŭn	______
fugue (937)	fūg	______
gender identity disorder (937)	GĔN-dĕr ī-DĔN-tĭ-tē dĭs-ŎR-dĕr	______
group therapy (938)	groop THĔR-ă-pē	______
hallucination (937)	hă-loo-sĭ-NĀ-shŭn	______
hallucinogen (939)	hă-LOO-sĭ-nō-jĕn	______
histrionic personality (928)	hĭs-trē-ŎN-ĭk pĕr-sŏn-ĂL-ĭ-tē	______
hypnosis (938)	hĭp-NŌ-sĭs	______
hypochondriasis (942)	hī-pō-kŏn-DRĪ-ă-sĭs	______
hypomania (942)	hī-pō-MĀ-nē-ă	______
iatrogenic (940)	ī-ă-trō-JĔN-ĭk	______
id (937)	ĭd	______

TERM	PRONUNCIATION	MEANING
insight-oriented therapy (939)	ĬN-sīt ŎR-ē-ĕn-tĕd THĔR-ă-pē	
kleptomania (940)	klĕp-tō-MĀ-nē-ă	
labile (937)	LĀ-bĭl	
lithium (939)	LĬTH-ē-ŭm	
mania (937)	MĀ-nē-ă	
mental (940)	MĔN-tăl	
mood disorders (937)	mood dĭs-ŎR-dĕrz	
mutism (937)	MŪ-tĭzm	
narcissistic personality (928)	năr-sĭ-SĬS-tĭk pĕr-sŏ-NĂL-ĭ-tē	
neuroleptic drug (940)	nōō-rō-LĔP-tĭk drŭg	
neurotransmitter (940)	nōō-rō-TRĂNZ-mĭt-ĕr	
obsession (924)	ŏb-SĔSH-ŭn	
obsessive-compulsive disorder (937)	ŏb-SĔS-ĭv cŏm-PŬL-sĭv dĭs-ŎR-dĕr	
opioids (931)	Ō-pē-ŏydz	
paranoia (937)	păr-ă-NŎY-ă	
paranoid personality (928)	PĂR-ă-nŏyd pĕr-sŏ-NĂL-ĭ-tē	
paraphilia (937)	păr-ă-FĬL-ē-ă	
pedophilia (929)	pē-dō-FĬL-ē-ă	
personality disorders (937)	pĕr-sŏ-NĂL-ĭ-tē dĭs-ŎR-dĕrz	
pervasive developmental disorders (937)	pĕr-VĀS-ĭv dĕ-VĔL-ŏp-mĕnt-ăl dĭs-ŎR-dĕrz	
phenothiazines (939)	fē-nō-THĪ-ă-zēnz	
phobia (937)	FŌ-bē-ă	
play therapy (939)	plā THĔR-ă-pē	
post-traumatic stress disorder (937)	pōst-traw-MĂT-ĭk strĕs dĭs-ŎR-dĕr	
projective test (937)	prō-JĔK-tĭv tĕst	
psychiatrist (937)	sī-KĪ-ă-trĭst	
psychiatry (922)	sī-KĪ-ă-trē	
psychoanalysis (939)	sī-kō-ă-NĂL-ĭ-sĭs	
psychodrama (939)	sī-kō-DRĂ-mă	

TERM	PRONUNCIATION	MEANING
psychogenic (940)	sī-kō-JĔN-ĭk	____________
psychologist (938)	sī-KŎL-ō-jĭst	____________
psychopharmacology (940)	sī-kō-făr-mă-KŎL-ō-jē	____________
psychosis (940)	sī-KŌ-sĭs	____________
psychosomatic (940)	sī-kō-sō-MĂT-ĭk	____________
psychotherapy (940)	sī-kō-THĔR-ă-pē	____________
pyromania (940)	pī-rō-MĀ-nē-ă	____________
reality testing (938)	rē-ĂL-ĭ-tē TĔS-tĭng	____________
repression (938)	rē-PRĔ-shŭn	____________
schizoid personality (928)	SKĬZ-ŏyd *or* SKĬT-sŏyd pĕr-sŏ-NĂL-ĭ-tē	____________
schizophrenia (938)	skĭz-ō-FRĔ-nē-ă	____________
sedatives (939)	SĔD-ă-tĭvz	____________
sexual disorders (938)	SĔX-ū-ăl dĭs-ŎR-dĕrz	____________
sexual masochism (929)	SĔX-ū-ăl MĂS-ō-kĭzm	____________
sexual sadism (929)	SĔX-ŭ-ăl SĀ-dĭzm	____________
somatoform disorders (938)	sō-MĂT-ō-fŏrm dĭs-ŎR-dĕrz	____________
substance-related disorder (938)	SŬB-stăns rē-LĀ-tĕd dĭs-ŎR-dĕr	____________
superego (938)	sū-pĕr-Ē-gō	____________
supportive psychotherapy (939)	sū-PŎR-tĭv sī-kō-THĔR-ă-pē	____________
tolerance (930)	TŎL-ĕr-ăns	____________
transference (939)	trăns-FŬR-ĕns	____________
transvestic fetishism (929)	trăns-VĔS-tĭk FĔT-ĭsh-ĭzm	____________
tricyclic antidepressants (939)	trī-SĬK-lĭk ăn-tĭ-dĕ-PRĔ-săntz	____________
voyeurism (929)	VŎY-yĕr-ĭzm	____________
xenophobia (940)	zĕn-ō-FŌ-bē-ă	____________

REVIEW SHEET

Write the meanings of the word parts in the spaces provided, and test yourself. Check your answers with the information in the chapter or in the Glossary (Medical Word Parts—English) at the end of the book.

Combining Forms

COMBINING FORM	MEANING	COMBINING FORM	MEANING
anxi/o	________________	phil/o	________________
aut/o	________________	phren/o	________________
cycl/o	________________	psych/o	________________
hallucin/o	________________	pyr/o	________________
hypn/o	________________	schiz/o	________________
iatr/o	________________	somat/o	________________
klept/o	________________	ton/o	________________
ment/o	________________	xen/o	________________
neur/o	________________		

Suffixes

SUFFIX	MEANING	SUFFIX	MEANING
-form	________________	-pathy	________________
-genic	________________	-phobia	________________
-kinesia	________________	-phoria	________________
-leptic	________________	-somnia	________________
-mania	________________	-thymia	________________
-oid	________________	-tropic	________________

Prefixes

PREFIX	MEANING	PREFIX	MEANING
a-, an-	________________	eu-	________________
agora-	________________	hypo-	________________
cata-	________________	para-	________________
dys-	________________		

evolve *Please refer to the Evolve website for additional exercises, games, and images related to this chapter.*

GLOSSARY

MEDICAL WORD PARTS—ENGLISH*

Combining Form, Suffix, or Prefix	Meaning
a-, an-	no; not; without
ab-	away from
abdomin/o	abdomen
-ac	pertaining to
acanth/o	spiny; thorny
acetabul/o	acetabulum (hip socket)
acous/o	hearing
acr/o	extremities; top; extreme point
acromi/o	acromion (extension of shoulder bone)
actin/o	light
acu/o	sharp; severe; sudden
-acusis	hearing
ad-	toward
-ad	toward
aden/o	gland
adenoid/o	adenoids
adip/o	fat
adren/o	adrenal gland
adrenal/o	adrenal gland
aer/o	air
af-	toward
agglutin/o	clumping; sticking together
-agon	assemble, gather
agora-	marketplace
-agra	excessive pain
-al	pertaining to
alb/o	white
albin/o	white
albumin/o	albumin (protein)
alges/o	sensitivity to pain
-algesia	sensitivity to pain
-algia	pain
all/o	other
alveol/o	alveolus; air sac; small sac
ambly/o	dim; dull
-amine	nitrogen compound
amni/o	amnion (sac surrounding the embryo)
amyl/o	starch
an/o	anus
-an	pertaining to
ana-	up; apart; backward; again, anew
andr/o	male
aneurysm/o	aneurysm (widened blood vessel)
angi/o	vessel (blood)
anis/o	unequal
ankyl/o	stiff
ante-	before; forward
anter/o	front
anthrac/o	coal
anthr/o	antrum of the stomach
anti-	against
anxi/o	uneasy; anxious
aort/o	aorta (largest artery)
-apheresis	removal
aphth/o	ulcer
apo-	off, away
aponeur/o	aponeurosis (type of tendon)
append/o	appendix
appendic/o	appendix
aque/o	water
-ar	pertaining to
-arche	beginning
arter/o	artery
arteri/o	artery
arteriol/o	arteriole (small artery)
arthr/o	joint
-arthria	articulate (speak distinctly)
articul/o	joint

*Page references for all word parts are listed in the index.

Combining Form, Suffix, or Prefix	Meaning
-ary	pertaining to
asbest/o	asbestos
-ase	enzyme
-asthenia	lack of strength
atel/o	incomplete
ather/o	plaque (fatty substance)
-ation	process; condition
atri/o	atrium (upper heart chamber)
audi/o	hearing
audit/o	hearing
aur/o	ear
auricul/o	ear
aut/o	self, own
aut-, auto-	self, own
axill/o	armpit
azot/o	urea; nitrogen
bacill/o	bacilli (bacteria)
bacteri/o	bacteria
balan/o	glans penis
bar/o	pressure; weight
bartholin/o	Bartholin glands
bas/o	base; opposite of acid
bi-	two
bi/o	life
bil/i	bile; gall
bilirubin/o	bilirubin
-blast	embryonic; immature cell
-blastoma	immature tumor (cells)
blephar/o	eyelid
bol/o	cast; throw
brachi/o	arm
brachy-	short
brady-	slow
bronch/o	bronchial tube
bronchi/o	bronchial tube
bronchiol/o	bronchiole
bucc/o	cheek
bunion/o	bunion
burs/o	bursa (sac of fluid near joints)
byssin/o	cotton dust
cac/o	bad
calc/o	calcium
calcane/o	calcaneus (heel bone)
calci/o	calcium
cali/o, calic/o	calyx (cup shaped)
capillar/o	capillary (tiniest blood vessel)
capn/o	carbon dioxide
-capnia	carbon dioxide
carcin/o	cancerous; cancer
cardi/o	heart
carp/o	wrist bones (carpals)
cata-	down
caud/o	tail; lower part of body

Combining Form, Suffix, or Prefix	Meaning
caus/o	burn; burning
cauter/o	heat; burn
cec/o	cecum (first part of the colon)
-cele	hernia
celi/o	belly; abdomen
-centesis	surgical puncture to remove fluid
cephal/o	head
cerebell/o	cerebellum (posterior part of the brain)
cerebr/o	cerebrum (largest part of the brain)
cerumin/o	cerumen
cervic/o	neck; cervix (neck of uterus)
-chalasia	relaxation
-chalasis	relaxation
cheil/o	lip
chem/o	drug; chemical
-chezia	defecation; elimination of wastes
chir/o	hand
chlor/o	green
chlorhydr/o	hydrochloric acid
chol/e	bile; gall
cholangi/o	bile vessel
cholecyst/o	gallbladder
choledoch/o	common bile duct
cholesterol/o	cholesterol
chondr/o	cartilage
chore/o	dance
chori/o	chorion (outermost membrane of the fetus)
chorion/o	chorion
choroid/o	choroid layer of eye
chrom/o	color
chron/o	time
chym/o	to pour
cib/o	meal
-cide	killing
-cidal	pertaining to killing
cine/o	movement
cirrh/o	orange-yellow
cis/o	to cut
-clasis	to break
-clast	to break
claustr/o	enclosed space
clavicul/o	clavicle (collar bone)
-clysis	irrigation; washing
coagul/o	coagulation (clotting)
-coccus (-cocci, *pl.*)	berry-shaped bacterium
coccyg/o	coccyx (tailbone)
cochle/o	cochlea (inner part of ear)
col/o	colon
coll/a	glue
colon/o	colon (large intestine)

Combining Form, Suffix, or Prefix	Meaning
colp/o	vagina
comat/o	deep sleep
comi/o	to care for
con-	together, with
coni/o	dust
conjunctiv/o	conjunctiva (lines the eyelids)
-constriction	narrowing
contra-	against; opposite
cor/o	pupil
core/o	pupil
corne/o	cornea
coron/o	heart (crown or circle)
corpor/o	body
cortic/o	cortex, outer region
cost/o	rib
crani/o	skull
cras/o	mixture; temperament
crin/o	secrete
-crine	secrete; separate
-crit	separate
cry/o	cold
crypt/o	hidden
culd/o	cul-de-sac
-cusis	hearing
cutane/o	skin
cyan/o	blue
cycl/o	ciliary body of eye; cycle; circle
-cyesis	pregnancy
cyst/o	urinary bladder; cyst; sac of fluid
cyt/o	cell
-cyte	cell
-cytosis	condition of cells; slight increase in numbers
dacry/o	tear
dacryoaden/o	tear gland
dacryocyst/o	tear sac; lacrimal sac
dactyl/o	fingers; toes
de-	lack of; down; less; removal of
dem/o	people
dent/i	tooth; teeth
derm/o	skin
-derma	skin
dermat/o	skin
desicc/o	drying
-desis	bind, tie together
dia-	complete; through
diaphor/o	sweat
-dilation	widening; stretching; expanding
dipl/o	double
dips/o	thirst
dist/o	far; distant
dors/o	back (of body)
dorsi-	back
-dote	to give
-drome	to run
duct/o	to lead, carry
duoden/o	duodenum
dur/o	dura mater
-dynia	pain
dys-	bad; painful; difficult; abnormal
-eal	pertaining to
ec-	out; outside
echo-	reflected sound
-ectasia	dilation; dilatation; widening
-ectasis	dilation; dilatation; widening
ecto-	out; outside
-ectomy	removal; excision; resection
-edema	swelling
-elasma	flat plate
electr/o	electricity
em-	in
-ema	condition
-emesis	vomiting
-emia	blood condition
-emic	pertaining to blood condition
emmetr/o	in due measure
en-	in; within
encephal/o	brain
end-	in; within
endo-	in; within
enter/o	intestines (usually small intestine)
eosin/o	red; rosy; dawn-colored
epi-	above; upon; on
epididym/o	epididymis
epiglott/o	epiglottis
episi/o	vulva (external female genitalia)
epitheli/o	skin; epithelium
equin/o	horse
-er	one who
erg/o	work
erythem/o	flushed; redness
erythr/o	red
-esis	action; condition; state of
eso-	inward
esophag/o	esophagus
esthes/o	nervous sensation (feeling)
esthesi/o	nervous sensation (feeling)
-esthesia	nervous sensation (feeling)
estr/o	female
ethm/o	sieve
eti/o	cause
eu-	good; normal; true
-eurysm	widening
ex-	out; away from
exanthemat/o	rash
exo-	out; away from

Combining Form, Suffix, or Prefix	Meaning
extra-	outside
faci/o	face
fasci/o	fascia (membrane supporting muscles)
femor/o	femur (thigh bone)
-ferent	to carry
fibrin/o	fiber
fibr/o, fibromat/o	fiber
fibros/o	fibrous connective tissue
fibul/o	fibula
-fication	process of making
-fida	split
flex/o	bend
fluor/o	luminous
follicul/o	follicle; small sac
-form	resembling; in the shape of
fung/i	fungus; mushroom (lower organism lacking chlorophyll)
furc/o	forking; branching
-fusion	to pour; to come together
galact/o	milk
ganglion/o	ganglion; collection of nerve cell bodies
gastr/o	stomach
-gen	substance that produces
-genesis	producing; forming
-genic	produced by or in
ger/o	old age
geront/o	old age
gest/o	pregnancy
gester/o	pregnancy
gingiv/o	gum
glauc/o	gray
gli/o	glial cells; neuroglial cells (supportive tissue of nervous system)
-globin	protein
-globulin	protein
glomerul/o	glomerulus
gloss/o	tongue
gluc/o	glucose; sugar
glyc/o	glucose; sugar
glycogen/o	glycogen; animal starch
glycos/o	glucose; sugar
gnos/o	knowledge
gon/o	seed
gonad/o	sex glands
goni/o	angle
-grade	to go
-gram	record
granul/o	granule(s)
-graph	instrument for recording
-graphy	process of recording
gravid/o	pregnancy
-gravida	pregnant woman
gynec/o	woman; female
hallucin/o	hallucination
hem/o	blood
hemat/o	blood
hemi-	half
hemoglobin/o	hemoglobin
hepat/o	liver
herni/o	hernia
-hexia	state of
hidr/o	sweat
hist/o, histi/o	tissue
home/o	sameness; unchanging; constant
hormon/o	hormone
humer/o	humerus (upper arm bone)
hydr/o	water
hyper-	above; excessive
hypn/o	sleep
hypo-	deficient; below; under; less than normal
hypophys/o	pituitary gland
hyster/o	uterus; womb
-ia	condition
-iac	pertaining to
-iasis	abnormal condition
iatr/o	physician; treatment
-ic	pertaining to
-ical	pertaining to
ichthy/o	dry; scaly
-icle	small
idi/o	unknown; individual; distinct
-ile	pertaining to
ile/o	ileum
ili/o	ilium
immun/o	immune; protection; safe
in-	in; into; not
-in, -ine	substance
-ine	pertaining to
infra-	below; inferior to; beneath
inguin/o	groin
insulin/o	insulin (pancreatic hormone)
inter-	between
intra-	within; into
iod/o	iodine
ion/o	ion; to wander
-ion	process
-ior	pertaining to
ipsi-	same
ir-	in
ir/o	iris (colored portion of eye)
irid/o	iris (colored portion of eye)
is/o	same; equal
isch/o	hold back; back

Combining Form, Suffix, or Prefix	Meaning
ischi/o	ischium (part of hip bone)
-ism	process; condition
-ist	specialist
-itis	inflammation
-itus	condition
-ium	structure; tissue
jaund/o	yellow
jejun/o	jejunum
kal/i	potassium
kary/o	nucleus
kerat/o	cornea; hard, horny tissue
kern-	nucleus (collection of nerve cells in the brain)
ket/o	ketones; acetones
keton/o	ketones; acetones
kines/o	movement
kinesi/o	movement
-kinesia	movement
-kinesis	movement
klept/o	to steal
kyph/o	humpback
labi/o	lip
lacrim/o	tear; tear duct; lacrimal duct
lact/o	milk
lamin/o	lamina (part of vertebral arch)
lapar/o	abdominal wall; abdomen
-lapse	slide, fall, sag
laryng/o	larynx (voice box)
later/o	side
leiomy/o	smooth (visceral) muscle
-lemma	sheath, covering
-lepsy	seizure
lept/o	thin, slender
-leptic	pertaining to seizing, taking hold of
leth/o	death
leuk/o	white
lex/o	word; phrase
-lexia	word; phrase
ligament/o	ligament
lingu/o	tongue
lip/o	fat (a type of lipid)
lipid/o	lipid
-listhesis	slipping
lith/o	stone; calculus
-lithiasis	condition of stones
-lithotomy	incision (for removal) of a stone
lob/o	lobe
log/o	study
-logy	study (process of)
lord/o	curve; swayback
-lucent	to shine
lumb/o	lower back; loin
lute/o	yellow
lux/o	slide
lymph/o	lymph
lymphaden/o	lymph gland (node)
lymphangi/o	lymph vessel
-lysis	breakdown; separation; destruction; loosening
-lytic	reducing, destroying; separating; breakdown
macro-	large
mal-	bad
-malacia	softening
malleol/o	malleolus
mamm/o	breast
mandibul/o	mandible (lower jaw bone)
-mania	obsessive preoccupation
mast/o	breast
mastoid/o	mastoid process (behind the ear)
maxill/o	maxilla (upper jaw bone)
meat/o	meatus (opening)
medi/o	middle
mediastin/o	mediastinum
medull/o	medulla (inner section); middle; soft, marrow
mega-	large
-megaly	enlargement
melan/o	black
men/o	menses; menstruation
mening/o	meninges (membranes covering the spinal cord and brain)
meningi/o	meninges
ment/o	mind; chin
meso-	middle
meta-	change; beyond
metacarp/o	metacarpals (hand bones)
metatars/o	metatarsals (foot bones)
-meter	measure
metr/o	uterus (womb); measure
metri/o	uterus (womb)
mi/o	smaller; less
micro-	small
-mimetic	mimic; copy
-mission	send
mon/o	one; single
morph/o	shape; form
mort/o	death
-mortem	death
-motor	movement
muc/o	mucus
mucos/o	mucous membrane (mucosa)
multi-	many
mut/a	genetic change
mutagen/o	causing genetic change
my/o	muscle

Combining Form, Suffix, or Prefix	Meaning
myc/o	fungus
mydr/o	wide
myel/o	spinal cord; bone marrow
myocardi/o	myocardium (heart muscle)
myom/o	muscle tumor
myos/o	muscle
myring/o	tympanic membrane (eardrum)
myx/o	mucus
narc/o	numbness; stupor; sleep
nas/o	nose
nat/i	birth
natr/o	sodium
necr/o	death
nect/o	bind, tie, connect
neo-	new
nephr/o	kidney
neur/o	nerve
neutr/o	neither; neutral; neutrophil
nid/o	nest
noct/o	night
norm/o	rule; order
nos/o	disease
nucle/o	nucleus
nulli-	none
nyct/o	night
obstetr/o	pregnancy; childbirth
ocul/o	eye
odont/o	tooth
odyn/o	pain
-oid	resembling; originating from
-ole	little; small
olecran/o	olecranon (elbow)
olig/o	scanty
om/o	shoulder
-oma	tumor; mass; fluid collection
omphal/o	umbilicus (navel)
onc/o	tumor
-one	hormone
onych/o	nail (of fingers or toes)
o/o	egg
oophor/o	ovary
-opaque	obscure
ophthalm/o	eye
-opia	vision condition
-opsia	vision condition
-opsy	view of
opt/o	eye; vision
optic/o	eye; vision
-or	one who
or/o	mouth
orch/o	testis
orchi/o	testis
orchid/o	testis
-orexia	appetite
orth/o	straight
-ose	full of; pertaining to; sugar
-osis	condition, usually abnormal
-osmia	smell
ossicul/o	ossicle (small bone)
oste/o	bone
-ostosis	condition of bone
ot/o	ear
-otia	ear condition
-ous	pertaining to
ov/o	egg
ovari/o	ovary
ovul/o	egg
ox/o	oxygen
-oxia	oxygen
oxy-	rapid; sharp; acid
oxysm/o	sudden
pachy-	heavy; thick
palat/o	palate (roof of the mouth)
palpebr/o	eyelid
pan-	all
pancreat/o	pancreas
papill/o	nipple-like; optic disc (disk)
par-	other than; abnormal
para-	near; beside; abnormal; apart from; along the side of
-para	to bear, bring forth (live births)
-parous	to bear, bring forth
parathyroid/o	parathyroid glands
-paresis	weakness
-pareunia	sexual intercourse
-partum	birth; labor
patell/a	patella
patell/o	patella
path/o	disease
-pathy	disease; emotion
pector/o	chest
ped/o	child; foot
pelv/i	pelvis; hip region
pelv/o	pelvis; hip region
pend/o	hang
-penia	deficiency
pen/o	penis
-pepsia	digestion
per-	through
peri-	surrounding
perine/o	perineum
peritone/o	peritoneum
perone/o	fibula
-pexy	fixation; to put in place
phac/o	lens of eye
phag/o	eat; swallow

Combining Form, Suffix, or Prefix	Meaning
-phage	eat; swallow
-phagia	condition of eating; swallowing
phak/o	lens of eye
phalang/o	phalanges (of fingers and toes)
phall/o	penis
pharmac/o	drug
pharmaceut/o	drug
pharyng/o	throat (pharynx)
phas/o	speech
-phasia	speech
phe/o	dusky; dark
-pheresis	removal
phil/o	like; love; attraction to
-phil	attraction for
-philia	attraction for
phim/o	muzzle
phleb/o	vein
phob/o	fear
-phobia	fear
phon/o	voice; sound
-phonia	voice; sound
phor/o	to bear
-phoresis	carrying; transmission
-phoria	to bear, carry; feeling (mental state)
phot/o	light
phren/o	diaphragm; mind
-phthisis	wasting away
-phylaxis	protection
physi/o	nature; function
phys/o	growing
-physis	to grow
phyt/o	plant
-phyte	plant
pil/o	hair
pineal/o	pineal gland
pituitar/o	pituitary gland
-plakia	plaque
plant/o	sole of the foot
plas/o	development; formation; growth
-plasia	development; formation; growth
-plasm	formation; structure
-plastic	pertaining to formation
-plasty	surgical repair
ple/o	more; many; varied
-plegia	paralysis; palsy
-plegic	pertaining to paralysis; palsy
pleur/o	pleura
plex/o	plexus; network (of nerves)
-pnea	breathing
pneum/o	lung; air; gas
pneumon/o	lung; air; gas
pod/o	foot
-poiesis	formation
-poietin	substance that forms
poikil/o	varied; irregular
pol/o	extreme
polio-	gray matter (of brain or spinal cord)
poly-	many; much; increased
polyp/o	polyp; small growth
pont/o	pons (a part of the brain)
-porosis	condition of pores (spaces)
post-	after; behind
poster/o	back (of body); behind
-prandial	pertaining to eating or mealtime
-praxia	action
pre-	before; in front of
presby/o	old age
primi-	first
pro-	before; forward
proct/o	anus and rectum
pros-	before; forward
prostat/o	prostate gland
prot/o	first
prote/o	protein
proxim/o	near
prurit/o	itching
pseudo-	false
psych/o	mind
-ptosis	falling; drooping; prolapse
-ptysis	spitting
pub/o	pubis (anterior part of hip bone)
pulmon/o	lung
pupill/o	pupil (dark center of the eye)
purul/o	pus
py/o	pus
pyel/o	renal pelvis
pylor/o	pylorus; pyloric sphincter
pyr/o	fever; fire
pyret/o	fever
pyrex/o	fever
quadri-	four
rachi/o	spinal column; vertebrae
radi/o	x-rays; radioactivity; radius (lateral lower arm bone)
radicul/o	nerve root
re-	back; again; backward
rect/o	rectum
ren/o	kidney
reticul/o	network
retin/o	retina
retro-	behind; back; backward
rhabdomy/o	striated (skeletal) muscle
rheumat/o	watery flow
rhin/o	nose
rhytid/o	wrinkle
roentgen/o	x-rays

Combining Form, Suffix, or Prefix	Meaning
-rrhage	bursting forth (of blood)
-rrhagia	bursting forth (of blood)
-rrhaphy	suture
-rrhea	flow; discharge
-rrhexis	rupture
rrhythm/o	rhythm
sacr/o	sacrum
salping/o	fallopian tube; auditory (eustachian) tube
-salpinx	fallopian tube; oviduct
sarc/o	flesh (connective tissue)
scapul/o	scapula; shoulder blade
-schisis	split
schiz/o	split
scint/i	spark
scirrh/o	hard
scler/o	sclera (white of eye); hard
-sclerosis	hardening
scoli/o	crooked; bent
-scope	instrument for visual examination
-scopy	visual examination
scot/o	darkness
seb/o	sebum
sebace/o	sebum
sect/o	to cut
semi-	half
semin/i	semen; seed
seps/o	infection
sial/o	saliva; salivary
sialaden/o	salivary gland
sider/o	iron
sigmoid/o	sigmoid colon
silic/o	glass
sinus/o	sinus
-sis	state of; condition
-sol	solution
somat/o	body
-some	body
somn/o	sleep
-somnia	sleep
son/o	sound
-spadia	to tear, cut
-spasm	sudden contraction of muscles
sperm/o	spermatozoa; sperm cells
spermat/o	spermatozoa; sperm cells
sphen/o	wedge; sphenoid bone
spher/o	globe-shaped; round
sphygm/o	pulse
-sphyxia	pulse
splanchn/o	viscera (internal organs)
spin/o	spine (backbone)
spir/o	to breathe
splen/o	spleen

Combining Form, Suffix, or Prefix	Meaning
spondyl/o	vertebra (backbone)
squam/o	scale
-stalsis	contraction
staped/o	stapes (middle ear bone)
staphyl/o	clusters; uvula
-stasis	stopping; controlling; placing
-static	pertaining to stopping or controlling
steat/o	fat, sebum
sten/o	narrowing
-stenosis	tightening; stricture
ster/o	solid structure; steroid
stere/o	solid; three-dimensional
stern/o	sternum (breastbone)
steth/o	chest
-sthenia	strength
-stitial	pertaining to standing or positioned
stomat/o	mouth
-stomia	condition of the mouth
-stomy	new opening (to form a mouth)
strept/o	twisted chains
styl/o	pole or stake
sub-	under; below
submaxill/o	mandible (lower jaw bone)
-suppression	stopping
supra-	above, upper
sym-	together; with
syn-	together; with
syncop/o	to cut off, cut short; faint
syndesm/o	ligament
synov/o	synovia; synovial membrane; sheath around a tendon
syring/o	tube
tachy-	fast
tars/o	tarsus; hindfoot or ankle (7 bones between the foot and the leg)
tax/o	order; coordination
tel/o	complete
tele/o	distant
ten/o	tendon
tendin/o	tendon
-tension	pressure
terat/o	monster; malformed fetus
test/o	testis (testicle)
tetra-	four
thalam/o	thalamus
thalass/o	sea
the/o	put; place
thec/o	sheath
thel/o, theli/o	nipple
therapeut/o	treatment
-therapy	treatment
therm/o	heat
thorac/o	chest

Combining Form, Suffix, or Prefix	Meaning
-thorax	chest; pleural cavity
thromb/o	clot
thym/o	thymus gland
-thymia	mind (condition of)
-thymic	pertaining to mind
thyr/o	thyroid gland; shield
thyroid/o	thyroid gland
tibi/o	tibia (shin bone)
-tic	pertaining to
toc/o	labor; birth
-tocia	labor; birth (condition of)
-tocin	labor; birth (a substance for)
tom/o	to cut
-tome	instrument to cut
-tomy	process of cutting
ton/o	tension
tone/o	to stretch
tonsill/o	tonsil
top/o	place; position; location
-tory	pertaining to
tox/o	poison
toxic/o	poison
trache/o	trachea (windpipe)
trans-	across; through
-tresia	opening
tri-	three
trich/o	hair
trigon/o	trigone (area within the bladder)
-tripsy	crushing
troph/o	nourishment; development
-trophy	nourishment; development (condition of)
-tropia	to turn
-tropic	pertaining to stimulating
-tropin	stimulate; act on
tympan/o	tympanic membrane (eardrum); middle ear
-type	classification; picture
-ule	little; small
uln/o	ulna (medial lower arm bone)
ultra-	beyond; excess
-um	structure; tissue; thing
umbilic/o	umbilicus (navel)
ungu/o	nail
uni-	one
ur/o	urine; urinary tract
ureter/o	ureter
urethr/o	urethra
-uria	urination; condition of urine
urin/o	urine
-us	structure; thing
uter/o	uterus (womb)
uve/o	uvea, vascular layer of eye (iris, choroid, ciliary body)
uvul/o	uvula
vag/o	vagus nerve
vagin/o	vagina
valv/o	valve
valvul/o	valve
varic/o	varicose veins
vas/o	vessel; duct; vas deferens
vascul/o	vessel (blood)
ven/o, ven/i	vein
vener/o	venereal (sexual contact)
ventr/o	belly side of body
ventricul/o	ventricle (of heart or brain)
venul/o	venule (small vein)
-verse	to turn
-version	turning (condition of)
vertebr/o	vertebra (backbone)
vesic/o	urinary bladder
vesicul/o	seminal vesicle
vestibul/o	vestibule of the inner ear
viscer/o	internal organs
vit/o	life
vitr/o	vitreous body (of the eye)
vitre/o	glass
viv/o	life
vol/o	to roll
vulv/o	vulva (female external genitalia)
xanth/o	yellow
xen/o	stranger
xer/o	dry
xiph/o	sword
-y	condition; process
zo/o	animal life

ENGLISH—MEDICAL WORD PARTS

Meaning	Combining Form, Suffix, or Prefix
abdomen	abdomin/o (*use with* -al, -centesis)
	celi/o (*use with* -ac)
	lapar/o (*use with* -scope, -scopy, -tomy)
abdominal wall	lapar/o
abnormal	dys-
	par-
	para-
abnormal condition	-iasis
	-osis
above	epi-
	hyper-
	supra-
acetabulum	acetabul/o
acetones	ket/o
	keton/o
acid	oxy-
acromion	acromi/o
across	trans-
action	-praxia
action	-esis
act on	-tropin
adenoids	adenoid/o
adrenal glands	adren/o
	adrenal/o
after	post-
again	ana-, re-
against	anti-
	contra-
air	aer/o
	pneum/o
	pneumon/o
air sac	alveol/o
albumin	albumin/o
all	pan-
along side of	para-
alveolus	alveol/o
anew	ana-
amnion	amni/o
aneurysm	aneurysm/o
angle	goni/o
animal life	zo/o
animal starch	glycogen/o
ankle	tars/o
antrum (of stomach)	anthr/o
anus	an/o
anus and rectum	proct/o
anxiety	anxi/o
aorta	aort/o
apart	ana-
apart from	para-
aponeurosis	aponeur/o
appendix	append/o (*use with* -ectomy)
	appendic/o (*use with* -itis)
appetite	-orexia
arm	brachi/o
arm bone, lower lateral	radi/o
arm bone, lower, medial	uln/o
arm bone, upper	humer/o
armpit	axill/o
arteriole	arteriol/o
artery	arter/o
	arteri/o
articulate (speak distinctly)	-arthria
asbestos	asbest/o
assemble	-agon
atrium	atri/o
attraction for	-phil
	-philia
attraction to	phil/o
auditory tube	salping/o
away from	ab-
	apo-
	ex-
	exo-
bacilli (rod-shaped bacteria)	bacill/o
back	re-
	retro-
back, lower	lumb/o
back portion of body	dorsi-
	dors/o
	poster/o
backbone	spin/o (*use with* -al)
	spondyl/o (*use with* -itis, -lithesis, -osis, -pathy)
	vertebr/o (*use with* -al)
backward	ana-
	retro-
bacteria	bacteri/o
bacterium (berry-shaped)	-coccus (-cocci, *pl.*)
bad	cac/o
	dys-
	mal-
barrier	claustr/o

Meaning	Combining Form, Suffix, or Prefix
base (not acidic)	bas/o
Bartholin glands	bartholin/o
bear, to	para-
	-parous
	-phobia
	phor/o
before	ante-
	pre-
	pro-
	pros-
beginning	-arche
behind	post-
	poster/o
	retro-
belly	celi/o
belly side of body	ventr/o
below, beneath	hypo-
	infra-
	sub-
bend, to	flex/o
bent	scoli/o
beside	para-
between	inter-
beyond	hyper-
	meta-
	ultra-
bile	bil/i
	chol/e
bile vessel	cholangi/o
bilirubin	bilirubin/o
bind	-desis
	nect/o
birth	nat/i
	-partum
	toc/o
	-tocia
birth, substance for	-tocin
births, live	-para
black	anthrac/o
	melan/o
bladder (urinary)	cyst/o (*use with* -ic, -itis, -cele, -gram, -scopy, -stomy, -tomy)
	vesic/o (*use with* -al)
blood	hem/o (*use with* -dialysis, -globin, lysis, -philia, -ptysis, -rrhage, -stasis, -stat)
	hemat/o (*use with* -crit, -emesis, -logist, -logy, -oma, -poiesis, -uria)
blood condition	-emia
	-emic

Meaning	Combining Form, Suffix, or Prefix
blood vessel	angi/o (*use with* -ectomy, -genesis, -gram, -graphy, -oma, -plasty, -spasm)
	vas/o (*use with* -constriction, -dilation, -motor)
	vascul/o (*use with* -ar, -itis)
blue	cyan/o
body	corpor/o
	somat/o
	-some
bone	oste/o
bone condition	-ostosis
bone marrow	myel/o
brain	encephal/o
branching	furc/o
break	-clasis
	-clast
breakdown	-lysis
breast	mamm/o (*use with* -ary, -gram, -graphy, -plasty)
	mast/o (*use with* -algia, -dynia, -ectomy, -itis)
breastbone	stern/o
breathe	spir/o
breathing	-pnea
bring forth	-para
	-parous
bronchial tube (bronchus)	bronch/o
	bronchi/o
bronchiole	bronchiol/o
bunion	bunion/o
burn	caus/o
	cauter/o
bursa	burs/o
bursting forth	-rrhage
	-rrhagia
calcaneus	calcane/o
calcium	calc/o
	calci/o
calyx	cali/o
	calic/o
cancerous	carcin/o
capillary	capillar/o
carbon dioxide	capn/o
	-capnia
care for, to	comi/o
carry	duct/o
	-phoresis
	-phoria
carrying	-ferent
cartilage	chondr/o

Meaning	Combining Form, Suffix, or Prefix
cast; throw	bol/o
cause	eti/o
causing genetic change	mutagen/o
cecum	cec/o
cell	cyt/o
	-cyte
cells, condition of	-cytosis
cerebellum	cerebell/o
cerebrum	cerebr/o
cerumen	cerumin/o
cervix	cervic/o
change	meta-
cheek	bucc/o
chemical	chem/o
chest	pector/o
	steth/o
	thorac/o
child	ped/o
childbirth	obstetr/o
chin	ment/o
cholesterol	cholesterol/o
chorion	chori/o
	chorion/o
choroid layer (of the eye)	choroid/o
ciliary body (of the eye)	cycl/o
circle or cycle	cycl/o
classification	-type
clavicle	clavicul/o
clot	thromb/o
clumping	agglutin/o
clusters	staphyl/o
coagulation	coagul/o
coal dust	anthrac/o
coccyx	coccyg/o
cochlea	cochle/o
cold	cry/o
collar bone	clavicul/o
colon	col/o (*use with* -ectomy, -itis, -pexy, -stomy)
	colon/o (*use with* -ic, -pathy, -scope, scopy)
color	chrom/o
come together	-fusion
common bile duct	choledoch/o
complete	dia-
	tel/o

Meaning	Combining Form, Suffix, or Prefix
condition	-ation
	-ema
	-esis
	-ia
	-ism
	-itus
	-sis
	-y
condition, abnormal	-iasis
	-osis
conjunctiva	conjunctiv/o
connect	nect/o
connective tissue	sarc/o
constant	home/o
control	-stasis, -stat
contraction	-stalsis
contraction of muscles, sudden	-spasm
coordination	tax/o
copy	-mimetic
cornea (of the eye)	corne/o
	kerat/o
cortex	cortic/o
cotton dust	byssin/o
crooked	scoli/o
crushing	-tripsy
cul-de-sac	culd/o
curve	lord/o
cut	cis/o
	sect/o, -section
	tom/o
cut off	syncop/o
cutting, process of	-tomy
cycle	cycl/o
cyst (sac of fluid)	cyst/o
dance	chore/o
dark	phe/o
darkness	scot/o
dawn-colored	eosin/o
death	leth/o
	mort/o, -mortem
	necr/o
deep sleep	comat/o
defecation (elimination of wastes)	-chezia
deficiency	-penia
deficient	hypo-
destroying	-lytic

Meaning	Combining Form, Suffix, or Prefix
destruction	-lysis
development	plas/o
	-plasia
	troph/o
	-trophy
diaphragm	phren/o
difficult	dys-
digestion	-pepsia
dilation	-ectasia
	-ectasis
dim	ambly/o
discharge	-rrhea
disease	nos/o
	path/o
	-pathy
distant	dist/o
	tele/o
distinct	idi/o
double	dipl/o
down	cata-
	de-
drooping	-ptosis
drug	chem/o
	pharmac/o
	pharmaceut/o
dry	ichthy/o
	xer/o
drying	desicc/o
duct	vas/o
dull	ambly/o
duodenum	duoden/o
dura mater	dur/o
dusky	phe/o
dust	coni/o
ear	aur/o (*use with* -al, -icle)
	auricul/o (*use with* -ar)
	ot/o (*use with* -algia, -ic, -itis, -logy, -mycosis, -rrhea, -sclerosis, -scope, -scopy
ear condition	-otia
eardrum	myring/o (*use with* -ectomy, -itis, -tomy)
	tympan/o (*use with* -ic, -metry, -plasty)
eat	phag/o
	-phage
eating	-phagia
egg cell	o/o
	ov/o
	ovul/o
elbow	olecran/o
electricity	electr/o
elimination of wastes	-chezia
embryonic	-blast
enclosed space	claustr/o
enlargement	-megaly
enzyme	-ase
epididymis	epididym/o
epiglottis	epiglott/o
equal	is/o
esophagus	esophag/o
eustachian tube	salping/o
excess	-ultra
excessive	hyper-
excessive pain	-agra
excision	-ectomy
expansion	-ectasia
	-ectasis
extreme	pol/o
extreme point	acr/o
extremities	acr/o
eye	ocul/o (*use with* -ar, -facial, -motor)
	ophthalm/o (*use with* -ia, -ic, -logist, -logy, -pathy, -plasty, -plegia, -scope, -scopy)
	opt/o (*use with* -ic, -metrist)
	optic/o (*use with* -al, -ian)
eyelid	blephar/o (*use with* -chalasis, -itis, -plasty, -plegia, -ptosis, -tomy)
	palpebr/o (*use with* -al)
face	faci/o
faint	syncop/o
falling	-ptosis
fallopian tube	salping/o
	-salpinx
false	pseudo-
far	dist/o
fascia	fasci/o
fast	tachy-
fat	adip/o (*use with* -ose, -osis)
	lip/o (*use with* -ase, -cyte, -genesis, -oid, -oma)
	steat/o (*use with* -oma, -rrhea)
fear	phob/o
	-phobia
feeling	esthesi/o
	-phoria
female	estr/o (*use with* -gen, -genic)
	gyenc/o (*use with* -logist, -logy, -mastia)

Meaning	Combining Form, Suffix, or Prefix
femur	femor/o
fever	pyr/o
	pyret/o
	pyrex/o
fiber	fibr/o, fibromat/o, fibrin/o
fibrous connective tissue	fibros/o
fibula	fibul/o (*use with* -ar)
	perone/o (*use with* -al)
finger and toe bones	phalang/o
fingers	dactyl/o
fire	pyr/o
first	primi-
	prot/o
fixation	-pexy
flat plate	-elasma
flesh	sarc/o
flow	-rrhea
fluid collection	-oma
flushed	erythem/o
follicle	follicul/o
foot	pod/o
foot bones	metatars/o
forking	furc/o
form	morph/o
formation	plas/o
	-plasia
	-plasm
	-poiesis
forming	-genesis
forward	ante-, pro-, pros-
four	quadri-
	tetra-
front	anter/o
full of	-ose
fungus	fung/i (*use* with -cide, -oid, -ous, -stasis)
	myc/o (*use with* -logist, -logy, -osis, -tic)
gall	bil/i (*use with* -ary)
	chol/e (*use with* -ary)
gallbladder	cholecyst/o
ganglion	gangli/o
	ganglion/o
gas	pneum/o
	pneumon/o
gather	-agon
genetic change	mut/a
	mutagen/o
give, to	-dote
given, what is	-dote
gland	aden/o
glans penis	balan/o

Meaning	Combining Form, Suffix, or Prefix
glass	silic/o
	vitre/o
glial cells	gli/o
globe-shaped	spher/o
glomerulus	glomerul/o
glucose	gluc/o
	glyc/o
	glycos/o
glue	coll/a
	gli/o
glycogen	glycogen/o
go, to	-grade
good	eu-
granule(s)	granul/o
gray	glauc/o
gray matter	polio-
green	chlor/o
groin	inguin/o
grow	-physis
growing	phys/o
growth	-plasia
gum	gingiv/o
habit	-hexia
hair	pil/o
	trich/o
half	hemi-
	semi-
hallucination	hallucin/o
hand	chir/o
hang	pend/o
hard	scirrh/o
hand bones	metacarp/o
hang, to	pend/o
hard	kerat/o
	scirrh/o
hardening	-sclerosis
	scler/o
head	cephal/o
hearing	acous/o
	audi/o
	audit/o
	-acusis
	-cusis
heart	cardi/o (*use with* -ac, -graphy, logy, logist, -megaly, -pathy, -vascular)
	coron/o (*use with* -ary)
heart muscle	myocardi/o
heat	cauter/o
	therm/o
heavy	pachy-
heel bone	calcane/o
hemoglobin	hemoglobin/o

Meaning	Combining Form, Suffix, or Prefix
hernia	-cele
	herni/o
hidden	crypt/o
hip region	pelv/i, pelv/o
holding back	isch/o
hormone	hormon/o
	-one
horn-like	kerat/o
horse	equin/o
humerus	humer/o
humpback	kyph/o
hydrochloric acid	chlorhydr/o
ileum	ile/o
ilium	ili/o
immature cells	-blast
immature tumor (cells)	-blastoma
immune	immun/o
in, into, within	em-
	en-
	endo-
	in-, intra-
	ir-
in due measure	emmetr/o
in front of	pre-
incomplete	atel/o
increased	poly-
increase in cell numbers (blood cells)	-cytosis
individual	idi/o
infection	seps/o
inferior to	infra-
inflammation	-itis
instrument for recording	-graph
instrument for visual examination	-scope
instrument to cut	-tome
insulin	insulin/o
internal organs	spanchn/o
	viscer/o
intestine, small	enter/o
inward	eso-
iodine	iod/o
ion	ion/o
iris	ir/o
	irid/o
iron	sider/o
irregular	poikil/o
irrigation	-clysis
ischium	ischi/o
itching	prurit/o
jaw, lower	mandibul/o
	submaxill/o
jaw, upper	maxill/o
jejunum	jejun/o
joint	arthr/o
	articul/o
ketones	ket/o
	keton/o
kidney	nephr/o (*use with* -algia, -ectomy, -ic, -itis, -lith, -megaly, -oma, -osis, -pathy, -ptosis, sclerosis, -stomy, -tomy)
	ren/o (*use with* -al, -gram, -vascular)
killing	-cidal
	-cide
knowledge	gnos/o, gno/o
labor	-partum
	toc/o
	-tocia
labor, substance for	-tocin
lack of	de-
lack of strength	-asthenia
lacrimal duct	dacry/o
	lacrim/o
lacrimal sac	dacryocyst/o
lamina	lamin/o
large	macro-
	mega-
larynx	laryng/o
lead	duct/o
lens of eye	phac/o
	phak/o
less	de-
	mi/o
less than normal	hypo-
life	bi/o
	vit/o
	viv/o
ligament	ligament/o
	syndesm/o
light	actin/o
	phot/o
like	phil/o
lip	cheil/o
	labi/o
lipid	lipid/o
little	-ole
	-ule
liver	hepat/o
lobe	lob/o
location	top/o

Meaning	Combining Form, Suffix, or Prefix
loin	lumb/o
loosening	-lysis
love	phil/o
luminous	fluor/o
lung	pulmon/o
lung	pneum/o (*use with* -coccus, -coniosis, -thorax)
	pneumon/o (*use with* -ectomy, -ia, -ic, -itis, -lysis)
	pulmon/o (*use with* -ary)
lymph	lymph/o
lymph gland	lymphaden/o
lymph vessel	lymphangi/o
make, to	-fication
male	andr/o
malformed fetus	terat/o
malleolus	malleol/o
mandible (lower jaw bone)	mandibul/o
	submaxill/o
many	multi-
	ple/o
	poly-
marketplace	agora-
marrow	medull/o
mass	-oma
mastoid process	mastoid/o
maxilla	maxill/o
meal	cib/o
	-prandial
measure	-meter
	metr/o
meatus	meat/o
mediastinum	mediastin/o
medulla oblongata	medull/o
meninges	mening/o
	meningi/o
menstruation; menses	men/o
metacarpals	metacarp/o
metatarsals (foot bones)	metatars/o
middle	medi/o
	medull/o
	meso-
middle ear	tympan/o
milk	galact/o
	lact/o
mimic	-mimetic
mind	ment/o
	phren/o
	psych/o
	-thymia
	-thymic
mixture	cras/o
monster	terat/o
mood	-thymia
	-thymic
more	ple/o
mouth	or/o (*use with* -al)
	stomat/o (*use with* -itis)
	-stomia
movement	cine/o
	kines/o
	kinesi/o
	-kinesia
	-kinesis
	-motor
much	poly-
mucous membrane	mucos/o
mucus	muc/o
	myx/o
muscle	muscul/o (*use* with -ar, -skeletal)
	my/o (*use with* -algia, -ectomy, -oma, -neutral, -pathy, -rrhaphy, -therapy)
	myos/o (*use with* -in, -itis)
muscle, smooth (visceral)	leiomy/o
muscle, striated (skeletal)	rhabdomy/o
muscle tumor	myom/o
muzzle	phim/o
myocardium	myocardi/o
nail	onych/o
	ungu/o
narrowing	-constriction
	sten/o
	-stenosis
nature	physi/o
navel	omphal/o
	umbilic/o
near	para-
	proxim/o
neck	cervic/o
neither	neutr/o
nerve	neur/o
nerve root	radicul/o
nervous sensation	esthes/o
	esthesi/o
	-esthesia
nest	nid/o
network	reticul/o
network of nerves	plex/o
neutral	neutr/o
neutrophil	neutr/o
new	neo-
night	noct/o
	nyct/o

Meaning	Combining Form, Suffix, or Prefix
nipple	thel/o, theli/o
nipple-like	papill/o
nitrogen	azot/o
nitrogen compound	-amine
no, not	a-, an-
none	nulli-
normal	eu-
nose	nas/o (*use with* -al)
	rhin/o (*use with* -itis, -rrhea, -plasty)
nourishment	troph/o
	-trophy
nucleus	kary/o
	nucle/o
nucleus (collection of nerve cells in the brain)	kern-
numbness	narc/o
obscure	-opaque
obsessive preoccupation	-mania
off	apo-
old age	ger/o
	geront/o
	presby/o
olecranon (elbow)	olecran/o
on	epi-
one	mon/o
	mono-
	uni-
one's own	aut/o
	auto-
one who	-er
	-or
opening	-tresia
opening, new	-stomy
opposite	contra-
optic disc (disk)	papill/o
orange-yellow	cirrh/o
order	norm/o
	tax/o
organs, internal	viscer/o
originating from	-oid
ossicle	ossicul/o
other	all/o
other than	par-
out, outside	ec-
	ex-
	exo-
	extra-
outer region	cortic/o
ovary	oophor/o (*use with* -itis, -ectomy, -pexy)
	ovari/o (*use with* -an)

Meaning	Combining Form, Suffix, or Prefix
own	aut-
oxygen	ox/o
	-oxia
pain	-algia (*use with* arthr/o, cephal/o, gastr/o, mast/o, my/o, neur/o, ot/o)
	-dynia (*use with* coccyg/o, pleur/o)
	odyn/o
pain, excessive	-agra
pain, sensitivity to	-algesia
	algesi/o
painful	dys-
palate	palat/o
palsy	-plegia
	-plegic
pancreas	pancreat/o
paralysis	-plegia
	-plegic
paralysis, slight	-paresis
parathyroid glands	parathyroid/o
patella	patell/a (*use with* -pexy)
	patell/o (*use with* -ar, -ectomy, -femoral)
pelvis	pelv/i
	pelv/o
penis	pen/o
	phall/o
people	dem/o
perineum	perine/o
peritoneum	peritone/o
pertaining to	-ac (*as in* cardiac)
	-al (*as in* inguinal)
	-an (*as in* ovarian)
	-ar (*as in* palmar)
	-ary (*as in* papillary)
	-eal (*as in* pharyngeal)
	-iac (*as in* hypocondriac)
	-ic (*as in* nucleic)
	-ical (*as in* psychological)
	-ile (*as in* penile)
	-ine (*as in* equine)
	-ior (*as in* superior)
	-ose (*as in* adipose)
	-ous (*as in* mucous)
	-tic (*as in* necrotic)
	-tory (*as in* secretory)
phalanges	phalang/o
pharynx (throat)	pharyng/o
phrase	-lexia
physician	iatr/o
pineal gland	pineal/o
pituitary gland	hypophys/o
	pituit/o
	pituitar/o

Meaning	Combining Form, Suffix, or Prefix
place	-stasis
	the/o
	top/o
plant	phyt/o
	-phyte
plaque	ather/o
	-plakia
pleura	pleur/o
pleural cavity	-thorax
plexus	plex/o
poison	tox/o
	toxic/o
pole	styl/o
polyp	polyp/o
pons	pont/o
pores, condition of	-porosis
position	top/o
potassium	kal/i
pour	chyme/o
	-fusion
pregnancy	-cyesis
	gest/o
	gester/o
	gravid/o
	-gravida
	obstetr/o
pressure	bar/o
	-tension
process	-ation
	-ion
	-ism
	-y
produced by *or* in	-genic
producing	-gen
	-genesis
prolapse	-ptosis
prostate gland	prostat/o
protection	immun/o
	-phylaxis
protein	albumin/o
	-globin
	-globulin
	prote/o
pubis	pub/o
pulse	sphygm/o
	-sphyxia
puncture to remove fluid	-centesis
pupil	cor/o
	core/o
	pupi/o
pus	purul/o
	py/o
put	the/o

Meaning	Combining Form, Suffix, or Prefix
put in place	-pexy
pyloric sphincter, pylorus	pylor/o
radioactivity	radi/o
radius (lower arm bone)	radi/o
rapid	oxy-
rash	exanthemat/o
record	-gram
recording, process of	-graphy
rectum	rect/o
recurring	cycl/o
red	eosin/o
	erythr/o
redness	erythem/o
	erythemat/o
reduce	-lytic
reflected sound	echo-
relaxation	-chalasia
	-chalasis
removal	-apheresis
	-ectomy
	-pheresis
renal pelvis	pyel/o
repair	-plasty
resembling	-form
	-oid
retina	retin/o
rhythm	rrhythm/o
rib	cost/o
roll, to	vol/o
rosy	eosin/o
round	spher/o
rule	norm/o
run	-drome
rupture	-rrhexis
sac, small	alveol/o
	follicul/o
sac of fluid	cyst/o
sacrum	sacr/o
safe	immun/o
sag, to	-ptosis
saliva	sial/o
salivary gland	sialaden/o
same	ipsi-
	is/o
sameness; unchanging; constant	home/o
scaly	ichthy/o
	squam/o
scanty	olig/o
scapula	scapul/o

Meaning	Combining Form, Suffix, or Prefix
sclera	scler/o
scrotum	scrot/o
sea	thalass/o
sebum	seb/o
	sebace/o
	steat/o
secrete	crin/o
	-crine
seed	gon/o
	semin/i
seizure	-lepsy
seizing, taking hold of (pertaining to)	-leptic
self	aut-
	auto-
semen	semin/i
seminal vesicle	vesicul/o
send, sending	-mission
sensation (nervous)	-esthesia
sensitivity to pain	alges/o
	-algesia
separate	-crine
	-crit
	-lytic
separation	-lysis
set, to	-stitial
severe	acu/o
sex glands	gonad/o
sexual intercourse	-pareunia
shape	-form
	morph/o
sharp	acu/o
	oxy-
sheath	-lemma
	thec/o
shield	thyr/o
shin bone	tibi/o
shine	-lucent
short	brachy-
shoulder	om/o
side	later/o
sieve	ethm/o
sigmoid colon	sigmoid/o
single	mon/o
sinus	sinus/o
skin	cutane/o (*use with* -ous)
	derm/o (*use with* -al)
	-derma (*use with* erythr/o, leuk/o)
	dermat/o (*use with* -itis, -logist, -logy, -osis)
	epitheli/o (*use with* -al, -lysis, -oid, -oma, -um)
skull	crani/o
sleep	hypn/o
	somn/o
	-somnia
sleep, deep	comat/o
slender	lept/o
slide, to	lux/o
sliding, condition of	-lapse
slipping	-listhesis
slow	brady-
small	-icle
	micro-
	-ole
	-ule
small intestine	enter/o
smaller	mi/o
smell	-osmia
smooth (visceral) muscle	leiomy/o
sodium	natr/o
soft	medull/o
softening	-malacia
sole (of the foot)	plant/o
solid	ster/o
	stere/o
solution	-sol
sound	echo-
	phon/o
	-phonia
	son/o
spark	scint/i
specialist	-ist
speech	phas/o
	-phasia
sperm cells (spermatozoa)	sperm/o
	spermat/o
spinal column (spine)	rachi/o
	spin/o
	vertebr/o
spinal cord	myel/o
spiny	acanth/o
spitting	-ptysis
spleen	splen/o
split	-fida
	-schisis
	schiz/o
stake (pole)	styl/o
stapes	staped/o
starch	amyl/o
state of	-hexia
	-sis
steal	klept/o
sternum	stern/o
steroid	ster/o

Meaning	Combining Form, Suffix, or Prefix
sticking together	agglutin/o
stiff	ankyl/o
stimulate	-tropic
	-tropin
stomach	gastr/o
stone	lith/o
stones, condition of	-lithiasis
stop	-suppression
stopping	-stasis
	-static
straight	orth/o
stranger	xen/o
strength	-sthenia
stretch	tone/o
stretching	-ectasia
	-ectasis
striated muscle	rhabdomy/o
stricture	-stenosis
structure	-ium
	-plasm
	-um, -us
structure, solid	ster/o
study of	log/o
	-logy
stupor	narc/o
substance	-in, -ine
substance that forms	-poietin
substance that produces	-gen
sudden	acu/o
	oxysm/o
sugar	gluc/o
	glyc/o
	glycos/o
	-ose
surgical repair	-plasty
surrounding	peri-
suture	-rrhaphy
swallow	phag/o
swallowing	-phagia
swayback	lord/o
sweat	diaphor/o (*use with* -esis)
	hidr/o (*use with* -osis)
swelling	-edema
sword	xiph/o
synovial (fluid)	synov/o
synovial membrane	synov/o
tail	caud/o
tailbone	coccyg/o
tarsus (ankle)	tars/o
tear	dacry/o (*use with* -genic, -rrhea)
	lacrim/o (*use with* -al, -ation)
tearing (cutting)	-spadia
tear gland	dacryoaden/o
tear sac	dacryocyst/o
temperament	cras/o
tendon	ten/o
	tend/o
	tendin/o
tension	ton/o
testis	orch/o (*use with* -itis)
	orchi/o (*use with* -algia, -dynia, -ectomy, -pathy, -pexy, -tomy)
	orchid/o (*use with* -ectomy, -pexy, -plasty, -ptosis, -tomy)
	test/o (*use with* -sterone)
thick	pachy-
thigh bone	femor/o
thalamus	thalam/o
thin	lept/o
thing	-um
	-us
thing that produces	-gen
thirst	dips/o
thorny	acanth/o
three	tri-
throat (pharynx)	pharyng/o
through	dia-
	per-
	trans-
throw, to	bol/o
thymus gland	thym/o
thyroid gland	thyr/o
	thyroid/o
tibia (shin bone)	tibi/o
tie	nect/o
tie together	-desis
tightening	-stenosis
time	chron/o
tissue	hist/o
	histi/o
	-ium
	-um
together	con-
	sym-
	syn-
tongue	gloss/o (*use with* -al, -dynia, -plasty, plegia, -rrhaphy, -spasm, -tomy)
	lingu/o (*use with* -al)
tonsil	tonsill/o
tooth	dent/i
	odont/o
top	acr/o
toward	ad-
	af-
	-ad

Meaning	Combining Form, Suffix, or Prefix
trachea (windpipe)	trache/o
transmission	-phoresis
treatment	iatr/o
	therapeut/o
	-therapy
trigone	trigon/o
true	eu-
tube	syring/o
tumor	-oma
	onc/o
turn	-tropia
	-verse
	-version
twisted chains	strept/o
two	bi-
tympanic membrane (eardrum)	myring/o
	tympan/o
ulcer	aphth/o
ulna	uln/o
umbilicus (navel)	omphal/o (*use with* -cele, -ectomy, -rrhagia, -rrhexis)
	umbilic/o (*use with* -al)
unchanging	home/o
under	hypo-
	sub-
uneasy	anxi/o
unequal	anis/o
unknown	idi/o
up	ana-
upon	epi-
urea	azot/o
ureter	ureter/o
urethra	urethr/o
urinary bladder	cyst/o (*use* with -cele, -ectomy, -itis, -pexy, -plasty, -plegia, -scope, -scopy, -stomy, -tomy)
	vesic/o (*use with* -al)
urinary tract	ur/o
urination	-uria
urine	ur/o
	-uria
	urin/o
uterus (womb)	hyster/o (*use* with -ectomy, -gram, -graphy, -tomy)
	metr/o (*use* with -rrhagia, -rrhea, -rrhexis)
	metri/o (*use with* -osis)
	uter/o (*use with* -ine)
uvea	uve/o
uvula	staphyl/o (*use with* -ectomy, -plasty, -tomy)
	uvul/o (*use with* -ar, -itis, -ptosis)

Meaning	Combining Form, Suffix, or Prefix
vas deferens	vas/o
vagina	colp/o (*use with* -pexy, -plasty, -scope, -scopy, -tomy)
	vagin/o (*use with* -al, -itis)
vagus nerve	vag/o
valve	valv/o
	valvul/o
varicose veins	varic/o
varied	ple/o
	poikil/o
vein	phleb/o (*use with* -ectomy, -itis, -tomy)
	ven/o (*use with* -ous, -gram)
	ven/i (*use with* -puncture)
vein, small	venul/o
venereal (sexual contact)	vener/o
ventricle	ventricul/o
vertebra (backbone)	rachi/o (*use* with -itis, -tomy)
	spondyl/o (*use with* -itis, -listhesis, -osis, -pathy)
	vertebr/o (*use with* -al)
vessel (blood)	angi/o (*use with* -ectomy, genesis, -gram, -graphy, -oma, -plasty, -spasm)
	vas/o (*use with* -constriction, -dilation, -motor)
	vascul/o (*use with* -ar, -itis)
vestibule of the inner ear	vestibul/o
view of	-opsy
viscera	splanchn/o
vision condition	-opia
	-opsia
	opt/o
	optic/o
visual examination	-scopy
vitreous body	vitr/o
voice	phon/o
	-phonia
voice box (larynx)	laryng/o
vomiting	-emesis
vulva	episi/o (*use with* -tomy)
	vulv/o (*use with* -ar)
wander	ion/o
washing	-clysis
wasting away	-phthisis
water	aque/o
	hydr/o
watery flow	rheumat/o
weakness	-paresis
wedge	sphen/o
weight	bar/o

Meaning	Combining Form, Suffix, or Prefix
white	alb/o
	albin/o
	leuk/o
wide	mydr/o
widening	-dilation
	-ectasia
	-ectasis
	-eurysm
windpipe (trachea)	trache/o
with	con-
	sym-
	syn-
within	en-, end-
	endo-
	intra-
woman	gynec/o
womb	hyster/o
	metr/o
	metri/o
	uter/o
word	lex/o
	-lexia
work	erg/o
wrinkle	rhytid/o
wrist bones (carpals)	carp/o
x-rays	radi/o
	roentgen/o
yellow	lute/o
	jaund/o
	xanth/o

APPENDIX I

Plurals

The rules commonly used to form plurals of medical terms are as follows:

1. For words ending in a, retain the a and add e.
   Examples:

Singular	Plural
bulla	bullae
bursa	bursae
vertebra	vertebrae

2. For words ending in is, drop the is and add es.
   Examples:

Singular	Plural
anastomosis	anastomoses
epiphysis	epiphyses
metastasis	metastases
prosthesis	prostheses
pubis	pubes

3. For words ending in ex and ix, drop the ex or ix and add ices.
   Examples:

Singular	Plural
apex	apices
varix	varices

4. For words ending in on, drop the on and add a.
   Examples:

Singular	Plural
ganglion	ganglia
spermatozoon	spermatozoa

5. For words ending in um, drop the um and add a.
   Examples:

Singular	Plural
bacterium	bacteria
diverticulum	diverticula
ovum	ova

6. For words ending in us, drop the us and add i.
   Examples:

Singular	Plural
bronchus	bronchi
calculus	calculi
nucleus	nuclei

Two exceptions to this rule are viruses and sinuses.

7. Additional rules are used to form plurals in other word families.
   Examples:

Singular	Plural
anomaly	anomalies
biopsy	biopsies
femur	femora
foramen	foramina
iris	irides
phalanx	phalanges
thorax	thoraces

evolve *Pronunciations for plural terms as well as other terms can be found on the Evolve website.*

APPENDIX II

Abbreviations, Acronyms, Eponyms, and Symbols

ABBREVIATIONS

Many of these abbreviations may appear with or without periods and with either a capital or a lowercase first letter. (Latin abbreviations are spelled out in *italics* in parentheses.)

A, B, AB, O blood types; may have subscript numbers
A2, A_2 aortic valve closure (a heart sound)
@ at
ā before
AAA abdominal aortic aneurysm
AAL anterior axillary line
AB, ab abortion
Ab antibody
ABCDE asymmetry (of shape), border (irregularity), color (variation with one lesion), diameter (greater than 6 mm), evolution (change)—characteristics associated with melanoma
abd abdomen; abduction
ABGs arterial blood gases
AC acromioclavicular (joint)
ac, a.c. before meals *(ante cibum)*
ACE angiotensin-converting enzyme (ACE inhibitors treat hypertension)
ACh acetylcholine (a neurotransmitter)
ACL anterior cruciate ligament (of knee)
ACLS advanced cardiac life support
ACS acute coronary syndrome(s)
ACTH adrenocorticotropic hormone (secreted by the anterior pituitary gland)
AD Alzheimer disease
AD right ear *(auris dextra)*; better to specify "right ear" rather than abbreviating
ad lib. as desired (*ad libitum,* "freely")
ADD attention deficit disorder
add adduction
ADH antidiuretic hormone; vasopressin (secreted by posterior pituitary gland)
ADHD attention-deficit hyperactivity disorder
ADL activities of daily living
ADT admission, discharge, transfer
AED automated external defibrillator
AF atrial fibrillation
AFB acid-fast bacillus/bacilli—the TB organism
AFO ankle-foot orthosis (device for stabilization)
AFP alpha-fetoprotein
Ag silver *(argentum)*
AGC absolute granulocyte count; atypical glandular cells (Pap smear)
AHF antihemophilic factor (same as coagulation factor XIII)
AICD automated implantable cardioverter defibrillator
AIDS acquired immunodeficiency syndrome
AIHA autoimmune hemolytic anemia
AIS adenocarcinoma in situ (precancerous cells are seen on Pap smear)
AKA above-knee amputation
alb albumin (protein)
alk phos alkaline phosphatase (elevated in liver disease)
ALL acute lymphocytic leukemia
ALS amyotrophic lateral sclerosis (Lou Gehrig disease)
ALT alanine aminotransferase (elevated in liver and heart disease); formerly called serum glutamic-pyruvic transaminase (SGPT)

AM, a.m., AM	in the morning *or* before noon *(ante meridiem)*
AMA	against medical advice; American Medical Association
amb	ambulate, ambulatory (walking)
AMD	age-related macular degeneration
AMI	acute myocardial infarction
AML	acute myelocytic/myelogenous leukemia
ANA	antinuclear antibody
ANC	absolute neutrophil count
AP, A/P	anteroposterior
A&P	auscultation and percussion
APAP	acetyl-*para*-aminophenol
APC	acetylsalicylic acid/aspirin, phenacetin, caffeine
aq.	water *(aqua)*; aqueous
ARDS	acute respiratory distress syndrome
AROM	active range of motion
AS	aortic stenosis
AS	left ear *(auris sinistra)*; better to specify "left ear," rather than abbreviating
ASA	acetylsalicylic acid (aspirin)
ASCUS	atypical squamous cells of undetermined significance (abnormal Pap smear finding that does not fully meet the criteria for a cancerous lesion)
ASD	atrial septal defect
ASHD	arteriosclerotic heart disease
AST	aspartate aminotransferase (elevated in liver and heart disease); formerly called serum glutamic-oxaloacetic transaminase (SGOT)
AU	both ears *(auris uterque)*; better to specify "in each ear/for both ears," rather than abbreviating
Au	gold *(aurum)*
AUB	abnormal uterine bleeding
AV	arteriovenous; atrioventricular
AVM	arteriovenous malformation
AVR	aortic valve replacement
AZT	azidothymidine
A&W	alive and well
B cells	lymphocytes produced in the bone marrow
Ba	barium
BAL	bronchoalveolar lavage
bands	immature white blood cells (granulocytes)
baso	basophils
BBB	bundle branch block
BC	bone conduction
BE	barium enema
bid, b.i.d.	twice a day *(bis in die)*
BKA	below-knee amputation
BM	bowel movement
BMD	bone mineral density
BMR	basal metabolic rate
BMT	bone marrow transplantation
BP, B/P	blood pressure
BPH	benign prostatic hyperplasia/hypertrophy
BPPV	benign paroxysmal positional vertigo
BRBPR	bright red blood per rectum (hematochezia)
BRCA1, BRCA2	breast cancer 1, breast cancer 2 (genetic markers for disease risk)
bs	blood sugar; breath sound(s)
BSE	breast self-examination
BSO	bilateral salpingo-oophorectomy
BSP	Bromsulphalein (bromosulfophthalein)—dye used in liver function testing; its retention is indicative of liver damage or disease
BT	bleeding time
BUN	blood urea nitrogen
bw, BW	birth weight
Bx, bx	biopsy
C	carbon; calorie
°C	degrees Celsius (on "metric" temperature scale); degrees centigrade
c̄	with *(cum)*
C1, C2	first cervical vertebra, second cervical vertebra (and so on)
CA	cancer; carcinoma; cardiac arrest; chronologic age
Ca	calcium
CABG	coronary artery bypass graft/grafting (cardiovascular surgery)
CAD	coronary artery disease
CAO	chronic airway obstruction
cap	capsule
CAPD	continuous ambulatory peritoneal dialysis
Cath	catheter; catheterization
CBC	complete blood (cell) count
CBT	cognitive behavioral therapy
CC	chief complaint
cc	cubic centimeter (same as mL: 1/1000 of a liter)
CCr, CrCl	creatinine clearance
CCU	coronary care unit; critical care unit
CDC	Centers for Disease Control and Prevention
CDH	congenital dislocated hip
CEA	carcinoembryonic antigen
cf.	compare *(confer)*
CF	cystic fibrosis; complement fixation (test)
c.gl	with *(cum)* glasses
CGMS	continuous glucose monitoring system
cGy	centigray (1/100 of a gray; a rad)
CHD	coronary heart disease; chronic heart disease
chemo	chemotherapy
CHF	congestive heart failure
chol	cholesterol
chr	chronic
μCi	microcurie
CIN	cervical intraepithelial neoplasia

CIS carcinoma in situ
CK creatine kinase
CKD chronic kidney disease
Cl chlorine
CLD chronic liver disease
CLL chronic lymphocytic leukemia
cm centimeter (1/100 of a meter)
CMA certified medical assistant
CMC carpometacarpal (joint)
CMG cystometrogram
CML chronic myelogenous leukemia
CMV cytomegalovirus
CNS central nervous system
CO carbon monoxide; cardiac output
CO_2 carbon dioxide
Co cobalt
c/o complains of
COD condition on discharge
COPD chronic obstructive pulmonary disease
CP cerebral palsy; chest pain
CPA costophrenic angle
CPAP continuous positive airway pressure
CPD cephalopelvic disproportion
CPR cardiopulmonary resuscitation
CR complete response; cardiorespiratory
CRBSI catheter-related bloodstream infection
CRF chronic renal failure
C&S culture and sensitivity (of sputum)
C-section cesarean section
CSF cerebrospinal fluid; colony-stimulating factor
C-spine cervical spine (films)
CT computed tomography (x-ray imaging in axial and other planes)
ct. count
CTPA CT pulmonary angiography
CTS carpal tunnel syndrome
Cu copper *(cuprum)*
CVA cerebrovascular accident; costovertebral angle
CVP central venous pressure
CVS cardiovascular system; chorionic villus sampling
c/w compare with; consistent with
CX, CXR chest x-ray (film)
Cx cervix
cysto cystoscopy
D&C dilatation/dilation and curettage
DCIS ductal carcinoma in situ
DD discharge diagnosis; differential diagnosis
Decub. decubitus (lying down)
Derm. dermatology
DES diethylstilbestrol; diffuse esophageal spasm
DEXA *or* DXA dual-energy x-ray absorptiometry (a test of bone mineral density)
DI diabetes insipidus; diagnostic imaging
DIC disseminated intravascular coagulation
DICOM digital image communication in medicine
diff. differential count (of kinds of white blood cells)
DIG digoxin; digitalis
DKA diabetic ketoacidosis
dL, dl deciliter (1/10 of a liter)
DLco diffusion capacity of the lung for carbon monoxide
DLE discoid lupus erythematosus
DM diabetes mellitus
DNA deoxyribonucleic acid
DNR do not resuscitate
D.O. doctor of osteopathy
DOA dead on arrival
DOB date of birth
DOE dyspnea on exertion
DPT diphtheria-pertussis-tetanus (vaccine)
DRE digital rectal examination
DRG diagnosis-related group
DSA digital subtraction angiography
DSM *Diagnostic and Statistical Manual of Mental Disorders*
DT delirium tremens (caused by alcohol withdrawal)
DTR deep tendon reflex(es)
DUB dysfunctional uterine bleeding
DVT deep vein thrombosis
D/W dextrose in water
Dx diagnosis
EBV Epstein-Barr virus (cause of mononucleosis)
ECC endocervical curettage; extracorporeal circulation; emergency cardiac care
ECF extended care facility
ECG electrocardiogram
ECHO echocardiography
ECMO extracorporeal membrane oxygenation
ECT electroconvulsive therapy
ED erectile dysfunction; emergency department
EDC estimated date of confinement
EEG electroencephalogram
EENT eyes, ears, nose, throat
EGD esophagogastroduodenoscopy
EKG electrocardiogram
ELISA enzyme-linked immunosorbent assay
EM electron microscope
EMB endometrial biopsy
EMG electromyogram
EMLA eutectic mixture of local anesthetics
EMT emergency medical technician
ENT ear, nose, throat
EOM extraocular movement; extraocular muscles
eos eosinophils (type of white blood cell)

EPO	erythropoietin
ER	emergency room; estrogen receptor
ERCP	endoscopic retrograde cholangiopancreatography
ERT	estrogen replacement therapy
ESR (sed rate)	erythrocyte sedimentation rate (increase indicates inflammation)
ESRD	end-stage renal disease
ESWL	extracorporeal shock wave lithotripsy
ETOH	ethyl alcohol
ETT	exercise tolerance test
EUS	endoscopic ultrasonography
F, °F	Fahrenheit, degrees Fahrenheit
FB	fingerbreadth; foreign body
FBS	fasting blood sugar
FDA	U.S. Food and Drug Administration
FDG-PET	2-deoxy-2[F-18]fluoro-D-glucose positron emission tomography
Fe	iron *(Latin, ferrum)*
FEF	forced expiratory flow
FEV_1	forced expiratory volume in first second
FH	family history
FHR	fetal heart rate
FPG	fasting plasma glucose
FROM	full range of movement/motion
FSH	follicle-stimulating hormone
F/U	follow-up
5-FU	5-fluorouracil (a chemotherapy drug)
FUO	fever of undetermined origin
Fx	fracture
G	gravida (pregnant)
g, gm	gram
μg	microgram (one millionth of a gram)
g/dL	grams per deciliter
Ga	gallium
GABA	gamma-aminobutyric acid; also spelled γ-aminobutyric acid—a neurotransmitter
GB	gallbladder
GBS	gallbladder series (an x-ray study)
GC	gonococcus
G-CSF	granulocyte colony-stimulating factor (promotes neutrophil production)
Gd	gadolinium
GERD	gastroesophageal reflux disease
GFR	glomerular filtration rate
GH	growth hormone
GI	gastrointestinal
GIST	gastrointestinal stromal tumor
G6PD	glucose-6-phosphate dehydrogenase (enzyme missing in an inherited red blood cell disorder)
GP	general practitioner
GM-CSF	granulocyte-macrophage colony-stimulating factor (promotes myeloid progenitor cells with differentiation to granulocytes)
grav. 1, 2, 3	*gravida* 1, 2 , 3—first, second, third pregnancy
gt, gtt	drop *(gutta),* drops *(guttae)*
GTT	glucose tolerance test
GU	genitourinary
Gy	gray—unit of radiation absorption (exposure); equal to 100 rad
GYN, gyn	gynecology
H	hydrogen
h., hr	hour
H_2 blocker	histamine type 2 receptor antagonist (inhibitor of gastric acid secretion)
HAART	highly active antiretroviral therapy (for AIDS)
HAI	hemagglutination inhibition
Hb, hgb	hemoglobin
HbA_{1c}	glycosylated hemoglobin test (for diabetes)
HBV	hepatitis B virus
hCG, HCG	human chorionic gonadotropin
HCl	hydrochloric acid
HCO_3	bicarbonate
Hct, HCT	hematocrit
HCV	hepatitis C virus
HCVD	hypertensive cardiovascular disease
HD	hemodialysis (performed by artificial kidney machine)
HDL	high-density lipoprotein
He	helium
HEENT	head, eyes, ears, nose, throat
Hg	mercury (Latin hydragyrum meaning "liquid silver")
H&H	hematocrit and hemoglobin (measurement)—red blood cell tests
HIPAA	Health Insurance Portability and Accountability Act (of 1996)
HIV	human immunodeficiency virus
HLA	histocompatibility locus antigen (identifies cells as "self")
HNP	herniated nucleus pulposus
h/o	history of
H_2O	water
H&P	history and physical (examination)
HPF; hpf	high-power field (in microscopy)
HPI	history of present illness
HPV	human papillomavirus
HRT	hormone replacement therapy
h.s.	at bedtime *(hora somni)*—write out so as not to confuse with hs (half-strength)
HSG	hysterosalpingography
HSV	herpes simplex virus
ht	height
HTN	hypertension (high blood pressure)
Hx	history
I	iodine
^{131}I	a radioactive isotope of iodine
IBD	inflammatory bowel disease (Crohn's and ulcerative colitis)

ICD implantable cardioverter-defibrillator
ICP intracranial pressure
ICSH interstitial cell–stimulating hormone
ICU intensive care unit
ID infectious disease
I&D incision and drainage
IgA, IgD, IgE, IgG, IgM immunoglobulins (type of antibodies)
IHD ischemic heart disease
IHSS idiopathic hypertrophic subaortic stenosis
IL-1 to IL-15 interleukins
IM intramuscular; infectious mononucleosis
inf. infusion; inferior
INH isoniazid (a drug used to treat tuberculosis)
inj. injection
INR international normalized ratio (measures the time it takes for blood to clot and compares it to an average)
I&O intake and output (measurement of patient's fluids)
IOL intraocular lens (implant)
IOP intraocular pressure
IPPB intermittent positive-pressure breathing
IQ intelligence quotient
ITP idiopathic thrombocytopenic purpura
IUD intrauterine device
IUP intrauterine pregnancy
IV intravenous
IVP intravenous pyelogram
K potassium
kg kilogram (equal to 1000 g)
KJ knee jerk
KS Kaposi sarcoma
KUB kidneys, ureters, bladder (x-ray study)
L, l liter; left; lower
μL microliter (one millionth of a liter)
L1, L2 first lumbar vertebra, second lumbar vertebra (and so on)
LA left atrium
LAD left anterior descending (coronary artery); lymphadenopathy
LADA latent autoimmune diabetes in adults
lat lateral
LB large bowel
LBBB left bundle branch block (a form of heart block)
LBW low birth weight
LD lethal dose
LDH lactate dehydrogenase
LDL low-density lipoprotein (high levels are associated with heart disease)
L-dopa levodopa (a drug used to treat Parkinson disease)
LE lupus erythematosus
LEEP loop electrocautery excision procedure
LES lower esophageal sphincter
LFTs liver function tests
LH luteinizing hormone
LLL left lower lobe (of lung)
LLQ left lower quadrant (of abdomen)
LMP last menstrual period
LMWH low-molecular-weight heparin
LOC loss of consciousness
LOS length of (hospital) stay
LP lumbar puncture
lpf low-power field (in microscopy)
LPN licensed practical nurse
LS lumbosacral (spine)
LSD lysergic acid diethylamide (a hallucinogen)
LSH laparoscopic supracervical hysterectomy
LSK liver, spleen, kidneys
LTB laryngotracheal bronchitis (croup)
LTC long-term care
LTH luteotropic hormone (same as prolactin)
LUL left upper lobe (of lung)
LUQ left upper quadrant (of abdomen)
LV left ventricle
LVAD left ventricular assist device
L&W living and well
lymphs lymphocytes
lytes electrolytes
MA mental age
MAC monitored anesthesia care; *Mycobacterium avium* complex (a common cause of opportunistic pneumonia)
MAI *Mycobacterium avium-intracellulare*
MAOI monoamine oxidase inhibitor (a type of antidepressant)
MBD minimal brain dysfunction
mcg microgram—also abbreviated μg; equal to one millionth of a gram
MCH mean corpuscular hemoglobin (average amount in each red blood cell)
MCHC mean corpuscular hemoglobin concentration (average concentration in a single red cell)
mCi millicurie
μCi microcurie
MCP metacarpophalangeal (joint)
MCV mean corpuscular volume (average size of a single red blood cell)
M.D., MD doctor of medicine
MDI multiple daily injections; metered-dose inhaler (used to deliver aerosolized medication to a patient)
MDR minimum daily requirement
MDS myelodysplastic syndrome (bone marrow disorder)
MED minimum effective dose

mEq	milliequivalent
mEq/L	milliequivalent per liter (unit of measure for the concentration of a solution)
mets	metastases
MG	myasthenia gravis
Mg	magnesium
mg	milligram (1/1000 of a gram)
mg/cc^3	milligram per cubic centimeter
mg/dL	milligram per deciliter
MH	marital history; mental health
MI	myocardial infarction; mitral insufficiency
mL, ml	milliliter (1/1000 of a liter)
mm	millimeter (1/1000 of a meter); 0.039 inch
mm Hg, mmHg	millimeters of mercury
MMPI	Minnesota Multiphasic Personality Inventory
MMR	measles-mumps-rubella (vaccine)
MMT	manual muscle testing
μm	micrometer (one millionth of a meter, or 1/1000 of a millimeter); sometimes seen in older sources as μ (for "micron," an outdated term)
MoAb	monoclonal antibody
MODS	multiple organ dysfunction syndrome
monos	monocytes (type of white blood cells)
MR	mitral regurgitation; magnetic resonance
MRA	magnetic resonance angiography
MRI	magnetic resonance imaging
mRNA	messenger RNA
MRSA	methicillin-resistant *Staphylococcus aureus*
MS	multiple sclerosis; mitral stenosis; morphine sulfate
MSL	midsternal line
MTD	maximum tolerated dose
MTX	methotrexate
MUGA	multiple-gated acquisition scan (of heart)
multip	multipara; multiparous
MVP	mitral valve prolapse
myop	myopia (nearsightedness)
N	nitrogen
NA, N/A	not applicable; not available
Na	sodium *(natrium)*
NB	newborn
NBS	normal bowel sounds; normal breath sounds
ND	normal delivery; normal development
NED	no evidence of disease
neg.	negative
NG tube	nasogastric tube
NHL	non-Hodgkin lymphoma
NICU	neonatal intensive care unit
NK cells	natural killer cells
NKA	no known allergies
NKDA	no known drug allergies
NOTES	natural orifice transluminal endoscopic surgery
NPO	nothing by mouth *(nil per os)*
NSAID	nonsteroidal anti-inflammatory drug (often prescribed to treat musculoskeletal disorders)
NSR	normal sinus rhythm (of heart)
NTP	normal temperature and pressure
O, O_2	oxygen
OA	osteoarthritis
OB/GYN	obstetrics and gynecology
OCPs	oral contraceptive pills
O.D.	doctor of optometry
OD	right eye *(oculus dexter)*; better to specify "right eye," rather than abbreviating
OD	overdose
OMT	osteopathic manipulative treatment
OR	operating room
ORIF	open reduction plus internal fixation
ORTH; Ortho.	orthopedics
OS	left eye (oculus sinister); better to specify "left eye," rather than abbreviating
os	opening; bone
OT	occupational therapy (helps patients perform activities of daily living and function in work-related situations)
OU	both eyes (oculus uterque); better to specify "both eyes," rather than abbreviating
oz	ounce
P	phosphorus; posterior; pressure; pulse; pupil
$\bar{p}$	after (post)
P2, P_2	pulmonary valve closure (a heart sound)
PA	pulmonary artery; posteroanterior
P-A	posteroanterior
P&A	percussion and auscultation
PAC	premature atrial contraction
$Paco_2$	partial pressure of carbon dioxide in arterial blood
PACS	picture archival communications system
PAD	peripheral arterial disease
palp.	palpable; palpation
PALS	pediatric advanced life support
Pao_2	partial pressure of oxygen in blood
Pap smear	Papanicolaou smear (from cervix and vagina)
para 1, 2, 3	unipara, bipara, tripara (number of viable births)
pc, p.c.	after meals *(post cibum)*
PCA	patient-controlled anesthesia
PCI	percutaneous coronary intervention
Pco_2, pCO_2	partial pressure of carbon dioxide
PCP	*Pneumocystis* pneumonia; phencyclidine (a hallucinogen)

PCR polymerase chain reaction (process that allows making copies of genes)
PD peritoneal dialysis
PDA patent ductus arteriosus
PDR *Physicians' Desk Reference*
PE physical examination; pulmonary embolus
PEEP positive end-expiratory pressure
PEG percutaneous endoscopic gastrostomy (feeding tube placed in stomach)
PEJ percutaneous endoscopic jejunostomy (feeding tube placed in small intestine)
per os by mouth
PERRLA pupils equal, round, reactive to light and accommodation
PET positron emission tomography
PE tube ventilating tube for eardrum
PFT pulmonary function test
PG prostaglandin
PH past history
pH potential hydrogen (scale to indicate degree of acidity or alkalinity)
PI present illness
PICC peripherally inserted central catheter
PID pelvic inflammatory disease
PIN prostatic intraepithelial neoplasia
PIP proximal interphalangeal (joint)
PKU phenylketonuria
PM, p.m. in the afternoon (post meridiem)
PMH past medical history
PMN polymorphonuclear leukocyte
PMS premenstrual syndrome
PND paroxysmal nocturnal dyspnea
PNS peripheral nervous system
PO, p.o. by mouth (per os)
p/o postoperative
Po_2, pO_2 partial pressure of oxygen
poly polymorphonuclear leukocyte
postop postoperative (after surgery)
PPBS postprandial blood sugar
PPD purified protein derivative (used in test for tuberculosis)
preop preoperative
prep prepare for
PR partial response
primip primipara
PRL prolactin
p.r.n. as needed; as necessary *(pro re nata)*
procto proctoscopy
prot. protocol
Pro. time prothrombin time (test of blood clotting)
PSA prostate-specific antigen
PT prothrombin time; physical therapy (helps patients regain use of muscles and joints after injury or surgery)
pt. patient
PTA prior to admission (to hospital)
PTC percutaneous transhepatic cholangiography
PTCA percutaneous transluminal coronary angioplasty
PTH parathyroid hormone
PTHC percutaneous transhepatic cholangiography
PTSD post-traumatic stress disorder
PTT partial thromboplastin time (a test of blood clotting)
PU pregnancy urine
PUVA psoralen ultraviolet A (a treatment for psoriasis)
PVC premature ventricular contraction
PVD peripheral vascular disease
PVT paroxysmal ventricular tachycardia
PWB partial weight-bearing
Px prognosis
Q blood volume; rate of blood flow (daily)
q every (*quaque,* "each")
qAM every morning; better to specify than to abbreviate
qd, q.d. every day *(quaque die)*; better to specify "each/every day," rather than confusing with qid or qod
qh every hour *(quaque hora)*; better to specify than to abbreviate
q2h every 2 hours; better to specify than to abbreviate
qid, q.i.d. four times daily *(quater in die)*; better to specify than to abbreviate
q.n.s. quantity not sufficient *(quantum non sufficit)*
qPM every evening; better to specify than to abbreviate
QRS a wave complex in an electrocardiographic study
q.s. sufficient quantity *(quantum sufficit)*
qt quart
R respiration; right
RA rheumatoid arthritis; right atrium
Ra radium
rad radiation absorbed dose
RAIU radioactive iodine uptake test
RBBB right bundle branch block
RBC, rbc red blood count; red blood cell
RDDA recommended daily dietary allowance
RDS respiratory distress syndrome
REM rapid eye movement
RF rheumatoid factor
Rh (factor) rhesus (monkey) factor in blood
RhoGAM drug to prevent Rh factor reaction in Rh-negative women
RIA radioimmunoassay (test for measuring minute quantities of a substance)
RLL right lower lobe/lung

RLQ right lower quadrant (abdomen)
RML right middle lobe (lung)
RNA ribonucleic acid
R/O rule out
ROM range of motion
ROS review of systems
RRR regular rate and rhythm (of heart)
RT right; radiation therapy
RUL right upper lobe (of lung)
RUQ right upper quadrant (of abdomen)
RV right ventricle
Rx treatment; therapy; prescription
$\bar{s}$ without *(sine)*
S1, S2 first sacral vertebra, second sacral vertebra (and so on)
S-A node sinoatrial node (pacemaker of heart)
SAD seasonal affective disorder
SARS severe acute respiratory syndrome
SBE subacute bacterial endocarditis
SBFT small bowel follow-through (x-ray study of small intestine function)
segs segmented, mature white blood cells (neutrophils)
SERM selective estrogen receptor modulator
s.gl without *(sine)* glasses
SGOT see AST
SGPT see ALT
SIADH syndrome of inappropriate antidiuretic hormone
SIDS sudden infant death syndrome
Sig. directions—medication instructions (*signa,* "mark")
SIRS systemic inflammatory response syndrome (severe bacteremia)
SL sublingual
SLE systemic lupus erythematosus
SMA-12 blood chemistry profile including 12 different studies/assays
SMAC sequential multiple analyzer computer (automated analytical device for testing blood)
SOAP subjective, objective, assessment, plan (used for patient notes)
SOB shortness of breath
s.o.s. if necessary (*si opus sit,* "if there should be [such a] necessity")
S/P status post (previous disease, condition, or procedure)
sp. gr. specific gravity
SPECT single photon emission computed tomography
SQ subcutaneous
S/S, Sx signs and symptoms
SSCP substernal chest pain
SSRI selective serotonin reuptake inhibitor (a type of antidepressant)
Staph. staphylococci (berry-shaped bacteria in clusters)
stat., stat immediately *(statim)*
STD sexually transmitted disease
STH somatotropic hormone (somatotropin) (a growth hormone)
STI sexually transmitted infection
Strep. streptococci (berry-shaped bacteria in twisted chains)
subcu, subcut subcutaneous
SQ subcutaneous
subQ, sub-Q subcutaneous
SVC superior vena cava
SVD spontaneous vaginal delivery
Sx symptoms; signs and symptoms
Sz seizure
T temperature; time
T cells lymphocytes produced in the thymus gland
T tube tube placed in biliary tract for drainage
T1, T2 first thoracic vertebra, second thoracic vertebra (and so on)
T_3 triiodothyronine (test)
T_4 thyroxine (test)
TA therapeutic abortion
T&A tonsillectomy and adenoidectomy
TAB therapeutic abortion
TAH total abdominal hysterectomy
TAT Thematic Apperception Test
TB tuberculosis
Tc technetium
TEE transesophageal echocardiogram
TENS transcutaneous electrical nerve stimulation
TFT thyroid function test
THR total hip replacement (an arthroplasty procedure)
TIA transient ischemic attack
tid, t.i.d. three times daily *(ter in die)*
TKR total knee replacement (an arthroplasty procedure)
TLC total lung capacity
TLE temporal lobe epilepsy
TM tympanic membrane
TMJ temporomandibular joint
TNF tumor necrosis factor
TNM tumor-node-metastasis (cancer staging system)
tPA tissue plasminogen activator
TPN total parenteral nutrition
TPR temperature, pulse, respirations
TRUS transrectal ultrasound (examination) (test to access the prostate and guide precise placement of a biopsy needle)
TSH thyroid-stimulating hormone

TSS	toxic shock syndrome
TUR, TURP	transurethral resection of the prostate
TVH	total vaginal hysterectomy
Tx	treatment
UA	unstable angina (chest pain at rest or of increasing frequency)
UAO	upper airway obstruction
UC	uterine contraction(s)
UE	upper extremity
UGI	upper gastrointestinal
umb.	navel (umbilicus)
U/O	urinary output
URI	upper respiratory infection
U/S	ultrasound; ultrasonography
UTI	urinary tract infection
UV	ultraviolet
VA	visual acuity
VATS	video-assisted thoracic surgery (a thorascopy procedure)
VC	vital capacity (of lungs)
VCUG	voiding cystourethrogram
VDRL	Venereal Disease Research Laboratory (test for syphilis)
VEGF	vascular endothelial growth factor
VF	visual field; ventricular fibrillation
V/Q scan	ventilation-perfusion scan (of lung)
V/S	vital signs; versus
VSD	ventricular septal defect
VT	ventricular tachycardia (an abnormal heart rhythm)
VTE	venous thromboembolism
WAIS	Wechsler Adult Intelligence Scale
WBC, wbc	white blood cell; white blood count
WDWN	well developed and well nourished
WISC	Wechsler Intelligence Scale for Children
WNL	within normal limits
wt	weight
XRT	radiation therapy
y/o, yr	year(s) old

ACRONYMS

An *acronym* is the name for an abbreviation that forms a pronounceable word.

ACE ("ace") angiotensin-converting enzyme
AIDS (ādz) acquired immunodeficiency syndrome
APGAR (ĂP-gahr) appearance, pulse, grimace, activity, respiration
BUN ("bun" *or* bē-yū-ĔN) blood urea nitrogen
CABG ("cabbage") coronary artery bypass graft/grafting
CAT ("cat") computerized axial tomography (outdated term; use CT)
CPAP ("see"-păap) continuous positive airway pressure
DEXA (DECKS-Ă) dual energy x-ray absorptometry
ELISA ("eliza") enzyme-linked immunosorbent assay
GERD (gĕrd) gastroesophageal reflux disease
GIST (jĭst) gastrointestinal stromal tumor
HAART ("heart") highly active antiretroviral therapy
HIPAA (HĬP-ă) Health Insurance Portability and Accountability Act of 1996
LASER (LĀ-zĕr) light amplification by stimulated emission of radiation
LASIK (LĀ-sĭk) laser in situ keratomileusis
LEEP ("leap") loop electrocautery excision procedure
MAC (măk) monitored anesthesia care; *Mycobacterium avium* complex
MICU (MĬK-yū) medical intensive care unit
MIS ("miss") minimally invasive surgery
MODS (mōdz) multiple organ dysfunction syndrome
MUGA (mū-gă) multiple-gated acquisition (scan)
NSAID (ĔN-sĕd) nonsteroidal anti-inflammatory drug
NICU (NĬK-yū) neonatal intensive care unit
PACS (păks) picture archival communications system
PALS (pălz) pediatric advanced life support
PANDAS (PĂN-dăz) Pediatric Autoimmune Neuropsychiatric Disorders Associated with Streptococcal Infections
PEEP ("peep") positive end-expiratory pressure
PEG ("peg") percutaneous endoscopic gastrostomy
PERRLA (PĔR-lă) pupils equal, round, reactive to light and accommodation
PET ("pet") positron emission tomography
PICU (PĬK-yŭ) pediatric intensive care unit
PIP ("pip") proximal interphalangeal (joint)
PUVA (poo-vă) psoralen ultraviolet A
REM (rĕm) rapid eye movement
SAD ("sad") seasonal affective disorder
SARS (sahrz) severe acute respiratory syndrome
SERM (sĕrm) selective estrogen receptor modulator
SIDS (sĭdz) sudden infant death syndrome
SIRS (sĕrz) systemic inflammatory response syndrome
SMAC ("smack") sequential multiple analyzer computer (blood testing)
SOAP ("soap") subjective, objective, assessment, plan
SPECT (spĕkt) single photon emission computed tomography
TENS (tĕnz) transcutaneous electrical nerve stimulation
TRUS ("truss") transrectal ultrasound
TURP (tŭerp) transurethral resection of the prostate
VATS (vătz) video-assisted thoracic surgery

EPONYMS

An *eponym* is a designation for a disorder, structure, or other medical entity derived from a person or place.

Achilles tendon (Achilles, Greek mythological hero)	This tendon connects the calf muscles to the heel. It lies at the only part of Achilles' body that was still vulnerable after his mother dipped him as an infant into the river Styx, when she held him by the heel.
Alzheimer disease (Alois Alzheimer, MD, German neurologist, 1864-1915)	Progressive mental deterioration marked by confusion, memory failure, and disorientation.
Apgar score (Virginia Apgar, MD, American anesthesiologist, 1909-1974)	Evaluation of an infant's physical condition, usually performed 1 minute and then 5 minutes after birth. Highest score is 10. An Apgar rating of 9/10 is a score of 9 at 1 minute and 10 at 5 minutes.
Asperger syndrome (Hans Asperger, Austrian psychiatrist, 1906-1980)	A developmental disorder characterized by impairment of social interactions (resembling autism) but lacking in delays in language development and mental functioning.
Barrett esophagus (Norman Barrett, English physician, 1903-1979)	The lining of the esophagus is damaged by acid reflux and may be a precancerous condition.
Bell palsy (Charles Bell, Scottish surgeon, 1774-1842)	Unilateral (one-sided) paralysis of the facial nerve.
Burkitt lymphoma (Denis Burkitt, English surgeon in Africa, 1911-1993)	Malignant tumor of lymph nodes; chiefly seen in central Africa. The Epstein-Barr virus is associated with this lymphoma.
Cheyne-Stokes respiration (John Cheyne, Scottish physician, 1777-1836; William Stokes, Irish physician 1804-1878)	Abnormal pattern of respirations with alternating periods of stoppage of breathing and deep, rapid breathing.
Colles fracture (Abraham Colles, Irish surgeon, 1773-1843)	A break (fracture) of the radius (outer forearm bone) near the wrist.
Crohn disease (Burrill B. Crohn, American physician, 1884-1983)	Chronic inflammatory bowel disease of unknown origin; usually affecting the ileum (last part of the small intestine), colon, or any part of the gastrointestinal tract.
Cushing syndrome (Harvey W. Cushing, American surgeon, 1869-1939)	A disorder resulting from chronic, excessive production of cortisol from the adrenal cortex. It can also result from administration of glucocorticoids (cortisone) in large doses for long periods of time.
Duchenne muscular dystrophy (Guillaume Benjamin Amand Duchenne, French neurologist, 1806-1875)	Abnormal, inherited condition marked by progressive hardening of muscles in the legs and hips (pelvis) beginning in infancy.
Epstein-Barr virus (Michael A. Epstein, English pathologist, born 1921; Yvonne M. Barr, English virologist, born 1932)	The herpesvirus that causes infectious mononucleosis and is associated with malignant conditions such as nose and throat cancer, Burkitt lymphoma, and Hodgkin disease.
eustachian tube (Bartolomeo Eustachio, Italian anatomist, 1524-1574)	Anatomic passageway that joins the throat and the middle ear cavity.
Ewing sarcoma (James Ewing, American pathologist, 1866-1943)	Malignant tumor that develops from bone marrow, usually in long bones or the hip (pelvis).
fallopian tube (Gabriele Falloppio, Italian anatomist, 1523-1562)	One of a pair of tubes or ducts leading from the ovary to the upper portion of the uterus.

Foley catheter (Frederic Foley, American physician, 1891-1966)	Rubber tube that is placed in the urethra to provide drainage of urine.
Giardia (Alfred Giardia, French biologist, 1846-1908)	One-celled organism (protozoan) that causes gastrointestinal infection with diarrhea, abdominal cramps, and weight loss. Cause of infection is usually fecally contaminated water.
Hodgkin disease (Thomas Hodgkin, English physician, 1798-1866)	Malignant tumor of the lymph nodes.
Huntington disease (George S. Huntington, American physician, 1851-1916)	Rare, hereditary condition marked by chronic, progressively worsening dance-like movements (chorea) and mental deterioration, resulting in dementia.
Kaposi sarcoma (Moricz Kaposi, Austrian dermatologist, 1837-1902)	Malignant neoplasm of cells that line blood and lymph vessels. Soft brownish or purple papules appear on the skin. The tumor can metastasize to lymph nodes and internal organs. It is often associated with AIDS.
Marfan syndrome (Bernard-Jean A. Marfan, French pediatrician, 1858-1942)	Hereditary condition that affects bones, muscles, the cardiovascular system (leading to aneurysms), and eyes (lens dislocation). Affected people have overlong extremities with "spider-like" fingers (arachnodactyly), underdeveloped muscles, and easily movable joints.
Meniere disease (Prosper Ménière, French physician, 1799-1862)	Chronic disease of the inner ear with recurrent episodes of dizziness (vertigo), hearing loss, and ringing in the ears (tinnitus).
Neisseria gonorrhoeae (Albert L. S. Neisser, Polish dermatologist, 1855-1916)	A type of bacterium that causes gonorrhea (a sexually transmitted disease).
Paget disease (James Paget, English surgeon, 1814-1899)	Disease of bone, often affecting middle-aged or elderly people; marked by bone destruction and poor bone repair.
Pap test (George Papanicolaou, Greek physician in the United States, 1883-1962)	Method of examining stained cells obtained from the cervix and vagina. It is a common way to detect cervical cancer.
Parkinson disease (James Parkinson, English physician, 1755-1824)	Slowly progressive degenerative neurologic disorder marked by tremors, mask-like facial appearance, shuffling gait (manner of walking), and muscle rigidity and weakness.
Raynaud phenomenon (Maurice Raynaud, French physician, 1834-1881)	Intermittent attacks of loss of blood flow (ischemia) of the extremities of the body (fingers, toes, ears, and nose). Episodes most often are caused by exposure to cold.
Reye syndrome (R. Douglas Reye, Austrian pathologist, 1912-1978)	Acute brain disease (encephalopathy) and disease of internal organs following an acute viral infection.
Rinne test (Heinrich A. Rinne, German otologist, 1819-1868)	Hearing test using a vibrating tuning fork placed against a bone behind the patient's ear (mastoid bone).
Rorschach test (Herman Rorschach, Swiss psychiatrist, 1884-1922)	Personality test based on a patient's interpretation of 10 standard ink blots.
Salmonella (Daniel E. Salmon, American pathologist, 1850-1914)	Type of bacteria (rod-shaped) that causes typhoid fever and types of gastroenteritis (inflammation of the stomach and intestines).
Shigella (Kiyoshi Shiga, Japanese bacteriologist, 1870-1957)	Type of bacteria that causes severe infectious gastroenteritis (inflammation of stomach and intestines) and dysentery (diarrhea, abdominal pain, and fever).

Sjögren syndrome (Heinrik S.C. Sjögren, Swedish ophthalmologist, 1899-1986)	Abnormal dryness of the mouth, eyes, and mucous membranes, caused by deficient fluid production. It is a disorder of the immune system.
Snellen test (Herman Snellen, Dutch ophthalmologist, 1834-1908)	Test of visual clarity (acuity) using a special chart. Letters, numbers, or symbols are arranged on the chart in decreasing size from top to bottom.
Tay-Sachs disease (Warren Tay, English ophthalmologist, 1843-1927; Bernard Sachs, American neurologist, 1858-1944)	Inherited disorder of nerve degeneration caused by deficiency of an enzyme. Most affected children die between the ages of 2 and 4 years.
Tourette syndrome (Georges Gilles de la Tourette, French neurologist, 1857-1927)	Condition marked by abnormal facial grimaces, inappropriate speech, and involuntary movements of eyes, arms, and shoulders (tics).
von Willebrand disease (Erick A. von Willebrand, Finnish physician, 1870-1949)	Inherited blood disorder marked by abnormally slow blood clotting; caused by deficiency in a blood clotting factor (factor VIII).
Weber tuning fork test (Hermann D. Weber, English physician, 1823-1918)	Test of hearing using a vibrating tuning fork with the stem placed in the center of the patient's forehead.
Whipple procedure (Allen O. Whipple, American surgeon, 1881-1963)	A surgical procedure to remove a portion of the pancreas and the stomach and the entire first part of the small intestine (duodenum). Used in the treatment of pancreatic cancer and other conditions.
Wilms tumor (Max Wilms, German surgeon, 1867-1918)	Malignant tumor of the kidney occurring in young children.

SYMBOLS

=	equals
≠	does not equal
+	positive
−	negative
↑	above, increase
↓	below, decrease
♀	female
♂	male
→	to (in direction of)
>	is greater than
<	is less than
1°	primary to
2°	secondary to
ʒ	dram
℥	ounce
%	percent
°	degree; hour
:	ratio; "is to"
±	plus or minus (either positive or negative)
′	foot
″	inch
∴	therefore
@	at, each
c̄	with
s̄	without
#	pound; number
≅	approximately equals, is about
Δ	change
p	short arm of a chromosome
q	long arm of a chromosome

APPENDIX III

Normal Hematologic Reference Values and Implications of Abnormal Results

The implications of abnormal results are major ones in each category. SI units are those used in the International System of Units, which generally are accepted for all scientific and technical uses. All laboratory values should be interpreted with caution because normal values differ widely among clinical laboratories.

cu mm = cubic millimeter (mm^3)
dL = deciliter (1/10 of a liter *or* 100 mL)
g = gram
L = liter
mg = milligram (1/1000 of a gram)
mL = milliliter
mEq = milliequivalent
mm = millimeter (1/1000 of a meter)
mmol = millimole
U = unit
mL = microliter
mmol = micromole (one millionth of a mole)

BLOOD CELL COUNTS

Cell Category	Conventional Units	SI Units	Implications	
Erythrocytes (RBCs)				
Females	4.0–5.5 million/mm³ *or* µL	$4.0–5.5 \times 10^{12}$/L	*High*	♦ Polycythemia ♦ Dehydration
Males	4.5–6.0 million/mm³ *or* µL	$4.5–6.0 \times 10^{12}$/L		
			Low	♦ Iron deficiency anemia ♦ Blood loss
Leukocytes (WBCs)				
Total	5000–10,000/mm³ *or* µL	$5.0–10.0 \times 10^{9}$/L	*High*	♦ Bacterial infection ♦ Leukemia ♦ Eosinophils high in allergy
Differential (%)				
Neutrophils	54–62			
Lymphocytes	20–40		*Low*	♦ Viral infection ♦ Aplastic anemia ♦ Chemotherapy
Monocytes	3–7			
Eosinophils	1–3			
Basophils	0–1			
Platelets	150,000–350,000/mm³ *or* µL	$200–400 \times 10^{9}$/L	*High*	♦ Hemorrhage ♦ Infections ♦ Malignancy ♦ Splenectomy
			Low	♦ Aplastic anemia ♦ Chemotherapy ♦ Hypersplenism

COAGULATION TESTS

Test	Conventional Units	SI Units	Implications	
Bleeding time (template method)	2.75–8.0 min	2.7–8.0 min	*Prolonged*	♦ Aspirin ingestion ♦ Low platelet count
Coagulation time	5–15 min	5–15 min	*Prolonged*	♦ Heparin therapy
Prothrombin time (PT)*	11–12.5 sec	11–12.5 sec	*Prolonged*	♦ Vitamin K deficiency ♦ Hepatic disease ♦ Oral anticoagulant therapy (warfarin)
Partial thromboplastin time (PTT)	25–34 sec	25–37 sec	*Prolonged*	♦ Intravenous heparin therapy

*The INR (international normalized ratio) is a standard tool for monitoring the effects of an anticoagulant, warfarin; the normal INR value is <1.5.

RED BLOOD CELL TESTS

Test	Conventional Units	SI Units	Implications	
Hematocrit (Hct)				
Females	37%–47%	0.37–0.47	*High*	♦ Polycythemia ♦ Dehydration
Males	40%–54%	0.40–0.54		
			Low	♦ Loss of blood ♦ Anemia
Hemoglobin (Hb, Hgb)				
Females	12.0–14.0 g/dL *or* 120–140 g/L	1.86–2.48 mmol/L	*High*	♦ Polycythemia ♦ Dehydration
Males	14.0–16.0 g/dL	2.17–2.79 mmol/L	*Low*	♦ Anemia ♦ Blood loss

SERUM TESTS

Test	Conventional Units	SI Units	Implications	
Alanine aminotransferase (ALT; SGPT)	5–30 U/L	5–30 U/L	*High*	♦ Hepatitis
Albumin	3.5–5.5 g/dL	35–55 g/L	*Low*	♦ Hepatic disease ♦ Malnutrition ♦ Nephritis and nephrosis
Alkaline phosphatase (ALP)	20–90 U/L	20–90 U/L	*High*	♦ Bone disease ♦ Hepatitis or tumor infiltration of liver ♦ Biliary obstruction
Aspartate aminotransferase (AST; SGOT)	10–30 U/L	10–30 U/L	*High*	♦ Hepatitis ♦ Cardiac and muscle injury
Bilirubin			*High*	♦ Hemolysis ♦ Neonatal hepatic immaturity ♦ Cirrhosis ♦ Biliary tract obstruction
Total	0.3–1.0 mg/dL	5.1–17 μmol/L		
Neonates	1–12 mg/dL	17–205 μmol/L		
Blood urea nitrogen (BUN)	10–20 mg/dL	3.6–7.1 mmol/L	*High*	♦ Renal disease ♦ Reduced renal blood flow ♦ Urinary tract obstruction
			Low	♦ Hepatic damage ♦ Malnutrition
Calcium	9.0–10.5 mg/dL	2.2–2.6 mmol/L	*High*	♦ Hyperparathyroidism ♦ Multiple myeloma ♦ Metastatic cancer
			Low	♦ Hypoparathyroidism ♦ Total parathyroidectomy
Cholesterol (desirable range)				
Total	<200 mg/dL	<5.2 mmol/L	*High*	♦ High-fat diet ♦ Inherited hypercholesterolemia
LDL cholesterol	<130 mg/dL	<3.36 mmol/L		
HDL cholesterol	>60 mg/dL	>1.55 mmol/L		
			Low	♦ Starvation

Test	Conventional Units	SI Units	Implications	
Creatine kinase (CK)				
Females	30–135 U/L	30–135 U/L	*High*	♦ Myocardial infarction
Males	55–170 U/L	55–170 U/L		♦ Muscle disease
Creatinine	<1.5 mg/dL	<133 µmol/L	*High*	♦ Renal disease
Glucose (fasting)	75–115 mg/dL	4.2–6.4 mmol/L	*High*	♦ Diabetes mellitus
			Low	♦ Hyperinsulinism
				♦ Fasting
				♦ Hypothyroidism
				♦ Addison disease
				♦ Pituitary insufficiency
Iron (Fe)				
Females	30-160 µg/dL	5.4-31.3 µmol/L	*High*	♦ Hemochromatosis
Males	45-160 µg/dL	8.1-31.3 µmol/L		♦ Transfusions
			Low	♦ Anemia
				♦ Bleeding
Lactate dehydrogenase (LDH)	100–190 U/L	100–190 U/L	*High*	♦ Tissue necrosis
				♦ Lymphomas
				♦ Muscle disease
Phosphate (PO_4^-)	3.0–4.5 mg/dL	1.0–1.5 mmol/L	*High*	♦ Renal failure
				♦ Bone metastases
				♦ Hypoparathyroidism
			Low	♦ Malnutrition
				♦ Malabsorption
				♦ Hyperparathyroidism
Potassium (K^+)	3.5–5.0 mEq/L	3.5–5.0 mmol/L	*High*	♦ Burn injury
				♦ Renal failure
				♦ Diabetic ketoacidosis
			Low	♦ Cushing syndrome
				♦ Loss of body fluids
Sodium (Na^+)	136–145 mEq/L	136–145 mmol/L	*High*	♦ Inadequate water intake
				♦ Water loss in excess of sodium
			Low	♦ Adrenal insufficiency
				♦ Inadequate sodium intake
				♦ Excessive sodium loss
Thyroxine (T4)	5–12 µg/dL	64–154 nmol/L	*High*	♦ Graves disease (hyperthyroidism)
			Low	♦ Hypothyroidism
Uric acid				
Females	2.5–8.0 mg/dL	150–480 µmol/L	*High*	♦ Gout
Males	1.5–6.0 mg/dL	90–360 µmol/L		♦ Leukemia

APPENDIX IV

Drugs

Following is an alphabetized list of the drugs referred to in Chapter 21 (tables), with brand name(s) in parentheses and explanation of use, including drug category and/or class. This Appendix, along with drugs listed alphabetically by brand name, appears on the Evolve website.

Generic Name (Brand Name)	Explanation of Use
abiraterone (Zytiga)	Endocrine/antiandrogen
acarbose (Precose)	Antidiabetic (type 2 diabetes)/alpha-glucosidase inhibitor
acetaminophen (Tylenol)	Analgesic/mild
acyclovir (Zovirax)	Antiviral
adalimumab (Humira)	Gastrointestinal/anti-TNF
albuterol (Proventil, Ventolin)	Bronchodilator
alendronate (Fosamax)	Antiosteoporosis/bisphosphonate
alprazolam (Xanax)	Tranquilizer/minor/benzodiazepine
aluminum antacid (Rolaids)	GI/antacid
aluminum + magnesium antacid (Gaviscon)	GI/antacid
amiodarone (Cordarone)	Cardiovascular/antiarrhythmic
amlodipine (Norvasc)	Cardiovascular/calcium antagonist
amoxicillin trihydrate (Amoxil, Trimox)	Antibiotic/penicillin
amoxicillin + clavulanate (Augmentin)	Antibiotic/penicillin
anastrozole (Arimidex)	Endocrine/aromatase inhibitor
aripiprazole (Abilify)	Tranquilizer/major
aspirin (Anacin, Ascription, Excedrin)	Analgesic/NSAID
atenolol (Tenormin)	Cardiovascular/beta-blocker
atorvastatin (Lipitor)	Cardiovascular/cholesterol-lowering
azithromycin (Zithromax)	Antibiotic/erythromycin class
budesonide (Pulmicort)	Respiratory/steroid inhaler
buspirone (BuSpar)	Tranquilizer/minor
butabarbital (Butisol)	Sedative-hypnotic
caffeine	Stimulant
calcitonin (Cibacalcin)	Endocrine/thyroid
carbamazepine (Tegretol)	Anticonvulsant
cefprozil (Cefzil)	Antibiotic/cephalosporin
ceftazidime (Fortaz)	Antibiotic/cephalosporin
cefuroxime axetil (Ceftin)	Antibiotic/cephalosporin
celecoxib (Celebrex)	Analgesic/NSAID
cephalexin (Keflex)	Antibiotic/cephalosporin
certolizumab pegol (Cimzia)	Gastrointestinal/anti-TNF

Generic Name (Brand Name)	Explanation of Use
cetirizine (Zyrtec)	Antihistamine
chlorpheniramine maleate (Chlor-Trimeton)	Antihistamine
chlorpromazine (Thorazine)	Tranquilizer, major/phenothiazine
cholestyramine (Questran)	Cardiovascular/cholesterol-binding
cimetidine (Tagamet)	GI/antiulcer/anti-GERD
ciprofloxacin (Cipro)	Antibiotic/quinolone
clarithromycin (Biaxin)	Antibiotic/erythromycin class
clopidogrel bisulfate (Plavix)	Antiplatelet
clotrimazole (Lotrimin, Mycelex)	Antifungal
codeine	Analgesic/narcotic
colestipol (Colestid)	Cardiovascular/cholesterol-binding
dalteparin (Fragmin)	Anticoagulant
denosumab (Prolia)	Antiosteoporosis/bisphosphonate
dexamethasone (Decadron)	Respiratory/steroid, intravenous or oral
dextroamphetamine and amphetamine (Adderall)	Stimulant
dextroamphetamine sulfate (Dexedrine)	Stimulant
diazepam (Valium)	Tranquilizer/minor/benzodiazepine
diclofenac sodium (Voltaren)	Analgesic/NSAID
digoxin (Lanoxin)	Cardiovascular/anti-CHF
diltiazem (Cardizem CD)	Cardiovascular/calcium antagonist
diphenhydramine (Benadryl)	Antihistamine
diphenoxylate + atropine (Lomotil)	GI/antidiarrheal
donepezil (Aricept)	Anti-Alzheimer disease
doxycycline	Antibiotic/tetracycline
econazole, topical (Spectazole)	Antifungal
efavirenz (Sustiva)	Anti-HIV
enalapril maleate (Vasotec)	Cardiovascular/ACE inhibitor
enoxaparin sodium (Lovenox)	Anticoagulant
epinephrine	Bronchodilator
erythromycin (Ery-Tab)	Antibiotic/erythromycin
escitalopram (Lexapro)	Antidepressant
estrogen (Premarin, Prempro, Estradiol)	Endocrine/estrogen
etanercept (Enbrel)	Gastrointestinal/anti-TNF
ethambutol (Myambutol)	Antitubercular
ether	Anesthetic/general
famotidine (Pepcid)	GI/antiulcer/anti-GERD
felbamate (Felbatol)	Anticonvulsant
fexofenadine (Allegra)	Antihistamine
fluconazole (Diflucan)	Antifungal
flunisolide (AeroBid)	Respiratory/steroid inhaler
fluoxymesterone (Halotestin)	Endocrine/androgen
flutamide (Eulexin)	Endocrine/antiandrogen
fluticasone propionate (Flovent)	Respiratory/steroid inhaler
formoterol (Foradil)	Bronchodilator
formoterol + budesonide (Symbicort)	Bronchodilator
fulvestrant (Faslodex)	Endocrine/aromatase inhibitor
furosemide (Lasix)	Cardiovascular/diuretic
gabapentin (Neurontin)	Anticonvulsant
glipizide (Glucotrol XL)	Antidiabetic (type 2 diabetes)/sulfonylurea
glyburide (Diabeta, Micronase)	Antidiabetic (type 2 diabetes)/sulfonylurea
goserelin (Zoladex)	Endocrine/antiandrogen

Generic Name (Brand Name)	Explanation of Use
haloperidol (Haldol)	Tranquilizer/major
halothane (Fluothane)	Anesthetic/general
hydrochlorothiazide (HydroDIURIL)	Cardiovascular/diuretic
hydrocodone w/APAP (Lortab, Vicodin)	Analgesic/narcotic
hydromorphone (Dilaudid)	Analgesic/narcotic
ibuprofen (Motrin, Advil)	Analgesic/NSAID
ibutilide (Corvert)	Antiarrhythmic
indinavir (Crixivan)	Antiviral/protease inhibitor/anti-HIV
infliximab (Remicade)	Gastrointestinal/anti-TNF
insulin aspart (NovoLog)	Antidiabetic (type 1 diabetes)
insulin detemir (Levemir)	Antidiabetic (type 1 diabetes)
insulin glargine (Lantus)	Antidiabetic (type 1 diabetes)
insulin glulisine (Apidra)	Antidiabetic (type 1 diabetes)
insulin lispro (Humalog)	Antidiabetic (type 1 diabetes)
insulin NPH (Humulin N)	Antidiabetic (type 1 diabetes)
insulin regular (Humulin R)	Antidiabetic (type 1 diabetes)
insulin zinc suspension (Ultralente)	Antidiabetic (type 1 diabetes)
interferon alfa-n1 (Wellferon)	Antiviral/anti-cancer drug
ipratropium bromide + albuterol (Combivent)	Bronchodilator
irbesartan (Avapro)	Cardiovascular/angiotensin II receptor antagonist
isoniazid *or* INH (Nydrazid)	Antitubercular
itraconazole (Sporanox)	Antifungal
ketorolac (Toradol)	Analgesic/NSAID
lamivudine (Epivir)	Antiviral/reverse transcriptase inhibitor/anti-HIV
lansoprazole (Prevacid)	GI/antiulcer/anti-GERD
lepirudin (Refludan)	Anticoagulant
letrozole (Femara)	Endocrine/aromatase inhibitor
leuprolide (Lupron)	Endocrine/antiandrogen
levalbuterol (Xopenex)	Bronchodilator
levetiracetam (Keppra)	Anticonvulsant
levofloxacin (Levaquin)	Antibiotic
levothyroxine (Levoxyl, Levothroid, Synthroid)	Endocrine/thyroid hormone
lidocaine (Xylocaine)	Anesthetic/local
lidocaine + prilocaine (EMLA)	Anesthetic/local
liothyronine (Cytomel)	Endocrine/thyroid hormone
lisinopril (Prinivil, Zestril)	Cardiovascular/ACE inhibitor
lithium carbonate (Eskalith)	Tranquilizer/major
loperamide (Imodium)	GI/antidiarrheal
loratadine (Claritin)	Antihistamine
lorazepam (Ativan)	Tranquilizer/minor/benzodiazepine
losartan (Cozaar)	Cardiovascular/angiotensin II receptor antagonist
lovastatin (Mevacor)	Cardiovascular/cholesterol-lowering
magnesium antacid (milk of magnesia)	GI/antacid
meclizine (Antivert)	Antihistamine
medroxyprogesterone acetate (Cycrin, Provera)	Endocrine/progestin
megestrol (Megace)	Endocrine/progestin
memantine (Namenda)	Anti-Alzheimer disease
meperidine (Demerol)	Analgesic/narcotic
metaproterenol (Alupent)	Bronchodilator
metformin (Glucophage)	Antidiabetic (type 2 diabetes)/biguanide

Generic Name (Brand Name)	Explanation of Use
methaqualone (Quaalude)	Sedative-hypnotic
methylphenidate (Ritalin)	Stimulant
methylprednisolone (Medrol)	Respiratory/steroid, intravenous or oral
methyltestosterone (Virilon)	Endocrine/androgen
metoclopramide (Reglan)	GI/antinauseant
metoprolol (Lopressor, Toprol-XL)	Cardiovascular/beta-blocker
miconazole (Monistat)	Antifungal
midazolam (Versed)	Sedative-hypnotic
modafinil (Provigil)	Stimulant/sleep antagonist
mometasone (Asmanex)	Respiratory/inhaler
montelukast sodium (Singulair)	Respiratory/leukotriene modifier
nafcillin (Unipen)	Antibiotic/penicillin
naproxen (Naprosyn)	Analgesic/NSAID
nifedipine (Adalat CC, Procardia)	Cardiovascular/calcium antagonist
nilutamide (Casodex)	Endocrine/antiandrogen
nitroglycerin	Cardiovascular/antianginal
nitrous oxide	Anesthetic/general
nystatin (Nilstat)	Antifungal
octreotide (Sandostatin)	Endocrine/growth
ofloxacin (Floxin)	Antibiotic/quinolone
olanzapine (Zyprexa)	Tranquilizer/major/antipsychotic
omeprazole (Prilosec)	GI/antiulcer/anti-GERD
ondansetron (Zofran)	GI/antinauseant
oxacillin (Bactocill)	Antibiotic/penicillin
oxycodone (OxyContin, Roxicodone)	Analgesic/narcotic
oxycodone with APAP (Roxicet, Endocet, Percocet)	Analgesic/narcotic
pamidronate disodium (Aredia)	Anti-osteoporosis/bisphosphonate
p-aminosalicylic acid granules (PASER)	Anitubercular
paregoric	GI/antidiarrheal
phenobarbital (Luminal)	Sedative-hypnotic/anticonvulsant
phenytoin sodium (Dilantin)	Anticonvulsant
pioglitazone (Actos)	Antidiabetic (type 2 diabetes)
pirbuterol (Maxair)	Bronchodilator
prasugrel (Effient)	Antiplatelet
pravastatin (Pravachol)	Cardiovascular/cholesterol-lowering
prednisone	Respiratory/steroid, intravenous or oral
promethazine (Phenergan)	Antihistamine
procaine (Novocain)	Anesthetic/local
prochlorperazine maleate (Compazine)	GI/antinauseant
propofol (Diprivan)	Anesthetic/general
propranolol (Inderal)	Cardiovascular/beta-blocker
quinapril (Accupril)	Cardiovascular/ACE inhibitor
raloxifene (Evista)	Endocrine/SERM/antiosteoporosis
ramipril (Altace)	Cardiovascular/ACE inhibitor
ranitidine (Zantac)	GI/antiulcer/anti-GERD
repaglinide (Prandin)	Antidiabetic (type 2 diabetes)/meglitinide
ribavirin (Copegus, Rebetol)	Antiviral
rifampin (Rifadin)	Antitubercular
risperidone (Risperdal)	Tranquilizer/major

Generic Name (Brand Name)	Explanation of Use
rivaroxaban (Xarelto)	Anticoagulant
rosiglitazone (Avandia)	Antidiabetic (type 2 diabetes)
rosuvastatin calcium (Crestor)	Cholesterol-lowering statin
salmeterol (Serevent)	Bronchodilator
salmeterol + fluticasone (Advair)	Corticosteroid anti-inflammatory–bronchodilator combination
simvastatin (Zocor)	Cardiovascular/cholesterol-lowering
sotalol (Betapace)	Cardiovascular/beta-blocker
spironolactone (Aldactone)	Cardiovascular/diuretic
sulfamethoxazole + trimethoprim (Bactrim)	Antibiotic/sulfonamide—antibacterial combination
sulfisoxazole (Gantrisin)	Antibiotic/sulfonamide
tamoxifen (Nolvadex)	Endocrine/SERM
temazepam (Restoril)	Sedative-hypnotic/benzodiazepine
terbinafine (Lamisil)	Antifungal
teriparatide (Forteo)	Antiosteoporosis/bisphosphonate
teriparatide (Forteo)	Endocrine/parathyroid
tetracycline (Sumycin, Terramycin)	Antibiotic/tetracycline
theophylline (Theo-Dur)	Bronchodilator
thiopental (Pentothal)	Anesthetic/general
thioridazine (Mellaril)	Tranquilizer/major/phenothiazine
ticagrelor (Brilinta)	Antiplatelet
tiotropium (Spiriva)	Bronchodilator
tissue plasminogen activator *or* tPA	Anticoagulant
tramadol (Ultram)	Analgesic/narcotic
triamcinolone (Aristocort)	Glucocorticoid
triamcinolone (Azmacort)	Respiratory/steroid inhaler
triamterene (Dyazide)	Cardiovascular/diuretic
triazolam (Halcion)	Sedative-hypnotic/benzodiazepine
trifluoperazine (Stelazine)	Tranquilizer/major/phenothiazine
valdecoxib (Bextra)	Analgesic/NSAID
valproic acid (Depakote)	Anticonvulsant
warfarin (Coumadin)	Anticoagulant
zafirlukast (Accolate)	Respiratory/leukotriene modifier
zidovudine *or* AZT (Retrovir)	Antiviral/reverse transcriptase inhibitor/anti-HIV
zidovudine + lamivudine (Combivir)	Anti-HIV
zileuton (Zyflo)	Respiratory/leukotriene modifier
zoledronic acid (Zometa)	Antiosteoporosis/bisphosphonate
zolpidem tartrate (Ambien)	Sedative-hypnotic

ILLUSTRATIONS CREDITS

Figure 10-19B, from Albert D: *Albert & Jakobiec's Principles & Practice of Ophthalmology*, ed 3, Philadelphia, 2008, Saunders.

Figure 11-10, from Applegate E: *The Anatomy and Physiology Learning System*, ed 2, Philadelphia, 2000, Saunders.

Figure 16-9A, from Barkauskas VH et al: *Health and Physical Assessment*, ed 2, St. Louis, 1998, Mosby.

Figure 20-15, from Beare PG, Myers JL: *Adult Health Nursing*, ed 3, St. Louis, 1998, Mosby.

Figure 5-20F, from Bird D, Robinson D: *Modern Dental Assisting*, ed 10, Philadelphia, 2012, Saunders.

Unnumbered Figure 2-3, Figures 6-8B, 12-13A, 12-18B, 13-15, 16-11, 17-14, 20-9C, from Black J, Hawks J: Medical-Surgical Nursing, 8th ed., Philadelphia, 2009, Elsevier/Saunders.

Figures 20-4, 20-8B, from Braunwald E: *Heart Disease: A Textbook of Cardiovascular Medicine*, ed 4, Philadelphia, 1992, Saunders.

Figures 5-20E, 9-6A, 10-19A, 16-5B, 16-6B, 16-8D, 16-10B, 16-12B, 16-13A, from Callen JP et al: *Color Atlas of Dermatology*, ed 2, Philadelphia, 2002, Saunders.

Figure 15-38B & E, from Canale ST, Beaty JH: *Campbell's Operative Orthopaedics*, ed 11, St. Louis, 2008, Mosby.

Figures 13-4, 13-6, from Carr JH, Rodak BF: *Clinical Hematology Atlas*, ed 2, St. Louis, 2004, Mosby.

Figures 12-13B, 21-2A, from Chabner DE: *Medical Terminology: A Short Course*, ed 5, Philadelphia, 2009, Saunders.

Figure 16-8C, from Cohen BA: *Atlas of Pediatric Dermatology*, London, 1993, Wolfe.

Figure 5-19, from Christensen B, Kockrow E: *Foundations and Adult Health Nursing*, ed 5, St. Louis, 2006, Elsevier/Mosby.

Figure 5-20A, from Christensen GJ: *A Consumer's Guide to Dentistry*, St. Louis, 2002, Mosby.

Figure 18-20, from Clinical Pathological Conference, *Am J Med* 20:133, 1956.

Figure 15-32, from Coughlin M et al: *Surgery of the Foot and Ankle*, ed 8, St. Louis, 2007, Mosby.

Figure 11-22B, from Crawford MH, DiMarco JP, Paulus WJ: *Cardiology*, ed 2, St. Louis, 2004, Mosby.

Figures 5-14, 5-21A, 5-23, 5-24, 5-26, 5-29B, 7-7, 7-12A, 8-15, 8-16A, 11-1, from Damjanov I: *Pathology for the Health-Related Professions*, ed 4, Philadelphia, 2012, Elsevier/Saunders.

Figure 15-16, from Dempster DW, Shane E, Horbert W, et al: A Simple Method for Correlative Light and Scanning Electron Microscopy Of Human Iliac Crest Bone Biopsies: Qualitative Observations in Normal and Osteoporotic Subjects, *J Bone Miner Res* 1:15, 1986.

Figure 16-8L, from Farrar WE: *Atlas of Infections of the Nervous System*, London, 1993, Mosby-Wolfe.

Figure 5-20B, from Feldman M et al: *Sleisenger and Fordtran's Gastrointestinal and Liver Disease*, ed 8, Philadelphia, 2006, Saunders.

Figure 17-25D, from Fireman P, Slavin RG: *Atlas of Allergies*, ed 2, London, 1996, Glower Medical Publishing.

Figure 11-21B, from Forbes CD, Jackson WF: *Color Atlas and Text of Clinical Medicine*, ed 3, London, 2003, Mosby.

Figures 8-24, 10-21, 20-13, from Frank ED et al: *Merrill's Atlas of Radiographic Positioning & Procedures*, ed 11, St. Louis, 2007, Mosby.

Figures 10-14B, 17-6A, from Frazier MS, Drzymkowski JW: *Essentials of Human Diseases and Conditions*, ed 3, Philadelphia, 2004, Saunders.

Figure 9-1B, from Gartner L: *Color Textbook of Histology*, ed 3, Philadelphia, 2007, Saunders.

Figure 20-8A, from Gill KA: *Abdominal Ultrasound: A Practitioner's Guide*, Philadelphia, 2001, Saunders.

Figure 22-2, from Gleitman H: *Psychology*, New York, 1991, WW Norton.

Figure 3-2, from Goering R et al: *Mims' Medical Microbiology*, ed 4, Edinburgh, 2008, Elsevier/Mosby Ltd.

Figures 2-3, 6-2A, 11-23A, from Goldman L, Schafer A: *Goldman's Cecil Medicine*, ed 24, Philadelphia, 2012, Elsevier/Saunders.

Figures 5-21B, 13-13, 16-8J, from Gould BE, Dyer R: *Pathophysiology for Health Professions*, ed 4, Philadelphia, 2011, Elsevier/Saunders.

Figure 15-35, from Greer I et al: *Mosby's Color Atlas and Text of Obstetrics and Gynecology*, London, 2001, Mosby.

Figures 2-14B, 10-16B, from Haaga J: *CT and MR Imaging of the Whole Body*, ed 4, St. Louis, 2003, Elsevier/Mosby.

Figures 16-8F, 16-15A, 16-18A, from Habif TP: *Clinical Dermatology*, ed 4, St. Louis, 2004, Mosby.

Figure 11-25, from Hicks GH: *Cardiopulmonary Anatomy and Physiology*, Philadelphia, 2000, Saunders.

Figure 13-5, from Hirsch JG: Cinemicrophotographic Observations of Granule Lysis in Polymorphonuclear Leucocytes during Phagocytosis, *J Exp Med*;116:827, 1962, by copyright permission of Rockefeller University Press.

Figure 1-5, from His E: *Hematopathology*, ed 1, Philadelphia, 2007, Elsevier/Churchill Livingstone.

Figures 6-3, 6-4A, 6-5, from Heuman DM, Mills AS, McGuire HH: *Gastroenterology*, Philadelphia, 1997, Elsevier/Saunders.

Figures 2-4B, 16-14A, from Huether S, McCance K: *Understanding Pathophysiology*, ed 5, St. Louis, 2012, Elsevier/Mosby.

Figures 10-20, 16-19B, 16-20A, 17-21, from Ignatavicius DD, Workman ML: *Medical-Surgical Nursing: Critical Thinking for Collaborative Care*, ed 4, Philadelphia, 2002, Saunders.

Figure 16-15B, from James W et al: *Andrews' Diseases of the Skin*, ed 11, Philadelphia, 2012, Saunders.

Figures 16-18B, 17-15, 17-17, 18-15A, from Jarvis C: *Physical Examination and Health Assessment*, ed 3, Philadelphia, 2000, Saunders.

Figure 15-33A, from Jebson LR, Coons DD: Total Hip Arthroplasty, *Surg Technol* October: 30(10):12-21, 1998.

Figure 7-5, from Joffe SA et al. *Radiographics* 23(6):1441-1455, 2003.

Figure 17-13A, from Kanski J, Bowling B: *Clinical Ophthalmology*, ed 7, Philadelphia, 2012, Saunders.

Figure 16-5A, from Kanski JJ: *Systemic Diseases and the Eye*, St. Louis, 2001, Mosby.

Figures 4-9, 6-8A, from Kliegman R et al: *Nelson Textbook of Pediatrics*, ed 19, Philadelphia, 2012, Elsevier/Saunders.

Figures 9-7, 10-15A, 11-17, 11-19A, 12-10, 12-11B, 12-12B, 19-2, 19-8B, from Kumar V, Cotran RS, Robbins SL: *Basic Pathology*, ed 8, Philadelphia, 2007, Saunders.

Figures 1-6B, 5-25C, 5-28B, 6-1, 7-12B, 8-18, 12-11A, 16-20C, 16-21B, 19-7B, 19-8A, 19-9, from Kumar V, Abbas A, Aster J: *Robbins & Cotran Pathologic Basis of Disease*, ed 8, Philadelphia, 2010, Elsevier/Saunders.

Figure 14-11B, from Lemmi FO, Lemmi CAE: *Physical Assessment Findings* CD-ROM, Philadelphia, 2000, Saunders.

Figures 5-18, 7-15A, 11-13, 11-19B & C, 12-8, 15-27, 16-17A, 16-22, 17-16, 17-20, 17-28B, 19-12, from Lewis SM et al: *Medical-Surgical Nursing*, ed 8, St. Louis, 2011, Elsevier/Mosby.

Figure 10-22, from Lundy-Ekman L: *Neuroscience*, ed 3, St. Louis, 2008, Mosby.

Figure 16-16, from Marcdante K et al: *Nelson Essentials of Pediatrics*, ed 5, Philadelphia, 2006, Saunders.

Figure 16-20B, from Marks J and Miller J: *Lookingbill and Marks' Principles of Dermatology*, ed 4, Philadelphia, 2007, Saunders.

Figure 15-33B, from Mercier LR: *Practical Orthopedics*, ed 5, St. Louis, 2000, Mosby.

Figure 20-3, from Mettler FA: *Essentials of Radiography*, ed 2, Philadelphia, 2004, Saunders.

Figure 15-34, from Miller MD, Howard RF, Plancher KD: *Surgical Atlas of Sports Medicine*, Philadelphia, 2003, Saunders.

Figures 15-38F, 18-17, from Moll JMH: *Rheumatology*, ed 2, London, 1997, Churchill Livingstone.

Figure 9-12A, from Morse SA et al: *Atlas of Sexually Transmitted Diseases and AIDS*, ed 2, 2003, London, Gower.

Figures 16-9C, 16-19A, 16-21A, from *Mosby's Medical, Nursing and Allied Health Dictionary*, ed 5, St. Louis, 1998, Mosby.

Figure 17-6B, from Newell FW: *Ophthalmology: Principles and Concepts*, ed 8, St. Louis, 1996, Mosby.

Figure 5-29A, from Odze R, Goldblum J: *Surgical Pathology of the GI Tract, Liver, Biliary Tract and Pancreas*, ed 2, Philadelphia, Saunders, 2009.

Figure 8-22, from O'Toole M [ed]: *Miller-Keane Encyclopedia & Dictionary of Medicine, Nursing & Allied Health*, ed 7, Philadelphia, 2003, Saunders.

Figure 17-13B, from Palay D and Krachmer J: *Primary Care Ophthalmology*, ed 2, St. Louis, 2006, Mosby.

Figure 16-14B, from Phipps WJ et al: *Medical-Surgical Nursing*, ed 7, St. Louis, 2003, Mosby.

Figure 6-2B, 7-10B, from Roberts J, Hedges J: *Clinical Procedures in Emergency Medicine*, ed 5, Philadelphia, 2010, Elsevier/Saunders.

Figure 8-16B, from Salvo S: *Mosby's Pathology for Massage Therapists*, ed 2, St. Louis, 2009, Mosby.

Figures 3-4, 16-3B, 16-7B, 16-8A, 18-15B, 18-16, from Seidel HM, et al: *Mosby's Guide to Physical Examination*, ed 5, St. Louis, 2003, Elsevier/Mosby.

Figure 1-3, from Soyer HP et al: *Dermoscopy*, ed 2, Philadelphia, 2012, Elsevier/Saunders.

Figures 5-20D, 9-12B, 14-10, 14-11A, 15-38A, from Swartz MH: *Textbook of Physical Diagnosis, History and Examination*, ed 5, Philadelphia, 2006, Saunders.

Figures 13-2A, 13-9, 16-2B, 17-2, 17-3, 17-7A, 19-1A, from Thibodeau GA, Patton KT: *Anatomy &Physiology*, ed 6, St. Louis, 2007, Mosby.

Figure 8-4, 12-9, from Thibodeau G, Patton K: *The Human Body in Health & Disease*, ed 4, St. Louis, 2005, Mosby.

Figure 13-10, from Tkachuk DC, Hirschmann JV, McArthur JR: *Atlas of Clinical Hematology*, Philadelphia, 2002, Saunders.

Figure 15-26B, US Centers for Disease Control and Prevention.

Figure 15-36, from Walter JB: *An Introduction to the Principles of Disease*, ed 3, Philadelphia, 1992, Saunders.

Figure 7-10A, from Warekois R and Robinson R: *Phlebotomy*, ed 2, Philadelphia, 2008, Saunders.

Figure 7-14B, from Wein A et al: *Campbell-Walsh Urology*, ed 10, Philadelphia, 2012, Saunders.

Figure 6-10, from Weinstein WM, Hawkey CJ, Bosch J: *Clinical Gastroenterology and Hepatology*, St. Louis, 2005, Mosby.

Unnumbered Figure 2-1, from Weir J et al: *An Imaging Atlas of Human Anatomy*, ed 4, Philadelphia, 2011, Elsevier/Mosby.

Figure 16-8E & I, from Weston WL et al: *Color Textbook of Pediatric Dermatology*, ed 3, 2002, St. Louis, Mosby.

Figure 16-8K, from White GM: *Color Atlas of Regional Dermatology*, London, 1994, Times-Mirror.

Figure 21-2, B to E, from Young AP, Kennedy DB: *Kinn's The Medical Assistant*, ed 9, Philadelphia, 2003, Saunders.

Figures 9-6B, 14-12, 15-13B & C, 15-38D, 16-6A, 16-8B, 16-12, from Zitelli BJ, Davis HW: *Atlas of Pediatric Physical Diagnosis*, ed 2, St. Louis, 1992, Mosby.

INDEX

A

Page numbers followed by f indicated figures; t, tables; b, boxes; and boldface pages are found on the Evolve website.

D

E

H

J

K

M

O

P

T